Sakshi Arora's

Self Assessment & Review GYNECOLOGY

Sakshi Arora's

Self Assessment & Review

GYNECOLOGY

Fourteenth Edition

Revised by

Roshini P

MBBS MS DNB

Consultant Obstetrician and Gynecologist

Bengaluru, Karnataka, India

Faculty at Kernel Series: DC Dutta's Textbook of Obstetrics

Faculty at DIGI NEET

NMC Certified NEET PG and Undergraduate Teacher

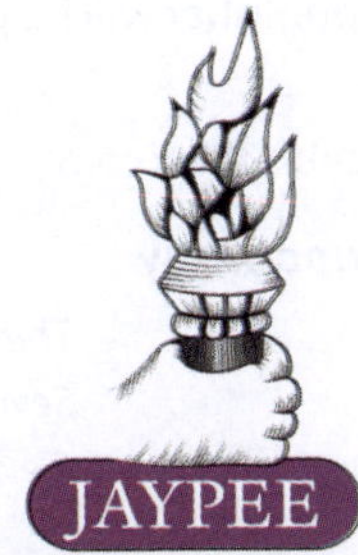

JAYPEE BROTHERS MEDICAL PUBLISHERS

The Health Sciences Publisher

New Delhi | London

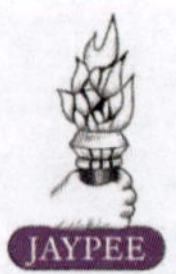

Jaypee Brothers Medical Publishers (P) Ltd

Headquarters
Jaypee Brothers Medical Publishers (P) Ltd
EMCA House, 23/23-B
Ansari Road, Daryaganj
New Delhi 110 002, India
Landline: +91-11-23272143, +91-11-23272703
+91-11-23282021, +91-11-23245672
Email: jaypee@jaypeebrothers.com

Corporate Office
Jaypee Brothers Medical Publishers (P) Ltd
4838/24, Ansari Road, Daryaganj
New Delhi 110 002, India
Phone: +91-11-43574357
Fax: +91-11-43574314
Email: jaypee@jaypeebrothers.com

Overseas Office
JP Medical Ltd.
83, Victoria Street, London
SW1H 0HW (UK)
Phone: +44 20 3170 8910
Fax: +44 (0)20 3008 6180
Email: info@jpmedpub.com

Website: www.jaypeebrothers.com
Website: www.jaypeedigital.com

© 2025, Jaypee Brothers Medical Publishers

The views and opinions expressed in this book are solely those of the original contributor(s)/author(s) and do not necessarily represent those of editor(s) or publisher of the book.

All rights reserved. No part of this publication may be reproduced, stored or transmitted in any form or by any means, electronic, mechanical, photocopying, recording or otherwise, without the prior permission in writing of the publishers.

All brand names and product names used in this book are trade names, service marks, trademarks or registered trademarks of their respective owners. The publisher is not associated with any product or vendor mentioned in this book.

Medical knowledge and practice change constantly. This book is designed to provide accurate, authoritative information about the subject matter in question. However, readers are advised to check the most current information available on procedures included and check information from the manufacturer of each product to be administered, to verify the recommended dose, formula, method and duration of administration, adverse effects and contraindications. It is the responsibility of the practitioner to take all appropriate safety precautions. Neither the publisher nor the author(s)/editor(s) assume any liability for any injury and/or damage to persons or property arising from or related to use of material in this book.

This book is sold on the understanding that the publisher is not engaged in providing professional medical services. If such advice or services are required, the services of a competent medical professional should be sought.

Every effort has been made where necessary to contact holders of copyright to obtain permission to reproduce copyright material. If any have been inadvertently overlooked, the publisher will be pleased to make the necessary arrangements at the first opportunity.

Inquiries for bulk sales may be solicited at: jaypee@jaypeebrothers.com

Sakshi Arora's Self Assessment & Review: Gynecology

First Edition: 2007 *Second Edition: 2009* *Third Edition: 2010* *Fourth Edition: 2011*
Fifth Edition: 2012 *Sixth Edition: 2013* *Seventh Edition: 2014* *Eighth Edition: 2015*
Ninth Edition: 2016 *Tenth Edition: 2017* *Eleventh Edition: 2018* *Twelfth Edition: 2019*
Thirteenth Edition: 2020

Fourteenth Edition: 2025

ISBN: 978-93-6616-268-3

Printed in India at Rajkamal Electric Press, Kundli, Haryana-131 028.

Dedicated to

The students of Gynecology and their families

A Letter to the Students

Dear Students,

As I write this, I imagine myself in you—an aspiring doctor with countless books, late-night coffee cups, and a heart full of hope.

Preparing for NEET-PG is no easy feat. But I want to assure you that you are not alone.

This book is more than just a guide; it is your companion through these challenging times. Each chapter, diagram, and question is curated with one goal in mind—your success. I understand the pressure you face, the self-doubt that creeps in, and the weight of expectations. But I also know your potential, your perseverance, and your passion.

Remember, Obstetrics and Gynecology are not just subjects—they are the stories of life itself. Many of you would pursue your career in this field. The knowledge you gain here would help you bring a new life into the world, cure illnesses, and give hope to those in despair.

Let this thought motivate you when the days feel long and the material feels overwhelming.

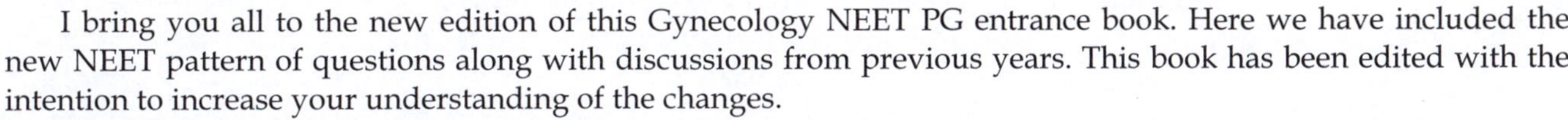

I bring you all to the new edition of this Gynecology NEET PG entrance book. Here we have included the new NEET pattern of questions along with discussions from previous years. This book has been edited with the intention to increase your understanding of the changes.

This 14/e includes:

- Most recent questions with explanation
- Theory and explanation of high-yield topics
- Image-based questions
- New diagnostic techniques
- Annexures for last minute revision
- INI-CET and NEET PG questions

I have given my best to incorporate the most important and must know questions for you. As this is my first attempt at this task, may I request you to kindly help me improvise this book better by notifying any typo errors or mistakes. I also want to inform you that for any doubts and clarification you can reach to me directly via following ways:

Emaild: drroshnip24@gmail.com

YouTube Channel: The Kernel Series: by Dr.Roshini P

/ The Kernel Series: by Dr.Roshini P

Looking forward for your support and cooperation.

Yours truly

Dr Roshini P

Acknowledgments

This book stands as a testament to teamwork and dedication. My deepest gratitude extends to:

- My mentors and teachers, for their invaluable guidance and support.
- My family, for their sacrifices, unconditional love, and belief in my endeavors.
- The students, for inspiring me every single day with your passion and perseverance.
- The publishing team, for their hard work and commitment to excellence.

Shri Jitendar P Vij (Group Chairman) for being my mentor. I will always remain indebted to him for his support.

Mr MS Mani (Group President) for his faith in me.

Mr Ankit Vij (Managing Director) for being so down-to-earth and always approachable.

Ms Chetna Malhotra (Senior Director—Professional Publishing, Marketing, and Business Development) for working hard with the team to achieve the deadlines.

Ms Ruby Sharma (Business Manager) for her continued and full support in managing the manuscript.

To all the students who have trusted me over the years, thank you. Your success is my greatest reward.

Dr Roshini P
drroshnip24@gmail.com
The Kernel Series: by Dr.Roshini P

How to Use this Book

- *Build strong foundations:* Begin with the theoretical portions to establish a solid base.
- *Chapter progression:* Follow the structured sequence to grasp concepts in a logical order.
- *Practice extensively:* Solve MCQs after each chapter to test and refine your understanding.
- *Leverage visual aids:* Use diagrams, flowcharts, and images to reinforce learning and improve retention.
- *Highlight key points:* Mark essential concepts and challenging questions for focused revision.
- *Utilize annexures:* Rely on the high-yield summaries and tables for rapid recall during exams.

1. FOR PRE-FINAL/FINAL YEAR STUDENTS

Obstetrics and Gynecology is a major subject not only for Final year but for all PG entrance examinations and supposedly for the Exit exam (if it comes). So you cannot take this subject lightly. I would suggest you all to start reading my book during your Third year MBBS to build your basics right from the beginning.

Sequence to Read Chapters

Now the sequence in which I want you read the chapters—(This will help you in understanding and building the concepts in a better way).

Entire Gynecology should be read in four parts

Part 1: Hormonal studies and menstrual cycle

Read the chapters in the following sequence:

1. Chapter 2: Reproductive Physiology and Hormones in Females
2. Chapter 4: PCOD
3. Chapter 11: Fibroid
4. Chapter 12: Endometriosis
5. Chapter 3: Menopause

Part 2: Development and sexual problems

1. Chapter 5: Congenital Malformations
2. Chapter 6: Sexuality and Intersexuality
3. Chapter 13: Disorders of Menstruation

Part 3: Anatomy and related chapters

1. Chapter 1: Anatomy
2. Chapter 8: Urogynecology
3. Chapter 7: Infections of the Genital Tract
4. Chapter 9: Infertility

Part 4: Remaining chapters

1. Chapter 10: Contraception
2. Chapter 14A: Cancer Endometrium
3. Chapter 14B: Cancer Ovary and Cervix

Sequence to follow while reading each chapter

Read the theory of a chapter from this book and then read the textbook. You will be able to easily understand the textbook now.

Now read the theory of that chapter once again.

Now solve the MCQ from the book.

Follow this with another reading from the textbook.

- This completes your chapter with one reading and revision.
- While reading the book, either make notes or mark in the book itself for quick revision. Mark the difficult and important MCQ for further revision.
- Do this for all the chapters.
- After completing the syllabus, start revising.
- Remember minimum 4–5 readings are required.

2. FOR INTERNS AND POST-INTERNS

- I do not recommend studying textbook now due to scarcity of time. However, textbook should be kept as a reference material
- Do not confuse yourself by studying many books.
- You should spend 10 days on both Obs and Gyne—6 for Obs and 4 for Gyne for first reading.

Read the theory of a chapter and solve MCQ of that chapter.
While solving MCQs, solve all questions at a stretch and only after this compare the answers.

↓

Re-read the theory of this chapter and now mark the important points for revision.
Remember, you should mark only that much so that the next reading of book can be finished in one third of the time. Similarly, encircle or mark the important MCQ for revision.
Just keep cutting those questions which you were able to solve at one go.

↓

Do same for all the chapters.

↓

During revision, study only marked portion with encircled MCQ only.
Second reading of entire Obs and Gyne should be finished in 4–5 days.

↓

Similarly third and fourth revision should be completed in 3 days each.

↓

Give one last revision just before exams in a day or two.

- Remember, Obs and Gyne is a very important subject. You can answer nearly all questions asked in any exam on Gynecology from this book if you concentrate.

In the end test yourself by attempting the 105 questions, question paper given of new pattern AIIMS exam and evaluate yourself.

I wish you all good luck for your exams and a very happy learning.

3. TIME MANAGEMENT TIPS

- *Plan strategically:* Allocate specific days to Obstetrics and Gynecology within your study plan:
  - *Obstetrics:* 6–7 days for a detailed reading and practice.
  - *Gynecology:* 4–5 days for focusing on oncology and high-yield topics.
- *Daily study plan:*
  - *Morning:* Focus on theory and understanding new topics.
  - *Afternoon:* Solve topic-specific MCQs to strengthen concepts.
  - *Evening:* Revise previously covered material or tackle weak areas.
- *Revisions:*
  - *First reading:* Read the theory thoroughly and solve MCQs.
  - *Second reading:* Focus on revision, aiming to cover material faster.
  - *Final review:* Use annexures, marked content, and tables for quick recall.

Dr Roshini P

Salient Features

- Fully colored edition
- Includes new AIIMS Pattern questions
- Includes latest staging and management of all cancers (Cervix and Vulva) as per FIGO guidelines
- Thoroughly revised and updated from William's Gynecology, 3/e
- Includes over 162 colored illustrations/USG/HSG images/Instruments & Specimens
- Includes image-based questions
- Includes Annexure Tables for Last Minute revision

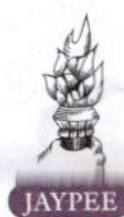

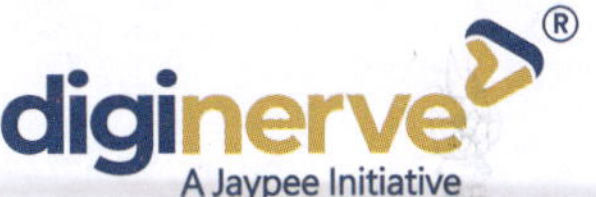

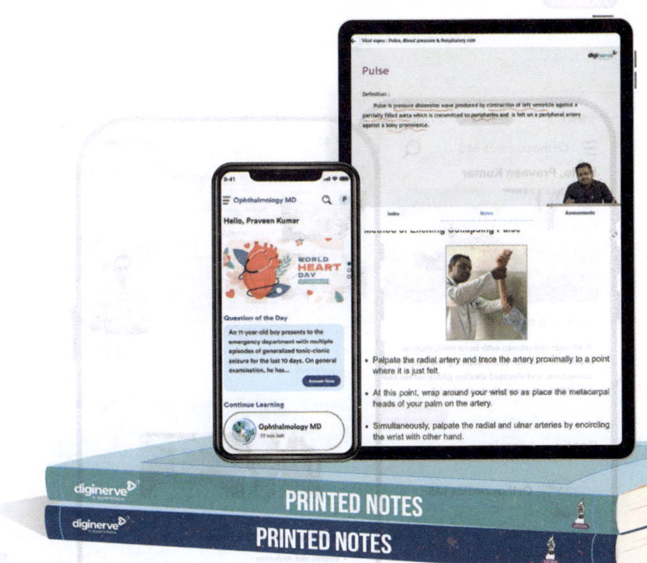

DigiNEET

Simplify your undergraduate studies and NEET PG preparation with this comprehensive program covering all 19 subjects. Crafted by India's top faculty, it includes video lectures, printed notes, OSCEs, a QBank, test series, and the innovative Dr. Wise AI Chatbot.

Course Features

1400+ hrs Video Lectures

1500+ Topics in Notes

15000+ Questions in QBank

1800+ GEMS

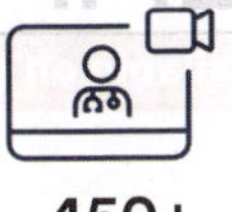

450+ OSCEs

Test Series

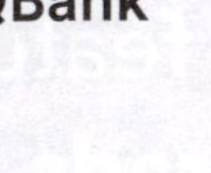

Dr. Wise AI Chatbot

Drug Chart

Regular Webinars by Esteemed Faculty

Access Anytime, Anywhere

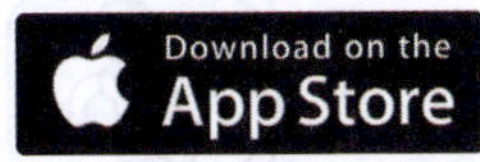

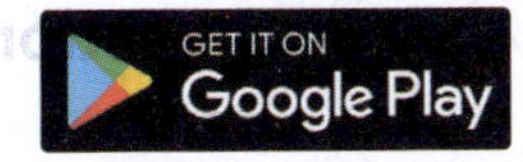

Scan to Download

+91-8800-418-418

marketing@diginerve.com

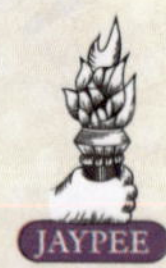

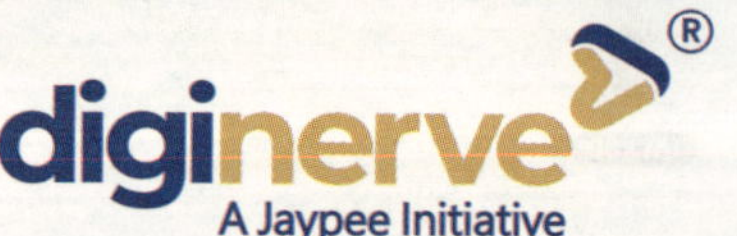

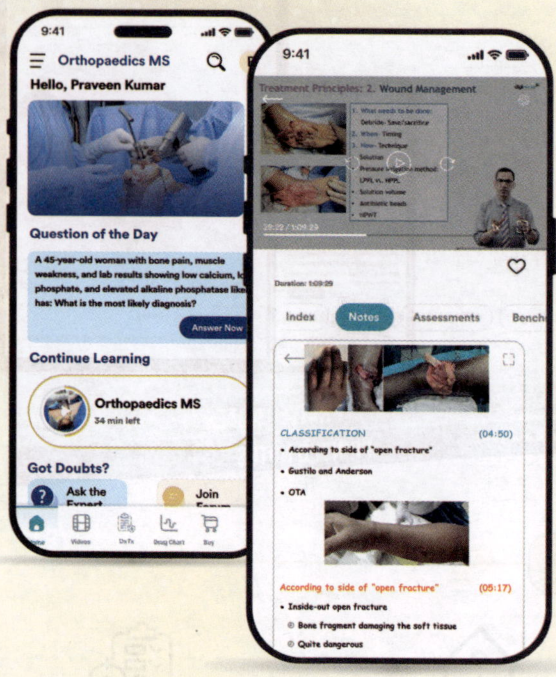

Premium Medical Content, Anytime, Anywhere

Trusted by 150K+ Users

20+ Courses

3600+ Hrs of Video Content

790+ Mentors

A host of features for **UnderGrads, PostGrads** and **Professionals**

Video Lectures

Notes

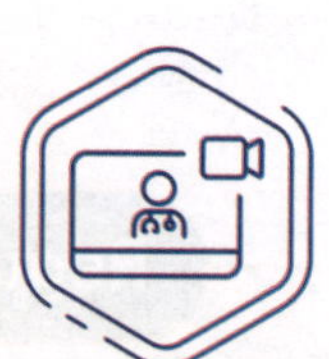

OSCEs

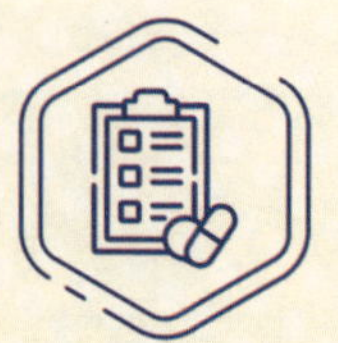

Drug Chart

Question Bank

Dr. Wise AI Chatbot

+91-8800-418-418 marketing@diginerve.com

Contents

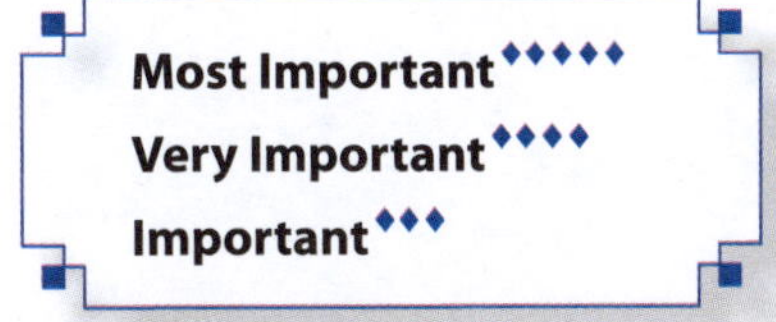

Symbols Used in the Book

Key points

Remember

Definition

Important One Liners

Mnemonic — Mnemonic

Important Topics: Vulval Cancer & Cancer of the Cervix Uteri

Vulval Cancer

Vulval Cancer

- It comprises of 4% of gynae cancers
- M/C variety of vulva cancer: Squamous cell carcinoma (in 90-92% cases) followed by melanoma (seen in 2-4% cases).
- M/c site is Hart line followed by Labia majora and then by Labia minora

Types of squamous variety of vulva cancer:

Warty/basaloid type	Keratinising type
• Seen in young females • Unifocal • Good prognosis • Associated with: – HPV infection – Smoking – Vulva intraepithelial lesion	• Seen in older females • Multifocal • Bad prognosis • Associated with – Lichen sclerosis – Squamous cell hyperplasia – Mutation in p 53 gene

Note: The gene mutation which can lead to vulva cancer: *Mutation in p 53 gene*

M/C age group for vulva cancer ≥ **65–70 years**

Vulval Cancer: Risk Factors and Clinical Presentation

a. HPV infection Most common HPV 16
Others – HPV 18, 31, 33 and 45

b. *Herpes simplex virus in smokers*
Note: Heifer simplex infection is not a risk factor in non-smokers

c. Smoking

d. Chronic immunosuppression

e. Lichen sclerosis

f. Squamous cell hyperplasia

g. Paget's disease (extra mammary): Leads to adenocarcinoma of vulva

h. Vulva intraepithelial neoplasia (within 4 years it can lead to vulva cancer).

Symptoms

M/C symptom: Pruritis

Others: Ulcer
Mass
Bleeding
Cachexia

Diagnosis

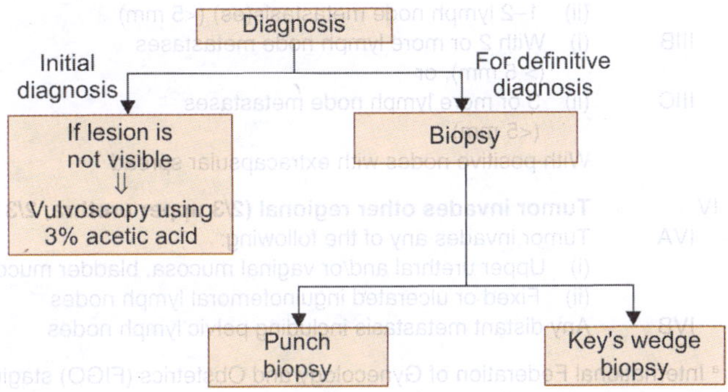

Spread

1. Direct spread: To vagina/urethra
2. Lymphatic spread:
   Note: Sentinel lymph node for vulval cancer: *Superficial inguinal lymph nodes*
   Lymph nodes which are not involved: Pelvic lymph nodes
3. Hematogenous spread

Prognostic Factors

a. Single most important prognostic factor: *Involvement of lymph nodes*

b. Depth of lesion

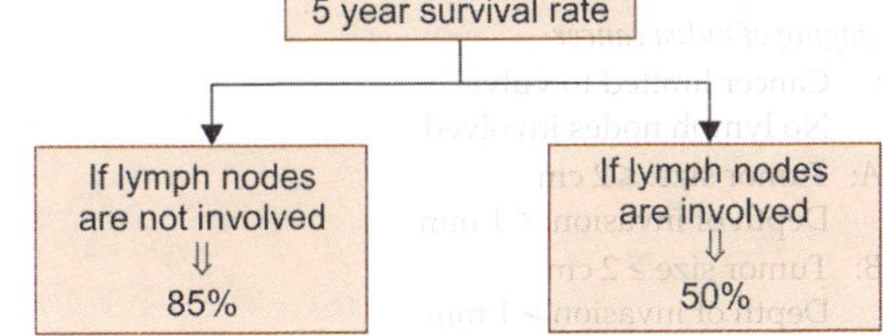

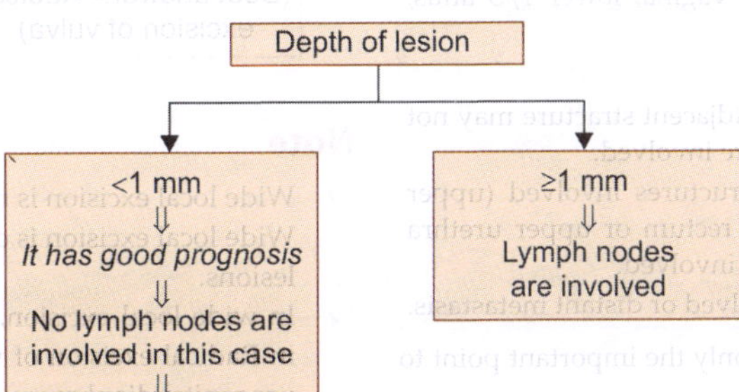

FIGO Staging of Vulval Cancer

Invasive Vulvar Cancer Staging

Stage[a]	*Characteristics*
I	**Tumor confined to the vulva**
IA	Lesions ≤2 cm in size, confined to the vulva or perineum and with stromal invasion ≤1.0 mm[b], no nodal metastasis
IB	Lesions >2 cm in size or with stromal invasion >1.0 mm[b], confined to the vulva or perineum, with negative nodes
II	**Tumor of any size with extension to adjacent perineal structure (1/3 lower urethra, 1/3 lower vagina, anus) with negative nodes**
III	**Tumor of any size with or without extension to adjacent perineal structures (1/3 lower urethra, 1/3 lower vagina, anus) with positive inguinofemoral lymph nodes**
IIIA	(i) With 1 lymph node metastasis (≥5 mm), or (ii) 1–2 lymph node metastasis(es) (<5 mm)
IIIB	(i) With 2 or more lymph node metastases (> 5 mm), or
IIIC	(ii) 3 or more lymph node metastases (<5 mm) With positive nodes with extracapsular spread
IV	**Tumor invades other regional (2/3 upper urethra, 2/3 upper vagina), or distant structures**
IVA	Tumor invades any of the following: (i) Upper urethral and/or vaginal mucosa, bladder mucosa, rectal mucosa, or fixed to pelvic bone, or (ii) Fixed or ulcerated inguinofemoral lymph nodes
IVB	Any distant metastasis including pelvic lymph nodes

[a] International Federation of Gynecology and Obstetrics (FIGO) staging.
[b] The *depth of invasion* is defined as the measurement of the tumor from the epithelial-stromal junction of the adjacent most superficial dermal papilla to the deepest point of invasion.

Important Points to Remember about Staging of Vulva Cancer

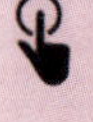

It is a clinical and surgical staging
Stage 1 and 2: Lymph nodes not involved
Stage 3 and 4: Lymph nodes are involved
Stage 3C: Lymph node involvement and there is extracapsular spread
Stage 4A2: Lymph nodes are fixed and ulcerated
Stage 4B: Pelvic node involved

Simple staging of vulva cancer

Stage 1: Cancer limited to vulva
No lymph nodes involved

Stage 1A: Tumor size: ≤ 2 cm
Depth of invasion: ≤ 1 mm

Stage 1B: Tumor size ≥ 2 cm
Depth of invasion: > 1 mm

Stage 2: Cancer of any size has involved lower part of adjacent structures lower (lower 1/3 of vagina, lower 1/3 anus, lower 1/3 urethra)

Lymph nodes are not involved

Stage 3: Any size of tumor or adjacent Adjacent stracture may not be involved and lymph nodes are involved.

Stage 4: 4A: Upper part of adjoining structures involved (upper vagina, upper anus, upper rectum or upper urethra involved) and lymph nodes involved.
4B: Pelvic lymph nodes are involved or distant metastasis.

Note: This is not complete staging, this is only the important point to be remembered in staging.

Management of Vulval Cancer

In vulva cancer: *Management means managing*
i. *Lesion*
ii. *The lymph nodes*

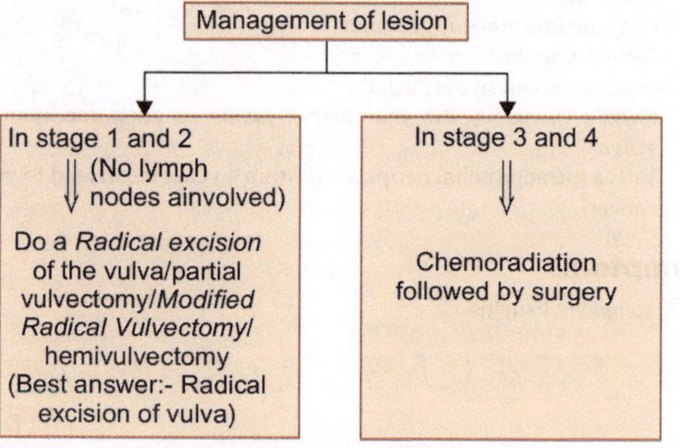

Note

- Wide local excision is not same as radical excision of vulva
- Wide local excision is done in benign conditions or premalignant lesions.
- In wide local excision, a superficial dissection is done, whereas in Radical excision of vulva, dissection is carried as deep as the urogenital diaphragm.

Management of Lymph Nodes in Vulval Cancer

Principles:

- Lymph node dissection done in vulva cancer is Inguinofemoral lymph node dissection
- **If lesion is within 2 cm of Midline:** A bilateral inguinofemoral lymph node dissection is done as vulval lymphatics cross on other side
- **If lesson is ≥2 cm away from Midline: A unilateral inguinofemoral lymph node dissection is done**

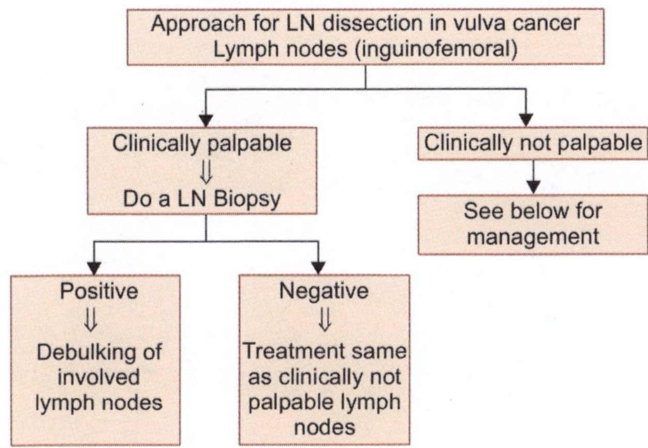

Approach to Clinically Not Palpable LN

- Only in stage IA (size of lesion <2 cm, depth of invasion is < 1 mm) no lymph node dissection is done
- **Rest in all stages:** Inguinofemoral LN dissection has to be done.

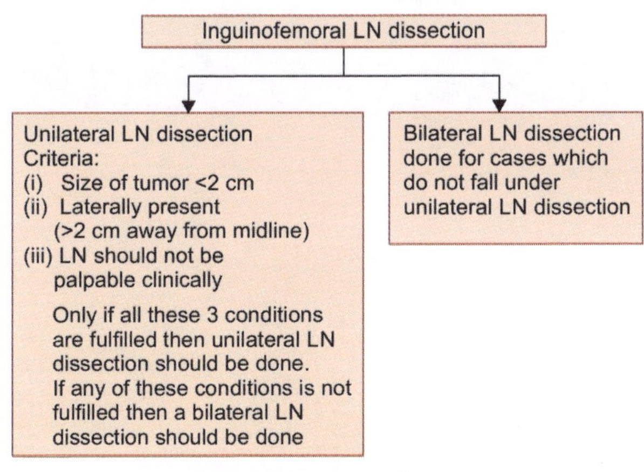

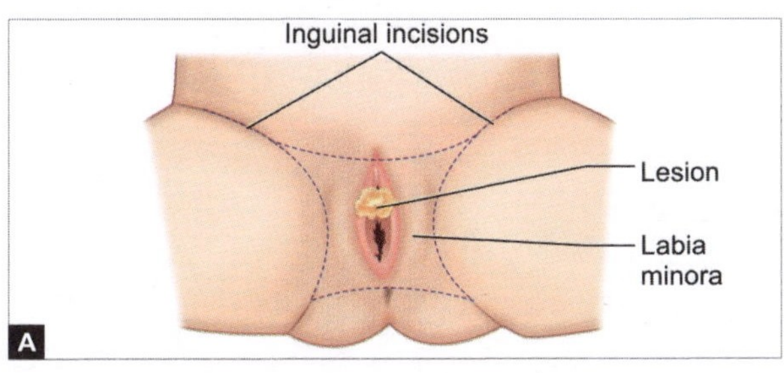

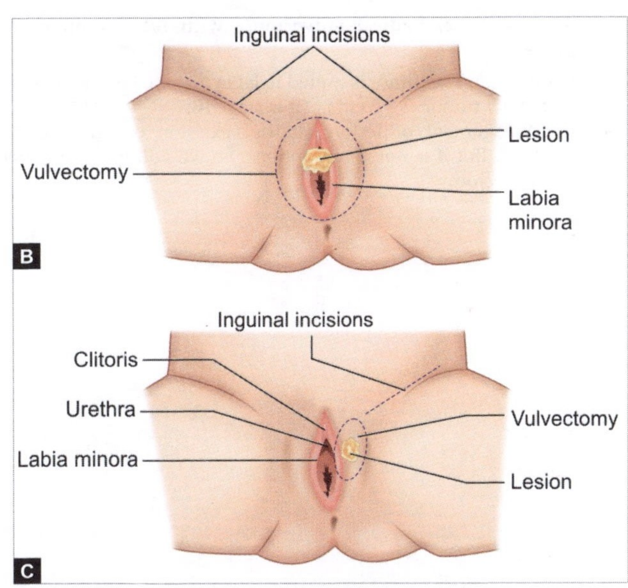

Types of vulvectomy used in the treatment of vulvar cancer. A. En bloc radical vulvectomy with bilateral inguinofemoral lymphadenectomy. B. Radical complete vulvectomy with bilateral inguinofemoral lymphadenectomy. C. Radical partial vulvectomy with ipsilateral inguinofemoral lymphadenectomy.

Questions:

1. **M/C variety of vulva cancer:**
   a. Melanoma
   b. Squamous cell carcinoma
   c. Melanoma
   d. Adenocarcinoma

   Ans. is b, i.e. Squamous cell carcinoma

   M/C variety of vulval cancer is squamous cell carcinoma (92%) followed by melanoma.
2. **All of the following are associated with vulval cancer except:**
   a. Lichen sclerosis
   b. Smoking
   c. Paget's disease
   d. OCP

   Ans. is d, i.e. OCP

   See the text for explanation.
3. **M/C HPV associated with vulva cancer:**
   a. HPV 16
   b. HPV 18
   c. HPV 6
   d. HPV 8

   Ans. is a, i.e. HPV16

   As discussed in text: M/C HPV associated with vulva cancer is HPV 16.
4. **A 76-year-old female presented with a non Healing ulcer on labia majora for 6 months measuring 2 × 3 cm with no palpable lymphadenopathy. Biopsy shows squamous cell carcinoma. Management includes:**
   a. Radical vulvectomy with U/L lymph node dissection
   b. Radical vulvectomy with B/L lymph node dissection
   c. Simple vulvectomy
   d. Chemoradiation with resection

Ans. is b, i.e. Radical vulvectomy with B/L lymph node dissection

Explanation: The tumor is united to labia majora, i.e. it is stage 1.

- Size of tumor: 2 × 3 cm i.e. it is stage IB.
- Management of lesion: Radical excision of vulva is to done. But it is not given options. So we will go for radical vulvectomy.

Management of Lymph Nodes

Stage of Tumor is IB: i.e. lymph node dissection has to be done. Now because size of tumor is 2 × 3 cm: (i.e. ≥ 2 cm) so a Bilateral inguinofemoral lymph node dissection has to be done. Hence complete management is: Option 'b' i.e. Radical vulvectomy with B/L lymph node dissection.

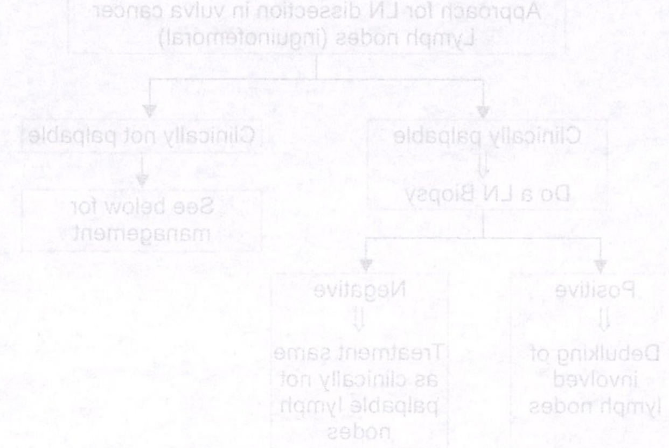

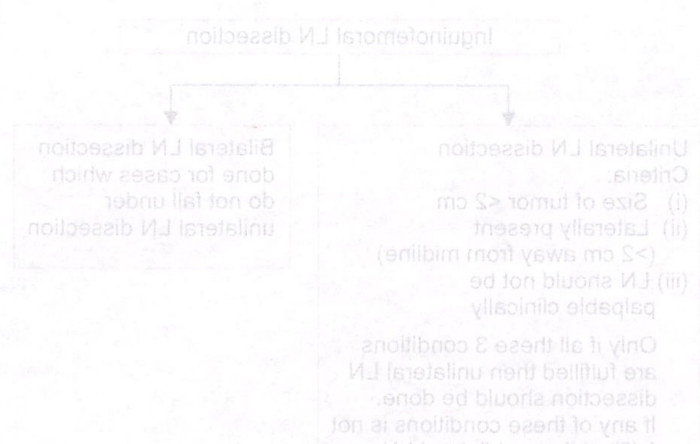

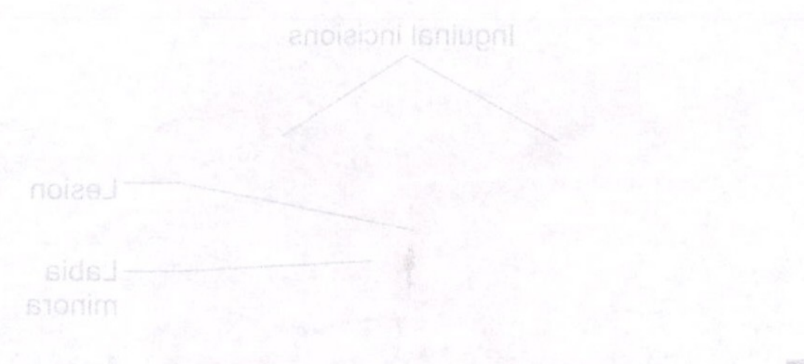

Cancer of the Cervix Uteri

Neerja Bhatla[1,*] Daisuke Aoki[2] Daya Nand Sharma[3] Rengaswamy Sankaranarayanan[4]

[1]Department of Obstetrics and Gynecology, All India Institute of Medical Sciences, New Delhi, India

[2]Department of Obstetrics and Gynecology, Keio University School of Medicine, Tokyo, Japan

[3]Department of Radiation Oncology, All India Institute of Medical Sciences, New Delhi, India

[4]Early Detection and Prevention Group, International Agency for Research on Cancer, Lyon, France

Introduction

Globally, cervical cancer continues to be one of the most common cancers among females, being the fourth most common after breast, colorectal, and lung cancer. In 2012, it was estimated that there were approximately 527 600 new cases of cervical cancer with 265 700 more common, being the second most common cancer in incidence among women and the third most common in terms of mortality.

Anatomical Considerations

The cervix, which is the lowermost part of the uterus, is a cylindrical-shaped structure composed of stroma and epithelium. The intravaginal part, the ectocervix, projects into the vagina and is lined by squamous epithelium. The endocervical canal extends from the internal os at the junction with the uterus to the external os which opens into the vagina and is lined by columnar epithelium. Almost all cases of cervical carcinoma originate in the transformation zone from the ecto- or endocervical mucosa. The transformation zone is the area of the cervix between the old and new squamocolumnar junction.

Early Detection and Prevention of Cervical Cancer

It is now recognized that cervical cancer is a rare long-term outcome of persistent infection of the lower genital tract by one of about 15 high-risk HPV types, which is termed the "necessary" cause of cervical cancer. HPV 16 and HPV 18 account for 71% of cases; while HPV types 31, 33, 45, 52, and 58 account for another 19% of cervical cancer cases 2, 3. It is well documented that nearly 90% of incident HPV infections are not detectable within a period of 2 years from the acquisition of infection and persist only in a small proportion. Persistent HPV infection denotes the presence of the same type-specific HPV DNA on repeated sampling after 6–12 months. Only one-tenth of all infections become persistent, and these women could develop cervical precancerous lesions.

This knowledge has resulted in the development of new initiatives for prevention and early detection. The two major approaches for control of cervical cancer involve: (1) prevention of invasive cancer by HPV vaccination; and (2) screening for precancerous lesions.

Primary Prevention of Cervical Cancer with HPV Vaccination

The fact that more than 80% of women followed over time will acquire at least one high-risk HPV infection suggests the ubiquitous nature of the HPV infection and reflects the ease of transmission. The estimated cross-sectional HPV prevalence worldwide among healthy women is around 11.7%, with the highest in Sub-Saharan Africa at around 24%, Age-specific cross-sectional HPV prevalence peaks at 25% in women aged less than 25 years, which suggests that the infection is predominantly transmitted through the sexual route following sexual debut. Thus, prophylactic HPV vaccination as a preventive strategy should target women before initiation of sexual activity, focusing on girls aged 10–14 years.

Three prophylactic HPV vaccines are currently available in many countries for use in females and males from the age of 9 years for the prevention of premalignant lesions and cancers affecting the cervix, vulva, vagina, and anus caused by high-risk HPV types: a bivalent vaccine targeting HPV16 and HPV18; a quadrivalent vaccine targeting HPV6 and HPV11 in addition to HPV16 and HPV18; and a nonavalent vaccine targeting HPV types 31, 33, 45, 52, and 58 in addition to HPV 6, 11, 16, and 18. The last two vaccines target anogenital warts caused by HPV 6 and 11 in addition to the above-mentioned malignant and premalignant lesions. All the vaccines are recombinant vaccines composed of virus-like particles (VLPs) and are not infectious since they do not contain viral DNA. For girls and boys aged 9–14 years, a two-dose schedule (0.5 mL at 0 and 5–13 months) is recommended. If the second vaccine dose is administered earlier than 5 months after the first dose, a third dose is recommended. For those aged 15 years and above, and for immunocompromised patients irrespective of age, the recommendation is for three doses (0.5 mL at 0, 1, 6 months). WHO has reviewed the latest data and concluded that there is no safety concern regarding HPV vaccines.

Secondary Prevention of Cervical Cancer by Early Detection and Treatment of Precancerous Lesions

Even with the advent of effective vaccines, screening will remain a priority for cervical cancer prevention for several decades. Cervical cancer screening has been successful in preventing cancer by detection and treatment of precursor lesions, namely, high-grade cervical intra-epithelial neoplasia (CIN 2 and 3) and adenocarcinoma in-situ (AIS).

Several cervical screening strategies have been found to be effective in varied settings. The tests used widely include conventional cytology (Pap smear), in recent years liquid-based cytology and HPV testing, and, in LMICs, visual inspection with acetic acid (VIA). While the Pap smear is still the major workhorse of screening and is associated with substantial declines in cervical cancer risk in high-income countries, it is a challenging and resource intensive technology that is not feasible in low-resource settings where poor organization, coverage, and lack of quality assurance result in suboptimal outcomes.

VIA involves detection of acetowhite lesions on the cervix 1 minute after application of 3%–5% freshly prepared acetic acid. In view of its feasibility, VIA screening has been widely implemented in opportunistic settings in many low-income countries in Sub-Saharan Africa. A single-visit approach (SVA) for screening with rapid diagnosis and treatment improves coverage, eliminates follow-up visits, and makes screening more time and cost-efficient in low-resource settings. VIA screening is particularly suitable for SVA and WHO has issued guidelines for implementing SVA in public health settings.

A single screening modality will never be universally applicable, but it is possible to adapt cost-effective means of cervical cancer screening to each country.

FIGO Staging

Cervical cancer spreads by direct extension into the parametrium, vagina, uterus and adjacent organs, i.e., bladder and rectum. It also spreads along the lymphatic channels to the regional lymph nodes, namely, obturator, external iliac and internal iliac, and thence to the common iliac and para-aortic nodes. Distant metastasis to lungs, liver, and skeleton by the hematogenous route is a late phenomenon.

Until now, the FIGO staging was based mainly on clinical examination with the addition of certain procedures that were allowed by FIGO to change the staging. In 2018, this has been revised by the FIGO Gynecologic Oncology Committee to allow imaging and pathological findings, where available, to assign the stage. The revised staging is shown in Table 1 (presented at the FIGO XXII World Congress of Gynecology and Obstetrics).

Table 1: FIGO staging of cancer of the cervix uteri (2018)

Stage	*Description*
I	The carcinoma is strictly confined to the cervix (extension to the uterine corpus should be disregarded)
IA	Invasive carcinoma that can be diagnosed only by microscopy, with maximum depth of invasion <5 mm[a]
IA1	Measured stromal invasion <3 mm in depth
IA2	Measured stromal invasion ≥3 mm and <5 mm in depth
IB	Invasive carcinoma with measured deepest invasion ≥5 mm (greater than Stage IA), lesion limited to the cervix uteri[b]
IB1	Invasive carcinoma ≥5 mm depth of stromal invasion, and <2 cm in greatest dimension
IB2	Invasive carcinoma ≥2 cm and <4 cm in greatest dimension
IB3	Invasive carcinoma ≥4 cm in greatest dimension
II	The carcinoma invades beyond the uterus, but has not extended onto the lower third of the vagina or to the pelvic wall
IIA	Involvement limited to the upper two-thirds of the vagina without parametrial involvement
IIA1	Invasive carcinoma <4 cm in greatest dimension
IIA2	Invasive carcinoma ≥4 cm in greatest dimension
IIB	With parametrial involvement but not up to the pelvic wall
III	The carcinoma involves the lower third of the vagina and/or extends to the pelvic wall and/or causes hydronephrosis or nonfunctioning kidney and/or involves pelvic and/or para-aortic lymph nodesc
IIIA	The carcinoma involves the lower third of the vagina, with no extension to the pelvic wall
IIIB	Extension to the pelvic wall and/or hydronephrosis or nonfunctioning kidney (unless known to be due to another cause)
IIIC	Involvement of pelvic and/or para-aortic lymph nodes, irrespective of tumor size and extent (with r and p notations)[c]
IIIC1	Pelvic lymph node metastasis only
IIIC2	Para-aortic lymph node metastasis
IV	The carcinoma has extended beyond the true pelvis or has involved (biopsy proven) the mucosa of the bladder or rectum. (A bullous edema, as such, does not permit a case to be allotted to Stage IV)
IVA	Spread to adjacent pelvic organs
IVB	Spread to distant organs

When in doubt, the lower staging should be assigned.

[a] Imaging and pathology can be used, where available, to supplement clinical findings with respect to tumor size and extent, in all stages.

[b] The involvement of vascular/lymphatic spaces does not change the staging. The lateral extent of the lesion is no longer considered.

[c] Adding notation of r (imaging) and p (pathology) to indicate the findings that are used to allocate the case to Stage IIIC. Example: If imaging indicates pelvic lymph node metastasis, the stage allocation would be Stage IIIC1r, and if confirmed by pathologic findings, it would be Stage IIIC1p. The type of imaging modality or pathology technique used should always be documented.

Source: Bhatla et al.[17]

Diagnosis and Evaluation of Cervical Cancer

Microinvasive Disease

Diagnosis of Stage IA1 and IA2 is made on microscopic examination of a LEEP (loop electrosurgical excision procedure) or cone biopsy specimen, which includes the entire lesion. It can also be made on a trachelectomy or hysterectomy specimen. The depth of invasion should not be greater than 3 mm or 5 mm, respectively, from the base of the epithelium, either squamous or glandular, from which it originates. The horizontal dimension is no longer considered in the 2018 revision as it is subject to many artefactual errors. Note must be made of lymphovascular space involvement, which does not alter the stage, but may affect the treatment plan. Extension to the uterine corpus is also disregarded for staging purposes as it does not in itself alter either the prognosis or management. The margins should be reported to be negative for disease. If the margins of the cone biopsy are positive for invasive cancer, the patient is allocated to Stage IB1.

Clinically visible lesions, and those with larger dimensions, are allocated to Stage IB, subdivided in the latest staging as IB1, IB2, and IB3 based on the maximum diameter of the lesion.

Invasive Disease

In the case of visible lesions, a punch biopsy may generally suffice, but if not satisfactory a small loop biopsy or cone may be required. Clinical assessment is the first step in allocation of staging.

Imaging evaluation may now be used in addition to clinical examination where resources permit. The revised staging permits the use of any of the imaging modalities according to available resources, i.e. ultrasound, CT, MRI, positron emission tomography (PET), to provide information on tumor size, nodal status, and local or systemic spread. The accuracy of various methods depends on the skill of the operator. MRI is the best method of radiologic assessment of primary tumors greater than 10 mm. However, ultrasound has also been shown to have good diagnostic accuracy in expert hands. The modality used in assigning staging should be noted for future evaluation.

For detection of nodal metastasis greater than 10 mm, PET-CT is more accurate than CT and MRI, with false-negative results in 4–15% of cases. In areas with a high prevalence of tuberculosis and inflammation, especially HIV-endemic areas, large lymph nodes are not necessarily metastatic. The clinician may make the decision on imaging or, when possible, can use fine needle aspiration or biopsy to establish or exclude metastases. This is especially true in advanced stages, where surgical assessment of para-aortic lymph nodes may be used to tailor treatment according to extent of disease. They can be accessed by minimally invasive surgery or laparotomy. Surgical exclusion of para-aortic lymph node involvement has been reported to have a better prognosis than radiographic exclusion alone.

A review of 22 articles that assessed the safety and impact of pretreatment para-aortic lymph node surgical staging (PALNS) found that 18% (range, 8%–42%) of patients with Stage IB–IVA cervical cancer had para-aortic lymph node metastases. The mean complication rate of PALNS was 9% (range 4–24%), with lymphocyst formation being the most common. In another study, up to 35% of clinically assessed Stage IIB and 20% of Stage III tumors were reported to have positive para-aortic nodes. In the revised staging, all these cases will be assigned to Stage IIIC as lymph node involvement confers a worse prognosis. If only pelvic nodes are positive, it is Stage IIIC1; if para-aortic nodes are also involved it is Stage IIIC2.

FIGO no longer mandates any biochemical investigations or investigative procedures; however, in patients with frank invasive carcinoma, a chest X-ray, and assessment of hydronephrosis (with renal ultrasound, intravenous pyelography, CT, or MRI) should be done. The bladder and rectum are evaluated by cystoscopy and sigmoidoscopy only if the patient is clinically symptomatic. Cystoscopy is also recommended in cases of a barrel-shaped endocervical growth and in cases where the growth has extended to the anterior vaginal wall. Suspected bladder or rectal involvement should be confirmed by biopsy and histologic evidence. Bullous edema alone does not warrant a case to be allocated to Stage IV.

Pathologic Staging

In case a surgical specimen is available or where image-guided fine-needle aspiration cytology has been done, the pathologic report is an important source for accurate assessment of the extent of disease. As in the case of imaging, the pathologic methods should also be recorded for future evaluation. The stage is to be allocated after all imaging and pathology reports are available. It cannot be altered later, for example at recurrence.

The FIGO and TNM classifications have been virtually identical in describing the anatomical extent of disease. The TNM nomenclature has hitherto been used for the purpose of documenting nodal and metastatic disease status. The revised FIGO classification is now more closely aligned with the TNM classification in this respect as well.

Histopathology

It is essential that all cancers must be confirmed by microscopic examination. Cases are classified as carcinomas of the cervix if the primary growth is in the cervix. All histologic types must be included. The histopathologic types, as described in the World Health Organization's 2014 Tumours of the Female Reproductive Organs are:

1. Squamous cell carcinoma (keratinizing; non-keratinizing; papillary, basaloid, warty, verrucous, squamotransitional, lymphoepithelioma-like)
2. Adenocarcinoma (endocervical; mucinous, villoglandular, endometrioid)
3. Clear cell adenocarcinoma
4. Serous carcinoma
5. Adenosquamous carcinoma
6. Glassy cell carcinoma
7. Adenoid cystic carcinoma
8. Adenoid basal carcinoma
9. Small cell carcinoma
10. Undifferentiated carcinoma

Grading by any of several methods is encouraged, but it is not a basis for modifying the stage groupings in cervical carcinoma. Histopathologic grades are as follows:

1. GX: Grade cannot be assessed
2. G1: Well differentiated
3. G2: Moderately differentiated
4. G3: Poorly or undifferentiated

Management of Cervical Cancer

Management of cervical cancer is primarily by surgery or radiation therapy, with chemotherapy a valuable adjunct.

Surgical Management

Surgery is suitable for early stages, where cervical conization, total simple hysterectomy, or radical hysterectomy may be selected according to the stage of disease and extent of spread of cervical cancer. Table 2 shows the types of radical hysterectomy. In Stage IVA, there is a place for pelvic exenteration in selected cases.

Table 2: Types of radical hysterectomy

	Simple extrafascial hysterectomy	*Modified radical hysterectomy*	*Radical hysterectomy*
Piver and Rutledge Classification	Type I	Type II	Type III
Querleu and Morrow classification	Type A	Type B	Type C
Uterus and cervix	Removed	Removed	Removed
Ovaries	Optional removal	Optional removal	Optional removal
Vaginal margin	None	1–2 cm	Upper one-quarter to one-third
Ureters	Not mobilized	Tunnel through broad ligament	Tunnel through broad ligament

Contd...

Contd...

	Simple extrafascial hysterectomy	*Modified radical hysterectomy*	*Radical hysterectomy*
Cardinal ligaments	Divided at uterine and cervical border	Divided where ureter transits broad ligaments	Divided at pelvic side wall
Uterosacral ligaments	Divided at cervical border	Partially removed	Divided near sacral origin
Urinary bladder	Mobilized to base of bladder	Mobilized to upper vagina	Mobilized to middle vagina
Rectum	Not mobilized	Mobilized below cervix	Mobilized below cervix
Surgical approach	Laparotomy or laparoscopy or robotic surgery	Laparotomy or laparoscopy or robotic surgery	Laparotomy or laparoscopy or robotic surgery

Microinvasive Cervical Carcinoma: FIGO Stage IA

Stage IA1

Young females: The treatment is completed with cervical conization unless there is lymphovascular space invasion (LVSI) or tumor cells are present at the surgical margin.

Older females: In women who have completed childbearing or elderly women, total extrafascial hysterectomy may also is recommended. Any route can be chosen, i.e. abdominal, vaginal, or laparoscopic.

Stage IA2

Older females: Since there is a small risk of lymph node metastases in these cases, pelvic lymphadenectomy is performed in addition to type 2 radical hysterectomy or more radical surgery. In low risk cases, simple hysterectomy or trachelectomy, with either pelvic lymphadenectomy or sentinel lymph node assessment, may be adequate surgical treatment. When the patient desires fertility, she may be offered a choice of the following: (1) cervical conization with laparoscopic (or extraperitoneal) pelvic lymphadenectomy; or (2) radical abdominal, vaginal, or laparoscopic trachelectomy with pelvic lymphadenectomy.

Post-treatment Follow-up

Follow-up with 3-monthly Pap smears for 2 years, then 6-monthly for the next 3 years is recommended after treatment of microinvasive carcinoma. With normal follow-up at 5 years, the patient can return to the routine screening schedule according to the national guidelines.

FIGO Stage IB1

FIGO Stage IB1 is considered as low risk with the following criteria: largest tumor diameter less than 2 cm, cervical stromal invasion less than 50%, and no suspicious lymph nodes on imaging in older females. The standard management is a type 3 radical hysterectomy, but modified radical hysterectomy may be considered in these cases. Pelvic lymphadenectomy should always be included on account of the high frequency of lymph node involvement.

A pelvic nerve-sparing surgical procedure is recommended in patients undergoing radical hysterectomy, in so far as radical curability is maintained, as intrapelvic injuries to the autonomic nerves (i.e. hypogastric nerve, splanchnic nerve, and pelvic plexus) often lead to impairment of urination, defecation, and sexual function, and consequent deterioration of the postoperative quality of life (QOL).

In young women desiring fertility sparing, a radical trachelectomy may be performed, indicated for Stage IA2–IB1 tumors measuring less than or equal to 2 cm in largest diameter. The cervix along with the parametrium is removed followed by anastomosis of the uterus with the vaginal end. Trachelectomy can be done by open abdominal, vaginal, or by minimally invasive routes. When a vaginal approach is planned, the pelvic nodes are first removed laparoscopically and sent for frozen section to confirm node negativity and then proceed with the radical trachelectomy vaginally. Alternatively, the nodes may be first be assessed by conventional pathologic methods and the radical trachelectomy done as a second surgery after 1 week.

FIGO Stage IB2 and IIA1

In FIGO Stage IB2 and IIA1 cervical cancer, surgery or radiotherapy can be chosen as the primary treatment depending on other patient factors and local resources, as both have similar outcomes. The advantages of surgical treatment are: (1) that it is feasible to determine the postoperative stage precisely on the basis of histopathologic findings, thereby enabling individualization of postoperative treatment for each patient; (2) that it is possible to treat cancers that are likely to be resistant to radiotherapy; and (3) that it is possible to conserve ovarian function. Intraoperative transpositioning of the ovaries high in the paracolic gutters away from the radiation field, in case it should be required subsequently, is also feasible. The preservation of ovarian and sexual function makes surgery the preferred mode in younger women. Type C radical hysterectomy represents a basic procedure for the treatment of cervical cancer, consisting of removal of the uterus, parametrium, upper vagina, and a part of the paracolpium, along with pelvic lymphadenectomy. As for the adjacent connective tissues, the anterior vesicouterine ligament (anterior and posterior leaf), lateral cardinal ligaments, and posterior sacrouterine and rectovaginal ligaments are cut from the uterus at sufficient distances from their attachments to the uterus. Lymphadenectomy constitutes one of the bases of this surgical procedure, and the extent of regional lymph node excision includes the parametrial nodes, obturator nodes, external, internal, and common iliac nodes.

The role of sentinel lymph node (SLN) mapping in cervical cancer is still experimental and needs more evidence to include into routine practice. It may have some role in early stage cervical cancer, i.e. FIGO Stage IA, IB1, and IB2. Dual labeling using blue dye and radiocolloid increases the accuracy of sentinel lymph nodes can be performed with. Indocyanine green dye with near infrared technique has been used in robotic surgery and laparoscopy. Pelvic lymphadenectomy needs to be considered if LVSI is present.

The route of surgery may be laparotomy or minimally invasive surgery, either laparoscopic or robotic. The LACC trial (Laparoscopic Approach to Cervical Cancer) compared the overall survival with open surgery versus laparoscopy or robotic surgery in early stage cervical cancer and showed a decreased overall survival. They concluded that hysterectomy by a minimally invasive route was associated with higher rates of recurrence than the open approach in early-stage cervical cancer patients. Further studies may be required to further confirm these findings.

FIGO Stage IB3 and IIA2

In Stage IB3 and IIA2, the tumors are larger and the likelihood of high risk factors such as positive lymph nodes, positive parametria, or positive surgical margins that increase the risk of recurrence and require adjuvant radiation after surgery are high. Other risk factors that increase the risk of pelvic recurrence even when nodes are not involved include: largest tumor diameter greater than 4 cm, LVSI, and invasion of outer one-third of the cervical stroma. In such cases, adjuvant whole pelvic irradiation reduces the local failure rate and improves progression-free survival compared with patients treated with surgery alone. However, the dual modality treatment increases the risk of major morbidity to the patient.

The treatment modality must, therefore, be determined based on the availability of resources and tumor- and patient-related factors. In all these cases concurrent platinum-based chemoradiation (CCRT) is the preferred treatment option for Stage IB3 to IIA2 lesions. It has been demonstrated that the prognosis is more favorable with CCRT, rather than radiotherapy alone, as postoperative adjuvant therapy as well in terms of overall survival, progression-free survival, and local and distant recurrences.

In areas where radiotherapy facilities are scarce, neoadjuvant chemotherapy (NACT) has been used with the goal of: (1) downstaging of the tumor to improve the radical curability and safety of surgery; and (2) inhibition of micrometastasis and distant metastasis. There is no unanimity of view as to whether it improves prognosis compared with the standard treatment.

The extent of surgery after NACT remains the same, i.e. radical hysterectomy and pelvic lymphadenectomy. The greater difficulty is in determining the indications for adjuvant therapy which are often kept the same as those after primary surgery. However, it must be remembered that NACT may give a false sense of security by masking the pathologic findings and thus affecting evaluation of indications for adjuvant radiotherapy/CCRT. NACT surgery is best reserved for research settings or those areas where radiotherapy is unavailable. This is especially true in patients with very large tumors or adenocarcinoma, which have lower response rates.

FIGO Stage IVA or Recurrence

Rarely, patients with Stage IVA disease may have only central disease without involvement to the pelvic sidewall or distant spread. Such cases, or in case of such a recurrence, pelvic exenteration can be considered but usually has a poor prognosis.

Radiation Management

In LMICs, the majority of patients present with locally advanced disease, where surgery plays a limited role, and radiotherapy has an important role. Over the last two decades, development of sophisticated planning and delivery techniques, and introduction of computer technology and imaging have galvanized the practice of radiotherapy, resulting in improved clinical outcome and reduced toxicity.

Apart from its curative role, radiotherapy can also be used as adjuvant therapy for operated patients to prevent locoregional recurrence, although the role of "dual modality" is discouraged, and as palliative therapy for alleviating distressing symptoms in patients with advanced incurable disease.

Radiation Therapy for Early Stage Disease (FIGO Stage IA, IB1, IB2, and IIA1)

Although surgery is preferred for early stage disease, in cases with contraindications for surgery or anesthesia, radiotherapy provides equally good results in terms of local control and survival. Treatment decision should be made on the basis of clinical, anatomic, and social factors. Patients with microinvasive disease have been treated by intracavitary radiation therapy (ICRT) alone with good results if surgery is contraindicated owing to medical problems. Selected patients with very small Stage IB1 disease (less than 1 cm) may also be treated with ICRT alone, particularly if there are relative contraindications to external beam radiation therapy (EBRT). A dose of 60–65 Gy equivalent is usually prescribed to Point A. Combination of EBRT and ICRT is also an option for such patients.

Adjuvant Radiotherapy

Following radical hysterectomy, Post Operative Radiotherapy (PORT) with or without chemotherapy is indicated for patients with adverse pathologic factors such as positive pelvic nodes, parametrial infiltration, positive margins, deep stromal invasion, etc. According to various prognostic factors, patients may be categorized into high-risk, intermediate-risk, or low-risk disease. High-risk disease includes patients with either positive surgical margins or lymph node metastases or parametrial spread, and such patients should be offered PORT with chemotherapy since the GOG 109 trial has shown overall survival advantage. Intermediate-risk patients with any two of three factors (tumor size more than 4 cm, lymphovascular invasion, deep stromal invasion) require PORT64, 81 and no chemotherapy should be offered to these patients. All other patients following radical hysterectomy are termed as low-risk disease patients and do not need any adjuvant therapy.

PORT consists of whole pelvic EBRT to cover the tumor bed and draining lymph node areas. A dose of 45–50 Gy is usually prescribed. Intensity modulated radiation therapy (IMRT), an advanced and refined technique of irradiation, has been explored in the postoperative setting to reduce the toxicity.

Radiation Therapy for FIGO Stage IB3 and IIA2

Although feasible, surgery as initial treatment is not encouraged for patients with Stage IB3 and IIA2 disease since 80% of them require PORT or CCRT. It is well known that the addition of adjuvant radiotherapy to surgery increases morbidity and thus compromises the quality of life. Additionally, combined modality treatment will unnecessarily overburden the surgical and radiation facilities, which are already inadequate in low-resource countries. Therefore, CCRT is the standard of care for Stage IB3 and IIA2 disease. CCRT includes external radiation and intracavitary brachytherapy.

Radiation Therapy for FIGO Stage IIB–IVA

Concurrent chemoradiation is considered the standard treatment for patients with locally advanced cervical cancer (LACC). The chemotherapy regimen is intravenous administration of weekly cisplatin during the course of EBRT.

A once-weekly infusion of cisplatin (40 mg/m^2 weekly with appropriate hydration) for 5–6 cycles during external beam therapy is a commonly used concurrent chemotherapy regimen. For patients who are unable to receive platinum chemotherapy, 5-fluorouracil-based regimens are an acceptable alternative.

The combination of EBRT and ICRT maximizes the likelihood of locoregional control while minimizing the risk of treatment complications. The primary goal of EBRT is to sterilize local disease and to shrink the tumor to facilitate subsequent ICRT. Standard EBRT should deliver a dose of 45–50 Gy to the whole pelvis by 2 or 4 field box technique (Table 3) encompassing uterus, cervix, adnexal structures, parametria, and pelvic lymph nodes. Although EBRT is commonly delivered by a Cobalt-60 teletherapy machine in several low-resource countries, linear accelerators are preferred nowadays as they provide higher energy beams resulting in more homogeneous dose delivery to deep tissues with relative sparing of superficial tissues. Recently, conformal radiotherapy techniques like 3D-CRT and IMRT are increasingly being used with encouraging results in terms of reduced toxicity owing to relative sparing of normal tissues.

Table 3: Field design for the pelvic radiotherapy

Field	Border	Landmark
AP-PA fields	Superior Inferior Lateral	L4–5 vertebral interspace 2 cm below the obturator foramen or 3 cm inferior to distal disease, whichever is lower 1.5–2 cm lateral to the pelvic brim

Contd...

Contd...

Table 3: Field design for the pelvic radiotherapy

Field	*Border*	*Landmark*
Lateral fields	Superior	Same as AP-PA field
	Inferior	Same as AP-PA field
	Anterior	Anterior to the pubic symphysis
	Posterior	0.5 cm posterior to the anterior border of the S2/3 vertebral junction. May include the entire sacrum to cover the disease extent

Although EBRT plays an important role in the treatment of cervical cancer, ICRT is also an extremely important component of curative treatment of cervical cancer since it delivers a high central dose to the primary tumor and reduced doses to adjacent normal organs owing to sharp dose fall-off.

Standard ICRT is usually performed using a tandem and two ovoids, or a tandem and ring. Any of the dose rate systems, namely low-dose-rate (LDR), high-dose-rate (HDR), or pulsed-dose-rate (PDR) may be practiced as all three yield comparable survival rates.108 The dose is usually prescribed to Point A or to high-risk clinical target volume (HRCTV) if image-based planning is used.

With an LDR system, a dose of 30–40 Gy is prescribed in one or two sessions. With HDR, various dose fraction schedules are used, employing a dose of 5.5–8 Gy by 3–5 weekly fractions.

If ICRT is not feasible either due to distorted anatomy or inadequate dosimetry, then interstitial brachytherapy should be considered. Interstitial brachytherapy consists of insertion of multiple needles/catheters into the primary tumor and parametria through the perineum with the help of a template. Due to the risk of trauma to normal structures like bowel and bladder, use of ultrasound imaging (especially transrectal) is suggested during the implant procedure.

Completion of the radiotherapy protocol within the stipulated time is an important goal as it has a direct correlation on the outcome. In retrospective analyses, patients whose radiotherapy treatment times exceeded 9–10 weeks had significantly higher rates of pelvic failure when compared with women whose treatment was completed in less than 6–7 weeks. Currently the recommendation is to complete the entire protocol of EBRT and brachytherapy within 8 weeks.

FIGO Stage IVB/Distant Metastases

Presentation with distant metastatic disease is rare, reported in about 2% of cases. A management plan should consider that the median duration of survival with distant metastatic disease is approximately 7 months.

Concurrent chemoradiation may have better response than systemic chemotherapy with overall and disease-free survivals of 69% and 57%, respectively, reported in patients with positive para-aortic and supraclavicular lymph nodes.

Recurrent Disease

Recurrences may occur locally in the pelvic or para-aortic, the patient may develop distant metastases, or there may be a combination. The risk of both pelvic and distant failure increases in proportion to tumor volume. Most recurrences are seen within 3 years and the prognosis is poor, as most patients die from progressive disease with uremia being the most common terminal event. The treatment plan depends on the patient's performance status, site and extent of recurrence and/or metastases, and prior treatment received.

If there is extensive local disease or distant metastatic disease, the patient is assigned to palliative therapy, with best supportive care and symptom control the recommended management.

Local Recurrence

The pelvis is the most common site of recurrence and patients who have only locally recurrent disease after definitive therapy, whether surgery or radiotherapy, are in a more favorable situation as the disease is potentially curable. Good prognostic factors are the presence of an isolated central pelvic recurrence with no involvement of the pelvic sidewall, a long disease-free interval from previous therapy, and the largest diameter of the recurrent tumor is less than 3 cm.

When the pelvic relapse follows primary surgery, it may be treated by either radical chemoradiation or pelvic exenteration. Confirmation of recurrence with a pathologic specimen obtained by biopsy is essential prior to proceeding with either therapy. The extent of recurrent disease and involvement of pelvic lymph nodes are prognostic factors for survival.

Concurrent chemotherapy with either cisplatin and/or 5-fluorouracil may improve outcome.

Pelvic exenteration may be feasible in some patients in whom there is no evidence of intraperitoneal or extrapelvic spread, and there is a clear tumor-free space between the recurrent disease and the pelvic sidewall. Owing to its high morbidity, it is reserved for those with expected curative potential and requires careful patient selection regarding the associated physical and psychological demands. A PET/CT scan is the most sensitive noninvasive test to determine any sites of distant disease, and should be performed prior to exenteration, if possible.

Special Situations

Cervical Cancer during Pregnancy

Adequate management of these patients requires a multidisciplinary team. The plan must be discussed with the patient and, preferably, her partner, as their wishes are to be respected.

Broadly, the management of cervical cancer in pregnancy follows the same principles as in the nonpregnant state. Before 16–20 weeks of pregnancy, patients are treated without delay. The mode of therapy can be either surgery or chemoradiation depending on the stage of the disease. Radiation often results in spontaneous abortion of the conceptus. From the late second trimester onward, surgery and chemotherapy can be used in selected cases while preserving the pregnancy. When the diagnosis is made after 20 weeks, delaying definitive treatment is a valid option for Stages IA2 and IB1 and 1B2, which has not been shown to have any negative impact on the prognosis compared with nonpregnant controls. Timing of delivery requires a balance between maternal and fetal health interests. When delivered at a tertiary center with appropriate neonatal care, delivery by classical cesarean and radical hysterectomy at the same time is undertaken not later than 34 weeks of pregnancy.

For more advanced disease, the impact of treatment delay on survival is not known. Neoadjuvant chemotherapy may be administered to prevent disease progression in women with locally advanced cervical cancer when a treatment delay is planned.

Annexures

Annexure 1

Hormones in Gynae

Ovarian cycle is initiated by	FSH
Ratio of FSH : LH in PCOD	1 : 2
FSH, LH Ratio checked on	Day 2–3 of menstrual cycle
LH surge is initiated by	Estrogen
Time between LH surge and ovulation	(32–36 hrs) Best answer (24–36 hrs) IInd best answer
Time between LH peak (serum) and ovulation	10–12 hrs
Time between LH peak (urinary) and ovulation	24 hrs
Peak levels of LH during menstrual cycle	75 ng/mL
Just before ovulation	Both LH and FSH surge
Progesterone synthesis begins	36 hrs before ovulation due to LH surge
Meiosis I is resumed due to	LH
Corpus luteum in non preg. females maintained by	LH
In pregnancy-maintained by	hCG
Maxm. function of corpus luteum/Maxm secretion of progesterone	D8/22nd day of menstrual cycle
Progesterone in viable pregnancy Progesterone in non viable pregnancy	> 25 ng/mL < 5 ng/mL
Total progesterone in single pregnancy	250 ng/dL
Total progesterone in multifetal pregnancy	600 ng/dL
Placenta takes over function of CL at	8–10 weeks
Life span of CL in non pregnant females	12–14 days
Life span of CL in pregnant females	10–12 weeks
Trigger for ovulation in Ⓝ cycle	LH
Trigger for ovulation in artificial cycle	hCG (5000–10,000 IU)
Ovum pickup done—hrs after hCG injection	36 hrs
1st cell division of embryo occurs	20 hrs after fertilisation
Stage of transfer of embryo in ART cycle	Blastocyst
Maxm number of embryo transferred	3
Site of transfer	2 cm below the fundus
What is the first stimulus the release of testosterone from Leydig cells of fetus	hCG (man) > ACTH
Sine a quanon for menopause	FSH ≥ 40 IU

Annexure 2

Lining of Female Genital Tract

Organ/Structure	Epithelial lining
• Bartholin's gland	Single layer of low columnar cell
• Bartholin's duct (Jeffcoate 7/e, p 24)	Multilayered columnar cells (Not transitional)
• Adult vagina	Stratified squamous epithelium
• Newborn vagina	Transitional epithelium
• Uterus	Columnar epithelium
• Cervix (endocervix, cervical canal)	High columnar epithelium
• Ectocervix	Squamous epithelium
• Fallopian tube	Ciliated columnar epithelium

Blood Supply of Genital Tract

Organ	Supplied by
Uterus	Uterine artery (branch of ant. div. of internal iliac artery) and ovarian artery.
Cervix	Descending cervical artery (branch of uterine artery).
Vagina	Vaginal artery (Separate branch of int. iliac artery or may come from uterine artery), branches of int. pudendal, middle and inferior rectal arteries.
Fallopian tube	Medial 2/3rd – uterine artery, lateral 1/3rd – ovarian artery.
Ovary	Ovarian artery (branch of aorta).
Vulva	Internal pudendal artery (terminal branch of int. iliac artery).

Annexure 3

Lymphatic Drainage of Female Genitalia

Organ	Lymphatic drainage
Ovaries	Para–aortic lymph node (lateral aortic nodes)
Fallopian Tube	• Along ovarian lymphatic • Along cornua • Lateral aortic lymph node • Superficial inguinal lymph node
Uterus • Fundus • Body • Cornus	 • Lateral aortic lymph node • External iliac lymph node • Superficial inguinal lymph node (along round ligament)
Cervix	• H – Hypogastric lymph node/internal iliac • O – Obturator lymph node • P – Presacral lymph node and parametrial lymph node (sentinel lymph node) • E – External iliac lymph node.
(***Note:*** Cervix does not drain into superficial inguinal lymph node So cancer cervix rarely involves inguinal lymph node). M/c lymph node involved in cancer cervix–obturator lymph node. Ist lymph node involved in cancer cervix–parametrial lymph node or paracervical lymph node (also called as ureteric lymph node).	
Vagina: • Upper part • Middle part • Lower	 • Same like cervix. • Internal iliac lymph node. • Superficial inguinal lymph node.
Vulva	• Superficial inguinal lymph node (sentinel lymph node) • Deep inguinal lymph node • Internal iliac nodes
Clitoris	• Superficial + deep inguinal lymph node (glansclitoris). • The anterior most lymph node of deep inguinal group is called as lymph node of cloquet/ Rosenmuller lymph node

Annexure 4

pH of Vagina at Different Ages

Age	Vaginal pH
Newborn infants	Between 5.5–6
6 weeks old child	6–8
Puberty	Charges from alkaline to acidic
Reproductive age group	4–5.5
Pregnancy	3.5–4.5
Menstruation	6–8
Menopause	6–8

Annexure 5

Some Important Measurements

Structure	Measurement
• Isthmus which forms lower uterine segment	5–6 mm^Q
• Female urethra	35–40 mm^Q
• Posterior vaginal wall	11.5 cm
• Anterior vaginal wall	9 cm
• Uterus (Nulliparous)	8 cm × 6 cm × 4 cm (3 × 2 × 1 inches)
Structure	**Measurement**
• Cervix	2.5–3.5 cm
• Ovary	3 × 2 × 1 cms
• Fallopian tube	10–12 cm
• Mature ovum	120–140 microns
• Mature/ripe graafian follicle	5–8 mm
Just before ovulation site of graafian follicle	16–24 mm (≈20 mm)
Some important angles to remember:	
• Angle of anteflexion (angle between cervix and uterus)	120–130°
• Angle of anteversion (angle between cervix and vagina)	90°
• Urethrovesical angle	100°

Annexure 6

Male and Female Derivatives of Embryonic Urogenital Structures

Embryonic structures	Derivatives	
	Male	**Females**
Genital swelling	Scrotum^Q	Labia majora^Q
Genital folds	Ventral aspect of penis	Labia minora
Genital tubercle^Q	Penis^Q	Clitoris^Q
Urogenital sinus	Urinary bladder Urethra except navicular fossa Prostate gland Prostatic utricle Bulbourethral glands	Urinary bladder Urethral and paraurethral glands Lower part of Vagina Bartholin's glands
Paramesonephric duct/Mullerian duct	Appendix of testes Prostatitis utriculus	Uterus, cervix, fallopian tubes, upper part of vagina
Mesonephric duct/Wolffian duct	Vas deferens Seminal vesicles, epididymis ejaculatory duct	Epoophoron, Paraoophoron Gartner's cyst, Organ of Rossenmuller
Genital ridge	Testis	Ovary

Annexure 7

Origin of Female Genital Tract

Part of female genital system	Originates from
Ovary	Genital ridge
Fallopian tubes	Mullerian/paramesonephric duct
Uterus	
Cervix	
Upper part of vagina	
Lower part of vagina	Sinovaginal bulb/Urogenital Sinus

Annexure 8

Culture Media and DOC of Various Organism

Culture Medium

Organism	Culture Medium
Trichomonas	Feinberg-Whittington media/Diamond media
Candida	Sabouraud's media
Chlamydia	McCoy cells/HeLa cells
Gonococci	Thayer Martin media
TB	LJ media/Bactec

DOC

Condition	Drug of choice
Trichomonas vaginitis	
Nonpregnant	Metronidazole (2 g single dose)
Pregnant	Metronidazole in 2nd & 3rd trimester
Candidiasis	Antifungals: Acyclovir or Fancyclovir
Bacterial vaginosis	Metronidazole
HSV	Acyclovir
Condition	**Drug of choice**
Syphilis	Benzathine penicillin
Chancroid	Azithromycin or Ceftriaxone or Erythromycin
Granuloma Inguinale/Donovanosis caused by *Calymmatobacterium* (*Klebsiella*) *granulomatis*	Doxycycline or Azithromycin Ciprofloxacin or Erythromycin
Gonococcal infection:	
Uncomplicated: Nonpregnant	Single dose = Ceftriaxone + Azithromycin or Doxycycline (100 mg B/D × 7 days)
Pregnant	Ceftriaxone or Cefixime. If patient is allergic to cephalosporin → Spectinomycin **Note:** for Gonococcal endocarditis antimicrobials should be continued for 4 weeks & for meningitis 10–14 days
Chlamydia	
Non pregnant	Ist Choice Single dose = Azithromycin + contact tracing 2nd choice = Doxycycline or Erythromycin
Pregnant	Ist Choice Azithromycin or Amoxicillin 2nd choice = Erythromycin
Scabies	
Non pregnant	Lindane
Pregnant & young children	10% Crotamine lotion cream or 5% Permethrin cream

Annexure 9

Clinical Features of Genital Ulcers

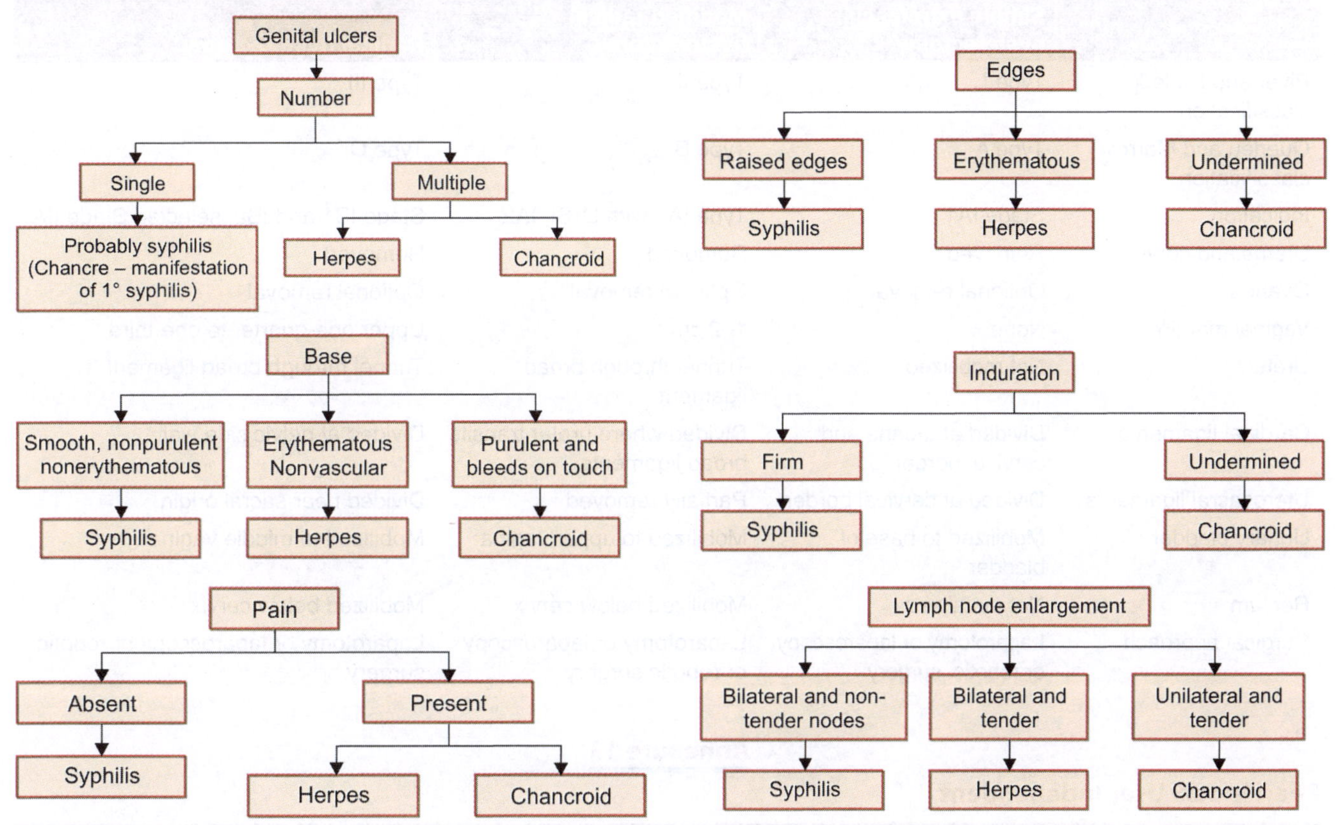

Annexure 10

Tests in Gynecology

Test	Use
GnRH stimulation test	Central precocious puberty
ACTH stimulation test	Non classical CAH
Sims Huhner test	Post coital test
Inslers test	Cervical mucus assessment
Miller Kurzrok test	Sperm mucus penetration test
Rubins test/tubal insufflation test	Fallopian tube potency
Q tip test, Bonney test	Urethral hypermobility test for SUI
Schiller's test	VILI
Whiff test	Bacterial vaginosis
Bonney test	SUI due to cystocele

Annexure 11

T1/2 of Hormones

Hormone	T1/2
LH	20 min
FSH	3–4 hours
hCG	36 hrs
HPL	10–13 mins
GnRH	2–4 mins
Oxytocin	3–5 mins

Annexure 12

Types of Radical Hysterectomy

	Simple extrafascial hysterectomy	Modified radical hysterectomy	Radical hysterectomy
Piver and Rutledge classification	Type I	Type II	Type III
Querleu and Morrow classification	Type A	Type B	Type C
Indication	Stage IA1	Type IA1 with LVSI, IA2	Stage IB1 and IB2, selected Stage IIA
Uterus and cervix	Removed	Removed	Removed
Ovaries	Optional removal	Optional removal	Optional removal
Vaginal margin	None	1–2 cm	Upper one-quarter to one-third
Ureters	Not mobilized	Tunnel through broad ligament	Tunnel through broad ligament
Cardinal ligaments	Divided at uterine and cervical border	Divided where ureter transits broad ligaments	Divided at pelvic side wall
Uterosacral ligaments	Divided at cervical border	Partially removed	Divided near sacral origin
Urinary bladder	Mobilized to base of bladder	Mobilized to upper vagina	Mobilized to middle vagina
Rectum	Not mobilized	Mobilized below cervix	Mobilized below cervix
Surgical approach	Laparotomy or laparoscopy or robotic surgery	Laparotomy or laparoscopy or robotic surgery	Laparotomy or laparoscopy or robotic surgery

Annexure 13

Pearl Index: User Independent

Contraception	Perfect use rate	Typical use
Implants	0.5%	.05%
Sterilization		
Male	0.1%	0.15%
Female	0.5%	0.5%
IUCD		
Mirena	0.2%	0.2%
CuT	0.6%	0.8%

User Dependent

Contraception	Perfect use rate	Typical use
OCP's	0.3%	8.7%
Vaginal ring	0.3%	8%
Transdermal path	0.3%	8%
DMPA	0.3%	3%
Diaphragm	20%	20%
Sponge		
Nullliparous	9	16
Parous	26	32
Condom		
Male	2	16
Female	5	21

Annexure 14

IOC and Gold Standards in Gynecology

	IOC	Gold standard
PID:	Laparoscopy	
Chlamydia	NAAT/PCR	Culture
Gonococcus infection	Saline microscopy	Gram stain
Candidiasis		Culture
Trichomonas vaginitis		Culture
Chancroid	Culture scrapings from ulcer	
Genital herpes	Electron microscopy of scrapings from ulcer	
LGV	ELISA test	
Syphilis	Screening = VDRL Confirmatory = Specific treponemal test	
Uterine malformation	MRI > 3D USG	Hysteroscopy
PCOD	Rotterdam criteria IOC–USG	
Fibroid	USG	
Endometriosis	Laparoscopy	HPE
Adenomyosis	USG > MRI	HPE
Congenital Adrenal Hyperplasia	17 hydroxy progesterone levels	ACTH stimulation challenge test

AIIMS New Pattern Questions with Answers

Gynecology

1. **Which of the following regarding development of female genital tract is not correct?**
   a. Uterus develops from Mullerian ducts
   b. Sinovaginal bulb contributes to development of vagina
   c. Ovaries arise from mesonephric tissue
   d. Fallopian tube arise from infused part of Mullerian ducts
2. **Day of ovulation is:**
   a. 14 days before next menstruation
   b. 14 days after menstruation
   c. 10 days after menstruation
   d. 18 days after menstruation
3. **Match list I (important events) and list II (main hormone responsible).**

	List I		List II
A.	Initiation of LH surge	1.	Progesterone
B.	Preventing luteolysis of corpus luteum	2.	LH
		3.	hcG
		4.	FSH
C.	Initiation of ovarian cycle	5.	Estrogen
D.	Luteal phase defect	6.	GnRH

	A	B	C	D
a.	5	1	6	2
b.	5	3	4	1
c.	5	2	4	1
d.	5	2	6	1

4. **All of the following changes occur after ovulation except:**
   a. Rise in basal body temperature
   b. Subnuclear Vacuolation
   c. LH surge
   d. Navicular cells in vaginal cytology
5. **Arrange the following events in order in which they occur during menstrual cycle.**
   a. Estrogen peak
   b. Maximum activity of corpus luteum
   c. Disappearance of ferning of cervical mucus
   d. Appearance of subnuclear vacuoles
   e. LH peak
   a. 1, 5, 4, 3, 2 b. 1, 5, 3, 4, 2
   c. 5, 1, 3, 4, 2 d. 5, 1, 4, 3, 2
6. **Which of the following statement is/are not correct:**
   a. FSH is necessary for development of granulosa cells
   b. Graffian follicle after ovulation becomes corpus luteum
   c. Atretic follicles are formed from atresia of corpus luteum
   d. Estradiol is formed from androgens in ovarian follicle
   e. Initial recruitment of follicles is hormone independent
7. **Arrange the following estrogens in order of potency:**
   a. $E_1 > E_2 > E_3 < E_4$ b. $E_2 > E_1 > E_3 > E_4$
   c. $E_2 > E_1 > E_4 > E_3$ d. $E_1 > E_2 > E_4 > E_3$
8. **In DUB for treatment of excessive bleeding, which of the following therapies is termed as medical curettage:**
   a. COC's b. Progestin
   c. NSAID d. Danazol
9. **A 17-year-old girl complains of heavy menstrual bleeding for 6 months. She has severe dysmenorrhoea on the first day of menstruation. She has 28-day regular cycles with excessive flow for 5 days. No abnormalities are detected on examination. The haemoglobin percentage is 9 g/dL. The coagulation profile and the ultrasound scan are normal. What is first line treatment?**
   a. Oral contraceptive pills for 3 cycles
   b. Mefenamic acid 500 mg 8 hourly during menstruation
   c. Norethisterone 5 mg three times daily for 7 days during menstruation
   d. Tranexamic acid 500 mg 8 hours during menstruation
   Note: When questions say first line treatment then use nonhormonal drugs
10. **A 17-year-old girl complains of continuous vaginal bleeding 3 weeks. She has had two previous similar episodes. Her BMI is 20. She has mild pallor of the mucus membranes, but no other abnormalities are detected. The haemoglobin percentage is 9 g/dL. The coagulation profile and the ultrasound scan are normal. What is the most Appropriate treatment?**
    a. Cyclical treatment with oral contraceptive pills for 3 months
    b. Norethisterone 5 mg thrice daily for 10 days
    c. Oral iron therapy
    d. Tranexamic acid 500 mg 8 hourly for 1 week
    Note: When questions say most appropriate treatment/ definitive treatment then use hormones
11. **A 35-year-old woman complains of heavy menstrual bleeding for 6 months. She has 28-days regular cycles which last for 7 days. Abdominal and vaginal examinations are normal. The haemoglobin percentage is 9 g/dL and the platelet count is within the normal range. The transvaginal ultrasound scan is normal. What is the most appropriate first line treatment?**
    a. Cyclical treatment with oral contraceptive pills for 3 months.
    b. Dilatation and curettage.
    c. Norethisterone 5 mg three times daily for 7 days during menstruation.
    d. Norethisterone 5 mg twice daily for 3 cycles of 21 days.
    e. Tranexamic acid 500 mg 8 hourly for 1 week during menstruation.
12. **A 36-years-old woman complains of irregular frequent menstrual bleeding for 6 months. Abdominal and vaginal examinations are normal. The haemoglobin level is 9 g/dL and the platelet count is normal. The transvaginal ultrasound scan is normal. Her BMI is 30. What is the first line treatment?**
    a. Cyclical treatment with oral contraceptive pills for 3 months
    b. Dilatation and curettage
    c. Norethisterone 5 mg three times daily for 7 days during menstruation
    d. Norethisterone 5 mg twice daily for 3 cycles of 21 days
    e. Tranexamic acid 500 mg 8 hourly for 1 week during menstruation

Ans: 1. c 2. a 3. b 4. c 5. a 6. a, b, d, e
7. b 8. b 9. b 10. a 11. e 12. a

13. A 44-year-old women complains of continuous vaginal bleeding for 6 months. She has had an endometrial biopsy 3 months ago and the histology report revealed proliferative endometrium. She responded to treatment with norethisterone 5 mg twice daily for 3 cycles of 21 days, but bleeding recurred soon after cessation of treatment. Transvaginal ultrasound scan reveals an endometrial thickness of 8 mm. The haemoglobin level is 9.5 gm/dL. The platelet count is normal. Her BMI is 22. She does not have any medical complications. What is the most appropriate method of treatment?

a. Insert a levonorgestrel-releasing intrauterine system
b. Perform a hysterectomy
c. Perform a dilatation and curettage
d. Treat with oral contraceptive pills for 3 cycles

14. A 44-year-old woman complains of continuous vaginal bleeding for 6 months. She has had endometrial biopsy 3 months ago and the histology report revealed proliferative endometrium. She did not respond to medical treatment with norethisterone 5 mg twice daily 21 days. Transvaginal ultrasound scan reveals an endometrial thickness of 7 mm. The haemoglobin level is 9 gm/dL. The platelet count is normal. What is the most appropriate method of treatment?

a. Insert a levonorgestrel-releasing intra-uterine system.
b. Perform a dilatation and curettage.
c. Perform a hysterectomy
d. Treat with oral contraceptive pills for 3 cycles.

Note: Patient is not responding to hormone therapy, hence surgery is the treatment.

15. A 45-year-old multiparous woman complains of irregular bleeding for two months. No abnormalities are detected on abdominal and vaginal examination. Transvaginal ultrasound scan reveals uniform thickening of the endometrium measuring 12 mm. What is the next step in the management?

a. Dilatation and curettage
b. Hysteroscopic visualization and biopsy
c. MRI scan
d. Outpatient endometrial biopsy (Pipelle aspiration)
e. Saline infusion sonohysterography.

16. A 46-year-old woman complains of irregular bleeding for two months. No abnormalities are detected on abdominal and vaginal examination. Transvaginal ultrasound scan reveals irregular thickening of the endometrium with a maximum thickness of 14 mm. What is the next step in the management?

a. Dilatation and curettage
b. Hysteroscopic visualisation and biopsy
c. MRI scan
d. Outpatient endometrial biopsy
e. Saline infusion sonohysterography

17. Ulliperistal acetate is a/an:

a. GnRH agonist
b. Androgen antagonist
c. Selective estrogen receptor modulator
d. Selective progesterone receptor modulator

18. Side effect of clomiphene citrate includes all except

a. Multiple pregnancy
b. Increase risk of ovarian cancer
c. Multiple polycystic ovary
d. Teratogenic effect on off springs

19. In a patient with DUB, with secretory endometrium on HPE, the initial treatment will be:

a. COC's b. Progestin
c. NSAIDs d. Danazol

20. For which of the following bleeding patterns are progesterone not recommended?

a. Anovulatory cyclical bleeding
b. Anovulatory prolonged cycle
c. Ovulatory heavy cycles
d. Premenstrual spotting

21. Match list I (scores) with the list II (condition in which it is used).

A.	Insler score	1.	Bacterial vaginosis
B.	Nugent score	2.	Trichomonas vaginitis
C.	Boer Meisel score	3.	Cervical mucus
D.	Ferrman Gallwey score	4.	Hirsutism
		5.	Alopecia
		6.	Pregnancy prognosis of tubal infertility

	A	B	C	D
a.	6	1	3	4
b.	6	2	3	5
c.	3	2	6	5
d.	3	1	6	4

22. According to Ferriman Gallwey Scoring system—hirsutism is diagnosed when score is more than:

a. 8 b. 12
c. 16 d. 20

23. A 20-year average weight female presented with oligomenorrhea and abnormal facial hair growth along with high serum free testosterone level. On USG the ovaries are normal. The diagnosis is:

a. Idiopathic hirsutism
b. PCOD
c. Testosterone secreting tumor
d. Adrenal hyperplasia

24. Identify the instrument shown:

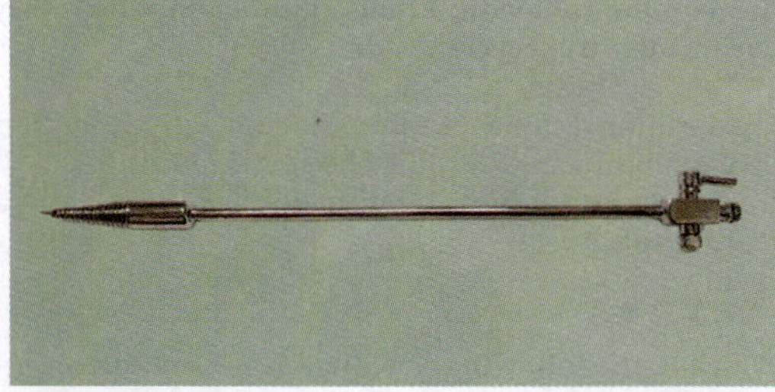

a. Hegar dilator b. Drew Smith Catheter
c. Leech Wilkinson Cannula
d. Visitor uterine Manipulator

25. A 58-year-old woman, post menopausal for last 8 years comes with H/o spotting per vagina. What is the most likely cause?

a. Endometrial hyperplasia b. Endometrial cancer
c. Atrophic endometrium d. ERT

26. HRT is C/I in:

a. Atherosclerosis b. Osteoporosis
c. Urogenital atrophy d. Venous thromboembolism

Ans: 13. a 14. c 15. d 16. b 17. d 18. d
19. a 20. c 21. d 22. a 23. b 24. c
25. c 26. d

27. Sexual precocity is often seen with:
a. Gauchers disease
b. Laurence Moon Biedl syndrome
c. Albright syndrome
d. Hand Schuller Christian disease

28. Consider the following features:
1. Presence of nonobstructive azoospermia
2. Tall undervirilized males with gynecomastia
3. Have small firm testis
4. Karyotype 47 XXY
5. Can be treated by TESE followed by ICSI

Features of Klinefelter's will include:
a. 1, 2, 3 b. 1, 2, 3, 4
c. 2, 3, 4 d. 1, 2, 3, 4, 5

Klinefelter syndrome:
- Incidence = 11–600 births
  1–2.1 of all males
- Males: Tall/undervirilized
  Have gynecomastia
  Have small; firm testes
- Increased risk of germ cell tumor, osteoporosis, hypothyroidism, diabetes and breast cancer
- MIC genotype 47 XXY
- But variation in number of X chromosome may occur
- Have Nonobstructive a azoospermia & can be treated by TESE followed by ICSI

29. Lower abdominal mass:
1. Chocolate cyst 2. Mature cystic teratoma
3. Fibroid 4. Cancer endometrium
5. Hematocalpos 6. Adenomyosis

Case 1: A 35-year-old nulliparous woman complains of menorrhagia:
O/E = Mass in abdomen palpable
P/V = Uterine size 16-18 weeks pregnancy
Tenderness present
Hb = 9 gm%
The most probable diagnosis of lower abdominal mass:
a. 1 b. 2
c. 3 d. 6

Note: Although fibroid are nontender but here due to large size it has undergone necrosis leading to pain.

Case 2: A 16-year-old female complains of pain in abdomen every month. She has not attained menarche.
O/E = Size of uterus is 14-16 weeks
P/A = No tenderness present
Secondary sexual characteristics are normal. On local examination tensed bluish hymen is seen.
Most probable diagnosis is
a. 1 b. 2
c. 4 d. 5

Note: She must be having imperforate hymen leading to hematocolpos

30. A 2-week-old neonate is diagnosed with ambiguous external genitalia at birth. Karyotype is 46 XX and examination under anesthesia does not reveal any other abnormality. Levels of 17 (OH) progesterone are raised. Most likely diagnosis is:
a. Turner syndrome b. CAH
c. MRKH syndrome d. Klinefelter syndrome

31. Match the description in list I with diagnosis in list II:

	List I		List II
A.	Hypoplastic uterus with streak gonads and short stature	1.	Testicular feminizing syndrome (complete)
B.	Hypoplastic uterus with streak gonads and normal stature	2.	MRKH syndrome
C.	Primary amenorrhea with anosmia	3.	Pure gonadal dysgenesis
D.	Primary amenorrhea with inguinal hernia with breast development corresponding to Tanner stage 5 and axillary hair corresponding to Tanner stage 1	4.	Kallman syndrome
		5.	Turner syndrome
		6.	Incomplete androgen insensitivity syndrome

	A	B	C	D
a.	5	3	4	1
b.	5	3	4	6
c.	3	2	4	1
d.	2	3	4	6

32. In which of following conditions Mullerian system is present?
a. MRKH syndrome b. Klinefelter syndrome
c. Swyers syndrome
d. Testicular feminization syndrome

33. Match list I (syndrome) with list II (associated condition) and detect correct answer.

	List I		List II
a.	Asherman syndrome	1.	Ascites, hydrothorax with fibroma of ovary
b.	Meigs syndrome	2.	Streak ovary with normal stature
c.	Kallmann syndrome	3.	Anosmia and color blindness with amenorrhea
d.	Swyer syndrome	4.	Streak gonads with short stature
		5.	Dysgenetic testis with amenorrhea
		6.	Intrauterine adhesions with amenorrhea

a. a-6, b-1, c-3, d-5 b. a-6, b-1, c-3, d-2
c. a-6, b-1, c-3, d-5 d. a-1, b-6, c-4, d-2

34. In testicular feminizing syndrome gonadectomy is indicated:
a. As soon as it is diagnosed
b. At puberty
c. Only when malignancy develops in it
d. When Hirsutism is evident

35. Consider the following findings:
1. Chromatin negative
2. Menorrhagia
3. Anovulatory cycles
4. Secondary amenorrhea

Which of the following is/are present in Turner syndrome?
a. 1 only b. 2 and 3
c. 2, 4 d. 1, 2, 3, 4

36. Primary amenorrhea can be caused by following Karyotypes *except*:
a. 45 XO b. 47 XXX
c. 46 XY d. 45 XO/46 XX

Ans: 27. c 28. d 29. Case 1 c, Case 2 d 30. b 31. a
32. c 33. a 34. b 35. a 36. b

37. In which of the following condition do the ovaries functions normally?
a. Turner's syndrome
b. Rokitansky-Kuster-Hauser syndrome
c. Androgen insensitivity syndrome
d. Swyer's syndrome

38. A mother brings her 19 years old daughter to your clinic complaint that she not started having menses. General examination reveals normally developed breasts and pubic hair. On pelvic examination, vaginal ending is blind and uterus is not palpable. Which of the following do you suspect?
a. Mullerian agenesis
b. Asherman syndrome
c. Gonadal dysgenesis
d. Turner's syndrome

39. A young female presented to you with primary amenorrhea. Examination reveals normal breast development and absent axillary hairs. Pelvic examination shows a normally developed vagina with clitoromegaly. On ultrasound, gonads are visible in the inguinal region. What is the most likely diagnosis?
a. Complete androgen insensitivity syndrome
b. Partial androgen insensitivity syndrome
c. Mayer Rokitansky Kuster Hauser syndrome
d. Gonadal dysgenesis

40. Consider the following statements:
1. The test should be done on Day 12-Day 13 of regular 28 day cycle
2. The cervical mucus is examined
3. In normal test, the sperms show rotatory motion
4. An abnormal test is followed by IVF

Which of the following statements pertain to postcoital test?
a. 1, 2, 3
b. 1, 2, 3, 4
c. 1, 2, 4
d. Only 1, 2

41. The nonavalent HPV vaccine .... against which strains of viruses:
a. 16, 18, 31, 33, 45, 52, 58, 68
b. 6, 8, 16, 18, 30, 32, 46, 53, 59, 69
c. Only 6, 8, 16, 18, 31, 33
d. Only 6, 8, 16, 18, 30, 32

42. Climacteric is related to:
a. Menstruation
b. Menarche
c. Menopause
d. None

43. Match the adult structure in list I with corresponding embryonic origin in list II:

List I	List II
a. Gartners duct	1. Mesonephric duct
b. Round ligament	2. Gubernaculum
c. Cower vagina	3. Genital ridge
d. Clitoris	4. Genital tubercle
	5. Müllerian duct
	6. Urogenital sinus

	A	B	C	D
a.	2	1	6	3
b.	2	1	5	3
c.	1	2	6	4
d.	1	2	5	4

44. Match list I (problem) with list II (IOC):

	List I		List II
A.	Endometriosis	1.	Laparoscopy
B.	Anovulation	2.	MAR test
C.	Ovarian failure	3.	Laparoscopic chromopertubation
D.	Antisperm antibody	4.	USG
		5.	Post coital test
		6.	AMH levels
		7.	Day 3 FSH
		8.	Hormonal study
		9.	Endometrial biopsy

	A	B	C	D
a.	1	9	6	5
b.	1	8	6	2
c.	3	4	7	5
d.	4	8	7	2

45. In azoospermia, the diagnostic test which can distinguish between testicular failure and obstruction of Vas deferens is:
a. Estimation of FSH level
b. Estimation of testosterone level
c. Karyotyping
d. FNAC of testis

46. In case of defect in level II De Lancey support the result is:
1. Cystocele
2. Enterocele
3. Rectocele
4. Urethrocele
a. Only 2
b. 1, 2
c. 1, 3
d. 1, 2, 3, 4

47. Match the following conditions of uterine prolapse in List I with surgery in List II

	List I		List II
a.	Young nulliparous female with 2° prolapse	1.	Colposuspension
b.	35 year old female with 2 children with 2° prolapse and cystocele and rectocele. She does not want pregnancy in future	2.	Gillians ventro suspension
c.	Prolapse in a 65 year old diabetic and Hypertensive female	3.	Fothergills surgery
d.	Vault prolapse	4.	Purandare cervicopexy
		5.	Le Forts colpocleisis
		6.	Uterosacral colposuspension

	a	b	c	d
A	4	3	5	2
B	2	3	6	1
C	2	6	1	3
D	4	3	5	6

48. Select the true statement regarding staging of cancer cervix.
a. Clinical examinations is the first step in staging
b. Biochemical investigation are included in staging
c. CT scan is best method to assess principal tumor less than 10 mm
d. Imaging and pathological fundings included in staging
e. For nodal metastasis more than 10 mm PET scan is best

Ans: 37. b 38. a 39. b 40. d 41. a 42. c
43. c 44. b 45. d 46. c 47. d 48. a, d, e

49. Dose of ulipristal as emergency contraceptive:
a. 3 mg b. 30 mg
c. 300 mg d. 300 mcg

50. Management of Retroverted uterus detected in routine examination in gynae clinic:
a. Pessary treatment
b. Ventral suspension surgery
c. Postural exercise
d. No treatment

51. Fitz-Hugh-Curtis syndrome is present in following:
a. Monoliasis b. Syphilis
c. TB d. Gonorrhea

52. Consider the following muscles:
1. Levator ani muscle
2. Ischiocavernosus
3. Bulbocavernosus
4. Obturator internus
5. Superficial transverse perenii

The muscles which do not attach to perineal body:
a. 2, 4 b. 2, 3, 4
c. 2, 3, 4, 5 d. only 4

53. Fistulas:
1. Vesicovaginal fistula
2. Ureterovaginal fistula
3. Uterovesical fistula
4. Urethrovaginal fistula
5. Rectovaginal fistula

Case 1: A case of obstructed labour which was delivered by cesarean section complains of cyclical passage of menstrual blood in urine. Which amongst the given options is the most likely site of fistula:
a. 1 b. 2
c. 3 d. 4

Case 2: A female complains of continuous passage of urine from vagina on methylene Blue 3 swab test, upper most cotton swab is wet with urine but is not stained with dye. The site of fistula is:
a. 1 b. 2
c. 4 d. 5

54. VVF due to obstructed labor occurs within:
a. 24 hrs b. 5 days
c. 48 hrs d. 2 weeks

55. An overweight hirsuit women of 30 years, with one live issue presented to the family planning clinic for advice for contraception. The best suited oral contraceptive will contain the following:
a. Norgestrel b. Noretisterone
c. Cyproterone acetate d. Medroxprogesterone acetate

56. Consider the following complication:
1. Cervical pregnancy
2. Cervical stenosis
3. Incompetent os
4. Cervical dystocia during labor
5. First trimester abortion

Which of the above complications occur after Fothergills repair?
a. 1, 2, 3, 4, 5 b. 1, 2, 3, 4
c. 2, 3, 4, 5 d. 2, 3, 4

57. Regarding de Lancey's level of support consider following parts:
1. Level I a. Support distal vagina, perineal body
2. Level II b. Support mid vagina
3. Level III c. Support apex

Which of the part given above is/are correctly matched:
a. 1 & 3 only b. 2 only
c. 2 & 3 only d. 1, 2 & 3

58. Which of the following conditions simulates most the menstrual pattern of pain:
a. Intramural fibroid b. Adenomyosis
c. Hematometra d. Granulosa cell tumor of ovary

59. With respect to Genuine stress incontinence, the treatment of choice is:
a. Kegels exercises
b. Busch colposuspension
c. TVT
d. Periurethral injection of bulking agent

60. Arrange the following steps of vaginal hysterectomy sequentially:
1. Clamping & cutting of uterine artery
2. Clamping & cutting of Tubo-ovarian round ligament pedicle
3. Clamping and cutting of cardinal ligament
4. Clamping & cutting of utero sacral ligament

a. 4, 3, 1, 2 b. 2, 1, 3, 4
c. 4, 1, 3, 2 d. 3, 4, 1, 2
(Remember its opposite in abdominal hysterectomy)

61. M/C organism leading to Bartholin abscess:
a. Treponema pallidum b. T. Vaginalis
c. N. gonorrhoeae d. Lymphoma venereum

62. Consider following statement regarding PID:
1. It prevalence is increasing all over the world
2. Infection of upper female genital factor females
3. Most important iatrogenic cause is IUCD
4. Cervical movement are painless
5. Always sexually transmitted

Correct statement are:
a. 1, 2, 3 b. 1, 2, 3, 4
c. 2, 3 d. 2, 3, 5

63. Match list I with list II:

	List I		List II
a.	Syphilis	1.	Donovan bodies
b.	Chancroid	2.	Chlamydia trachomatis
c.	Granuloma inguinale	3.	N. gonorrhoeae
d.	LGV	4.	Hemophilus ducreyi
		5.	Treponema pallidum

	a	b	c	d
A.	5	4	2	3
B.	5	4	1	2
C.	4	1	2	3
D.	3	5	1	2

64. Which of the following cause Bacterial vaginosis:
1. Gardnerella
2. Mycoplasma
3. Ureaplasma urealyticum

a. only 1 b. 1, 2
c. 1, 3 d. 1, 2, 3

BV is replacement of doderlein bacilli by gardnerella vaginalis, ureaplasma urealyticum, mobiluncus, mycoplasma hominis & prevotella

Ans: 49. b 50. d 51. d 52. a 53. Case 1 b, Case 2 b
54. b 55. c 56. d 57. b 58. c 59. c
60. a 61. c 62. a 63. b 64. d

65. Consider the following HSG a appearances:
1. Lead pipe appearance
2. Cog wheel appearance
3. Waist sign appearance
4. Tobacco pouch appearance
5. Beaded appearance

The HSG appearance seen in genital TB patients are:
a. 1, 2, 3, 4, 5 b. 1, 2, 4, 5
c. 1, 4, 5 d. 2, 3, 4, 5

66. Arrange the following sites in order of increasing frequency of genital TB (least frequent to most frequent):
1. Endometrium
2. Fallopian tube
3. Ovary
4. Cervix

a. 2, 1, 3, 4 b. 2, 3, 1, 4
c. 4, 1, 3, 2 d. 4, 3, 1, 2

67. See the image and answer question:

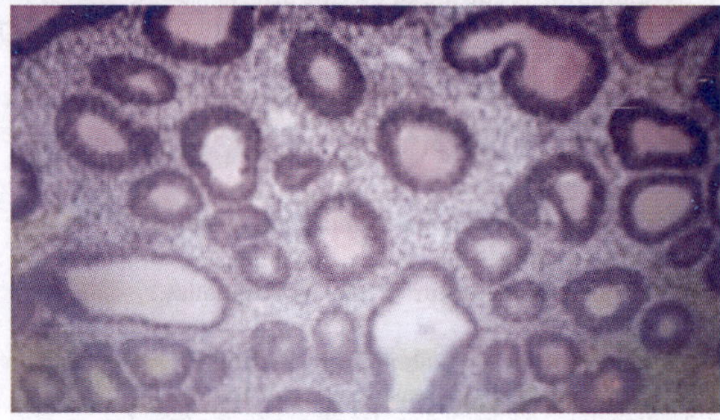

I: Histopathological pattern shown in image is
a. Proliferative endometrium
b. Secretory endometrium
c. Cytic glandular hyperplasia
d. Endometrial cancer

II: TOC of in a female of 30 years in this condition
a. Observation b. Clomiphene citrate
c. Progestine d. Hysterectomy

68. Consider the following abnormalities:
1. Defective oocyte pickup
2. Luteinized unruptured follicle
3. Luteal phase defect
4. Impaired tubal motility
5. Anovulation

The abnormalities which may be responsible for infertility in a case of endometriosis of ovary include:
a. 1, 4 b. 1, 2, 4
c. 1, 2, 3, 4 d. 1, 2, 3, 4, 5

69. Consider the following malignant ovarian tumors:
1. Dysgerminoma
2. Serous cystadenocarcinoma
3. Malignant teratoma
4. Brenner tumor
5. Endodermal sinus tumor

Which of the following occur were commonly in children and adolescent as compared to older women
a. 1, 2, 3 b. 1, 3, 5
c. 1, 2, 4, 5 d. 1, 3, 4, 5

70. In endometriosis arrange the following sites from least common to most common:
1. Uterosacral ligament
2. Broad ligament
3. Pouch of Douglas
4. Fallopian tube

a. 4 < 2 < 1 < 3 b. 2 < 4 < 1 < 3
c. 1 < 4 < 2 < 3 d. 4 < 1 < 3 < 2

71. All of the following may occur in a female exposed to DES in utero except:
a. T shaped uterus b. Clean cell carcinoma
c. Vaginal adenosis d. Renal anomalies

72. Arrange the following steps involved in formation of female genital tract organs sequentially:
1. Fundus becomes dome shaped
2. Fusion of Mullerian duct
3. Downward extension of Mullerian duct
4. Dissolution of intervening septum

a. 3, 2, 4, 1 b. 2, 3, 1, 4
c. 3, 2, 1, 4 d. 2, 3, 4, 1

73. Consider the following progesterone:
1. Levonorgestrel
2. MPA
3. Norethisterone acetate
4. Desogestrel
5. Gestodene

Third generation progesterone are:
a. 1, 2, 3 b. 4, 5
c. 1, 4, 5 d. 1, 2, 3, 4, 5

74. If 20 women become pregnant out of 100 women using a contraceptive agent for 2 years. Pearl index is:
a. 10 b. 20
c. 30 d. 40

75. Consider the following contraceptives:
1. OCP 2. Copper T
3. Condom male 4. Spermicide
5. Diaphragm

Which of these is conventional contraceptive:
a. 3, 4, 5 b. 3, 4
c. 2, 3, 4, 5 d. 1, 2, 3, 4, 5

76. A 54-year old female who had attained menopause 2 years back, complains of single episode of bleeding. TVS show endometrial thickness of 4 mm with an area of focal thickness of 6 mm. What is the most appropriate next step in management?
a. Perform fractional curettage
b. Perform hysteroscopy and biopsy
c. Perform Pipelle aspiration
d. Renew in 3 months of earlier if bleeding recurs

77. A 65-years-old women presents with postmenopausal bleeding. Biopsy shows grade 2 endometrioid carcinoma at the fundus of uterus. She has uncontrolled diabetes and hypertension. What is the most appropriate next step in management?
a. Perform MRI scan
b. Perform TAH + BSO
c. Perform TAH + BSO + pelvic and paraaortic lymph node dissection
d. Surgery followed by RT

Ans: 65. c 66. d 67. (I) c, (II) c 68. d 69. b 70. a
71. d 72. a 73. b 74. a 75. b 76. b
77. a

78. A 54-year-old female presents with postmenopausal bleeding. Biopsy shows endometrioid variety of endometrial cancer of 1 cm in the uterine fundus histology show grade I tumor. MRI shows <50% of myometrial involvement. Next step in management is:
a. TAH + BSO
b. TAH + BSO with pelvic lymphadenectomy
c. TAH = BSO with pelvic and paraaortic lymphadenectomy
d. TAH 4-BSO followed by RT

79. A 52-years-old female has endometrial cancer of endometrioid variety stage Ia grade II limited to endometrium. The tumor has not spread outside the uterus. Size of tumor is 3-4 cm. What is the most appropriate management?
a. TAH = BSO
b. TAH+ BSO with pelvic lymphadenectomy
c. TAH + BSO with pelvic and paraaortic lymphadenectomy
d. TAH + BSO followed by RT

80. Presence of signet ring cells in a cellular or myxomatous stroma is diagnostic of:
a. Gonadoblastoma b. Hilus cell tumor
c. Struma ovarii d. Krukenberg tumor

81. All are complications of fibroid in pregnancy except:
a. Red degeneration b. Obstructed labor
c. PPH d. Placenta previa

82. A 36-year-old female presents with heavy menstrual bleeding. She has one child of 7 years. USG shows a single 3 × 3 cm submucosal fibroid. Hemoglobin is 10.5 gm/dL. What is the best treatment option for her?
a. GnRH injection b. UAE
c. Hysteroscopic myomectomy
d. Laparoscopic myomectomy
e. TAH

83. A patient complaints of post coital bleed; no growth is seen, on per speculum examination; next step should be:
a. Colposcopy biopsy b. Conization
c. Repeat pap smear d. Culdoscopy

84. Site of placement of tension free vaginal Tapes in stress urinary incontinence:
a. At ureterovaginal junction
b. At ureterovaginal junction
c. At upper part of urethra
d. At middle part of urethra
e. At lower part of urethra

85. A 45-year-old P2L2 female has CIN grade III confirmed on papsmear and colposcopy. Best management:
a. Conization b. LEEP
c. Cryosurgery d. Hysterectomy

86. A 35-year-old multiparous woman is found to have preclinical invasive disease of the cervix penetrating to a depth of 2 mm with a width of 5 mm. She has no fertility wishes. What is the most appropriate treatment?
a. Knife cone biopsy
b. Loop electrosurgical excision of the transformation zone
c. Repeat colposcopy in three months.
d. Total hysterectomy
e. Wertheim's hysterectomy

87. A 42-year-old multiparous woman found to have preclinical invasive disease of the cervix penetrating to a depth 4 mm with a width of 7 mm. What is the most appropriate treatment?
a. Chemoradiotherapy
b. Modified radical hysterectomy
c. Radical trachelectomy
d. Knife cone biopsy e. Total hysterectomy

88. A 45-year-old woman with one child is found to have visible cervical lesion measuring 7 cm. Biopsy of the lesion reveals a squamous carcinoma of the cervix. The lesion is confined to the cervix. She wishes to preserve her fertility. What is the most appropriate treatment?
a. TAH
b. Radical hysterectomy with pelvic node dissection
c. Radical Trachelectomy with pelvic node dissection
d. Chemoradiation

89. Assertion: When pregnancy occurs with Copper T in position, it should be left in situ.

Reason: Copper in situ does not lead to increased risk of congenital malformation
a. Both Assertion and Reason are correct and Reason is correct explanation of Assertion
b. Both Assertion and Reason are correct but Reason is not correct explanation of Assertion
c. Assertion is correct. Reason is incorrect
d. Reason is correct. Assertion is incorrect
e. Both are incorrect

90. Match the corpus: cervix ratio at various ages:

List I (age group)		List II (corpus: Cervix ratio)	
A.	Before puberty	1.	1:1
B.	Reproductive age	2.	2:1
C.	Menopause	3.	3:1
D.	At puberty	4.	1:2
		5.	1:3

	A	B	C	D
a.	2	5	1	4
b.	5	3	1	4
c.	4	3	1	2
d.	5	3	1	2

91. Assertion: Uterine artery runs transversally while the ureter runs in AP direction through ureteric canal of parametrium where they cross each other.

Reason: The ureter may get injured during TAH if precaution is not taken while cramping uterine artery.
a. Both Assertion and Reason are correct and Reason is correct explanation of Assertion
b. Both Assertion and Reason are correct but Reason is not correct explanation of Assertion
c. Assertion is correct. Reason is incorrect
d. Reason is correct. Assertion is incorrect
e. Both are incorrect

92. A man is found to have a sperm concentration of 2 million/mL on one occasion. What is the next step in the management?
a. Estimate serum FSH and testosterone levels
b. Perform testicular aspiration
c. Repeat the test in three months
d. Repeat the test in three weeks
e. Test for antisperm antibodies

Ans: 78. a 79. b 80. d 81. d 82. c 83. a
84. d 85. b 86. d 87. b 88. d 89. e
90. c 91. a 92. c

93. A man is found to have azoospermia on two occasions three months apart. What is the next step in the management?
a. Estimate serum FSH and LH levels
b. Perform karyotyping
c. Perform a testicular biopsy
d. Perform testicular aspiration

94. An adolescent girl with dysgerminoma stage 1a is managed by:
a. Unilateral salpingo-oophorectomy
b. TAH + unilateral salpingo-oophorectomy
c. BSO alone
d. Chemotherapy

95. Cytoscopy done in a diagnosed patient of cancer cervix shows bullous edema. IVP shows hydroureter staging of patient is:
a. Stage 3b b. Stage 3C
c. Stage 4a d. Stage 4b

96. A woman with which of the following health problem should avoid centchroman
a. PCOS b. Endometrial hyperplasia
c. Woman with DUB d. Endometriosis

97. A 55-year-old woman is diagnosed with invasive cervical carcinoma by cone biopsy. Pelvic examination and rectal examination reveal the parametrium is free of disease but upper part of vagina is involved with tumor. IVP and sigmoidoscopy are negative but CT scan of abdomen and pelvis shows grossly enlarged pelvic and paraaortic nodes. This patient is classified as stage:
a. IIa b. IIb
c. IIIc1 d. IIIc2

98. A 26-year-old woman who has been infertile for 2 years attends the clinic. She has 28 day regular menstrual cycles. Day 21 progesterone level is 30 nmol/L. The seminal fluid analysis is normal She has no other complaints.

Which of the following investigations should be performed next?
a. Hydrotubation
b. Hysterosalpingogram
c. Laparoscopy and dye test.
d. Transvaginal ultrasound scanning follicular tracking
e. Tubal insufflation

99. A 26-year-old woman who has been infertile for 2 years attends the clinic. She has frequent periods with dysmenorrhea which is worst on the third day. She also complains of deep dyspareunia. Day 21 progesterone level is 30 nmol/L. The seminal fluid analysis is normal. Which of the following investigations should be performed next?
a. Hysterosalpingogram
b. Hysteroscopy
c. Laparoscopy and dye test
d. Transvaginal ultrasound scan for follicular tracking
e. Tubal insufflation

100. Which of the following is not a characteristic of MRKH syndrome:
a. Cardiac anomalies
b. Mullerian duct aplasia
c. Renal anomalies
d. Skeletal anomalies

101. Match list I (nomenclature) with list (II) characteristic and select correct answer:

List I		List II	
A.	Serous cyst adenoma	1.	Cystic with Cebacious maternal
B.	Mucinous cystadenoma	2	Multilocular cyst
C.	Simple serous cyst	3.	Unilocular cyst
D.	Cystic Teratoma	4.	Few cystic compartment
		5.	Variegated cystic and solid

A B C D A B C D
a. 3, 2, 4, 1 b. 4, 2, 3, 1
c. 4, 2, 3, 5 d. 3, 2, 4, 5

102. Assertion: Supravaginal elongation of cervix occurs in uterovaginal prolapse.
Reason: There is gaping genital hiatus but ligamentous support of uterus is strong:
a. Both Assertion and Reason are correct. Reason is right explanation of Assertion
b. Both Assertion and Reason are correct. Reason is not correct explanation of Assertion
c. Assertion is correct, Reason incorrect
d. Reason is correct, Assertion is not correct
e. Both Assertion and Reason incorrect

Ans: 93. a 94. a 95. a 96. a 97. d
98. b 99. c 100. a 101. b 102. a

CHAPTER 1

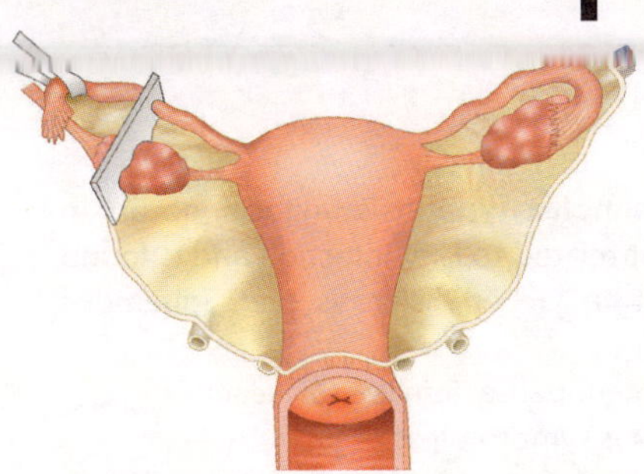

Anatomy of the Female Genital Tract

External Genital Organs (Syn: Vulva, Pudendum)

Definition

Vulva

Composite name for female external genitalia.

The vulva includes all structures visible externally, i.e. Mons Pubis, Labia Majora, Labia Minora, Clitoris, Vestibule, Bartholin glands, Minor Vestibular glands, Paraurethral glands (Fig. 1.1).

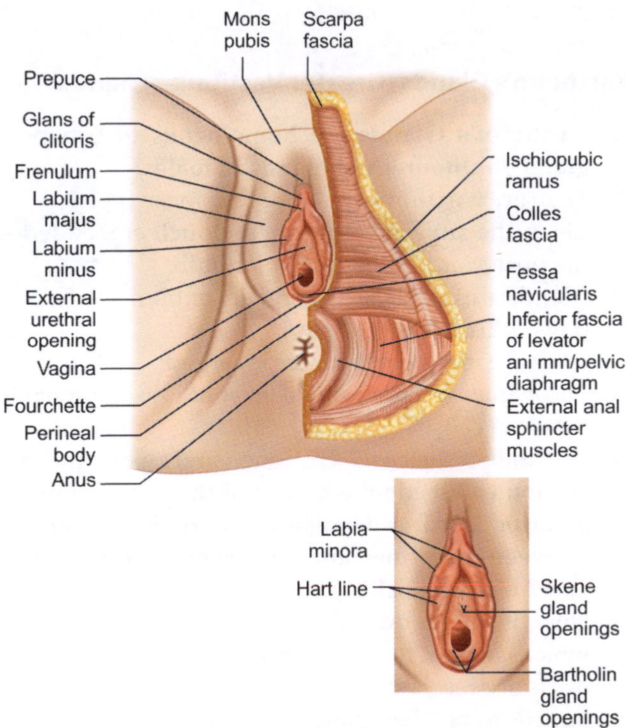

Fig. 1.1: Vulva

- **Mons Pubis** (Veneris): Pad of subcutaneous adipose connective tissue lying in front of the pubis and in the adult females covered by hair.
- **Labia Majora:** Lie on either side and join posteriorly to form **the posterior commissure.** Their inner side is hairless. **It is homologous to the scrotum in a male.** The round ligament terminates **at its anterior third**[Q]. (V Imp)

  The labia majora and the mons veneris contain:
  - The hair follicles.
  - The sebaceous glands.
  - Modified sweat glands known as the apocrine glands.

The hidradenoma of vulva arises from the apocrine glands of labia majora and mons veneris.

- **Labia Minora:** They are two thick folds of skin, devoid of fat, lying within the labia majora. Anteriorly, they **enclose the clitoris** and unite with each other in front and behind the clitoris to form the **prepuce** and the **frenulum**, respectively. Lower portion of the labia fuses across the midline to form a fold of skin called the **fourchette. It is homologous to the ventral aspect of the penis.**
- The Labia Minora is covered by keratinized squamous epithelium on their outer surface. On the inner surface the lateral part is covered by the same epithelium uptil 'Hart line'. Medial to Hart line it is covered by nonkeratinized squamous epithelium.

  Labia Minora lacks hair follicles, eccrine glands & apocrine glands. But it has numerous sebaceous glands.
- **Clitoris:** It is a small erectile body (2.0 cm) lying in the anteriormost part of the vulva. **It is homologous to the male penis.** It consists of glans, a body and two crura. Glans is covered by stratified squamous epithelium. Clitoris rarely exceeds 20 cm in length. Clitoris receives its blood supply from internal pudendal artery. **Deep artery of clitoris supplies clitoral body. Dorsal artery of clitoris supplies glans and prepuce.**
- **Vestibule:** It is a Triangular space bounded **anteriorly by the clitoris, posteriorly by the**

fourchette, and on either side by the labia minora. It has 4 openings, namely (Fig. 1.1):

1. Urethral opening.
2. Vaginal orifice opening.
3. Bartholin's ducts on either side.
4. Ducts of paraurethral glands, also known as **Skene's ducts** on the posterior surface of urethra.

Extra Edge

- The posterior part of vestibule between fourchette and vaginal opening is called **fossa navicularis**.
- Hymen is thin fold of mucous membrane attached to vaginal orifice all around.
- It is lined by stratified squamous epithelium on both sides.
- The hymen is most commonly torn posterolaterally or posteriorly.
- It is replaced by tags after childbirth, called **carunculae myrtiformes**.

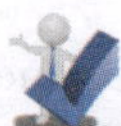

KEY POINTS

Annular hymen: Hymen with one opening.
Cribriform hymen: Hymen with multiple openings.
Septate hymen: Hymen with 2 openings and a band in between.

Development of Vulva
Clitoris develops from genital tubercle.
Labia minora → genital folds.
Labia majora → genital (labioscrotal) swellings.
Vestibule → urogenital sinus.

Important Concept

Vulva

- **Blood supply** → Internal Pudendal Artery
- **Sensory innervation** → Pudendal Nerve ($S_2 - S_4$)
- **Lymphatic drainage** → Inguinal Nodes

First to superficial inguinal LN **(sentinel LN) and** then to deep inguinal LN).
Lymphatic drainage of clitoris is deep inguinal nodes or **LN of cloquet (Rosenmüller LN).**

Extra Edge

Vulvar Carcinoma:

- **M/C Variety** - Squamous cell carcinoma
- In squamous cell carcinoma of vulva. There are 2 varieties:
  - **Basaloid or Warty type**: It is multifocal, occurs in younger patients and is related to HPV infection and smoking. Risk factors are similar to cancer cervix.

Contd...

Contd...

  - **Keratinizing or simplex type:** It is unifocal, occurs in older patients, not related to HPV infection and is found in areas adjacent to Lichen Sclerosis and Squamous Hyperplasia.
    Age: M/C in postmenopausal females (65 years)
    Symptoms: M/C it is symptomless
    Diagnosis: Made by Keys punch biopsy or Wedge Biopsy
    M/C route of spread: Lymphatic (Sentinel lymph nodes = Superficial Inguinal Lymph Nodes)

Management:

Microinvasive Stage T_{1a} = Tumor size ≤ 2 cm in diameter with 1 mm or less of stromal invasion (in these cases inguinal metastasis is rare).

It is a Managed by wide local excision.

Early vulvar cancer = (Stage T_{1b}, Early T_2) - Treatment should be individualized, mostly radical local excision is done.

Advanced T_2 cancer or T_3 cancer: Chemoradiation.

Homologous Glands in Males and Females (V. Imp)

Males	Females
Prostate gland	Skene glands/paraurethral glands
Cowpers gland	Bartholin gland
Glands of Littre (in penile urethra)	Glands of labia minora and labia majora

Bartholin's Glands (Greater Vestibular Glands)

- **Bartholin's Glands are homologous to Cowper's gland^Q/bulbourethral glands in males.**
- They are 2 in number and of Racemose type^Q
- Lie in the **superficial perineal pouch** embedded in the posterior part of vestibular bulb.
- Glands are oval in shape and are of the size of a pea^Q (Figs. 1.2A to C)
- They are impalpable unless enlarged.
- The acini is lined by single layer of low columnar or cuboidal cells.^Q
- Bartholin's duct is 2 cm long^Q and opens into the vestibule, outside the hymen at the **junction of the anterior 2/3rd and posterior 1/3rd in the groove between the hymen and labium minora at 5 o'clock and 7 o'clock position.**^Q
- Duct is lined by stratified squamous epithelium which changes to transitional epithelium as terminal ducts are reached.
- Function of the gland is to produce abundant alkaline mucus during sexual excitement.

Note: Bartholin's glands are Greater Vestibular glands. The Minor Vestibular glands are simple mucus secreting and open along Hart line.

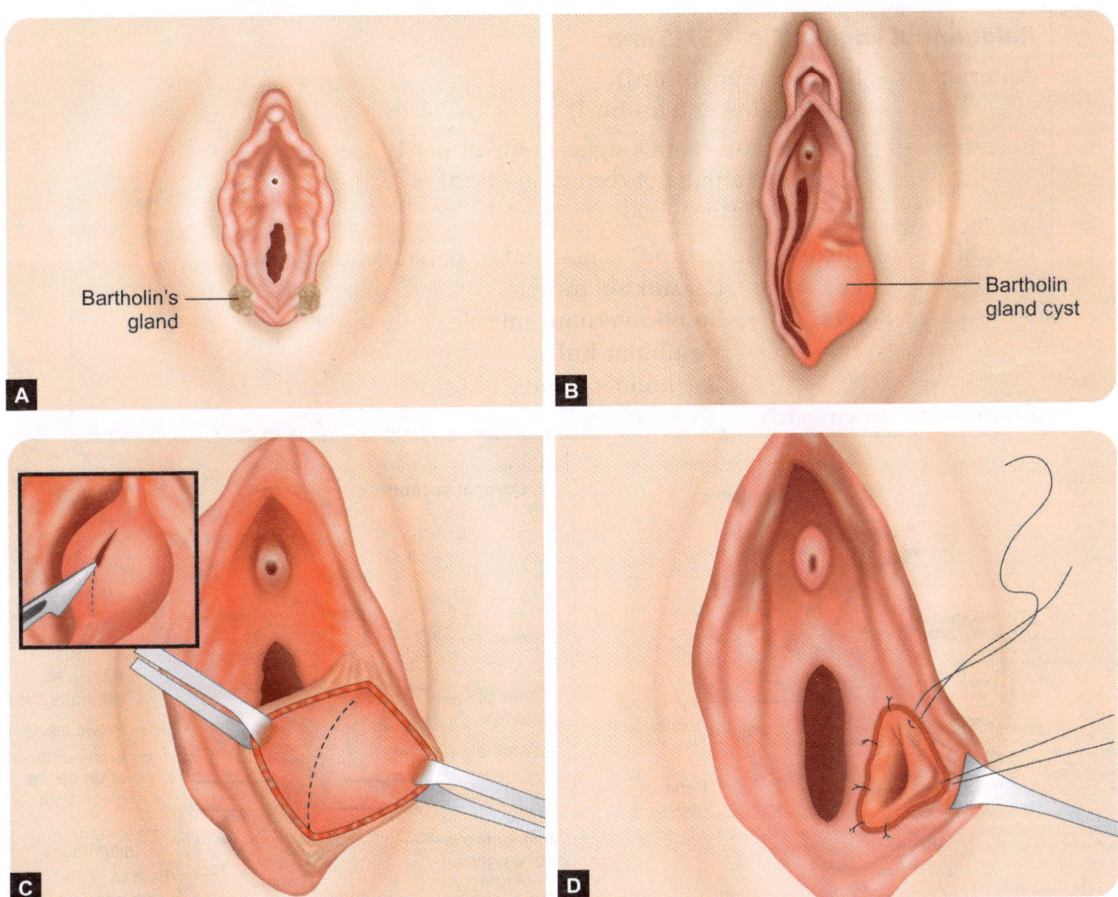

Figs. 1.2A to D: (A) Location of Bartholin Gland; (B) Bartholin cyst; (C and D) Steps of Marsupilization

KEY POINTS

Bartholin's cyst – formed when Bartholin's duct is blocked.

- M/c cyst of vulva.
- M/c cause = gonococcal infection (earlier), Now = *E.Coli*.
- M/c site = fluctuant, non-tender, swelling present on inner side of junction of anterior 2/3rd with posterior 1/3rd of the labium majora.
- TOC = Marsupialization.

Bartholin abscess.

- Management = Incision and drainage.
- M/C cause: *E.coli* > N. gonorrhoeae

Bartholin Gland Carcinoma

- Primary carcinoma of Bartholin Gland is rare
- It can be adenocarcinoma/ squamous cell carcinoma/ Transitional cell carcinoma or adenoid cystic carcinoma (better prognosis)
- M/C symptom - Vulvar mass or perineal pain
- Management - Radical vulvectomy with bilateral groin and pelvic node dissection.

Skene's Tubules

Skene's tubules are the paraurethral glands equivalent to **prostrate in males**. Both Bartholin's glands and Skene's tubules arise as downgrowths of urogenital sinus.

Internal Genital Organs

The internal genital organs in a female include vagina, uterus, fallopian tubes, and the ovaries.

Vagina

- Distensible fibromuscular canal connecting the uterine cavity with the exterior at the vulva.
- Anterior wall = 7.5 cm, posterior wall = 9 cm in length.
- Upper vagina is separated by cervix into anterior, posterior and lateral fornices.
- Deepest fornix = posterior fornix; Shallowest fornix = anterior fornix
- On cut section = It is H-shaped.

Relations of Vagina (Fig. 1.3) V. Imp

Anterior → Bladder (upper third)
Urethra (lower two-third)

Posterior → **P** = Pouch of Douglas in the upper 1/3rd
A = Ampulla of rectum in middle 1/3rd
P = Perineal body in lower 1/3rd

Lateral → **Medicos** = Mackenrodt's ligament or pelvic cellular tissue
Love = Levator ani muscle
Books = Bulbocavernous muscle
Vestibular **bulb**
Bartholin's glands

From above downwards

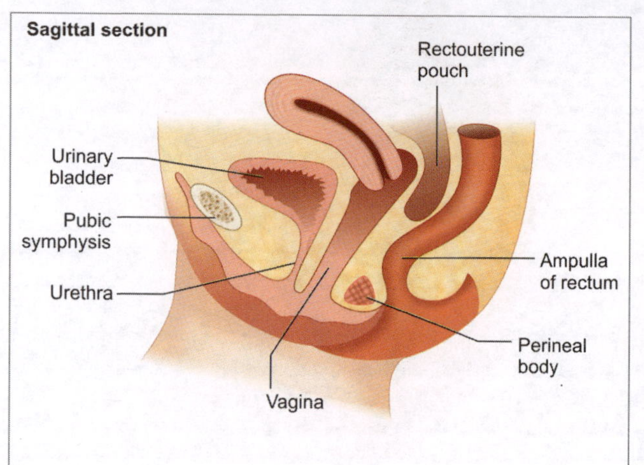

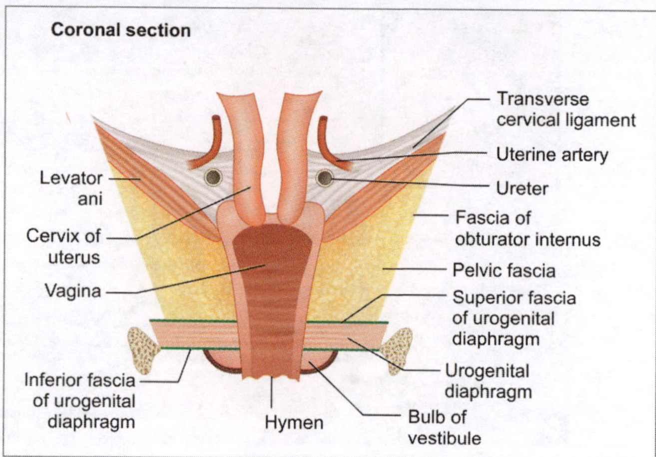

Fig. 1.3: Relations of vagina

The cervix and all 4 fornices are related to[Q]:
- Uterine vessels
- Mackenrodt's ligament
- Ureter[Q]

- Vagina has inhabitant bacteria called **Doderlein's bacteria** which is a **lactobacilli**[Q] and converts the glycogen present in vaginal epithelium into lactic acid[Q] under the influence of estrogen.
  Thus, pH of vagina is acidic.

Doderlein's Bacilli (Figs. 1.4 and 1.5)

- Gram positive, rod shaped bacilli
- They are the only organism which will grow at pH 4–4.5 in vagina
- Sugar fermenting and convert glycogen of vaginal epithelial into lactic acid
- Grows anaerobically in acidic medium
- Is the only organism in upper 2/3 vagina
- Generally appears within 15 hours of birth in newborn.

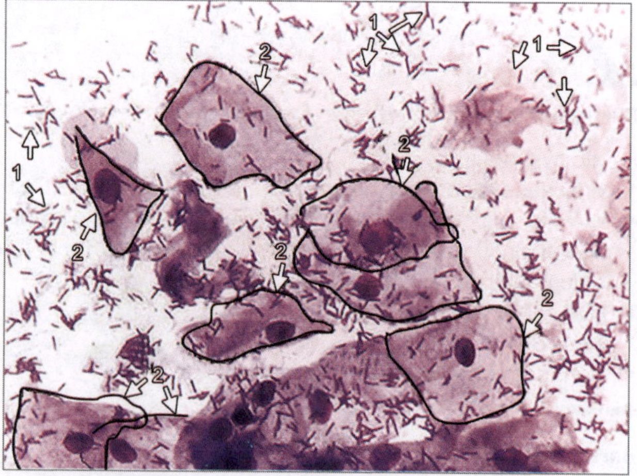

Fig. 1.4: Doderlein's Bacilli in vagina

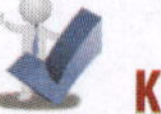

KEY POINTS

Note: They are present in a newborn female's then they disappear (after 10–14 days) to reappear at puberty and then again disappear after menopause.

- The pH of vagina in an adult woman is 4–5.5 with an average of 4.5.
- The pH of vagina varies with age.

Age	Vaginal pH
• In a newborn infant[Q]	Between 5.5–6
• 6 weeks old child[Q] until before puberty	Changes from acidic to alkaline[Q] (6–8)
• Puberty[Q]	Changes from alkaline to acidic (as Doderlein's bacteria appear)
• Reproductive age group[Q]	4–5.5[Q]
• Pregnancy[Q]	3.5–4.5[Q]
• During menstruation	6–8 (as blood is alkaline)
• Menopause	6–8[Q] (Doderlein's bacteria disappear)

Note: pH of vagina also varies along its length, being highest in the upper part because of admixture of alkaline cervical mucus.

- Vagina does not have any mucus-secreting glands.[Q] Since vagina does not have any glands, vaginal discharge is not actually derived from vagina.
  The components of vaginal secretion are derived from:
  - Endocervical glands (mainly)
  - Endometrial glands
  - Bartholin's glands (it gives secretions at the time of intercourse only)

- Vagina does not have any serosal covering except for the area covered by cul de sac posteriorly.[Q]
- Apart from Doderlein's bacilli, it contains many other pathogenic organisms including Cl. welchii.

Vaginal Epithelium

Vagina is lined by nonkeratinized **stratified squamous epithelium** which is composed of the following types of cells (Figs. 1.6A to D):

- **Parabasal/basal cells:** These are basophilic cells (blue in color) with indistinct outline and large nuclei which are predominant when there is no hormonal dominance[Q], e.g. menopause.
- **Intermediate cells:** These are basophilic cells, blue in color, with distinct outline and little larger nuclei than superficial cells which are predominant when there is progesterone predominance[Q], i.e. in luteal phase/later half of menstrual cycle.

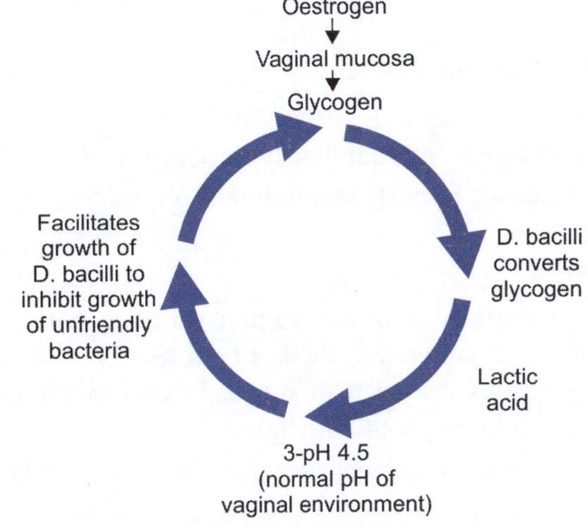

Fig. 1.5: Doderlein cycle

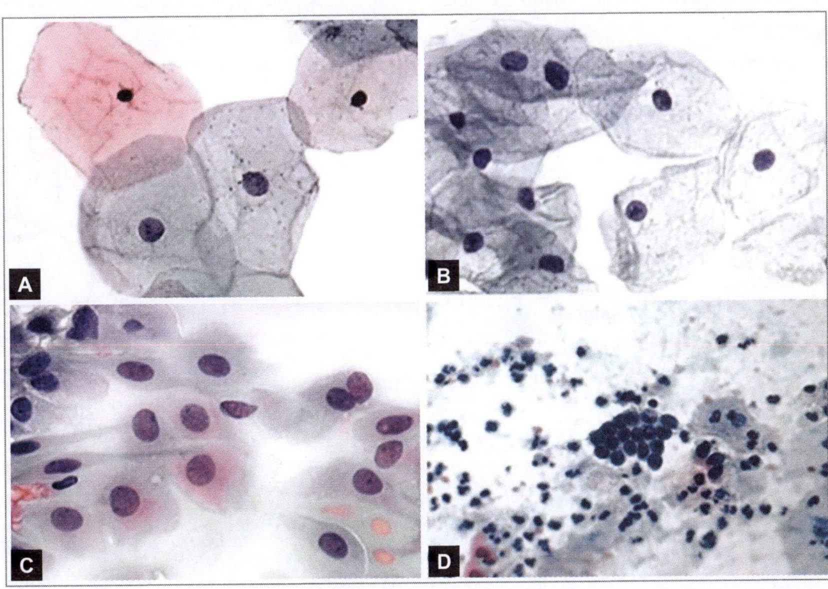

Figs. 1.6A to D: Cells of vagina. (A) Superficial cells; (B) Intermediate cells; (C) Parabasal cells; (D) Basal cells

KEY POINTS

In newborn females, vagina is lined by transitional epithelium.[Q] Squamous epithelium is resistant to gonococcal infection hence theoretically gonococcal vaginitis can occur in new born females but not in young females

- **Superficial cells:** These are eosinophilic cells, (pink in color) with pyknotic nuclei which are predominant when there is estrogen predominance, i.e. in follicular phase/first half of menstrual cycle.

Blood supply is from 3 arteries:

1. **Descending vaginal artery:** Branch of either uterine A or a direct branch of internal iliac A
2. **Internal pudendal artery**
3. **Middle rectal artery**

Lymphatic Drainage

Upper vagina: Same as cervix (see below)
Middle vagina: Internal iliac lymph nodes
Lower vagina: Superficial inguinal LN

Nerves

The innervation of upper vagina contains both sympathetic and parasympathetic fibers (S_2-S_4). Only free nerve endings are seen in mucosa. No other type of nerve endings are noted in vagina.

Lower part of vagina is supplied by pudendal nerve.

Angle of Anteversion (Figs. 1.7)
Angle between cervix and vagina (Remember V for version and V for vagina) = 90°
Angle of Anteflexion (at the level of internal os)
Angle between cervix and uterus = 120°–130°
Angle which vagina makes with horizontal = 45°

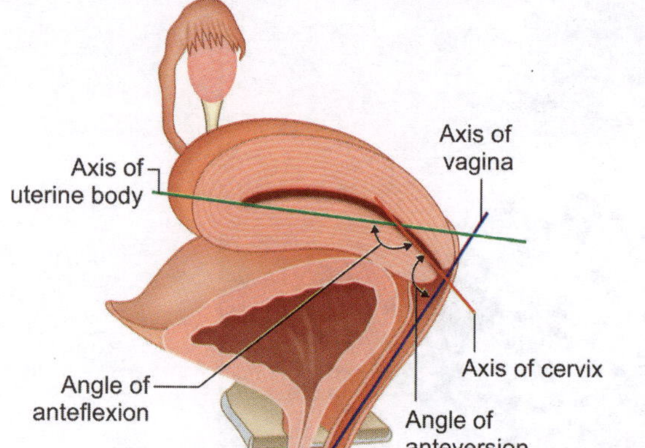

Fig. 1.7: Angle of anteversion and angle of anteflexion

Uterus

- It is pyriform in shape
- Weight of nonpregnant uterus in nulliparous females = 50–70 gm
- Weight of nonpregnant uterus in multiparous females = 80 gm
- Weight of pregnant uterus = 1000 gm
- Length of nonpregnant uterus in nulliparous females = 6–8 cm (7.5 cm)
- Length of nonpregnant uterus in multiparous females = 9–10 cm
- Length of pregnant uterus = 35 cm
- Capacity of nonpregnant uterus = 10 ml
- Capacity of pregnant uterus = 5000 ml
- Position of uterus: Most common is **anteverted** and **anteflexed (Fig. 1.7)**. **Anteflexion is at the level of the Internal os.**

Note: In inches, size of uterus is 3.25 × 2.5 × 1.5 inches.

Uterus consists of: A. Body; B. Isthmus; C. Cervix.

(A) Body

The wall of body consists of three layers:

1. **Serosa**: Visceral Peritoneum covers the posterior part of uterus and posterior cervix. Only the upper part of anterior uterus is covered by visceral peritoneum.
2. **Myometrium:** Consisting of thick bundle of muscle which forms 3 distinct layers during pregnancy:
   - Outer longitudinal.
   - Inner circular.
   - Middle interlacing fibers **called living ligature** (Fig. 1.8).

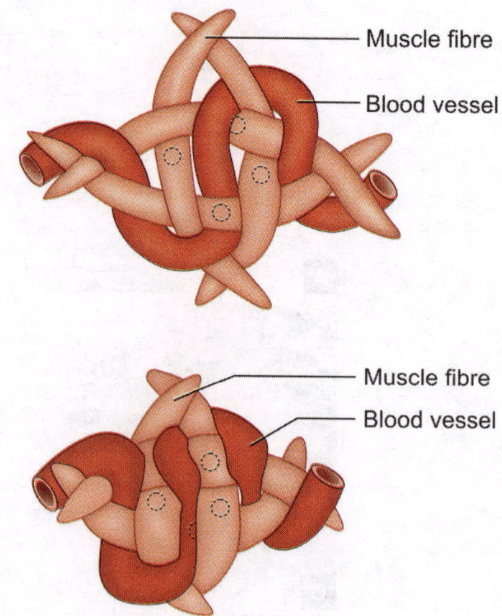

Fig. 1.8: The middle layer of myometrium acting as living ligature

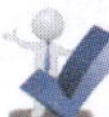

KEY POINTS

Middle layer of uterus is called **living ligature**, since it has fibers in criss-cross manner. Therefore, after the delivery of placenta, uterus contracts and these fibers occlude the blood vessels preventing postpartum hemorrhage (PPH). This is the reason when tone of uterus is lost (atonic uterus), this action cannot take place and PPH occurs.

3. **Endometrium:** It is the mucous lining of the cavity. As there is no submucous layer, the endometrium is directly attached to the muscle coat. It consists of lamina propria and surface epithelium. **The surface epithelium is a single layer of ciliated columnar epithelium** but cilia are lost once menstruation begins at puberty:

- Endometrial cavity is triangular in shape.
- The body of uterus is further divided into **fundus** and **body proper** (Fig. 1.9).
  - Fundus is the part which lies above the opening of the uterine tubes (or fallopian tubes)
  - The body proper is triangular and lies between the openings of the tube at the cornua and isthmus
  - The site of uterus at which the fallopian tube opens in the uterus is called **cornua**.

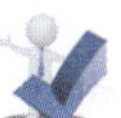

KEY POINTS

The structures attached at the cornua are (Fig. 1.9): **(Mnemonic RTO).**

1. **R**ound ligament (R)
2. Fallopian **T**ube (T)
3. **O**varian ligament (O)

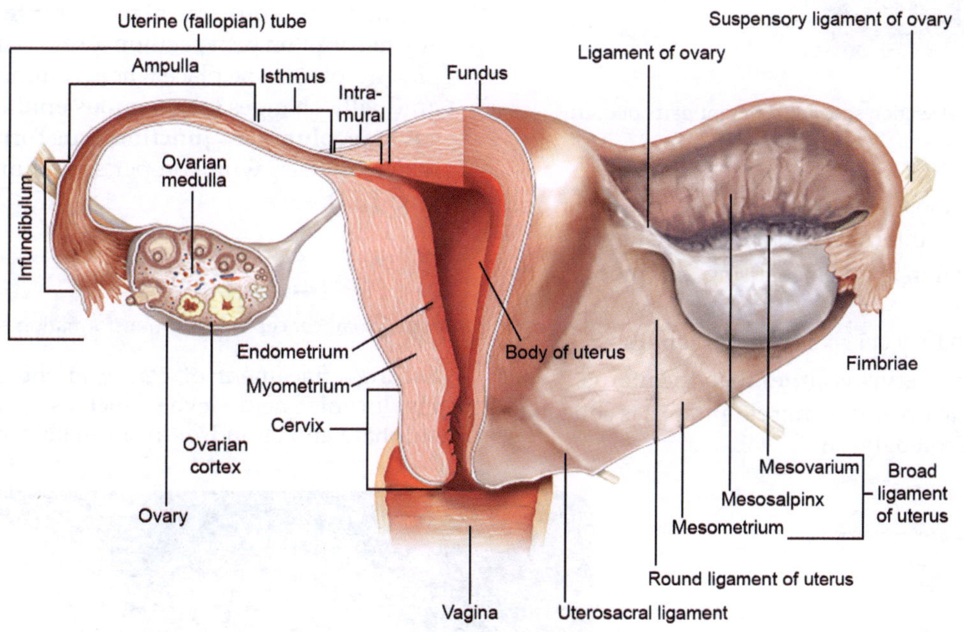

Fig. 1.9: Diagrammatic representation of Structures attached at cornua of uterus

Note: In Figure 1.9, the posterior view is seen as ovaries are clearly visible. So from posterior to anterior, there is ovarian ligament/fallopian tube/round ligament.

Fallopian tube is superiormost and then ovarian and round ligament are at the same level.

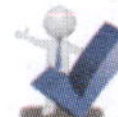

KEY POINTS

Structures attached at cornua of uterus

From anterior to posterior, they are: R ⇒ T ⇒ O

From superior to inferior: Fallopian tube is the superiormost. Round ligament and ovarian ligament lie inferior to it at the same level.

Hence, **most common cause of failure of ligation**—identification of wrong structure.

(B) Isthmus

- Constricted (0.5 cm) part of uterus situated between body of uterus and cervix.
- It extends from anatomical internal os above to the histological os below (Fig. 1.10).
- Isthmus forms the lower uterine segment (LUS) after the 12th week of pregnancy (in the second trimester).
- It is best formed in late pregnancy.
- At term, LUS is formed by isthmus–70% and cervix–30%

- At cesarean, LUS can be identified by a loose fold of peritoneum (uterovesical fold)
- Length of LUS at term = 5 cm
- At the time of labor it becomes 10 cm, due to taking up of cervix.

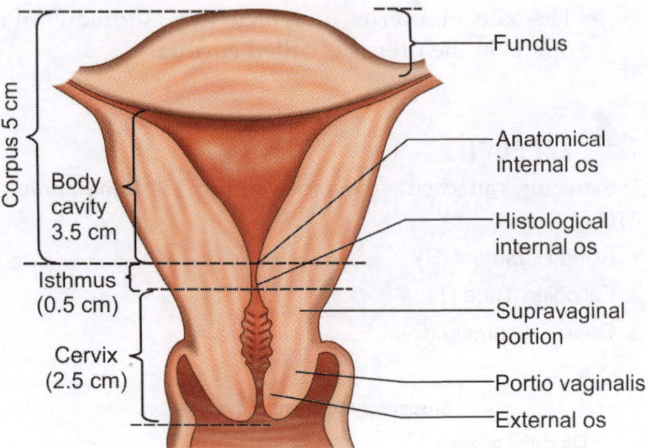

Fig. 1.10: Coronal section showing different parts of uterus

(C) Cervix

- It is the lowermost part of the uterus extending from the histological internal os to the external os.
- It is cylindrical in shape measuring 2.5 cm in length and **diameter**.
- During pregnancy cervix is **4 cm in length**.
- Before puberty cervix is larger than the uterus.
- Cervix is made up of 10% muscle and rest is collagen, Elastin and Proteoglycan

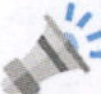

Important One Liners

Age	Corpus/Cervix ratio
Before puberty	1:2
At puberty	2:1
In adults/Reproductive age	3:1 or 4:1
After menopause	Whole of uterus and cervix atrophy

- Cervical canal is fusiform in shape
- The cervix is divided into a supravaginal part (**Endocervix**) – the part lying above the vagina and a vaginal part (**Portio vaginalis** or **exocervix**) which lies within the vagina, each measuring 1.25 cm (Fig. 1.11).
- **Endocervix** is lined by **single layer of tall columnar epithelium**[Q]. On per speculum examination it appears red in color. **Portio vaginalis** or **exocervix** is lined by **nonkeratinized stratified squamous epithelium**[Q] on per speculum examination it appears pink in colour. The place where columnar epithelium gradually changes to squamous epithelium is called **squamocolumnar junction/transformation zone,** which appears white on per speculum examination (Fig. 1.11).

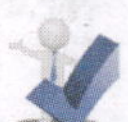

KEY POINT

M/c site for cancer cervix/CIN is transformation zone.

- During effacement of cervix at the time of labor: Hyaluronic acid levels increase and dermatan sulphate and chondroitin sulphate decreases.

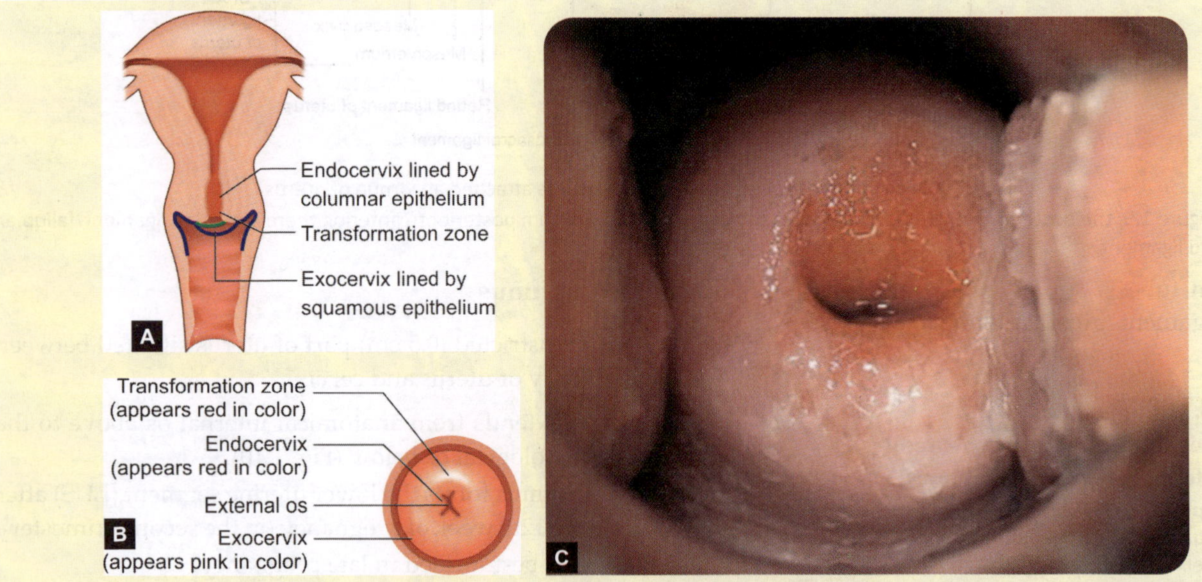

Figs. 1.11A to C: Cervix diagrams (A): Showing endocervix and Exocervix; (B): P/S view; (C): Photograph of P/S

Contd...

Contd…

External os (Figs. 1.11A to C)
Where cervix opens into vagina

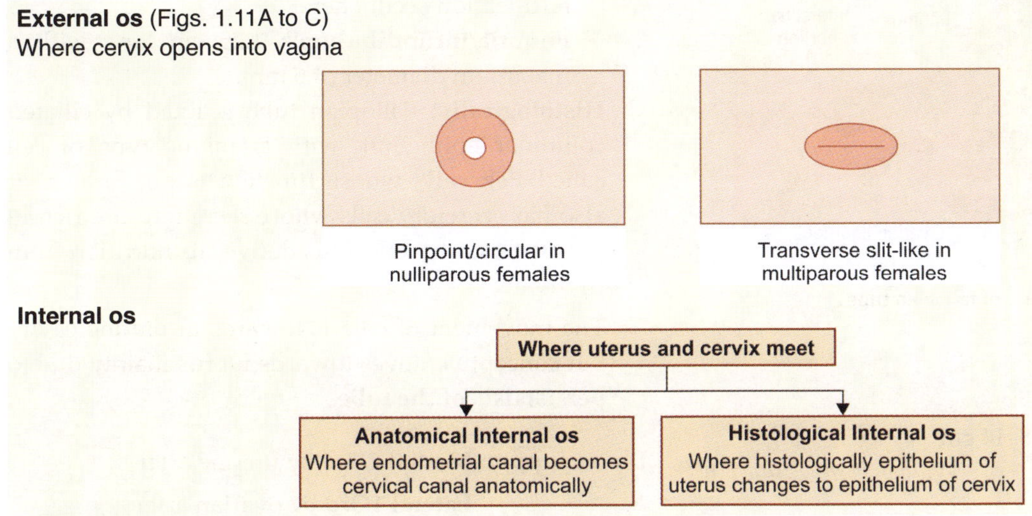

Significance of internal os

- Area between anatomical and histological internal os is called **isthmus**.
- At the level of internal os, uterine artery moves upwards.
- Peritoneum is reflected at this level on to the bladder. This is the point of identification of internal os during lower segment cesarean sections (LSCS).
- Uterosacral ligaments lie at this level and Mackenrodt's ligament lies below this level.

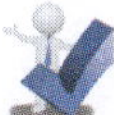

KEY POINTS

In erect posture, the internal os lies on the upper border of the symphysis pubis and the external os lies at the level of ischial spines.

Blood Supply: The blood supply of uterus is from the uterine artery (branch of anterior division of internal iliac artery) and ovarian artery of **cervix** is from descending cervical artery (branch of uterine artery).

Lymphatic Drainage

(A) Uterus

Fundus: Drains into para-aortic/lateral aortic lymph nodes.
Body: Drains into external iliac lymph nodes
Cornua: Drains into superficial inguinal nodes along with round ligament (Remember: Superficial not Deep).

(B) Cervix

Mnemonic

HOPE
H–Hypogastric lymph nodes/ Internal iliac lymph nodes
O–Obturator lymph nodes
P–Paracervical lymph nodes or ureteric lymph nodes
E–External iliac lymph nodes

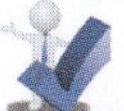

KEY POINTS

Remember:

- MC lymph node involved in Ca cervix – Obturator LN
- 1st lymph node involved in Ca cervix – Paracervical LN (Ureteric LN)
- Ca cervix does not involve superficial inguinal LN.

Sensory supply:

Uterus: T_{10}–L_1
Cervix: S_2–S_4

Clinical Correlation

Pain during labor

During early labor: Pain is due to uterine contraction therefore felt along segment T_{10}–L_1 (nerve supply of uterus)
During late labor: Pain is due to cervical dilatation therefore felt along segment S_2–S_4 (nerve supply of cervix and upper vagina)
For painless labor—blockage to be given from T_{10} segment
For instrumental delivery: Pudendal nerve block given (as lower vagina and perineum is supplied by pudendal nerve)
For cesarean section—blockage given from T_4 segment (to block the peritoneum also).

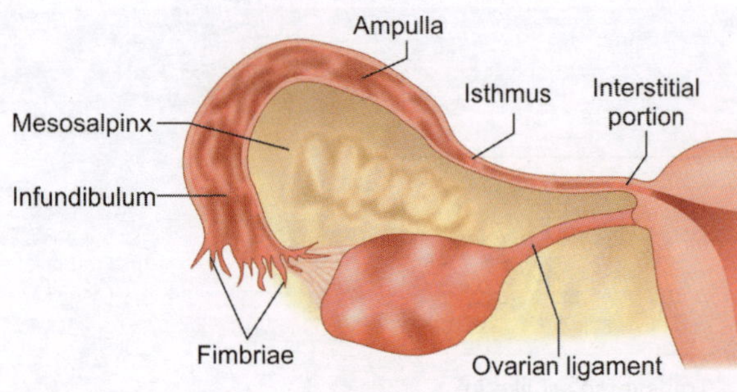

Fig. 1.12: Parts of fallopian tube

Fallopian Tube

- **Length** = 4 inches or 8–14 cm
  – Williams Obs 25th/ed, p28
- **Parts of tube are:**
  - **Interstitium (Intramural):** 1.25 cm long and 1 mm diameter (**narrowest part**[Q] of the tube). It has no longitudinal muscles, only circular muscles are present and acts as **anatomical sphincter**[Q] by forming tubal ostia. This part lies within the uterine wall.
  - **Isthmus:** 2.5 cm long and 2 mm in diameter[Q] (second narrowest part[Q]); It lies closest to uterine wall and acts as **physiologic sphincter.**
  - **Ampulla:** Widest[Q] and longest part[Q] (5 cm) and fertilization occurs here.[Q]
  - **Fimbria/infundibulum**[Q]: 1.25 cm long with a maximum diameter of 6 mm.
- **Histologically:** Fallopian tube is lined by ciliated columnar epithelium with a unique type of cell called **Peg cell**[Q] whose function is not known.[Q] It also has secretory cells whose secretions are rich in pyruvate. Early conceptus derives its nutrition from pyruvate.[Q]
- The movement of cilia is towards at uterine cavity but conceptus moves towards uterus mainly due to **persistalsis of the tube.**

Blood supply: Medial 2/3rd by uterine artery
Lateral 1/3rd by ovarian artery

Lymphatic drainage:

- Lateral part along with ovarian lymphatic drains into lateral aortic LN/ or Para-aortic LN.
- Medial part along with cornua drains into superficial inguinal LN.

Nerve Supply: T_{11}, T_{12}, L_1

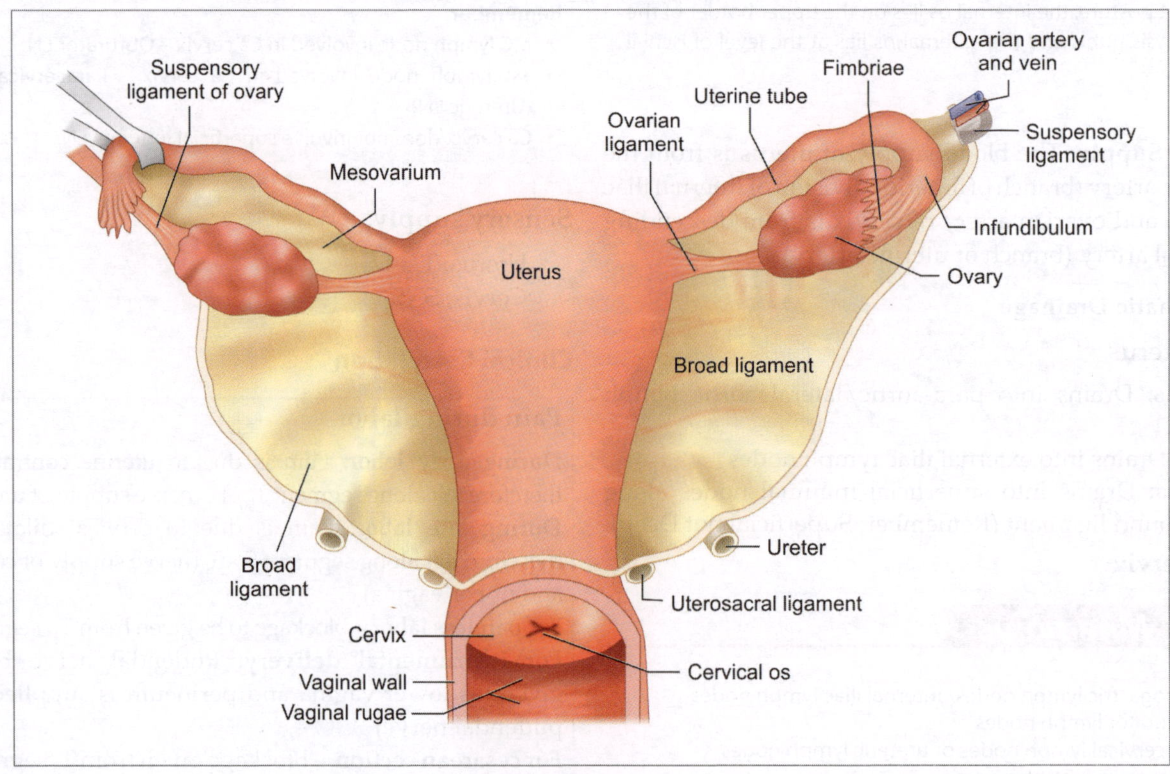

Fig. 1.13: Ovary: Anatomy as seen posteriorly

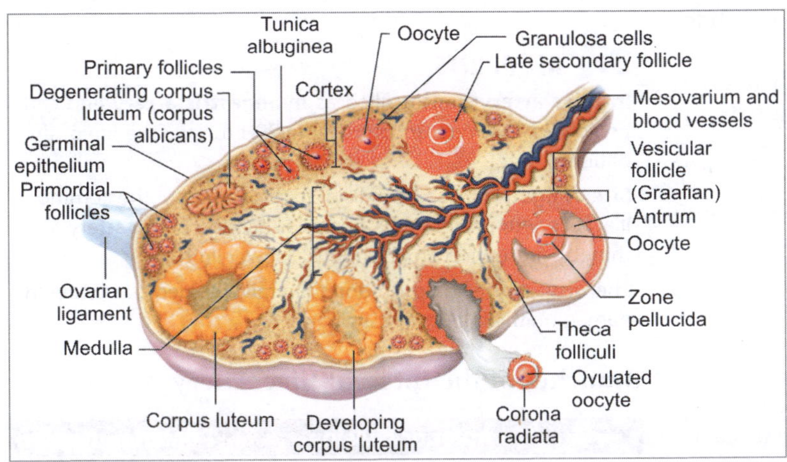

Fig. 1.15: Histology of ovary

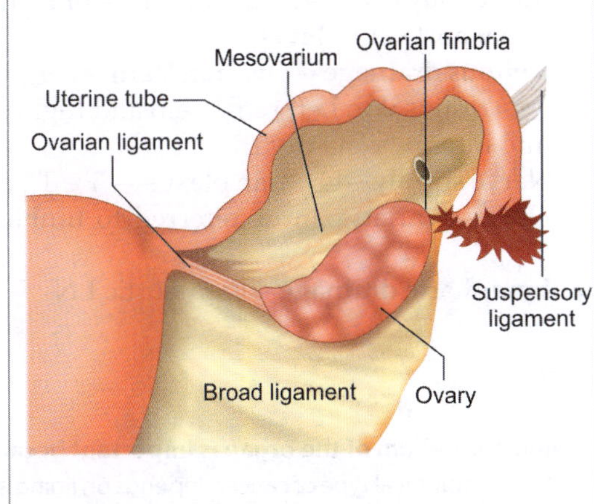

Fig. 1.14: Ligaments related to ovary

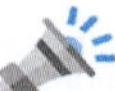

Important One Liners

Important questions on fallopian tube:

- **M/c site for fertilization**: Ampulla of fallopian tube.
- **M/c site for ectopic pregnancy**: Ampulla of fallopian tube.
- **M/c site for tubal abortion**: Ampulla of fallopian tube.
- **M/c site for tubal rupture**: Isthmus of fallopian tube.
- **M/c site for tubectomy**: Isthmus.
- Best prognosis for reversibility/recanalization of tube is if there is isthmo-isthmic anastomosis.
- **Anatomical sphincter**: interstitial part
- **Physiological sphincter**: isthmus

Also Know

- **TB causes block in:** Cornual part of uterus
- **Gonococcus causes block in:** Fimbrial end of tube

Ovary

- Measures = 3.5 × 2.5 × 2 cms
- Menopause = 2 × 1 × 1.5 cms
- **Mean ovarian volume:**
  - In premenarchal females = 3 ml
  - In menstruating females = 9.8 ml
  - In postmenopausal females = 5.8 ml
- The surface of active ovary is corrugated and pale.
- Ovary is only structure in abdomen which is not covered by peritoneum.
- The part of ovary attached to mesovarium is called as Hilum All nerves and vessels leave at this part.
- They lie in the **ovarian fossa of Waldeyer** on the lateral pelvic wall.
- Ovary is formed **at T_{10}** segment and then descends down in the pelvis with the help of **Gubernaculum.** Uterus **divides the Gubernaculum into ovarian ligament** and **round ligament**.
- The ovary is attached to the posterior layer of the broad ligament by **the mesovarium,** to the lateral pelvic wall by **infundibulopelvic ligament** and to the uterus by **the ovarian ligament.**

KEY POINTS

Ligaments in relation to ovary (Figs. 1.9 and 1.14)

- **Ovarian ligament**—connects ovary to uterus
- **Infundibulopelvic ligament (suspensory ligament of ovary)** connects ovary to lateral pelvic wall.
- It has ovarian nerves and vessels
- **Mesovarium**—It connects ovary to broad ligament posteriorly.

Relations of the ovary

Anteriar: External iliac vessels.

Posterior: Internal iliac vessels and ureter.

Floor: Obturator nerve.

Histology of Ovary

- **The ovary is covered by a single layer of cubical cells called as Germinal Epithelium of Waldeyer.**
- It is now recognized that germinal epithelium does not give rise to germ cells so now it is called as surface epithelium. The epithelium is present only in early age. Later, the ovary is coated only by connective tissue Tunica albuginea. The subepithelial connective tissue gives rise to tunica albuginea (Figs. 1.14 and 1.15).
- **The cortex of ovary** has follicles in various stages of development:
  - It has Germ cells: derived **from Epiblast**[Q]
  - Follicular cells, i.e. Granulosa and Theca cells
  - The cortex is separated from Germinal epithelium by Tunica Albuginea. But at some places, follicles are directly in contact with Germinal Epithelium called as **Cords of Pflueger**
- **In the medulla** are present blood vessels and **Hilus cells** (secreting androgens).
- This is the reason why Hilus cell tumor is masculinizing tumor of ovary.

- **Blood supply**—Ovarian artery—Branch of abdominal aorta at **L_2 level**
- **Venous drainage—Ovarian Vein**—Left side ovarian vein drains into Left renal vein and Right side drains into inferior vena cava.
- **Nerve supply**—Ovarian plexus — T_{10}, T_{11} (not T_9–T_{10}). Hence ovarian pain is referred to umbilical region (T_{10}).
- **Lymphatic drainage**—Para-aortic LN.

KEY POINTS

Lining epithelium of the organ is important because

- M/C histological type of cancer depends on lining epithelium, e.g. M/C variety of Fallopian Tube Cancer is Adenocarcinoma as the tube is lined by columnar epithelium.
- M/C variety of **Uterine Cancer** (endometrial cancer) is Adenocarcinoma (lining epithelium of uterus is columnar).
- M/C variety of **Vaginal Cancer** is Squamous Cell Carcinoma (lining epithelium is squamous cell).
- In cervix, endocervix is lined by columnar epithelium and exocervix by squamous epithelium. Hence, in all females, there is an area in cervix where one epithelium changes into other, this is called **Transformation Zone**. Since here one type of epithelium is changing into other type, it is the **M/C site for cancer cervix.**
- M/C variety of cancer cervix is Squamous Cell Cancer.
- Now since endocervix is lined by columnar epithelium, hence adenocarcinoma can also occur in cervix. **The M/C site for adenocarcinoma of cervix is endocervix** (not Transformation Zone).

Lining of Female Genital Tract (See Annexure 2)

Blood Supply of Genital Tract

Ovarian Artery

- Arises from Aorta at L_2 level below the renal artery
- Branches in pelvis other than the ovary are:
  - Branch to ureter
  - Fallopian tube
  - Uterine anastomosis.

Note: In the abdomen, just at its origin, it gives branch to ureter.

Ovarian vein drains into inferior vena cava on right side and left renal vein on left side.

Internal Iliac Artery

It is the main feeding vessel of the pelvis and pelvic organs. It divides into anterior and posterior divisions.

Note: Only the anterior division supplies the pelvic viscera.

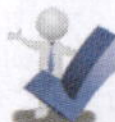

KEY POINTS

Int iliac artery is also called as **hypogastric artery** and can be ligated in severe uncontrollable PPH to save the life of the patient.

Site of ligation: 2.5–3 cm distal to bifurcation of the common iliac artery to preserve the posterior division of the artery and thereby preserving blood supply to lower limb.

The dissection should be done laterally to medially to avoid damaging the hypogastric vein.

Branches of the Internal Iliac Artery

	Anterior division	Posterior division
Visceral branches	Superior vesical Obliterated umbilical Inferior vesical Middle rectal Uterine	Nil
Parietal branches	Vaginal Obturator Inferior gluteal Internal pudendal	Iliolumbar Sacral Superior gluteal

Uterine Artery

- As a terminal branch of anterior division of internal iliac artery, uterine artery runs downwards and medially to cross the ureter near the cervix (2 cm lateral to cervix). It then ascends along the lateral border of the uterus in a tortuous course giving branches to both uterine surfaces.
- 2 cm lateral to internal os (or cervix), where it crosses the ureter, is called **water under bridge** (bride-artery, water-urine in ureter). **This is the most common site of ureteric injury during hysterectomy followed by pelvic brim (Figs. 1.16 and 1.23).**

Mnemonic

Branches of uterine artery to uterus (Fig. 1.17):

U = **Uterine artery**—from outside to inside
A = **Arcuate artery**—supplies outer 1/3rd of myometrium
R = **Radial artery**—supplies inner 2/3rd of myometrium
B = **Basal artery**—supplies basal endometrium
S = **Spiral artery**—supplies superficial endometrium

Besides giving branches to uterus, uterine artery gives:

- **Sampson Artery** - branch to round ligament
- Ovarian branch
- Tubal branch
- Descending cervico vaginal artery—supplies lower cervix and upper vagina.

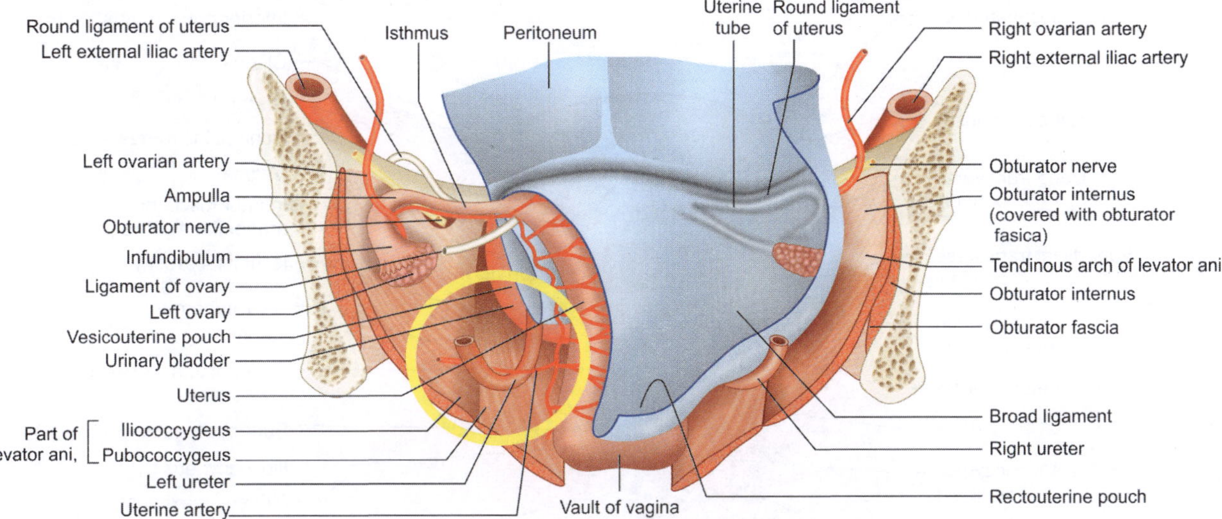

Fig. 1.16: Image showing water under bridge

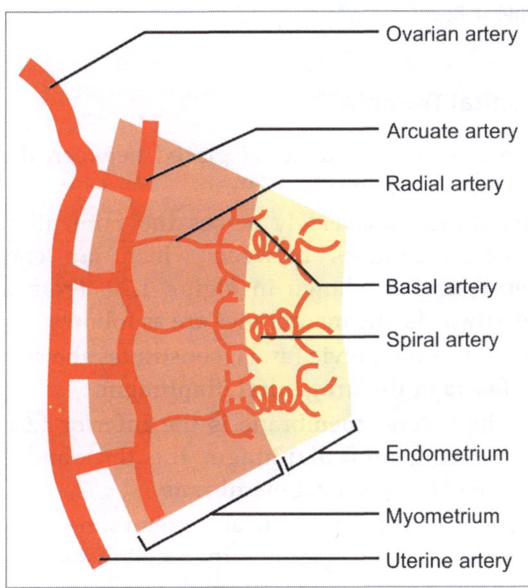

Fig. 1.17: Branches of uterine artery to uterus

Pelvic Floor (Syn: Pelvic Diaphragm)

Pelvic floor is a muscular partition which separates the pelvic cavity from the anatomical perineum. Pelvic diaphragm consists of **the two levator ani muscles** (composed of Pubococcygeus, Iliococcygeus, Puborectalis) **and Ischiococcygeus muscles** (also called simply **coccygeus muscles**).

Levator Ani Muscle (Fig. 1.18)

- **The levator ani muscles are composed of the pubococcygeus (including the pubovaginalis and pubourethralis), puborectalis, and the iliococcygeus.**
- The levator ani is a broad, curved sheet of muscle stretching anteriorly from the pubis and posteriorly from the coccyx and from one side of the pelvis to the other. It hangs like a hammock.
- Its origin is from the tendinous arch called **Arcus Tendinous** extending from the body of the pubis to the ischial spine.
- The levator ani is inserted into the central tendon of the perineum, the wall of the anal canal, the anococcygeal ligament, the coccyx, and the vaginal wall.
- It is perforated by the urethera, vagina, and anal canal.
- **The levator ani assists the anterior abdominal wall muscles in containing the abdominal and pelvic contents.**

Note: Levator ani muscle includes Pubococcygeus, Puborectalis, Iliococcygeus but not Ischiococcygeus. (V Imp)

Innervation

- Traditional teaching is that the levator ani muscles are innervated by the pudendal nerve on the perineal surface and direct branches of the sacral nerves on the pelvic surface. Evidence indicates that the levator ani muscles are innervated solely by a nerve travelling on the superior (intrapelvic) surface of the muscles without the contribution of the pudendal nerve. This nerve, referred to as the levator ani nerve, originates from S_3, S_4, and/or S_5 and innervates both the coccygeus and the levator ani muscle complex.

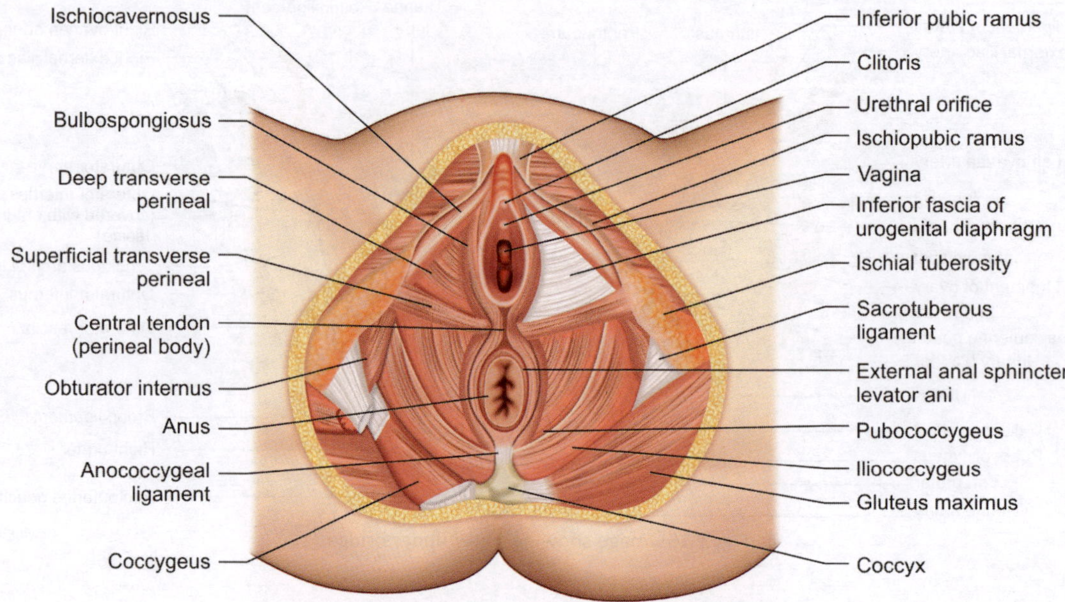

Fig. 1.18: Muscles forming pelvic floor

Perineum

As seen on the surface of the body, the perineum is the region where the external genitalia and the anus are located. Anatomically, the perineum is bounded above by the inferior surface of the pelvic floor, below by the skin between the buttocks and thighs. Laterally, it is bounded by the ischiopubic rami, ischial tuberosities and sacrotuberous ligaments and posteriorly, by the coccyx.

Perineum is rhomboid in shape, and can be divided into anterior and posterior triangular areas. These are the urogenital triangle placed anteriorly, and **the anal triangle placed posteriorly** (Fig. 1.19).

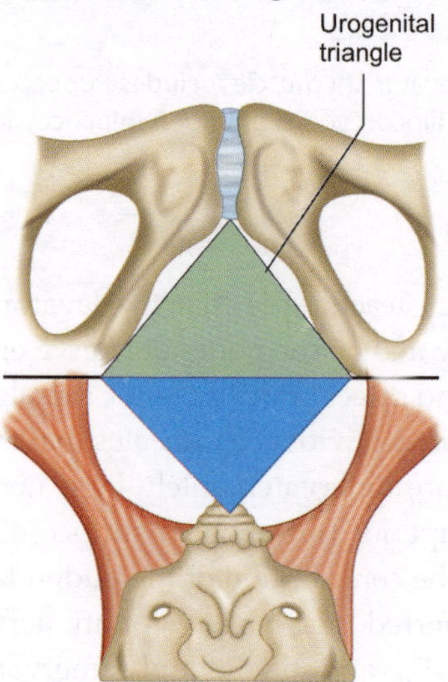

Fig. 1.19: Boundaries of the perineum

Urogenital Triangle

- The urogenital triangle is placed between the two ischiopubic rami (Fig. 1.19).
- Stretching transversely across the rami, there are three membranes between which are enclosed two spaces as shown in Figure 1.20. From above downwards, the membranes are as follows:
  - Part of the pelvic fascia, constitutes the **superior fascia of the urogenital diaphragm.**
  - The second membrane is the **inferior fascia of the urogenital diaphragm**. It is thick and is also called the **perineal membrane**.
  - The most superficial membrane is **the membranous layer of superficial fascia.**
- Between the upper and middle membranes, there is the **deep perineal space (or pouch)**. The deep perineal has pouch the following muscles—**deep transverse perinei (paired) and sphincter urethrae (Fig. 1.18)**.
- Between the middle and lower membranes, there is the **superficial perineal space (or pouch). The superficial perineal pouch has superficial transverse perinei (paired), bulbospongiosus, the ischiocavernosus (paired) covering the crura of the clitoris and the Bartholin's gland (paired). These are called as Muscles of Vulva**.
- **Posteriorly, all the three membranes are attached to the perineal body and to each other thus closing the superficial and deep perineal spaces behind**.

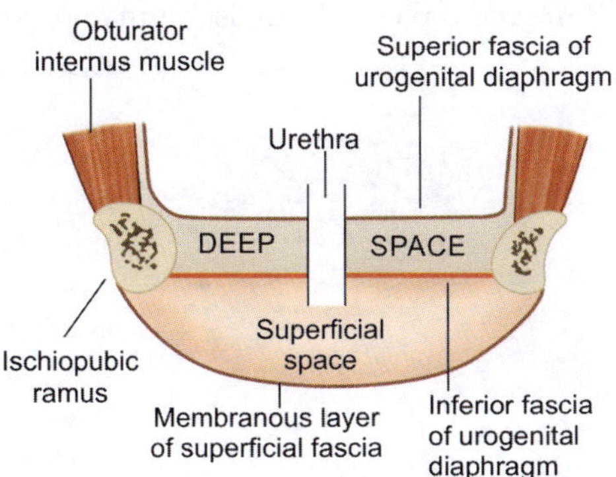

Fig. 1.20: Schematic coronal section through urogenital triangle to show formation of superficial and deep perineal spaces

Perineal Body

The perineal body (or central tendon of the perineum) is a fibromuscular body placed in the median plane at the junction of the anal and urogenital triangles.

It is pyramidal in shape and has all the 3 layers of muscles, i.e. *(See Fig. 1.19)*
- Levator ani
- Deep transverse perinei
- Superficial transverse perinei
- Fibers of external anal sphincter.
- External urinary sphincter
- Bulbospongiosus (bulbocavernosus)

Mnemonic

Muscles attached on perineal body
BLESSD
B = Bulbospongiousus
L = Levator ani
E = External anal sphincter (some fibres)
S = Urinary Sphincter
S = Superficial transverse perinei
D = Deep transverse perinei

Now before going further see Figure 1.18

In the figure: See that superficially in the perineum there are 3 muscles present:
- Superficial Transverse perinei muscles.
- Bulbospongiosus
- Ischiocavernosus

Another muscle present in superficial pouch is anal sphincter. So total there are 4 muscles. Also see, Ischiocavernosus is a muscle present on the sides & not in midline, hence it is not attached to perineal body. Thus it is not included in muscles attached to perineal body.

Note: Levator ani & Ischiococcygeus are muscles of pelvic floor not of perineum.

Broad Ligament

- It is a double fold of peritoneum extending from side of uterus to lateral pelvic wall.
- Does not support the uterus[Q].
- Does not contain ovary but is attached to ovary through the mesovarium.
- Parts of broad ligament (Flowchart 1.1).

Flowchart 1.1: Parts of Broad ligament

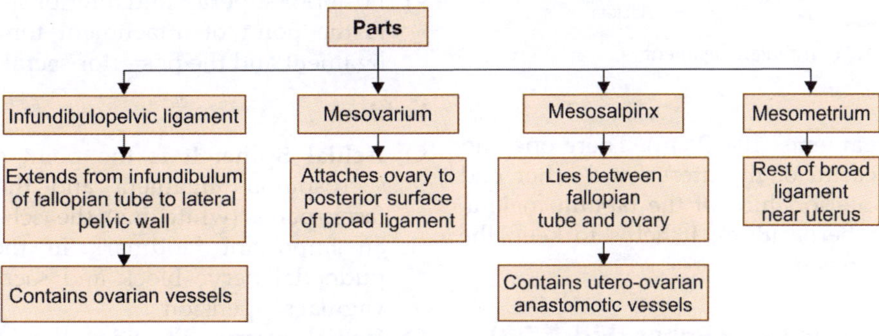

Flowchart 1.2: Contents of broad ligament

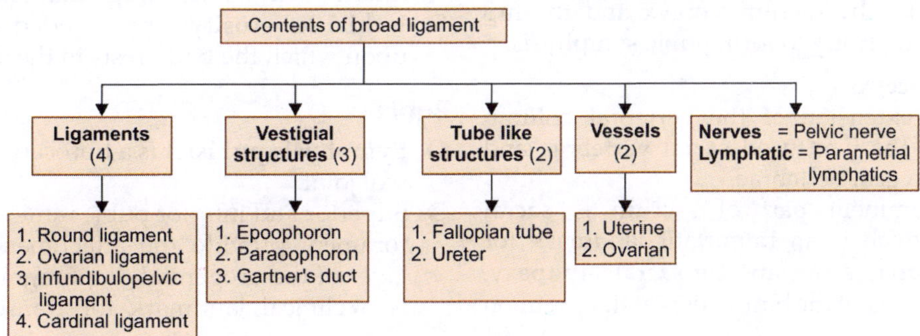

Pelvic Cellular Tissue

- The pelvic cellular tissue condenses at many places and gives rise to (Fig. 1.21):
  - **Uterosacral ligament** that extends from S_2, S_3, and S_4 to the posterior and lateral part of supravaginal cervix.
  - **Cardinal liagments/Mackenrodts ligaments/ transverse cervical ligaments** that extends in fan-shaped manner from pelvic wall and inserted into the lateral supravaginal cervix. **It is the main support of uterus.**
  - **Pubocervical ligament** extend from anterolateral aspect of cervix to the back of pubic bone lateral to pubic symphysis.

  Note: Together these 3 ligaments are called as **Triradiate ligament**.

Importance

- Support the pelvic organs.
- Form a protective sheath for blood vessels and ureter.

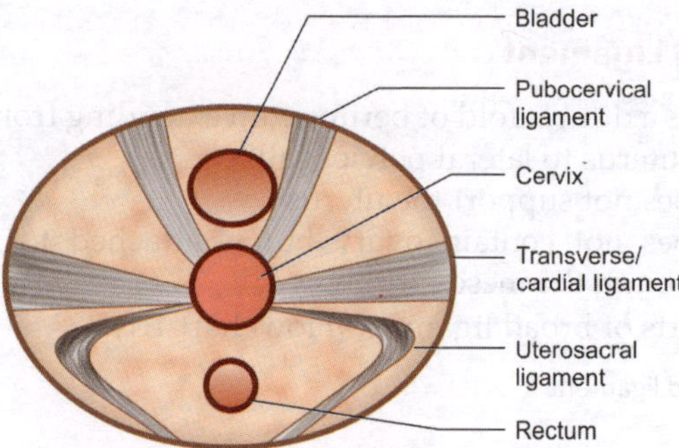

Fig. 1.21: Triradiate ligament

Round Ligament

These are paired ligaments (10–12 cm). There one end is attached at the cornu of the uterus and other end terminates in the anterior third of the labium majora. It develops from gubernaculum. It helps to keep the uterus in anteverted position.

Important Points on Bony Pelvis (Fig. 1.22)

The pelvis is formed by sacrum, coccyx and the hip bones which fuse anteriorly to form pubic symphysis.

The sacrum and coccyx:

- These are an extension of the vertebral column resulting from the five fused sacral vertebrae and four fused coccygeal vertebrae.
- The most prominent part of sacrum is **sacral promontory** which is an important landmark for insertion of a laparoscope and **for sacralcolpopexy**. It is located just below the bifurcation of the common iliac arteries.

Hip Bone has 3 parts: ilium, ischium and pubis.

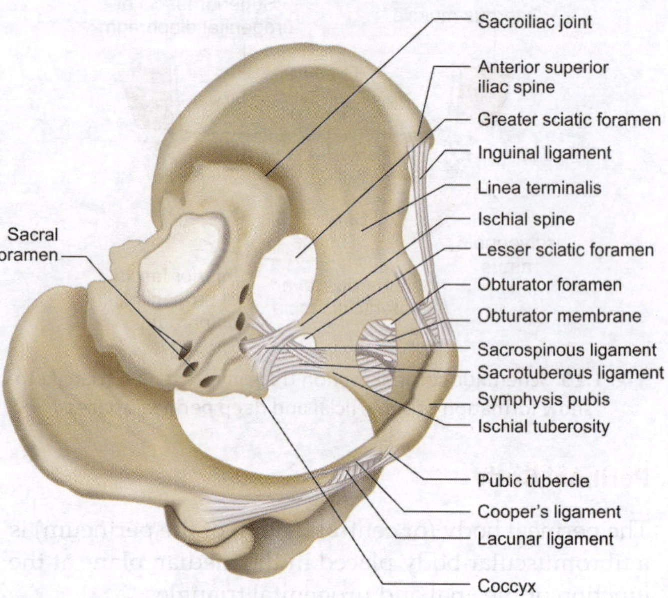

Fig. 1.22: The female pelvis. The pelvic bones (the innominate bone, sacrum, and coccyx) and their joints, ligaments, and foramina

Ilium

- Iliac crest - provides attachments to the iliac fascia, abdominal muscles and fascia lata.
- Anterior superior and inferior spine: It is the place where inguinal ligament is attached and **is clinically important as a lateral landmark for laparoscopic entry.**
- Posterior superior and inferior spine - superior spine is the point of attachment for the sacrotuberous ligament and the posterior sacral iliac ligament.

Ischium

- **Ischial Spine:** It is the point of fixation for the sacrospinous ligament and the arcus tendineus fascia pelvis (white line); the ischial spine represents an important landmark in the performance of pudendal nerve block and sacrospinous ligament vaginal suspension
- **Ischial ramus:** Provides the attachment for the inferior fascia of the urogenital diaphragm
- **Ischial tuberosity:** The rounded bony prominence upon which the body rests in the sitting position.

Pubis

- **Symphysis pubis:** It is a fibrocartilaginous symphyseal joint.
- Superior and inferior pubic rami - encircle obturator foramen; provide the attachment for the inferior layer of the urogenital diaphragm; the inferior rami is a clinical landmark for transobturator tape in urinary incontinence.

Joints in Pelvis

Name	Type
Sacrococcygeal joint	Cartilaginous Joint
Symphysis pubis	Cartilaginous Joint
Sacroiliac joint	Synovial Joint

Ureter

- Extends from kidney to bladder
- Measurement in females = 2.5 cm
- Totally retroperitoneal in location
- The lower half of each ureter transverses the pelvis after crossing the common iliac vessels at their bifurcation, just medial to the ovarian vessels.

In its pelvic path in the retroperitoneum, several relationships are of significance and are areas of greatest vulnerability to injury of the ureter (Fig. 1.23).

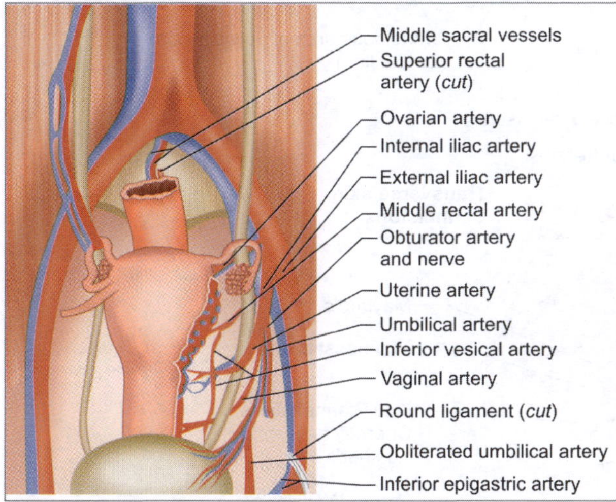

Fig. 1.23: Cause of ureter

1. The ovarian vessels cross over the ureter as it approaches the pelvic brim and lie in lateral proximity to the ureter as it enters the pelvis.
   This is the **2nd M/C site of ureteric injury** during hysterectomy.
2. As the ureter descends into the pelvis, it runs within the broad ligament just lateral to the uterosacral ligament, separating the uterosacral ligament from the mesosalpinx, mesovarium, and ovarian fossa.
3. At about the level of the ischial spine, the ureter crosses under the uterine artery in its course through the cardinal ligament. **This site is called as** water **under bridge and is 2 cm lateral to internal os (See Figs. 1.16 and 1.23). This is the M/C site of ureteric injury during hysterectomy**.
4. The ureter then turns medially to cross the anterior upper vagina as it traverses the bladder wall.
   Note: About 75% of all iatrogenic injuries to the ureter result from gynecological procedures, **most commonly abdominal hysterectomy**[Q]**.** Hysterectomy with highest risk of injuring the ureter is **Wertheim's hysterectomy**[Q]**.**

Retroperitoneal Surgical Spaces

Important Retroperitoneal surgical spaces are:

- Retroperitoneal space of pelvic sidewall
- Presacral space
- Prevesical/Retropubic/Space of Retzius

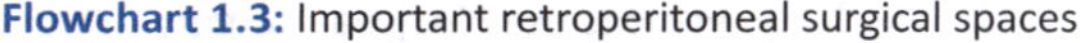

Flowchart 1.3: Important retroperitoneal surgical spaces

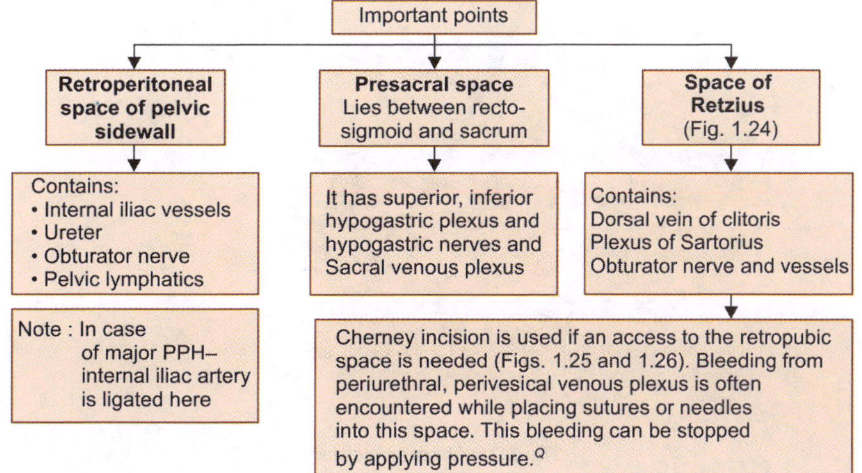

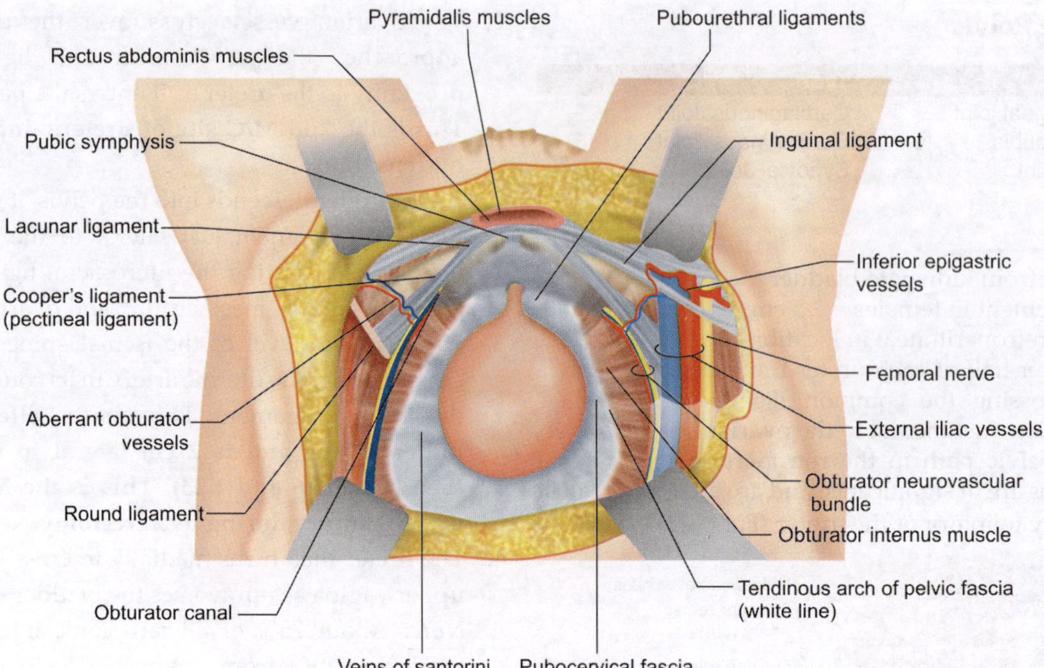

Fig. 1.24: Space of Retzius

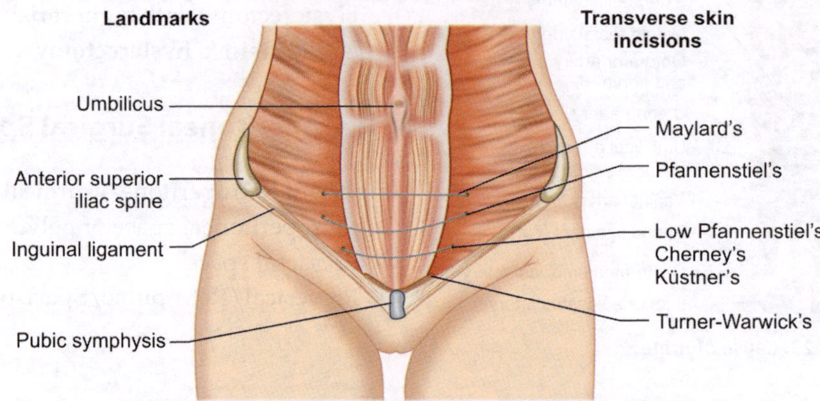

Fig. 1.25: Incisions used in gynae surgery

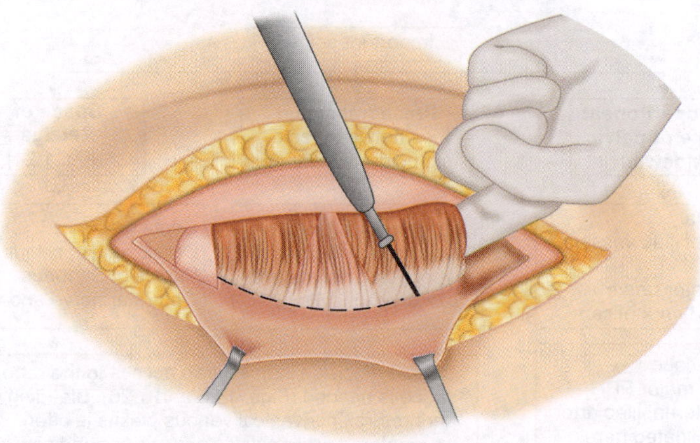

Fig. 1.26: Cherney incision

NEW PATTERN QUESTIONS

N1. With regards to labia majora all are correct *except*:
a. Is homologous to scrotum in males
b. Is supplied by branches of internal and external pudendal arteries
c. Drains into superficial inguinal lymph nodes
d. The broad ligament terminates at its anterior end

N2. The triangular area bounded by clitoris, fourchette and labia minora is:
a. Fossa navicularis b. Ventricle
c. Vestibule d. Vulva

N3. Identify the structure 'X' marked on the figure:
a. Fossa navicularis b. Fourchette
c. Posterior commissure d. Vestibule TM

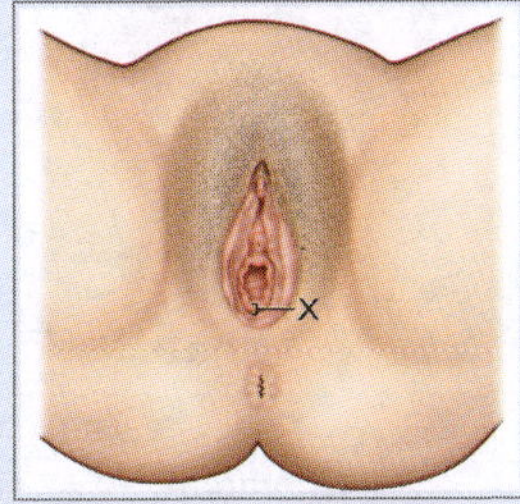

N4. Prostate glands is homologous to:
a. Bartholin's gland b. Cowper's gland
c. Skene glands d. Bulbourethral glands

N5. Fourchette is where:
a. Both labia minora meet posteriorly
b. Both labia minora meet posteriorly
c. Labia minora and majora meet
d. Distance between vulva and labia minora

N6. TOC of Bartholin cyst:
a. Incision and drainage b. Marsupilization
c. Cystectomy d. Antibiotics

N7. For hormonal study, sample should be taken from which wall of vagina:
a. Anterior wall b. Posterior wall
c. Lateral wall d. Any wall

N8. Vaginal defence is lost:
a. Within 10 days of birth
b. After 10 days of birth
c. During pregnancy d. At puberty

N9. With regards to vagina all are correct *except*:
a. Makes an angle of 45° with the horizontal in erect posture
b. Looks like letter 'H' on cross section
c. Vaginal axis lies parallel to the uterus and at right angles to the plane axis of inlet
d. Is lined by stratified squamous epithelium

N10. Theoretically, Gonococcal vaginitis can be seen:
a. In puberty
b. In newborn females
c. In reproductive age females
d. Sex workers

N11. Angle of anteflexion occurs at the level of:
a. External os b. Internal os
c. Cervix d. Isthmus *(JIPMER 2012)*

N12. Size of uterus in inches:
a. 5 × 4 × 2 b. 4 × 3 × 1
c. 3 × 2 × 1 d. 4 × 2 × 1

N13. Identify the structure 'X' shown in figure:
a. Fallopian tube b. Round ligament
c. Ovarian ligament d. Broad ligament

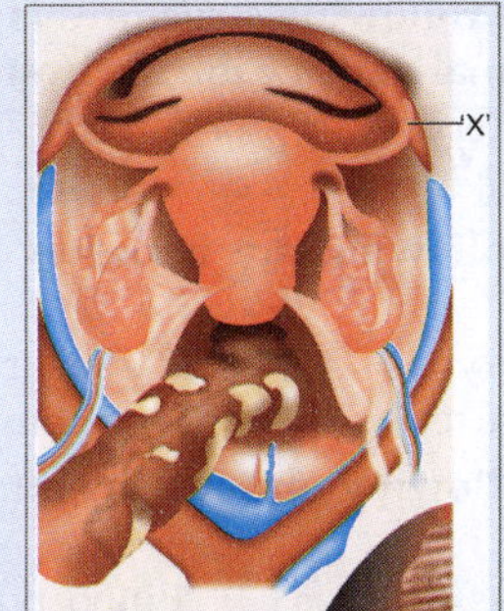

N14. Isthmus is the area of uterus:
a. Bounded by histological internal os above and anatomical internal os below
b. Bounded by anatomical internal os above and histological internal os below
c. Bounded by uterus above and anatomical internal os below
d. Bounded by histological internal os above and external os below

N15. Cervix: Corpus ratio before puberty is:
a. 1:2 b. 2:1
c. 1:3 d. 3:1

N16. M/C lymph node involved Ca Cervix:
a. Obturator lymph node
b. Inguinal
c. Internal iliac d. External iliac

N17. Longest part of fallopian tube is:
a. Isthmus b. Interstitial
c. Ampulla d. Fimbriae

N18. M/c cause of B/L cornual block is:
a. TB b. Gonococcal infection
c. Physiological spasm d. Chlamydia

N19. Which ligament carries ovarian artery in lateral wall:
a. Ovarian ligament
b. Suspensory ligament of ovary
c. Broad ligament d. Round ligament

N20. Ovary is:
a. Is attached to the posterior layer of the broad ligament by mesovarium
b. Has hilus cells in the cortex
c. Ovarian veins drain into inferior vena cava
d. Is connected to the uterus by infundibulopelvic ligament

N21. In uncontrollable PPH, all of the following arteries can be ligated *except*:
a. Uterine artery
b. Anterior division of internal iliac artery
c. Posterior division of internal iliac artery
d. Ovarian artery

N22. All of the following are true with respect to ligation of internal iliac artery *except*:
a. For hemostasis, anterior division is to be ligated
b. Collateral circulation is established later between middle sacral and lateral sacral arteries
c. Bleeding is always controlled with it
d. The artery should be ligated and not transected

N23. Which of the following structures is most susceptible to unintentional damage during hysterectomy:
a. Uterine artery b. Ureter
c. Urinary bladder d. Urethra

N24. All of the following are branches of uterine artery *except*:
a. Spiral artery b. Radial artery
c. Sampson artery d. Obturator artery

N25. All of the following muscles are attached to perineal body *except*:
a. Levator ani b. Bulbospongiosus
c. Ischiocavernosus d. Ext. anal sphincter

N26. The ligament connecting ovary to lateral pelvic wall is:
a. Infundibulo pelvic ligament
b. Ovarian ligament
c. Round ligament d. Broad ligament

N27. The ureter is recognized by the following features during surgery *except*:
a. Pale glistening appearance
b. Longitudinal vessels on the surface
c. Peristalsis d. Distal end

N28. M/C site of ureteric injury during hysterectomy:
a. Pelvic brin
b. Where it is crossed by uterine artery
c. Where it enters the bladder
d. Where it is over obturator vessels

N29. All of the following support the uterus *except*:
a. Uterosacral ligament b. Pubocervical ligament
c. Broad ligament d. Cardinal ligament

N30. Round ligament is supplied by:
a. Ovarian artery b. Interior iliac artery
c. Sampson artery d. Vaginal artery

N31. Canal of Nuck contains:
a. Ovarian ligament b. Round ligament
c. Based ligament d. Fallopian tube

N32. The ligament which helps to keep the uterus in anteverted and anteflexed position:
a. Round ligament b. Broad ligament
c. Pubocervical ligament d. Cardinal ligament

N33. The ligament which prevents retroversion of uterus:
a. Round ligament b. Uterosacral ligament
c. Pubocervical ligament d. Cardinal ligament

N34. The vessel most susceptible for injury while inserting umbilical laparoscopic trocar and during dissection for sacral colpopexy:
a. Inferior epigastric artery
b. Left common iliac vein
c. Left common iliac artery
d. Aorta

N35. Identify the type of hymen given in figure:
a. Septate hymen b. Cribriform hymen
c. Imperforate hymen d. Vaginal hymen

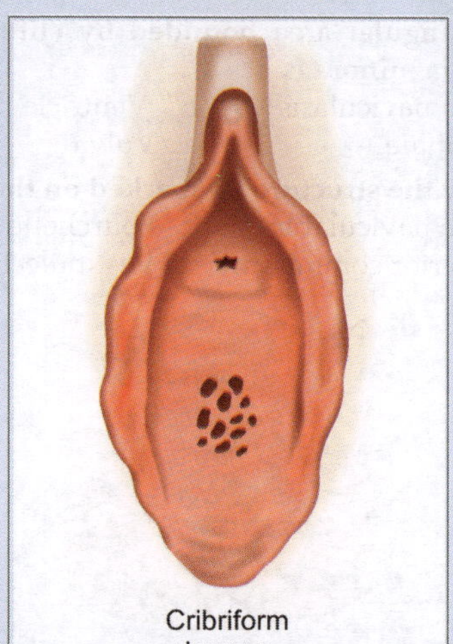
Cribriform hymen

N36. Maximum number of mucosal folds are seen in which part of fallopian tube:
a. Infundibulum b. Ampulla
c. Isthmus d. Interstitial part

N37. Arrange the parts of fallopian tube from medial to lateral:
a. Isthmus>Interstitium>Ampulla>Infundibulum
b. Isthmus>Ampulla>Interstitium>Infundibulum
c. Interstitium>Isthmus>Ampulla>Infundibulum
d. Infundibulum>Interstitium>Ampulla>Isthmus

N38. Superficial muscles of perineum are:
a. Sphincter urethrae b. Ischiocavernosus
c. Levator ani d. Ischiococcygeus

N39. All of the following muscles are attached to perineal body *except*:
a. Superficial transverse perinei muscle
b. Iliococcygeus
c. Bulbospongiosus d. Ischiocavernosus

N40. Nerve supply of perineum is:
a. Pudendal nerve b. Inferior rectal nerve
c. Pelvic splanchnic nerve
d. Hypogastric plexus

N41. Contents of blood ligament are all except:
a. Ovarian vessels in its infundibulo pelvic part
b. Fallopian tube in its upper part
c. Ovarian ligament in its anterior fold
d. Gartner's duct

N42. Labia Minora lacks all *except*
a. Hair follicles b. Sebaceous glands
c. Eccrine glands d. Apocrine glands

PREVIOUS YEAR QUESTIONS

1. **All of the following pelvic structures support the vagina, *except*:** *(AIIMS May 04)*
   a. Perineal body b. Pelvic diaphragm
   c. Levator ani muscle
   d. Infundibulopelvic ligament
2. **All are related to lateral vaginal fornix** *except:* *(JIPMER 90)*
   a. Ureters b. Mackenrodt's
   c. Inferior vesical artery d. Uterine artery
3. **The pH of vagina in adults is:** *(Delhi 98, DNB 00 95)*
   a. 3.5 - 4.5 b. 4.5 - 5.5
   c. 5.5 - 6.5 d. 6.5 - 7.5
4. **Protective bacterium in normal vagina is:** *(J and K 01)*
   a. Peptostreptococcus b. Lactobacillus
   c. Gardenella vaginalis d. E. coli
5. **The main source of physiological secretion found in the vagina is:** *(AIIMS 98)*
   a. Bartholin's glands b. Gartner's duct
   c. Vagina d. Cervix
6. **With reference to vagina which of the following statement is not correct:** *(UPSC 07)*
   a. It has mucus secreting gland
   b. It is supplied by uterine artery
   c. It is lined by stratified squamous epithelium
   d. Its posterior wall is covered by peritoneum
7. **Which of the following about lymphatics of vulva is true:** *(AI 98)*
   a. Do not cross the labiocrural fold
   b. Traverse labia from medial to lateral
   c. Drain directly into deep femoral glands
   d. Do not freely communicate with each other
8. **Uterine: cervix ratio upto 10 years of age:**
   a. 3:2 b. 2:1 *(JIPMER 2011)*
   c. 3:1 d. 1:2
9. **The epithelial lining of cervical canal is:** *(TN 90)*
   a. Low columnar b. High columnar
   c. Stratified squamous d. Ciliated columnar
10. **Nabothian follicles occur in:** *(TN 91)*
    a. Erosion of cervix b. Ca endometrium
    c. Ca cervix d. Ca vagina
11. **Bartholin's duct opens into:** *(DNB 99)*
    a. Labia majora and minora
    b. A groove between labia minora and hymen
    c. The lower vagina d. The upper vagina
12. **A woman presents with a fluctuant non tender swelling at the introitus. The best treatment is:** *(AI 08)*
    a. Marsupilization b. Incision and drainage
    c. Surgical resection d. Aspiration
13. **Bartholin's cyst is caused by:** *(DNB 04)*
    a. Candida b. Anaerobes
    c. Gonococcus d. Trichomonas
14. **Narrowest part of fallopian tube is:** *(Delhi 93)*
    a. Interstitial portion b. Isthmus
    c. Infundibulum d. Ampulla
15. **'Peg cells' are seen in:** *(DNB 00)*
    a. Vagina b. Vulva
    c. Ovary d. Fallopian tubes
16. **The length of fallopian tube is:** *(DNB 95)*
    a. 8 - 12 cm b. 12 - 15 cm
    c. 15 - 18 cm d. 18 - 20 cm
17. **Uterine artery is a branch of:** *(DNB 00, 95)*
    a. Aorta b. Common iliac
    c. Internal iliac d. External iliac
18. **Vaginal epithelium is derived from:** *(AIIMS Nov 13)*
    a. Endoderm of urogenital sinus
    b. Mesoderm of urogenital sinus
    c. Endoderm of genital ridge
    d. Mesoderm of genital ridge
19. **Anatomical sphincter of fallopian tubes?** *(AIIMS Nov 13)*
    a. Ampulla b. Isthmus
    c. Intramural d. Infundibulum
20. **Incorrect statement about uterus:** *(PGI Nov 2011)*
    a. Length of uterine cervix > length of corpus in nulliparous women
    b. Length of uterine cervix > length of corpus in multiparous women
    c. Uterus is 7 cm long in adult multiparous
    d. Uterus is 25 cm long in multiparous women
    e. Epithelium in corpus is ciliated columnar
21. **Which of the following is true about vulvodynia:**
    a. Surgery is usually done for localized vulval lesion
    b. Pain without any significant lesion
    c. Tricyclic antidepressant is useful
    d. Psychological factor is associated
22. **True about anatomy of vagina:**
    a. Covered by columnar epithelium
    b. Covered by non keratinized stratified squamous epithelium
    c. Vaginal secretion is from transudation of endometrial epithelium
    d. Supplied by cervicovaginal branch of the uterine artery
    e. Anterior wall is longer than posterior wall
23. **True about anatomy of Fallopian Tube:**
    a. Length is 20 cms *(PGI May 2012)*
    b. Medial to lateral structures are – isthmus, interstitial part, ampulla and fimbriae
    c. Ovary is attached to uterus by ovarian ligament
    d. Uterine artery supplies medial 2/3 of tube
    e. Ampulla is longest part

24. Ovarian pathology is referred to: *(AIIMs 2010)*
a. Gluteal region b. Anterior thigh
c. Medial part of thigh d. Back of thigh

25. The following lymph nodes receive lymphatics from the uterus *except*: *(AIIPG 2005)*
a. External iliac b. Internal iliac
c. Superficial inguinal lymph nodes
d. Deep inguinal lymph nodes

26. Lymphatic drainage of cervix is by all lymph nodes *except*:
a. Parametrial lymph nodes *(AIIPG 2006)*
b. Deep inguinal lymph nodes
c. Obturator lymph nodes
d. External iliac lymph nodes

27. Cervix is/are drained by: *(PGI Nov 2015)*
a. External iliac LN b. Internal iliac LN
c. Aortic LN d. Inguinal LN
e. Sacral LN

28. Pudendal nerve block abolishes pain from: *(JIPMER May 2016)*
a. Upper cervix b. Lower cervix
c. Upper vagina d. Lower vagina

29. Which is true regarding ovary:
a. Mesovarium contains ovarian vessels
b. Ovarian ligament connects ovaries to uterus
c. Ovarian fossa is related to ilioinguinal
d. Suspensory ligament of ovary connects ovaries to uterus

30. False regarding anatomy of cervix is: *(JIPMER May 2014)*
a. Cervix is 2 times longer in size than uterus in children
b. Cervix is equal in size to uterus in puberty
c. Fundus of uterus drains into para-aortic lymph nodes
d. Uterine artery is lateral to cervix & passes anterior to uterus

31. Which of the following muscle is attained to perineal body: *(JIPMER 2013)*
a. Pubocervical b. Bulbospongiosus
c. Ischiocavernous d. Ischiococcygeus

32. Cortex of ovary consists of all of the following except:
a. Graafian follicle *(JIPMER 2011)*
b. Hilus cells
c. Primordial follicle
d. Corpus luteum

ANSWERS TO NEW PATTERN QUESTIONS

N1. Ans. is d, i.e. The broad ligament terminates at its anterior end *Ref: Dutta Gynae 6th/ed, p1*

All options are correct with respect to labia except: Option d because it is round ligament and not broad ligament which terminates at its anterior end.

N2. Ans. is c, i.e. Vestibule *Ref: COGDT 11th/ed, p26*

Vestibule is the triangular area bounded anteriorly by the clitoris, posteriorly by Fourchette and on either side by labia minora.

N3. Ans. is a, i.e. Fossa navicularis

The structure marked is the distance between fourchette (place where posterior end of labia minora join) and hymen i.e. it is fossa navicularis.

N4. Ans. is c, i.e. Skene glands *Ref: COGDT 11th/ed, p24*

Glands in male	Homologous glands in females
• Prostate gland	• Skene glands/paraurethral glands
• Cowper's gland	• Bartholin gland
• Glands of Littre (in penile urethra)	• Glands of labia majora • Glands of labia minora

N5. Ans. is a, i.e. Both labia minora meet posteriorly *Ref: COGDT 11th/ed, p24*

Remember: Mnemonic FFP: from anterior to posterior
- **F** = Fossa Navicular is: Distance between hymen and fourchette
- **F** = Fourchette—Posteriorly where labia minora meet
- **P** = Posterior Commissure—Posteriorly where labia majora meet

N6. Ans. is b i.e. Marsupialization

TOC for Bartholin cyst—Marsupialization.
TOC for Bartholin abscess—Incision and drainage.

N7. Ans. is c, i.e. Lateral wall

Vaginal study gives a fair idea about the hormonal status and, in turn, about ovulation/ovarian cycle.

- For hormonal study, sample should be taken from: Lateral wall
- For cytological study (Papsmear), sample should be taken from: Posterior wall

N8. Ans. is b, i.e. After 10 days of birth *Ref: Dutta Gynae 6th/ed, p5*

Vaginal defense is lost at 10 days after birth. The maternal estrogen circulating the newborn maintains the vaginal defense for 10 days. Thereafter it is lost upto pre-puberty. High level of circulating estrogen increase the vaginal defense during puberty, pregnancy and in premenstrual phase. Again after Menopause, vaginal defense is lost.

N9. Ans. is c, i.e. Vaginal axis lies parallel to the uterus and at right angles to the plane axis of inlet *Ref: Dutta Gynae 6th/ed, p4,5*

The vaginal canal is directed upwards and backwards forming an angle of 45° with the horizontal in erect posture. **The long axis of the vagina almost lies parallel to the plane of the pelvic inlet and at right angles to that of the uterus (not vice versa).** Vagina has got an anterior, a posterior, and two lateral walls. The anterior and posterior walls are apposed together but the lateral walls are comparatively stiffer especially at its middle, hence it looks 'H' shaped on transverse section.

N10. Ans. is b, i.e. In newborn females

Squamous epithelium is resistant to Gonococcal infection, and since in all adult females, vagina is lined by stratified squamous epithelium. Hence, gonococcal vaginitis does not occur.

In newborn females, vagina is lined by transitional epithelium. Therefore, theoretically speaking, gonococcal vaginitis can occur in newborn females.

N11. Ans. is b, i.e. Internal os

Angle of anteflexion between uterus and cervix, at the level of internal os.

N12. Ans. is c, i.e. 3 × 2 × 1 inches *Ref: Jeffcoates Principle of Gynae 9/ed, pg 32*

Remember, best answer to this question is 3.25 × 2.5 × 1.5 inches.

N13. Ans. is b, i.e. Round ligament

At the cornua structures attached from anterior are to posterior
- Round ligament (R)
- Fallopian Tube (T)
- Ovarian ligament (O)

N14. Ans. is b, i.e. Bounded by anatomical internal os above and histological internal os below

See the text for explanation

N15. Ans. is b, i.e. 2:1.

See the text for explanation.

N16. Ans. is a, i.e. Obturator lymph node

- M/c Lymphnode involved in Ca cervix: obturator LN
- 1st Lymphnode involved in Ca cervix: ureteric/paracervical LN

N17. Ans. is c, i.e. Ampulla

Fallopian tube

• Longest part	Ampulla
• Widest part	Ampulla
• Narrowest part	Interstitium
• 2nd Narrowest part	Isthmus
• Anatomical sphincter	Interstitium
• Physiological sphincter	Isthmus

N18. Ans. is c, i.e. Physiological spasm

M/c cause of bilateral cornual block at the time of HSG is physiological spasm.

N19. Ans. is b, i.e. Suspensory ligament of ovary *Ref: COGDT 11th/ed, p36*

The suspensory ligament of ovary (infundibulopelvic ligament) contains the ovarian artery, veins and nerves.

N20. Ans. is a, i.e. Is attached to the posterior layer of the broad ligament by mesovarium *Ref: Dutta Gynae 6th/ed, p11,12*

- Ovary measures about 3.5 cm in length, 2.5 cm in breadth and 2 cm in thickness. In nulliparae, the ovary lies in the ovarian fossa on the lateral pelvic wall. The ovary is attached to the posterior layer of the broad ligament by the mesovarium, to the lateral pelvic wall by infundibulopelvic ligament and to the uterus by the ovarian ligament.
- The substance of the gland consists of outer cortex and inner medulla.

- **Medulla:** It consists of loose connective tissues. There are small collection of cells called "hilus cells" which are homologous to the interstitial cells of the testes.
- **Arterial supply** is from the ovarian artery.
- **Venous drainage** is through pampiniform plexus, to form the ovarian veins which drain into inferior vena cava on the right side and left renal vein on the left side.
- Sympathetic supply comes down along the ovarian artery from T_{10} segment. Ovaries are sensitive to manual squeezing.

N21. Ans is c, i.e. Posterior division of internal iliac artery

All the arteries supplying the uterus, can be ligated to control PPH.
1. Uterine artery
2. Ovarian artery
3. Anterior division of internal iliac artery (uterine artery arises from it).

N22. Ans. is c, i.e. Bleeding is always controlled with it *Ref: Dutta Gynae 6th/ed, p33*

Only the **anterior division of internal iliac artery** supplies the pelvic viscera and **hence should be ligated for controlling** severe PPH. **The artery should not be transected.** Hemostasis is effective due to temporary lowering of pulse pressure by 85%. On ligation of internal iliac artery → **collateral circulation develops between systemic arteries and internal iliac artery.**

Ligation of internal iliac artery and development of collateral circulation

Systemic artery		Internal iliac artery
Lumbar (aorta) →	with	← Iliolumbar
Middle sacral (aorta) →	with	← Lateral sacral
Superior rectal (inferior mesenteric) →	with	← Middle rectal
Ovarian (aorta) →	with	← Uterine

Bleeding does not always stop after ligation due to presence of aberrant vessels or it could be venous bleeding.

N23. Ans. is b, i.e. Ureter.

M/C structure to be damaged during hysterectomy is ureter
M/C site of ureteric injury – where it crossed by uterine artery.
2nd M/C of ureteric injury – at the pelvic brain

N24. Ans. is d, i.e. Obturator artery

Branches of uterine artery are:

To the uterus:
- A = Arcuate artery
- R = Radial artery
- B = Basal artery
- S = Spiral artery

To the cervix
- Descending cervical artery

To the round ligament
- Samson artery

Ovarian artery
Arcuate artery
Radial artery
Basal artery
Spiral artery
Endometrium
Myometrium
Uterine artery

N25. Ans. is c, i.e. Ischiocavernous

The following muscles are attached to perineal body.

B = Bulbospongiosus **L** = Levator ani **E** = External anal sphincter **S** = Urinary sphincter **S** = Superficial transverse perinei **D** = Deep transverse perinei

Ischiocavernous is not attached to perineal body
See the Figure below.

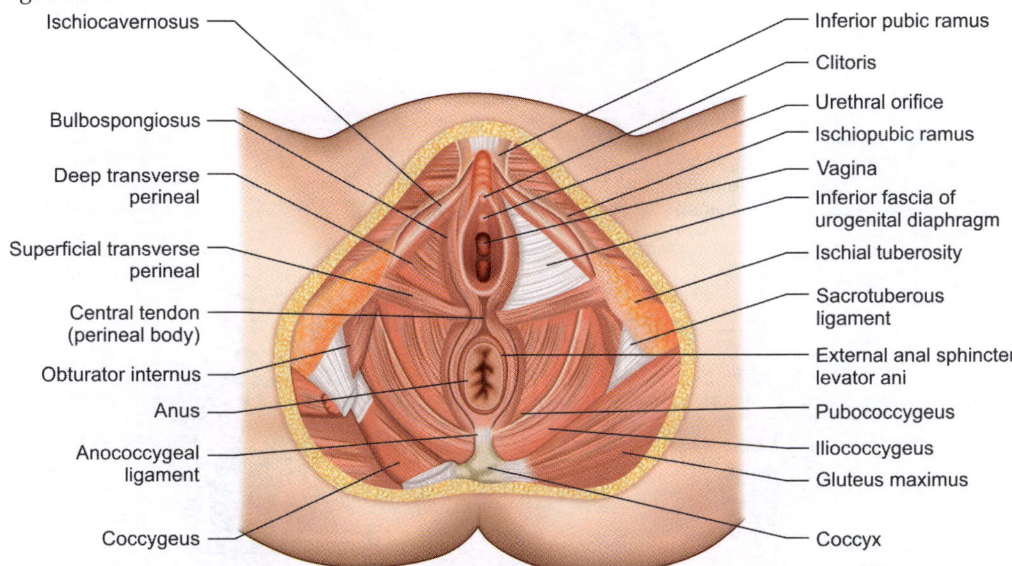

N26. Ans. is a, i.e. Infundibulo pelvic ligament
See the text for explanation

N27. Ans. is d, i.e. Distal end

Ureter is recognised during surgery by: 1. Pale glistering appearance 2. Longitudinal vessels on surface 3. Peristalsis

Note: The fallopian tube is identified by distal end (due to presence of fimbria) not ureter.

N28. Ans. is b, i.e. Where it is crossed by uterine artery
Site of ureteric injury during hysterectomy
1st M/C = where it is crossed by uterine artery
2nd M/C = Near pelvic brim

N29. Ans. is c, i.e. Broad ligament
Broad ligament does not support the uterus.

N30. Ans. is c, i.e. Sampson artery
Round ligament is supplied by sampson artery, which is a branch of uterine artery.

N31. Ans. is b, i.e. Round ligament
The Canal of nuck is an abnormal patent pouch of peritoneum extending into the labia majora of women. It is analogous to **patent processes vaginalis in males.** It is attached to the uterus by the round ligament through the internal inguinal ring into the inguinal canal. Normally it obliterates and disappears by 1st year of life.

N32. Ans. is a, i.e. Round ligament.

N33. Ans. is b, i.e. Uterosacral ligament.

Remember

- The ligament which keeps the uterus in anteverted and anteflexed position—Round ligament.
- The ligament which prevents retroversion—uterosacral ligament.

N34. Ans. is b, i.e. Left common iliac vein *Ref: Novaks 15th/ed, p74*

The left common iliac vein lies medial to the artery and is at the risk of injury during umbilical laparoscopic trocar insertion and during dissection for sacral colpopexy.

N35. Ans. is b, i.e. Cribriform hymen

The following images show various types of Hymen.

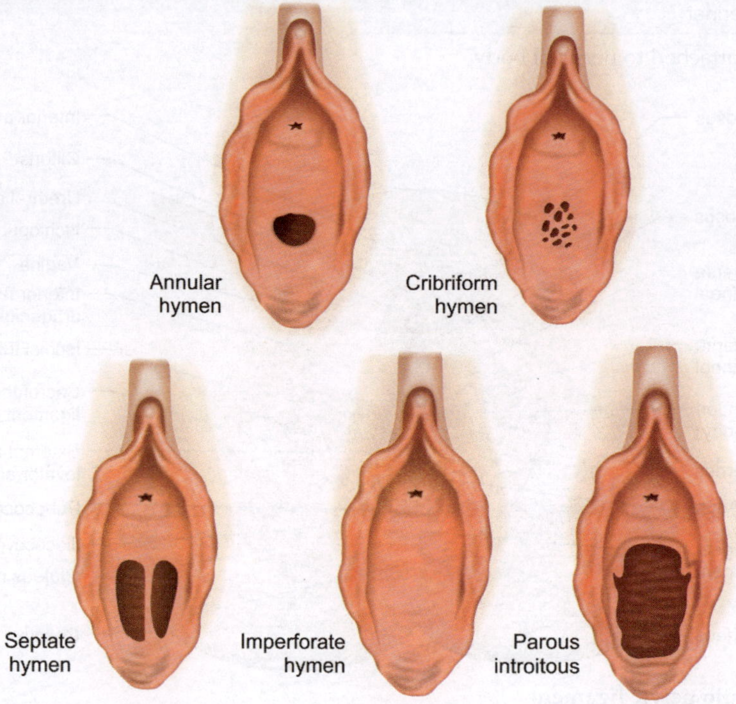

N36. Ans. is a, i.e. Infundibulum

The mucosa of fallopian tube is thrown into longitudinal folds, which are more pronounced distally in the infundibulum and are very few in intramural part.

N37. Ans. is c, i.e. Interstitium>Isthmus>Ampulla>Infundibulum

See the text for explanation

N38. Ans. is a, i.e. Sphincter urethrae *Ref: Shaws TB of Gynaecology 15th/ed, p17*

The muscles present superficially are:

- Superficial transverse perinei muscles
- Bulbospongiosus (sometimes called as sphincter vaginae)
- Ischiocavernous
- External sphincter muscle of anus

N39. Ans. is d, i.e. Ischiocavernosus

Ischiocavernosus is not present in midline, it is not attached to perineal body.

N40. Ans. is a, i.e. Pudendal nerve

N41. Ans. is c, i.e. Ovarian ligament in its anterior fold

Now in the question, all the options which are given are contents of broad ligament.

Now before you regard the question as dummy question-read the options again carefully.

Option a: Ovarian vessels in its infundibulopelvic part-correct.

Option b: Fallopian tube in its upper part- correct.

Option c: Ovarian ligament in its anterior fold- now ovarian ligament is a part of broad ligament that's right, but its not present in its anterior fold-it is present in its posterior fold

Option d: Gartner's duct- yes, it is a part of broad ligament.

So here the incorrect answer is option c

N42. Ans. is b, i.e. Sebaceous glands. *Ref: Williams Obs 25th/ed, p17*

See the text for explanation.

ANSWERS TO PREVIOUS YEAR QUESTIONS

1. **Ans. is d, i.e. Infundibulopelvic ligament** *Ref: Jeffcoate 7th/ed, p46; CGDT 10th/ed, p49*
   - Friends our question is related to the supports of vagina. Before going into its details lets have a second look at the options. All the options given in the question are somehow related to vagina, therefore may have a role in supporting vagina except the infundibulopelvic ligaments.
   - *Infundibulopelvic ligament attach the ovary to the lateral pelvic wall and supporta the ovary, but has no connection to the vagina or uterus, therefore does not support either structures.*

   So, by exclusion, our answer is infundibulopelvic ligament.

   Now, coming on to the details of supports of vagina.

   Vagina is supported in the lower part by:
   - Bulbocavernosus muscle (at the level of introitus)
   - Urogenital diaphragm
   - Perineal muscles
   - Levator ani muscles (known as pelvic diaphragm) support the lower 1/3rd of vagina

   In its upper part: vagina is supported by: Cardinal ligament (also called as transverse cervical ligament)

   The anterior wall of vagina, urethra and bladder base are supported by: Pubocervical fascia

   The posterior wall of vagina is supported by: Perineal body

2. **Ans. is c, i.e. Inferior vesical artery** *Ref: Shaw 15th/ed, p5*

   Vagina is supported in the lower part by:

   The cervix and all 4 fornices are related to
   - *Uterine Vessels*[Q]
   - *Mackenrodt's ligament*[Q]
   - *Ureter*[Q]

   Posteriorly surrounding the pouch of douglas lie the uterosacral ligaments.[Q]

3. **Ans. is b, i.e. 4.5–5.5**
4. **Ans. is b, i.e. Lactobacillus** *Ref: Jeffcoate 7th/ed, p27-28; Dutta Gynae 5th/ed, p7*
5. **Ans. is d, i.e. Cervix** *Ref: Shaw 15th/ed, p128; Dutta Gynae 5th/ed, p6*

   See the text of explanation.

6. **Ans. is a, i.e. It has mucus secreting glands** *Ref: Shaw 15th/ed, p4,20,18 for blood supply*

   Lets analyse each option separately:

   Option a: It has mucus secreting glands – incorrect as

   No glands open into vagina[Q] *and vaginal secretion is mainly derived from mucous discharge of cervix and partly from transudate through vaginal epithilium.*[Q]
   - The vaginal mucosa is lined by stratified squamous epithelium.[Q]
   - In newborn, the epithelium is transitional in nature and cornified cells are scanty until puberty and this is the reason why gonococcal vaginitis can occur in newborns.

   Option b: Supplied by uterine artery – correct as vagina is supplied by vaginal artery which arises either from uterine artery or can sometimes be a direct branch of internal iliac artery.

   Option c: It is lined by stratified squamous epithelium – correct.

   Option d: Posterior wall is covered by peritoneum.

   "There is no serosal covering (on vagina) except for the area covered by cul de sac and we all know that cul de sac is related to posterior wall of vagina". *Ref: Shiela Balakrishnan, 1st/ed, p5*

7. **Ans. is b, i.e. Traverse labia from medial to lateral** *Ref: Dutta Gynae 5th/ed, p29-30; CGDT 10th/ed, p18*

   Special features of vulval lymphatics are as follows:
   - *The lymphatics of each side freely communicate with each other.*
   - *The lymphatics hardly cross beyond labiocrural fold.*
   - Vulval lymphatics also anastomose with lymphatics of lower 1/3rd of vagina and drain into external iliac nodes.
   - *Superficial lymph nodes are the primary lymph nodes that act as sentinel glands of vulva. Deep inguinal nodes are secondarily involved. It is unusual to find pelvic glands without metastasis in inguinal nodes.*

   "From the upper 2/3rd of the left and right labia majora superficial lymphatics pass towards the Symphysis and turn laterally to joint the medial superficial inguinal nodes." *Ref: CGDT 10th/ed, p18*

   Hence, they traverse labia from medial to lateral side.

8. Ans. is d, i.e. 1:2 *Ref: Shaw 15th/ed, p8*

The relationship of the length of the cervix and that of the body of uterus varies with age.

Age	Uterus to cervix ratio (Corpus/Cervix ratio)
• Before puberty	1:2
• At puberty	2:1
• In adults/Reproductive age	3:1 or 4:1
• After menopause	Whole of uterus and cervix atrophy

9. Ans. is b, i.e. High columnar *Ref: Shaw 15th/ed, p7*

Read the text for explanation.

10. Ans. is a, i.e. Erosion of cervix *Ref: Shaw 15th/ed, p325; Dutta Gynae 5th/ed, p259*

Cervical erosion: Condition where squamous epithelium of ectocervix is replaced by columnar epithelium which is continuous with endocervix. It occurs when estrogen levels are high as in pregnancy and use of oral contraceptives (ocp's).
As a result of healing of an erosion, the mouth of cervical gland is blocked. The blocked gland becomes distended with secretion and forms small cysts which can be seen with naked eye and so called *Nabothian cyst*.

11. Ans. is b, i.e. A groove between labia minora and hymen *Ref: Dutta Gynae 5th/ed, p2; Jeffcoate 7th/ed, p24*

See the text of explanation

12. Ans. is a, i.e. Marsupilization

13. Ans. is c, i.e. Gonococcus *Ref: Jeffcoates 7th/ed, p450-1; William Gynae 1st/ed, p96*

Fluctuant non-tender swelling at the introitus suggests a diagnosis of Bartholin's, cyst.

Bartholin's cyst:

- It is the most common cyst of vulva.
- Bartholins' cyst are produced from accumulation of secretions of Bartholin's gland.
- The cyst may develops either in the duct (more common) or in the gland
- **Etiology**: Cyst formation occurs due to the obstruction of the main duct or opening of an acinus.
- The cause of obstruction is usually fibrosis which follows either infection or trauma.
- **It was formerly believed that the infection was invariably gonococcal but now M/C organism is *E. coli*.**
- Left Bartholins' gland is more often affected than the right.

Presentation:

- Usually presents as a unilateral swelling that bulges across the vaginal introitus.
- Size of the cyst rarely exceeds hen's egg.
- Swelling is present characteristically on the inner side of the junction of the anterior 2/3rd with posterior 1/3rd of the labium majus.
- The swelling is fluctuant and usually non tender
- Patient may present with discomfort, dyspareunia, or infection.
- **Treatment of choice is Marsupialization: It is preferred over traditional excision operations.**

14. Ans. is a, i.e. Interstitial portion

15. Ans. is d, i.e. Fallopian tubes *Ref: Shaw 15th/ed, p11*

16. Ans. is b, i.e. 12–15 cm *Ref: Shaw 15th/ed, p11*

The length of tubes varies from 7–12 cms. *Novaks 15th/ed, p90*

17. Ans. is c, i.e. Internal iliac artery *Ref: Shaw 14th/ed, p17*

As discussed in text uterine artery is a branch of anterior division of internal iliac artery

18. Ans. is a, i.e. Endoderm of urogenital sinus *Ref: Shaw's Textbook of Gynecology 15th/ed, p91; Dutta Gynae 6th/ed, p35*

Development of vagina is composite, partly from the mullerian ducts (paramesonephric ducts) and partly from the urogenital sinus.

Part of vagina	Development
Upper 3/5th	Mullerian ducts
Lower 2/5th	Urogenital sinus
Hymen	Junction of mullerian ducts and urogenital sinus
Epithelium of the vagina and portio vaginalis part of cervix	Endoderm of urogenital sinus
Fibromuscular layer of vagina	Mesoderm of fused caudal part of mullerian ducts
Vaginal introitus	Ectoderm of genital folds

19. Ans. is c, i.e. Intramural part *Ref: John Hopkins manual of human functional anatomy p144*

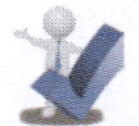

KEY POINTS

Anatomical sphincter of fallopian tube is intramural part

Physiological sphincter is Isthmus part

20. Ans. is a, b and d, i.e. Length of uterine cervix > length of corpus in nulliparous women, Length of uterine cervix > length of corpus in multiparous women, Uterus is 25 cm long in multiparous women.

In uterus:

- The cervix is to corpus ratio is 2:1 before puberty.
- Length of nonpregnant uterus in nulliparous females = 6 to 8 cm (7.5 cm)
- Length of nonpregnant uterus in multiparous females = 9 to 10 cm
- Length of pregnant uterus = 35 cm

21. Ans. is b, c and d, i.e. Pain without any significant lesion, Tricyclic antidepressant is useful and Psychological factor is associated *Ref: COGST 10K p635-638*

Vulvodynia

- Vulvar pain in absence of relevant visible physical finding is vulvodynia

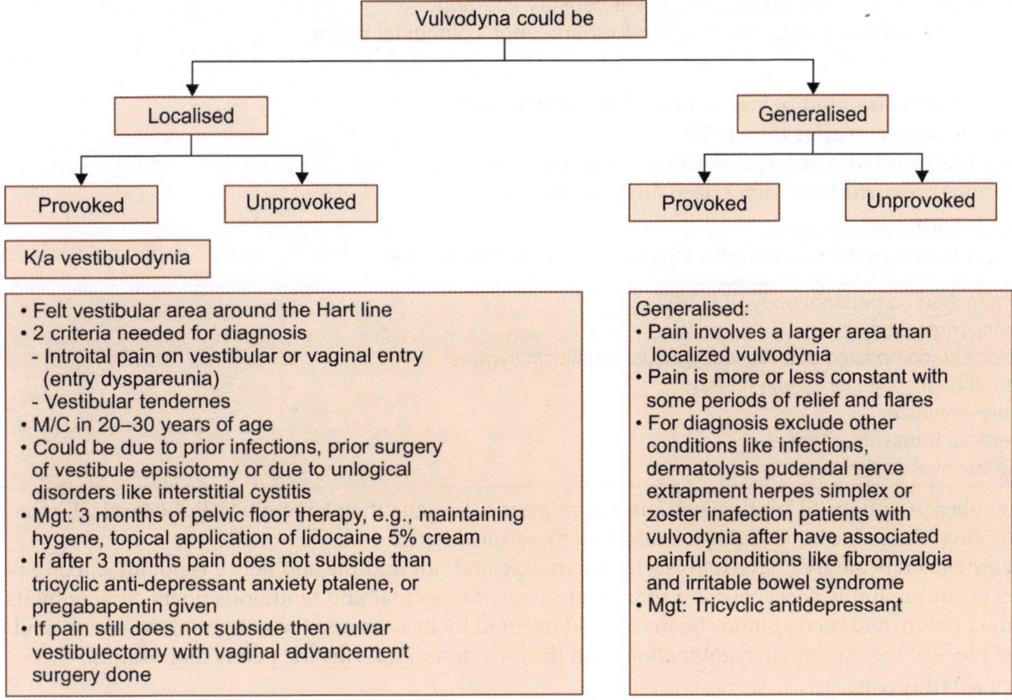

22. Ans. is b, c and d, i.e Covered by non keraterized stratified squamous epithelium, Vaginal secretion is from trasudation of endometrial epithelium and Supplied by cervicovaginal branch of the uterine artery

23. Ans. is c, d and e, i.e. Ovary is attached to uterus by ovarian ligament, Uterine artery supplies medial 2/3rd of the tube, Ampulla is the longest part.

- Length of tube is 8-12 cm, not 20 cm
- Medial to lateral parts of the tube are: interstitial>isthmus>ampulla and fimbriae

24. Ans. is c, i.e. Medial part of thigh

Ovarian pathology may irritate the obturator nerve which lies close to the ovary. Obturator nerve supplies the medial side of thigh and thus ovarian pathology can lead to pain in medial side of thigh, by phenomenon of **Somatic referred pain**.

25. Ans. is d, i.e. Deep inguinal lymph nodes

- Lymphatics from fundus reach para-aortic lymph nodes
- Lymphatics from cornua reach superficial inguinal lymph nodes along with those from Round ligament
- Lymphatics from body of uterus reach external iliac lymph nodes.
- Hence the answer is Deep inguinal lymph nodes.

26. Ans. is b, i.e. Deep inguinal lymph nodes

27. Ans. is a, b and e, i.e. External iliac lymph nodes, Internal iliac lymph nodes and Sacral lymph nodes.

Lymphatic drainage of cervix

HOPE

H–Hypogastric lymph nodes/Internal iliac lymph nodes

O–Obturator lymph nodes

P–Paracervical lymph nodes, Parametrial or ureteric lymph nodes

E–External iliac lymph nodes

28. Ans. is d, i.e. Lower vagina

- The innervation of upper vagina contains both sympathetic and parasympathetic fibers (S2–S4).
- Lower part of vagina is supplied by pudendal nerve.

29. Ans. is b, i.e. Ovarian ligament connects ovar ovaries to uterus.

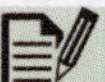 **Remember**

Mesovarium connects ovary posteriorly to the broad ligament.
Ovarian ligament connects ovary to uterus (option b)
Suspensory ligament or infundibulopelvic ligament connects ovary to lateral pelvic wall.
Ovarian vessels and nerves are present in suspensory ligament.
Ovarian fossa is related posteriorly to obturator nerve, not ilioinguinal nerve.

30. Ans. is b, i.e. Cervix is equal in size to uterus at puberty.

At puberty the cervix : corpus ratio is 1:2.
That means uterus is twice as large as cervix not equal.
Rest all options are correct and don't need any explanation.

31. Ans. is b, i.e. Bulbospongiosus

As discussed earlier in the text muscles attached to Perineal body are:

Muscles attached on perineal body BLESSD
B = Bulbospongiousus
L = Levator ani (comprising of pubococcygeous and iliococcygeus)
E = External anal sphincter (some fibres)
S = Urinary Sphincter
S = Superficial transverse perinei
D = Deep transverse perinei

Now remember in options to confuse you instead of pubococcygeus they have given **Pubocervical**, which is a ligament connecting cervix to pubic bone and is not attached to perineal body.

Ischiocavernosus repeatedly I have told is a lateral muscle and not midline and hence is not attached to perineal body.

Ischiococcygeus or simply coccygeus is a triangular plane of muscular and tendinous fibers, arising by its apex from the spine of the ischium and sacrospinous ligament, and inserted by its base into the margin of the coccyx and into the side of the lowest piece of the sacrum. In combination with the levator ani, it forms the pelvic diaphragm.

32. Ans. is b, i.e. Hilus cells

As discussed in the text of the chapter, Hilus cells are the only cells present in Medulla of ovary. They resemble Leydig cells of testis and hence their tumor is masculinizing tumor of the ovary.

REVIEW/PRACTICE QUESTIONS

1. **Vulva is:**
   a. Vaginal opening
   b. Area enclosed by Labia Minora, clitoris and fourchette.
   c. Female external genital organs
   d. Male external genital organs
2. **All of the following are correctly matched *except*:**
   a. Clitoris: Penis
   b. Labia majora: Scrotum
   c. Skene gland: Prostate gland
   d. Bartholin gland: Prostate gland
3. **All of the following statement are correct regarding Labia Majora *except*:**
   a. It contains hair follicles, sebaceous gland and apocrine glands
   b. Round ligament terminates at its anterior end
   c. It posteriorly meets to form the fourchette
   d. It is homologous to scrotum in males
4. **Hidradenoma of vulva arises from:**
   a. Sweat glands of Labia Majora
   b. Sweat glands of Labia Minora
   c. Apocrine glands of Labia Majora
   d. Apocrine glands of Labia Minora
5. **All are true regarding relations of vagina *except*:**
   a. Bladder–anterior
   b. Levator ani–laterally
   c. Bartholin gland–posterior
   d. Perineal body–posterior
6. **All are parts of vulva *except*:**
   a. Labia Minora
   b. Labia Majora
   c. Perineal body
   d. Clitoris
7. **All are true about Bartholin's glands *except*:**
   a. Homologous of male bulbourethral glands
   b. Present in superficial perineal pouch
   c. Located at junction of anterior 1/3rd and middle 1/3rd of labia majora
   d. Opens into the vestibule between hymen & labia minora
8. **Name the muscle forming the pelvic diaphragm:**
   a. Deep transverse perinei
   b. Sphincter urethrae
   c. Levator ani
   d. None
9. **Levator ani muscle includes all *except*:**
   a. Puborectalis
   b. Pubococcygeus
   c. Iliococcygeus
   d. Ischiococcygeus
10. **Ureter lies in which wall of ovary fossa?**
    a. Anterior
    b. Posterior
    c. Medial
    d. Lateral
11. **All of the following pairs are correct concerning lymphatics of uterus *except*:**
    a. Fundus: Para-aortic
    b. Mid uterus: External iliac
    c. Cervix: Superficial inguinal lymph nodes
    d. Cervix: Sacral nodes
12. **Portio vaginalis is the other name for:**
    a. Supravaginal part of cervix
    b. Vaginal part of cervix
    c. Outer half of vagina
    d None
13. **All of the following pairs are correctly matched *except*:**
    a. Ovary: T_{10}-T_{11}
    b. Uterus: T_{10}-L_1
    c. Vulva: L_1-L_2
    d. Cervix: S_2-S_4
14. **Incision used for gaining access to space of Retzius:**
    a. Pfannenstiel incision
    b. Cherney incision
    c. Maylard incision
    d. Rutherford-Morrison incision
15. **All are correct *except*:**
    a. Vestibule has 6 openings
    b. Greater vestibular glands ducts open distal to hymenal ring, one at 5 o'clock and other at 7 o'clock position
    c. Skene glands lie near the urinary meatus
    d. Minor vestibular glands open along the hymen

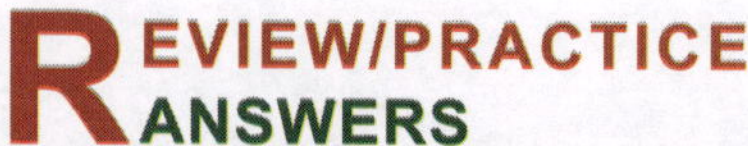

REVIEW/PRACTICE ANSWERS

1. **Ans. is c, i.e. Female external genital organs** *Ref: Jeffcoates Gynae 9th/ed, p23*
2. **Ans. is d, i.e. Bartholin gland: Prostate gland** *Ref: Williams Obs 25th/ed, p38, Table 3.1 and Jeffcoates Gynae 9th/ed, p25*
3. **Ans. is a, i.e. It contains hair follicles, sebaceous gland and apocrine glands** *Ref Jeffcoates Gynae 9th/ed, p23-24,*
4. **Ans. is c, i.e. Apocrine glands of Labia Majora** *Ref: Shaw Gynae 15th/ed, p2*
5. **Ans. is c, i.e. Bartholin gland–posterior** *Ref: Shaw Gynae 15th/ed, p5*
6. **Ans. is c, i.e. Perineal body** *Ref: Williams OBS 25th/ed, p16.*
   Some books say perineum is a part of vulva, others don't. So, best answer here is 'c'.
7. **Ans. is c, i.e. Located at junction of anterior 1/3rd and middle 1/3rd of labia majora**
   Located at junction of anterior 2/3rd and posterior 1/3rd, and not junction middle 1/3rd and posterior 1/3rd.
8. **Ans. is c, i.e. Levator ani** *Ref: Shaw 15th/ed, p15 and Jeffcoates Gynae 9th/ed, p46*
9. **Ans. is d, i.e. Ischiococcygeus** *Ref: Williams Gynae 3rd/e p802*
10. **Ans. is b, i.e. Posterior** *Ref: Jeffcoates Gynae 9th/ed, p38*
11. **Ans. is c, i.e. Cervix: superficial inguinal lymph nodes**
    Cervix does not drain into inguinal lymph nodes.
12. **Ans. is b, i.e. Vaginal part of cervix** *Ref: Jeffcoates Gynae 9th/ed, p32*
13. **Ans. is c, i.e. Vulva: L_1–L_2**

Also Know

Organ	Spinal segment
Ovaries	$T_{10} - T_{11}$
Fallopian tube	T_{10}
Uterus	$T_{10} - L_1$
Cervix & upper vagina	$S_2 - S_4$
Lower vagina and Perineum	Pudendal Nerve

14. **Ans. is b, i.e Cherney incision**
15. **Ans. is d, i.e. Minor vestibular glands open along the hymen** *Ref: Williams OBS 25th/ed, p17*

CHAPTER 2

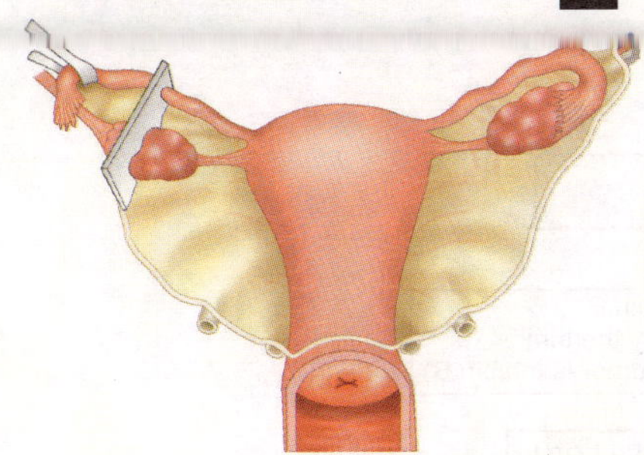

Reproductive Physiology and Hormones in Females

Ovarian Cycle

At puberty, the hypothalamo pituitary ovarian axis becomes functional and releases GnRH in a pulsatile manner. GnRH in turn leads to the release of FSH.

- **Ovarian cycle begins with hormone Follicle-stimulating Hormone (FSH).**♀ **(See flowchart 2.1)**
- Primary oocytes in intrauterine life get surrounded by follicular cells and are called as **primordial follicle**. (Measurement 0.03–0.05 mm).
- Under the influence of FSH, the follicular cells of the dominant primordial follicle differentiate into an outer layer of cells called as **Theca cells** and an inner layer called as **Granulosa cells**.

Menstrual Cycle

- In intrauterine life—oogenesis begins
- Oogonia undergoes mitosis to become Primary Oocyte.
- Then primary oocyte undergoes Meiosis I but it gets *arrested* in intrauterine life in **Diplotene stage of Prophase** and it is unable to get converted to secondary oocyte. It remains in this arrested stage i.e. **Dictyate stage till puberty**
- The arrest is over at puberty
- At puberty, the primary oocyte gets converted to secondary oocyte (23X) and 1st polar body is released. This conversion is called *ovulation*.
- Until puberty, in the ovary, all the primary oocytes remain in arrested stage. These primary oocytes get surrounded by the follicular cells of ovary and this structure is called as *primordial follicle* (present in the cortex of ovary) (Figs. 2.1A and B)
- Thus ovary is a reservoir of many such follicles.
- In other words, where in infertility, we do tests for ovarian reserve, we actually are trying to find whether ovary has follicles or not.
- At puberty, the hypothalamo pituitary ovarian axis becomes functional and releases GnRH in a pulsatile manner.

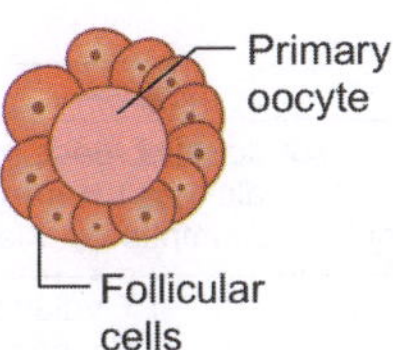

Fig. 2.1A: Primordial follicle—Primary oocyte surrounded by follicular cells

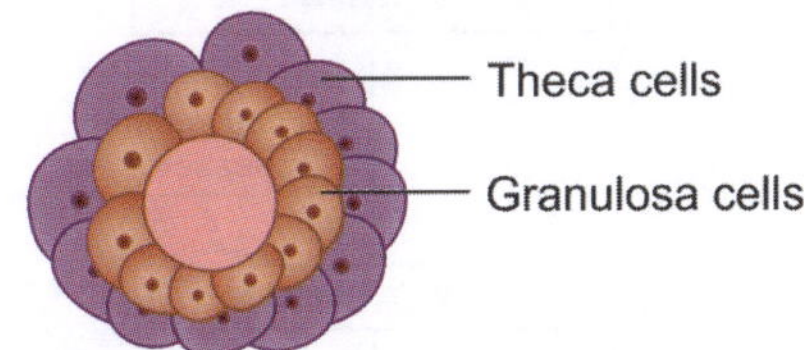

Fig. 2.1B: The follicular cells differentiate into two types of cells—Theca cells and Granulosa cells

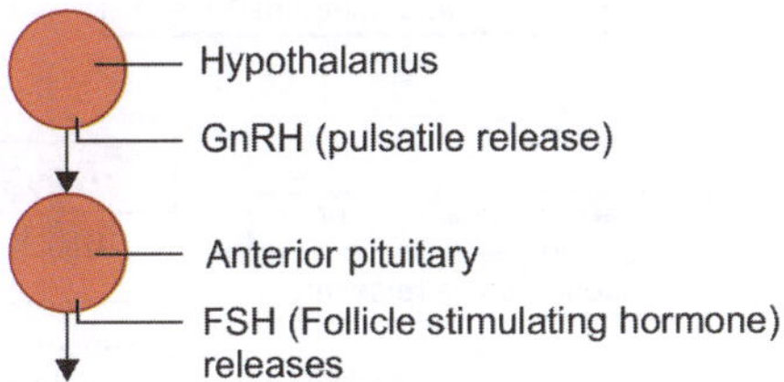

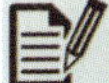

Remember

The number of follicles keep decreasing, i.e. the follicles undergo atresia every month.

- That is why the number of follicles is maximum at 20 weeks of gestation and then decreases.
- Now at puberty when FSH is released it prevents the follicles from apoptosis and stimulates them instead.

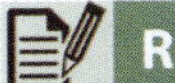

Remember

The initial recruitment of follicles is hormone independent.

- Now to understand what happens when FSH is released—see flowchart 2.1

Flowchart 2.1: Menstrual cycle

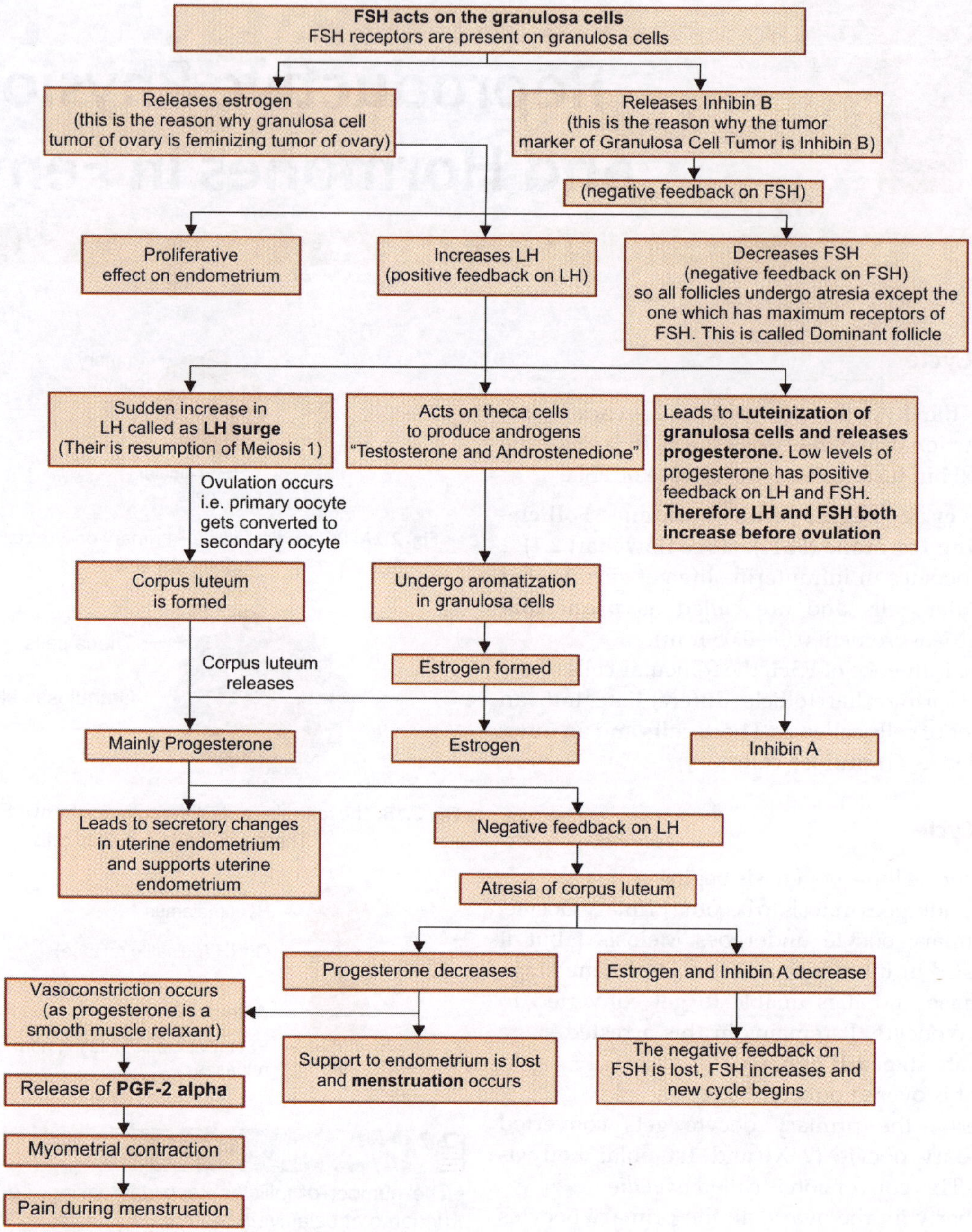

- **FSH acts on the granulosa cells** — FSH receptors are present on granulosa cells
  - Releases estrogen (this is the reason why granulosa cell tumor of ovary is feminizing tumor of ovary)
  - Releases Inhibin B (this is the reason why the tumor marker of Granulosa Cell Tumor is Inhibin B) → (negative feedback on FSH)
- Proliferative effect on endometrium
- Increases LH (positive feedback on LH)
- Decreases FSH (negative feedback on FSH) so all follicles undergo atresia except the one which has maximum receptors of FSH. This is called Dominant follicle
- Sudden increase in LH called as **LH surge** (Their is resumption of Meiosis 1) → Ovulation occurs i.e. primary oocyte gets converted to secondary oocyte → Corpus luteum is formed → Corpus luteum releases → Mainly Progesterone
- Acts on theca cells to produce androgens "Testosterone and Androstenedione" → Undergo aromatization in granulosa cells → Estrogen formed → Estrogen, Inhibin A
- Leads to **Luteinization of granulosa cells and releases progesterone.** Low levels of progesterone has positive feedback on LH and FSH. **Therefore LH and FSH both increase before ovulation**
- Mainly Progesterone → Leads to secretory changes in uterine endometrium and supports uterine endometrium
- Progesterone, Estrogen, Inhibin A → Negative feedback on LH → Atresia of corpus luteum
  - Progesterone decreases → Vasoconstriction occurs (as progesterone is a smooth muscle relaxant) → Release of **PGF-2 alpha** → Myometrial contraction → Pain during menstruation
  - Progesterone decreases → Support to endometrium is lost and **menstruation** occurs
  - Estrogen and Inhibin A decrease → The negative feedback on FSH is lost, FSH increases and new cycle begins

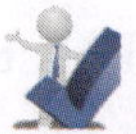

KEY POINTS

- Ovarian cycle is initiated by FSH
- As early as 5–7 days, dominant follicle is selected. The rest of the follicles become atretic by Day 8
- The basic prerequisite in ovulatory cycle is fluctuating levels of E_2. If for any reason, the E_2 levels become static, anovulation is a rule (as in PCOS)
- The two-cell theory of steroidogenesis suggests that FSH acts on Granulosa cells to produce estrogen, and LH acts on Theca cells to produce androgens (Fig. 2.2).

Note:

i. Testosterone gets converted to Estradiol (E_2)
ii. Androstenedione gets converted to Esterone (E_1) (Fig. 2.2)

Reaction (i) and (ii) occur both in Granulosa cells, whereas reaction (ii) can occur in adipose tissue also.

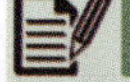

Remember

FSH receptors are present only on Ganulosa cells LH receptors are present both on Granulosa and Theca cells.

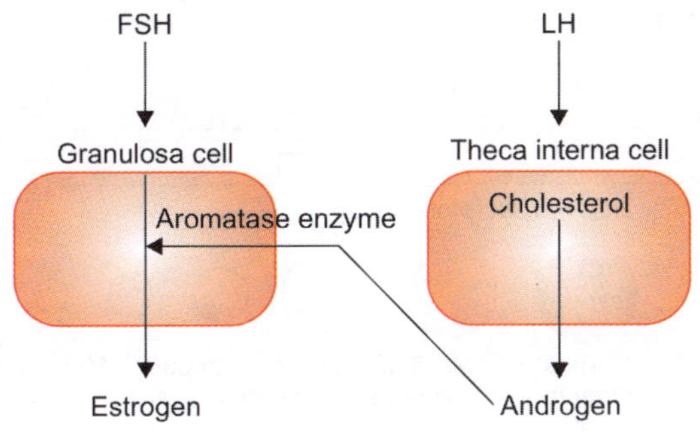

Fig. 2.2: 2-cell 2-gonadotropin theory

Ovulation

Important Points

- Peak level of estradiol is **200 pg/ml** seen on D10–D11. LH surge occurs after estradiol peak is sustained for 48 hours. Thus LH surge occurs due to estrogen surge.
- The increase in LH leads to production of small amount of progesterone from the Theca cells. This causes a positive feedback on FSH.
- Time between LH surge $\xrightarrow{\text{32–36 hrs}}$ ovulation
  LH peak $\xrightarrow{\text{10–12 hrs}}$ ovulation
  - Time between estrogen peak and LH peak = 14–24 hours
  - Time between estrogen peak and ovulation = 24–36 hrs
  - Mean duration of LH Surge = 48 hrs.
- What initiates LH surge: Estradiol-levels 200 pg/mL for 48 hours initiates LH surge.
- LH leads to luteinization of granulosa cells and progesterone is released by granulosa cells. Therefore progesterone **synthesis begins 36 hours before ovulation.**[Q]
- LH surge is initiated by estrogen but for maintenance of LH surge both estrogen and progesterone are required.
- Hormone responsible for resumption of meiosis I—LH
- When is Meiosis I resumed —36 hours before ovulation (because of LH surge)
- Just before ovulation there is both LH & FSH surge (*See* Fig. 2.4) but ovulation is due to LH surge
- Just before ovulation size of graffian follicle is 18–20 mm.
- Ovulation occurs 14 days before the first day of succeeding cycle. Therefore, in a 26-day cycle, ovulation will occur 14 days prior to 26th day, i.e. 26 - 14 = 12th day.

> Therefore, **Day of ovulation = Length of menstrual cycle - 14**

- 1st sign of ovulation on endometrial biopsy is **appearance of subnuclear vacuoles**[Q]**.**

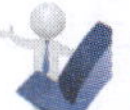

KEY CONCEPT

How ovulation occurs and oocyte is extruded:

The exact mechanism of this expulsion is not known but it is not due to increase in follicular pressure.

- **Possible mechanisms are:**
  - Follicular wall thinning due to enzymes like plasmin and collagenase
  - Increase in plasminogen activator
  - Increase in prostaglandin which in turn lead to increased smooth muscle contractions in ovary leading to ovulation.

This is the reason why women undergoing infertility treatments are advised to avoid prostaglandin synthetase inhibitors in preovulatory period, to avoid luteinized unruptured follicle syndrome.

- Minimum levels of LH & FSH are seen in Luteal phase (as high conc. of progesterone has a -ve feedback on LH & FSH) (*See* Fig. 2.4)
- After ovulation, the ruptured Graafian follicle becomes Corpus luteum.
- The yellowish color is due to lipid and pigment carotene.
- Progesterone attains its highest peak about 8 days after the LH peak, i.e. day when corpus luteum has maximum function.
- **Luteal–Placental shift** is the turnover of function from corpus luteum of pregnancy to placenta. This transition period continues from eight weeks to ten weeks.
- **Luteal–Follicular shift** is the period that extends from the demise of corpus luteum to the selection of a new dominant follicle for the next cycle. It is due to fall in the levels of estradiol, progesterone and inhibin. There is simultaneous rise in the levels of GnRH and FSH.

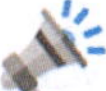

Important One Liners

Corpus luteum:

- In non-pregnant state it is maintained by **hormone LH**
- Life span: of **corpus luteum** in non pregnant females: 10–12 days
- Maximum activity occurs 8 days after ovulation, i.e. day 22 of menstrual cycle, **i.e. maximum progesterone secretion occurs on 22nd day (that is why all tests of ovulation are** done on day 22 of cycle). Maximum progesterone is 40 mg/day
- In pregnant state, corpus luteum is maintained **by hormone hCG.**
- Life span of corpus luteum pregnant state ≈ 10–12 weeks.
- Hormone which rescues corpus luteum from undergoing luteolysis = hCG

Line Diagram Showing Ovarian and Menstrual Cycle (Fig. 2.3)

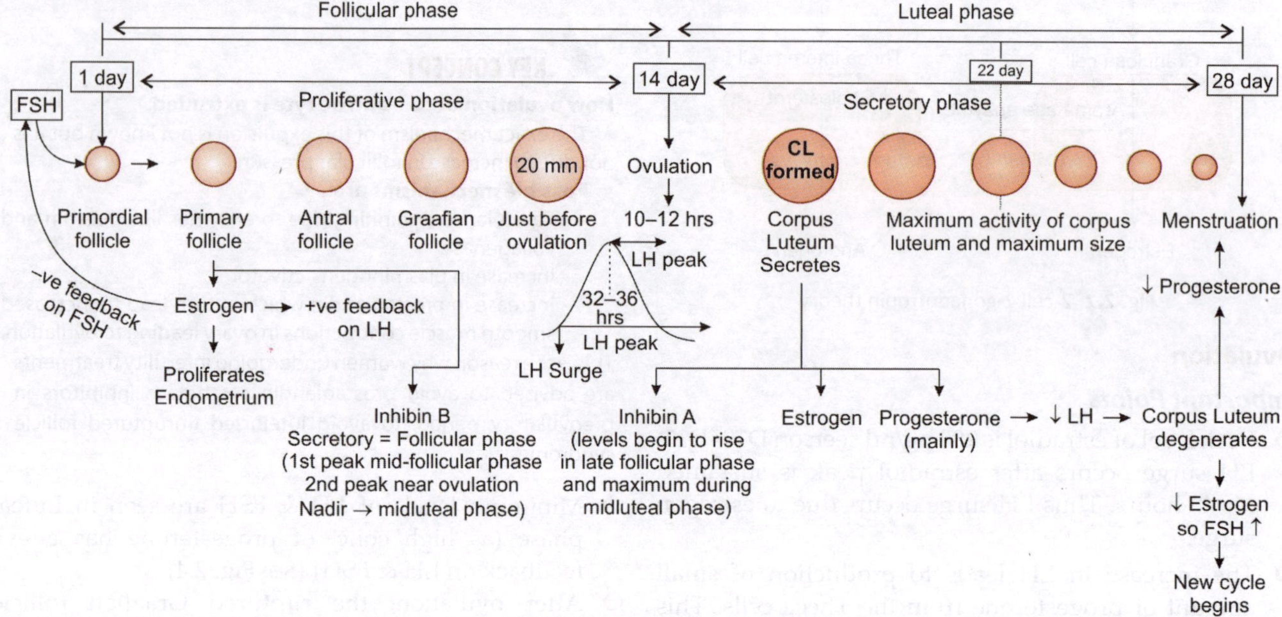

Fig. 2.3: Line diagram showing menstrual cycle

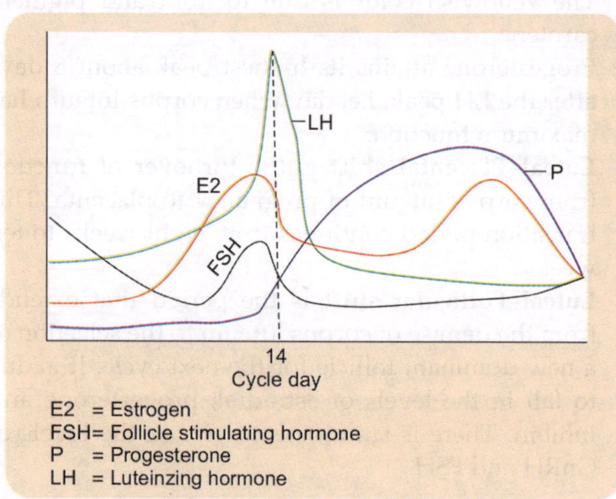

Fig. 2.4: The hormonal changes occurring during menstrual cycle

Structure of a Mature/Antral Follicle

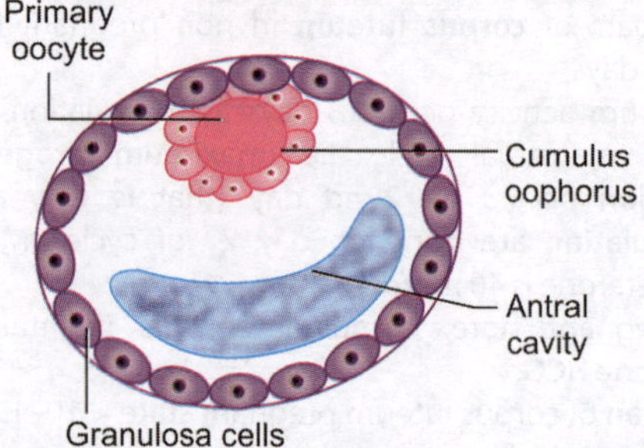

- Antral follicles form from ongoing development in selected oocytes.
- In these, follicular fluid collects between the granulosa cells, ultimately producing a fluid filled space known as Antrum
- Granulosa cells in the antral follicle are divided into 2 types:
  - The cells surrounding the oocyte are called as ***Cumulus Oophorus*** and the ones surrounding the antrum are called *mural* granulosa cells
  - The antral follicular fluid consists of plasma filtrate factors secreted by granulosa cells like estrogen and growth factors. LH is secreted in fluid in mid of cycle. If LH is present from very beginning of cycle as in patients of PCOD it leads to degeneration of granulosa cells and thus anovulation occurs.

Gonadal Peptides

The most important gonadal peptides include:

i. Inhibin
ii. Activin
iii. Follistatin

- These peptides are secreted and expressed in ovary, pituitary, test, placenta, brain, adrenal, liver, kidney and bone marrow
- Inhibin decreases FSH secretion
- Activin increases FSH secretion
- Follistatin suppresses FSH β gene expression by binding to it and preventing the interaction of activin with its receptors
- Activin and follistatin have paracrine action, i.e. they act locally but not Inhibin.

Inhibin

- Consists of 2 dissimilar peptides (called as α- and β- subunits). There are 2 forms of Inhibin viz. Inhibin A and Inhibin B.
- In both of them α- subunit is identical, whereas β- subunit is specific but inhibin structure is dissimilar to LH and FSH (Details in Table 2.1).

Table 2.1: Inhibin

Inhibin A	Inhibin B
Secreted by corpus luteum in luteal phase under the effect of LH	Secreted by granulosa cells in proliferative phase under the effect of FSH
Peak levels—Midluteal phase	1st peak at midfollicular phase and second at LH surge
During pregnancy placenta produces inhibin A	Inhibin B levels are low during pregnancy

Endometrium

Menstruation is shedding of uterine endometrium, hence it is important to know structure of endometrium Details in Table 2.2

Table 2.2: Endometrium

Superficial layer (2/3rd)	Deep layer (1/3rd)
It consists of stratum compactum and stratum spongiosum	It consists of Stratum Basalis
These layers are supplied by spiral arteries which undergo vasoconstriction during secretory phase due to release **of PFG-2α**	It is supplied by basilar arteries which donot undergo vasoconstriction
This causes necrosis or sloughing of these layers at the time of menstruation	During secretory phase these basilar arteries remain straight, so the blood supply of stratum basale remains intact. *Therefore, this layer is not shed during menstruation and during secretory phase it causes regeneration of whole endometrium*

Menstruation and Pain

- Progesterone is a smooth muscle relaxant.
- During luteal phase, when corpus luteum degenerates, levels of progesterone decrease.
  This leads to vasoconstriction, release of PGF-2α and dysmenorrhea

Flowchart 2.2: Mechanism of Dysmenorrhea

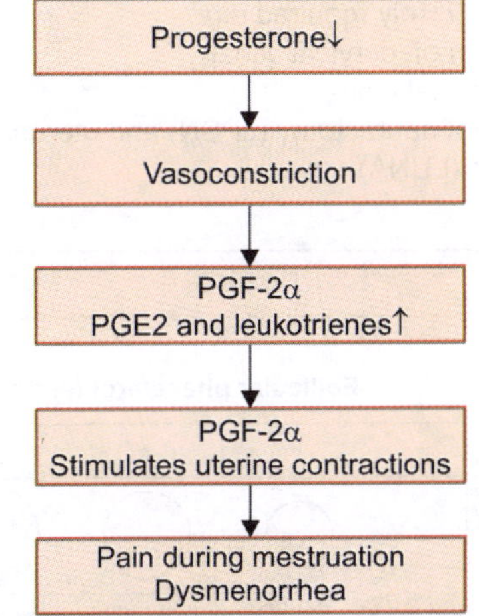

Important Concept

- Dysmenorrhea in other words signifies that levels of progesterone decrease in a female in whom earlier they were normal, i.e. dysmenorrhea occurs only in ovulatory cycles and not in anovulatory cycles.
- Endometrial concentration of PGF-2α correlate with the severity of dysmenorrhea.

Dysmenorrhea

Dysmenorrhea means painful menstruation of sufficient magnitude so as to incapacitate day to day activities.
It can be of 2 types (Table 2.3)

Table 2.3: Dysmenorrhea

Primary/Spasmodic	Secondary/Congestive
• No pelvic pathology is responsible for the pain • Mostly seen in adolescents • M/C in affluent society • Almost always confined to ovulatory cycle, hence pain appears within 6 months–1 year after onset of menarche (when cycles become ovulatory)	• Pain is due to presence of pelvic pathology. • Pain seen many years after menarche (females) • Can be seen in anovulatory cycles also • Generally seen in reproductive age females.
• Pain appears on 1st day of menstrual period and usually lasts for 12 hours. • Pain never persists beyond 48 hours	• Pain appears 3–5 days prior to the period and is not relieved completely with the start of the period.
• Pain is spasmodic and confined to lower abdomen. May radiate to back and medial aspect of thigh	• Patients mainly complain of deep seated, pelvic pain. Pain is dull, situated in back and front without any radiation

Contd...

Contd…

Primary/Spasmodic	Secondary/Congestive
• Systemic discomfort present Treatment of spasmodic dysmenorrhea- 1. Prostaglandin synthetase inhibitor- M/C used drug. 2. OCP's × 3 – 6 cycles- if pain is not relieved by analgesics and antispasmodics then OCP's are given **Principle**- OCP's make the cycles anovulatory and hence pain is relieved. 3. Surgery – rarely required e.g. – Dilatation of cervical canal – Paracervical block. – Presacral neurectomy (LPSN) and uterosacral nerve ablation (LUNA)	• No systemic discomfort seen Important causes are • PID • Endometriosis • Adenomyosis • IUCD in utero • Uterine fibroid • Polyps • Cervical stenosis • Congenital malformation of uterus like bicornuate uterus **Management:** Treatment of the underlying cause.

MENSTRUAL CYCLE

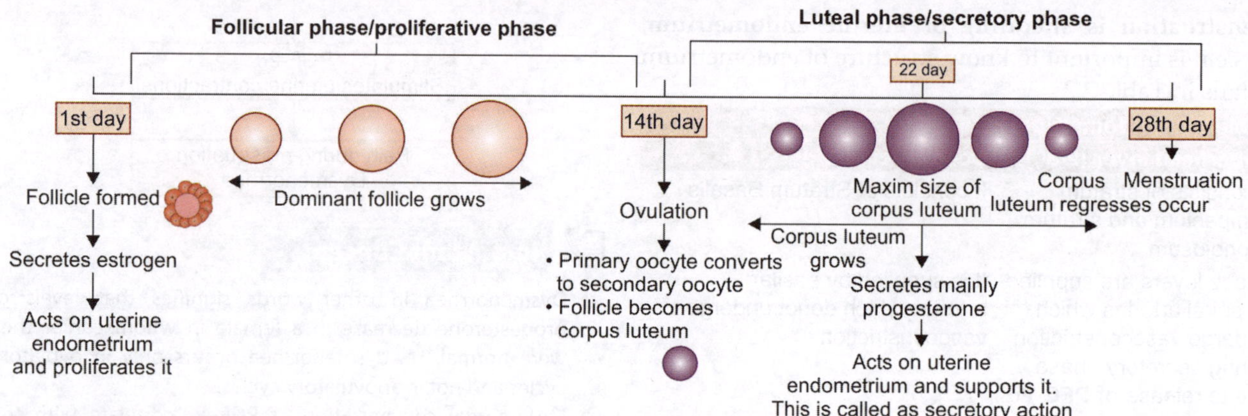

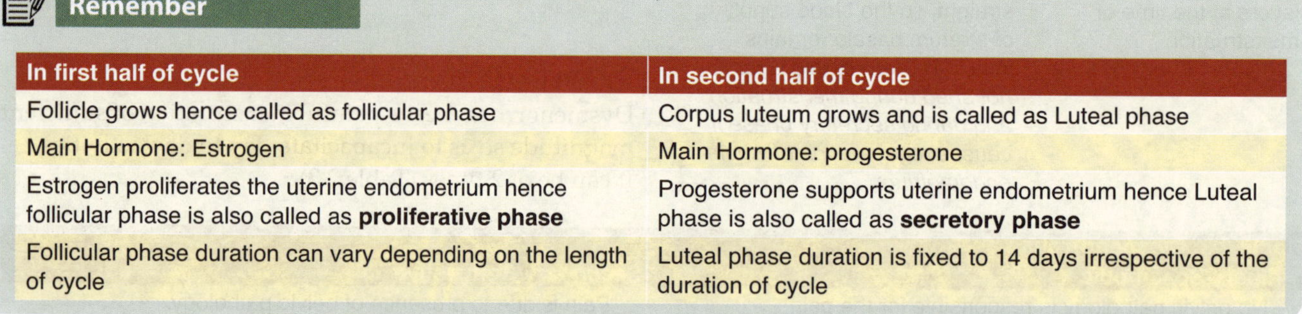

Remember

In first half of cycle	In second half of cycle
Follicle grows hence called as follicular phase	Corpus luteum grows and is called as Luteal phase
Main Hormone: Estrogen	Main Hormone: progesterone
Estrogen proliferates the uterine endometrium hence follicular phase is also called as **proliferative phase**	Progesterone supports uterine endometrium hence Luteal phase is also called as **secretory phase**
Follicular phase duration can vary depending on the length of cycle	Luteal phase duration is fixed to 14 days irrespective of the duration of cycle

- Menstruation basically is due to decrease in levels of progesterone, as the levels of progesterone decrease suddenly, the support to endometrium is lost and it is shed.

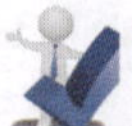

KEY CONCEPT

- If a female wants to postpone her menstruation due to some family function or pilgrimage, then her progesterone levels should not drop. Hence, we advise them to start taking tablet progesterone 3–4 days before menstruation and continue taking it till she wants to postpone.
- The day her family function/pilgrimage is over, she should stop taking the tablets. So the level of progesterone decreases and support to endometrium is lost and she menstruates.

Table 2.4: Menstrual cycle

Feature	Menstrual Phase	Proliferative Phase (Fig. 2.3)	Secretory Phase (Fig. 2.4)
Thickness of stratum functionale	Absent	Thin to thick	Thickest
Appearance of endometrial glands	Portions of glands in stratum basale	Straight	Highly coiled (cork screw appearance with secretions in glands)
Degree of coiling of coiled arteries	Absent	Less coiled	Highly coiled
Predominant gonadotropin	Falling LH, rising FSH	FSH	LH
Predominant ovarian hormone	Transition from progesterone to estrogen	Estrogen	Progesterone
Days of idealized 28-day cycle	1–5	5–14	14–28
Viscosity of cervical secretions	Difficult to determine	Thinnest at day 14	Increasing viscosity

Remember

For menstruation to occur, initially the levels of progesterone should be high and then they should drop suddenly.
If a female has low levels of progesterone from beginning, then menstruation will not occur like in anovulation/ PCOS.

KEY CONCEPT

Then what are anovulatory cycles

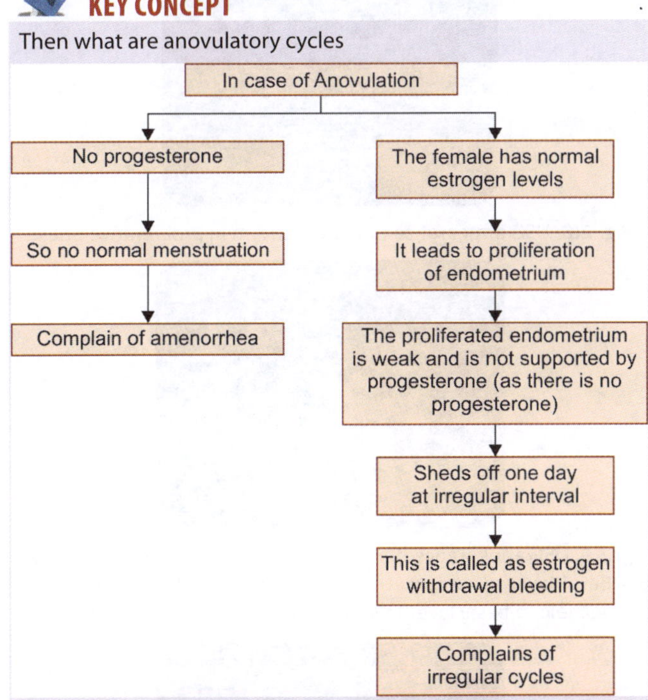

Also Know

- We did that in ovulatory cycles, pain was due to PGF-2α and PGF-2α was released due to vasoconstriction which was brought about by sudden decrease in levels of progesterone
- In anovulatory cycles, bleeding is due to increased estrogen and not decreased, progesterone, hence anovulatory cycles are painless.

Characteristics of anovulatory cycles:

1. Irregular
2. Painless

Menstrual blood is mainly arterial blood.

Appearance of Endometrium

Remember

The menstrual cycle can be divided into 2 phases:

- Follicular phase/Proliferative phase: Main hormone is Estrogen
- Luteal phase/secretory phase: Main hormones is progesterone

In both these phases, on endometrial biopsy and on doing USG – different typical appearances are seen as discussed below

Proliferative Phase

From around day 5, the menstrual cycle enters the proliferative stage. During this phase, which lasts approximately 9 days, the endometrium is thick, stoma compact and short straight glands are present (Fig. 2.5).

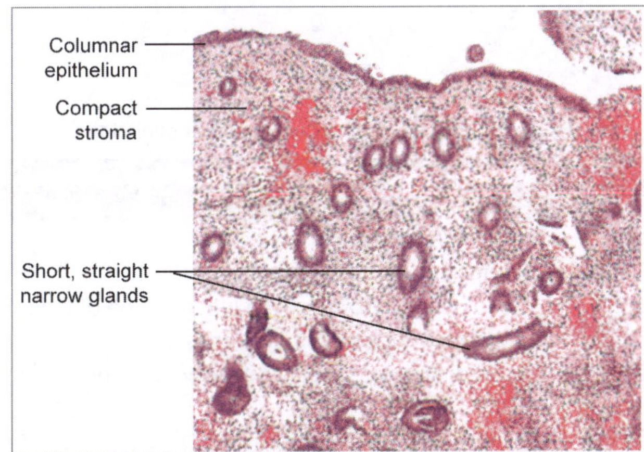

Fig. 2.5: Appearance of endometrium in proliferative phase

Secretory Phase

The secretory phase lasts approximately 13 days and, during this time, the endometrium is now preparing for the implantation of an embryo. The glands start to appear like deflated balloons or **"saw-toothed"**, the glandular **epithelium become vacuolated as they begin to accumulate glycogen, and the lumen becomes filled with glycogen/glycoprotein secretions.** The surrounding blood vessels become large, and the lamina propria becomes even more oedematous (Fig. 2.6).

Under the effect of progesterone, these glycogen near vacuoles move from base of glandular cells towards there lumen.

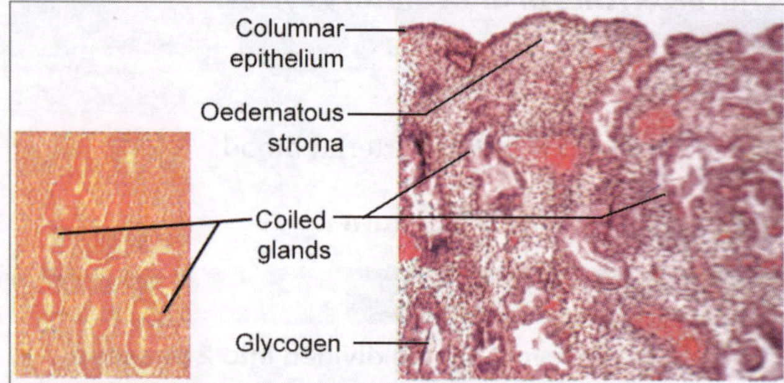

Fig. 2.6: Appearance of endometrium in secretory phase

Ovulation

Figure 2.7 shows changes at the time of ovulation, characterized by subnuclear vacuolation.

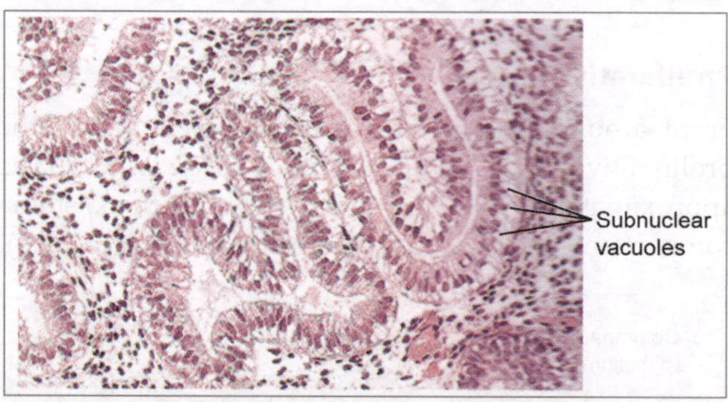

Fig. 2.7: Appearance of endometrium at ovulation

Table 2.5: Daywise changes in histopathology of endometrium

Day	Endometrial changes
D–16	Subnucleus vacuolation
D–18	Vacuoles move towards the lumen of the glands
D–20	Corkscrew appearance of Glands
D–22	Maximal stroma oedema due to VEGF and mitoses seen
D–24	Perivascular filling
D–26	Lymphocytic infiltration

USG Appearances of Endometrium in Different Phases

The endometrium is a thin echo genic strip composed of a superficial layer (zona functionalis) and deep basal layer. The thickness and sonographic appearance of the endometrium change cyclically with the menstrual cycle

- In the **menstrual phase**, endometrium is thin and brightly echogenic, as superficial layer is shed.
- During **early proliferative phase** (Day 5–9), endometrium appears as a bright echogenic line and late proliferative phase, its thickness increases (Fig. 2.8).
- During **secretory phase**, the functional layer becomes thickened, soft and endomatous under the influence of progesterone. The functional layer becomes isoechoic to basal layer (Fig. 2.9)

Note: At the time of ovulation, endometrium gives a typical **Trilaminar appearance** (Fig. 2.10).

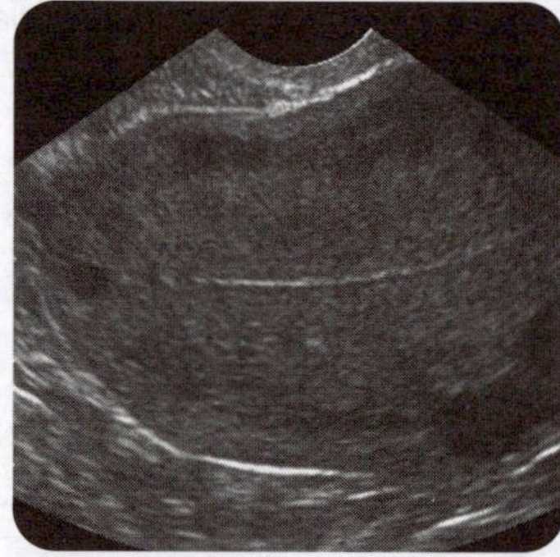

Fig. 2.8: USG appearance of endometrium in proliferative phase

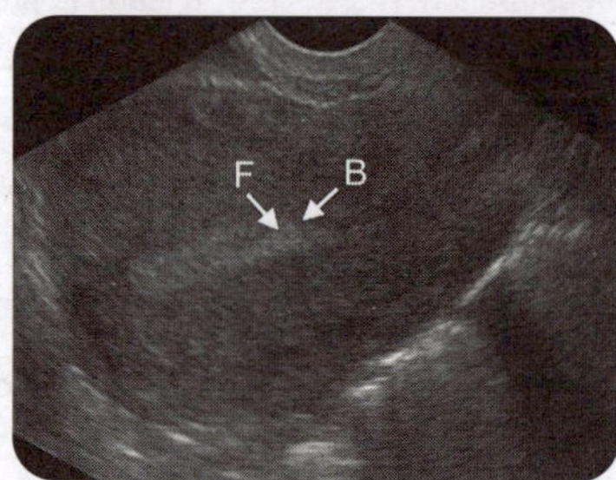

Fig. 2.9: USG appearance during secretory phase F = functional layer B = Basal layer of endometrium. The functional layer has become ischoechoic to basal layer in secretory phase

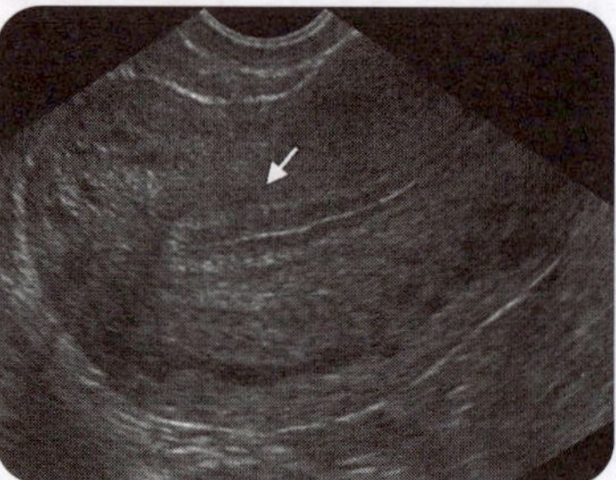

Fig. 2.10: USG appearance of ovulation showing trilaminar appearance of endometrium at the time of ovulation

Thickness of Endometrium

–Callen USG in Obs & Gynae 5/e, Page 910

- Immediately after menstruation = 0.5–2 mm
- Proliferative phase = 4–8 mm
- Periovulatory phase = 6–10 mm
- Secretory phase = 7–14 mm
- In postmenopausal females in 80% cases it is < 8 mm. (in normal asymptomatic patients)
- In patients with post menopausal bleeding– investigations should begin if it is > 4 mm

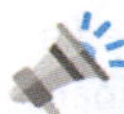

Important One Liners

- Stratum Basalis is responsible for regeneration of endometrium during next menstrual cycle.
- Menstrual blood is mainly arterial blood.
- Prostaglandin released at menstruation = PFG-2α.
- Release of PGF-2α is due to withdrawal of progesterone and causes vasoconstriction of spiral arterioles and also causes constriction of myometrium which leads to dysmenorrhea.
- Therefore, pain is always present in ovulatory cycles.

HORMONES

Hypothalamo pituitary ovarian axis in females:

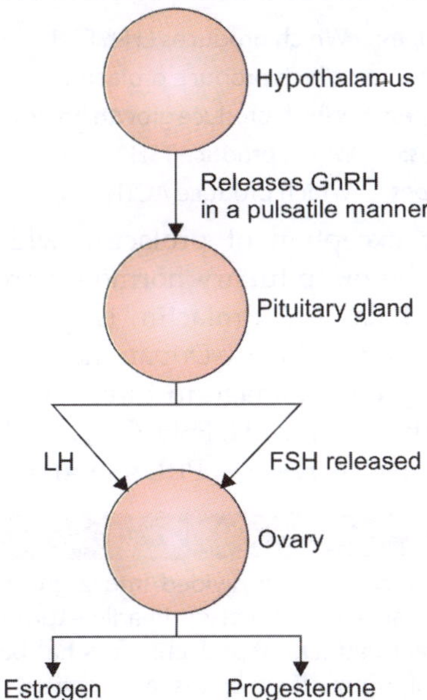

Hypothalamic-pituitary-ovarian (HPO) axis is not developed before puberty. It becomes sensitive around 8-12 years and is fully established by 13–14 years. Initially due to release of GnRH, only LH is released from pituitary. Later as the axis matures both LH and FSH are released. That is why initial few cycles are anovulatory. (So painless)

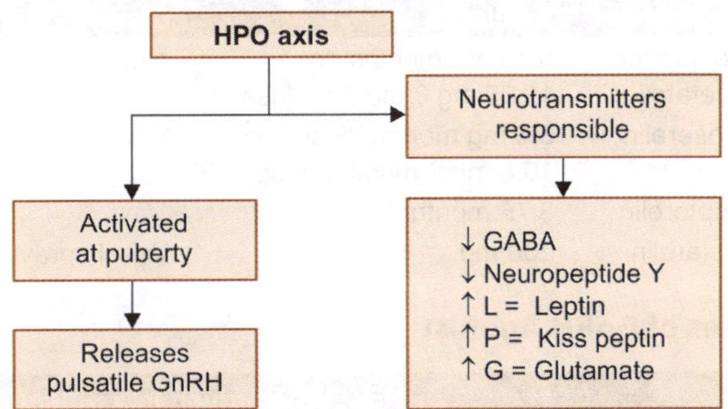

Note: In obese females, pubertal changes occur early due to increased levels of leptin.

GnRH

Natural GnRH

- Decapeptide
- Synthesised by Arcuate nucleus
- Released by hypothalamus at puberty in a pulsatile manner
- T1/2 < 10 minutes
- Secreted in a pulsatile manner at different times of menstrual cycle
- Initially secreted only at night
- 1st hormone which releases after GnRH secretion at puberty – LH
- When GnRH pulse frequency is high: LH is preferentially released and when low, FSH is released, predominantly.

Synthetic GnRH

Synthetic GnRH action depends on the manner in which it is given:

1. *If given in pulsatile manner*: It will act like natural GnRH and increase LH, FSH, estrogen and progesterone, that in turn leads to ovulation.
2. *When synthetic GnRH is given continuously*: Initially, there is release of LH, FSH, i.e. flare reaction occurs which typically lasts for 1 week but later continuous, non-pulsatile GnRH administration results in pituitary desensitization and subsequent loss of ovarian steroidogenesis. In other words, there is decreased estrogen. Hence, continuous GnRH can be used in treatment of all hyperestrogen conditions

Also Know

- GnRH antagonist are inactive if taken orally but intramuscular, subcutaneous and intranasal preparations are available.

Examples	Available as	Given
Leuprolide acetate	3.75 mg months dose 11.25 mg 3 months dose	1/m
Goserelin	3.6 mg months dose 10.8 mg 3 months dose	S/C
Triptorelin	3.75 months	1/m
Nafarelin	200 mg	Nasal spray

Uses of GnRH Agonist

When given continuously	When given in a pulsatile manner
Used in all hyperestrogenic conditions like: • Precocious puberty • Endometeriosis • Fibroid • ER positive breast cancer	• Delayed, puberty • To bring about ovulation • Sexual infertilism
In males it used in Prostate Cancer	
Adverse effect	**Adverse effect**
Leads to menopause like symptoms: • Osteoporosis • Hot flushes • Vaginal dryness • Depression	• Leads to multiple ovulation/Twin pregnancy
In males it can lead to impotence, Gynaecomastia and osteoporosis	• Can lead its scarring of ovary due to excessive ovulation leading to ovarian cancer

Note: Leuprolide is FDA approved for leiomyoma treatment whereas all except Triptorelin are FDA approved for treating endometriosis.

Important Concept

Osteoporosis due to GnRH

- The decrease in Bone mineral density associated with treatment with GnRH for 6 months is significant.
- Bone loss occurs both in lumbar spine (trabecular bone) and femoral neck (cortical bone) and approaches 1% per month
- After discontinuation of treatment, bone loss is slowly recovered but not completely.
- To prevent osteoporosis whenever GnRH is used for ≥ 6 months **'add back'** therapy is given in the form of conjugated estrogen 0.625 mg and MPA 2.5 mg daily (or norethindrone 5 mg daily). Add back therapy has added advantage of preventing hot flushes and genitourinary atrophy.

GnRH Antagonist

- In contrast to agonists, GnRH antagonists are also available.
- Two agents in this class are cetrorelix and ganirelix are currently FDA approved for infertility use in women undergoing controlled ovarian hyperstimulation.
- However, a limitation of these drugs is that they are daily injectables.
- A new agent *elagolix*, is a nonpeptide oral GnRH antagonist that is currently being evaluated for both endometriosis and leiomyoma treatment.

Also Know

- The neurons which release GnRH are derived from medial olfactory placode and migrate upwards via nervus terminalis to the hypothalamus. If this transport is defective, it leads to **KALLMANN syndrome.**
- Gene responsible for this migration is **Anosmin 1.** It is defective in Kallmann syndrome.
- **Kallman syndrome:** Triad of **anosmia, hypogonadism** and **color blindness** in men. Women may be affected and other associated defects may include cleft lip, cleft palate, cerebellar ataxia, nerve deafness and abnormalities of thirst.
- **Height of individual is normal.**
- Primary amenorrhea is a rule.

Anterior Pituitary Hormones

The anterior pituitary gland contains 5 hormones producing cell types and their products. These include:

- *Gonadotropes*: Which produces LH & FSH
- *Lactotropes*: Which produce prolactin
- *Somatotropes*: Which produce growth hormone
- *Thyrotropes*: Which produce TSH
- *Adrenotropes*: Which produce ACTH

- With the exception of prolactin, which is under tonic inhibition, pituitary hormones are stimulated by hypothalamus. Prolactin is primarily under inhibitory regulation by Dopamine.
- Thus in case of damage to pituitary stalk, their is hypopituitarism for LH, FSH, GH, ACTH & TSH but an associated increase in PRL secretion.

Also Know

Dopamine receptors are divided into 2 groups D_1 and D_2. Cells in the anterior pituitary primarily express D_2 subtype. The medical treatment of prolactinomas has been improved in terms of both effectiveness and patient tolerance by development of D_2 specific ligands. For e.g., Dopamine agonist cabergoline is a D_2 specific ligand whereas Bromocriptine is non-specific.

Natural FSH and LH/Gonadotropins

- Released from anterior pituitary in a pulsatile manner.

- Produced by basophils
- FSH T½ = 3-4 hours
- LH T½ = 20 minutes
- It has membrane bound cytoplasmic receptors
- FSH receptors are present on Granulosa cells in females and Sertoli cells in males.
- LH receptors are present on Theca cells and granulosa cells in females and Leydig cells in males.

Functions of FSH – Females

- Promotes gametogenesis in females and spermatogenesis in males
- Production of estrogen in females

Functions of LH

- Ovulation induction
- Formation and maintenance of corpus luteum in non-pregnant states
- Progesterone production
- Regulation of menstrual cycle

Synthetic FSH and LH

- The most commonly used commercial preparation of FSH is **Human Menopausal Gonadotropin** (HMG ampule contains 75 IU FSH and 75 IU LH).

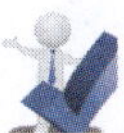

KEY POINTS

Human menopausal gonadotropin (HMG) is obtained from urine of postmenopausal females.

- Recently highly purified FSH (Metrodin–75 IU/amp) has been made available.
- It is administered subcutaneously.
- Human chorionic gonadotropin (hCG) has biological action like LH and is available in 1000–5000 ampoules obtained from urine of pregnant woman. Recombinant hCG is now available.

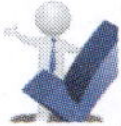

KEY POINTS

Chances with gonadotropins:
- Multiple pregnancy = 30%
- Ovarian Hyperstimulation Syndrome (OHSS) = 5%

Prolactin

- Polypeptide hormone secreted by anterior pituitary gland
- Acts on breast and is responsible for milk secretion[Q]
- Acts on pituitary to reduce secretion of GnRH and brings about anovulation[Q] and lactation amenorrhea.

KEY POINTS

In Prolactinomas levels of prolactin increases and females complain of:
- Galactorrhea
- Amenorrhea (due to ↓ GnRH)

In Sheehan's syndrome – There is post partum necrosis of anterior pituitary gland

∴ ↓ FSH, ↓ LH } → Amenorrhea

↓ Prolactin which leads to failure to lactate baby.

Important Concept

- Prolactin in inhibited by: Dopamine
- Prolactin is increased by: Serotonin, norepinephrine opioid, estrogen and TRH.

Hyperprolactinemia

Etiology

- **Physiological causes**:
  - Pregnancy
  - Sleep
  - Eating
  - Coitus
  - Chest wall simulation like breast examination
- **Conditions which damage pituitary stalk and prevent dopamine mediated inhibition of PRL** secretion, e.g.:
  - **Tumor**: Prolactinoma
  - Radiation
  - Infiltrative disease like TB, sarcoidosis
- **Low thyroid**, i.e. primary hypothyroidism (as it reflexely increases TRH & TRH stimulates prolactin). So, in all patients of hyperprolactinemia always do thyroid testing.
- **Drugs which block dopamine e.g.**, phenothiazines
- **Drugs which deplete catecholamines** (monoamine oxidase inhibitor).

Prolactinoma

Important Points

- Pituitary adenomas are the most common cause of acquired, pituitary dysfunction and comprise approximately 15% of all intracranial tumors.
- Adenomas may be microadenoma (<10 mm in diameter) or microadenoma (>10 mm in diameter).

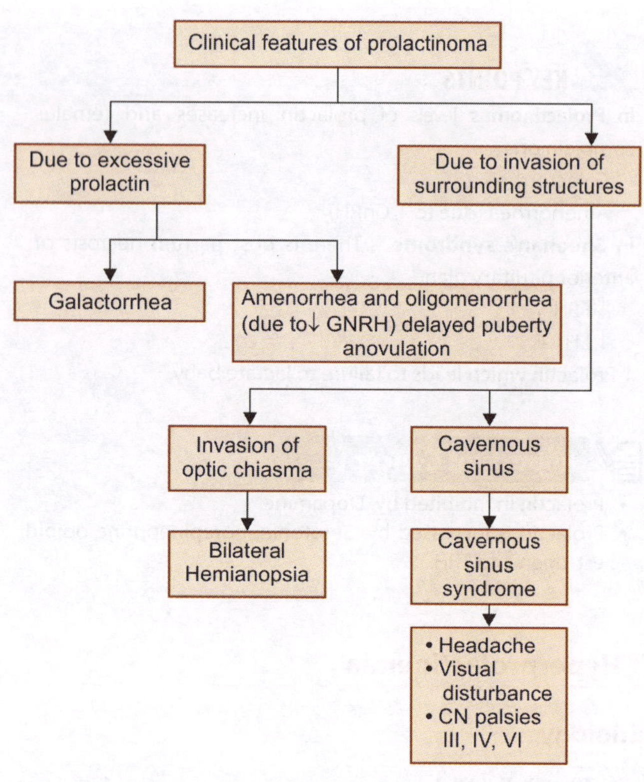

Algorithm Describing Evaluation & Treatment of Pituitary Adenoma

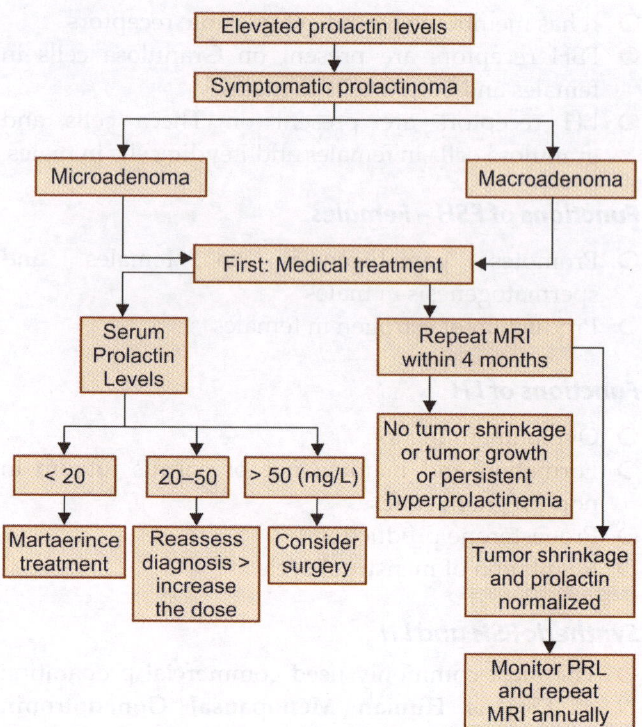

Treatment

- Most pituitary tumors grow slowly and many cease to grow after attaining a certain size. Thus, asymptomatic patients with microadenoma may be managed conservatively with serial MRI & serum PRL levels every 1 to 2 years as the risk of progression to a macroadenoma is <10%.
- Therapy should be considered if it is associated with amenorrhea or galactorrhea.
- Neurosurgical evaluation is mandatory when visual field defects or severe headache are present.
- In general, **first line treatment is medication for both** micro- and macroadenoma.
- **Drug of choice** = Cabergoline (less side effects, longer half life allowing once-twice weekly dosing) and is more effective.
- **Dose** = 0.25 mg orally twice weekly
- **Drawback**: It is expensive
- **Alternative** *drug*: Bromocriptine
- **Drawback**: Headache, postural hypotension, blurred vision, drowsiness & leg cramps.
- Neurosurgery is required for refractory tumors or those causing acute worsening of symptoms.
- Approach for pituitary – Transsphenoidal Route.

Oxytocin

- Naturally occurring oxytocin is nonapeptide
- Synthetic oxytocin is octapeptide
- It is synthesised in periventricular nucleus of hypothalamus.

Route	Time of onset	Duration of action
I/m bolus	3 mins	3 hours
I/v infusion	Immediate	1 hour

Management: If female wants pregnancy→ pulsatile GnRH and if not then estrogen and progesterone.

- **It should never be given I/V bolus as it can lead to hypotension and cardiac arrest.**
- T1/2 = 3 mins
- Storage = Ideal temperature – 2 to 8°C
  Room temperature – shelf life = 3 months
- Responsible for **milk ejection**
- **Note: Hormone responsible for milk ejection:** Oxytocin
- **Hormone responsible for milk secretion: Prolactin.**

Steroid Hormones

Table 2.6: Steroid Hormones

	Estrogen	Progesterone
Composition	C_{18} compounds with phenolicring E_1 = Estrone E_2 = Estradiol (17β-estradiol) E_3 = Estriol E_4 = Estrone (See Flowchart 2.3 for details)	Natural progesterone: C_{21} compound Synthetic Progesterone is 19-nortestosterone derivative and is similar to androgens. Hence they have androgenic side effects. **Remember**: As generation increases ⇒ androgenic side effects decrease and adverse effects like alteration in lipid profile decreases (See Flowchart 2.4 for details)
Receptor	• Nuclear receptors • Estrogen receptor upregulate progesterone receptor	Nuclear receptors Progesterone receptor down regulate estrogen receptor
Source	1. Granulosa cells (E_2) with the help of aromatase enzyme 2. Theca cells (produce androgens which are converted to estrogen by enzyme aromatase in granulosa cells) E_1 3. Placenta-(with the help of precursors obtained from fetus) (E_3 and E_4) 4. Corpus luteum (E_2)	1. Corpus luteum 2. Placenta (with the help of maternal LDL)
State	• Mostly present in bound form • Only 1% free • Mostly bound to sex hormone binding globulin (69%) and albumin (30%) • **Estrogen increases sex hormone binding globulin synthesis**	• Mostly present in bound form • Only 2% free • Mostly bound to albumin and cortisol binding globulin
End product	Glucuronides (sulfonamides)	Pregnanediol
Effect on uterus	• Proliferation of endometrium • Growth of uterus in nonpregnant state **Note:** This is the reason why in Turner's syndrome (where estrogen is deficient) uterus and vagina are underdeveloped.	• Secretory effect on endometrium • Growth of uterus in pregnancy • Smooth muscle relaxation during pregnancy
Effect on cervix	Cervical mucus is • Copious • Clear and watery • Elastic (can be stretched between fingers-called as **spinbarkeitt**) • Has increased water and electrolyte content, decreased, protein content • When dried and seen under microscop, shows a characteristic **fern like** pattern	Cervical mucus is • Scanty • Thick, tenacious • Loses its stretchability (fractures on stretching, called as **'tack'**) • Has increased, protein content and decreased water and electrolyte • On drying and seeing under microscope it loses its fern like pattern
Effect on vagina	• Superficial cells predominate • High karyopyknotic index	• Intermediate cells predominate • Low karyopyknotic index
Effect on fallopian tube	Increases motility Decreases secretion	Decreases motility Increases secretion
Effect on salt & water	Retention	Excretion
Lipid profile	↑ HDL ↑ TG ↓ LDL (This estrogen is cardioprotective)	↓ HDL ↓ TG ↑ LDL
Breast development	• Promotes ductular development	Promotes Glandular development

Contd…

Contd…

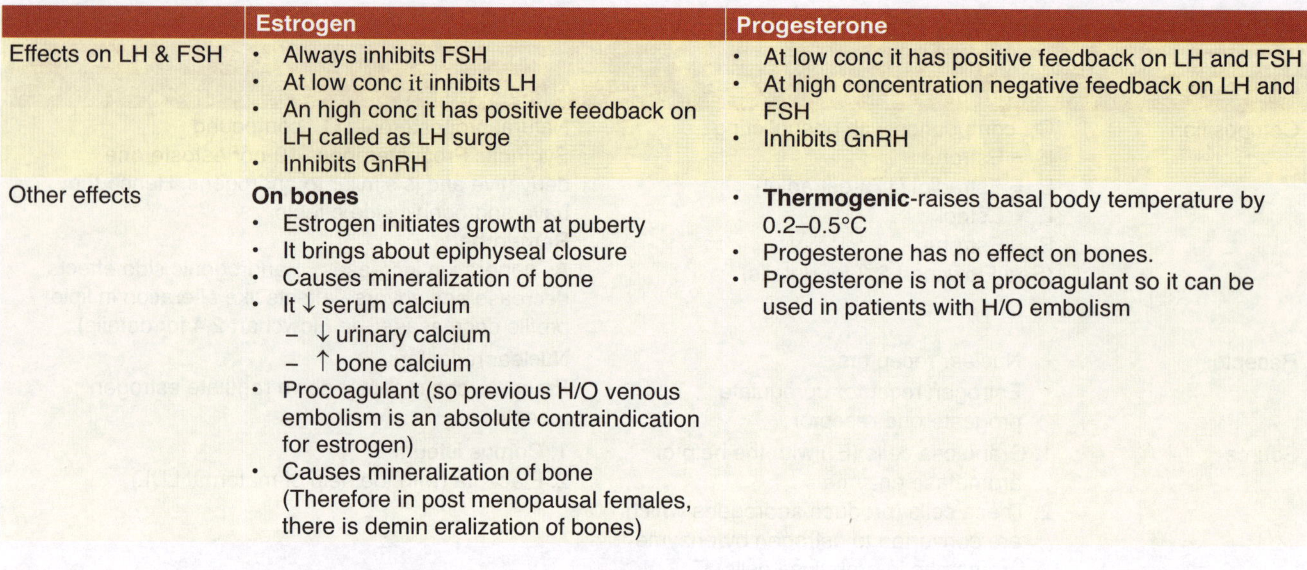

	Estrogen	Progesterone
Effects on LH & FSH	• Always inhibits FSH • At low conc it inhibits LH • An high conc it has positive feedback on LH called as LH surge • Inhibits GnRH	• At low conc it has positive feedback on LH and FSH • At high concentration negative feedback on LH and FSH • Inhibits GnRH
Other effects	**On bones** • Estrogen initiates growth at puberty • It brings about epiphyseal closure • Causes mineralization of bone • It ↓ serum calcium – ↓ urinary calcium – ↑ bone calcium • Procoagulant (so previous H/O venous embolism is an absolute contraindication for estrogen) • Causes mineralization of bone (Therefore in post menopausal females, there is demin eralization of bones)	• **Thermogenic**-raises basal body temperature by 0.2–0.5°C • Progesterone has no effect on bones. • Progesterone is not a procoagulant so it can be used in patients with H/O embolism

Estrogen

Flowchart 2.3: Estrogen

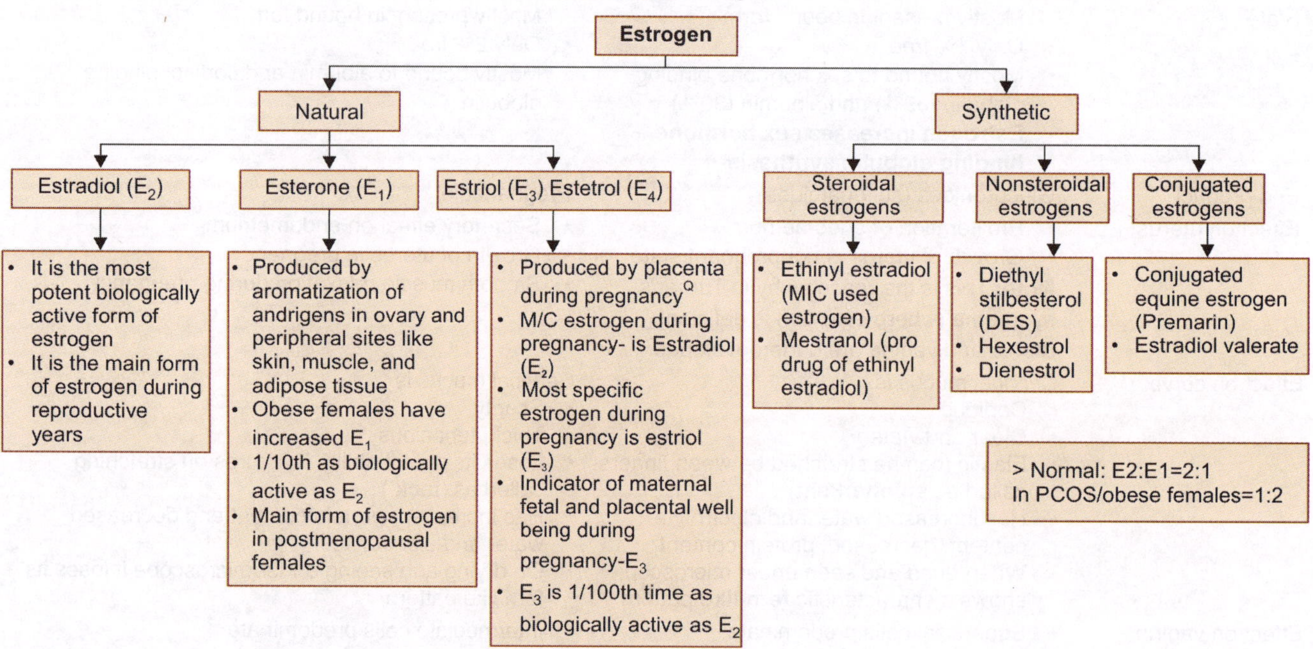

Note: One of the markers of estrogen potency is levels of sex hormone binding globulin.

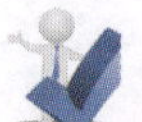

KEY POINTS

- **Natural estrogens** are ineffective orally due to extensive first pass metabolism. Estrogens undergo enterohepatic circulation that is also responsible for hepatic adverse effects (hepatic adenoma and thromboembolism).
- As the generation increases in progesterone, androgenic side effects decrease and effect on lipid profile decreases.

Indications of Estrogen Therapy

- **Delayed, puberty:** If breast development does not start even at 14 years of age then, 10 µg estrogen may be of help.
- **Lactation suppression:** Estrogen suppress lactation effectively (mixogen) but there is a risk of thromboembolism

- **Hostile cervical mucus:** In infertility to improve the quality of cervical mucus and with clomiphene citrate therapy, low dose estrogens are added.
- **DUB and polymenorrhea:**
  - Given for acute bleeding episodes
  - Conjugated equine estrogen in a dose of 10 mg/day. Bleeding stops in 24 hours
  - Combined OCPS can also be given for maintenance therapy
- **Menopausal symptoms:**
  - Short term for hot flushes (This is the most important aim of estrogen when given in HRT)
  - Give topical estrogen cream for senile vaginitis
  - Give long-term for prevention and treatment of osteoporosis
  - In Turner's syndrome.
- **OCP's:** Contain estrogen and progesterone (as estrogen alone can lead to endometrial cancer).
  - Estrogen alone can be used as a post coital pill.
- For treating vulvovaginitis in children
- **Intersex:** In Turner's syndrome or gonadal dysgenesis (46, XY) estrogens are given for the growth of secondary sex characters. In androgen insensitivity syndrome (TFS), estrogen replacement therapy is indicated to prevent regression of breast development after gonadectomy.

Side Effects

- Nausea vomiting.
- Retention of water results in painful breast and weight gain.
- It can also in over migraine and hypertension.
- Endometrial carcinoma with unopposed estrogen given for a long time.
- Probably an increased risk of breast carcinoma.
- Thromboembolism and cerebral thrombosis.
- Gall bladder and liver disease (cholestatic jaundice and gallstones).

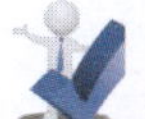

KEY POINTS

- When estrogen is administered alone, it can lead to endometrial hyperplasia and endometrial cancer. Therefore in reproductive age females, if prolonged use is desired – progesterone (Medroxy progesterone) is added.
- **Contraindications to use of estrogen**
  - History of thromboembolism
  - Liver disease
  - Severe hypertension
  - Heart disease
  - Estrogen dependent tumor, e.g. breast adenoma

Progesterone

Flowchart 2.4: Progesterone

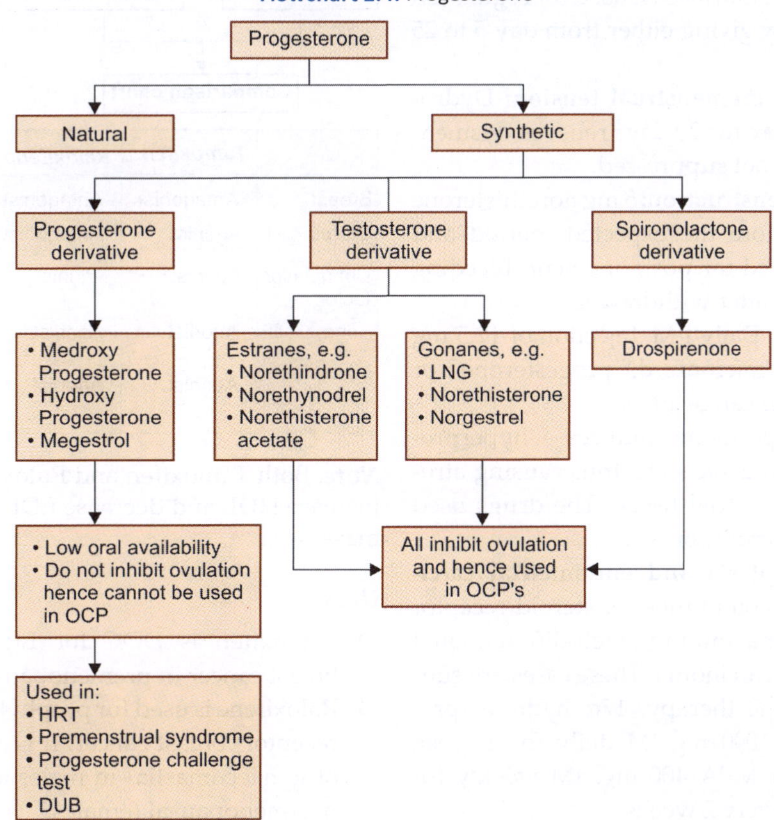

The progesterones used in OCP's can be categorized into 4 generations (1st, 2nd, 3rd & 4th generation). As the generation increases, androgenic side effects decreases.

- *1st generation*: Estranes (have androgenic side effects like acne, increased HDL)
- *2nd generation*: Gonanes (have androgenic side effects like acne, increased HDL)
- *3rd generation*: Least androgenic activity, e.g., Desogestrel, gestodene, norgestimate
- *4th generation*: Antiandrogenic e.g. drospirenone dienogest

Side Effects of Progesterone

A = Acne
B = Break through bleeding
C = Irregular cycle
D = Decreased libido, depression
E = Edema

Uses of Progesterone

- **Progesterone challenge test:** Details in chapter on amenorrhea.
- **Contraception:** Progesterone alone is used as mini pill. DMPA, NET EN, implants, vaginal ring, LNG IUCD are also available.
- **DUB:** To stop acute bleeding episode Norethisterone 5 mg TDS is effective. Can also be used for regulation of menstrual cycle by giving either from day 5 to 25 or day 15 to 25.
- **Dysmenorrhea and Premenstrual tension:** Dydrogesterone from 5th day for 20 days relieves dysmenorrhea. Ovulation is not suppressed.
- **Postponement of menstruation:** 5 mg norethisterone TDS for 3 days before the expected, period and continued till the need for postponement. Bleeding occurs 48 – 72 hours after withdrawal.
- **Luteal phase defect:** Daily I M. Injection of 12.5 mg progesterone, oral micronized, progesterone, or vaginal suppositories can be given.
- **Endometriosis:** Progesterone induces a hyperprogestogenic, hypoestrogenic state, thus causing atrophy of ectopic endometrial tissue. The drugs used are MPA, dydrogesterone, or NE.
- **Endometrial hyperplasia and endometrial carcinoma:** Role depends on number of steroid receptor on tumor which is maximum in well-differentiated grade I endometrial carcinoma. These cases are suitable for progesterone therapy. 17α hydroxy progesterone caproate 1000 mg IM daily for 1 week and then weekly or MPA 400 mg, IM weekly for 3 months and then every 2 weeks.
- **Hormone replacement therapy (HRT):** Progestins are combined with estrogen as an HRT for post menopausal woman where uterus is present. Can be used cyclically or continuously.

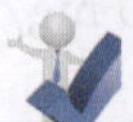

KEY POINTS

Progesterone, unless specially formulated in micronised, progesterone, is inactive orally because of high first pass metabolism in liver.

Selective Estrogen-Receptor Modulators (SERMs) (Flowchart 2.5)

These are the agents that act as estrogen agonists in some tissues and antagonists in other tissues. *Agonistic action is beneficial in tissues like bone (decreased resorption) and blood (better lipid profile) whereas it is deleterious in endometrium, breast (increased risk of carcinoma) and liver (predisposition to thromboembolism).*

Flowchart 2.5: SERMs

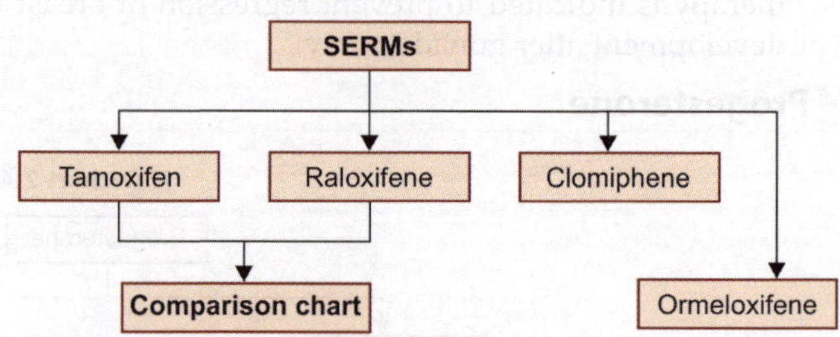

	Tamoxifen	*Raloxifene*
Breast	Antagonist	Antagonist
Uterus	Agonist	Antagonist
Coagulation factor	Agonist	Agonist
Bone	Agonist	Agonist
Lipid profile	Agonist	Agonist

Note: Both Tamoxifen and Raloxifene like estrogen will increase HDL and decrease LDL and will increase bone mass.

Uses:

- Tamoxifen is DOC for ER^{+ve} (Estrogen receptor) breast cancer in premenopausal females
- Raloxifene is used for prophylaxis for ER^{+ve} (Estrogen receptor) breast cancer, It is also used for treatment of gynaecomastia in males and for osteoporosis in postmenopausal females.

Side Effects

Both these cause:

- Hot flushes
- Thrombosis
- Tamoxifen can lead to endometrial cancer as it is agonist on Endometrium (not raloxifene)

Note: Some other SERMs

- *Toremifene*: Can be used for treating Tamoxifene resistant ER+ breast cancer
- *Clomiphene*: Used for ovulation induction
- *Ormeloxifene*: Used as a non steroidal hormonal OCP—Saheli (centchroman).

Also Know

- **Fulvestrant** is the first FDA approved agent in the new class of drugs that are called **selective estrogen-receptor downregulators (SERDs)**. These have an improved safety profile, faster onset, and longer duration of action than the SERMs due to their pure ER antagonist activity. It was approved for postmenopausal women with **hormone receptor-positive metastatic breast cancer that has progressed despite tamoxifen therapy. It is 100 times more potent than Tamoxifen but still it is less toxic than Tamoxifen Route = S/C (250 mg once a month).**

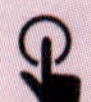

Recently approved (in 2013)

- SERM by FDA is: **Bazedoxifene**
  - Combination of **Bazedoxifene and estrogen** is approved by FDA. (BZA: 20 mg + estrogen = 0.45 mg)
  - The combination has estrogenic effects on bone (hence is used to prevent & treat osteopososis) and is anti estrogenic on uterus and breast
  - The drug combination is to be given in females with intact uterus

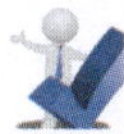

KEY POINTS

All SERM's have hot flushes as their side effect, hence cannot be used in the management of hot flushes but bazedoxifene + estrogen combination can be used for treating hot flushes

Clomiphene Citrate

- Was first used in gynecology in 1956
- It is non steroidal triphenylethylene compound related to diethylstilbestrol (DES).
- It is an isomer of cis and trans form. Enclomiphene is more potent isomer and anti estrogenic whereas zuclomiphene is weak antiestrogenic.

Mechanism of Action (Flowchart 2.6)

Flowchart 2.6: Mechanism of action of clomiphene

Clomiphene binds to estrogen receptors
⇓
Decrease levels of estrogen
⇓
Hence negative feedback on FSH is lost
⇓
Therefore FSH increases
⇓
It stimulates a number of follicles to grow
(So side effect of clomiphene is Multiple pregnancy)

- So for the action of clomiphene, **Hypothalamic Pituitary Ovarian Axis should be intact.**

Indications

- Anovulation, as in PCOS (DOC is letrozole followed by clomiphene).
- Anovulatory DUB with infertility.
- Amenorrhea and anovulation following the use of OCP's (Post pill amenorrhea).
- In vitro fertilisation, GIFT technique and assisted reproduction technique.
- Male infertility (Role doubtful).

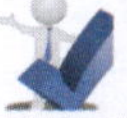

KEY POINTS

- Clomiphene can be given from D_2–D_6 or Day $_5$–Day $_9$
- Initial dose = 50 mg/day
- Maximum dose = 100 mg/day
- Follicular monitoring is done from Day 10 onwards. When follicle reaches a size of 16 mm to 20 mm, Inj hCG (**which acts as ovulation trigger**) is given.
- Dose: 5000 to 10,000 IU I/m or subcutaneous 250 mcg.
- Inj hCG acts like LH surge as hCG and LH are functionally the same
- Ovulation occurs after 32–36 hrs of Inj hCG.

Result

80% ovulate but only 30–40% conceive because of anti-estrogenic effect of clomiphene in cervical mucus leading to thick cervical mucus.

Note: Clomiphene

Side Effects

- Multiple pregnancy (mostly twin pregnancy)—5 to 8% (chances are always < 10%)
- Most dreaded side effect = Ovarian Hyper Stimulation Syndrome (< 1%)
- Due to decreased estrogen, Menopausal symptoms like Hot flushes (vasomotor symptoms are seen). This is M/C side effect of clomiphene.

- Side effects because of which its use should be stopped immediately are **visual symptoms.**
- **Ovarian cancer incidence is increased.**

Aromatase Inhibitors

- Androgen (androstenedione) are converted to estrogen E1 in the peripheral tissue in females with the help of an enzyme, aromatase. The drugs inhibiting this enzyme will decrease the formation of estrogen.
- Aromatase inhibitors are divided into first and second generation compounds. **First generation drugs include aminoglutethimide and second generation agents are letrozole, anastrozole, both these are nonsteroidal competitive inhibitor and exemestane (steroidal noncompetitive inhibitor)**
- Aromatase inhibitors are useful in all those conditions where there is hyperestrogenemia like fibroids, endometriosis and breast cancer.
- Letrozole is now the DOC for ovulation induction, in obese PCOD females. Principle is same like clomiphene.
- They are DOC for ER + breast cancer in post menopausal female
- Common side effects of these drugs include bone pain, hot flushes and vaginal dryness.

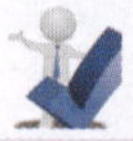

KEY POINTS

Letrozole: for ovulation induction

- Pregnancy rates similar to clomiphene
- Multiple pregnancy rates: less
- NO congenital malformation seen in fetus.
- Also used in precocious puberty.

Antiprogesterone

Mifepristone RU 486

- Derivative of 19 nortestosterone.
- Competitive antagonist of progesterone and glucocorticoid receptors.
- Binds to progesterone receptors and nullifies the effects of endogenous progesterone.
- There is release of prostaglandins from the endometrium and early termination of pregnancy.
- It leads to softening of cervix
- 85% drug is absorbed after oral therapy, peak is reached in 1–2 hours. Half life is 24 hours and excreted in bile and feces.
- In the absence of progesterone, it acts as weakly progesteronic.

Uses of Mifepristone

- As postcoital pill (600 mg given within 72 hours of unprotected sex).
- To induce abortion upto 7 weeks of amenorrhea along with misoprostol (medical abortion).
- Ripening of cervix prior to prostaglandin induction of mid-trimester abortion.
- Management of ectopic pregnancy.
- Cushing's syndrome: because of its antiglucocorticoid action.
- Medical management of uterine fibroid.
- As an emergency contraceptive (Once in a month: Single dose of 10 mg is taken on 27th day of cycle irrespective of day and number of times intercourse).

Side Effects

- Headache
- GI upset
- Abdominal cramps with diarrhea
- Adrenal failure
- Teratogenecity (If medical methods of abortion fails with RU – 486, pregnancy should be terminated any how).

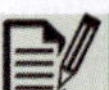

Remember

Moebius syndrome occurs due to the use of misoprostol and not mifepristone during pregnancy.

Selective Progesterone Receptor Modulator

Ulipristal

- It is a selective progesterone receptor modulator
- Its main use is in emergency contraception

Mechanism of action: It blocks or delays ovulation and delays maturation of endometrium

Brand name: Ella (not available in India)

Uses

- Emergency contraception (30 mg tablet to be used within 5 days of unprotected intercourse). More effective than levonorgestrel.
- Used for decreasing size and bleeding in fibroid

Side effects: Nause. vomiting, dysmenorrhea, abdominal pain

C/I: Severe liver disease pregnancy.

Androgens in the Female

Circulating androgens found in the blood of premenopausal women include dehydroepiandrosterone

(DHEA), DHEA sulfate (DHEA-S), androstenedione, and testosterone. Androgens are produced by the adrenal glands, the ovary, and from peripheral conversion of estrogen (with the help of enzyme aromatase) (Fig. 2.12).

Androstenedione

- Produced in equal amounts by the adrenal glands (50%) and the ovaries (50%)
- Majority of androstenedione is converted to testosterone
- Normal serum concentration ranges from 60 to 300 ng/dL

Testosterone

- Second most potent androgenic hormone.[Q] *(first being DHT)*
- In women, nearly 25% of testosterone is secreted from the ovaries and 25% is from the adrenal glands. The remaining one-half is produced from peripheral conversion of androstenedione to testosterone in the skin, muscle kidneys, liver, and adipose tissue.
- Normal circulating concentrations range from 20 to 80 ng/dL.
- Mostly bound to Albumen and sex hormone binding globulin.
- 1% free in females (2% in males)
- Receptors–Intra cytoplasmic
- Endproduct–Oxosteroid (ketosteroid)
- Testosterone has good oral absorption but has high first pass metabolism.

DHEA and DHEA-S

- Androgen precursors, much less potent than testosterone and produced, predominantly by the adrenal glands (DHEA-S is produced only by adrenal).

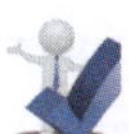

KEY POINTS

Measurement of DHEA-S is used to assess adrenal function as it is produced exclusively by adrenals

- DHEA is metabolized quickly, thus measurement of its serum concentration does not reflect adrenal gland activity. **DHEA-S has a much** longer half-life than DHEA, and measurement of its **serum level is used to assess adrenal function.**[Q]

Dihydrotestosterone (DHT)

- Testosterone is converted to dihydrotestosterone (DHT) by **5-alpha-reductase,** an enzyme found in many androgen-sensitive tissues.
- Very potent androgen primarily responsible for the androgenic effects on hair follicles.
- 3 α androstenediol glucoronide (3α–AG) is an important metabolite of DHT.

Important Concept

- **M/C Androgen produced by ovary**: Androstenedione > Testosterone > DHEA
- **Most potent androgen**: Dihydrotestosterone > Testosterone
- Androgen produced only by adrenal gland DHEA–Sulphate.

Sex Hormone Binding Globulin (SHBG)

- It is synthesised in liver
- Testosterone and Insulin inhibits its synthesis
- Estrogen promotes its synthesis
- Low levels of SHBG is a marker of insulin resistance.

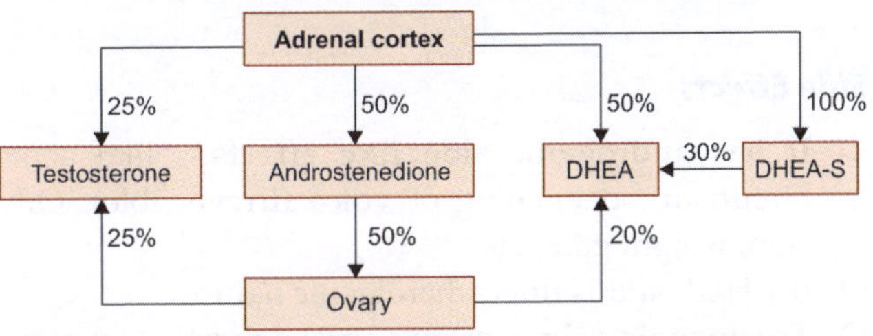

Fig. 2.11: Androgens in the females

Danazol

- It is a 17α ethinyl testosterone derivative.
- It is a compound with weak androgenic, progestational and antigonadotropic activity (Table 2.7).

Table 2.7

Antigonadotropic agent	Androgenic
Acts on HPO axis and decreases frequency of GnRH pulses ↓ No LH surge (no change in basal gonadotropin levels) ↓ ↓ estrogen (endometrial atrophy) ↓ Pseudomenopause like state	As it decreases synthesis of sex hormone binding globulin hence level of free testosterone increases and thus it has virilising side effects

- It acts directly on ovaries and inhibits steroidogenesis.

Uses (Table 2.8)

Table 2.8: Uses

In females		In males
Uterus: • **Endometriosis** (as it causes endometrial atrophy) • DUB in old females • Fibromyoma (to ↓ its size and vascularity) • Infertility	*In Breast for:* • Cyclical mastalgia • **Fibrocystic breast disease**	• Precocious puberty • Gynecomastia • Improves libido (as it a testosterone derivative)

Other uses

In hereditary angioneurotic edema.
(It is the DOC for its prophylaxis)
Dose = 400–800 mg OD

Side Effects

- **It has androgenic side like effects**[Q] like acne, hirsutism[Q], deepening of voice (irreversible), Oily skin, weight gain, etc.
- It ↓ HDL and is thus athero genic nature
- **Teratogenic in early pregnancy**[Q] (causing masculinization of female fetus), therefore it should not be used in young females.
- ***Danazol should not be given for more than 6–9 months at a time because of its antiestrogenic action and virilizing effects.***[Q]
- It is hepatotoxic and can lead to hepatocellular cancer.

Contraindications

- Liver disease (as it is hepatotoxic)
- Carcinoma prostrate

Gestrinone

It is a 19–Nortestosterone derivative. Gestrinone has actions and uses similar to danazol but has **longer t½ (28 hours) so is used in biweekly doses. Dose** = 2.5 mg twice weekly. Its side effects are milder to danazol and thus it is preferred over danazol.

Antiandrogens

Drugs in this group can act **by inhibiting the synthesis, activation or action of androgens.**

- **Steroid synthesis inhibitors: Ketoconazole** inhibits the synthesis of adrenal and gonadal hormones but its usefulness in the treatment of prostatic carcinoma is limited by serious toxicity on prolonged use. It can cause **gynaecomastia** due to increase in estradiol: testosterone ratio. **Abiraterone** is an **orally active prodrug** that acts by inhibiting 17-α-hydroxylase and 17, 20-lyase.
- **5-α reductase inhibitors:** Most of the actions of testosterone are mediated by its conversion to DHT by 5-α reductase. Important amongst these are growth of prostate, male pattern baldness and hirsutism in females. **Finasteride (It selectively inhibits 5α reductase II) and dutasteride (it is a non selective inhibitor of 5α** reductase) are 5α reductase inhibitors useful in the *treatment of BPH (decrease size and weight of prostate), DOC for male pattern baldness and androgenic hirsutism* by reducing the production of DHT.
- **Androgen receptor inhibitors: Cyproterone and cyproterone acetate** act as antagonists of androgen receptors. Latter compound has marked, progestational activity that inhibits feedback enhancement of LH and FSH. These drugs are useful in the **treatment of hirsutism** and as a component of **contraceptive** pills. **Flutamide, bicalutamide and nilutamide** are other antiandrogens that act by same mechanism. ***These are useful for the treatment of prostatic carcinoma****. Flutamide can cause gynaecomastia and reversible liver damage.* These drugs *can also be combined with GnRH agonists (like leuprolide) to reduce the initial flare up reaction. Nilutamide can cause interstitial pneumonitis.*

Note: All antiandrogens can lead to impotence and gynecomastia. These risks are much more with androgen receptors inhibitors than with 5 alpha reductase.

- **Diane 35 or Ginette has** EE 35 mg and cyproterone acetate 2 mg. It is the DOC in teenagers with irregular periods and hirsutism.
- **Spironolactone**: It is an aldosterone antagonist that also competes with DHT for its receptor. It can be used for the *treatment of hirsutism.*

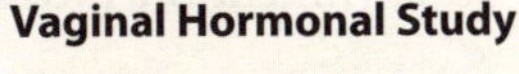

Extra Edge

Vaginal Hormonal Study

Flowchart 2.7

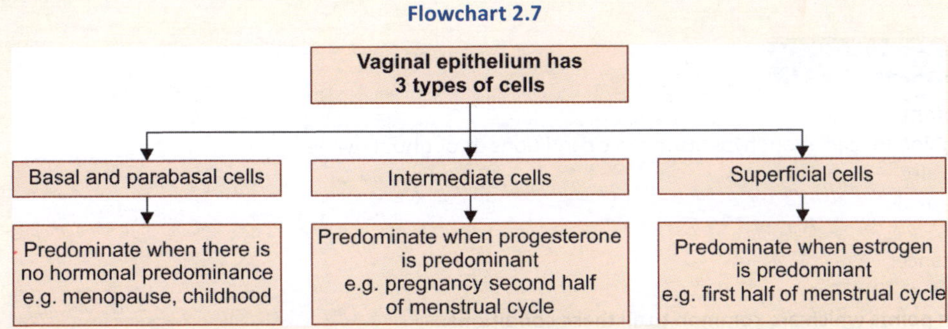

See Fig. 1.6A to C for images of cells

- The ovarian hormones estrogen and progesterone thus influence vagina.

Note: For hormonal study – smear should be taken from lateral wall of upper third of vagina[Q].

Maturation Index (Table 2.9)

- It is the relative percentage of parabasal, intermediate and superficial cells per 100 cells counted.
- It is expressed in 3 numbers, a/b/c.
  - 'a' represents number of parabasal cells per 100 cells counted.
  - 'b' represents number of intermediate cells per 100 cells counted.
  - 'c' represents number of superficial cells per 100 cells counted.
- It indirectly reflects the endocrine status of the cervix.
- See Table 2.10 for Maturation index at different ages.

Table 2.9: Maturation index from birth to menopause

	MI	Smear features	Inference
At birth	0/95/5	—	Combined effect of circulating maternal hormones: oestrogen, progesterone & corticoids.
Childhood	80/20/0	—	MI shifting to left because of diminished steroid hormones.
Reproductive period: Preovulatory	0/40/60	Smear clear, cells are discrete	Oestrogen ++
Mid secretory	0/70/30	Smear dirty, cells in clusters	Oestrogen + Progesterone ++
During pregnancy	0/95/5	Marked folding of the intermediate cells : 'navicular cells'	Oestrogen ++ Progesterone ++ Corticosteroids +
Postpartum	100/0/0	—	Parabasal maturation
Postmenopausal	100/0/0	—	Lack of oestrogen.

Important Facts

- The intermediate and superficial cells contain glycogen under the influence of oestrogen and therefore vagina stains deep brown in colour after painting with iodine solution (called as Positive schillers test).[Q]
- The glycogen content is highest in vaginal fornix and lowest in lower one third of vagina.
- Estrogen dominant smears appear clear and show discrete cornified, polygonal eosinophilic cells.
- Progesterone dominated smears are dirty as intermediate cells predominate.

- **Cornification index/karyopyknotic index**: It is the ratio of cornified cells (mature squamous cells) per 100 cells counted since epithelial cells are cornified under the influence of hormone estrogen, so cornification index indicates estrogenic effect.

Important Concept

Hyperestrogenism

Friends you are going to read about hyperestrogenic conditions throughout gynae.

These conditions are:

- Fibroid
- Endometriosis
- Endometrial cancer
- Ovarian cancer

There are certain points which are common to all these conditions:

These are:

- All these conditions are M/C in nulliparous females
- Hence Pregnancy and Multiparity is a protective factor in all these conditions.
- Since androgens are converted to estrogens in adipose tissue, all these conditions are **M/C in obese females**
- **Hence exercise or physical activity is a protective factor** for all these conditions.
- Androgens are converted to estrogens in adipose tissue with the help of enzyme aromatase

$$\text{Androgens} \xrightarrow[\text{in adipose tissue}]{\text{Aromatase}} \text{Estrogens}$$

- Smoking inhibits enzyme aromatase, so it is protective in all these conditions.
- Letrozole inhibits enzyme aromatase can be used in the management of fibroid and endometriosis
- Early menarche and Late menopause is a risk factor for all these conditions.

NEW PATTERN QUESTIONS

N1. Ovarian cycle is initiated by:
a. LH b. FSH
c. Estrogen d. GRH

N2. Just before ovulation there is:
a. LH surge b. FSH surge
c. LH and FSH surge d. None

N3. Granulosa cells produces estrogen with the help of the enzyme:
a. Alkaline phosphatase b. Aromatase
c. Acid phosphatase d. Glucuronidase

N4. The following are related to granulosa cells *except*:
a. It has got no blood supply
b. In the first half of the cycle, it has no steroidogenic function
c. Granulosa cells produce activin and inhibin
d. Estrogen stimulates the proliferation of granulosa cells

N5. All of the following statements are correct *except*:
a. LH surge is initiated due to sustained levels of 200 pg of estrogen for 48 hours
b. LH surge is maintained by esterogen and progestrone both
c. Meilosis I is hormone dependent
d. Meilosis II is hormone dependent

N6. Maximum progesterone synthesis occurs on—day of the cycle
a. 16th day b. 20th day
c. 22nd day d. 24th day

N7. All are true regarding folliculogenesis and ovulation *except*:
a. Chronic elevation of androgens is detrimental to the follicles
b. AMH supports monofollicular development
c. First phase of follicular growth is gonadotropin insensitive
d. Elevated and static level of estradiol is essential for ovulation.

N8. The following are related to corpus luteum *except*:
a. Luteinised granulosa cells produce progesterone
b. Estrogen continues to be produced by the luteinised theca cells
c. Luteolysis is due to estrogen, PGF2α and endothelin
d. The peak steroid production is between 23rd and 25th day

N9. The earliest morphological evidence of ovulation on endometrial biopsy is:
a. Pseudostratification
b. Basal vacuolation
c. Decrease in glycogen content
d. Predecidual reaction

N10. All of the following statements are correct *except*:
a. Menstrual blood is mainly arterial
b. Prostaglandin released at the time of menstruation is PGE2
c. Zona basalis regenerates the endometrium during next cycle
d. Anovulatory cycles are painless

N11. All of the following are produced by ovary *except*:
a. Estrone b. Androstenedione
c. Testosterone d. 17 hydroxy progesterone
e. DHEA-S

N12. Luteal phase defect is due to:
a. Uterine scaring
b. Chromosomal abnormality
c. Abnormal release of GnRH
d. Absence of oocytes in ovary

N13. On examination of endometrial tissues obtained from a biopsy reveals simple columnar epithelium with no subnuclear vacuoles. The stroma is edematous and a tortuous gland contains secretions. Thus findings are consistent with which stage of menstrual cycle?
a. Non ovulatory cycle
b. Mid secretory
c. Early secretory
d. Late proliferative phase

N14. Pulsatile GnRH is used for managing:
a. Precocious puberty b. Fibroid
c. DUB d. Anovulatory infertility

N15. Following are seen in Kallmann syndrome *except*:
a. Hypogonadism b. Night blindness
c. Anosmia d. Normal height

N16. All of the following changes are seen in puberty *except*:
a. ↑ Leptin b. ↓ GABA
c. ↑ Glutamate d. ↑ Neuropeptide Y

N17. HMG can lead to multiple pregnancy is:
a. 5% b. 10%
c. 20% d. 30%

N18. All of the following statements are true regarding estrogen *except*:
a. Responsible for pre-ovulatory LH surge
b. Causes negative feedback on FSH
c. Produces proliferative endometrium
d. Secreted by theca cells

N19. Sensitivity of uterine musculature is:
a. Enhanced by Estrogen
b. Enhanced by Progesterone
c. Enhanced by E and inhibited by P
d. Enhanced by P and inhibited by E

N20. The increasing order of potency of estrogen is:
a. E1, E2, E3 b. E1, E3, E2
c. E3, E1, E2 d. E2, E1, E3

N21. 3rd generation progesterone includes all *except*:
a. Desogestrel b. Norgestrel
c. Norgestimate d. Gestodene

N22. A sample of cervical mucus is taken on Day 12 of the menstrual cycle: The mucus is thin, clear, elastic. It is placed on a slide and allowed to air dry. When placed under microscope, what would you *expect*:
a. Clear field devoid of bacteria
b. Thick mucus with back ground bacteria
c. A fern pattern characteristic of estrogen
d. Clearly defined, parabasal cells

N23. All of the following SERM can be used for ovulation induction *except*:
a. Clomifene b. Raloxifene
c. Tamoxifen d. Droloxifene

N24. SERM used for contraception:
a. Raloxifene b. Ormeloxifene
c. Clomifene d. Toremifene

N25. The most serious complication of clomiphene therapy for induction of ovulation is:
a. Bone marrow depression
b. Hyperstimulation syndrome
c. Secondary amenorrhea
d. Multiple pregnancy

N26. The side effect of clomiphene because of which its use should be immediately stopped:
a. Hotflashes b. Multiple pregnancy
c. Terato genecity
d. Visual symptoms

N27. In clomiphene induced cycle, what acts as ovulation trigger?
a. LH b. FSH
c. GnRH d. hCG

N28. Major sources of androgen in females are all *except*:
a. Adrenals
b. Ovaries
c. Peripheral conversion to androgen precursors in the liver, gastro-intestinal tract and adipose tissue
d. Corpus luteum

N29. Vaginal smear in old lady shows:
a. Atropic cells on smear
b. Basal and parabasal cells
c. Superficial cells
d. Few intermediate cells seen

N30. The maturation index on vaginal cytology is a diagnostic method for evaluating the:
a. Adequacy of cytotoxic drug therapy
b. Gender of an anatomically abnormal child
c. Malignant change at squamo columnar junction of cervix
d. Endocrine status of cervix

N31. Vaginal cytology for hormonal change is best taken from:
a. Posterior wall b. Anterior wall
c. Lateral wall d. Any wall

N32. Cornification index or eosinophilic index indicates:
a. Progesterone effect b. Estrogenic effect
c. Effect of LH d. All of the above

N33. Before ovulation, which of the following is seen:
a. ↑ LH, ↓FSH b. ↓ LH, ↑FSH
c. ↑ LH, ↑FSH d. ↓ LH, ↓FSH

N34. Main source of testosterone in females is:
a. Adrenal gland
b. Ovary
c. Both a and b
d. Peripheral conversion of androstenediane

N35. False statement regarding spasmodic dysmenorrhea is:
a. Often cured by delivery of a child
b. Pain usually appears on the first day of menstruation
c. Pain persists for 2–3 days
d. Rare above age of 35 years

N36. All are used in treating spasmodic dysmenorrhea *except*:
a. Bromocriptine
b. Ibuprofen
c. Mefenamic acid
d. Norethisterone and ethinyl estradiol

N37. A 20-year-old woman gives a history of sharp pain in the lower abdomen for 2–3 days every month approximately 2 weeks before the menses. The most probable etiology for her pain is:
a. Endometriosis b. Dysmenorrhea
c. Pelvic tuberculosis d. Mittelschmerz syndrome

N38. Which of the following modalities have shown best result for pre menstrual syndrome?
a. SSRI b. Progesterone
c. Oestrogen d. Anxiolyties

N39. Which of the following is NOT to be given in cyclic mastalgia is:
a. Evening primrose oil b. Danazol
c. Tamoxifen d. Estrogen

N40. The Gene present in theca cell and absent in granulosa cell which enables theca cell to produce androgens:
a. CYP17 gene b. CYP12 gene
c. p53 d. KRAS

N41. Fetal ovary can produce estrogen by:
a. 6 weeks b. 8 weeks
c. 10 weeks d. 12 weeks

N42. All are correctly matched *except*:
a. GnRH receptor—G protein coupled receptor
b. LH/CG receptor—G protein coupled receptor
c. Estrogen—Nuclear receptor
d. FSH—Cytoplasmic receptor

PREVIOUS YEAR QUESTIONS

Ovarian Cycle

1. **Which of the following is seen in the ovulatory phase?** *(AIIMS May 11)*
   a. Stimulation of continuation of reduction division of oocytes
   b. Inhibin A is increased
   c. FSH increases steroid synthesis in granulosa cells
   d. Activin causes FSH to act on granulosa cells
2. **In ovarian cycle increased levels of LH are due to:**
   a. Increased, progesterone *(AIIMS May 11)*
   b. Increased Estrogen
   c. Increased FSH d. Increased androgens
3. **In 40 days of menstrual cycle the ovulation occurs at:**
   a. 14th day b. 20th day *(UP 03)*
   c. 26th day d. 30th day
4. **The ovarian cycle is initiated by:** *(DNB 96)*
   a. FSH b. Estrogen
   c. LH d. Progesterone
5. **The corpus luteum secretes:** *(DNB 04)*
   a. Estrogens b. Progesterone
   c. Both d. None
6. **Apoptosis can occur by change in hormone levels in the ovarian cycle. When there is no fertilization of the ovum, the endometrial cells die because:** *(AIIMS Nov 03)*
   a. The involution of corpus luteum causes estradiol and progesterone levels to fall dramatically
   b. LH levels rise after ovulation
   c. Estradiol levels are not involved in the LH surge phenomenon
   d. Estradiol inhibits the induction of the progesterone receptor in the endometrium
7. **Corpus luteum functions maximally without an implantation for ...... days** *(PGI June 00)*
   a. 9 b. 12
   c. 6 d. 15
8. **Maximum function of corpus luteum occurs:**
   a. At ovulation b. Before ovulation
   c. 3 days after ovulation
   d. 8–9 days after ovulation
9. **In a study it is observed that the right ovary ovulates more than the left, all are possible explanations for the cause *except*:** *(AIIMS Nov 2010, AIIMS Nov 2012)*
   a. Anatomical asymmetry
   b. Difference in blood supply to both sides
   c. Right handedness is more common in population
   d. Some embryological basis
10. **Ovulation occurs:** *(AIIMS May 2013)*
    a. Before LH surge
    b. After biphasic rise in body temperature
    c. After ripening of follicle by FSH
    d. Before estrogen peak
11. **True about timing of LH surge:** *(PGI May 2013)*
    a. Occur 12 hour before ovulation
    b. Occur 24 hour before ovulation
    c. Occur 12 hour after ovulation
    d. Occur 24 hour after ovulation
    e. Occur at time of ovulation
12. **Which of the following is not related with menstrual cycle?** *(AI 2011)*
    a. Hormonal changes b. Vaginal cytology
    c. Estrous cycle d. Endometrial sampling
13. **True about ovulation and menstruation:** *(PGI Nov 2014)*
    a. Temperature decreases at time of ovulation
    b. Estrogen has a role in proliferative phase
    c. LH surge occurs before ovulation
    d. 80 ml blood loss is normal
14. **True about ovulation and menstruation:** *(PGI Nov 2014)*
    a. Temperature decreases at time of ovulation
    b. Estrogen has a role in proliferative phase
    c. LH surge occurs before ovulation
    d. 100 mL blood loss is normal
15. **Serum levels of different hormones estimated on day of ovulation will depict:** *(JIPMER May 2016)*
    a. ↑ FSH, LH, Estrogen and progesterone
    b. ↑ FSH, LH, Estrogen and ↓ progesterone
    c. ↑ FSH, LH, ↓ Estrogen and Progesterone
    d. ↑ FSH, LH, ↓ Estrogen and ↑ Progesterone

Hormones – Estrogen/Progesterone

16. **Naturally occurring estrogens are:** *(PGI Dec 08, May 2011)*
    a. Estrone b. Estradiol
    c. Estriol d. Diethylstilbestrol
    e. Pregnanediol
17. **The production of cervical mucus is stimulated by:** *(AIIMS Nov 02)*
    a. Progesterone b. Estradiol
    c. Estriol d. Pregnenolone
18. **Ferning of cervical mucus depends on:** *(DNB 96)*
    a. Estrogen b. Progesterone
    c. LH d. FS
19. **In an infertile woman, endometrial biopsy reveals proliferative changes. Which hormone should be preferred?** *(AI 01)*
    a. MDPA b. Desogestrel
    c. Norethisterone d. None of the above
20. **End product of progesterone metabolism found in urine is:** *(AIIMS May 2013)*
    a. Pregnenolone
    b. 17-OH pregnenolone exerected in urine
    c. Pregnanediol
    d. Pregnanetriol

21. True about testosterone in females: *(PGI May 2015)*
a. > 50% testosterone secreted from ovary
b. > 80% testosterone secreted from ovary
c. ~ .05% ng/ml is plasma concentration
d. Slight decrease in the secretion at time 0/5 ovulation
e. Daily production of testosterone is 0.2–0.3% mg

22. Secretory phase of endometrium is due to: *(JIPMER May 2014)*
a. Estrogen b. Progesterone
c. Prolactin d. Pregnanediol

23. M/C progesterone metabolite is were: *(JIPMER May 2014)*
a. Pregnenolone b. 17 hydroxy Pregnenolone
c. Pregnanetriol d. Pregnanediol

24. All are correct regarding estrogen, *except*: *(JIPMER 2012)*
a. Responsible for preovulatory surge of LH
b. Causes negative feedback on FSH
c. Produces proliferative endometrium
d. Secreted by Theca cells

Clomiphene

25. Clomiphene citrate is: *(AP 97)*
a. Antiandrogen b. Synthetic steroid
c. Antiestrogen d. GnRH analogue

26. Clomiphene citrate is indicated in: *(AI 98)*
a. Stein–Leventhal syndrome
b. Ovarian cyst
c. Asherman's syndrome
d. Carcinoma endometrium

27. True about Clomiphene citrate : *(PGI June 07)*
a. Commonly causes hyperstimulation syndrome
b. Used for ovulation induction
c. Multiple pregnancies seen in 3–8% cases

28. True about clomiphene citrate is: *(AIIMS May 09/May 10)*
a. Enclomiphene has antiestrogenic affect
b. Chance of pregnancy is three fold as compared to placebo
c. Risk of multiple pregnancy is 2–4%
d. It can also be used for male infertility with oligozoospermia

29. Side effect of clomephene citrate includes all *except*: *(AIIMS Nov 07)*
a. Multiple pregnancy
b. Increase risk of ovarian cancer
c. Multiple polycystic ovary
d. Teratogenic effect on off springs

30. A patient treated for infertility with clomiphene citrate presents with sudden onset of abdominal pain and distension with ascites, the probable cause is:
a. Uterine repture
b. Ectopic pregnancy rupture
c. Multifetal pregnancy
d. Hyperstimulation syndrome

GnRH

31. GnRH analogue may be given in all of the following *except*: *(AI 99)*
a. Prostate Ca b. Endometrial Ca
c. Fibromyoma - uterus d. Precocious puberty

32. GnRH analogues are useful in all *except* : *(AP 97)*
a. Endometriosis b. Hyperprolactinemia
c. Precocious puberty d. Menstrual disturbances

Danazol

33. Danazol is used in the treatment of: *(AIIMS May 02)*
a. Cyclical mastalgia b. Breast cyst
c. Noncyclical mastalgia
d. Epithelial changes in breast

34. Danazol is used in all *except*: *(JIPMER 91)*
a. Hirsutism
b. Endometriosis
c. Dysfunctional uterine bleeding
d. Fibroid

Mifepristone

35. Which of the following statements are true about mifepristone? *(PGI Dec 01)*
a. Also called RU - 486 b. It is a 19 - norsteroid
c. Acts on receptors d. Given only intravenously
e. Used for menstrual regulation

Inhibin/Relaxin

36. Following are the features of inhibin *except*: *(Karnataka 06)*
a. Non steroidal water soluble protein
b. Secreted by Graafian follicle
c. Stimulates FSH secretion
d. Increased secretion of inhibin occurs in polycystic ovarian disease

37. The probable source of relaxin is: *(JIPMER 91; DNB 98)*
a. Ovary b. Adrenal cortex
c. Liver d. Bartholin's gland
e. Anterior pituitary

Others

38. Ulipristal acetate is a/an: *(AIIMS Nov 2015)*
a. GnRH agonist
b. Androgen antagonist
c. Selective estrogen receptor modulator
d. Selective progesterone receptor modulator

39. Cause of secondary dysmenorrhea in a young female: *(PGI June 05)*
a. Tuberculosis b. Adenomyosis
c. CIN d. Endometriosis
e. Subserous fibroid

ANSWERS TO NEW PATTERN QUESTIONS

N1. Ans. is b, i.e. FSH

FSH: Important questions
Ovarian cycle is initiated by–FSH
Marker of menopause – FSH (≥ 40 IU)
Test for ovarian reserve = Day 3 FSH levels
Test to distinguish between causes of male infertility – FSH levels
In PCOD LH: FSH = 2:1 or 3:1
Test for FSH and LH should be done on Day 2 or 3 of cycle

N2. Ans. is c, i.e. LH and FSH surge
Just before ovulation both LH and FSH surge occur
Mainly responsible for ovulation = LH surge.

N3. Ans. is b, i.e. Aromatase
Androgen produced by theca cells is converted to estrogen in granulosa cells with the help of enzyme aromatase.

N4. Ans. is b, i.e. In the first half of the cycle, it has no steroidogenic function
As discussed in the text; primordial follicle has granulosa cells and theca cells.
In the Dominant follicle, there is marked enlargement of granulosa cells with lipid inclusion under the influence of FSH and estrogen. (i.e. option d is correct)
Granulosa cells produce estrogen and inhibin B in the first half of the menstrual cycle. (So option b is incorrect). The granulosa cells do not have a blood supply. The granulosa cells layer become vascularised only after ovulation with the formation of corpus luteum.

N5. Ans. is d, i.e. Meiosis II is hormone dependant

Remember

- Meiosis I is hormone dependant (due to LH surge)
- Meiosis I is resumed 32–36 hrs before ovulation due to LH surge
- Meiosis II is not hormone dependant

N6. Ans. is c, i.e. 22nd day
Maximum progesterone production will coincide to maximum activity of corpus luteum = 8 days after ovulation, i.e. Day 22 of menstrual cycle.

N7. Ans. is d, i.e. Elevated and static level of estradiol is essential for ovulation *Ref: Novack 15th/ed, p157*
Till now we have studied ovarian cycle. Now know a few more details:

- Follicular development is a dynamic process that continues from menarche until menopause. The process is desgined to allow the monthly recruitment of a of follicles and ultimately, to release a single, mature dominant follicle during ovulation each month.
- **The initial recruitment and growth of the primordial follicle is Gonadotropin independent** and affects a chort over several months. (i.e. option c is correct, novak 15/e pg 152)
- Shortly after this, it becomes gonadotropin dependant & FSH initiates ovarian cycle

Role of AMH (anti mullerian hormone)
AMH inhibits initial recruitment of primordial follicles into the pool of growing follicles. It also decreases responsiveness of follicles to FSH. AMH plays an important role for monofollicular development and ovulation.

The probable mechanisms for monofollicular development and ovulation

1. All the primordial follicles that reach the preantral stage, produce AMH.
2. AMH inhibits further growth of primordial follicles by decreasing the responsiveness of follicles to FSH.
3. The growth of dominant follicle is uninhibited as the dominant follicle has maximum number of FSH receptors, and it produces less AMH, i.e. option c is correct.

Coming to option 'd'
As discussed in the preceding text:
The basic prerequisite in ovulatory cycle is fluctuating levels of E_2. If for any reason the E_2 levels become static, anovulation is a rule (as in PCOS). Thus option d is incorrect.
Now option 'a':
Chronic elevation of androgens suppresses Hypothalamic– pituitary secretion of FSH, a detriment to the development and maturation of a dominant follicle. Thus clinically, androgen excess results in chronic anovulation, as seen in PCOS.

N8. Ans. is d, i.e. The peak steroid production is between 23rd and 25th day. *Ref: Dutta Gynae 6th/ed, p72,73*
In corpus luteum: The granulosa cells whose basic role in the follicular phase was aromatisation of androgens to estrogens, undergo a change in role and become predominantly progesterone synthesising cells (**option a is correct**). Although they continue to aromatase androgen produced by theca cells.

The theca cells continue to produce androgens which are converted to become estrogen (option b is correct).

The size and activity of corpus luteum reaches peak by 7th–8th day post ovulation (i.e. 14 + 8 = 22nd Day of menstrual cycle), this also correlates with peak luteal phase estrogen and progesterone (i.e. option d is incorrect it should 20–22 days and not 23-25th day).

Corpus luteum has a life span of 12–14 days, From day 23 of cycle, regression begins. The cause of degeneration is prostaglandin F2α, estrogen and endothelin.

N9. Ans. is b, i.e. Basal vacuolation *Ref: Leon speroff 7th/ed, p120,190; Dutta Gynae 6th/ed, p91*

Endometrial biopsy was used in the past to find out whether the female has ovulated or not. Nowadays USG follicular monitoring is being done

Subnuclear basal vacuolation is characterized by glandular growth and presence of vacuoles due to secretion of glycogen between nuclei and basement membrane. It is due to the effect of progesterone. **Basal vacuolization is the earliest evidence of ovulation (36–48 hours after ovulation) and persists until about 21st day of the cycle.**

Pseudostratification of nuclei is characteristic of proliferation phase but persists until active progesterone secretion begins. Hence, it is noted until 18th - 19th day of the menstrual cycle.

Predecidual reaction is first evident on day 23 of the menstrual cycle.

N10. Ans. is b, i.e. Prostaglandin released at the time of menstruation is PGE_2

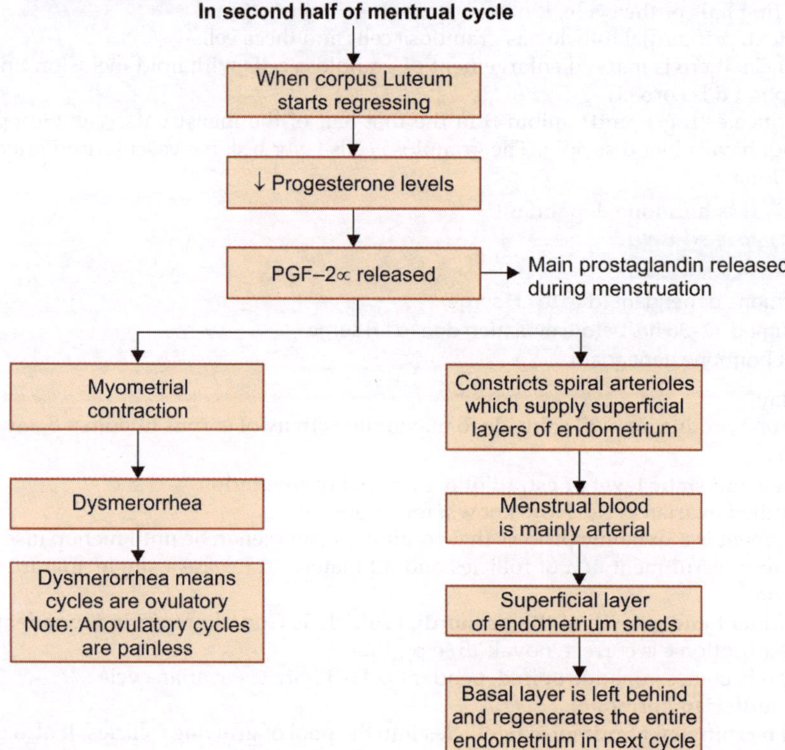

N11. Ans. is e, i.e. DHEA-S *Ref: Williams gynae 3rd/ed, p350*

"The most important secretory products of ovarian steroid biosynthesis are progesterone and estradiol. However, ovary also secretes esterone, androstenedione, testosterone and 17 a hydroxy progesterone".

DHEA-S is produced exclusively by adrenal gland.

N12. Ans. is c, i.e. Abnormal release of GnRH

In the luteal phase, i.e. second half of menstrual cycle, main hormone is progesterone.

Luteal phase defect is a condition in which there is insufficient progesterone. This can occur due to any cause like abnormal GnRH secretion.

Diagnosis is made on Endometrial biopsy (≥ 2 day lag in the endometrial dating and actual day of cycle).

N13. Ans. is b, i.e. Mid secretory

As we know subnuclear vacuolation is the earliest histopathological change in secretory phase. These secretory vacuoles then move upwards towards the apex. Since subnuclear vacuolation is absent it is not early secretory phase.

The edematous stroma and tortuous gland point towards mid secretory phase.

N14. Ans. is d, i.e. Anovulatory infertility

Pulsatile GnRH is used for:

- Ovulation induction (in managing anovulatory infertility)
- Delayed, puberty

N15. Ans. is b, i.e. Night blindness

Kallmann syndrome is condition where there is hypogonadism (d/t hypothalamic failure), anosmia and **color** blindness (not night blindness) in males.

Height remains normal

Females with this syndrome will complain of primary amenorrhea and infertility.

N16. Ans. is d, i.e. ↑ Neuropeptide Y.

See the text for explanation.

N17. Ans. is d, i.e. 30% cases *(Ref: Novat 15th/ed, p1155)*

Chances of multiple pregnancy with	Chances of OHSS
Clomiphene = 5–8% (< 10%)	< 1%
HMG = 35% (here 30% being closest)	5%

N18. Ans. is d, i.e. Secreted by theca cells

Estrogen is produced by:

- Granulosa cells
- Theca cells form androgen which are converted to estrogen by enzyme aromatase under the influence of enzyme FSH (It is not secreted by Theca cells)
- Corpus luteum
- By peripheral conversion of androgens in adipose tissue.

N19. Ans. is c, i.e. Enhanced by E and inhibited by P

N20. Ans. is c, i.e. E_3, E_1, E_2

Least potent = $E_3 > E_1 > E_2$ (Most potent).

N21. Ans. is b, i.e. Norgestrel

See the text for explanation.

N22. Ans. is c, i.e. A fern pattern characteristic of estrogen.

On day 12, when cervical mucus is viewed under microscope, it shows a fern like pattern under the effect of estrogen.

N23. Ans. is b, i.e. Raloxifene

See the text for explanation.

N24. Ans. is b, i.e. Ormeloxifene

Ormeloxifene is the active ingredient of **centchroman** or saheli.

N25. Ans. is b, i.e. Hyperstimulation syndrome *Ref: Shaw 15th/ed, p315*

Ovarian hyperstimulation syndrome is the most dreaded complication of Clomiphene (discussed in detail in chapter 9 on infertility).

N26. Ans. is d, i.e. Visual symptoms

Remember: For clomiphene

- M/C side effect of clomiphene
  - Menopausal symptom-hot flashes
  - Ovarian cyst formation
- Side effect for which its use should be immediately stopped—visual symptoms
- Most dreaded side effect
  - OHSS
- Chances of OHSS = <1%
- Chances of multiple pregnancy -
- < 10% (5–8%)
- Maximum dose = 100 mg
- Maximum duration of use = 12 months.

N27. Ans. is d, i.e. hCG

HCG acts as ovulation trigger in clomiphene induced cycles.

N28. Ans. is d, i.e. Corpus luteum

Read the preceding text for explanation.

N29. Ans. is b, i.e. Basal and parabasal cells

N30. Ans. is d, i.e. Endocrine status of cervix

N31. Ans. is c, i.e. Lateral wall of vagina *Ref: Dutta Gynae 5th/ed, p110*

Read the text for explanation.

N32. Ans. is b, i.e. Estrogenic effect *Ref: Taber's Dictionary 19th/ed, p714*

Estrous: It is cyclical period of sexual activity in non human female mammals, marked by congestion of and secretion by the uterine mucosa, proliferation of vaginal epithelium, swelling of the vulva, ovulation, and acceptance of the male by the female. During estrus, the animal is said to be "in heat".

Also Know

Estrus cycle: The sequence from the beginning of one estrus period to the beginning of the next.

It includes:

- Proestrus
- Estrus
- Metestrus followed by
- Diestrus (period of quiescence).

N33. Ans. is c, i.e. ↑ LH and ↑ FSH

Before ovulation, there is both LH and FSH surge

N34. Ans. is d, i.e. peripheral conversion of androstenedione

The major source of testosterone in females is from peripheral conversion of androstenedione to testosterone

N35. Ans. is c, i.e. Pain persists for 2–3 days

Spasmodic dysmenorrhoea is another name for primary dysnenorrhoea. (i.e. no pelvic pathology is responsible for pain)

Characteristics of spasmodic dysmenorrhoea

- Seen in adolescent girls
- Pain appears within 2 years of menarche
- Family history may be present
- Pain is spasmodic nature. It is located in lower abdomen and may radiate to back and medial aspect of thigh.
- Associated systemic discomfort seen
- Pain begins few hours before a rest of menstruation and losts for 12–24 hours, but never 48 hours more than
- Pain is often cured after child birth
- Management: NSAIDs or OCPs

N36. Ans. is a, i.e. Bromocriptine

See the text for explanation.

N37. Ans. is d, i.e. Mittelschmerz syndrome *Ref: Dutta Gynae 4th/ed, p172, 5th/ed, p178*

- A female giving history of sharp pain in lower abdomen, every month, 2 weeks before the menstruation suggests mittelschmerz as the diagnosis.
- Mittelschmerz is synonymous to painful ovulation. Pain is associated with rupture of ovarian follicle at the time of ovulation.

For more details refer to the preceeding text.

N38. Ans. is a, i.e. SSRI *Ref: William's Gynae 1st/ed, p300; Jeffcoate 7th/ed, p629; Novaks 15th/ed, p311,312; Leon speroff 8th/ed, p578; John hopkins manual of obs and gynae 4th/ed, p462*

Premenstrual disorders:

- Frequently women of reproductive age experience symptoms during the late luteal phase of their menstrual cycle, and collectively these complaints are termed, **premenstrual syndrome (PMS) or premenstrual dysphoric disorder (PMDD)**
- It is mostly seen in women aged to 30–45 years

Treatment of PMS:

Conservative measures	Inhibition of ovulation	Medications directed at symptoms
• Elimination of caffeine from diet • Smoking cessation • Counselling, emotional support • Low-fat, high-fiber diet and essential fatty acids in diet. • Regular exercise • Adequate sleep • Stress reduction	• Oral contraceptives (especially drospirenone containing) • GnRH agonist	• For fluid retention: diuretics • For pain: Prostaglandin synthetase • For mastalgia: evening primrose oil and pyridoxine • For anxiety/depression: SSRI like fluoxetine preferred • Tricyclic antidepressants can also be used

Choice of treatment in PMS

Amongst all the drugs used-SSRI's have shown the best results

"For premenstrual dysphoric disorder, selective serotonin re uptake inhibitor (SSRI'S) proved effective in clinical trials".
Ref: Novak 15th/ed, p312

"Women who meet strict criteria for diagnosis of PMS or PMDD, including socioeconomic dysfunction, are candidates for treatment with an SSRI (fluoxetine, sertraline, paroxetine, verlaflexine), administered daily or only during the luteal phase" Ref: Leon speroff 8th/ed, p578

"SSRIs are the most effective pharmacologic treatment for moderate to severe PMS and PMDD"
Ref: John hopkins manual of obs and gynae 4th/ed, p462

Remember: The most significant side effect of SSRI is sexual dysfunction including decreased libido and anorgasmia.

N39. Ans. is d, i.e. Estrogen *Ref: Shaw 15th/ed, p477,478*

Mastalgia is painful breast:
It can be:

Cyclical	Non-cyclical
• Mostly seen in young women • It occurs for a few days before menstruation • It is usually bilateral diffuse and most severe during luteal phase of menstrual	• Mostly seen in older women • May be a symptom of breast carcinoma, cyst Tietze syndrome (Chest wall pain) • It has no relation to menstrual cycle • It is often focal.

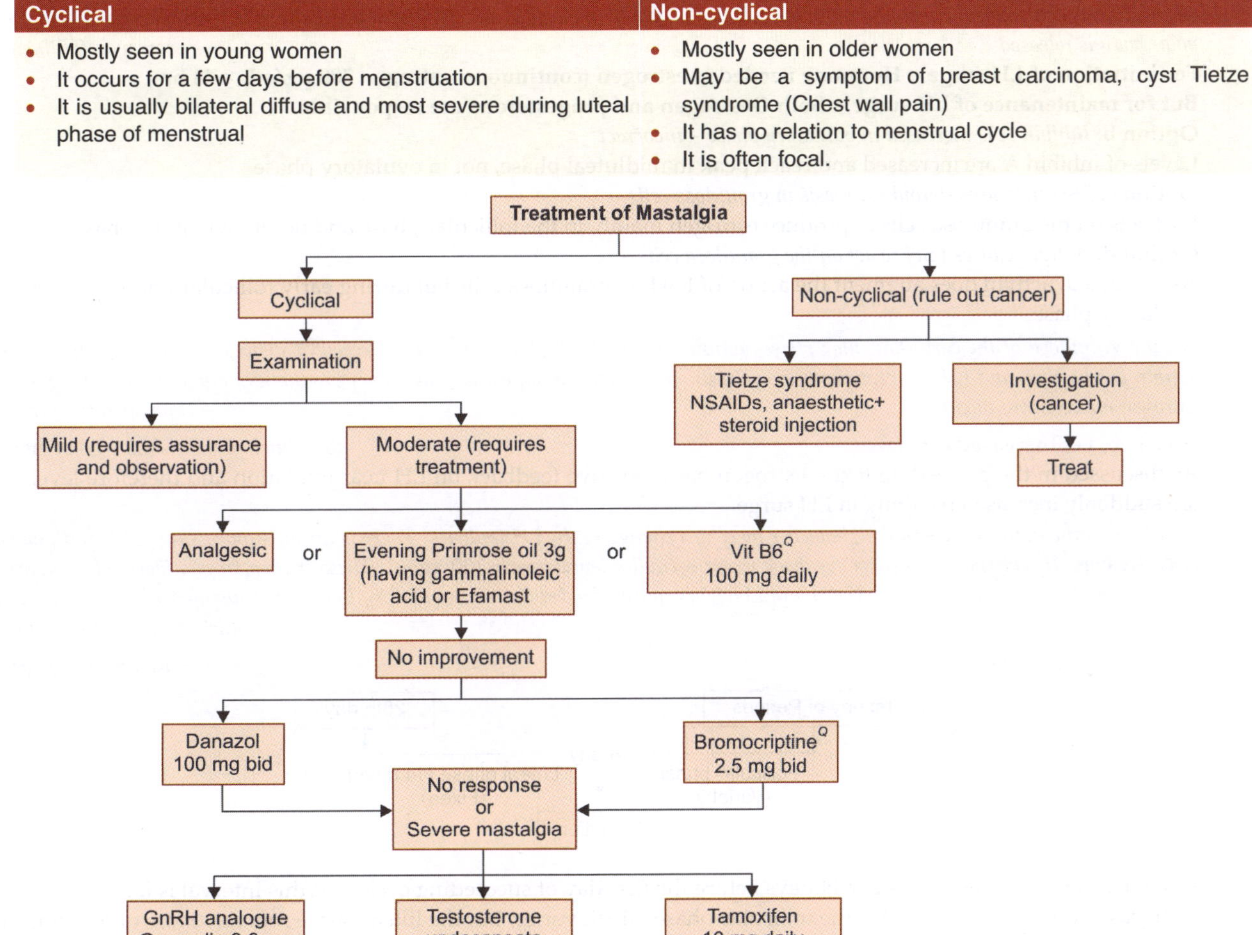

N40. Ans. is a, i.e. CYP 17 gene *Ref: Williams Gynae 3rd/ed, p350*

"Theca cells express all of the enzymes needed to produce androstenedione. This includes high levels of CYP17 gene expression, whose enzyme product catalyzes 17-hydroxylation. This is the rate limiting step in the conversion of progesterones to androgens."

N41. Ans. is b, i.e. 8 weeks *Ref: William Gynae 3rd/ed, p350*

"In utero, the fetal human ovary has the capacity to produce estrogen by 8 weeks of gestation".

N42. Ans. is d, i.e. FSH-cytoplasmic receptor *Ref: William Gynae 3rd/ed, p339*

- GnRH receptors, LH and hCG receptors are G protein coupled receptor (present in cell membrane)
- FSH also binds to G protein coupled receptor located on granulosa cell membrane.
- Estrogen, Progesterone and Androgens are nuclear receptors. These nuclear hormone receptors are localized in cytoplasm. Following ligand binding they are translocated to nucleus to exerts to effect

ANSWERS TO PREVIOUS YEAR QUESTIONS

Ovarian Cycle

1. **Ans. is a, i.e. Stimulation of continuation of reduction division of oocytes**

Ref: Leon Speroff 8th/ed, p213,223,226,229; Jeffcoate 7th/ed, p60-63

Lets analyse each option – In ovulatory phase.

Option a: *Stimulation of continuation of reduction division of oocytes – correct*

During oogenesis the primary oocyte is arrested in prophase of meiosis 1. Just before ovulation, the LH surge initiates the continuation of meiosis, forming secondary oocyte and 1st polar body.

"The LH surge initiates the resumption of meiosis in the oocyte (meiosis is not completed until after the sperm has entered and second polar body is released." – *Leon speroff 8th/ed, p229*

For initiation of LH surge = Hormone needed is estrogen (continuous estrogen 200 pg/mL × 48 hrs)

But for maintenance of LH surge = Both Oestrogen and progesterone are responsible.

Option b: *Inhibin A is increased in ovulatory phase – incorrect*

Levels of inhibin A are increased and reach peak in midluteal phase, not in ovulatory phase.

Option c: *FSH increases steroid synthesis in granulosa cells –*

FSH acts on the granulosa cells to produce estrogen mainly in the follicular phase and not in ovulatory phase.

Option d: *Activin causes FSH to act on the granulosa cells –*

As discussed, activin does augment the action of FSH on granulosa cells but during early follicular phase and not during ovulatory phase.

"In the granulosa of the early follicular phase, activin augments FSH activities: FSH receptor expression, aromatization, inhibin/activin production, and LH receptor expression. In the theca, activin suppresses androgen production, allowing the emergence of an estrogen microenvironment." – *Leon speroff 8th/ed, p226.*

2. **Ans. is b, i.e. Increased estrogen** *Ref: Shiela Balakrishnan TB of gynae p34*

As discussed in the preceeding text - Estrogen has a positive feedback on LH near ovulation and therefore levels of LH are suddenly increased resulting in LH surge.

"With dramatic increase in estradiol, however there is a change in the LH feedback. There is initial suppression of LH with low levels of oestradiols. It switches to positive feedback when estradiol levels reach 200 pg/ml. These high estrogen levels also increase the production of more bioactive form of FSH and LH. This causes the dramatic bioovulatory LH surge causing 10 fold increase in LH."

– *Shiela Balakrishnan 1st/ed, p34*

3. **Ans. is c, i.e. 26th day** *Ref: Shaw 15th/ed, p30*

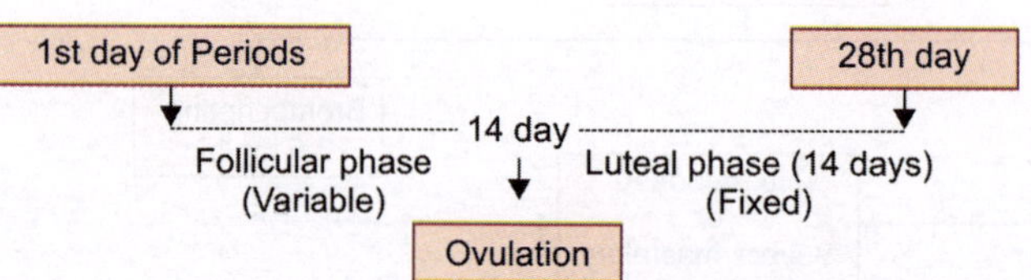

- Ovulation is estimated to occur 14 days before the first day of succeeding cycle and this interval is fixed.
- In case of irregular cycles, it is the follicular phase which varies, but the luteal phase remains more or less constant at 14 days, therefore day of ovulation can be estimated by counting 14 days backward.
- *As in the question* the cycle is of 40 days, ovulation will occur 14 days prior to next menstruation i.e. (40-14) = 26 day

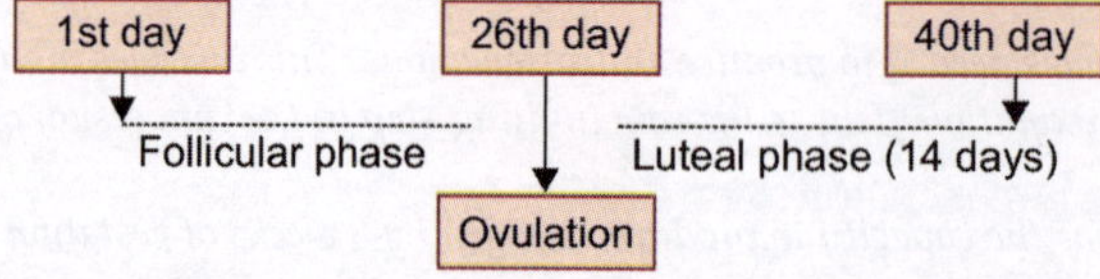

Remember = Day of ovulation = Length of Menstrual cycle – 14

4. **Ans. is a, i.e. FSH** *Ref: Shaw 14th/ed, p41, Dutta Gynae 5th/ed, p82*

As discussed in text–

Ovarian cycle is initiated by FSH

Remember: Following questions asked, previously on FSH

FSH

i. It is the hormone which initiates ovarian cycle
ii. In menopausal females- Since primordial follicles are decreased so levels of estrogen is decreased, so negative feedback on FSH is decreased, hence levels of FSH are increased and increased FSH levels are a sine qua non of menopause.
iii. Human menopausal gonadotropin (HMG) is FSH and LH obtained from the urine of postmenopausal females
iv. FSH levels can help in differentiating the causes of male infertility viz
In pretesticular cause of male infertility = FSH decreases
In testicular cause = FSH levels increase
In posttesticular cause = FSH is normal

5. **Ans. is c, i.e. Both** *Ref: Dutta Gynae 5th/ed, p85*

6. **Ans. is a, i.e. The involution of corpus luteum causes estradiol and progesterone levels to fall dramatically** *Ref: Jeffcoates 7th/ed, p83-84; Leon speroff 7th/ed, p121-122*

7. **Ans. is a, i.e. 9 days** *Ref: Leon speroff 8th/ed, p236*

8. **Ans. is d, i.e. 8–9 days after ovulation** *Ref: Shaw 14th/ed, p28*

Corpus luteum: After ovulation, the ruptured Graafian follicle develops into corpus luteum.

- Corpus luteum reaches it maximum maturity by 22nd day of cycle (Size = 2 cms or more), ovulation occurs on day 14, i.e. 8th days after ovulation corpus luteum reaches its maximum maturity.
- Colour of corpus luteum in early stages is greyish yellow[Q] due to presence of lipids and later is distinctive yellow due to pigment carotene.[Q]
- Corpus luteum secretes:

a. Progesterone (mainly)
b. Estrogen
c. Inhibin
d. Relaxin - secreted by corpus luteum of pregnancy

- In non-pregnant states activity of corpus luteui is maintained by hormone LH whereas in pregnant states by hormone hCG.[Q]
- The corpus luteum rapidly declines 9–11 days after ovulation and starts forming corpus albicans if pregnancy does not occur
- In the first half of the secretory phase, acid phosphatase and potent lytic enzymes are confined to lysosomes. Their release is inhibited by progesterone stabilization of the lysosomal membranes. With the involution of corpus luteum levels of estrogen and progesterone fall, the lysosomal membranes are not maintained and enzymes are released which cause apoptosis of the endometrial cells.
- *"The withdrawl of estrogen and progesterone initiates important endometrial events, vasoconstriction, the process of apoptosis, tissue loss and finally menstruation." – Leon Speroff 7th/ed, p121*
- If pregnancy occurs, hCG similar to LH stimulates corpus luteum to secrete progesterone. It's growth reaches a peak at 8th week of gestation and it remains functionally active till 10–12 weeks of gestation, whereby the placenta takes over its function of producing progesterone.

9. **Ans. is c, i.e., Right handedness is more common in population** *Ref: humrep.oxfordjournal.org/content/12/8/1730.full.pdf*

- In the primate it is suggested that ovulations occur with equal frequency in the left and right ovary.
- In the humans there is some controversy about the frequency of ovulation on each side.
- It is believed that in normally menstruating women ovulation was significantly higher in right ovary.
- It is believed that right sided, predominance was either **genetically determined** or due to **difference in the vasculature of the ovaries.**
- **The anatomical asymmetry** between the left and right side are also thought to be the reason.
- The left ovarian vein drains to the left renal vein and the right ovarian vein to the inferior venacava.
- The left renal vein is thought to be under high pressure than the right and therefore drain slower. Because the left ovary drains slower, the collapsed follicle (corpus luteum) takes longer to clean and thereby diminishes the chances that ovulation will occur on that side the following month.
  - No such condition exists on the right side which is why successive right side ovulation is more common.

10. **Ans. is c, i.e. After ripening of follicle by FSH**

We have discussed ovarian cycle in detail in preceding text.
The question is very simple as ovulation occurs after LH surge and estrogen peak and because of ovulation there is biphasic rise in temperature.

11. **Ans. is b, i.e. Occur 24 hours before ovulation** *Ref: Dutta gynae 6th/ed, p93*

Best answer is 32–36 hours; second best answer is 24–36 hours

12. **Ans. is c, i.e. Estrous cycle** *Ref: Leon speroff 7th/ed, p116-120*

13. **Ans. is b, c, and d, i.e. Estrogen has a role in proliferative phase, LH surge occurs before ovulation and 80 mL blood loss is normal**

- With these changes in the ovary there are simultaneous changes in the uterine endometrium, i.e. in the menstrual cycle. In a 28 day menstrual cycle.

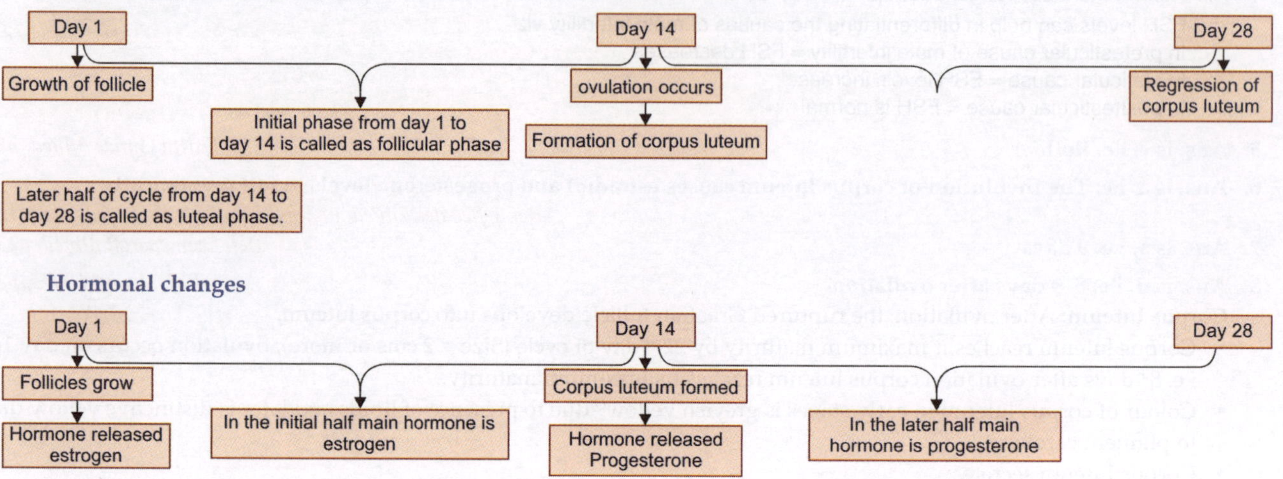

Thus, hormonal levels coincide with ovarian cycle.

Endometrial sampling

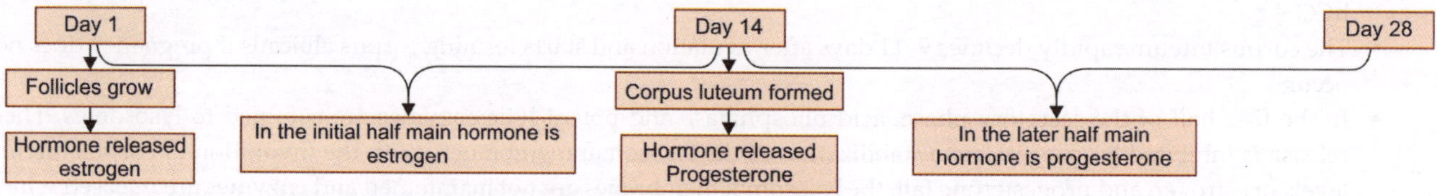

Thus endometrial sampling reveals whether the endometrium is in proliferative or secretory phase and thus indirectly indicates whether ovulation has occurred or not and so endometrial sampling also coincides with ovarian cycle.

Vaginal cytology *Ref: Dutta Gynae 5th/ed, p110*

Vaginal squamous epithelium is composed of following types of cells:

Parabasal/ basal cells	Which are predominant when there is no hormonal dominance.
Intermediate cells	Which are predominant when there is progesterone predominance i.e. in luteal phase/later half of menstrual cycle.
Superficial cells	Which are predominate when there is estrogen predominance i.e. in follicular phase first half of menstrual cycle. Vaginal cytology gives a fair idea about the hormonal status and in turn about ovulation/ ovarian cycle.

Cervical changes

Cyclical changes occur in the cervix in response to the changes in estrogen and progesterone.

Under the influence of estrogen cervical mucus is thin, profuse, watery, more alkaline, promoting the ascent of sperms.

The cervical mucus is thinnest at the time of ovulation and its elasticity increases (spinnbarkeit)

Progesterone makes cervical mucus scanty, thick, viscous and it loses its stretching ability (Tack). So cervical changes also correspond to the ovarian cycle.

14. **Ans. is b and c, i.e. Estrogen has a role in proliferative phase and LH surge occurs before ovulation**

Well options a, b, c do not need further explanation

Bleeding of 100 mL is not normal.

Bleeding exceeding 80 mL is taken as heavy menstrual bleeding/ **Menorrhagia**.

15. **Ans. is a, i.e. ↑ FSH, ↑ LH, ↑ Estrogen and ↑ Progesterone**

Now we know that just before ovulation there is LH & FSH surge so LH and FSH increase at the time of ovulation. Level of estrogen & progesterone are also raised. The levels of progesterone begin to rise and are maximum by Day 22 of cycle. See the graph below:

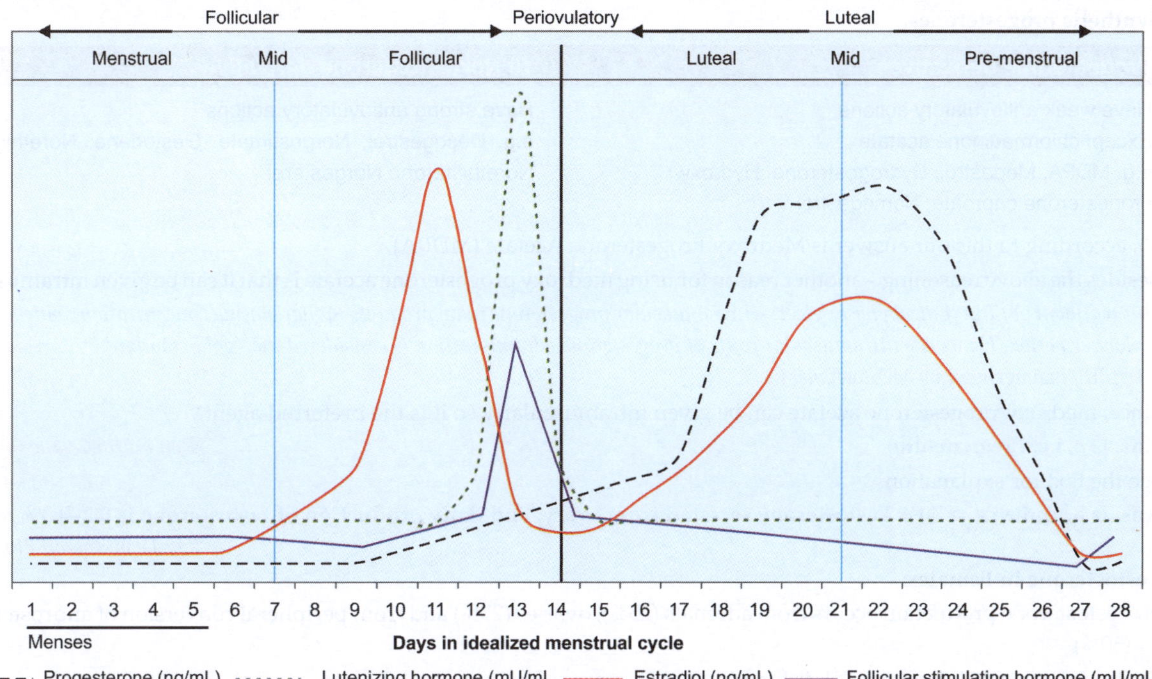

"Immediately prior to ovulation, when theca interna begins to luteinize, and during luteal phase, the plasma progesterone level rises from 6 nmol/L to 63 nmol/L". *Ref: Jeffcoates 9th/ed, p75*

Hormones – Estrogen/Progesterone

16. Ans. is a, b and c, i.e. Estrone, Estradiol and Estriol *Ref: Shaw 15th/ed, p42; Jeffcoate 7th/ed, p67; KDT 6th/ed, p297*

Estrogens :

- Natural estrogens are C18 steroids
- Main Source - Theca and Granulosa cells of Graafian follicle and corpus luteum.
- Secondary source - Adrenal cortex

Naturally occurring estrogen
Estradiol – Main estrogen during reproductive years.
Esterone (Produced by peripheral aromatization of androstenedione) – Main estrogen after menopause
Estriol (main source is placenta) – Most specific estrogen during pregnancy.

17. Ans. is b, i.e. Estradiol *Ref: Shaw 15th/ed, p42-43,216*

18. Ans is a, i.e. Estrogen

Estrogen is responsible for the secretion of cervical mucus and progesterone is responsible for making it thick and viscid. Under the influence of estrogen cervical mucus is copious, watery elastic (can be stretched) and when dried it shows a characteristic fern pattern. Under the influence of progesterone cervical mucus is thick, scarly, loses its stretchability and an drying does not show fern like pattern.

In Q 17.

- Now we have to choose between option b and c as both estradiol and estriol are derivatives of estrogen.
- I have mentioned earlier that estradiol is the more potent form of estrogen, in fact it is the most potent estrogen and estriol the least. So obviously estradiol will be responsible for most of the physiological action of estrogen and is therefore the option of choice.

19. Ans. is a, i.e MDPA *Ref: KDT 6th/ed, p307*

In the question, the infertile woman's endometrial biopsy shows proliferative changes. Endometrial biopsy for infertility is taken on D 25 of cycle with the aim to rule out anovulation. Normally on these days, endometrial biopsy should show secretory changes (as ovulation occurs on D-14 and subsequently there is an increase in progesterone levels in body). But in case of anovulation, endometrial biopsy shows proliferative changes.

The hormone which should be administered here is obviously progesterone, but that derivative of progesterone which has a weak antiovulatory effect so that it would not further inhibit ovulation.

Synthetic progesterones:

Progesterone derivatives	19 Nortestosterone derivatives
Have weak antiovulatory actions. Except chlormadinone acetate e.g. MDPA, Megestrol, Dydrogesterone, Hydroxy progesterone caproate, Nomegestrol	Have strong antiovulatory actions e.g. Desogestrel, Norgestimate, Gestodene, Norethindrone, Norethisterone Norgesterel

So, according to this our answer is Medroxy Progesterone Acetate (MDPA).

Besides the above reasoning – another reason for using medroxy progesterone acetate is that it can be given intramuscularly.

"In treatment of LPD (Luteal phase defect) – Intramuscular progesterone in oil produces higher plasma concentration, which sustained for longer period. Hence the intramuscular route of progesterone administration is considered the "gold standard." – Advanced infertility management by Mehroohansotia

Since, medroxy progesterone acetate can be given intramuscularly so it is the preferred agent.

20. **Ans. is c, i.e. Pregnanediol** *Ref: Dutta Gyane 6th/ed, p75*

See the text for explanation.

21. **Ans. is a, and e i.e. > 50% Testosterone secreted from ovary, and daily production of testosterone is 0.2–0.3% mg** *Ref: Leon Speroff 8th/ed, p537*

Testosterone in Females:

- Testosterone production occurs from adrenals (25%), ovaries (25%) and from peripheral conversion of androstenedione (50%)
- Production rate is between 0.1–0.4 mg/day
- Normal serum concentration is 20–80 mg/dL
- 80% of circulating testosterone is bound to sex hormone binding globulin, 19% to albumin, Thus only 1% is free.

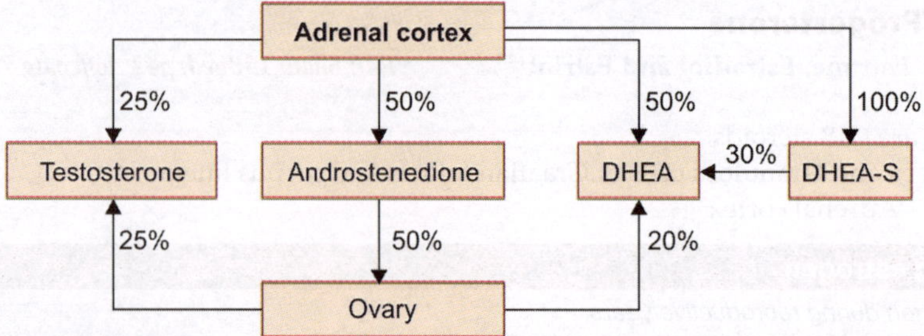

22. **Ans. is b, i.e. Progesterone**

Remember

All the effects on endometrium are due to estrogen and progesterone, not due to their urinary metabolites. So secretory endometrium is due to progesterone and don't confuse your concepts just because pregnanediol is given in the options.

23. **Ans. is d, i.e. Pregnanediol**
24. **Ans is d, i.e. Secreted by Theca cells**

Clomiphene

25. **Ans. is c, i.e. Antiestrogen** *Ref: Shaw 15th/ed, p314*

Clomiphene is an antiestrogen.

Category	Drug
Antiestrogen/SERM	Clomiphene, Tamoxifen
Antiprogesterone	Mifepristone
Antiandrogen	*Cyproterone acetate, Spironolactone, Flutamide, Finasteride*

26. **Ans. is a, i.e. Stein-Leventhal Syndrome** *Ref: Shaw 15th/ed, p314*
27. **Ans. is b and c, i.e. Used for ovulation induction and Multiple pregnancy seen in 3–8% cases** *Ref: Shaw 15th/ed, p314*

28. Ans is a, i.e. Enclomiphene has antiestrogenic effect. *Ref: Novak 15th/ed, p1153-1154; Shaw 15th/ed, p314; Jeffcoates 7th/ed, p104-105; Leon speroff 8th/ed, p1294-1295,1281*

Indications of clomiphene:

- Anovulatory infertility in case of PCOS (Stein-Leventhal syndrome), Chiari frommel syndrome.
- Amenorrhea and anovulation following the use of OCP's (Post pill amenorrhea).
- In vitro fertilization, GIFT technique and Assisted Reproduction Technique.

"It is the usual first choice for ovulation induction in most patients because of relative safety, efficacy, route of administration and relative low cost". – Novak 14th/ed, p64

Results: 80–85% treated women ovulate and 40-50% conceive after the use of Clomiphene.

Ref: Novak 14th/ed, p1064; Shaw 14th/ed, p284

Side effects:

Clomiphene and multiple pregnancy

"*Multiple ovulation and multiple pregnancy in* (case of clomiphene) *is 10%*" .... *Shaw 15th/ed, p 314.*

"Multi follicular development is relatively common and the overall risk of multiple pregnancy is increased approximately 7-10%" *– Leon speroff 8th/ed, p1302*

Novak 14th/ed, p 1064 says – "Incidence of multiple pregnancies ranges from 6.25 to 12.3%."

Jeffcoates 7th/ed, p105 says –

"Pregnancy occurs in 40 - 50% of women following treatment and even though the dosage is carefully monitored, 5-10% of the conceptions are multiple."

Clomiphene for the management of oligospermia in males with idiopathic male infertility.

– Leon speroff 8th/ed, p1281

- Most infertile men are eugonadotropic, normally virilized, and otherwise normal, but have low sperm density. Empiric treatment with either clomiphene citrate or tamoxifen is commonly offered to stimulate increased, pituitary gonadotropin secretion and spermatogenesis in men with idiopathic subfertility. Whereas treatment appears to benefit some men, there is no reliable method for identifying those who might respond. Overall antiestrogenic treatment is not effective.

"A randomized clinical trial conducted by WHO involving nearly 200 men and over 1300 couple months of observation found no differences among men treated with clomiphene or placebo. Moreover a meta analysis including 10 randomized trials involving over 700 men concluded that evidence is inefficient to indicate that anti estrogen treatment improves semen quality or male fertility."

– Leon speroff 8th/ed, p 1281

From the above lines it is clear - It has shown to increase fertility in oligospermic males in randomized controlled trials is incorrect.

29. Ans. is d, i.e. Teratogenic effect on offsprings *Ref: Jeffcoates 7th/ed, p105; Leon Speroff 7th/ed, p1182*

Side effects of clomiphene: *Ref: Textbook Gynecology Show 4th/ed, p281*

- Increased risk of multiple pregnancy
- Hot flushes
- Nausea, vomiting
- Headache
- Visual disturbances like scotoma
- Ovarian hyperstimulation syndrome
- Increase chances of enlargement, pain, cystic changes, haemorrhage and multiple ovulation in the ovaries.
- Increase risk of ovarian cancer
- Increase rate of abortion
- Alopecia (rare) and galactorrhoea (rare).

"There is no substantial evidence that clomiphene treatment increases the overall risk of birth defects or any one anomaly in particular" – Leon Speroff 7th/ed, p1182

There is no evidence to indicate that cc treatment is associated with a higher incidence of congenial abnormalities

30. Ans. is d, i.e. Hyperstimulation syndrome

Read the text for explanation.

GnRH

31. Ans. is b, i.e Endometrial Ca *Ref: Jeffcoate 7th/ed, p652*

32. Ans. is b, i.e. Hyperprolactinemia *Ref: Shaw 15th/ed, p319-320,653*

Read the text for explanation.

Danazol

33. Ans. is a, i.e Cyclical mastalgia *Ref: Shaw 15th/ed, p313; KDT 5th/ed, p271*

34. Ans. is a, i.e. Hirsutism *Ref: Shaw 15th/ed, p313*

Read the text for explanation.

Mifepristone

35. **Ans. is a, b, c and e, i.e. Also called RU – 486; It is a 19 Norsteroid; Acts on receptors; Used for menstrual regulation** *Ref: Shaw 15th/ed, p237,246,317*

RU 486 (Mifepristone) is a 19 Norsteroid synthetic derivative of progesterone. It has affinity for progesterone receptors and therefore blocks its actions.

Route of administration: Oral

Uses:

- As post coital pill (600 mg given within 72 hours of unprotected sex).
- To induce abortion upto 7 weeks of amenorrhea along with misoprostol (medical abortion).
- Ripening of cervix prior to prostaglandin induction of mid trimester abortion.
- Management of ectopic pregnancy.
- Cushing's syndrome : because of its antiglucocorticoid action.
- Medical management of uterine fibroid.

Side effects:

- Headache
- GI upset
- Adrenal failure
- Teratogenecity (If medical methods of abortion fails with RU – 486, pregnancy should be terminated any how).

Inhibin/Relaxin

36. **Ans. is c, i.e. Stimulates FSH secretion** *Ref: Shaw 15th/ed, p45; Dutta Gynae 5th/ed, p72; Leon Speroff 7th/ed, p197, 8th/ed, p212,213,172*

Inhibin:

- Inhibin is a *non-steroidal water soluble protein.*[Q]
- It is secreted by Graffian follicle.[Q]
- It is of two types - Inhibin A and B. In the early and midfollicular phase Inhibin B is the predominant form secreted whereas Inhibin A begins to rise in late follicular phase to reach a peak in mid luteal phase.

Inhibin suppresses FSH secretion and not LH

- In PCOS inhibin secretion increases.[Q]

37. **Ans. is a, i.e. Ovary** *Ref: Clinical Gynecology Endocrinology and Infertility by Leon Speroff 7th/ed, p284-285, 8th/ed, p299; Shaw 15th/ed, p45*

- Relaxin is a peptide hormone.[Q] It is produced by the ovary[Q] to be specific by the corpus luteum of pregnancy[Q] If corpus luteum is in options, it should be the answer of choice. It has also been identified in:
  - placenta[Q]
  - decidua[Q]
  - chorion[Q]
- It is not detected in men[Q] and non pregnant women.[Q]
- Levels of Relaxin rise during 1st trimester when corpus luteum is dominant and declines in the second trimester. This suggests a role in maintaining early pregnancy.[Q]
- In animals, relaxin softens the cervix, inhibits uterine contractions and relaxes public symphysis.[Q]
- It has no effect on prolactin secretion but enhances growth hormone secretion by the pituitary.[Q]

Others

38. **Ans. is d, i.e. Selective progesterone receptor modulator** *Ref: Harrison's Principles of Internal medicine 19th/ed, p2391*

Ulipristal acetate (trade name EllaOne in the European Union, Ella in the US for contraception, and Esmya for uterine fibroid) is a selective progesterone receptor modulator (SPRM).

Pharmacodynamics

As an SPRM, ulipristal acetate has partial agonistic as well as antagonistic effects on the progesterone receptor. It also binds to the glucocorticoid receptor, but is only a weak antiglucocorticoid relative to mifepristone, and has no relevant affinity to the estrogen, androgen and mineralocorticoid receptors. Phase II clinical trials suggest that the mechanism might consist of blocking or delaying ovulation and of **delaying the maturation of the endometrium**.

Medical Uses

- **Emergency contraception:** For emergency contraception, a 30 mg tablet is used within 120 hours (5 days) after an unprotected intercourse or contraceptive failure. It has been shown to prevent about 60% of expected, pregnancies, and prevents more pregnancies than emergency contraception with levonorgestrel.
- **Treatment of uterine fibroids:** Ulipristal acetate is used for preoperative treatment of moderate to severe symptoms of uterine fibroids in adult women of reproductive age in a daily dose of a 5 mg tablet. Treatment of uterine fibroids with ulipristal acetate for 13 weeks effectively controlled excessive bleeding due to uterine fibroids and reduced the size of the fibroids.

Interactions

Ulipristal acetate is metabolized by CYP3A4 in vitro. Ulipristal acetate is likely to interact with substrates of CYP3A4, like rifampicin, phenytoin, St John's wort, carbamazepine or ritonavir. Therefore, concomitant use with these agents is not recommended. It might also interact with hormonal contraceptives and progestogens such as levonorgestrel and other substrates of the progesterone receptor, as well as with glucocorticoids.

Adverse Effects

Common side effects include abdominal pain and temporary menstrual irregularity or disruption. Headache and nausea were observed under long-term administration (12 weeks), but not after a single dose.

Contraindications

Ulipristal acetate should not be taken by women with severe liver diseases because of its CYP-mediated metabolism. It has not been studied in women under the age of 18.

Pregnancy: Unlike levonorgestrel, and like mifepristone, ulipristal acetate is embryotoxic in animal studies. Before taking the drug, a pregnancy must be excluded.

39. **Ans. is a, d and e, i.e. Tuberculosis, Endometriosis and Subserous fibroid**

Ref: Dutta Gynae 5th/ed, p174-5; Jeffcoate 7th/ed, p622-3; Textbook of Gynae sheila Balakrishnan 1st/ed, p203

Causes of secondary dysmenorrhea:
- **Endometriosis**–(M/C cause)
- **PID–(2nd M/C cause) (i.e. TB in options)**
- Adenomyosis
- IUCD
- **Uterine fibroid (i.e. Subserous fibroid in option)**
- Polyps
- Cervical stenosis
- Congenital malformation of uterus like bicornuate uterus

Management: Treatment of the underlying cause.

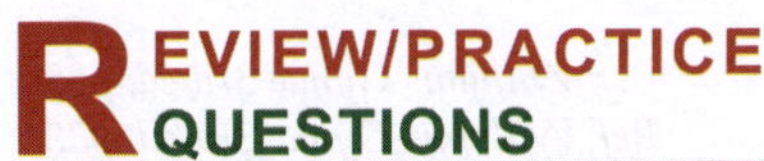

REVIEW/PRACTICE QUESTIONS

1. **At Puberty – First event is:**
   a. Sleep associated increase in LH
   b. Sleep associated increase in FSH
   c. Early morning associated increase in LH
   d. Early morning associated increase in FSH
2. **Major site for conversion of androstenedione to estrone:**
   a. Granulosa cells b. Theca cells
   c. Adipose Tissue d. Breasts
3. **Testosterone is converted to _________ granulosa cells with the help of enzyme aromatase:**
   a. E1 b. E2
   c. E3 d. E4
4. **Androstenedione is converted to _____ granulosa cells and adipose tissue with the help of enzyme aromatase:**
   a. E1 b. E2
   c. E3 d. E4
5. **The peptides secreted by ovary are:**
   a. Inhibin b. Activin
   c. Follistatin d. All of the above
6. **The figure shows graphical representation of levels of progesterone during the cycle. Identify the Day X when it is reaching its peak:**

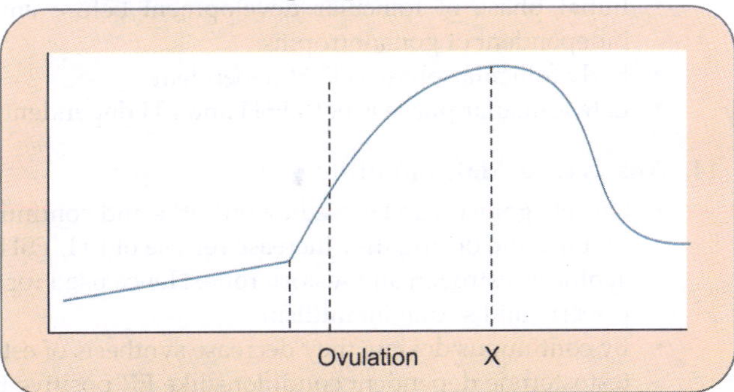

   a. Day 6 after ovulation
   b. Day 8 after ovulation
   c. Day 10 after ovulation
   d. Day 12 after ovulation

7. Inhibin produced by placenta during pregnancy:
a. Inhibin A b. Inhibin B
c. Both d. None

8. Inhibin and activin are expressed in:
a. Ovary
b. Placenta
c. Pituitary
d. All of the above

9. Mean duration of LH surge:
a. 24 hours b. 32 hours
c. 36 hours d. 48 hours

10. All of the following are possible mechanisms for extrusion of oocyte during ovulation *except*:
a. Enzyme collagenase thins the follicular wall
b. Increase in follicular pressure
c. Tissue plasminogen activity is increased
d. Prostaglandins stimulate smooth muscle contraction in ovary

11. Ovulation is said to have occurred if progesterone levels exceed ________on day 21 of cycle:
a. 1 ng/mL b. 2 ng/mL
c. 3 ng/mL d. 5 ng/mL

12. Hormone rescuing corpus luteum from atresia/luteolysis:
a. LH
b. Progesterone
c. FSH
d. HCG

13. Before ovulation development of granulosa cell is dependent on: *(AIIMS November 2018)*
a. Estrogen b. Progesterone
c. FSH d. LH

14. Continuous GnRH is useful in all except:
a. Precautious puberty *(AIIMS November 2019)*
b. Prostate cancer
c. Male infertility
d. Endometriosis

REVIEW/PRACTICE ANSWERS

1. **Ans. is a, i.e. Sleep associated increase in LH** *Ref: Williams Gynae 3rd/ed*
2. **Ans. is c, i.e. Adipose tissue** *Ref: Williams Gynae 3rd/ed, p351*
3. **Ans. is b, i.e. E2**
4. **Ans. is a, i.e. E1**
5. **Ans. is d, i.e. All of the above** *Ref: Williams Gynae 3rd/ed, p351*
6. **Ans. is b, i.e. Day 8 after ovulation**
7. **Ans. is a, i.e. Inhibin A**
8. **Ans. is d, i.e. All of the above** *Ref: Williams Gynae 3rd/ed, p351*
9. **Ans. is d, i.e. 48 hours** *Ref: Williams Gynae 3rd/ed, p353*
10. **Ans. is b, i.e. Increase in follicular pressure** *Ref: Williams Gynae 3rd/ed, p354*
11. **Ans. is c, i.e. 3 ng/mL** *Ref: Williams Gynae 3rd/ed, p354*
12. **Ans. is d, i.e. HCG** *Ref: Williams Gynae 3rd/ed, p355*
13. **Ans. is c i.e. FSH**
    - Initial phase of follicular development before enter in menstrual cycle i.e. from primordial to antral follicle is independent of gonadotropins.
    - Early follicular phase is FSH dependent
    - Late follicular phase is both FSH and LH dependent

14. **Ans. is c, i.e. Male infertility** *Ref: Goodman Gilman 13th/ed, p781*
    - GnRH agonists can be used by pulsatile and continuous dosing.
    - By pulsatile dosing they increase release of LH/FSH and estrogen and cause ovulation, spermatogenesis and increase synthesis estrogen and testosterone. Hence used for treatment of anovulation, oligospermia (male infertility), delayed puberty and sexual infantilism.
    - By continuous dosing, they decrease synthesis of estrogen and testosterone. Hence used for treatment of estrogen and testosterone dependent conditions like ER positive breast cancer, endometriosis, uterine fibroids, precocious puberty and prostate cancer.

CHAPTER 3

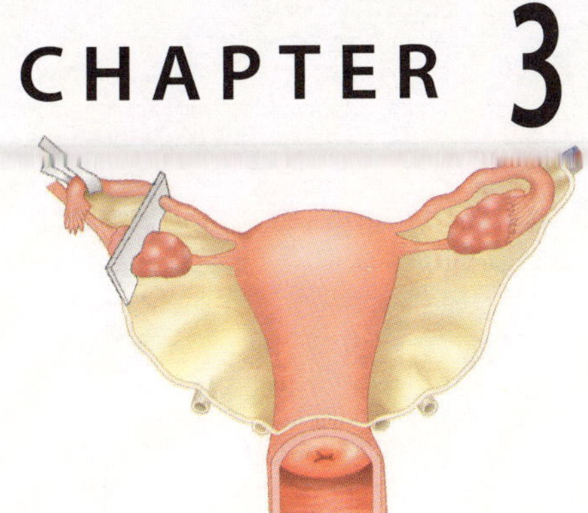

Menopause and HRT

Menopause and HRT

Menopause is derived from the Greek words 'men' (month) and 'pausis' (cessation)

It is permanent cessation of menses dated by the last menstrual period followed by 12 months of amenorrhea due to loss of ovarian activity

Perimenopause: Period of time surrounding menopause characterized by fluctuating hormone levels, irregular menstrual cycle and symptom asset.

- The average age of menopause is 51.5 years (with a normal range is 43–57) years.
- In India, age of menopause is 47 years.
- Menopause transition is seen between 40 to 51 years (average age of onset of menopause transition = 47 years) and it typically spans 4 to 7 years.

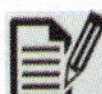

Important Concept

- Smoking is one of the major causes of early menopause.
- Increase in FSH (≥ 40 IU/L) is sine quanon for menopause
- Premature menopause—If menopause occurs at an age of 40 or earlier in a female
- Delayed menopause—If menopause fails to occur by 55 years or more.

Also Know

- Reproductive age , Menopause and Postmenopause period in a female life can be staged by STRAW system
- In the Straw system, the anchor stage (main event) is final menopause period (FMP).

5 stages precede FMP and 2 stages follow FMP (See Table 3.1 for details).

Table 3.1: Straw system of staging

Stage	Period	Important points
–5	Early reproductive period	
–4	Reproductive peak	
–3	Late reproductive period	FSH levels begin to increase from stage–3, not because of decreasing estrogen but due to decreasing inhibin levels.
–2	Early menopause transition	Variable cycle length (>7 days different from normal)
–1	Late menopause transition	• Estrogen production decreases significantly • Vasomotor symptoms—Hot flushes experienced in stage –1 and + 1 • ≥ / = 2 skipped cycles and at least one intermenstrual interval of • ≥ / = 60 days
Final Menopause Period		Vasomotor symptoms—Hot flushes experienced in stage s–1, 0 and + 1
+1a	1 year following menopause	Vasomotor symptoms—Hot flushes experienced in stages –1, 0 and + 1
+1b	2–5 years post menopause	
+2	Remaining life	

Pathophysiology

Flowchart 3.1

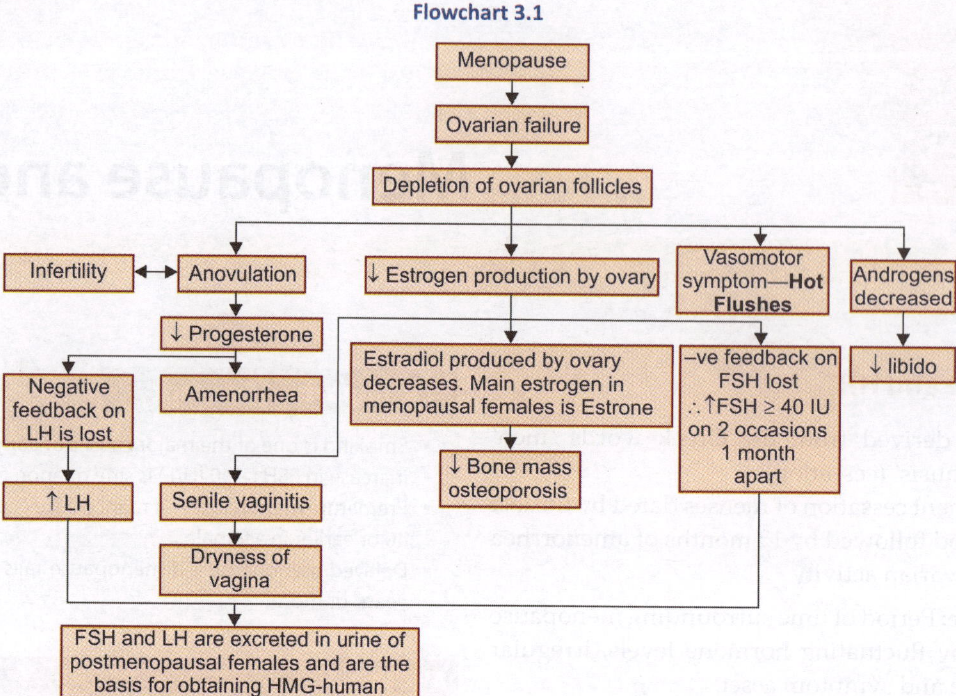

Pathology

Hypothalamic Pituitary Ovarian Axis

- The levels of FSH and LH increase and become ≥ 40 IU. Initially FSH levels increase, later on LH increases. The increase in FSH is 10–20 times whereas of LH is 3 times. This is because LH is cleared from blood more faster (half life of LH is 20 mins) than FSH (half life is 3 hrs) and perhaps because there is no specific negative feedback peptide like inhibin for LH .
- **Serum estradiol** decreases (as the number of follicles decrease in ovary) = <20 pg/mL
- **Levels of Inhibin** decrease
- **Levels of Anti Mullerian hormone**—decrease

Anti Mullerian hormone is a glycoprotein secreted by Granulosa cells of secondary and preantral follicles. AMH levels decrease progressively and markedly across menopause transition as the number of follicles decrease.
As AMH levels correlate with the number of follicles, hence it is also used as a test for ovarian reserve (which you will read about in chapter on Infertility)

Androgen production by ovary:

- **Androstenedione** decreases by 50% in post menopausal females. The main source of this hormone after menopause is adrenal gland.
- Testosterone levels in premenop a usal and post menopausal females is roughly same. On one side all hormones are decreasing on other side testosterone remains normal—this is because gonadal cells present in ovary produce more testosterone because of increased GnRH as estrogen is low so negative feedback of estrogen is gone. Also as estrogen decreases so SHBG decreases, free testosterone increases and this explains hirsutism, defeminisation and even virilisation seen in menopausal females.
- **Levels of androgens** produced by adrenal also decrease especially DHEAS and DHEA by 80% and 60% respectively. This is called as Adrenopause. The mechanism responsible for it is unknown.

Note

At menopause ovarian function completely stops, so levels of estradiol decrease. But adrenal function does not stop, it decreases. So whatever androgens are produced by adrenal are converted to esterone in adipose tissue with the help of enzyme aromatase.

- M/C estrogen during menopause is E1 (Esterone)

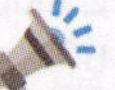

Important One Liners on FSH

It is the hormone which initiates ovarian cycle

- In menopausal females—levels of FSH are increased
- Human menopausal gonadotropin (hMG)—is FSH and LH obtained from the urine of postmenopausal females
- FSH levels can help in differentiating the causes of male infertility viz:
  - In pretesticular cause of male infertility = FSH ↓
  - In testicular cause = FSH ↑
  - In post testicular cause = FSH is normal

Ovary

- As we know at 20 weeks of intrauterine life the number of follicles are maximum i.e. 6 to 7 million
- At time of birth, they decrease and become 1-2 million
- From birth onwards, primordial follicles constantly are activated, mature partially and then regress.
- A more depletion of ovarian follicles starts in the late 30s and early 40s and continues until a point at which the menopausal ovary is completely devoid of follicles.

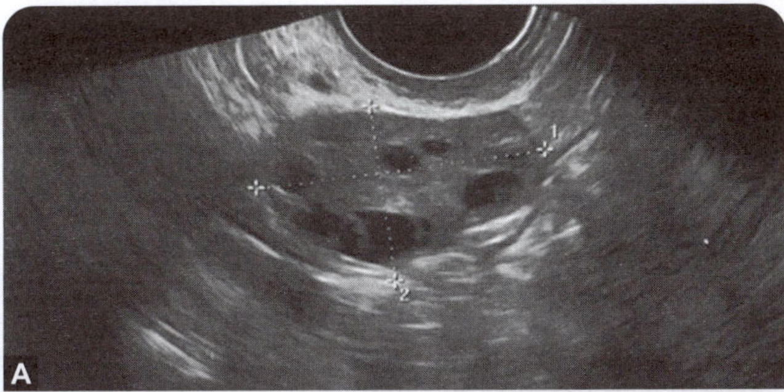

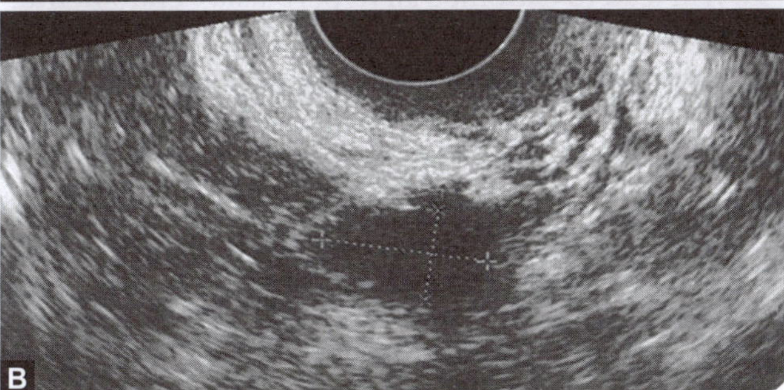

Figs. 3.1A and B: Transvaginal sonographic images of a pre-and postmenopausal ovary. (A) In general, premenopausal ovaries have greater volume and contain follicles, which are seen as multiple, small, anechoic smooth-walled cysts, (B) In comparison, post menopausal ovaries have smaller volume and are characteristically devoid of follicular structures

Endometrium

- During menopause transition (MT), abnormal uterine bleeding (AUB) is common. Anovulation is the most common cause of erratic bleeding during MT. However, because the time interval surrounding menopause is characterized by relatively high, cyclic estrogen levels and relatively low progesterone production, women in MT are at increased risk for developing endometrial hyperplasia or carcinoma. Estrogen-sensitive neoplasms, such as endometrial polyps and uterine leiomyomas, and pregnancy-related events are also considered. Many woman in their late 40s do not consider themselves fertile and will cease contraception but will still have occasional ovulatory cycles. Contraception can be discontinued by all women at age 55. No spontaneous pregnancies above that age have been reported. Some women may still have menstrual bleeding above age 55, but ovulation is rare and any oocytes are likely poor quality and not viable.
- In all women, regardless of menopausal status, the etiology of AUB should be determined as outlined in Chapter 8. As noted, endometrial cancer is suspected in any woman in menopause transition with AUB. The overall incidence of endometrial cancer is approximately 0.1 percent of women in this group per year, but in women with AUB in MT, the risk increases to 10 percent. Thus endometrial biopsy is done to exclude malignancy.

Vaginal Cytology

- Vaginal epithelium shows predominance of Basal and Parabasal cells.
- Maturation index- 100/0/0
- Doderlein bacilli are lost, so vaginal pH increases and becomes alkaline.
- Without estrogen's trophic influence, the vagina loses collagen, adipose tissue, and ability to retain water. As vaginal walls shrink, rugae flatten, and the vagina attains smooth-walled, pale-pink appearance. The thin vaginal surface is friable and prone to submucosal petechial hemorrhages or bleeding with minimal trauma. The blood vessels in the vaginal walls narrow, and over time the vagina itself contracts and loses flexibility.

Genitourinary Syndrome of Menopause

- Oestrogen deficiency has deleterious effects on the urogenital system. It has been reported that as many as one-third of women aged 50 years and older experience urogenital problems. Oestrogen deficiency results in a:
  - Thin and paler vaginal mucosa
  - Loss of normal rugosities
  - The moisture content is low
  - The pH increases (usually pH > 5)
  - May exhibit inflammation and small petechiae
  - Cytology reveals a loss in superficial cells and an increase of basal and parabasal cells
  - In reproductive age women, the vaginal flora is dominated by lactobacilli. In post-menopausal women, the vagina is gradually repopulated with diverse flora, including pathogenic organisms commonly found in urinary tract infections (e.g. coliform bacteria), as a result of the reduced acidity. The decrease in lactobacilli, yeast, and

bacterial vaginosis-associated bacteria also may explain the lower incidence of bacterial vaginosis and yeast vaginitis in post-menopausal women than in women of reproductive age.
  - The lower urinary tract and the genital tract in females have a common embryological origin. Oestrogen receptors have been reported in the trigone of the bladder and the proximal and distal urethra.
- Functional changes, which have been noted, include the following:
  - Elderly women have lower flow rates
  - Higher bladder volume at the first sensation to void
  - Increasing urinary residue
- Similarly, changes in collagen in the endopelvic fascial and periurethral tissue account for the hypermobility. and reduced urethral closure pressure and may thus explain the prevalence of stress incontinence.
- Dry and atrophic vaginal and urethral epithelium can cause:
  - Vaginal discomfort
  - Itching
  - Dyspareunia
  - Recurrent vaginitis.
- International Society for Study of Women's Sexual Health and North American Menopause Society came to a consensus to replace atrophic vaginitis with new terminology of GSM–genitourinary syndrome of menopause.

> GSM is defined as a collection of symptoms and signs associated with a decrease in oestrogen and other sex steroids involving changes to the labia majora/minora, clitoris, vestibule/introitus, vagina, urethra, and bladder. The syndrome may include but is not limited to genital symptoms of dryness, but lubrication, discomfort or pain, and impaired function; and urinary symptoms of urgency, dysuria and recurrent urinary tract infections. Women may present with some or all of the signs and symptoms, which must be bothersome and should not be better accounted for by another diagnosis.

Transvaginal Route and Drugs Available as

- Vaginal creams: Creams for local benefits are available and their absorption is limited and mainly used for local effects
- Oestradiol ring releases 8 mg oestradiol per 24 hours at a constant rate. The ring is easy to insert and remove, as it is soft and flexible. Each ring is to be used continuously for 90 days and is well tolerated giving significant relief from vaginal dryness, itching, dyspareunia, and dysuria. Vaginal tablets of oestradiol are also available.
- Local oestrogen therapy is effective for symptoms of vaginal atrophy, although it is not effective for the management of vasomotor symptoms and cannot reduce the risk for osteoporosis.
- Vaginal estrogen therapy reduces vaginal pH by restoring lactobacilli.
- When low-dose oestrogen is administered locally for vaginal atrophy, progestogen is generally not indicated.

Menopausal Symptoms and Treatment

As seen in Pathophysiology of menopause, basic problem in menopause is due to decreased estrogen levels.

Hence replacing estrogen, i.e, HRT is the mainstay of therapy in Menopause.

Rules for HRT

- **If females uterus is intact**– give estrogen and progesterone (because if you give estrogen alone, it will lead to endometrial hyperplasia/ endometrial cancer).
- **If females uterus is removed**–give only estrogen

Benefits of HRT

- Increased bone mineral density
- Decreased risk of fractures
- Decreased vasomotor symptoms
- Decreased rates of colorectal cancer

Indications of HRT

- Main indication for prescribing HRT is hot flushes
- Prevention of osteoporosis

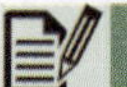

Important Concept

Special groups of women who require HRT:
- Premature ovarian failure
- Gonadal dysgenesis
- Surgical or radiation menopause

Types	
Estrogen • Can be given oral or transdermal • Transdermal is preferred for women with hypertriglyceridemia or impaired hepatic function • Given alone in women who have undergone hysterectomy	Estrogen and Progestin • Women with an intact uterus to decrease the risk of endometrial cancer

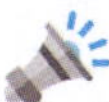

Important One Liners

Risk of coronary heart disease does not decrease by giving HRT but rather risk increases after giving HRT

Hormonal Treatment Options

- Estrogen should be given continuously. The estrogen commonly used is conjugated estrogen (0.625 mg), micronized estradiol (1-2 mg), ethinyl estradiol (5 mcg).
- Progestogen is given in addition to estrogen in women who have an intact uterus, to reduce the risk of endometrial hyperplasia.
- Earlier sequential combined regime was used, whereby estrogen was administered daily & progestone for 2 weeks, every month. This results in withdrawal cyclical bleeding. These days continuous combined therapy is used as it provides 'period-free' therapy for patients.
- Progestin IUD (Mirena) can also be used in post-menopausal women.
- Transdermal estrogen therapy is the method of choice for the following patients:
  - Women at high risk for thromboembolism
  - Women with hypertriglyceridemia
  - Obese women with metabolic syndrome

Absolute contraindications to HRT ABCD

A = Acute liver disease or current gallbladder disease
B = Undiagnosed vaginal bleeding
C = Cancer (breast/uterine)
D = DVT (thrombo-embolic disease) or its history

Also Know

HRT is associated with increased risk of:
S = stroke
V = venous thromboembolism
C = cholecystitis
H = coronary heart disease
Bharat= Breast cancer (Breast cancer appears only to be a risk factor with long term use of > 5 years).

Vasomotor Symptoms

- Thermoregulatory and cardiovascular changes that accompany a hot flush are well documented. An individual hot flush generally lasts 1 to 5 minutes, and skin temperatures rise because of peripheral vasodilation. This change is particularly marked in the fingers and toes, where skin temperature can increase 10 to 15°C. Most women sense a sudden wave of heat that spreads over the body, particularly the upper body and face. Sweating begins primarily on the upper body, and corresponds closely in time with an increases in skin conductance.
- So at the time of hot flush temperature increases , but 5 to 9 minutes after a hot flush temperature decreases due to sweating.
- Hot flushes can also be accompanied by palpitations, anxiety, irritability and panic.
- The flush coincides with a surge of LH (not FSH)

Cause of Vasomotor Symptoms

- Sudden decrease in levels of estrogen. This is the main cause of vasomotor symptoms. But remember if levels of estrogen are already low like in Turners syndrome, such females do not experience hot flushes unless first exposed to estrogen and then withdrawn from treatment.
- Norepinephrine and serotonin are the neurotransmitters which trigger hot flushes .

Management of Vasomotor Symptoms

The mainstay of management/first line treatment of vasomotor symptoms is HRT.

Rules for HRT

If females uterus is intact—give estrogen and progesterone (because if you give estrogen alone, it will lead to endometrial hyperplasia/endometrial cancer).
If females uterus is removed—give only estrogen.

- Tibolone[Q] (it is STEAR-selective tissue estrogen activity regulator, which has estrogenic, progestogenic, and androgenic properties)
- **Non-hormonal prescription medicines:** (not approved by FDA)
  - Clonidine[Q]
  - Selective serotonin reuptake inhibitor: paroxetine, fluoxetine
  - Serotonin and norepinephrine[Q] reuptake inhibitor: venlafaxine[Q]
  - Dopamine antagonist : Veralipride[Q]
  - Gabapentin[Q]
  - Bellergal (combination of ergotamines, phenobarbital and belladona, approved for the treatment of migrain).[Q]
  - Mirtazapine
  - Trazodone

Non-prescription Medicines

- Isoflavones (100 mg/day)[Q]
- Soy products (60 g/d)[Q]
- Vitamin E (800 IU/day)

Osteoporosis

It is the single most important health hazard associated with menopause

- Osteoporosis is loss of bone strength resulting in an increased risk of fracture

- Diagnosis is made by determining Bone Mineral Density (BMD) by Dual Energy X-ray Absorptiometry (DEXA) scan
- **BMD is best measured at hip** (and predictive of hip fracture and fracture at other sites)

T scores: Standard deviation between patient and average young adult bone mass. The more negative the score is, the greater is the risk of fracture
Z scores: It corresponds to the same measurements using women of same age as the reference. Definitions based on Bone Mineral Density normal T score –0 to –1 SD Osteopenia–T score –1 to –2.5; SD Osteoporosis–T score below –2.5 SD

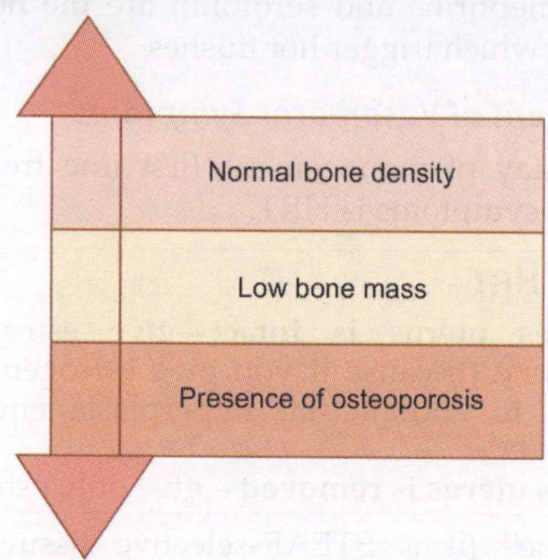

Fig. 3.2: T-score normal, osteopenia, and osteoporosis

The clinical relevance of a BMD in a postmenopausal woman is estimated by using the T score. For younger women, interpretation utilizes the Z score.

Markers of Bone formation: Serum Bone specific Alkaline Phosphatase and Osteocalcin
Markers of bone resorption: Serum C- telopeptide (CTX) and urinary N telopeptide (NTX)

Screening for Osteoporosis

- Screening for osteoporosis should be offered to any postmenopausal patient who presents with a fracture.
- Other candidates for bone mineral density determination are women older than age of 65
- The US Preventive Services Task Force recommends screening at the age of 60 for women who have risk factors for osteoporosis. The strongest risk factors for osteoporosis are:
  - Older age >65 years
  - Early menopause
  - Malabsorption syndrome
  - Systemic glucocorticoid therapy > 3 months
  - Hypogonadism
  - Primary Hyperparathyroidism
  - Body weight <57 kg
  - Excessive caffeine or alcohol intake
  - Smoker
  - Sedentary life style

Bone losing medications are:
- Chronic and excessive exposure to thyroxine
- Glucocorticoid therapy
- SSRI therapy
- Proton pump inhibiting drugs
- Aromatase inhibitors

Physiology of Bones

- Bone is constantly being remodelled in a dynamic process where osteoblasts are responsible for bone formation and osteoclasts for its resorption.
- Osteoblast regulate the activity of osteoclast by producing a **Rank ligand** which binds to its receptor, **Rank**, on the surface of osteoclast cells, inducing their differentiation and helping them to bring about bone resorption.
- On the other hand, osteoblasts secrete a soluble **protein osteoprotegerin**, (OPG) that blocks **Rank/Rank** ligand interaction and, thus, brings about osteoclast apoptosis.
- Now estrogen promotes the formation of OPG and that is how it increases bone mass by decreasing bone resorption.
- Thus if we have to treat osteoporosis , either the drug has to act on osteoblast and increase bone formation or it has to act on osteoclast i.e. enhance its apoptosis and decrease bone resorption.

Drugs acting on osteoblast- i.e. act by promoting bone formation	Drugs acting on osteoclast i.e they act by preventing bone resorption
Teriparatide: It is recombinant PTH	**Bisphosphonates** (Alendronate 10 mg, Risedronate, Ibandronate)
Strontium Ranelate: inhibits bone resorption as well as stimulates bone formation	**Estrogen/ SERM e.g. Raloxifene (60 mg), Bazedoxifene (20 mg)**
	Calcitonin/Salcalcitonin
	Denosumab: monoclonal antibody against RANK ligand

Drugs acting on osteoclast
- **B**- Bisphosphonates
- **C**-Calcitonin/Salcalcitonin
- **D**-Denosumab
- **E**-Estrogen/SERM

Another way of classifying these drugs is:

Drugs to prevent osteoporosis	Drug to prevent and treat osteoporosis	Drugs to treat osteoporosis
Calcium	Estrogen	Denosumab
Vitamin D	SERM	Teriparatide
Calcitonin	Bisphosphonate	Strontium Ranelate
	Tibolone	

Management Protocol for Osteoporosis

1st line – Bisphosphonate

2nd line

- Combined estrogen and progestin therapy (if uterus is intact)
- Only estrogen (if female is hysterectomised)
- Tibolone (STEAR)
- Raloxifene (SERM)

Bisphosphonates

- They are 1st line of treatment of osteoporosis.
- These agents are used for the treatment of osteoporosis due to their inhibitory effect on osteoclast mediated bone resorption. These drugs accelerate apoptosis of osteoclasts and also suppress differentiation of osteoclast precursors to mature osteoclasts (by inhibiting IL-6).

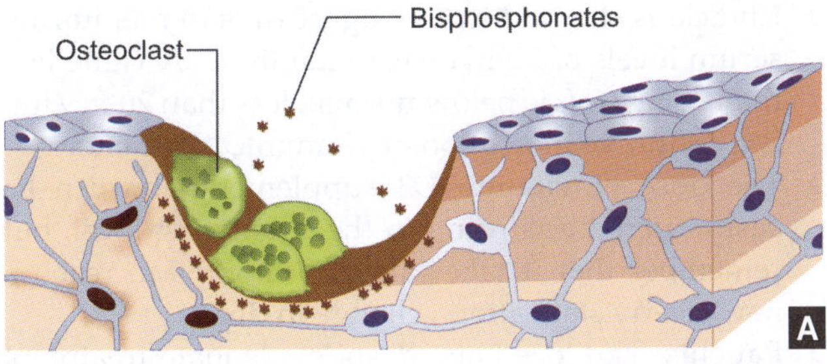

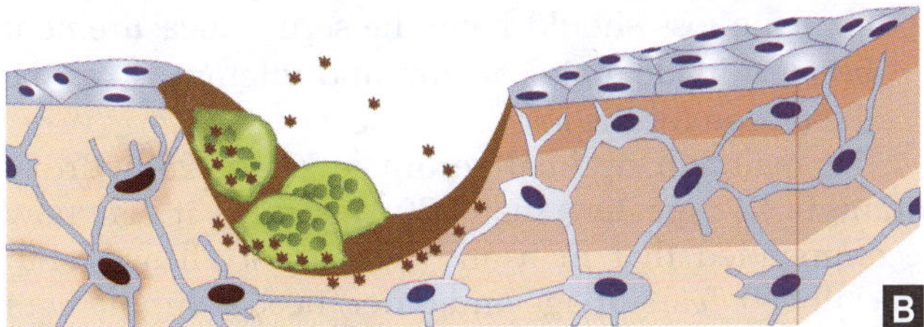

Figs. 3.3A and B: Bisphosphonates reduce fractures by suppressing bone resorption by osteoclasts. The molecular structure of the bisphosphonates is analogous to that of the naturally occurring pyrophosphates. (A) Bisphosphonate concentrations is increased eightfold at sites of active bone resorption. (B) The bisphosphonates enter osteoclasts and reduce resorption through inhibition **of farnesyl pyrophosphate synthase**. Inhibition of this enzyme leads to disruption of osteoclast attachment to the bone surface. This halts resorption and promotes early osteoclast cell death.

- Drugs in the group include Alendronate/Risedronate/Ibandronate which are all given orally and Zolendronate which is given IV.
- Side effects are heart burn, esophageal irritation, esophagitis, diarrhea and **its long term side effects are osteonecrosis of jaw and atypical femur fracture**.
- The onset of severe pain at any site is an indication to discontinue bisphosphonate treatment.
- Maximum it should be used for 5 years.

Patient should take each dose after an overnight fast, while sitting in the upright position and should follow by drinking a glass of water and should remain upright and not eat for 30 minutes after administration.

Main contraindications of bisphosphonates are renal dysfunction, esophageal motility disorders and peptic ulcer.

Raloxifene

- Raloxifene is a Selective Estrogen Receptor Modulator (SERM)[Q].
- SERM are compounds that act as both estrogen agonist and antagonists depending on the tissue.
- Raloxifene exercises estrogen-like action on both bones and lipids and estrogen antagonist on breast or endometrium.
- Reduces the risk of vertebral fracture by 50%. *Note:* Raloxifene has least effect on the reduction rate of hip fracture.
- It causes 10% reduction in total and low density lipoprotein and raises HDL.
- It does not raise the level of triglycerides, hence it is cardioprotective in long term.
- It does not have a proliferative effect on endometrium, so raloxifene is not associated with an increase in the risk of uterine cancer.

It decreases the risk of breast cancer

Side Effects: Hot flushes (so it cannot be used in managing hot flushes), cramps, increased incidence of retinopathy, and venous thrombosis.[Q]

KEY POINTS

- Hot flushes are a side effect of raloxifene therapy, hence raloxifene cannot be used to treat it.

Contraindications

- Venous thrombosis
- It should not be given with estrogen
- Hepatic dysfunction
- Stop the drug 72 hours before surgery
- Not to be given with drugs such as indomethacin, naproxen, ibuprofen, and diazepam.

Note: **Bazedoxine** is like Raloxifene but can be combined with estrogen—TSEC i.e. Tissue selective estrogen complex. The idea is to gain benefits of estrogen (as bazedoxifene has little effect on hot flushes), protect the endometrium and possibly breast, and enhance some actions of estrogen, such as reduction in fractures. This approach to postmenopausal therapy may eliminate the need for progestational agents.

Hence this combination can be used both for managing osteoporosis and hot flushes.

Teriparatide

- It has been noted that PTH in low and pulsatile dose stimulates bone formation whereas in excess it causes resorption of bones.
- So Teriparatide which is recombinant parathyroid hormone when given in low pulsatile doses, can increase bone formation.
- It is given in daily subcutaneous injection and is approved by FDA for treatment of postmenopusal women with established osteoporosis who are at increased risk of fracture.
- Its rare side effect is osteosarcoma of bones and its use is not recommended for more than 2 years.

Denosumab

- It is a fully human monoclonal antibody to RANK ligand.
- This inhibits osteoclast development and activity. And in turn decreases bone resorption and increases BMD.
- Dose: 60 mcg subcutaneous once every 6 months.

Calcitonin

- **Calcitonin** is a hormone that is produced in humans by the parafollicular cells (commonly known as C-cells) of the thyroid gland.
- **Calcitonin** is involved in helping to regulate levels of calcium and phosphate in the blood, opposing the action of parathyroid hormone.
- More specifically, calcitonin lowers blood Ca^{2+} levels in two ways:
  - **Major effect:** Inhibits *osteoclast* activity in bones
  - **Minor effect:** Inhibits *renal tubular cell* reabsorption of Ca^{2+} and phosphate, allowing them to be excreted in the *urine*
  - Salcalcitonin or synthetic calcitonin can be taken only by women who are at least five years post menopause .
  - Patients with severe osteoporosis seem to do the best with this drug.
  - It is a protein so its oral administration leads to its digestion.
  - It can be given by Nasal spray or by injection.
  - Salmon calcitonin nasal spray has been associated with reduction in vertebral fracture risk amongst post menopausal women with osteoporosis.
  - 200 IU of nasal spray daily for up to 5 years reduces the risk of vertebral fracture by 33%.
  - Nasal or I/V calcitonin is associated with 10% incidence of nausea or gastric discomfort, 10% chances of local site reaction and 3% chance of RHINITIS.

Role and dose of Vitamin D

Osteoporosis releated to aging is due significantly to age-related changes in Vitamin D and calcium metabolism. There is an age-related decrease in the ability of tissues to convert the major circulating form of vitamin, 25-hydroxy vitamin D, to the active from of vitamin D (1,25 dihydroxycholecalciferol, better known as 1,25 dithydroxy vitamin D), and there is a decrease in the ability of the intestine to absorb dietary vitamin D. Exposure of the skin to ultraviolet rays in sunlight stimulates the formation of cholecalciferol (vitamin D3).

Because adequate and active vitamin D depends on cutaneous generation mediated by sun exposure, women in the winter months can easily be relatively vitamin D deficient and lose bone. In far northern and southern areas, the winter sunlight is inadequate to stimulate dermal activation. But even, in areas of the world where there is adequate sun exposure, Inadequate dietary intake and an indoor lifestyle yield a significant number of women with abnormally low levels of circulating 25-hydroxy vitamin D. In addition, clothing and sunscreens prevent the cutaneous production of vitamin D3.

Measurement of 25-hydroxyvitamin D

- Clinicians should be more aggressive in monitoring serum levels of 25-hydroxy vitamin D. A value less than 30 ng/mL is below normal; less than 20 ng/mL is a definitive indication of vitamin D deficiency.
- The dose of vitamin D3 supplementation can be easily titered according to the circulating level, but remember that it takes about 3 months to reach a new steady state after a change in dose.
- Patients who lose bone despite adequate treatment for bone loss should have the serum measurement because inadequate calcium and vitamin D can be the reason for the loss.

To maintain optimal serum levels of 25-hydroxy vitamin D, greater than 30 ng/mL, it is now recommended that men and women of all ages, but specially 60 years of age and older, need a supplement of 1000 to 2000 IU vitamin D3 daily.

Calcium Supplementation

- There has been considerable confusion over whether calcium supplementation by itself can offer protection against postmenopausal osteoporosis.
- Calcium absorption decreases with age because of a decrease in biologically active vitamin D and

becomes significantly impaired after menopause. A positive calcium balance is mandatory to achieve adequate prevention against osteopororis.

- Calcium supplementation (1,000 mg/day) reduces bone loss and decreases fractures, especially in individuals with low daily intakes.
- Estrogen acts to improve calcium absorption by increasing the levels of 1, 25-dihydroxy vitamin D and makes it possible to utilize effective supplemental calcium in lower doses.
- In order to remain in zero calcium balance, women on estrogen therapy require total of 1,000 mg elemental calcium per day.
- Because the average woman receives about 500 mg of calcium in her diet, the minimal daily supplement for women on estrogen equals an additional 500 mg.
- Women not on estrogen require a daily supplement of at least 1,000 mg calcium reach the recommended intake of 1,500 mg/day.

Also Know

Women's Health Initiative (WHI)

- The study investigated health risks and benefits of hormone therapy in healthy postmenopausal women aged 50–79 old.
- **In the study** continuous combined HRT (estrogen 0.625 mg + medroxy progesterone acetate 2.5 mg OD) was given to 16,608 women with an intact uterus—Originally designed to run for 8.5 years but stopped early after 5.2 years (July 2002) because the evidence for harm (breast cancer, CHD, stroke, pulmonary embolism) outweighed benefit (fracture reduction and colon cancer reduction)

Contd...

Contd...

- Estrogen alone (0.625 mg) was given alone to 10,732 women with a previous hysterectomy—This arm was also stopped early (February 2004 instead of March 2005) because of increased stroke risk and no heart disease benefit.

Denosumab

- Osteoclasts express a receptor called **receptor for activated nuclear factor k B** (RANK) on its surface. When this receptor is stimulated by RANK ligand, bone resorption results due to activation of osteoclasts. Denosumab is monoclonal antibody against this ligand and is useful for the treatment of osteoporosis.

Strontium Ranelate

- It has a novel mechanism of action as it inhibits bone resorption as well as stimulates bone formation. Strontium is incorporated into hydroxyapatite, replacium. Small increased risk of venous thrombosis, seizures are abnormal cognition have been seen with them.
- Strontium ranelate inhibits bone resorption as well as stimulates bone formation.

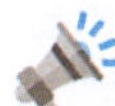

Important One Liners

Special groups of women who require HRT:

- Premature ovarian failure
- Gonadal dysgenesis
- Surgical or radiation menopause

NEW PATTERN QUESTIONS

N1. Marker for menopause transition is:
a. Menstrual irregularity
b. Hot flushes
c. ↓ bone mass
d. Cessation of menstruation

N2. Menopause transition of a female is from:
a. 30–49 years b. 35–49 years
c. 40–51 years d. 40–60 years

N3. Main estrogenic hormone in postmenopausal females is:
a. Estradiol b. Estrone
c. Estriol d. Estetrol

N4. The cut-off point of serum estrogen level for the diagnosis of ovarian failure:
a. 10 pg/mL b. 20 pg/mL
c. 30 pg/mL d. 40 pg/mL

N5. All of the following are related to hormonal changes in postmenopausal females *except:*
a. Hot flushes b. Weight gain
c. Osteoporosis d. Coronary heart disease

N6. Contraception can be discontinued by all women at age:
a. ≥ 45 years age b. ≥ 50 years
c. ≥ 55 years d. ≥ 60 years

N7. A 56-year-old post-menopausal on HRT, minimal daily supplement of calcium is:
a. 500 mg b. 1000 mg
c. 1500 mg d. 2000 mg

N8. Recommended daily supplement of vitamin D3 for females is:
a. 200–500 IU b. 500–1000 IU
c. 1000–2000 IU d. 2000–2500 IU

N9. Best predictor of heart disease in menopausal females:
a. Total cholesterol
b. Estrogen levels
c. HDL-cholesterol levels
d. Total LHDL levels

N10. Indication for using estrogen and progesterone in a hysterectomized female are all *except:*
a. Females undergone supracervical hysterotomy
b. Females with endometriosis
c. Females with endometrioid tumors of the ovary
d. Females with fibroid of uterus

N11. All of the following tests are recommended for preventive health screening in postmenopausal females *except:*
a. Mammography b. Colonoscopy
c. TSH levels d. Estrogen levels

N12. A 45-year-old female who had total abdominal hysterectomy and bilateral salpingo-oophorectomy for endometriosis attends the clinic after 1 year with vasomotor symptoms. What is the best management option?
a. Continuous combined HRT
b. Estrogen only HRT
c. Raloxifene
d. Tibolone

N13. Best time to check levels of FSH to detect menopausal transition:
a. Day 2–5 after LMP b. Day 7–10 after LMP
c. Day 11–14 after LMP d. Just before mestruation

N14. Average age of menopause is:
a. 45 years b. 47 years
c. 49 years d. 51 years

N15. Best treatment for hot flushes:
a. OCP b. Estrogen
c. Clonidine d. Vitamin E

N16. Contraindication for estrogen therapy nearly are all *except:*
a. Uterine cancer b. Breast cancer
c. Hypertension
d. Previous H/O thromboembolism

N17. Hot flushes are experienced by a menopause female in stage:
a. –4 b. –3
c. –2 d. –1

N18. All of the following drugs are used in managing osteoporosis *except:*
a. Alendronate b. Teriparatide
c. Denosumab d. Fluoxetine

N19. Drug active on osteoblast:
a. Alendronate b. Strontium
c. Calcitonin d. Denosumab

N20. Bisphosphonates act by inhibition of enzyme:
a. Aromatase b. Carbonic anhydrase
c. Pyrophosphate synthetase
d. Hydroxylase

PREVIOUS YEAR QUESTIONS

1. **Which of these is diagnostic of menopause?** *(AIIMS Nov 2015)*
   a. Serum FSH > 40 b. Serum LH > 20
   c. Serum FSH < 40 d. Serum estradiol < 30
2. **HRT is helpful in all of the following *except*:** *(AIIMS Nov 06, AIIMS May 2013, JIPMER May 2014)*
   a. Vaginal atrophy b. Flushing
   c. Osteoporosis d. Coronary heart disease
3. **Hormone replacement therapy (HRT) is indicated in:** *(PGI Nov 2012)*
   a. Cardiovascular disease
   b. Osteoporosis
   c. Hot flushes
   d. Atrophic vaginitis
4. **Estrogen administration in a menopausal woman increases the:** *(AIIMS May 06)*
   a. Gonadotropin secretion
   b. LDL - cholesterol
   c. Bone mass
   d. Muscle mass
5. **True regarding postmenopausal osteoporosis is:** *(PGI May 00)*
   a. Decreased vitamin D
   b. Decreased serum calcium
   c. Normal serum chemistries
   d. Decreased vitamin C
   e. Smoking
6. **Non-hormonal drug to prevent post menopausal osteoporosis is:** *(Delhi 99)*
   a. Alendronate b. Estrogen
   c. Raloxifene d. Parathyroid
7. **All of the following are the advantages of using Raloxifene over estrogen in postmenopausal women *except*:** *(AI 04)*
   a. Reduces fracture rates
   b. Avoids endometrial hyperplasia
   c. Reduces the incidence of venous thrombosis
   d. No increase in incidence of breast carcinoma
8. **A 48-year-old female suffering from severe menorrhagia (DUB) underwent hysterectomy. She wishes to take hormone replacement therapy. Physical examination and breast are normal but X-ray shows osteoporosis. The treatment of choice is:** *(AIIMS May 01)*
   a. Progesterone
   b. Estrogen and progesterone
   c. Estrogen
   d. None
9. **Basanti Devi, a 45 years old woman, presents with hot flushes after stopping of menstruation. 'Hot Flush' can be relieved by administration of following agents:** *(AI 02)*
   a. Ethinyl estradiol b. Testosterone
   c. Fluoxymesteron d. Danazol
10. **All of the following appear to decrease hot flushes in menopausal women *except*:** *(AI 05)*
    a. Androgens b. Raloxifene
    c. Isoflavones d. Tibolone
11. **Absolute contraindication of hormone replacement therapy is:** *(AIIMS Dec 98)*
    a. Thrombosis b. Fibrocystic disease
    c. Fibroadenoma d. Hemorrhage
12. **True statement related to HRT:** *(PGI May 2012)*
    a. ↓ Chance of Hip fracture
    b. ↓ Chance of Breast cancer
    c. ↓ Chance of Colon cancer
    d. ↓ Chance of Endometrial cancer
    e. ↑ Chance of DVT
13. **Finding(s) of atrophic vaginitis is/are:**
    a. Low pH of vagina
    b. Occur due to estrogen deficiency
    c. Frequent intercourse is useful
    d. Intercourse causes painless bleeding
    e. Estradiol vaginal ring is helpful
14. **Drugs used in HRT:** *(PGI Nov 2013)*
    a. Estrogen b. Corticosteroid
    c. Calcitonine d. Bisphosphonate
    e. Clomipnene citrate

ANSWERS TO NEW PATTERN QUESTIONS

N1. Ans. is a, i.e. Menstrual irregularity *Ref: Williams gynae 3rd/ed, p472*

There is only one marker of menopausal transition, is menstrual irregularity. The cycles have long intervals (greater than 60 days).

N2. Ans. is c, i.e. 40–51 years *Ref: Williams gynae 3rd/ed, p471*

> **Menopause:**
> Transition is between 40–51 years.
> Average duration = 4–7 years
> Average age of menopause = 41.5 years.

N3. Ans. is b, i.e. Estrone *Ref: Leon Speroff 8th/ed, p689*

Main estrogenic hormone during menopause = estrone

It is mainly derived from the peripheral conversion of androstenedione.

Levels of estrone in menopausal females = 30-70 pg/mL

Levels of estradiol in menopausal females = 10-20 pg/mL

N4. Ans. is b, i.e. 20 pg/mL *Ref: Dutta Gynae 6th/ed, p57,65*

Diagnosis of menopause or ovarian failure is made from classical symptom of hot flush (50%) confirmed by elevated FSH levels to more than 40 IU/mL and serum estradiol <20 pg/mL.

N5. Ans. is b, i.e. Weight gain

Weight gain in postmenopausal females is not due to any hormonal change but due to lifestyle changes.

N6. Ans. is c, i.e. ≥ 55 years *Ref: Williams gynae 3/e, p474)*

Contraception can be discontinued by all women at ≥ 55 years of age.

N7. Ans. is a, i.e. 500 mg *Ref: Leon Speroff 8th/ed, p729*

- In order to maintain zero calcium balance, women on estrogen therapy require a total of 1000 mg elemental calcium daily.
- Because the average woman receives about 500 mg of calcium in her diet, the minimal daily supplement for woman on estrogen equals additional 500 mg
- Women not on estrogen require a daily supplement of at least 1000 mg calcium to reach recommended intake of 1500 mg/day

Calcium Requirement for Zero Balance

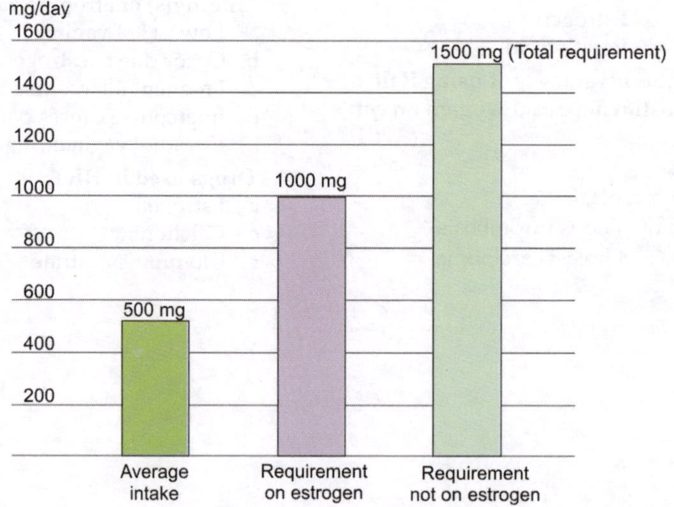

N8. Ans. is c, i.e. 1000–2000 IU *Ref: Leon Speroff 8th/ed, p731,734*

Recommended vitamin D supplementation of both males and females is 1000-2000 IU/day

Note: Levels of 25-hydroxy vitamin D should be measured annually in older individuals

> Values less than 30 ng/ml are below normal
> Values less than 20 ng/ml is an indication of definite vitamin D deficiency

N9. Ans. is c, i.e. HDL-cholesterol levels *Ref: Leon Speroff 8th/ed, p707*

The strongest prediction of coronary heart disease in woman is a low HDL-cholesterol.
Average HDL-cholesterol in women is 55-60 mg/dL.
If HDL-cholesterol is 10 mg/dL, it increases the risk of coronary heart disease by 40-50%

N10. Ans is d, i.e. Females with fibroid of uterus. *Ref: Leon Speroff 8th/ed, p762*

Normally in females who have undergone hysterectomy, only estrogen is given for HRT. But there are certain conditions in which, in spite of hysterectomy, both Estrogen and Progesterone are given (this is because these females have very high estrogen levels in their bodies).

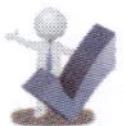

KEY POINTS

Indications of Estrogen and progesterone in hysterectomized women

1. Females with past history of endometriosis (due to the risk of adenocarcinoma if treated with only estrogen in such females)
2. Females who have undergone supracervical hysterectomy (as there is residual endometrium)
3. Females with adenocarcinoma of the endometrium
4. Females with history of endometroid tumors of the ovary.

N11. Ans. is d, i.e. Estrogen levels *Ref: Leon Speroff 8th/ed, p685*

Preventive Health Screening of Healthy Postmenopausal Women

1. A complete medical history and physical examination should be performed every 5 years, at age 40, 45, 50 & 55
2. Annual visits should include a breast and pelvic examination (including a rectovaginal examination), recording of BMI, screening for sexually transmitted infections, TSH assessment at 40 years & then every 2 yearly from 60 years (because hypothyroidism increases with age).
3. Bone mass should be measured in females over 65 years/females with fractures or females who have one or more risk factor for osteoporosis.
4. Annual screening mammography from 40 years
5. Colonoscopy is recommended at 50 and 55 years.

N12. Ans. is a, i.e. Continuous combined HRT

As discussed earlier in females who have had hysterectomy, then only estrogen can be used for HRT. But point to be noted here is the reason for hysterectomy is endometriosis and, as discussed in Q. N10, in such females even after hysterectomy, both endrogen and progesterone are used. So the answer is continuous combined HRT as HRT is first line of management for hot flushes.

N13. Ans. is a, i.e. Day 2–5 after LMP *Ref: Shaw gynae 16th/ed, p66*

Always Remember: for detecting FSH & LH due to any reason, best time is Day 2–3 of the cycle.

N14. Ans. is d, i.e. 51 years *Ref: Williams Gynae 3rd/ed, p471*

"The average age of women experiencing their final menstrual period (FMP) is 51.5 years, but a halt to menses from ovarian failure may occur at any age."

N15. Ans. is b, i.e. Estrogen *Ref: Williams gynae 3rd/ed, p495*

"Systemic estrogen therapy is the most effective treatment for vasomotor symptoms and the value of such treatments has been demonstrate in numerous RCTs" *Ref: Williams gynae 3rd/ed, p495*

Now one very important thing regarding HRT which has to be remembered is:
"It has to be given in lowest possible doses"
In the question there are 2 options:
OCP's and estrogen
Although in females whose uterus is intact estrogen is given along with progesterone but that does not mean we give OCP's

Now why not OCP's
In low dose OCP's the dosage of estrogen (ethinyl estradiol) is 20 mcg whereas for HRT the dose of daily estrogen is 5 mcg and now a days even 2.5 mcg is used.

So the best answer is option b, i.e. Estrogen (and not option a - OCP's)

N16. Ans. is c, i.e. Hypertension *Ref: Williams Gynae 3rd/ed, p495*

Absolute C/I for use of Estrogen:

1. Undiagnosed abnormal genital bleeding
2. Known/suspected or H/O breast cancer
3. Known/suspected estrogen dependent tumor
4. Active or prior venous thromboembolism or any thromboembolic disease
5. Liver dysfunction or disease
6. Known or suspected pregnancy.

N17. Ans. is d, i.e. –1

Hot flushes are experienced in stages –1, Menopause and + 1, see text for explanation)

N18. Ans. is d, i.e. Fluoxetine

Fluoxetine is SSRI used for managing flushes not osteoporosis

N19. Ans. is b, i.e. Strontium

Only 2 drugs act on osteoblast

1. Teriparatide
2. Strontrium

N20. Ans. is c, i.e. Pyrophosphate synthetase

See the text Fig. 3.3 for explanation

ANSWERS TO PREVIOUS YEAR QUESTIONS

1. Ans. is a, i.e. Serum FSH > 40 *Ref: Shaw's Textbook of Gynecology 15th/ed, p62*

Diagnostic Criteria for Menopause

- Estrogen (E2) low at 10–20 pg/mL
- Estrone (E1) – 30–70 pg/mL
- E2/E1 < 1
- Urine FSH > 40 IU/L

2. Ans. is d, i.e. Coronary heart disease

3. Ans. is b, c and d, i.e. Osteoporosis; Hot flushes; and Atrophic vaginitis

Ref: Harsision 16th/ed, p30, 18th/ed, p3043; Williams Gynae 1st/ed, p494; Jeffcoate 6th/ed, p105-106

- Friends, *(Harrison 16th/ed, p30)* breaks a popular myth of using HRT for prevention of coronary Heart disease. Until recently, it was believed that the sex specific effect of gonadal steroids on CVS and lipid metabolism accounted for the different rates of coronary heart disease (CHD) in women as compared to men.
- Estrogen increases HDL and decreases LDL whereas androgens have the opposite effect and this was further supported by the increase in incidence of CHD after menopause.
- These findings led to the widespread use of HRT for primary and secondary prevention of CHD.

But recent trials have shown an increase in the incidence of CHD in women placed on HRT as compared to those not on HRT. *Ref: Harrison 16th/ed, p30*

This fact is supported by *Williams Gynae. 3rd/ed, p494* which says—

"In the many reviews and discussions following WHI (Women Health Initiative), most clinicians agree that Hormone Therapy is associated with an increased risk of CHD in older menopausal women and an increased risk of breast cancer, stroke, venous thromboembolism and cholecystitis."

"The WHI randomized controlled trial of combination hormone therapy versus placebo shoed that hormone therapy didnot prevent heart disease in healthy women, but instead it increased the risk of cardiovascular events in older women" *Ref: Novak 15th/ed, p1242*

4. Ans. is c, i.e. Bone mass *Ref: Harrison 18th/ed, p3041; Novak 13th/ed, p1124; KDT 6th/ed, p298*

Before seeing any reference for the question let's rule out some options.

- Estrogen administration will exert a negative feedback on gonadotropin secretion and decreases gonadotropin secretion rather than increasing it (***Option 'a' ruled out***).

Option 'c', i.e. Bone mass

- Estrogen given as hormone replacement therapy is most beneficial in preventing osteoporosis, i.e. it must be increasing bone mass.

So, Option 'c' is correct.

Now have a look what texts have to say :

"Estrogen helps to maintain bone mass and skeletal integrity thereby protecting against osteoporosis." *Ref: Novak 13th/ed, p1124*

"Estrogen is important in maintaining bone mass primarily by retarding bone resorption." *Ref: KDT 6th/ed, p298*

Now for option b *Ref: Leon spent 8th/ed, p755*

Both oral and traditional estrogen: reduce
- Total cholesterol
- LDL
- Lipoprotein (a)

Compared to transdermal estrogen the oral estrogen significantly increases:
- HDL
- Triglycerides

Whereas transdermal estrogen decreases triglyceride. That is why transdermal estrogen is preferred in females with increased triglycerides level.

5. **Ans. is a, b and e, i.e. Decreased vitamin D; and Decreased serum calcium and smoking** *Ref: Leon speroff 8th/ed, p716*
   - During perimenopausal and postmenopausal period there is decrease in bone mass called as osteoporosis.
   - Main cause of osteoporosis in perimenopausal and postmenopausal period is decreased estrogen.

Other causes of decreased bone mass are shown in figure.

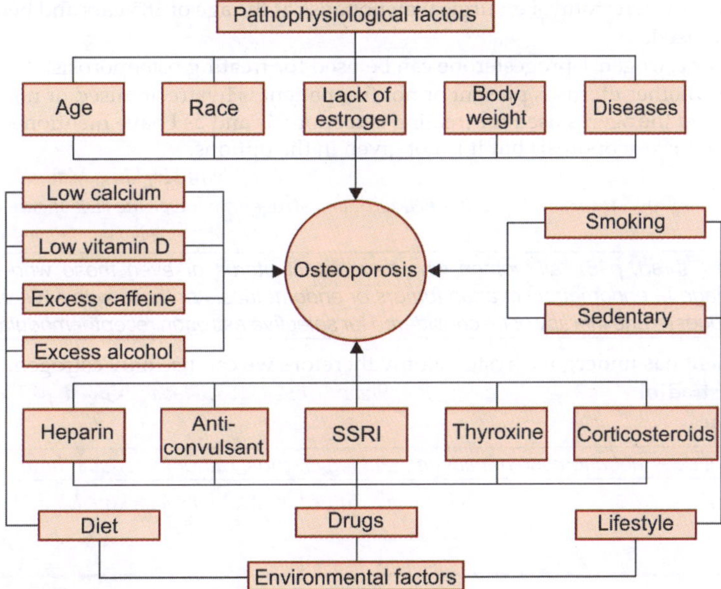

- Decreased calcium absorption
- Decrease in conversion of 25-hydroxy D3 to 1,25-dihydroxy D3, as a result of age-related decrease in hydroxylase activity.
- Amenorrhea (i.e. hypoestrogenism) is another cause of decreased bone mass.

6. **Ans. is a, i.e. Alendronate** *Ref: Novak 14th/ed, p1130*

Alenderonate, etidronate, pamidronate, and Ibandronate are bisphosphonates which inhibit bone resorption, and are very effective for both osteoporosis prevention and treatment.

Uses:
- First line drugs for treating postmenopausal osteoporosis
- Paget's disease
- Osteolytic bone metastasis.

Caution: *Patient should be instructed to take these drugs on an empty stomach with a large glass of water and then to remain upright for at least 30 minutes as its major side effect is GI upset.*

Route of administration: Oral or IV infusion

Now let's have a look at other options:
- *Raloxifene:* It is a selective estrogen receptor modulator which is also useful in management of osteoporosis but it is a hormonal preparation.
- *Parathyroid hormone:* It is a novel therapy for osteoporosis. Unlike most of the treatments for osteoporosis that inhibit bone resorption, parathyroid hormone stimulates new bone formation. It is given by daily subcutaneous injection.

Also Know

Other non-hormonal drugs used in osteoporosis:
a. Calcium
b. Vitamin D
c. Slow releasing sodium fluoride.

7. **Ans. is c, i.e. Reduces the incidence of venous thrombosis** *Ref: Shaw 15th/ed, p69*

Raloxifene increases the incidence of venous thrombosis rather than decreasing it.

It does not have a proliferative effect on endometrium, so it is not associated with an increase in the risk of uterine cancer.

Role of raloxifene in breast cancer.

"The SERM tamoxifen is an estrogen antagonist in the breast that is used in the treatment of estrogen-receptor positive breast cancer. Raloxifene also may reduce the risk of breast cancer. Postmenopausal women receiving raloxifene as part of a large osteoporosis treatment trial, experienced a 76% reduction in the risk of invasive breast cancer compared with placebo-treated women."

Ref: Novak 14th/ed, p1333

8. **Ans. is c, i.e. Estrogen** *Ref: Jeffcoate 7th/ed, p95 onwards; Williams Gynae 1st/ed, p495,499-500*

- The female underwent hysterectomy, i.e. surgical menopause at the age of 48 years and her X-ray shows osteoporosis—hence HRT can be advised.
- Both estrogen alone or estrogen + progesterone can be used for treating osteoporosis.

The choice depends on whether uterus is present or not (i.e. patient is hystrectomised or not).

We have already discussed the agents used for treating osteoporosis and as I have mentioned earlier bisphosphonates are the first line of treatment for osteoporosis but it is not given in the options.

(Ref: John Hopkin's Manual of Obs and Gynae 4th/ed, p513)

"For women with a uterus, a progestin should be combined with an estrogen, to lower the risk of endometrial cancer."

Ref: William Gynae 3rd/ed, p495

According to Jeffcoate (7th/ed, p96) "all women who have intact uterus or even those who underwent hysterectomy for endometrial Cancer (Stage I), endometroid ovarian tumors or endometriosis or those with severe osteoporosis should receive combined estrogen - progesterone therapy or be considered for selective estrogen receptor modulator therapy (SERM therapy)."

In the question the patient has undergone hysterectomy therefore we can use only estrogen.

9. **Ans. is a, i.e. Ethinyl estradiol** *Ref: Shaw 15th/ed, p67; Novak 14th/ed, p1326; Williams Gynae 1st/ed, p495*
10. **Ans. is b, i.e. Raloxifene** *Ref: Jeffcoates 7th/ed, p98*

Raloxifene is a SERM. It does not decrease hot flushes and leg cramps, rather increases them.

11. **Ans. is a, i.e. Thrombosis** *Ref: Novak 15th/ed, p1245; John Hopkins Manual of Obs and Gynae 4th/ed, p510*

Mnemonic

A = **A**ctive liver disease/or Gallbladder disease
B = Undiagnosed vaginal **b**leeding
C = **C**ancers of endometrium and breast
D = **D**eep vein thrombosis

12. **Ans. is a, c and e, i.e. Decreased chances of hip fracture, Decreased chances of colon cancer, Increased chance of Deep venous Thrombosis**

Hormone Replacement Therapy:-

Benefits	Risks
• Increased bone mineral density • Decreased risk of fractures. • Decreased incidence of colorectal cancer • Decreased vasomotor symptoms like Hot flushes	• Increased risk of **s**troke • Increased chances of **V**enous Thromboembolism • Increased chances of choleceptitis • Increased risk of coronary **h**eart disease • Increased risk of **b**reast cancer (if used for ≥ 5 years) • (m) Svch Bharat (Read—LoPN Hkkjr)

13. **Ans. is b, c and e, i.e Occurs due to estrogen deficiency, Frequent intercourse is useful and Estradiol vaginal ring is helpful** *Ref: Leon speroff 8th/ed, p688*

Example:

"There are 2 main sexual changes in the aging women. There is a reduction in the rate of production and volume of vaginal lubricating fluid and there is some loss of vaginal elasticity and thickness of epithelium. Less vaginal atrophy is noted in sexually active women than in inactive women; presumably the activity maintains vaginal vasculature and circulation. (i.e. option c is correct – frequent intercourse is useful)"

Leon speroff 8th/ed, p688

The changes which occur in urogenital symptom due to menopause i.e **urogenital syndrome of menopause:**

Jeffcoate's Principles of gynaecology 9th/ed, p1081

Estrogen deficiency has deleterious effects on urogenital system (i.e. option b is correct). These are:
- Thin & pale vaginal mucosa
- Loss of normal rugosities
- Decreased moisture content
- **The pH increases (pH > 5)** i.e. option a i.e. low pH of vagina is incorrect
- Histology reveals loss in superficial cells and an increase in basal and parabasal cells

- Dry and atrophic vaginal and urethral epithelium can cause:
- Vaginal discomfort
- Itching
- Dyspareunia (i.e. there is pain during intercourse)
- Recurrent vaginitis

Note: International Society for Study of Women's Sexual Health has replaced atrophic vaginitis with new terminology genito urinary syndrome of Menopause (GSM)

Management of atrophic vaginitis

Local estrogen therapy either in form of cream or vaginal ring *Ref: Jeffcoate's 9th/ed, p1091*

14. Ans. is a, i.e. Estrogen

See the text for details.

REVIEW/PRACTICE QUESTIONS

1. All of the following hormones decrease in menopause *except*:
a. Estradiol b. FSH
c. DHEA - sulphate d. Inhibin

2. Premature menopause is before age of:
a. 40 years b. 45 years
c. 30 years d. 35 years

3. Genitourinary syndrome of menopause includes all *except:*
a. Vaginal dryness b. Decreased vaginal pH
c. Recurrent UTI d. Urinary urgency

4. Age of senescence as per WHO is:
a. Above 55 years b. Above 58 years
c. Above 60 years d. Above 65 years

5. All of the following drugs act osteoclast *except*:
a. Teriparatide b. Bisphosphonates
c. Calcitonin d. Denosumab

6. Maturation index at menopause:
a. 40:60:0 b. 100:0:0
c. 0:100:0 d. 0:0:100

7. First line management of osteoporosis:
a. HRT b. SERM
c. Bisphosphonates d. Vitamin D

8. HRT increases the risk of all *except:*
a. Venous thromboembolism
b. Colorectal cancer
c. Stroke
d. Cholecystitis

9. Natural product which is helpful in alleviating symptoms of Hot flushes:
a. Milk b. Fish
c. Soy product d. Vitamin E

10. Leading cause of death in females more than 65 years:
a. Heart disease
b. Cancer
c. Cerebrovascular disease
d. Alzheimer disease

11. Mark the following statements as true or false with respect to the indications of hormone replacement therapy after menopause: *(AIIMS May 2019)*
a. It is effective for vasomotor symptoms during perimenopausal period
b. It should be given for young women with premature menopause
c. It is useful for primary prevention of heart disease
d. Cyclical HRT is preferred over continuous HRT in perimenopausal women
e. None

12. Assertion: Hot flushes are common after menopause
Reason: Estrogen withdrawal happens in menopause *(AIIMS May 2019)*
a. Both Assertion and Reasoning are independently true/correct and Reason is the correct explanation of the Assertion
b. Both Assertion and Reasoning are independently true/correct and Reason is not the correct explanation of the Assertion
c. Assertion is independently a true/correct statement but the Reason is independently an incorrect/false statement
d. Assertion is independently a false/incorrect statement but the Reason is independently a true/correct statement
e. Both Assertion and Reason are independently a false/incorrect statement

REVIEW/PRACTICE ANSWERS

1. **Ans. is b, i.e. FSH**
2. **Ans. is a, i.e. 40 years**
3. **Ans. is b, i.e. Decreased vaginal pH** *Ref: Jeffcoates 9th/ed, p1082, Williams gynae 3rd/ed, p505*
4. **Ans. is d, i.e. Above 65 years** *Ref: Jeffcoates 9th/ed, p1075*
5. **Ans. is a, i.e. Teriparatide**
6. **Ans. is b, i.e. 100:0:0**
7. **Ans. is c, i.e. Bisphosphonates**
8. **Ans. is b, i.e. Colorectal cancer** *Ref: Williams gynae 3rd/ed, p474*
9. **Ans. is c, i.e. Soy product** *Ref: Williams gynae 3rd/ed, p498*

Note: phytoestrogens are plant derived compounds that bind to estrogen receptors and have both estrogen agonist and antagonist Properties. They are found in soy products and Red lover.

Flax seed is rich in alpha linolenic acid, a form of omega – 3 fatty acid. It helps in decreasing vasomotor symptoms. Vitamin E provides minimal or no vasomotor symptom improvement.

10. **Ans. is a, i.e. Heart disease** *Ref: Williams 3rd/ed, p507*

> Example: M/C cause of death ≥ 65 years in females:
> Heart disease > cancer > CVA.
> M/C cause of death between 45 and 54 years in females:
> Cancer > Heart disease > Accidents.

11. **Ans. is a-T, b-T, c-F, d-T**

Hormone replacement therapy

- The main indication of HRT is vasomotor and other symptoms in the perimenopausal period.
- It should be used at the smallest effective dose and for the shortest duration.
- Young women with premature menopause clearly deserve HRT.
- Hysterectomized women should receive estrogen alone, while those with intact uterus should be given estrogen + progestin.
- Perimenopausal women should be given cyclic HRT rather than continuous HRT.
- First line management for osteoporosis in postmenopausal females is bisphosphonates
- HRT is not the best option to prevent osteoporosis and fractures.
- HRT affords no protection against cardiovascular diseases conventional dose combined HRT. It may even increase the risk of venous thromboembolism, MI and stroke.
- HRT does not protect against cognitive decline; may increase the risk of dementia.
- Combined HRT increases the risk of breast cancer, gallstones and migraine.
- Transdermal HRT may have certain advantages over oral HRT.
- The need for HRT should be assessed in individual women, and not prescribed routinely.

12. **Ans. is a, i.e. Both Assertion and Reasoning are independently true/correct and Reason is the correct explanation of the Assertion**

Hot flushes are due to estrogen deficiency. This can be seen from following lines of *Leon Speroff.*

"The correlation between most of flushes and estrogen reduction can be clinically supported by effectiveness of estrogen therapy and absence of flushes in hypoestrogenic states like gonadal dysgeneses."

CHAPTER 4

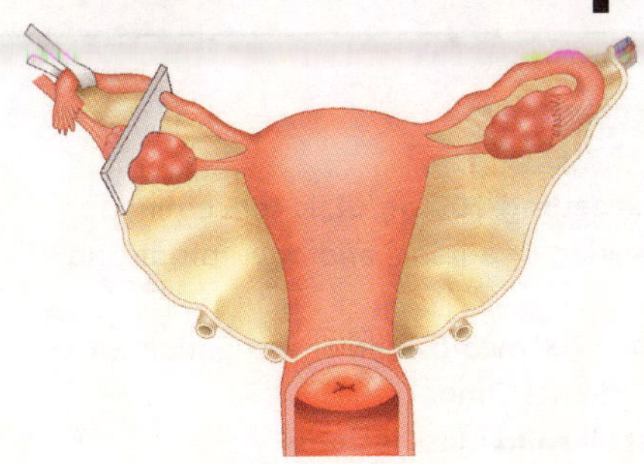

PCOD, Hirsutism and Galactorrhea

Hyperandrogenism

It is characterised by an abnormally elevated serum concentration of androgen or physical findings consistent with androgen excess. Androgenic hormones in female can stimulate abnormal terminal hair growth, i.e. hirsutism.

Hirsutism	Virilization	Hypertrichosis
• Excessive growth of androgen-dependent sexual hair or male distribution of hair in females.	• It is characterized by more extensive androgen induced changes than hirsutism alone, like acne, increased oily skin, temporal balding, **clitoromegaly**, deepening of voice, development of male muscular pattern and body habitus with atrophy of breasts.	• Excessive growth of nonsexual hair, i.e. lanugo hair
• Hair are coarse, dark and terminal hair		• Hair are soft and lightly pigmented

Note: For details of androgens in females, refer to chapter 2 of this book.

Clitoromegaly

For detecting clitoromegaly—clitoral index is useful, i.e. clitoral length (in mm) and width (in mm) are multiplied. Values ≥ 35 mm^2 are abnormal.

Causes of Hyperandrogenism

- PCOS
- Late Onset Congenital Adrenal Hyperplasia (CAH)
- Tumors of ovary and adrenal gland
- Cushing's syndrome
- Idiopathic or drug induced process

Note: Hyperprolactinemia can be associated with hyperandrogenism as it is likely that prolactin receptors are located on adrenal glands. When prolactin binds to these adrenal receptors, it stimulates the release of DHEAS.

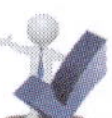

KEY POINTS

- DHEA-S > 700 ng/dL is consistent with abnormal adrenal function.
- **17 alpha hydroxy progesterone:** Normal range = 100 – 300 ng/dL
- Prolactin = Normal range is 1–20 ng/mL

Late-Onset or "Nonclassical" Congenital Adrenal Hyperplasia (CAH)

- Excess androgen production is a common feature shared by most forms of CAH (details of CAH are discussed in Chapter 5).
- Unlike typical CAH, symptoms of late-onset CAH are not evident until late childhood or adolescence.
- It is an autosomal recessive disorder with an enzyme defect.
- The most common adrenal enzyme defect is 21-hydroxylase (21-OH) deficiency.

Signs and Symptoms

- No genital ambiguity at birth (unlike classical CAH)
- They present with androgen excess at puberty in the form of premature pubarche, acne, hirsutism, heterosexual precocious puberty and menstrual irregularity.

Diagnosis

Although it seems that non-classical CAH should be excluded specifically in all women with hirsutism, the yield from routine testing is quite low as the disease itself is very uncommon.

Therefore, specific testing for non-classical CAH can be reserved for females
i. With early onset hirsutism (pre- or perimenarcheal including girls with premature adrenarche)
ii. With family history of the disorder
iii. Or high-risk ethnic group (hispanic, mediterranean, Jewish, etc.)

- **Screening test for CAH:** Measure the basal levels of 17-OHP (hydroxy progesterone) in the morning. If the levels of 17-OHP are between 200 and 800 ng/dL, then confirmatory test should be done, i.e. ACTH stimulation test. If levels are initially ≥ 800 ng/dL no need to do confirmatory test.

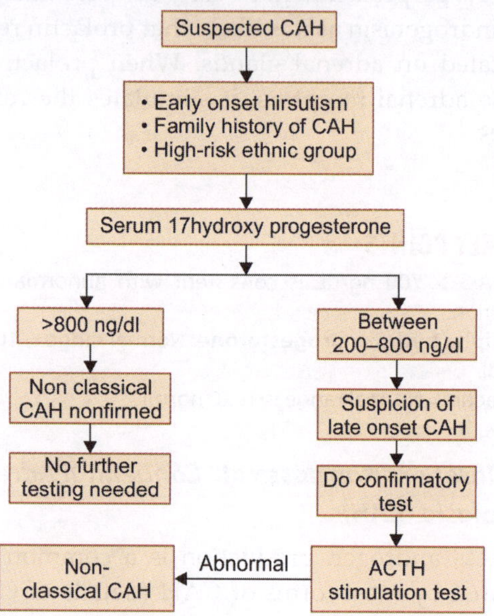

Fig. 4.1: Algorithm for diagnosis of non-classical CAH

- If levels are ≥ 800 ng/dL. They are virtually diagnostic of CAH (Fig. 4.1).
- **Confirmatory test:** It is ACTH Stimulation test. Patients with late-onset hyperplasia have 17-OHP levels **more than 1,500 ng/dL after 1 hour in response to a 250-µg I/V ACTH stimulation challenge.**

Treatment

- **Glucocorticoids:** Restore ovulation by reducing circulating androgen levels.

Androgen-Producing Ovarian or Adrenal Tumors

- Tumors of the ovary or adrenal gland that secrete androgens although rare, can lead to hirsutism.
- The presence of an androgen-producing tumor is suspected on the basis of clinical findings.
- **Palpation of an adnexal mass in** a patient with symptoms of hyperandrogenism or **rapid onset of virilization even** in the presence of normal testosterone levels should prompt a workup for a pelvic tumor.

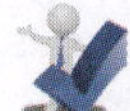

Important Concept

- Testosterone levels **exceeding 200 ng/dL** is concerning for the presence of an ovarian or adrenal androgen-producing tumor.
- DHEA-S levels more than 700 mcg/dl merit investigation with MRI/CT of adrenal for adrenal tumor.
- **TVS identifies almost all solid mass lesions.**

Note: In Figure 4.2 the values of testosterone > 150 ng/dL are taken as androgen secreting tumor, whereas latest is value as per *Williams gynae* 3rd/ed > 200 ng/dL taken as androgen secreting tumor.

Idiopathic Hirsutism

It is presence of hirsutism in absence of hyperandrogenism, i.e. androgen levels are normal.

KEY POINTS

In a Nutshell

- Levels of 17-OHP - ≥ 200 ng/dL may be CAH
- Levels ≥ 800 ng/dL-confirm CAH
- Testosterone = > 200 ng/dL - indicate androgen secreting tumor
- DHEAS = > 700 mEg/dL - indicate adrenal tumor
- **1st test to be done when a female presents with hirsutism is level of Serum testosterone**

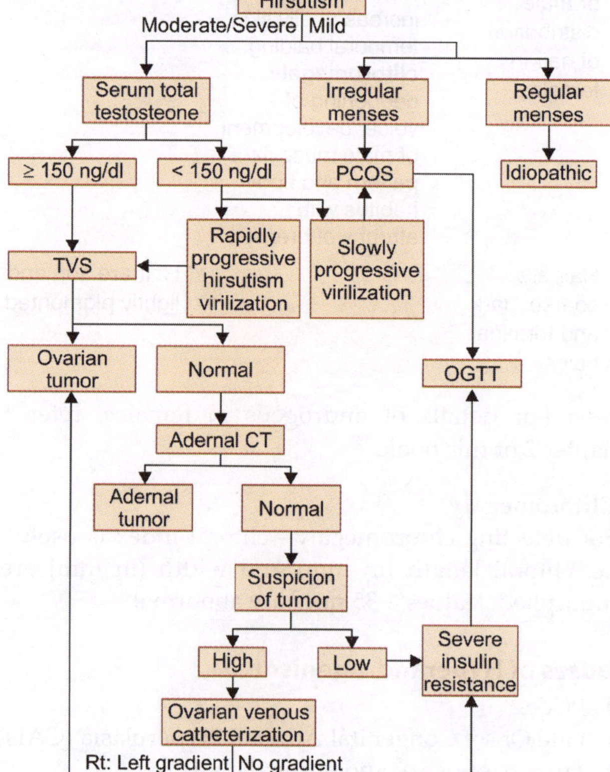

Fig. 4.2: Algorithm for differential diagnosis of hirsutism (***Source:*** Leon Speroff 8/e pg 549)

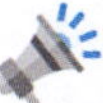

Important One Liners

- **M/C cause of hirsutism in a young female:** PCOS
- **M/c pathological cause of hirsutism in young female:** PCOS
- **2nd M/C cause of hirsutism in young females:** Idiopathic hirsutism.
- **M/c cause of rapid onset hirsutism in a young female:** Testosterone producing tumor.

Anovulation

Anovulation can be due to any cause which disrupts the normal hypothalamic pituitary ovarian axis (Fig. 4.3).

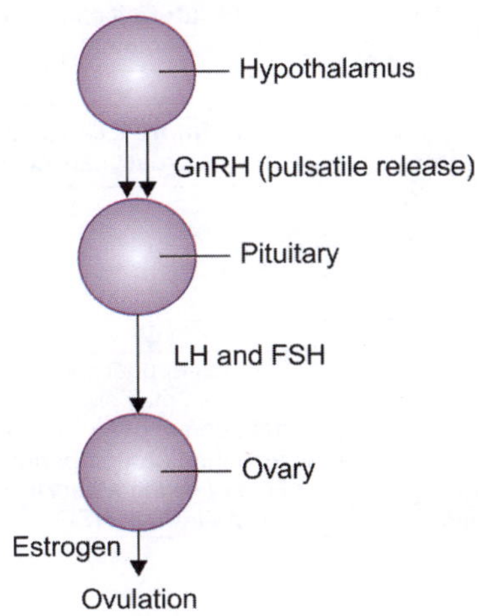

Fig. 4.3: Hypothalamic pituitary ovarian axis

Table 4.1: Causes of anovulation

Central Defects	
• Hypothalamus	• Emotional causes-weight loss, eating disorders, excessive exercise
• Pituitary	• Pituitary tumors, hyperprolactinemia
• Ovary	• PCOS
Peripheral Defects	
• Abnormal estrogen levels	• High levels of estrogen have a negative feedback on FSH. Therefore, levels of FSH are decreased, which leads to anovulation; e.g.: • Pregnancy • Estrogen secreting tumor of ovary: Granulosa cell tumor • Obesity (increased conversion of androgen to estrogen)

Contd...

Contd...

Central Defects	
• Abnormal Thyroid levels	• As it leads to hyperprolactinemia
• Ovarian dysgenesis/ Gonadal failure	• No follicles, ∴ anovulation occurs
• Abnormal androgen levels	• When levels of androgen are very high in females, it is converted to 5 ∝ androgens which inhibits aromatase activity & stops conversion of androgen to estrogen (Fig. 4.4)
• Abnormal prolactin levels	• Hyperprolactinemia leads to anovulation and amenorrhea

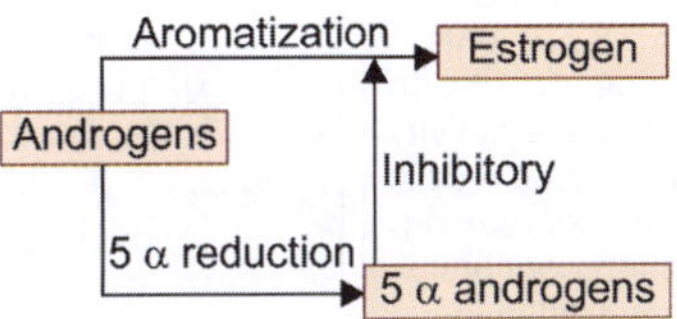

Fig. 4.4: Effect of high androgen

Polycystic Ovary Syndrome (PCOS)

- PCOD/PCOS is the M/C Endocrine disorder of reproductive age females affecting 4-12% females.
- The condition was first described in 1935 by Irving F. Stein and Michael L. Leventhal so also called Stein-Leventhal syndrome.
- Familial inheritance is seen in PCOS. Some suggest autosomal dominant mode of inheritance (Gene *CYP21* mutation has been discovered in this connection).
- PCOS/PCOD is a syndrome manifested by amenorrhea, hirsutism, obesity and enlarged ovaries.
- M/C age = Reproductive age.

- PCOS occasionally is seen in prepubertal females.
- Risk factors for prepubertal PCOS are:
  - Low birth weight
  - Premature adrenarche
  - Atypical sexual precocity
  - Obesity with acanthosis nigricans.
- Diagnosis of PCOS in adolescent age group is difficult.

Pathophysiology of PCOS (Fig. 4.5)

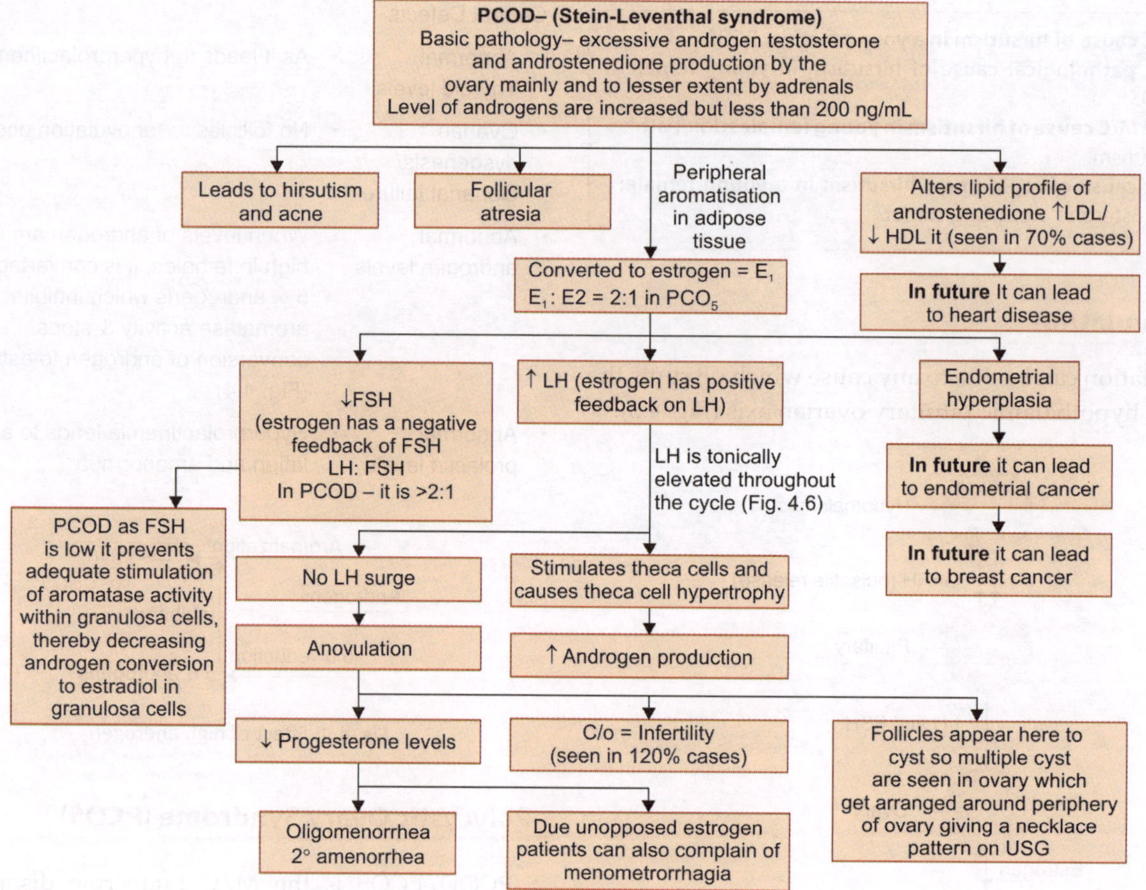

Fig. 4.5: Pathophysiology of PCOS

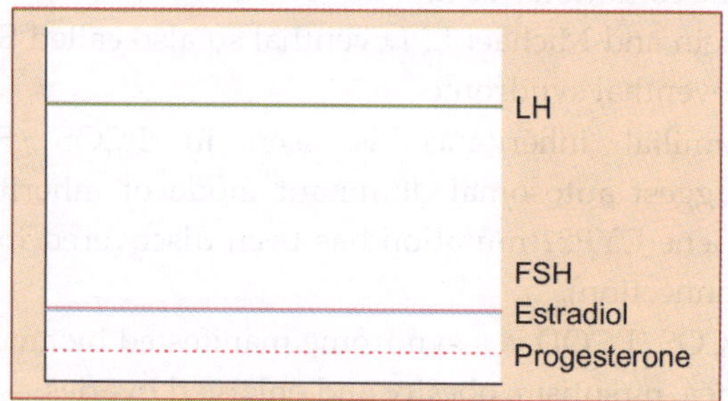

Fig. 4.6: Hormonal mileu in PCOS female

Features of PCOD/PCOS

Apart from the pathophysiology explained, there are other features of PCOD like

Obesity: Most patients of PCOD are obese (BMI ≥ 30 kg/m²) but PCOD can also occur in thin females. The risk for PCOS increases with obesity.

Insulin resistance/Hyperinsulinemia: Insulin resistance is defined as reduced glucose uptake response to a given amount of insulin 70–75% PCOS patients will have hyperinsulinemia which itself contributes to hyperandrogenism in two ways:

i. By stimulating synthesis of androgens from ovary along with LH.
ii. By decreasing sex hormone-biding globulin. Amongst insulin resistance patients –15% will have PCOS,

Insulin Resistance can be detected by:

$$\frac{\text{Sr. Fasting blood sugar}}{\text{Sr. Fasting insulin}} < 4.5$$

Fasting serum insulin >25 m IU/mL

- Insulin resistance appears to stem from a post binding abnormality in Insulin Receptor mediated signal transduction
- Both lean and obese women with PCOS are found to be insulin resistant.
- But Insulin resistivity is decreased more in obese women with PCOS than lean women with PCOS (Fig. 4.7)

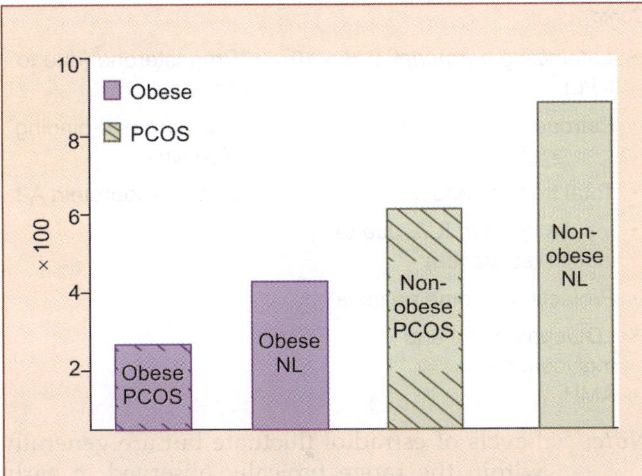

Fig. 4.7: Insulin sensitivity is decreased in obese women with PCOS (NL: Normal without PCOS)

- Insulin resistance can also lead to hyperpigmented velvety patches of skin in neck/axilla/below breast or in thigh, called as **acanthosis nigricans** (Fig. 4.8).
- Acanthosis nigricans is more common in obese females with PCOS than normal weight females with PCOS.

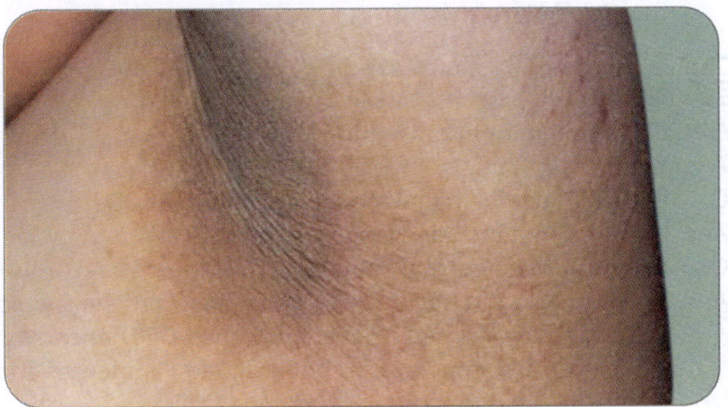

Fig. 4.8: Acanthosis nigricans in a PCOS patient

Note: Insulin resistance and hyperinsulinemia are the cause of hyperandrogenism and not its result. Hence, treatment with a GnRH agonist can normalize elevated serum testosterone and androstenedione in PCOD patients but has no effect on insulin resistance.

- **A baseline 2 hr** OGTT is **recommended by ACOG after 75 gms of glucose in all** PCOS patients as upto 30–35% have impaired glucose tolerance and upto 10% have diabetes mellitus.

Hyperandrogenemia

- Excessive androgen production in PCOS is primarily due to excessive synthesis by ovaries & to a lesser extent by the adrenal.
- Excessive androgens can either be detected biochemically or clinically by hirsutism, acne and alopecia.

- Hirsutism can be graded by **Modified Ferriman-Gallwey score.** In original scoring, 11 sites were noted & given a score from 0-4.
  In modified score, 2 sites are removed, viz. forearms and legs.
  ∴ Now 9 sites are seen for hirsutism.
  Maximum Score - 36
  If score ≥ 8: Hirsutism is present (mild)
  If score ≥ 15: Moderate/severe hirsutism is present

Anovulation

In PCOS there is anovulation: The causes of anovulation are:

- In appropriate Gonadotropin secretion (i.e. absent LH surge) and presence of LH from the beginning of cycle
- Insulin resistance
- Large number of antral follicles with increased ovarian androgens.

This is the reason why Laparoscopic ovarian drilling/wedge resection is helpful in PCOS as theca cells are destroyed so there is less androgen production.

Menstrual Dysfunction

In women with PCOS, menstrual dysfunction ranges from amenorrhea (25% cases) to oligomenorrhea (<8 periods in 1 year) (85% cases) to menometrorrhagia with associated iron deficiency anemia.

Acne

- Acne vulgaris is a frequent clinical finding in adolescents. However, acne that is persistent or has late onset suggests PCOS.
- The pathogenesis of acne involves 4 factors.
  1. Blockage of follicular opening by hyperkeratosis
  2. Sebum overproduction
  3. Proliferation of commensal PROPIONIBACTERIUM ACNES
  4. Inflammation
- In sebaceous gland, testosterone is converted to DHT (more active metabolite). In women with androgen excess there is overstimulation of androgen receptors in pilosebaceous unit that leads to increased sebum production, inflammation and comedone formation. Inflammation leads to scarring.

Syndromes associated with PCOD/PCOS are:

1. **HAIR-AN syndrome**

H, A — Hyperandrogenism
I, R — Insulin resistance
A, N — Acanthosis nigricans

2. **Metabolic X syndrome**

Any 3 of the following 5 should be present to diagnose Metabolic 'X' Syndrome:

iv. Abdominal obesity (waist circumference > 88 cm or 35 inches)
v. Triglycerides > 150 mg/dl
vi. HDL - cholesterol < 50 mg/dl
vii. BP = ≥ 130/85 mm of Hg
viii. Fasting blood sugar = 110–126 mg/dl
2 hour postprandial sugar - 140-199 mg/dl

Diagnostic Criteria

Rotterdam criteria (2003). Any two of the following three criteria should be present to diagnose a patient having PCOD after excluding other etiologies.

(Novak 15th/ed, p1076)

- Ovulatory dysfunction such as oligomenorrhea or amenorrhea
- Clinical (hirsutism/acne/alopecia) or biochemical evidence of hyperandrogenism i.e. S. testosterone between 70-150 ng/dl (levels >200 indicate testosterone secreting ovarian tumor not PCOS)
- Polycystic ovarian morphology on USG scan defined as presence of 12 or more cysts size: (2–9 mm) in any one ovary or both ovaries, with enlarged ovaries (>10 ml) and other criterias being excluded (like cushing disease, adrenal hyperplasia)

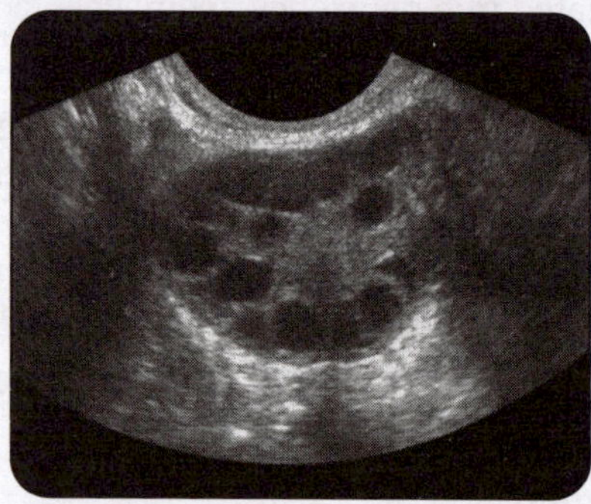

Fig. 4.9: Ultrasonography picture of polycystic ovary

- Historically, a polycystic ovary displays increase in the number of ripening and atretic follicles, cortical stromal thickness and number of hilar cells nest.
- Also remember as per Rotterdam criteria, any 2 criteria are needed to make a diagnosis of PCOS, hence in PCOS patients ovaries can be normal.

Hormonal Changes in PCOS

Hormonal changes in PCOS

Hormones Increased	Hormones Decreased
• Androgens[Q] (Testosterone, Androstenedione, DHEA, DHEAS)	• Follicle stimulating hormone (FSH)
• *Luteinizing hormone*[Q] (LH > 10 IU/L)	• Progesterone (due to anovulation)
• Estrone	• Sex hormone-binding globulin
• Total free estrone	• HDL & Apoprotein A-I
• Insulin (> 10 m IU/L due to insulin resistance)	
• Prolactin (in some patients)	
• LDL/cholesterol and triglycerides	
• AMH	

Note:
- Levels of estradiol fluctuate but are generally within the range typically observed in early follicular phase
- Levels of inhibin B are normal or mildly elevated.
- The classical PCOS contains 2–3 fold more growing preantral and antral follicles (the smaller follicles) than normal ovaries.
- These antral follicles produce anti-Müllerian hormone. Hence in PCOS patients levels of AMH are raised.

Important Concept

Q. **Can a thin patient have PCOS?**
Ans. Yes
Q. **Is LH/FSH useful in making a diagnosis of PCOD?**
Ans. No, as it is not included in Rotterdam criteria
Q. **Can ovaries be normal in PCOS**
Ans. Yes (According to Rotterdam criteria, any 2 criteria should be fulfilled to diagnose a patient having PCOD) hence even if patient has normal ovaries but has irregular menses and hirsutism, she is diagnosed as having PCOD.

Management of PCOS

Management of PCOS depends on the problem with which patient comes. The first step is weight reduction.

Conservative Treatment

Women with PCOS who have fairly regular cycle intervals (8 to 12 menses per year) and mild hyperandrogenism may choose not to be treated. In these women, however, periodic screening for dyslipidemia, diabetes mellitus, and metabolic syndrome is prudent.

For obese women with PCOS, important lifestyle changes focus on diet and exercise. Even modest weight loss (5 percent of body weight) can result in restoration of normal ovulatory cycles in some women. This improvement results from reductions in insulin and androgen levels, the latter mediated through increases in SHBG levels (Huber-Buchholz, 1999; Kiddy, 1992; Pasquali, 1989).

Treatment of Oligo and Anovulation

Hormonal Agents

Women with oligo- or anovulation typically have fewer than eight menses per year, often skip menses for several months at a time, or simply have amenorrhea.

A first-line treatment for menstrual irregularities is combination oral contraceptive pills (COCs) which induce regular menstrual cycles, lower androgen levels, and thin the endometrium.

Theoretically, COCs that contain progestins with fewer androgenic properties are preferred. Such progestins include a third-generation progestin, such as norgestimate or desogestrel; or the newer progestin, drospirenone. Alternative combination hormonal contraceptive options include the contraceptive patch and vaginal ring. Before COC initiation, if a woman's last menses was more than 4 weeks prior, a pregnancy test is indicated.

In patients who are not candidates for combination hormonal contraception, progesterone withdrawal is recommended every 1 to 3 months. Examples of regimens used include: medroxyprogesterone acetate (MPA), 5 to 10 mg orally daily for 12 days, or micronized progesterone, 200 mg orally each evening for 12 days.

For Insulin Resistance

Insulin Sensitizing Agents

Metformin is the most commonly prescribed particularly in women with impaired glucose tolerance and insulin resistance. In clinical studies, 1500 to 2000 mg in divided doses daily with meals is typically used. More common side effects are gastrointestinal, and these can be minimum by starting at a low dose and gradually increasing the dose several weeks to an optimal level.

Metformin decreases androgen levels in both lean and obese women with PCOS, leading to increased rates of spontaneous ovulation. Several studies demonstrate that up to 40 percent of anovulatory women with PCOS will ovulate, and many will achieve pregnancy with metformin alone. Metformin is a category B drug and is safe use as an ovulatory induction agent.

- **Sponsored PCOS consensus Workshop Group (2008) amends against the routine use of metformin for ovulation induction, and first-line treatment remains letrozole or citrate clomiphene note that the addition of metformin to clomiphene is indicated for women with PCOS and glucose intolerance.**
- The **thiazolidinediones** are another class of medication used for patients with diabetes mellitus. Similar to metformin, rosiglitazone and pioglitazone improve ovulation rates some. However, the glitazones are category C drugs and should be discontinued if pregnancy is achieved.

Hirsutism

With hirsutism treatment primary goal is lowering androgen level to halt further conversion of Vellus hairs to terminal ones. However, medical therapies will not eliminate hair already present.

- Best drug: OCP's
- They should be given for 6 months. If response does not come then add spironolactone (Androgen receptor antagonist).
- In patients not responding to any treatment. GnRH agonist are given.
- Post menopausal females with hirsutism can be advised to use Eflornithine Hydrochloride applied twice daily.
- **Eflornithine** is an irreversible inhibitor of ornithine decarboxylase. This enzyme is necessary for hair follicle cell division and function and its inhibition results in slower hair growth. It does not remove hair permanently. It requires 4-8 weeks of use before changes are noticed.

Drugs used in managing Hirsutism in PCOS

- OCP (DOC)
- 5 α reductase inhibitor
  - Finasteride (5 mg daily)
- Androgen receptor antagonist
  - Spironolactone (50-100 mg oral)
  - Cyproterone acetate
  - Flutamide
- GnRH
- Efornithine Hydrochloride
- Permanent hair removal using laser.

Consequences of PCOS

Short-term Consequences of PCOS

- Hirsutism
- Irregular cycles
- Infertility (easily treatable)

Long-term Consequences of PCOS/Anovulation

Increased Risk of:

- Cardiovascular disease
- Diabetes (Type 2) (10% cases)
- Endometrial cancer
- Breast Ca
- Ovarian Ca (+/–)
- Depression and mood disorder
- Metabolic X syndrome
- Sleep apnea syndrome (30–40 times increased chances)
- Non-alcoholic steatohepatitis

(Depression and mood disorder, Metabolic X syndrome, Sleep apnea syndrome: due to obesity)

A COG (2012) recommends endometrial assessment in any woman older than 45 years with abnormal bleeding and in those younger than 45 years with a history of unopposed estrogen exposure such as seen in obesity or PCOS, failed medical management and persistent bleeding.

Pregnancy Complications in PCOS

- Women with PCOS who become pregnant experience an increased rate (30–50%) of early miscarriage
- Other pregnancy complications are:
  - Gestational diabetes
  - PIH
  - Preterm birth
  - Penatal mortality
  - Increased pregnancy loss in the form of abortions.

Hirsutism

Causes of Hirsutism

Hirsutism is associated with excess androgen production (either from ovaries or adrenals), so any cause which increases androgens causes hirsutism.

Note: • Most of the testosterone is bound to sex hormone binding globulin (SHBG) and is considered biologically inactive.

• Testosterone which is not bound to SHBG is considered biologically active, therefore any factor which decreases SHBG; cause increase in free testosterone and therefore causes hirsutism.

- Sex Hormone binding globulin is a glycoprotein produced by liver
- SHBG Synthesis is suppressed by:
  - All = androgen
  - India = Insulin
  - P = Progestin
  - G = Growth hormone
  - Council = Corticoids.

Mnemonic

All India PG council

- Low SHBG means more of free testosterone & hence it can lead to:
  - Hyperandrogenism
  - Impaired Glucose tolerance
  - Diabetes mellitus

- SHBG Synthesis is increased by estrogen

Factors	
• **Increase SHBG**	• **Decrease SHBG**
• *(Therefore, ↓free Testosterone)*	*(Therefore, ↑free Testosterone)*
• High estrogens like in OCP's	• PCOD[Q]
• Pregnancy	• Adrenal hyperplasia[Q]
• Liver cirrhosis	• Cushing syndrome[Q]
• Elevated thyroid hormone	• Growth hormone[Q]
	• Insulin[Q]
	• Prolactin[Q]
	• Increase in Androgens itself[Q]

Causes of Hirsutism

Ovary Related	Adrenal Related	Medications	Others
• PCOD (M/C)[Q]	• Congenital adrenal[Q] hyperplasia		• Acromegaly[Q]
• Masculinizing tumors of ovary[Q]	• Adrenal tumor[Q]		Hyperprolactinemia[Q]
• Theca lutein cyst[Q]	• Cushing syndrome[Q]		• Hypothyroidism[Q]
• Luteoma of pregnancy[Q]			

Medications that may cause hirsutism and/or hypertrichosis

Hirsutism	Hypertrichosis
• Anabolic steroids	• Cyclosporine
• Danazol	• Diazoxide
• Metoclopramide	• Hydro cortisone
• Methyldopa	• Minoxidil
• Phenothiazines	• Penicillamine
• Progestins	• Phenytoin
• Reserpine	• Psoralens
• Testosterone	• Streptomycin

Pathophysiology of Hirsutism

- Elevated androgen levels play a major role in hirsutism
- Within a hair follicle, testosterone is converted to DHT by enzyme 5α-reductase
- Both DHT & Tests sterone convert soft, short vellus hair to coarse terminal hair.
- This conversion is irreversible and occurs only in androgen resistive areas, e.g. lips, chin sideburns, chest.

Medical Management of Hirsutism

- **Combined oral contraceptives:** First and most effective treatment for hirsutism is low-dose OCP's. It is preferable to use COCs with drospirenone, desogestrel or cyproterone acetate. Hormone therapy must be continued for 6 months to see its effects.

For undergraduates

How are OCPs helpful in hirsutism:

- Androgen production in hirsute women is an LH-dependant process. LH acts on theca cells to produce androgens. Estrogen-progestin contraceptives suppress LH secretion & so suppress androgen production.
- The high level of estrogen in OCP's stimulates hepatic SHBG production. (∴ Less of free testosterone)
- Directly or indirectly E-P contraceptives can decrease adrenal DHEA-S secretion.
- Contraceptive progestin inhibits 5 alpha reductase activity in other words reduces the production of dihydrotestosterone.

- **Antiandrogens:** They are effective treatment for hirsutism. They should be used with contraceptives as they have the potential to adversely affect sexual development in a male fetus if patient conceives during treatment. Examples of antiandrogens are spironolactone, cyproterone acetate, flutamide and finasteride.

Treatment box

- 1st line treatment for hirsutism is always = **low dose OCPs for at least 6 months**
- If desired response is not achieved with OCPs alone after 6 months—antiandrogen should be added, with spironolactone being the first choice
- The use of GnRH agonist should be reserved for patients who fail to respond to or cannot tolerate more traditional methods
- Permanent hair removal using electrolysis or photoepilation techniques (laser, pulsed light) when necessary is best postponed until hormonal suppression has achieved its maximum benefit

Contd...

- For mild facial hair in menopausal females: **Eflornithine hydrochloride** (13.9%) cream is used, it is an inhibitor of enzyme ornithine decarboxylase which is found in dermal papilla that is essential for hair growth.

Galactorrhea

- **Galactorrhea is the secretion of a milky fluid which is inappropriate (unrelated to child birth).** The secretion contains fat globules when examined under microscope and is confirmatory for milk.
- Prolactin (PRL) is the most important hormone involved in the **pathophysiology of amenorrhea and/or galactorrhea**. Prolactin is under tonic hypothalamic inhibitory control of prolactin inhibitory factor (PIF).
- **Prolactin inhibits GnRH pulse secretion.** So gonadotropin levels are suppressed. Hyperprolactinemia inhibits ovarian steroidogenesis. Thus, it results in hypogonadotropic hypogonadism, oligomenorrhea, amenorrhea, anovulation and many other clinical effects of hypoestrogenism.
- PRL levels should be estimated in all women with galactorrhea, oligomenorrhea or amenorrhea. TSH level should also be measured to rule out primary hypothyroidism.
- Prolactinoma is present in about 50 percent of women with hyperprolactinemia. Serum prolactin level when raised on repeat assay beyond 20 ng/mL, suggests evaluation of sella turcica. Level beyond 100 ng/mL is associated with high incidence of prolactinoma. Most of the prolactinomas are microadenomas. **About 33 percent of women with high prolactin levels, have galactorrhea.** However, galactorrhea can be seen in women with normal serum prolactin.

Important One Liners

In patients presenting with galactorrhea, amenorrhea and visual symptoms or headache, always measure prolactin levels to rule out prolactinoma.

- Bromocriptine was the drug used for galactorrhea. Cabergoline is more effective and well tolerated as compared to bromocriptine and has become the DOC for treating hyperprolactinemia.
- If an infertile female comes with increased prolactin, then DOC is Bromocriptine as it is an ovulation-inducing drug also.

NEW PATTERN QUESTIONS

N1. M/C cause of hirsutism in a young female:
a. Ovarian tumor b. Adrenal tumor
c. CAH d. PCOS

N2. A 30-year-old female complains of facial hair growth and oligomenorrhea. 1st investigation needed in this case is:
a. TVS
b. S. testosterone levels
c. S. DhEAs level
d. 17-OH progesterone levels

N3. Measuring 17-OHP is useful in all of the following cases of hirsutism *except*:
a. Rapid onset hirsutism
b. Early onset hirsutism
c. Family H/O CAH
d. Hirsutism in a premenarcheal female

N4. All are true with regards to pregnancy luteoma *except*:
a. Can lead to virilization
b. True tumor
c. Bilateral usually
d. Regress spontaneously after delivery

N5. Clitoromegaly is defined if clitoris is:
a. ≥ 5 mm b. ≥ 7 mm
c. > 10 mm d. 15 mm

N6. The biochemical changes in established cases of Stein-Leventhal syndrome are as mentioned *except*:
a. Marked elevation of LH in contrast to FSH
b. Insulin resistance
c. Elevation of plasma testosterone
d. Elevation in the level of sex hormone binding globulin (SHBG) level

N7. Scoring system used for hirsutism is:
a. Danforth and Trotter score
b. Halter score
c. Ferriman-Gallway score
d. MC knight score

N8. According to Ferriman- Gallwey scoring system—hirsutism is diagnosed when score is more than:
a. 8 b. 12
c. 16 d. 20

N9. % of PCOS patients having diabetes mellitus:
a. 50% b. 30%
c. 20% d. 10%

N10. BMI of an overweight female is:
a. 19–24 b. 25–29
c. 30–34 d. Less than 19

N11. Figure shows a 22-year-old female complaining of irregular cycles, weight gain and discoloration of neck. USG revealed multiple cysts in both the ovaries. The metabolic abnormalities which need to be ruled out in this patient are:
a. Hyperinsulinism b. Hyperandrogenism
c. Diabetes mellitus d. Diabetes insipidus

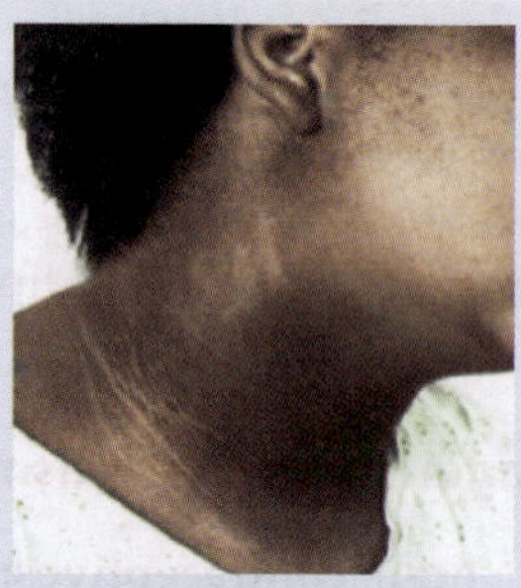

N12. The following are related to bromocriptine therapy *except*:
a. It is used to inhibit inappropriate lactation with secondary amenorrhoea
b. It is specific in suppressing only the prolactin secretion
c. If pregnancy occurs, there is increased incidence of multiple pregnancy
d. Its teratogenic effect on the fetus is inconclusive

N13. Ovarian cause of hirsutism is:
a. PCOD b. Ovarian cancer
c. Dysgerminoma d. Endometriotic cyst

N14. DOC for Hirsutism:
a. OCPs b. Progesterone
c. Danazol d. Spironolactone

N15. All of the following are used in management of hirsutism *except*:
a. Spironolactone b. GnRH
c. Danazol d. OCPs

N16. Percentage of females with oligomenorrhea in PCOs:
a. 50% b. 60%
c. 70% d. 80%

N17. All of the following are features of virilization *except*:
a. Acne b. Clitoromegaly
c. Increased breast size d. Increased muscle mass

N18. All of the following are raised in PCOS *except*:
a. E_2:E_1 b. LH:FSH
c. LDL: HDL d. Fasting serum insulin

N19. Prepubertal PCOS, risk factors are all *except*:
a. Increased birth weight
b. Premature Adrenarche
c. Obesity with acanthosis nigricans
d. Atypical sexual precocity

N20. All of the following complications can occur in pregnant females with PCOS *except*:
a. PIH b. Preterm birth
c. Abruptio placenta d. Gestational diabetes

N21. Gene involved in PCOS:
a. CYP 19 b. CYP 20
c. CYP 21 d. CYP 36

N22. Skin manifestations of PCOS are all *except*:
a. Acne b. Hirsutism
c. Seborrheic dermatitis d. Alopecia

PREVIOUS YEAR QUESTIONS

1. **Which of the following statements is incorrect regarding polycystic ovarian disease?** *(AI 06)*
   a. Elevated LH hormone
   b. Can cause infertility
   c. May be associated with abnormal glucose tolerance test
   d. Results in postdated pregnancy
2. **The following hormone is raised in polycystic ovarian syndrome:** *(AI 06)*
   a. 17 - OH progesterone
   b. Follicular stimulating hormone
   c. Luteinizing hormone
   d. Thyroid stimulating hormone
3. **PCOD—Hormonal Status:** *(PGI Dec 08)*
   a. LH decreased
   b. LH increased, FSH normal to low
   c. FSH increased
   d. 17 OH progesterone normal
   e. Testosterone increased >2 ng/mL
4. **True about PCOD:** *(PGI June 09)*
   a. ↑ LH & ↓ FSH b. ↑ FSH & ↓ LH
   c. ↑ LH & ↓ FSH d. Hyperinsulinemia
   e. ↑ TSH
5. **All are true about polycystic ovarian disease (PCOD)** *except*: *(PGI May 2015)*
   a. Testosterone >200 ng/mL
   b. Infertility
   c. High FSH/LH ratio
   d. ↑ Insulin level
   e. ↑E2/oestrone (E1) ratio
6. **Which of the following is the most likely diagnosis in a 27-year-old obese woman presenting with Oligomenorrhea, infertility and hirsutism?** *(AI 04)*
   a. Polycystic ovaries
   b. Endometriosis
   c. Pelvic inflammatory disease
   d. Turner's syndrome
7. **In PCOD symptoms and signs seen are:** *(PGI June 07)*
   a. Amenorrhoea
   b. Alopecia
   c. Theca cell hyperplasia
   d. Hyperandrogenism
   e. Anovulation
8. **A 28-year-old lady, Rani, is suspected to have polycystic ovarian disease. Sample for testing LH & FSH are best taken on the following days of menstrual cycle:** *(AI 02)*
   a. 1–4 b. 8–10
   c. 13–15 d. 24–26
9. **True about Stein-Leventhal syndrome is/are:** *(PGI June 03)*
   a. Oligomenorrhea and amenorrhea
   b. Seen in postmenopausal women
   c. Innumerate cysts in ovary
   d. BRCA - 1 is associated
   e. Theca cell hypertrophy
10. **PCOD which of the following is seen:** *(PGI Dec 02)*
    a. Hirsutism b. Secondary amenorrhoea
    c. Streak ovaries d. ↑ FSH/LH
    e. ↑ Oestrogen
11. **In Polycystic ovarian diseases, all of the following are seen** ***except*****:** *(PGI Dec 01)*
    a. Endometrial carcinoma
    b. Increased FSH c. Streak ovaries
    d. Insulin resistance e. Hirsutism
12. **All are true about polycystic ovarian disease** ***except*****:** *(AIIMS Nov 08)*
    a. Persistently elevated LH
    b. Increased LH/FSH ratio
    c. Increased Dheas
    d. Increased prolactin
13. **The first step in the management of hirsutism due to Stein-Leventhal syndrome is:** *(PGI June 99)*
    a. OCP b. HMG
    c. Spironolactone d. Bromocriptine
14. **Treatment of Hirsutism in PCOD, drugs used are:** *(PGI Dec 08)*
    a. Menopausal Gonadotropin
    b. GnRH
    c. Spironolactone
    d. Hcg
15. **A hirsuite lady with PCOD treatment is:** *(Kolkata 2009)*
    a. Ethinyl estradiol + Levonorgestrel
    b. Ethinyl estradiol + Desogestrel
    c. Levonorgestrel
    d. None
16. **Most common cause of hirsutism:** *(AIIMS Dec 97)*
    a. Polycystic ovary disease
    b. Arrhenoblastoma
    c. Cushing syndrome
    d. Congenital adrenal hyperplasia
17. **Most common cause of hirsutism in a teenage girl:** *(AIIMS June 97)*
    a. Ovarian disease b. Pheochromocytoma
    c. Obesity d. Adrenogenital syndrome
18. **A 16-year-old girl presents with rapid onset hirsutism and amenorrhea. Best investigation is:** *(AIIMS June)*
    a. Testosterone estimation
    b. Dihydroepiandrosterone
    c. Adrenocorticoids
    d. LH and FSH estimation
19. **Kali Rani, a 20-year-old girl presents with history of rapidly developing hirsutism and amenorrhea. To establish the diagnosis you would like to proceed with which of the following tests in blood:** *(AI 02)*
    a. 17 - OH progesterone
    b. DHEA
    c. Testosterone
    d. LH: FSH ratio

20. A 22-year-old woman comes for treatment of hirsutism. She is obese and has facial acne and hirsutism on her face. Serum LH level is 36 mIU/mL and FSH is 9 mIU/mL. Androstenedione and testosterone levels are mildly elevated, but serum DHEAS is normal. The patient does not wish to conceive at this time. Which of the following is the most appropriate treatment of her condition? *(All India 2002)*

a. Oral contraceptives pills
b. Corticosteroids
c. GnRH analog
d. Wedge resection of ovary

21. Persistent anovulation not treated leads to all *except*: *(PGI June 99)*

a. Hirsutism
b. Osteoporosis
c. Endometrial carcinoma
d. Increased risk of CVS disease

22. A 20-year average weight female presented with oligomenorrhea and abnormal facial hair growth along with high serum free testosterone level. On USG the ovaries are normal. The diagnosis: *(AIIMS Nov 2010, AIIMS Nov 2012)*

a. Idiopathic hirsutism
b. PCOD
c. Testosterone secreting tumor
d. Adrenal hyperplasia

23. All of the following are associated with polycystic ovarian syndrome *except*: *(AI 2010)*

a. Ovarian carcinoma
b. Endometrial carcinoma
c. Insulin resistance
d. Osteoporosis

24. True about PCOS: *(PGI May 2010)*

a. High FSH/LH ratio
b. Unilateral large ovarian cyst
c. Hirsutism
d. Increased risk of diabetes mellitus
e. OCP is given for treatment

25. In PCOD, which of the following drugs is not used for infertility? *(AIIMS Nov 2013, May 2015)*

a. Spironolactone b. Tamoxifen
c. Clomiphene d. OC pill

26. All are true about PCOD *except*: *(PGI May 2014)*

a. Metformin is used for treatment
b. Acanthosis nigricans may be associated
c. Occurs in post menopausal females only
d. Associated with obesity
e. Infertility may be present

27. Testosterone is/are secreted by: *(PGI Nov 2013*

a. Leydig cells
b. Sertoli cells
c. Zona reticularis of adrenal cortex
d. Zona glomerulosa
e. Interstitial cells of Leydig

28. In PCOD true is: *(PGI Nov 2013)*

a. ↑ LH
b. ↑ FSH
c. ↓ Oesterone
d. ↑ Insulin
e. ↑ Androgens

29. All are true about PCOD: *(PGI May 15)*

a. Testosterone >2 ng/mL
b. Infertility
c. High TSH/LH ratio
d. ↑ Insulin
e. ↑ E_2/E_1 ratio

30. Ovarian cause of Hirsutism: *(JIPMER 2012)*

a. PCOD
b. Ovarian cancer
c. Dysgerminoma
d. Endometriotic cyst

31. Adult woman has H/O amenorrhea, hirsutism and acne. She is at risk of developing which of the following conditions? *(JIPMER Nov 2014)*

a. Endometrial carcinoma
b. Ovarian carcinoma
c. Multiple pregnancy
d. Infertility

32. Hirsutism is caused by all *except*: *(JIPMER 2013)*

a. PCOD
b. CAH
c. Obesity
d. Testicular pregnancy syndrome

33. Ultrasonographic criteria for the diagnosis of PCOD include: *(PGI May 2019)*

a. Number of follicles
b. Stromal volume
c. Ovarian volume
d. Stromal echogenicity
e. Stromal blood flow

34. False regarding PCOS is/are: *(PGI December 2018)*

a. Different criteria used at different places
b. Rotterdam criteria is used
c. More common in Caucasians as compared to South Asians
d. Prevalence in China is 5%
e. More common in monozygotic twins

ANSWERS TO NEW PATTERN QUESTIONS

N1. Ans. is d, i.e. PCOS *Ref: Leon Speroff 8th/ed, p545*

M/C cause of hirsutism in young females PCOD/PCOS

M/C pathological cause of hirsutism in young females—PCOS/PCOD.

2nd M/C cause of hirsutism in young females is Idiopathic hirsutism

N2. Ans. is b, i.e. S. testosterone levels *Ref: Leon Speroff 8th/ed, p544*

N3. Ans. is a, i.e. Rapid onset hirsutism

In any female who comes with hirsutism, first & foremost it is necessary to understand that laboratory evaluation is indicated for many but not all women with hirsutism. Laboratory evaluation is to be recommended for women with moderate or severe hirsutism or hirsutism that is sudden in onset, rapidly progressive or associated with symptoms or signs of virilization. The first **and most important investigation to be done in case of hirsutism is S. testosterone levels.** Testing for nonclassical CAH, i.e. serum hydroxyprogesterone should be reserved for patients with early onset of hirsutism (premenarcheal females) women with a family history of the disorder and those in high-risk ethinic groups. In rapid onset hirsutism—there is suspicion of estrogen secreting ovarian/adrenal tumor (not CAH—Ans N3).

N4. Ans. is b, i.e. True tumor *Ref: Leon Speroff 8th/ed, p540-541*

Pregnancy luteoma

- It is a hyperplastic mass of luteinized ovarian cells.
- Not a true tumor
- Size of luteomas = 6-10 cm
- Usually bilateral
- Virilization during pregnancy can raise the suspicion of pregnancy luteoma
- Only one-third of pregnancy luteomas are associated with maternal hirsutism or virilization (This is because any increase in serum-free testosterone is accompanied by an increase in sex hormone-binding globulin (SHBG)
- It regresses promptly after delivery

N5. Ans. is c, i.e. > 10 mm

Clitoromegaly is defined as clitoris ≥ 10 mm is size or clitoral index (length multiplied width) greater than 35 mm

Note: Normal length = 5.0 ± 1.4 mm

N6. Ans. is d, i.e. Elevation in the level of sex hormone binding globulin (SHBG) level *Ref: Dutta Gynae 6th/ed, p460*

In PCOS (stein leventhal syndrome) the levels of SHBG decrease.

N7. Ans is c, i.e. Ferriman-Gallway score

N8. Ans. is a, i.e. 8 *Ref: Internet Search*

Ferriman-Gallway scoring is a scoring method for detecting hirsutism. In the original system—hair growth at 11 sites was noted:

1. Upper lip
2. Chin
3. Chest
4. Upper back
5. Lower back
6. Upper abdomen
7. Lower abdomen
8. Upper arms
9. Forearms
10. Thighs
11. Legs

In the modified method—2 sites were deleted-forearms and legs. Thus in the modified scoring system–hair growth is seen at 9 sites. In each of the nine locations-a score between 0-4 is given depending on growth of terminal hair

Maximum score = 36

In caucasian women a score of 8 or higher is regarded as indicative of androgen excess.

N9. Ans. is d, i.e. 10% *Ref: Leon Speroff 8th/ed, p517*

PCOS: Up to 35% exhibit impaired glucose tolerance and upto 10% have diabetes mellitus.
In all PCOS patients, a baseline 2-hour OGTT is recommended.

N10. Ans. is b, i.e. 25–29 *Ref: Leon Speroff 7th/ed, p470-475,780*

BMI (kg/m²)	Category
<19	Underweight
19.1-24.9	Normal
25-29.9	Overweight
30-34.9	Obese
> 35	Morbidly obese

N11. Ans. is a, i.e. Hyperinsulinism

The condition shown in the image is acanthosis nigricans seen in cases of insulin resistance. This patient is having PCOD/PCOS as suggested by acanthosis nigricans, irregular cycles, weight gain and multiple cyst in the ovary.

N12. Ans. is c, i.e. If pregnancy occurs, there is increased incidence of multiple pregnancy *Ref: Leon Speroff 7th/ed, p460-470*

Bromocriptine:

It is a dopamine agonist, used in the management of galactorrhea.

Peak of Bromocriptine occurs 1-3 hours after oral administration but very little remains in circulation after 14 hours.

Pregnancy following bromocriptine has got no teratogenic effects on off spring.

There is no increased incidence of multiple pregnancy.

Side effect of bromocriptine: Giddiness, dizziness and postural hypotension

Cabergoline: It is longer acting. A single dose of cabergoline can inhibit prolactin secretion for 7 days. Thus it has become DOC in case of hyperprolactinemia.

A newer dopamine agonist licensed for treatment of hyperprolactinemia is Guinagolide (non ergot dopamine D_2 agonist).

N13. Ans. is a, i.e. PCOD

See the text for explanation.

N14. Ans. is a, i.e. OCPs

OCPs are the DOC for hirsutism.

N15. Ans. is c, i.e. Danazol

Management of Hirsutism

- OCPs (best & most effective)
- Medroxyprogesterone acetate (150 mg/m every 3 months or 10-20 mg orally daily)
- Spironolactone (50-100 mg B/D)
- Cyproterone acetate (is a part of Diane-Diane has; 2 mg cyproterone acetate and 50 mg ethinyl estradiol)
- Flutamide (not preferred due to its hepatotoxicity)
- Finasteride
- GnRH agonist
- Topical eflornithine hydrochloride

Note: Danazol's side effect is hirsutism, hence it can never be used in managing hirsutism.

N16. Ans. is d, i.e. 80% *Ref: Shaw 15th/ed, p370*

Patients of PCOS develop early oligomenorrhea (87%) or short period of amenorrhea (26%) followed by prolonged periods.

N17. Ans. is c, i.e. Increased breast size *Ref: Williams gynae 3rd/ed, p395*

Clinical features of Virilization	
Acne	Androgenic alopecia
Hirsutism	Decreased breast size
Amenorrhea	Deepening of voice
Clitoromegaly	Increased muscle mass

N18. Ans. is a, i.e. E_2:E_1 *Ref: Shaw gynae 15th/ed, p370 Table 38.1*

In PCOS:

- E_1:E_2 Ratio is increased not E_2:E_1
- LDL:HDL Ratio is increased
- LH:FSH Ratio is increased
- Fasting insulin levels were raised
- Fasting glucose/insulin ratio is decreased <4.5.

N19. Ans. is a, i.e. Increased birth weight *Ref: Williams gynae 3rd/ed, p397*

Risk factors for PCOS in adolescent girls

- Low birth weight
- Premature adrenarche
- Obesity with acanthosis nigricans
- Atypical sexual precocity

N20. Ans. is c, i.e. Abruptio placenta *Ref: Williams gynae 3rd/ed, p393*

See the text for explanation

N21. Ans. is c, i.e. CYP 21 *Ref: Shaw 15th/ed, p369*

The gene mutation involved in PCOS is CYP 21.

N22. Ans. is c, i.e. Seborrheic dermatitis *Ref: Jeffcoates 9th/ed, p467*

Skin manifestations of PCOS are:

- Acne
- Hirsutism
- Alopecia (androgenic alopecia)
- Acanthosis nigricans

ANSWERS TO PREVIOUS YEAR QUESTIONS

1. **Ans. is d, i.e. Results in postdated pregnancy**

   Ref: Dutta Gynae 4th/ed, p421-425; Shaw 15th/ed, p369-371; Williams Gynae 1st/ed, p383 Onwards

   As discussed in the preceding text PCOD
   - Leads to increase in LH (option a correct)
   - Associated with glucose intolerance (due to insulin resistance).
   - Can cause infertility.
   - Postdated pregnancy is not a complication of PCOD/PCOS. Rather PCOS leads to preterm labour.
2. **Ans. is c, i.e. Luteinizing hormone**
3. **Ans. is b and e, i.e. LH increased, FSH normal to low and Testosterone increased > 2 ng/ml**
4. **Ans. is a and d, i.e. ↑ LH & ↓ FSH and Hyperinsulinemia**

   Ref: Shaw 15th/ed, p370; Dutta Gynae 5th/ed, p440-441; Williams Gynae 1st/ed, p384-386

   Lab Abnormalities

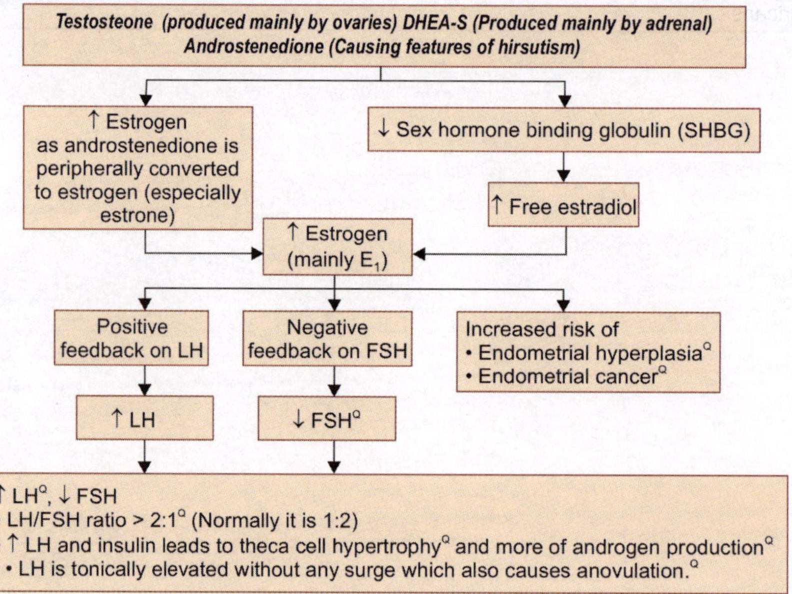

   - Ratio of Fasting Glucose: Fasting insulin in PCOS < 4.5
5. **Ans. is a, c and e, i.e. Testosterone > 200 ng/ml; High FSH/LH ratio and ↑E_2/oestrone (E_1) ratio**

   As discussed in the above question

   In PCOS: LH is increased and FSH decreased (i.e. option c is incorrect).

   ∴ FSH/LH ratio will be low(opposite will be true i.e. LH/FSH will be high)

   Similarly in PCOD= levels of E_2 are less but E_1 which is mainly formed by conversion of testosterone to estrogen is high.

   ∴ E_2/E_1 ratio will low (i.e. option e is incorrect)

   In PCOD: levels of testosterone are increased but never more than 200 ng/ml (i.e. option a is incorrect).

   Rest all options are correct, and discussed in detail in the preceding text.
6. **Ans. is a, i.e. Polycystic ovaries** *Ref: Shaw 15th/ed, p371; Novak 14th/ed, p1076*

   A young woman presenting in the third decade with obesity, oligomenorrhea, infertility and hirsutism leaves no doubt for the diagnosis of PCOS.

   According to Rotterdam criteria → PCOD is diagnosed if any 2 of the following criteria are being fulfilled:

   i. Ovulatory dysfunction such as oligomenorrhea or hyperandrogenism.

   ii. Clinical or biochemical evidence of hyperandrogenism.

   iii. USG criteria

   Since this female, has oligomenorrhea and hirsutism, so 2 of the criteria are being fulfilled.
7. **Ans. is a, b, c, d and e, i.e. All are correct options** *Ref: Shaw 15th/ed, p369-371; Williams Gynae 1st/ed, p386*

   In a patient of PCOD, amenorrhea, hyperandrogenism, anovulation and theca cell hyperplasia will be seen as discussed in the preceding text.

Hyperandrogenism: It is manifested clinically by:

- Hirsutism (i.e. presence of coarse, dark terminal hair distributed in male pattern).
- Acne (Acne that is persistent or is late in onset) and/or[Q]
- Androgenic alopecia.[Q]

Therefore alopecia can also be seen in PCOD patient

Note: In contrast signs of virilization such as increased muscle mass, deepening of the voice and clitoromegaly are not typical of PCOS. Virilization reflects much higher androgen levels and should prompt investigation for an androgen producing tumor of ovary or the adrenal gland.[Q]

8. **Ans. is a, i.e. 1–4 days** *Ref: Jeffcoate 6th/ed, p205*

In PCOS: *"Determination of the follicle stimulating hormone (FSH) and luteinizing hormone (LH) levels may help to confirm the diagnosis of polycystic ovaries. These are assayed on the second or third day of the cycle".*

Ref: Jeffcoate 6th/ed, p205

9. **Ans. is a, c and e, i.e. Oligomenorrhea and amenorrhea; Innumerate cysts in ovary; and Theca cell hypertrophy**

Ref: Shaw 15th/ed, p369-371

- There is no doubt that PCOD causes oligomenorrhea/amenorrhea, i.e. ***option 'a'*** is correct.
- PCOS is seen in young females. Most common age affected is 15–25 years[Q]. and not postmenopausal, so ***option 'b'*** is incorrect.
- *Pathologically* – Ovaries are enlarged (2–5 times the normal size). Tunical albuginea is thickened. There is Theca cell hypertrophy (stromal hyperthecosis) and multiple follicular cysts are localized along the surface of ovary (i.e. ***options 'c'*** and ***'e'*** are correct).
- BRCA-1 is not associated with PCOD.[Q] (i.e. ***options 'd'*** is incorrect)
- BRCA-1 gene has been located at the chromosomal locus *17q21*; women who inherit a mutated allele of this gene from either parent have an approx. 60-80% lifetime chance of developing *Breast Ca* and about 33% chance of developing *Ovarian Ca.*
- Men who carry a mutant allele of the gene of BRCA-1 have an increased incidence of Prostate Ca, but not usually of
- Breast Ca.
- BRCA-2 gene which has been located to chromosome 11, is associated with an increased incidence of Breast Ca in both men and women.

Also Know

Sonographic findings in case of PCOS include: (See Fig. 4.9)

- > 12 small cysts (2 to 9 mm in diameter)
- Increased ovarian volume (> 10 ml).
- Increased amount of stroma relative to the number of follicles.
  - Only one ovary with these findings is sufficient to define PCOS.
  - Other findings like Pearl necklace appearance in which follicles are distributed underneath the capsule in a row and increase in stromal echogenicity have been eliminated as diagnostic criteria.

10. **Ans. is a, b, and e, i.e. Hirsutism; Secondary amenorrhoea; and ↑ Oestrogen**

Ref: Novak 14th/ed, p1078–1079; Williams Gynae 1st/ed, p385-386

Friends, here I would like to point out that in ***option "e"*** it is mentioned oestrogen : which is correct in cases of PCOS.

In PCOS:

"Patients with PCOS, E1, levels are increased E2 is at a follicular phase level." *__Novak 14th/ed, p1078; 15th/ed, p1079*

Therefore, in PCOS = E1 > E2, i.e. Reversal of E2 : E1 ratio.

"Elevated androstenedione levels contribute to an increase in estrone levels through peripheral conversion."

__Williams Gynae 1st/ed, p386

Note:

- Streak ovaries are seen when genetic material is missing either from the long or short arm of X-chromosome or complete X-chromosome is missing as in Turner's syndrome.
- Streak ovaries are not seen in PCOS patients.

11. **Ans. is b and c, i.e. Increased FSH; and Streak ovaries**

Ref: Shaw 15th/ed, p369-371; Jeffcoate 7th/ed, p385-386,390; Williams Gynae 1th/ed, p390 for Option 'a'

"In women with PCOS, a threefold increased risk of endometrial cancer has been reported. Endometrial hyperplasia and endometrial cancer are long-term risks of chronic anovulation, and neoplastic changes in the endometrium are felt to arise from chronic unopposed estrogen." *__ Williams Gynae 1st/ed, p390*

Rest all options have been explained earlier

12. Ans. is d, i.e. Increase prolactin *Ref: Jeffcoate 9th/ed, p463; Leon Speroff 7th/ed, p472*

Leon Speroff specifically mentions:

"In contrast to the characteristic picture of fluctuating hormone levels in the normal cycle, a 'steady state' of Gonadotropins and sex steroids can be depicted in association with persistent anovulation." *Ref: Leon Speroff 7th/ed, p471*

This is depicted clearly in the following graph from *Leon Speroff 7th/ed, p 472.*

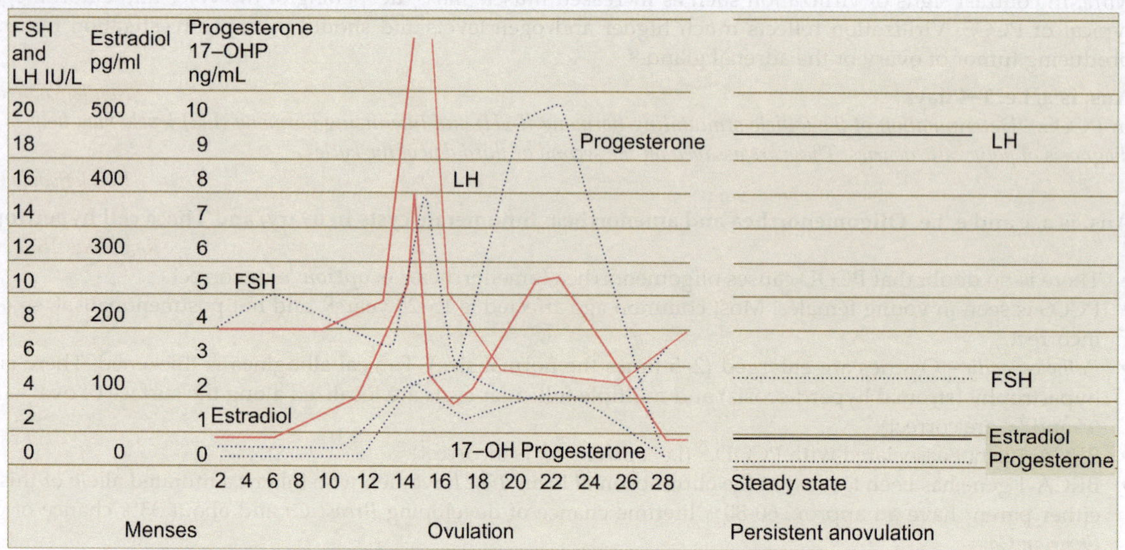

So now there is no doubt that ***option 'a'*** is correct.

"Approximately 70-80% of women with PCOS demonstrate frank elevations in circulating androgens particularly free testosterone, and 25-30% will have elevated levels of adrenal androgen metabolite, DHEAS" *– Jeffcoate 9th/ed, p463*

"The serum DHEA-S concentration is moderately elevated in over half of the woman with PCOS."

i.e., ***option 'c'*** is correct.

"Prolactin levels are usually normal, although they may be slightly elevated (generally < 40 ng / ml in a small fraction of patients." *– Jeffocate 9th/ed, p463*

According to *Williams Gynae 1st/ed, p 392* – If in a patient of hirsutism with irregular menses (i.e., anovulation) –

Prolactin levels	
Are normal ↓	***If elevated*** ↓
PCOS / congenital adrenal hyperplasia should be considered	Pituitary/ovarian neoplasm should be considered

Thus, increase prolactin levels are not a diagnostic feature of PCOS. So it is the answer of choice here.

13. Ans. is a, i.e. OCP

14. Ans. is b and c, i.e. GnRH and Spironolactone *Ref: Novak 14th/ed, p1082-1083; 15th/ed, p1085-1089; Williams Gynae 1st/ed, p396-397; Shaw 15th/ed, p117-118; John Hopkins Manual of Obs and Gynae 4th/ed, p491-492*

See the text for explanation

15. Ans. is b, i.e. Ethinyl estradiol + Desogestrel *Ref: Novak 14th/ed, p 1083, 15th/ed, p 1086 KDT Pharma 6th/ed, p 307*

As discussed earlier—OCPs decrease adrenal and ovarian androgen production and reduce hair growth in nearly two thirds of hirsute patients. When an OCP is used to treat hirsutism, a balance must be maintained between the decrease in free testosterone levels and the intrinsic androgenicity of the progestin.

Progesterones with:

High androgenic bioactivity	Newer progestins with low androgenic bioactivity
• Norgestrel • Norethindrone • Norethindrone acetate • Drospirenone	• *Desogestrel i.e. class III* • Gestodene • Norgestimate

Thus, newer progestins with minimal androgenic activity are preferred for management of hirsutism in a patient of PCOD/PCOS (i.e. option b is correct).

16. Ans. is a, i.e. Polycystic ovary disease (PCOD)

Ref: CGDT 10th/ed, p937; Williams Gynae 1st/ed, p387; Leon Speroff 7th/ed, p501

See the text for explanation.

17. Ans. is a, i.e. Ovarian disease

See the text for explanation.

18. Ans. is a, i.e. Testosterone estimation

19. Ans. is c, i.e. Testosterone *Ref: Dutta Gynae 4th/ed, p524; Leon Speroff 7th/ed, p502-511,515; Williams Gynae 1st/ed, p391*

"A variety of ovarian neoplasms, both benign and malignant may produce testosterone and lead to virilization. Specifically, women with an abrupt onset, typically within several months, or sudden worsening of virilizing signs should prompt concern for a hormone producing ovarian or adrenal tumor. Symptoms may include deepening of voice, frontal balding, severe acne or hirsutism or both, increased muscle mass and clitoromegaly. Accordingly, serum testosterone levels may be used to exclude these tumors. Free testosterone levels are more sensitive than total testosterone levels as an indicator of hyperandrogenism. Although improving, current free testosterone assays lack a uniform laboratory standard. For this reason, total testosterone levels remain the best approach for excluding a tumor. Threshold values beyond 200 ng /dl of total testosterone warrant evaluation for an ovarian lesion."

– Williams Gynae 1st/ed, p391

So now I do not need to explain that testosterone estimation is the best investigation in case of rapid onset hirsutism and amenorrhea.

Lines of Leon Speroff further support the answer—

"A serum testosterone concentration greater than 150 mg/dl identifies almost all woman with a potential androgen producing tumor. However, a tumor still should be suspected and excluded in a woman with rapidly progressive hirsutism or signs and symptoms of virilization, even when the serum testosterone concentration is below the threshold value." *– Leon Speroff 8th/ed, p52*

- M/C cause of rapid onset hirsutism in young females = Testosterone producing tumor

DHEA sulphate is produced exclusively by the adrenal gland. Therefore, serum DHEAS levels above 700 mcg/dl are highly sensitive for the presence of an adrenal neoplasm.

Adrenal imaging with abdominal CT or MRI is indicated for any patient with DHEAS levels that exceed this value.

20. Ans. is a, i.e. Oral contraceptive pills

This patient is having hirsutism with altered LH: FSH ratio. Most probably it is a case of PCOS

1st line management of hirsutism in PCOS is OCPs.

21. Ans. is b, i.e. Osteoporosis

In PCOS patients: Estrogen levels are high, hence it never leads to osteoporosis.

Ref: Clinical Gynaecologic Endocrinology & Infertility by Leon Speroff 7th/ed, p484; Novak 1083 15th/ed, p1085

22. Ans. is b, i.e. PCOD *Ref: Leon Speroff 8th/ed, p508,518,519,520; Williams Gynae 1st/ed, p383,384*

In the question patient is presenting with oligomenorrhea, abnormal facial hair growth and high serum free testosterone level.

All these features can be seen in PCOD, Testosterone secreting tumors and adrenal hyperplasia. So lets consider each option separately:

Option 'a'- Idiopathic hirsutism: It is defined classically as hirsutism accompanied by normal ovulatory and menstrual function in absence of hyperandrogenemia i.e. androgen levels are normal. Idiopathic hirsutism is ruled out because patient in the question has oligomenorrhea and high serum free testosterone levels.

Option 'c'- Testosterone secreting tumor–It is rare condition, which is almost always accompanied by severe or rapidly progressive hirsutism and symptoms or signs of virilisation (deepening of voice, temporal or male pattern baldness, breast atrophy, increased muscle mass and clitoromegaly).

"The possibility of a tumor is excluded primarily by the clinical history and physical examination. Very few women will require specific evaluation to exclude the diagnosis." *Ref: Leon Speroff 8th/ed, p520*

Since other features of virilization are absent and hirsutism is not rapid in onset, so testosterone producing tumor is excluded in this patient.

Another point which goes against if testosterone producing tumor is, in ovaries, the ovaries are normal on ultrasound in this patient whereas in case of testosterone producing tumors, solid ovarian mass lesion should be identified in most of the cases.

"Transvaginal ultrasonography will identify almost all solid ovarian mass lesions, although very small tumors located in the hilar region can escape detection." *Ref: Leon Speroff 8th/ed, p520*

Coming to Option 'd'- Congenital Adrenal Hyperplasia- Congenital Adrenal Hyperplasia (CAH) is caused by adrenal steroidogenic enzyme defects that result in excessive adrenal androgen production.

M/C cause is 21 hydroxylase enzyme deficiency other rare causes are Defect in 11b hydroxylase, 3b hydroxysteroid dehydrogenase.

Females with classical CAH typically present at birth with ambiguous genitalia and this would rarely be confused with PCOS, but those with non-classical or late onset form of CAH present later, during childhood or early adolescence with precocious puberty or as young adults with signs of hyperandrogenism, very much like those of PCOS.

"Whereas it is logical to recommend that non-classical CAH be excluded specifically in all women with hyperandrogenism, we believe that specific testing can be safely reserved for those having an early onset of hirsutism (pre or perimenarcheal, including girls with premature adrenarche), women with a family history of the disorder, and those in high risk ethanic groups (Hispanic, medittaraneaen slavic, Ashkenazi jewish or yupic eskimo heritage. The yield from routine screening is very low as the disorder is uncommon."

Ref: Leon Speroff 8th/ed, p319

Thus from above discussion- it is clear that classical congenital adrenal hyperplasia is ruled out completely; non classical hyperplasia may be a possibility but since it is not common in general population but in hispanic, meditaranean, groups, etc. it can be kept in +/– status.

Option 'b'- PCOD

A 20-year-old female presenting with oligomenorrhea and hirsutism- chances of PCOD are high.

According to **Rotterdam criteria** (2003) adopted for the diagnosis of PCOD.

Any 2 out of the three should be present for diagnosing PCOD

1. Oligoanovulation
2. Clinical and/or biochemical signs of hyperandrogenism
3. Polycystic ovaries on USG

In the question, patient is presenting with oligomenorrhea (anovulation) and increased free serum testosterone levels as well as hirsutism (biochemical and clinical signs of hyperandrogenism), two criteria are being fulfilled and we have also excluded androgen secreting tumor and congenital adrenal hyperplasia, so PCOD can be diagnosed.

Some of you may argue that ovaries are normal in USG in this patient, whereas in PCOD- multiple cysts (≥12 in number, 2-9 mm in diam) are seen in one or both ovaries and ovarian volume is ≥ 10 ml.

Read what Leon speroff 8/e, p 514 has to say on this issue–.

"Again, the important point is that PCOS is a functional disorder in which polycystic ovaries result from chronic anovulation. Although present in most women with chronic diagnosis hyper androgenic anovulation, polycystic ovaries donot establish and are not required for diagnosis of PCOS." *Ref: Leon Speroff 8th/ed, p515, 522*

So it is clear in PCOD- Polycystic ovaries are not required for diagnosis. Another point is that this female is average weight whereas in PCOD- females are obese- so now let us read what Leon Speroff has to say on this issue:

"Observations indicate that obesity relates primarily to genetic and environmental factors and is a common but not essential feature of PCOS. Obesity contributes modestly to the risk for developing PCOS and adds to the patho physiology in already affected women by aggravating the degrees of insulin resistance and hyperinsulinemia."

Ref: Leon Speroff 8th/ed, p508

Now this leaves us with no doubt that diagnosis of the patient in the question is PCOD.

23. Ans. is d, i.e. Osteoporosis *Ref: Leon Speroff 7th/ed, p470-480, 8th/ed, p500-518; Novak 14th/ed, p1082, 15th/ed, p1085*

Relationship between bone mineral density and Insulin resistance in PCOS Journal of Bone mineral metabolism vol 19, Number 4, July 2001, p 257-262

This was definitely one of the most controversial questions in AIPG 2010. As explained earlier endometrial cancer and insulin resistance are seen in PCOD. Osteoporosis is never seen in PCOD patients.

What about ovarian cancer?

The main theory for development of epithelial ovarian cancer (which accounts for 85-90% of all ovarian CA) is the "Theory of incessant ovulation" which means "more the ovulation, more the risk".

But in PCOS there is anovulation and hence per say it is protective for CA ovary.

But, PCOS patients are infertile and ovulation induction is required for treatment of infertility. Use of ovulation inducing agents like gonadotrophins, clomiphene letrozole, etc. is one of the risk factors for development of ovarian cancer. This is how PCOS can be associated CA ovary. So the studies are still going on whether ovarian cancer leads to PCOS or not:

"The risk of ovarian cancer is increased two to three fold in woman with PCOS." *Ref: Novak 15th/ed, p1085*

24. Ans. is c, d, and e, i.e. Hirsutism; Increased risk of diabetes mellitus; and OCP is given for treatment

See the text for explanation.

25. Ans. is a, i.e. Spironolactone *Ref: Shaw's Textbook of Gynecology 15th/ed, p371; Dutta Gynae 6th/ed, p470*

There is no confusion with regards to the use of clomiphene citrate or Tamoxifen for infertility. The confusion is between OCP's and spironolactone. Spironolactone is not used for treating infertility. OCPs used for sometime, can lead to suppression of gonadotropins and then exogenous gonadotropins can be given to increase fertility.

26. Ans. is a, b, d and c, i.e. Metformin is used for treatment, Acanthosis nigricans may be associated, Associated with obesity and infertility may be present

See the text for explanation.

27. **Ans. is a, c and e, i.e. Leydig cells, Zona reticularis of adrenal cortex and Interstitial cells of Leydig.**
"Testosterone is also formed by the adrenal cortex from zona reticularis layer. *Ref: AK Jain 5th/ed, p821*
"Interstitial on laydig cells secrete testosterone at about the time of puberty" *Ref: AK Jain 5th/ed, p815*
Another source of testosterone is Androstenedione.
Androstenedione is converted to testosterone

28. **Ans. is a, d and e, i.e. ↑ LH, ↑ Insulin and ↑ Androgen**
"While oesterone levels increases, oestradiol levels remain normal with the result that oesterone/estradiol ratio rises."
Ref: Shaw 16th/ed, p43

Rest see the text for explanation.

29. **Ans. is c and e, i.e. High FSH/LH ratio and ↑ E_2/E_1 ratio**
As discussed earlier in PCOS
- LH: FSH ratio is increased to 2 or 3:1. The reverse is not true i.e. FSH:LH ratio is decreased.
- Levels of testosterone are > 2 ng/mL. (most androgens are from ovary).
- E_1:E_2 ratio is increased. The reverse is not true.

Remember
- All androgens Testosterone/epiandrosteredione, DHEA are raised
- Fasting insulin is raised and more than 10 m IU/L
- F. glucose/insulin ratio < 4.5.
- Sex hormone binding globulin is decreased.

30. **Ans. is a, i.e. PCOD**
See the text for explanation

31. **Ans. is a, i.e. Endometrial carcinoma**
This adult female is having amenorrhea, hirsutism and acne. In other words 2 out of 3 criteria are fulfilled as per the Rotterdam criteria. So we can say she has PCOD/PCOS.
Now both Endometrial cancer and infertility are seen in PCOS.
But Infertility due to PCOS is most easily treated and is never a long term consequence, whereas due to excessive estrogen secretion—Endometrial cancer is a long term consequence and hence our option of choice.

32. **Ans. is d, i.e. Testicular feminization syndrome** *Ref: Dutta Gynae 5th/ed, p546, Jeffecoates 9th/ed, p476*

Causes of hirsutism		
Ovarian	Adrenal	Others
PCOS	Congenital adrenal Hyperplasia	Obesity
HAIR-AN syndrome	Cushing syndrome	
Androgen secreting tumor	Adrenal Tumor	
Sertoli Leydig cell Tumor		

33. **Ans. is a and c, i.e. Number of follicles and Ovarian volume** *Ref: Leon Speroff 9th/ed, p414.*
According to **Rotterdam guideline, only follicle number per ovary** and **ovarian volume are included** in ultrasonographic criteria for the diagnosis of PCOD.
As per Rotterdam criteria:
To diagnose polycystic ovary on USG.
i. Number of follicles should be ≥12. and size of follicles should be between 2 to 9 mm, or
ii. Volume of ovary >10 mL
Presence of any one of these two morphologic USG finding in a single ovary serves as meeting the criteria.
Note: The AE-PCOS Society has recommended that in order to characterize ovarian appearance as PCOS, the minimal number of small follicles should be increased from a threshold of 12, as is specified by Rotterdam criteria, to a minimum of 25. But till now this is only a recommendation.

34. **Ans. is c, i.e. More common in Caucasians as compared to South Asians** *Ref: Various references*
"The prevalence of PCOS varies depending on which criteria are used to make the diagnosis."
https://www.ncbi.nlm.nih.gov/pmc/articles/PMC3872139
- Diagnostic criteria for PCOS have been offered by three groups: the National Institutes of Health/National Institute of Child Health and Human Disease (NIH/NICHD); the European Society for Human Reproduction and ***Embryology/American Society for Reproductive Medicine ESHRE/ASRM (Rotterdam criteria)***; and the Androgen Excess and PCOS Society.

"It has been reported that the prevalence of PCOS is considered to be higher in South Asians than in Caucasians residing in the United Kingdom, but prevalence is not necessarily higher in non-United Kingdom Caucasians. Fifty-two percent of Asian women who reside in the Indian subcontinent present with polycystic ovaries, which is considered to the highest reported prevalence"

https://www.ncbi.nlm.nih.gov/pmc/articles/PMC6266413/

"The prevalence of PCOS in Chinese women aged 19–45 years is 5.6%."

https://www.ncbi.nlm.nih.gov/pubmed/23814096

"Greater concordance has been reported in monozygotic twins versus dizygotic twins."

https://www.ncbi.nlm.nih.gov/pmc/articles/PMC3872139/

PCOD diagnostic criteria and prevalence

- The clinical presentation of PCOS varies widely. Women with PCOS often seek care for menstrual disturbances, clinical manifestations of hyperandrogenism, and infertility.
- ***The prevalence of diagnosis of PCOS may vary in different regions depending upon the criteria used for making the diagnosis, as there are more than one criteria to make the diagnosis.***
- Diagnostic criteria for PCOS have been offered by three groups: the National Institutes of Health/National Institute of Child Health and Human Disease (NIH/NICHD); the European Society for Human Reproduction and Embryology/American Society for Reproductive Medicine (ESHRE/ASRM); and the Androgen Excess and PCOS Society.

Criteria for the diagnosis of polycystic ovary syndrome

NIH/NICHD 1992	ESHRE/ASRM (Rotterdam criteria) 2004	Androgen Excess Society 2006
• Exclusion of other androgen excess or related disorders • Includes all of the following: – Clinical and/or biochemical hyperandrogenism – Menstrual dysfunction	• Exclusion of other androgen excess or related disorders • Includes two of the following: – Clinical and/or biochemical hyperandrogenism – Oligo-ovulation or anovulation – Polycystic ovaries	• Exclusion of other androgen excess or related disorders • Includes all of the following: – Clinical and/or biochemical hyperandrogenism – Ovarian dysfunction and/or polycystic ovaries

Abbreviations: ESHRE/ASRM, European Society for Human Reproduction and Embryology/American Society for Reproductive Medicine; NIH/NICH, National Institute of Child Health and Human Disease

- While there are certain consistencies between the criteria offered by the different groups, important differences exist.
- ***The diagnosis of PCOS using the Rotterdam*** and AES criteria depends on the use of a reliable method to describe polycystic ovarian morphology. The criteria for polycystic ovarian morphology proposed by the Rotterdam consensus group includes the presence of 12 or more follicles measuring between 2 and 9 mm in diameter and/or an increased ovarian volume of greater than 10 cm^3. This presentation in one ovary sufficiently defines the polycystic ovary.
- Prevalence estimates for PCOS, as defined by the NIH/NICHD criteria, indicate that PCOS is a common endocrinopathy affecting 4–8% of women of reproductive age. ***Recently, several groups have demonstrated that the prevalence of PCOS varies depending on the diagnostic criteria used*** These studies consistently report that the prevalence estimates using the Rotterdam criteria are two to three times greater than those obtained using the NIH/NICHD criteria.
- A high prevalence of PCOS or its features among first-degree relatives is suggestive of genetic influences. ***In addition, greater concordance has been reported in monozygotic twins versus dizygotic twins.***
- Caucasian females living in the US and Europe are less likely to develop PCOS compared with females residing in the Middle East whereas Black women (the majority are African-Americans and Afro-Brazilians) tend to have the highest risks of developing PCOS.
- In general, we would expect that under the same diagnostic criterion of PCOS, Chinese women are at a lowest risk of developing PCOS, and then in an ascending order through Caucasian women and females residing in the Middle East, with Black women having the highest risks of developing this syndrome.

CHAPTER 5

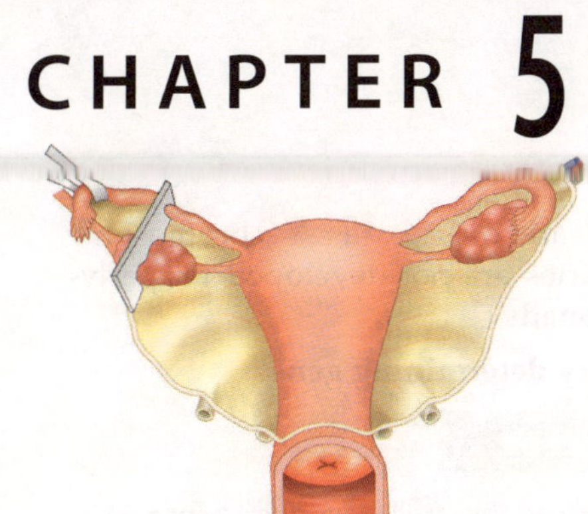

Congenital Malformations

Embryology Related to Development in Males and Females

- Sex of a fetus is determined by **S**ex **R**elated **R**egion present in short arm of **Y** chromosome
- SRY region is also called as Testis Determining factor

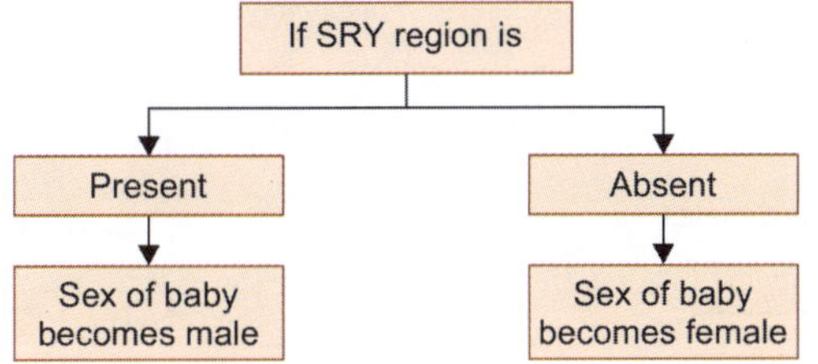

Revision of Embryology

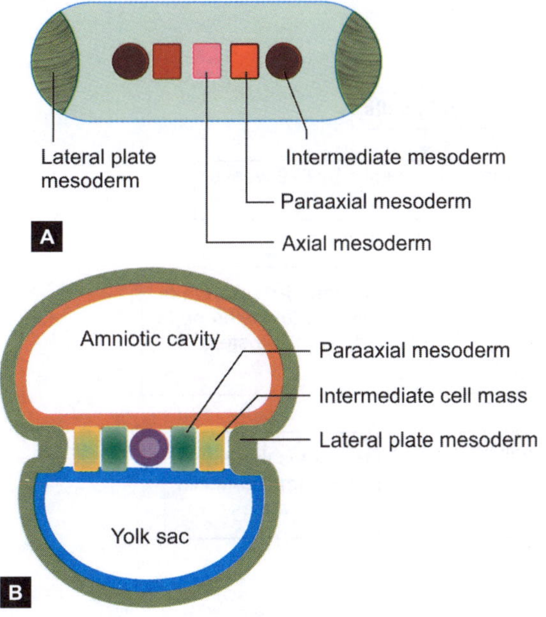

Figs. 5.1A and B: Parts of Mesoderm

- Intermediate Mesoderm forms the ducts (i.e. Mullerian and Wolffian duct) and forms the Urogenital Ridge which forms Gonads and kidneys
- The Dorso somatic part of Lateral plate mesoderm forms the External Genitalia.

Embryological Origin of Various Structures in both Sexes at a Glance

- Gonads: Arise from Genital Ridge (mesodermal in origin)
- Ducts: Also mesodermal in origin
- Germ cells: Originate from Epiblast
- Ext: Genitalia: Arise from dorso somatic part of Lateral plate mesoderm

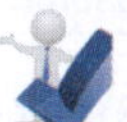

KEY POINTS

Major part of genito-urinary system arise from mesoderm **except** the parts which are arising from urogenital sinus which are endodermal in origin.

Development of Gonads

- Gonads (both testis and ovaries) develop from the genital ridge (which is formed by 5th week of gestation)
- Initially gonads are bipotential, i.e. they can form either testis or ovaries. Epithelial cords grow into the mesenchyme (primary sex cords) and the biopotential gonads now possess an outer cortex and inner medulla.
- **The sexual differentiation depends on Sex Determining Region (SRY region) present on short arm of Y-chromosome.**[Q]
- **If Y-chromosome is present** → the medulla of the gonads develop into testes (7 weeks) and cortex regresses.
- **If SRY region is absent, i.e. Y chromosome is absent** → the cortex of gonads develop into ovaries (8 weeks) and the medulla regresses.

Development of Testis

In males:

The primary sex cords become concentrated on the medulla of the gonad and proliferate (to form Testicular cords) and their ends anastomose to form the Rete Testis (Figs. 5.1A and B).

 **Important Concept**

- The first feature which distinguishes between testis and ovaries: is formation of Testicular cords.

- The testicular cords, become the **seminiferous tubules** and get a capsule called **tunica albuginea**. Mesenchyme grows between the tubes to separate them (Leydig cells).
- The seminiferous tubules are composed of 2 layers of cells – supporting cells (sertoli cells) derived from germinal epithelium and spermatogonia derived from the primordial germ cells.

Development of Ovary

- Ovaries are formed because of absence of 'Y' chromosome but for proper development of ovaries-presence of two X chromosomes is required. This is the reason why in Turner's syndrome (45X0) although Gonads are ovaries (as Y chromosome is absent) but ovaries are not developed properly-called **as streak gonads**.
- **WNT-4 is the ovary determining gene.**

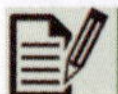 **Important Concept**

- Ovaries are not formed by Mullerian duct hence in Mullerian agenesis – ovaries/ovulation is normal

Development of Duct

In Embryonic life, 2 pairs of ducts are present in both males & females.

1. Mesonephric duct
2. Paramesonephric duct

These ducts arise from Intermediate mesoderm. Further development of ducts in both sexes is shown in Flowchart 5.1 (in males) and in Flowchart 5.2 (in females).

In males:

Flowchart 5.1: Development in males

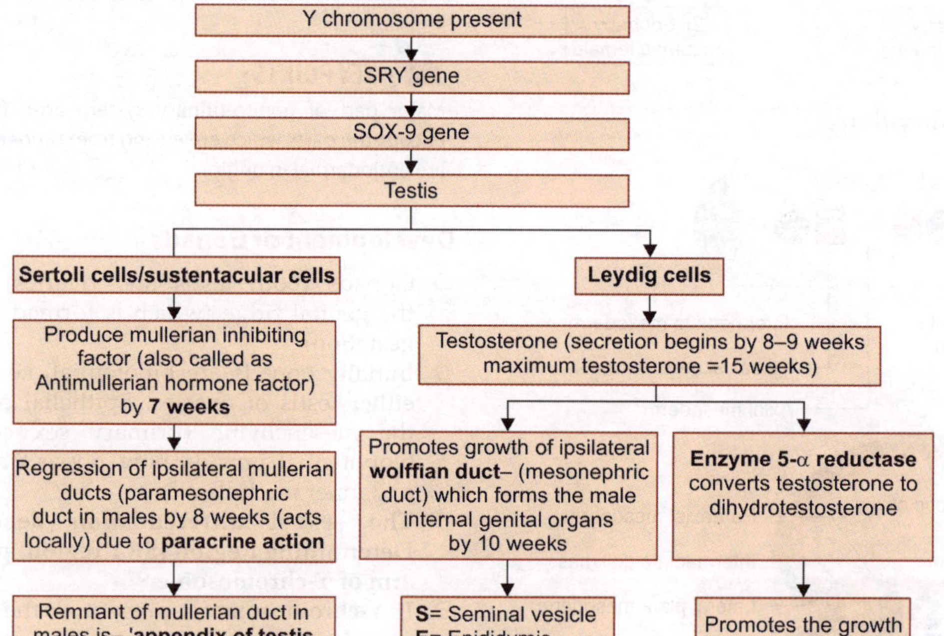

Blood Testis Barrier (Fig. 5.2)

It is formed by Sertoli cells or Sustentacular cells.

- These cells surround the growing germ cells i.e. sperms in its various stages of development and prevent it from coming in contact with the toxins present in blood
- Thus they (Sertoli cells) form a blood testis barrier.
- The Leydig cells lie outside this barrier

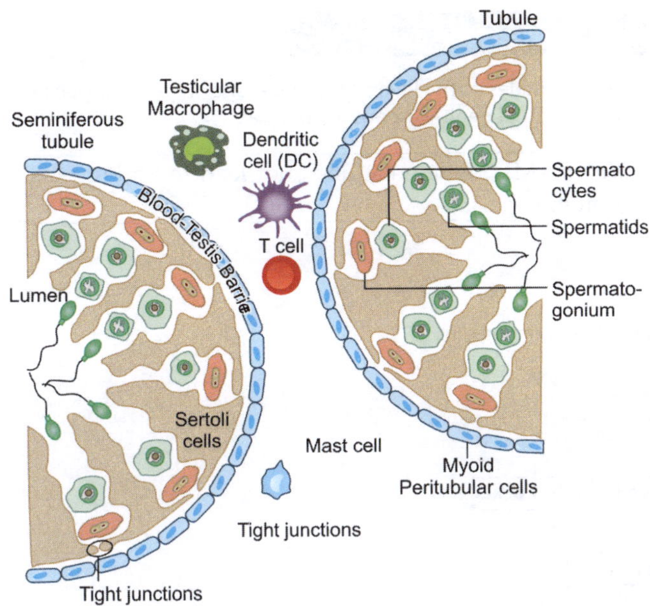

Figs. 5.2: Blood Testis Barrier

Extra Edge

- In males & females there is: Pronephros, Mesonephros and metanephros.

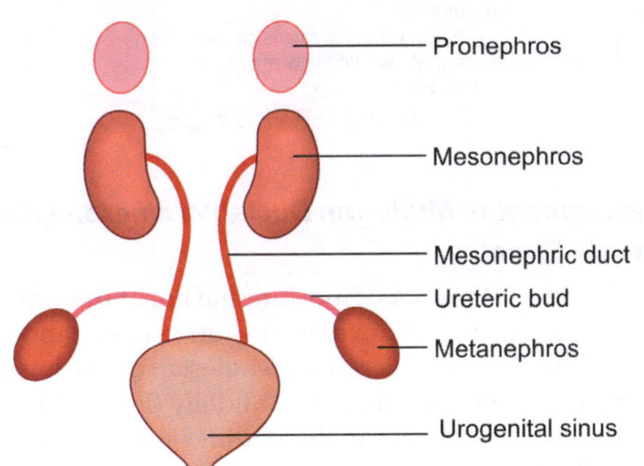

Fig. 5.3: Pronephros, Mesonephros and Metanephros

- The mesonephros gives mesonephric duct which opens in the Urogenital Sinus & forms the Trigone of the bladder Mesonephric duct also gives the ureteric bud stimulates the Metanephros to form the Renal System
- Now after all this has happened, the Mesonephric Duct will be called as Wolffian Duct, which in males will form the internal genital organs and in females will disappear.
- In males the Mesonephros forms the efferent ductules or tubules (see Fig. 5.4).

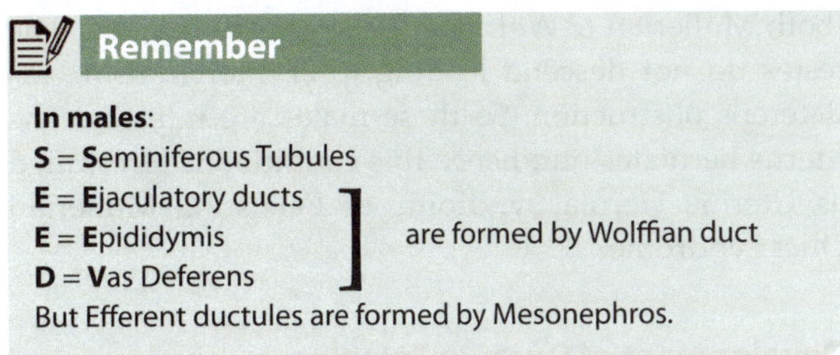

Remember

In males:
S = **S**eminiferous Tubules
E = **E**jaculatory ducts
E = **E**pididymis
D = **V**as Deferens
] are formed by Wolffian duct
But Efferent ductules are formed by Mesonephros.

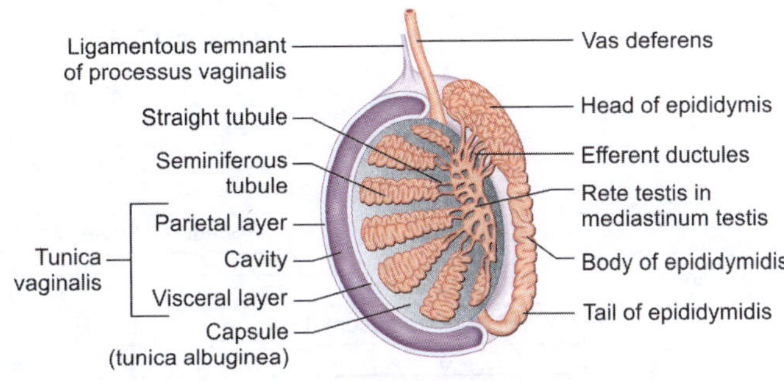

Fig. 5.4: Testis section to show seminiferous tubules, straight tubules & Efferent ductules

Development of Male External Genitalia

Under the influence of dihydrotestosterone:

- Genital tubercle forms glans penis
- Genital swellings forms scrotum
- Genital folds forms penile urethra
- Male genital development is complete by 12–14 weeks.

Clinical Correlation

Anti-Mullerian Hormone Deficiency (AMH deficiency)

Flowchart 5.2: Anti-Mullerian hormone deficiency

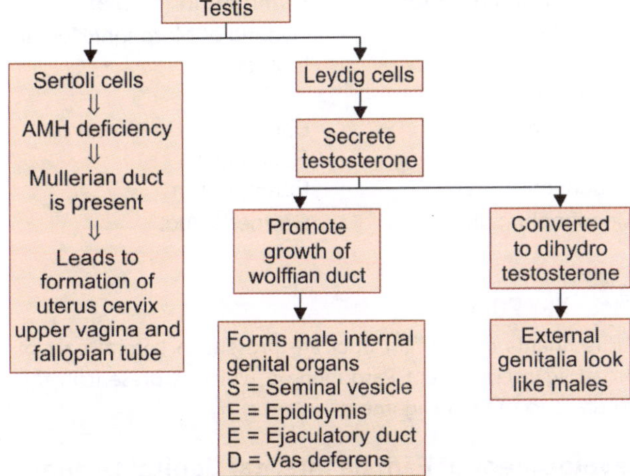

So in males with AMH deficiency both male and female internal genital organs are present. The ducts (both Mullerian & Wolffian ducts/get intertwined. The testes do not descend leading to cryptorchidism, vas deferens obstruction. So these males are infertile. The uterus herniates out: hence this condition is also called as Uterine Hernia Syndrome or Persisting Mullerian Duct Syndrome.

Remember

In these males as the levels of testosterone are normal, hence their external genital organs are normal.

Note: AMH deficiency does not lead to ambiguous genitalia.

Development of Ducts in Females

Flowchart 5.3: Development of ducts in females

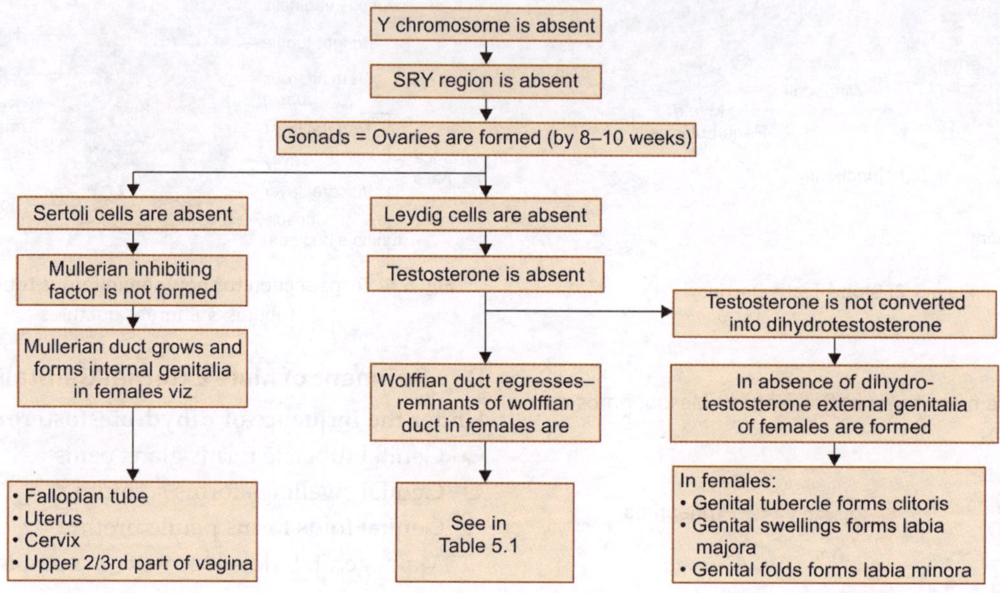

Remnants of Wolffian Duct (Mesonephric Duct) in Females

Table 5.1: Remnants of Wolffian Duct (Mesonephric Duct) in Females

Part of Wolffian duct	Remnant in females
Pronephros	Hydatid of Morgagni/Kobelt tubercle
Mesonephros:	
Cranial end	Epoophoron or Organ of Rosenmuller
Caudal end	Paroophoron
Mesonephric duct	Gartner's duct

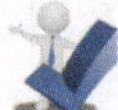

KEY POINTS

All remnants of Wolffian duct are present in Lateral part of Broad ligament except Paroophoron which is present in the Medial part of Broad ligament.

Development of Female Internal Genital Organs

The major part of the female genital tract develops from the **Mullerian ducts**.

Development of Mullerian Ducts/Paramesonephric Ducts in Females

- In the 5th-6th week of intrauterine life of the embryo, Mullerian ducts develop as an invagination of intermediate cell mass. Two Mullerian ducts develop, one on either side and grow caudally (Fig. 5.5B). They approach each other in the midline after crossing the Wolffian duct and fuse (Fig. 5.5C). Fusion begins by 7-8 weeks and is completed by 12 weeks.[Q]
- Fusion proceeds in below upwards direction (Fig. 5.5C).
- Initially when the two Mullerian ducts fuse, an intervening septum is present (Fig. 5.5D), but later by 5th month[Q] of intrauterine life, it also disappears (Fig. 5.5E).
- Thus each side Mullerian duct forms each side Fallopian tube, each half of uterus, each half of cervix, each half of upper vagina.
- When by 5th month (20 weeks) septa disappears, single uterine cavity is formed (Fig. 5.5E).
- Till now the fundus of uterus is flat. In the last step fundus of uterus becomes dome shaped (Fig. 5.5F).

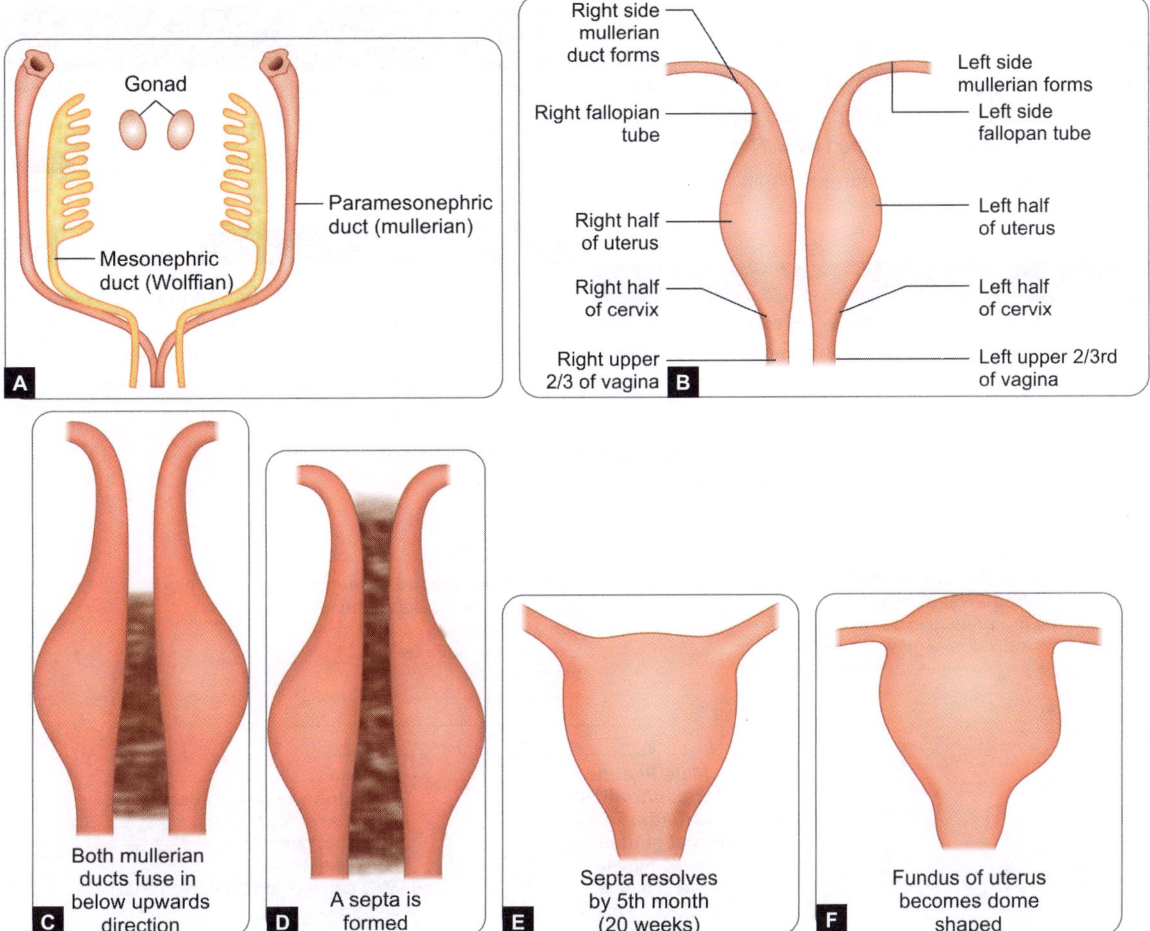

Figs. 5.5A to F: Differentiation of Mullerian duct. (A): Mesonephric duct and para mesonephric duct; (B): Parts formed by Mullerian duct; (C): Fusion of ducts; (D): Septa formed; (E): Resolution of septa; (F): Fundus of uterus becomes dome-shaped

Development of Vagina

Vagina develops from two sources:

- Mainly from the Mullerian duct which forms upper 2/3 part of vagina (i.e. it is mesodermal in origin)
- Partly from the urogenital sinus/sinovaginal bulb which forms lower 1/3rd part of vagina. The lower third thus to endodermal in origin
- Hymen represents the remnant of sinovaginal bulb
- Together they form a solid vaginal plate.
- Canalization of the solid vaginal plate occurs at 20 weeks
- If this canalization fails to occur it leads to **Transverse Vaginal Septum.**
- The mucous membrane or epithelium of **vagina is derived from endoderm of urogenital sinus**[Q] and muscles from mesoderm of mullerian duct.

Development of External Genitalia

External genitalia are derived from dorso somatic part of lateral part mesoderm.

Important Concept

- **In males:** External genitalia look like male genitalia due to the presence of testosterone in Intrauterine life. If testosterone is absent in intrauterine life or males are resistant to testosterone, their genitalia start resembling female genitalia (called as **Ambiguous Genitalia**)
- **M/C cause of ambiguous genitalia in males is:** Androgen Insensitivity Syndrome (Testicular feminizing syndrome).
- **In females**: External genitalia look like females due to absence of testosterone in intrauterine life. If due to any reason female is exposed to testosterone in intrauterine life her genitalia will start resembling male genitalia.
- **M/C cause of ambiguous genitalia in females is:** Congenital Adrenal Hyperplasia.
- For ipsilateral development of wolffian duct, high local concentration of testosterone is required, this is the reason why wolffian ducts do not develop in female fetuses exposed to excess endogenous adrenal androgens as in congenital adrenal hyperplasia.

Note:

In Males	**In Females**
Testes formation = 7 weak	Ovary formation = 8 weeks,
External genitalia formed by = 14 weeks	External genitalia are formed by = 11 weeks

Hence the sex of fetus can be confirmed 100% by USG by 14 weeks.

Also Know

Homologous organ: Those organs which have same embryological origin both in males and females are called Homologous organs.

Embryological origin	Male	Females
Genital Tubercle	Penis	Clitoris
Genital swellings	Scrotum	Labia Majora
Genital folds	Dorsal side of urethra	Labia Minora

Remember

- Prostate Glands in male in homologous to Skene Glands or para urethral Glands in females.[Q]
- Cowpers Gland or Bulbourethral Glands in males is homologous to Bartholin glands in females.[Q]

Flowchart 5.4: Hermaphroditism

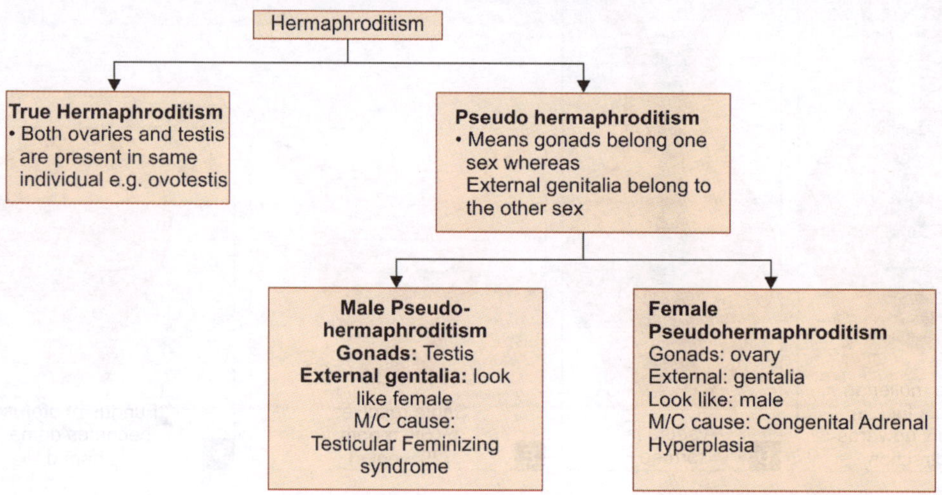

Anomalies of Internal Genital Organs

Gartner's Cyst

Gartner's cyst are cysts of the remnants of wolffian duct. Main location : Anterolateral wall of vagina, hence are often confused with cystocele.

Features differentiating them are seen in Table 5.2:

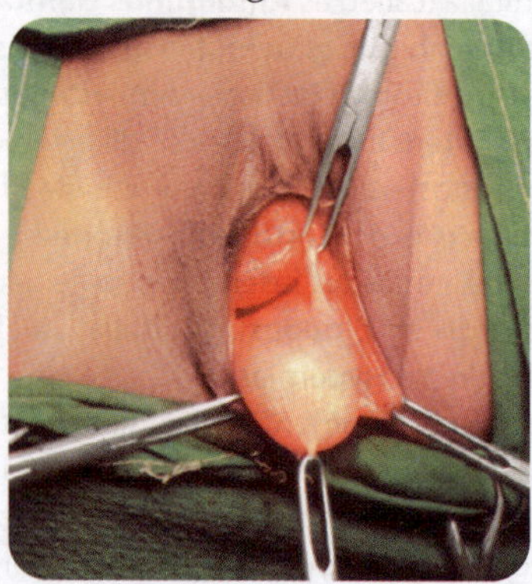

Fig. 5.6: Gartner's cyst. Note the shiny appearance of mucosa

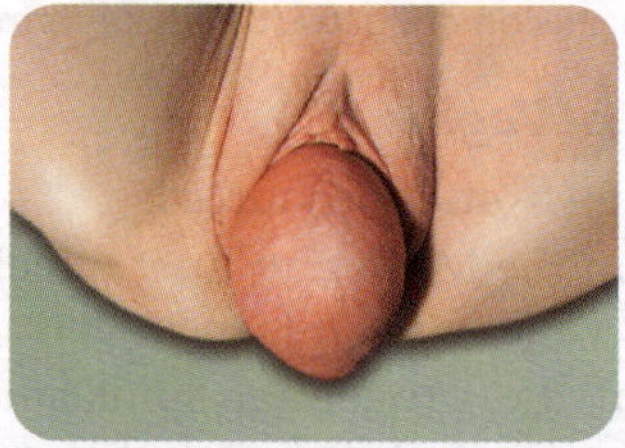

Fig. 5.7: Second degree uterine prolapse showing cystocele. Note the rugosities of vaginal mucosa

Table 5.2: Differences between the features of Gartner's cyst and cystocele.

Features of Gartner's cyst	Cystocele
Rugosities of the overlying vaginal mucosa are lost and vaginal mucosa over it becomes tense and shiny (Fig. 5.6)	Rugosities present (Fig. 5.7)
Margins are well defined	Margins not well defined
Not reducible	Reducible
No impulse on coughing	Impulse on coughing present

Remember

- Bartholin cyst is not present in anterolateral wall of vagina. It is present in vulva between Labia Majora and Minora.
- M/C vaginal cyst: Inclusion cyst (not Bartholin cyst)

Vertical Fusion Defects of Vagina

If there is a disorder in fusion of downgrowing Mullerian duct and upgrowing derivative of urogenital sinus, it results in **Transverse Vaginal Septum.**

Location

Transverse vagina septum can be located in (Fig. 5.8):

i. 46% septa are located in upper part.[Q]
ii. 40% septa are located in middle part.[Q]
iii. 14% septa are located in lower part.[Q]

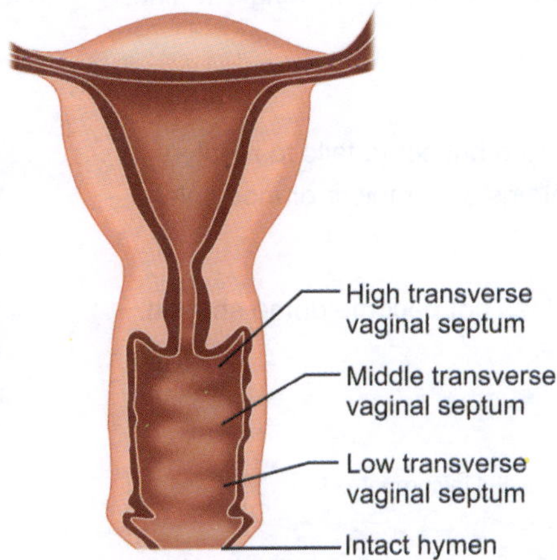

Fig. 5.8: Transverse vaginal septa-location

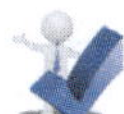

KEY POINTS

Transverse vaginal septum mostly corresponds to the level of external os (as most of them are located in the upper part)

Presentation

Transverse vaginal septum can present either in:

Neonatal Age-group

- The placental transfer of estrogen results in stimulating the glands of the endocervix which results in formation of mucocolpos, and can present as:
  - Abdominal tumor.[Q]
  - Can compress the ureter resulting in hydroureter followed by hydronephrosis.[Q]
  - Can compress the rectum resulting in obstipation/ intestinal obstruction.[Q]

At Puberty

- Patient can present with primary amenorrhea (actually called as cryptomenorrhea[Q] as uterus menstruates normally but blood does not come out due to outflow tract obstruction).[Q]
- Secondary sexual characteristics are normal.[Q]
- Due to cryptomenorrhea, blood gradually collects and distends first the vagina (hematocolpos)[Q], then cervix, uterus (hematocervix and hematometra) and finally the tube (hematosalpinx)[Q]. All these present as pelvic/abdominal tumor.
- The abdominal tumor can irritate the bladder followed by compression of internal urinary meatus leading to complete retention of urine (This occurs 3–4 years after the onset of hidden menstruation and therefore, patient is generally aged 15–18 years[Q]).
- Patient may complain of monthly cyclic pain (backache/lower abdomen pain).[Q]
- D/D = Imperforate Hymen

Management

- In case of septa in lower and middle part of vagina- surgical removal of septa vaginally followed by reanastomosis.
- In case of upper septa (in inner 1/3), abdominal surgery is required.

Note: Successful pregnancy following resection of the septa is inversely related to the level of septa in vagina.

Mullerian Duct Anomalies/Lateral Fusion Defects

They are due to failure of mullerian ducts either to unite or defect in dessostuning of septa.

Mullerian Duct Anomalies (Table 5.3)

Table 5.3: Mullerian duct anomalies

S. No.	Anomaly	Defect	
1.	**Mullerian agenesis**	Here both Mullerian ducts are absent. Hence both Fallopian tubes, uterus cervix and upper vagina are absent. The Ovary and lower vagina are present	

Contd...

Contd...

	Anomaly	Defect	
2.	**Unicornuate uterus**	It does not represent a defect in the fusion of the ducts, rather here one of Mullerian ducts is completely absent and so there is only 1 fallopian tube. Uterus, cervix, and vagina though appear to be normal are only half of the fully developed organ[Q] ***Note:*** Patients with unicornuate uterus have increased incidence of infertility, endometriosis and dysmenorrhea.	
3.	**Uterus didelphys**	It is a condition where there is a failure of fusion along the whole length of mullerian duct resulting **in 2 vagina,** 2 cervix, and 2 uterus[Q] ***Note:*** This is the only condition where 2 vaginas are present	
4.	**Bicornuate uterus** *a. Uterus bicornis unicollis*	In this condition only the lower part of the ducts fuse leaving the cornua separate, so **always there is a single vagina** Here vagina and cervix are fused, i.e. single vagina, single cervix but 2 uterus[Q]	
	b. Uterus bicornis bicollis	Here vagina is fused but cervix and uterus are not fused, i.e. single vagina, 2 cervix and 2 uterus[Q]	
5.	Septate/Subseptate uterus	In this condition; both MD fuse & form a septa but septa fails to resolve. So the uterus is outwardly normal but contains a complete or incomplete septum inside.	
6.	Arcuate uterus	Here the fundus of uterus remains flat & does not become dome shaped.	

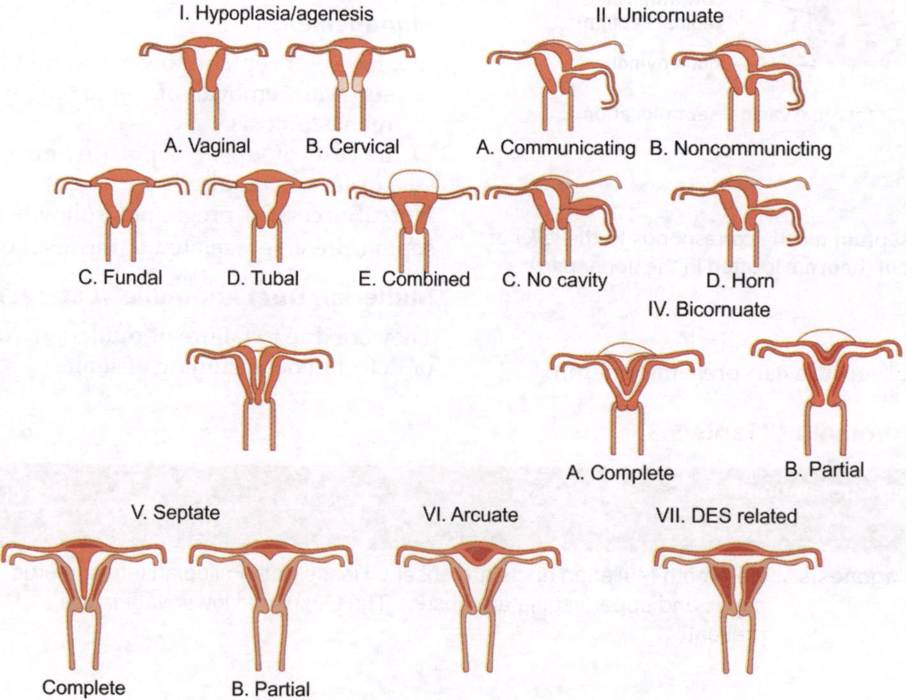

Fig. 5.9: WHO classification of Mullerian duct anomalies

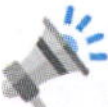

Important One Liners

- **M/C congenital anomaly of uterus:** Septate > Bicornuate uterus
- **M/C problem associated with them** Second trimester recurrent abortions
- **M/C anomaly causing abortion:** Septate uterus
- **M/C anomaly associated with infertility:** Septate uterus
- Anomaly with best reproductive outcome arcuate uterus.

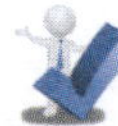

KEY POINTS

WHO classification of Mullerian duct anomalies

Class I	Mullerian agenesis (MRKH syndrome)
Class II	Unicornuate uterus
Class III	Didelphys uterus
Class IV	Bicornuate uterus
Class V	Septate uterus
Class VI	Arcuate uterus
Class VII	DES related abnormalities/T shaped uterus

Also Know

Mullarian malformations are also related with renal amomalies in 30 – 50% cases

Diagnosis of Mullerian Duct Anomalies

- **HSG:** Hysterosalpingogram (HSG) is mainly preferred in uterine anomalies but it cannot distinguish between a septate and bicornuate uterus. Hence it is not the ICO.

HSG: Hysterosalpingography

Done between day 5 and day 11 of the menstrual cycle (Best done on D-10)—In the preovulatory phase:

- It is an OPD procedure
- No anesthesia is required
- Water soluble radiopaque dye is injected into the cervical canal. Its passage is seen through the uterus and fallopian tube by doing serial X-rays.
- Instrument used during HSG is Leech Wilkinson cannula (Fig. 5.10).

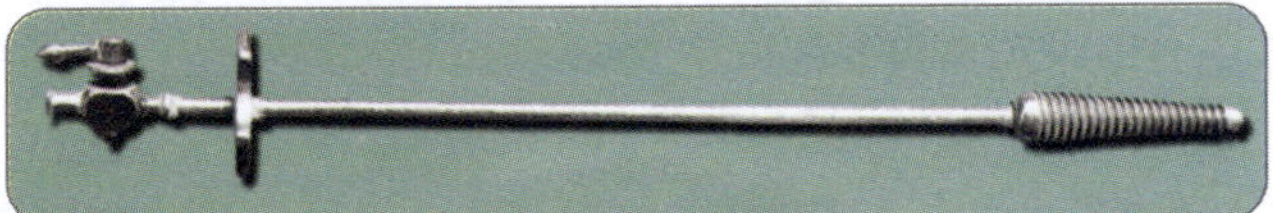

Fig. 5.10: Leech Wilkinson cannula used for performing HSG

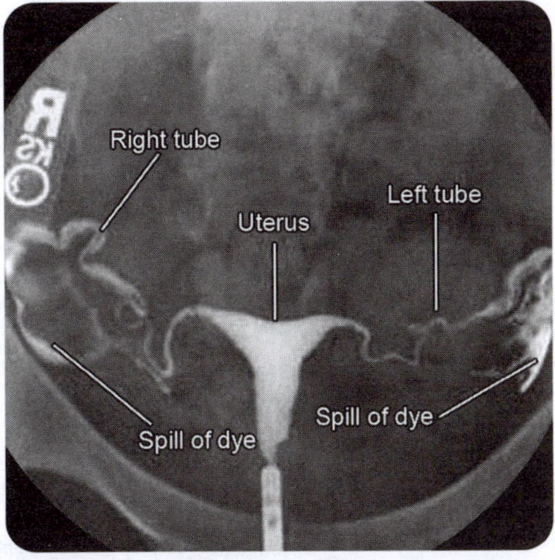

Fig. 5.11: HSG showing normal spillage from tubes and normal anatomy

HSG is not the Investigation of choice for Mullerian malformations. It cannot distinguish between bicornuate and septate uterus.

Note: Although HSG cannot differentiate between bicornuate and septate uterus, still they can be differentiated by the features discussed in Flowchart 5.5.

Indications of HSG

- IOC for Tubal patency
- For mullerian malformations
- For space occupying lesions under uterus

Absolute contraindications for HSG

- Genital TB
- Current pelvic infection
- Pregnancy
- Allergy to dye.

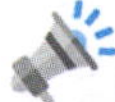

Important One Liners

In congenital malformation

IOC: MRI, If MRI is not given in options then 3D USG

Gold Standard—Laparoscopy + Hysteroscopy

2nd best = Laparoscopy

HSG: Tips for Identification

In exams be it PGME or spotters in final year exams, HSG of uterine anomalies is one of the favorites of examiners.

Wherever you get an HSG—identify the condition with the help of the following points:

Flowchart 5.5

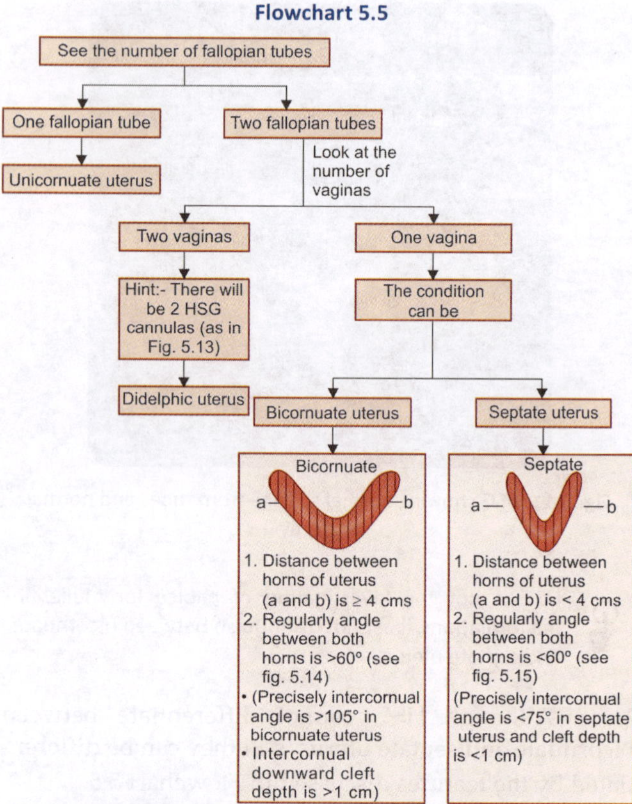

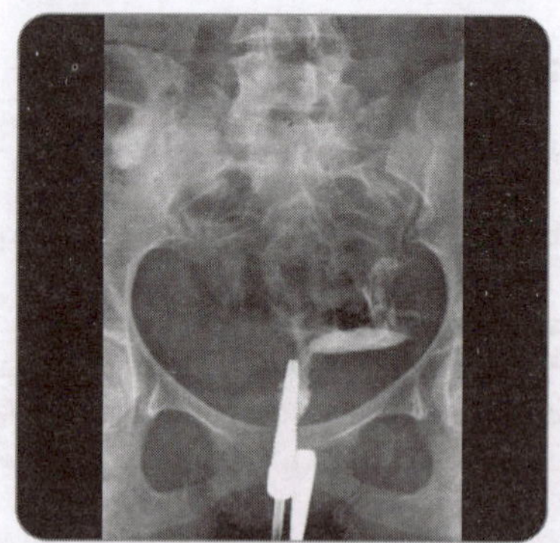

Fig. 5.12: Unicornuate uterus

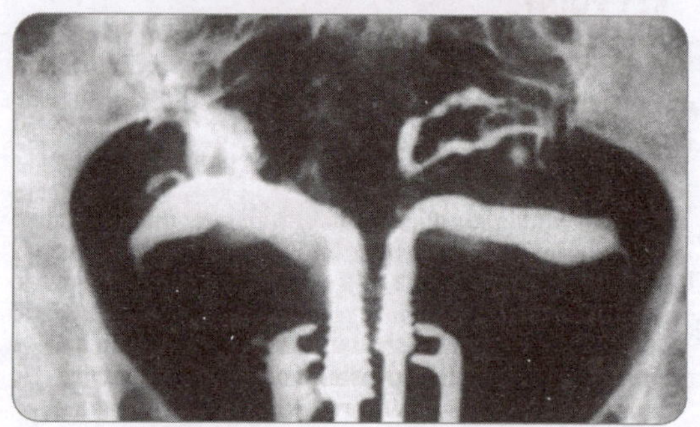

Fig. 5.13: HSG of uterus didelphys
(***Note***: See 2 vagina, 2 cannula it means didelphysic uterus)

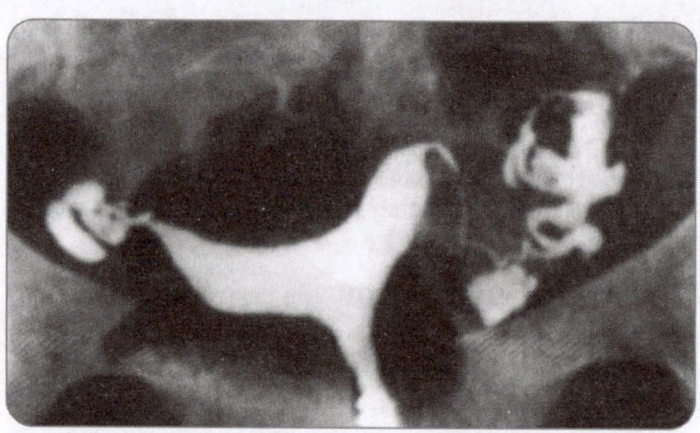

Fig. 5.14: HSG of bicornuate uterus
(***Note***: Distance between both the horns is ≥ 4 cm and angle > 60°)

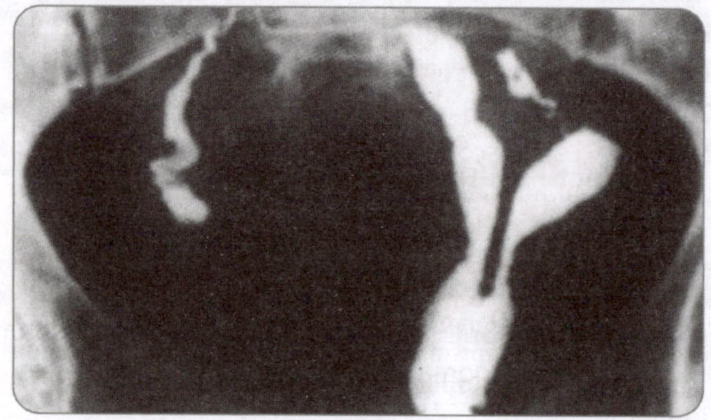

Fig. 5.15: HSG of septate uterus
(***Note***: Distance between both the horns is < 4 cm and < 60°)

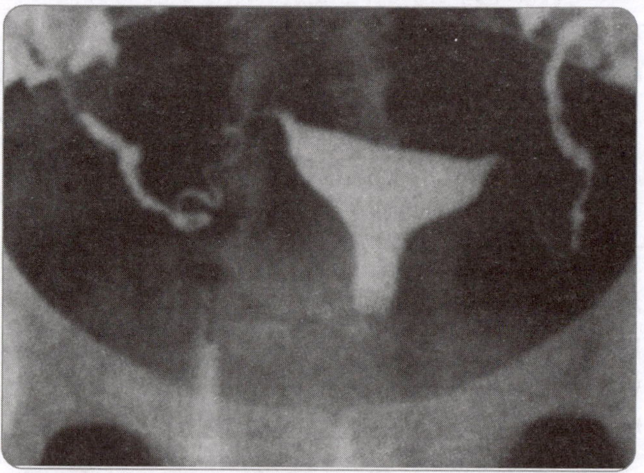

Fig. 5.16: HSG of arcuate uterus (flat topped uterus)

Management of Bicornuate or Septate Uterus

Presence of uterine malformation per se is not an indication of surgical correction. **Unification operation is indicated in otherwise unexplained cases of infertility or if it has lead to ≥ 3 abortions.**[Q]

Options Include

- **For bicornuate uterus:** (and if needed for Didelphys uterus)

- ➢ **Unification surgery done either hysteroscopically (preferred) or by abdominal route, e.g. Straussman metroplasty (Fig. 5.16).**
- **For septate uterus:**
  - ➢ **Earlier**: Jones/Tompkins Metroplasty was done.
  - ➢ **Nowadays: Hysteroscopic resection of septa** is being done after inducing endometrial atrophy by administering GnRH analogue for 2 months.
  - ➢ **Main complications:** Uterus perforation and fluid overload.

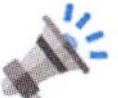

Important One Liners

- **Best reproductive outcome:** Seen in Arcuate uterus > Didelphic uterus > Bicornuate uterus.
- **Worst reproductive outcome** seen in Unicornuate uterus
- **Uterine anomaly M/C associated with renal anomalies** Unicornuate uterus (40%)
- **Surgical correction not needed in uterus:** Arcuate > didelphic uterus

Mullerian Agenesis/Mayer Rokitansky Kuster Hauser Syndrome

- Congenital absence of both the uterus and vagina due to absence of both Mullerian ducts is termed as Mullerian Agenesis on MRKH syndrome.
- In classic mullerian agenesis, patients have shallow vaginal pouch measuring only 1 or 2 inches deep.
- In addition uterus, cervix and upper vagina are absent.
- Typically ovaries are normal as they arise from genital ridge and a part of distal fallopian tubes is present.
  Karyotype = 46 XX[Q]
  Phenotype = Female

Associated Abnormalities

- Renal anomalies (M/C Renal anomaly, it is associated with: Renal agenesis followed by Horse-shoe shaped kidney)[Q].
- Skeletal abnormalities[Q] (most common hemivertebrae leading to Scoliosis and Klippel-Feil syndrome.
- Ear anomalies & hearing loss which is unilateral.

When mullerian agenesis is associated with Renal anomalies and skeletal anomalies-it is called **Mayer-Rokitansky-Kuster-Hauser syndrome.**

Clinical Features

- Patient presents between 15–18 years of age with primary amenorrhea[Q] (due to absence of uterus).
- Secondary sexual characteristics are normal[Q] as ovaries are normal (because ovaries do not develop from mullerian duct but from genital ridge, so ovulation is also normal) i.e. breast, pubic hair and axillary hair all are normal.
- On Per Rectal examination: Vagina is felt like a blind pouch and uterus is absent[Q].
- *"Although in MRKH fallopian tube should be absent, typically a part of the distal tube is present* (distal 1/3rd present)." *–William Gynae 1st/ed, p416*
- Findings are confirmed by USG[Q].

Management

- These females cannot menstruate, we cannot treat this symptom as uterus is absent. But because upper part of vagina is absent, ∴ their coital function is hampered. Thus these females can be made capable of getting married by doing vaginoplasty.

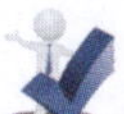

KEY POINTS

- Vaginoplasty should only be performed when the girl is just married or about to be married[Q].
- Vaginoplasty is done either by **McIndoe Reed Procedure**[Q] or **Williams vaginoplasty**[Q] or laparoscopically by **Modified Vecchietti operation.**
- Main complication of vaginoplasty–Restenosis and dyspareunia.

Note: These females are capable of having their genetic offspring because their ovaries are normal hence - oocyte can be picked up and with husbands semen, IVF can be done. Zygotes are then transferred to surrogate mothers uterus.

India's Recent Advance

First successful uterine transplant has been done in Galaxy Care Laparoscopy Institute in Pune under Dr Shailesh Puntambekar on May 18, 2017 on a patient of MRKH.

The patient received uterus from her mother and was scheduled for an IVF in January.

Differential Diagnosis of MRKH

- Cryptomenorrhea: Imperforate hymen (Here fallopian tube, uterus and cervix are present).
- Testicular feminization syndrome (Karyotype is 46 XY).
  Best test to differentiate between MRKH and Testicular Feminizing syndrome is Karyotyping.

Also Know

- **DES Related Anomalies**—DES was an estrogen which was used earlier but has now been withdrawn, as it leads to a number of problems.
- Cancers due to DES exposure:
  - i. Vaginal clear cell carcinoma
  - ii. Adenocarcinoma of cervix/CIN
- *In Uterus:* M/c problem associated with DES uterus *Exposure:* Hypoplastic uterus
- *Most characteristic:* T shaped uterus
- *In cervix:* Cervical Hood, cervical collars.
- *In vagina*: vaginal adenosis

(During normal development, vagina is originally lined by glandular epithelium derived from mullerian ducts.

By end of 2nd trimester, this layer is replaced by squamous epithelium extending up from urogenital sinus.

Failure of squamous epithelium to completely line the vagina is called as **Adenosis**. It appears Red in colour & adenosis can lead to vaginal Clean Cell Adeno-Carcinoma).

Note: *In females DES exposure does not lead to Renal anomalies*

In males in utero DES exposure leads to

- Cryptorchidism
- Hypospadias
- Testicular Hypoplasia

NEW PATTERN QUESTIONS

N1. SRY region is present on:
a. Short arm of Y chromosome
b. Long arm of Y chromosome
c. Short arm of X chromosome
d. Long arm of X chromosome

N2. The concentration of testosterone is maximum in IU life in males at:
a. 7–10 weeks b. 14–18 weeks
c. 20–24 weeks d. At term

N3. Which of the following is formed by Mullerian duct in males?
a. Testis b. Hydatid of Morgagni
c. Seminal vesicle d. Epoophoron

N4. The target gene for SRY which favors testis differentiation is:
a. SOX-9 gene b. RS po 1 gene
c. Dax 1 gene d. WNT-4 gene

N5. All of the following take part in male genital tract development *except*:
a. SRY b. SOX-9
c. FGF-9 d. WNT-4

N6. Regression of Mullerian duct in males occurs at:
a. 5 weeks b. 6 weeks
c. 7 weeks d. 8 weeks

N7. All of the following structures are homologous *except*:
a. Labia majora and scrotum
b. Labia minora and penile urethra
c. Epoophoron and caudal end of wolffian duct
d. Clitoris and glans penis

N8. All are derivatives of paramesonephric duct *except*:
a. Appendix of testis b. Hydatid of morgagni
c. Uterus d. Gartner's duct

N9. Gartner's cyst can be differentiated from cystocele by all *except*:
a. Not reducible
b. No impulse on coughing
c. Presence of rugosities of overlying vaginal mucosa
d. None of above

N10. Vertical fusion defect can result in:
a. Septate uterus
b. Didelphic uterus
c. Bicornuate uterus
d. Transverse vaginal septum

N11. Unicollis bicornis means:
a. Two uterine cavity with one cervix
b. Single vagina with double uterus
c. Incomplete septum of uterus
d. Double uterus and double cervix

N12. M/C uterine malformation associated with renal anomalies:
a. Bicornuate b. Unicornuate
c. Septate d. Didelphys

N13. M/C uterine malformation associated with infertility:
a. Bicornuate b. Unicornuate
c. Septate
d. Didelphys

N14. While evaluating a 30-year-old woman for infertility, you diagnosed a bicornuate uterus. You explain that additional testing is needed because of the womans risk of increased risk of congenital anomalies in which system?
a. Skeletal b. Haematopoietic
c. Urinary d. CNS

N15. A 16-year-old girl presents with primary amenorrhea. Her secondary sexual characteristics are well developed with good axillary and pubic hair. Examination of external genitalia reveals absence of vagina. USG reveals absence of uterus. Most likely diagnosis is:
a. Androgen insensitivity syndrome
b. Gonadal agenesis
c. Mayer-Rokitansky-Kuster-Hauser syndrome
d. True hermaphrodite

N16. Diethylstilbestrol causes the following defects *except*:
a. Renal anomalies b. Perifimbrial cysts
c. T shaped uterus d. Vaginal adenosis

N17. Identify the condition shown in HSG: F1 shows
a. Septate uterus b. Bicornuate uterus
c. Didelphys uterus d. Unicornuate uterus

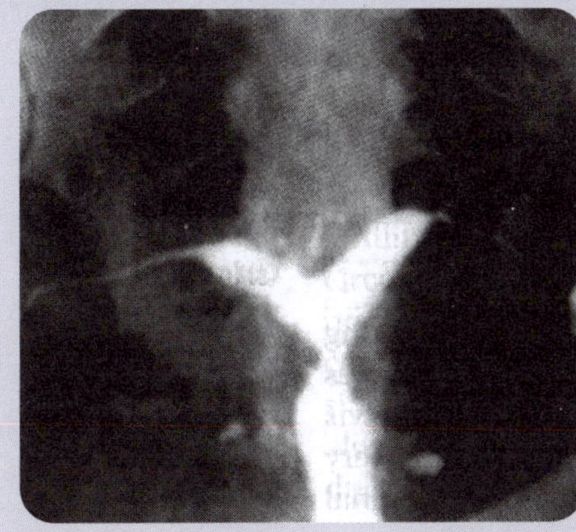

Fig. F1

N18. Hysteroscopic view shown in figure F2: shows
a. Normal uterine cavity
b. Asherman syndrome
c. Septate uterus
d. Uterus perforation

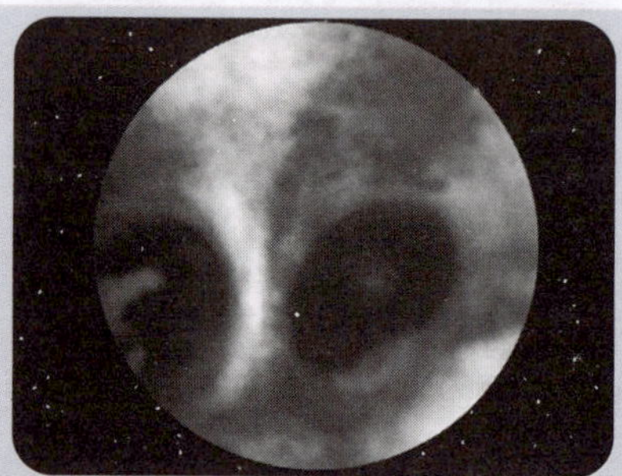

Fig. F2

N19. Identify the condition shown in Figure F3

a. Ambiguous genitalia
b. Bifid clitoric
c. Clitoromegaly
d. Normal genitalia of females

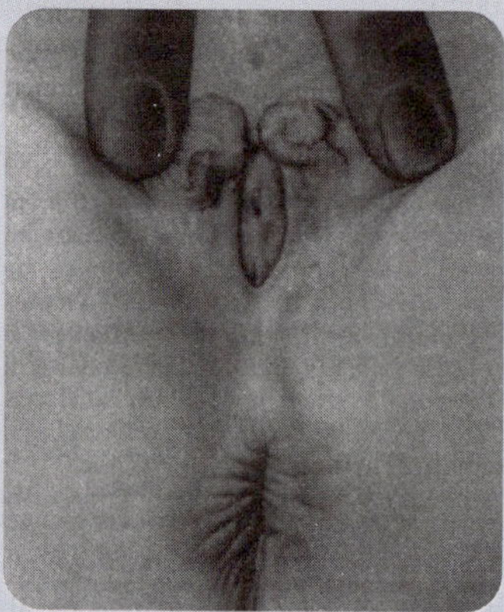

Fig. F3

N20. Identify the condition shown in HSG:-F4

a. Bicornuate uterus b. Normal uterus
c. Arcuate uterus d. Septate uterus

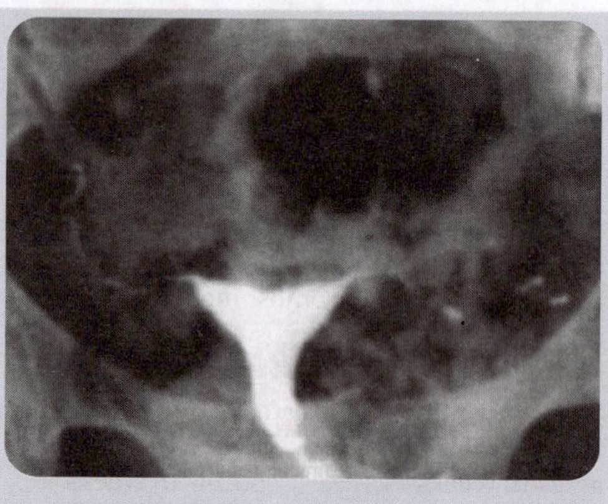

Fig. F4

N21. Paramesonephric duct forms:

a. Seminal vesicle b. Ureter
c. Uterus d. Vas deferens

N22. Gartners duct is present in

a. Cervix b. Vulva
c. Vagina d. Labia Minora

N23. Complete failure of mullerian duct fusion will result in:

a. Arcuate uterus b. Septate uterus
c. Bicornuate uterus d. Didelphys uterus

N24. Diagnostic workup in septate uterus before surgery includes:

a. HSG
b. USG
c. Laparoscopy
d. All of the above

N25. Vaginal atresia is associated with all *except*:

a. Lack of development of lower part of vagina
b. Normal secondary sexual characteristic
c. Female external genitalia
d. Presence of cervix

PREVIOUS YEAR QUESTIONS

1. **To diagnose uterus didelphys, procedure of choice is:** *(AIIMS 92, AI 95)*
   a. Laparoscopy
   b. IVP
   c. HSG
   d. USG
2. **The most important indication for surgical repair of a bicornuate uterus is:** *(AIIMS Nov. 05)*
   a. Infertility
   b. Dysmenorrhea
   c. Menorrhagia
   d. Habitual abortion
3. **Vaginal atresia is associated with:** *(AIIMS June 98)*
   a. Uterine atresia
   b. Exstrophy of bladder
   c. Imperforate hymen
   d. Ovarian atrophy
4. **Ideal age for repair of vaginal agenesis is:** *(AIIMS 92)*
   a. 6 months
   b. 3 years
   c. At puberty
   d. Before marriage
5. **Ovary develop from:** *(PGI June 02)*
   a. Mullerian duct
   b. Genital ridge
   c. Genital tubercle
   d. Mesonephric duct
   e. Sinovaginal bulbs
6. **Diagnosis of septate uterus done by:** *(PGI Dec 04)*
   a. USG
   b. Uterine sound
   c. Hysteroscopy
   d. Hysterosalpingography
   e. Laparoscopy
7. **MC congenital abnormality of uterus is:** *(PGI Dec 05)*
   a. Uterus didelphys
   b. Arcuate
   c. Unicornuate
   d. Septate
   e. Bicornuate
8. **Transverse vaginal septum corresponds to:** *(PGI Dec 04; June 04)*
   a. External os
   b. Vesical neck
   c. Bladder base
   d. Hymen
   e. Above the external meatus
9. **All of the following are features of mullerian agenesis *except*:** *(PGI Dec 04)*
   a. 46 XX karyotype
   b. Normal breast development
   c. Absent vagina
   d. Ovarian agenesis
10. **True about MRKH syndrome:** *(PGI May 2010)*
    a Absent uterus
    b. Absent ovary
    c. Absent vagina
    d. XX phenotype
    e. XY phenotype
11. **Characteristic features of Rokitansky Kuster Hauser syndrome are all of the following *except*:** *(AI 99; Delhi 05)*
    a. Absent uterus
    b. Absent vagina
    c. Anovulation
    d. 46 XX
12. **In complete mullerian duct aplasia all of the following are likely to be absent *except*:** *(AI 07)*
    a. Ovaries
    b. Fallopian tubes
    c. Uterus
    d. Vagina
13. **Rokitansky Kuster Hauser syndrome is associated with:** *(AI 01)*
    a. Ovarian agenesis
    b. Absent fallopian tube
    c. Vaginal atresia
    d. Bicornuate uterus
14. **Mayer-Rokitansky-Kuster-Hauser syndrome consists of:** *(AIIMS May 09)*
    a. Ovaries, uterus, fallopian tubes present
    b. Uterus absent, fallopian tube ovaries present
    c. All absent
    d. Uterus present, tubes and ovaries absent
15. **Which of the following condition does not present with both mullerian and wolffian duct structures?** *(AI 2010)*
    a. Antimullerian hormone deficiency
    b. FSH receptor mutation
    c. Ovotesticular syndrome
    d. Mixed gonadal dysgenesis
16. **Vaginal epithelium is derived from:** *(AIIMS May, Nov 2013)*
    a. Endoderm of urogenital sinus
    b. Mesoderm of urogenital sinus
    c. Endoderm of genital ridge
    d. Mesoderm of genital ridge
17. **Complete failure of mullerian duct fusion will result in:** *(AI 02; UP 04)*
    a. Uterus didelphys
    b. Arcuate uterus
    c. Subseptate uterus
    d. Bicornuate uterus
18. **Bicornuate uterus is due to:** *(PGI Dec. 98)*
    a. Incomplete fusion of uterine cavity
    b. Incomplete fusion of paramesonephric duct
    c. Incomplete fusion of mesonephric duct
    d. Incomplete formation of vagina
19. **A 16-year-old girl presents with primary amenorrhea. She has well developed breast, public hair and axillary hair. Examination shows absent vagina and an USG uterus is absent. What is the most likely diagnosis?**
    a. Androgen insensitivity syndrome
    b. Congenital adrenal hyperplasia
    c. Mullerian agenesis
    d. Turner syndrome

20. Labia minora is homologus to: *(MCI pattern Q)*
a. Penis
b. Scrotum
c. Penile urethra
d. Corpus cavernosa

21. Inferior 1/3rd of vagina is derived from: *(MCI pattern Q)*
a. Genital fold
b. Urogenital sinus
c. Mullerian duct
d. Wolffian duct

22. Unicornuate uterus belongs to class-------- of American Fertility Society classification
a. Class I
b. Class II
c. Class III
d. Class IV

23. The cranial end of Wolffian duct forms: *(JIPMER 2012)*
a. Epo-ophoron
b. Para oophoron
c. Gartner's duct
d. Uterine canal

24. All of the following develop from Wolffian duct: *(JIPMER 2011)*
a. Epoophoron
b. Paraoophoron
c. Gartner's duct
d. Bartholin duct

25. In mullerian agenesis, there is absence of: *(PGI Nov 2013)*
a. Ovary
b. Vagina
c. Uterus
d. Cervix
e. Fallopian tube

26. True about MRKH syndrome:
a. 46 XY
b. Upper 2/3 vagina absent
c. Ovary atrophic
d. Uterus abnormal
e. Amenorrhea

27. Ejaculatory duct developes from: *(JIPMER 2017)*
a. Ureteric bud
b. Mesonephric duct
c. Mullerian duct
d. Wolffian duct

28. Imperforate hymen is associated with: *(PGI May 2019)*
a. Secondary amenorrhea
b. Cyclic abdominal pain
c. Reduced secondary sexual characters
d. Short stature
e. Urine retention

ANSWERS TO NEW PATTERN QUESTIONS

N1. Ans. is a, i.e. Short arm of Y chromosome

See the text for explanation

N2. Ans. is b, i.e. 14–18 weeks *Ref: Leon Speroff 8th/ed, p339*

Testosterone production in males begins by 8 weeks of intrauterine life and is maximum by 15–18 weeks of intrauterine life

N3. Ans. is b, i.e. Hydatid of Morgagni

Remnants of Mullerian duct (paramesonephric duct) in males are:

(i) Prostatic utriculus

(ii) Appendix of testis (Hydatid of Morgagni)

N4. Ans. is a, i.e. SOX-9 gene *Ref: Leon Speroff 8th/ed, p334*

The target gene for SRY which favours testis differentiation is SOX-9 gene

The genes which favour ovary differentiation are:
WnT4
Rspo1
Dax 1

N5. Ans. is d, i.e. WNT-4 *Ref: Langman Embryology 12th/ed, p46-247*

Genes for male development

SRY gene	Master Gene for testis development
SOX 9	SRY and SOX 9 induce testis to form FGF-9 (chemotactic factor). FGF-9 causes tubules from mesonephric duct to penetrate gonadal ridge
SF1 (steroidogenic factor)	It stimulates differentiation of sertoli or leydig cells

WNT-4 is ovary determining gene. This gene upregulates DAXI which inhibits the function of SOX 9 in females.

N6. Ans. is d, i.e. 8 weeks *Ref: Leon Speroff 8th/ed, p342*

"AMH gene expression is induced by SOX-9 in sertoli cells and results in the ipsilateral regression of mullerian ducts by 8 weeks in males". *Ref: Leon Speroff 8th/ed, p342*

N7. Ans. is c, i.e. Epoophoron and caudal end of wolffian duct

Epoophoron is the remnant of cranial end of wolffian duct and not caudal end. Also it is a remnant, not homologous organ.

N8. Ans. is d, i.e. Gartner's duct *Ref: Dutta Gynae 5th/ed, p38*

Gartner's duct is a remnant of Wolffian duct (mesonephric duct) in females and not paramesonephric duct (Mullerian duct). **Hydatid of Morgagni is a term used both for Appendix of testis in males and kobelt tubercle in females.**

N9. Ans. is c, i.e. Presence of rugosities of overlying vaginal mucosa *Ref: Dutta Gynae 6th/ed, p210*

Gartner's cyst – are cysts of the remnants of Wolffian duct.

M/C location = Anterolateral aspect of vagina and hence are often confused with cystocele.

Features of Gartner's cyst are:
- Rugosities of the overlying vaginal mucosa are lost.
- Vaginal mucosa over it becomes tense and shiny.
- Margins are well defined.
- Not reducible.
- No impulse on coughing.

N10. Ans. is d, i.e. Transverse vaginal septum

Vertical fusion defect results in Transverse Vaginal Septum

N11. Ans is a, i.e. Two uterine cavity with cervix *Ref: Shaw 14th/ed, p85; Jeffcoate 7th/ed, p199; Williams Gynae 1st/ed, p417*

Unicollis means single cervix

Bicornis means two uterine cavities.

N12. Ans. is b, i.e. Unicornuate *Ref: Leon Speroff 8th/ed, p146*

"Approximately 40% of patients with a unicornuate uterus will have a urinary tract anomaly (usually of kidney) *Ref: Leon Speroff 8th/ed, p146*

N13. Ans. is c, i.e. Septate *Ref: Jeffoates 8th/ed, p188*

"The only form of malfusion deformity which may lower fertility significantly is a fully septate vagina." *Ref: Jeffoates, 8th/ed, p188*
"Septate anomaly is the anomaly most highly associated with reproductive failure and obstetrical complications including first and second trimester miscarriage, preterm delivery, fetal malpresentation, IUGR and infertility. *Ref: Leon Spercoff 8th/ed, p1172*

N14. Ans. is c, i.e. Urinary system

Mullerian anomalies have a 30% association with urinary anomalies

N15. Ans. is c, i.e. Mayer-Rokitansky-Kuster-Hauser syndrome

16-year-old girl with primary amenorrhea **and**
Normal secondary characteristics (Rules out gonadal dysgenesis)
Normal axillary hair and pubic hair (Rules out Androgen insensitivity syndrome)
USG shows absent uterus
This leaves no doubt for MRKH as the diagnosis.

N16. Ans. is a, i.e. Renal anomalies *Ref: Jeffcoate 7th/ed, p202*

Diethylstilbestrol exposure *in utero* leads to **varied anomalies** of female genital tract.
But remember simply:
"Unlike all other congenital uterine malformations, the DES uterus is not associated with an increase in renal anomalies." *Ref: Jeffcoate 7th/ed, p202*

Even if you do not remember all the anomalies caused by DES, just remember the above line and your MCQ will be solved.
In males it leads to- hypospadias cryptorchidism, testicular hypoplasia.

Other important points

Anomalies due to DES exposure
Cervix: Cervical collar
Cervical hood
CIN
Adenocarcinoma of cervix
Vagina: Vaginal adenosis
Clear cell cancer
Uterine anomalies = M/C : Hypoplastic uterus
Most characteristic = T shaped uterine cavity

In males it leads to:
- Hypospadias
- Cryptorchidism
- Testicular hypoplasia

N17. Ans. is b, i.e. Bicornuate uterus *Ref: Ieffwates 8th/ed, p190*

The HSG shown-shows single vagina as there is single cannula seen. This could be a case of **Bicornuate uterus** or **Septate uterus.** Although both are difficult to differentiate on HSG-still there are a few ways by which they can be differentiated.

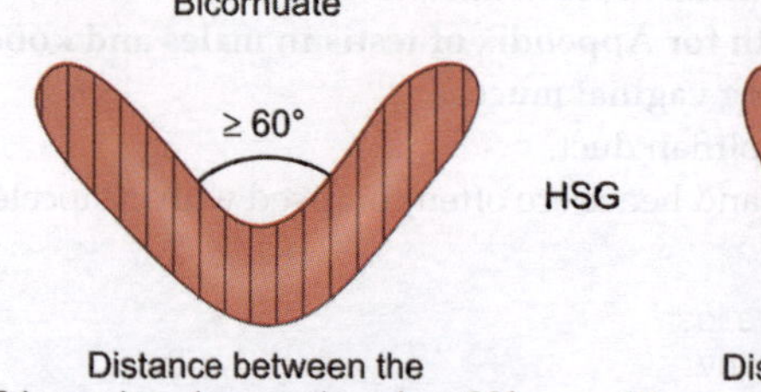

According to *Williams gynae 3rd/e pg422. "Widely diverging horns seen on HSG may suggest a bicornuate uterus. An intercornual angle <105 degrees suggests bicornuate uterus, whereas one <75 degrees indicates septate uterus."*
Now as seen in figure: Angle between the 2 horns is more than 60°, hence it is an HSG of bicornuate uterus.

N18. Ans. is c, i.e. Septate uterus

The image is a hysteroscopic view of uterine cavity. As seen, the uterine cavity is divided into 2 by a septa, hence it is a hysteroscopic view of septate uterus.

N19. Ans. is b, i.e. Bifid clitoric *Ref: Ieffcoates 8th/ed, p198*

The genital tubercle is formed from two mesodermal bands which grows round from the dorsal aspect of the fetus in the 3rd week. These also provide for the musculature of the abdominal wall, musculature of the anterior wall of the bladder and urethra and pubic symphysis. Failure of these bands to develop properly or to fuse result in **a bifid clitoris,** ectopic vesicle, divarication of the foreparts of the labia majora, absence of hair bearing skin of the pubes and a split pelvis.

N20. Ans. is c, i.e. Arcuate uterus *Ref: Ieffcoates 8th/ed, p186*

Arcuate uterus is a flat topped uterus as seen in the HSG. Here the fundal bulge fails to develop after fusion of the ducts. The fundal myometrium is extremely thin in this case.

N21. Ans. is c, i.e Uterus

Para mesonephric duct is the other name for Mullerian duct so now we don't need any explanation for this one.

N22. Ans. is c, i.e Vagina

Gartner's duct is present in anterolateral wall of vagina.

N23. Ans. is d, i.e Didelphys uterus

	Condition	Called as
1.	Complete absence of both mullerian ducts	Mullerian agenesis
2.	Absence of one side mullerian duct	Unicornuate uterus
3.	Complete failure of fusion of both mullerian ducts	Uterus Didelphys
4.	Partial fusion of both side mullerian ducts.	Biocornuate uterus
5.	If both sides Mullerian duct fuse septa forms but septa fails to resolve	Septate uterus

N24. Ans. is d, i.e. All of the above *Ref: Williams gynae 3/e, pg 422*

For septate uterus:

"Sonography and HSG seen acceptable imaging technique in the initial investigation when the presumptive diagnosis is a septate uterus, laparoscopy may be performed for a definitive diagnosis and before hysteroscopic resection of septa is initiated".

Ref: Williams gynae 3/e, pg 422

N25. Ans. is d, i.e Presence of cervix *Ref: Williams gynae 3/e, pg 419*

- Vaginal atresia is a condition where the urogenital sinus fails to develop hence lower part of vagina is absent & is replaced by a fibrous strand.
- Genotype of female = 46XX
- Gonads = Normal ovaries
- Secondary sexual characteristics are normal
- Upper reproductive tract is normal (uterus, cervix, etc.)

IOC: MRI

Note: Presence of cervix distinguishes this condition from mullerian agenesis.

ANSWERS TO PREVIOUS YEAR QUESTIONS

1. Ans. is d, i.e. USG *Ref: Williams Gynae 1st/ed, p417; Leon Speroff 8th/ed, p147*

IOC for uterine anomalies = MRI or 3D USG

Gold standard is = Laparoscopy

"Today, vaginal USG, especially three dimensional ultrasound, sonohysterography and MRI are highly accurate. HSG alone can yield inaccurate result due to failure to perfuse both uterine horns on either side of a midline division and cannot reliably distinguish between bicornuate and septate uterus" *Ref: Leon Speroff 8th/ed, p147*

2. Ans. is d, i.e. Habitual abortion

Ref: Munrokers Operative Obstetrics 10th/ed, p192-193; Jeffcoate 7th/ed, p204; Williams Gynae 1st/ed, p418

Management: Bicornuate uterus requires surgical treatment only when it causes habitual abortions.Q

"When a bicornuate or septate uterus has caused not less than 3 miscarriages and no pregnancy has resulted in a viable child, surgery may be indicated." *Ref: Jeffcoate 7th/ed, p204*

"Surgical reconstruction of the bicornuate uterus has been advocated in women with multiple spontaneous abortions and in whom no other causative factors are identified." *Ref: William Gynae 1st/ed, p418*

Surgery done is: Unification surgery where an incision is made over the uterus and the 2 horns are sutured together to form a single cavity.

After such a surgery: If woman conceives she should be taken up for elective LSCS at 38 weeks of gestation.Q These days hysteroscopic metroplasty is being done.

3. **Ans. is a, i.e. Uterine atresia** *Ref: Shaw 15th/ed, p95; Williams Gynae 1st/ed, p416*

Vaginal atresia is associated with uterine atresia and syndrome is called as *Mayer Rokitansky Kuster Hauser syndrome* (for details, see the preceding text).

4. **Ans. is d, i.e. Before marriage** *Ref: Shaw 15th/ed, p96*
   - Repair of vaginal agenesis (in testicular feminization syndrome and Mayer Rokitansky-Kuster Hauser syndrome) is done by vaginoplasty.
   - Vaginoplasty should only be performed when the girl is just married or about to be married.

Techniques:
- Construction of artificial vagina by *McIndoe operation* (procedure of choice).
- *Williams vaginoplasty* – creates a pouch out of labia majora dissection.
- Amnion vaginoplasty.

5. **Ans. is b, i.e. Genital ridge** *Ref: Dutta Gynae 5th/ed, p38*

Male and female derivatives of embryonic urogenital structures.

Part of female genital system	Originates from
Ovary	Genital ridge
Fallopian tubes Uterus Cervix Upper part of vagina	Mullerian/paramesonephric duct
Lower part of vagina	Sinovaginal bulb/urogenital Sinus

6. **Ans. is a, b, c and e, i.e. USG; Uterine sound; and Hysteroscopy; Laparoscopy**
Ref: Jeffcoate 7th/ed, p203; Williams Gynae 1st/ed, p418

Friends here it is first important to understand that septate uterus is confused with bicornuate uterus.

In septate uterus, after lateral fusion of Mullerian ducts, their is failure of their medial segments to regress which creates a permanent septum within the uterine cavity. The septum passes down from the uterine fundus. The fundus is normal in appearance.

In bicornuate uterus, the 2 halves of Mullerian duct do not fuse and there is defect in fusion of fundus as well.

So, both these conditions are different.

Septate uterus can be distinguished:

Clinically by:
- *P/V examination* - Septate vagina and 2 cervix may be felt.
- *By passing a sound.*

Investigations:
- **HSG:** HSG is mainly preferred in uterine anomalies but it cannot distinguish between a septate and bicornuate uterus. This is because in order to distinguish between the 2, uterine fundus should be visible.
- **Transvaginal USG:** It is the best method to distinguish between a septate and bicornuate uterus. As it reveals the shape of the fundal contour. *Ref: Williams Gynae 1st/ed, p418*
- **Hysteroscopy:** It is both diagnostic and curative.
- **MRI:** Expensive technique but provides the most accurate diagnosis.
- **Sonohysterography** (involves transvaginal ultrasound during or after introduction of sterile saline).

It can also distinguish between a septate and bicornuate uterus by revealing both the double uterine cavity and the shape of fundal contour.

Laparoscopy and laparotomy (per se) fail to reveal septate uterus. *Ref: Jeffcoate 7th/ed, p203*

This is quite obvious as outward appearance of a septate uterus is normal.

7. **Ans. is d, i.e. Septate** *Ref: Clinical Gynecological Endocrinology & Infertility by Leon Speroff 7th/ed, p132*

See the text

8. **Ans. is a, i.e. External os** *Ref: Williams Gynae 1st/ed, p413*

If there is a disorder in fusion of downgrowing Mullerian duct and upgrowing derivative of urogenital sinus, it results in transverse vaginal septum which causes imperforate vagina (or vaginal agenesis).

In a series reported:
- 46% septa were located in upper part.[Q]
- 40% septa were located in middle part.[Q]
- 14% septa were located in lower part.[Q]

The upper part corresponds to external os, therefore it is the option of choice. For further details on transverse vaginal septum see the preceding text.

9. **Ans. is d, i.e. Ovarian agenesis**
10. **Ans. is a, c and d, i.e. Absent uterus; Absent vagina and XX phenotype**
Ref: Jeffcoate 7th/ed, p197-198; Shaw 15th/ed, p95-96; COGDT 10th/ed, p549; Williams Gynae 3rd/ed, p420
11. **Ans. is c, i.e. Anovulation**
12. **Ans. is a, i.e. Ovaries**

13. Ans. is b, i.e. Absent fallopian tube

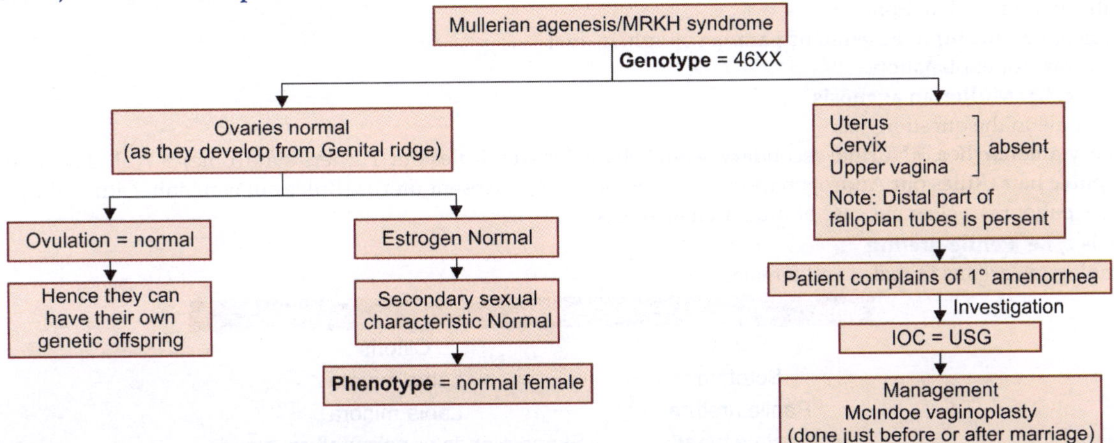

To understand why distal part of fallopian tube is present:
Mullerian ducts grow downward, therefore there will be cases where there will be well formed abdominal ostia associated with hypoplasia or absence of the remainder of the tubes, uterus and vagina or the tubes and uterus may be present and the vagina absent.
As discussed in Answer N25. vaginal atresia means urogenital sinus fails to develop. Hence both vaginal atresia and mullerian agenesis are different.
"Typically, a portion of the distal fallopian tube are present".

14. Ans. is b, i.e. Uterus absent, fallopian tube and ovaries present *Ref: Shaw 15th/ed, p95; Jeffcoate 7th/ed, p196*
In MRICH/mullerian agenesis
"Typically, normal ovaries present given their separate embryonic source and a part of distal fallopian tubes is present."

15. Ans. is b, i.e. FSH receptor mutation *Ref: Leon Speroff 7th/ed, p344,348, 8th/ed, p342,347,365*
Antimullerian hormone deficiency = persistent mullerian duct syndrome = uterine hernia syndrome
- Karyotype is 46 XY
- Since Y chromosome is present gonads are testis, i.e. they are males. In this syndrome, in males - sertoli cells fail to secrete Mullerian inhibiting factor and Mullerian duct is present.
- Since Leydig cell are also present, they secrete testosterone normally, thus Wolffian duct is also present. So in anti-Mullerian hormone deficiency both mullerian and wolffian ducts are present.
- **Ovotestis:** It is seen in true hermaphroditism. Both ovaries and testis are present. There is ambiguity of external genitalia. The internal structures depend on the degree of differentiation of the gonads.
- **Mixed Gonadal dysgenesis** Karyotype = 45XO/46XY.
- In this situation, the gonadal pattern on one side is streak gonad ovary (corresponding to karyotype 45 XO) and a normal testis on the other side (corresponding to karyotype 46 XY)
- Mullerian duct and Wolffian duct development correlates with the character of ipsilateral gonad, i.e.

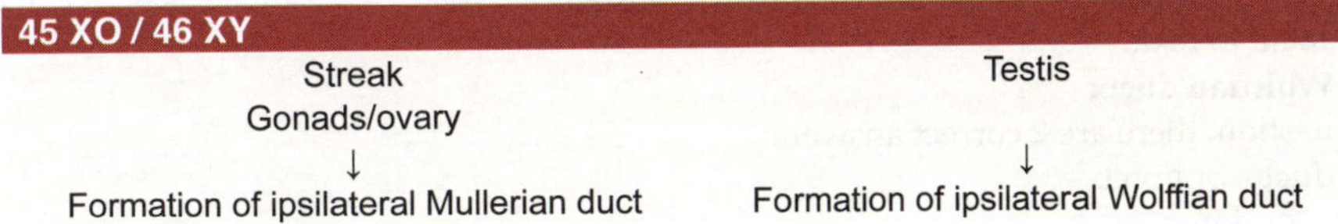

Thus, both Mullerian duct and wolffian ducts are present
In case of FSH receptor mutation in females, Mullerian ducts develop normally, the problem is in the binding of FSH to its receptors. The patient presents with primary or early secondary amenorrhea, variable development of secondary sexual characters and high levels of FSH and LH. Thus here only mullerian duct would be present as the karyotype of females is normal, i.e. 46(XX). So, answer to our question is FSH receptor mutation.

16. Ans. is a, i.e. Endoderm of urogenital sinus *Ref: Dutta Gyane 6th/ed, p37*

Vagina is developed mainly from the Müllerian ducts and partly from the urogenital sinus.
- Upper three-fifth of vagina above the hymen, develops from the fused uterovaginal canal of the Müllerian ducts.
  - Mucous membrane is developed from the endoderm of the canalized (vaginal plate) sinovaginal bulb (urogenital sinus).
  - The musculature is developed from the mesoderm of the fused caudal vertical part of the Müllerian ducts.
  - The hymen is developed from the junction of the Müllerian tubercle (mesodermal) and the urogenital sinus (endodermal).
- Lower one-fifth of vagina below the hymen is developed entirely from the endoderm of the urogenital sinus.
- Vaginal introitus is developed from the ectoderm of the genital folds after rupture of the bilaminar urogenital membrane.

17. Ans. is a, i.e. Uterus didelphys
See the text for explanation.

18. Ans. is b, i.e. Incomplete fusion of paramesonephric duct
See the text for explanation.

19. Ans. is c, i.e. Mullerian agenesis.
The female in the question has:
Primary amenorrhea + Normal secondary sexual characteristic (Rules out Turners syndrome) + Well developed axillary and pubic hair (Rules out Androgen Insensitivity Syndrome) + Absent uterus (Rules out congenital adrenal hyperplasia).
Hence, patient is a clear cut case of mullerian agenesis.

20. Ans. is c, i.e. Penile urethra
Homologous organs in males and females

Male	Female
Penis	Clitoris
Scrotum	Labia majora
Penile urethra	Labia minora
Prostate glands	Skene glands or paraurethral glands
Cowpers glands	Bartholins glands

21. Ans. is b, i.e. Urogenital sinus
See the text for explanation

22. Ans. is b, i.e. class II

WHO Classification of Mullerian Duct Anomalies.

Class I	: Mullerian agenesis
Class II	: Unicornuate uterus
Class III	: Didelphic uterus
Class IV	: Bicornuate uterus
Class V	: Septate uterus
Class VI	: Arcuate uterus
Class VII	: DES related anomalies

23. Ans. is a, i.e. Epo-ophoron
The cranial end of Wolffian duct form the Epoophoron.

24. Ans. is d, i.e., Bartholin duct
See the text for explanation

25. Ans. is b, c, and d i.e. Vagina, Uterus and Cervix *Ref: Williams Gyane 3/ed, p420*
"Congenital absence of both the uterus and vagina is termed as mullerian aplasia, mullerian agenesis or MRKH syndrome. In classic mullerian agenesis, patients have shallow vaginal pouch, measuring only 1 to 2 inches deep. In addition, the uterus, cervix and upper vagina are absent. Typically, normal ovaries persist given their separate embryonic source and a portion of distal fallopian tubes is present." *Ref: Williams Gyane 3rd/ed, p420*

26. Ans. is, b and e, i.e. Upper 2/3 vagina absent and Amenorrhea *Ref: Williams Gyane 3/ed, p420*
Discussed in detail in text.

27. Ans. is d, i.e. Wolffian ductx
Now in this question, there are 2 correct answers:
Mesonephric duct – option b
Wolffian duct – option d
Like I have explained in text, the Mesonephric duct after giving rise to ureteric bud is called as wolffian duct.
It is this wolffian duct which forms
S = seminal vesicle
E = ejaculatory duct
E = Epididymis
D = Vas deferens.
Hence better answer here is Wolffian duct.

28. Ans. is b and e, i.e. Cyclic abdominal pain, and Urine retention
Imperforate hymen *causes* ***primary amenorrhea***
- Secondary sexual characters are normal in imperforate hymen.
- Height of patient is normal.

CHAPTER 6

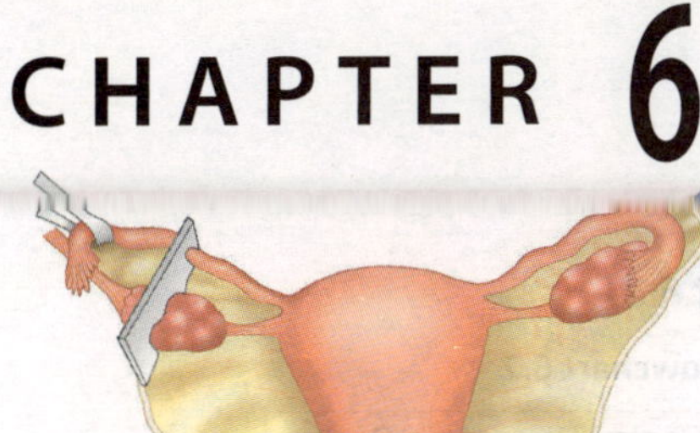

Puberty (Including Issues Related to Sexuality and Intersexuality)

Puberty

Normally there is a negative feedback on the hypothalamus in childhood. With the onset of puberty, this negative feedback is removed and there is a significant increase in the amplitude of pulsatile release of GnRH by the hypothalamus leading to puberty.

- Age of puberty in girls: 8 to 12 years.
- Mean age: 10.5 years

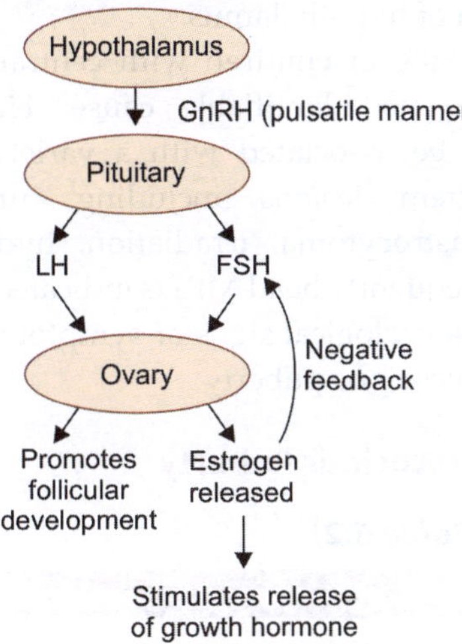

Fig. 6.1: HPO axis in females

Mnemonic

Sequence of puberty in girls.

- Gross = Accelerated **g**rowth or growth spurt (1st sign) of puberty)
- B = Breast budding/Thelarche **(1st visible sign of puberty)**
- P = Development of **p**ubic hair—Pubarche
- H = Increase in **H**eight/peak growth velocity attained
  Males = In **M**enstruation (menarche) (12.5 years)

Gross BPH in males.

- On an average, the entire time taken for all events to occur in puberty is 4.6 years.
- Menarche occurs 2.6 years after onset of puberty.

In males—Sequence of puberty

- Mean age of pubertal, onset = 11.5 years (Range = 9 to 13 years)

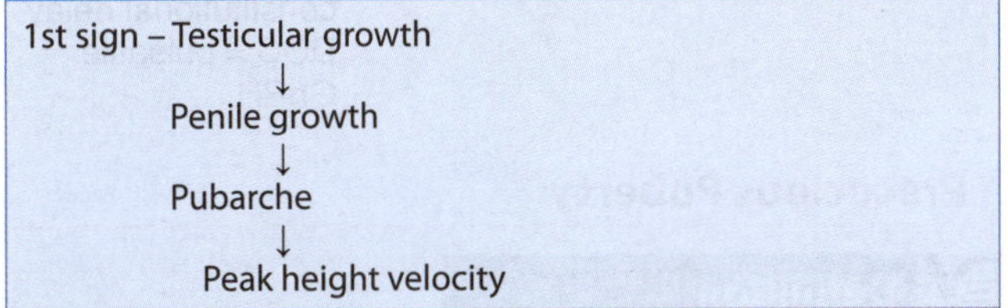

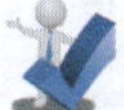

KEY POINTS

Estrogen is mainly responsible for breast growth and epiphyseal closure in females.

Development of pubic hair and axillary hair in girls is dependent on androgen.

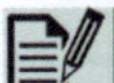

Remember

Breast is secondary sexual characteristic in females so if any question says secondary sexual characteristic format it means breast present

- In girls, development of breast and pubic hair occurs in 5 stages as described by Tanner, called as **Tanner staging** for breast and pubic hair development.

Note: There is no need to know complete Tanner staging, so just remember:

Tanner stages 1 and 2: refer to initial stage of breast development or less developed breast or pubic hair.

Tanner stages 4 and 5: refer to advanced stages of breast and pubic hair development or fully developed breast and pubic hair.

Also Know

Growth rate of boys and girls are similar till age of 10.5 years. The growth spurt in girls overtakes that of boys for 1–2 years then plateaus.

Precocious & Delayed Puberty

See Table 6.1 for brief about these issues

Table 6.1: Precocious and delayed puberty

	Females	*Males*
Precocious puberty	< 8 years M/c in females M/c cause:- Idiopathic DOC = Continues GnRH DOC = Continuous GnRH *Note*: CNS tumours like Hamartomas can lead to precocious puberty so always do MRI in patients of precocious puberty	< 9 years
Delayed puberty	No secondary sexual characteristic by 13 years of age	No testicular growth by 14 years of age M/c in boys M/c cause = constitutional delay DOC = pulsatile GnRH

Precocious Puberty

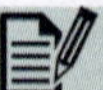

Definition

Precocious puberty: is onset of menstruation before the age of 10 years or appearance of breast budding before the age of 8 years in females.
In males: If puberty occurs before 9 years — it is precocious.

Important One Liners

M/C cause of precocious puberty in females is Idiopathic

Central Precocious Puberty

Precocious puberty can be central (TRUE) on peripheral (PSEUDO) precocious puberty.

Flowchart 6.1

Precocious puberty

→ **Central/True precocious puberty (M/C)**
- It is due to excessive GnRH, gonadotropins and sex hormones because of premature activation of hypothalamic pituitary ovarian axis.
- Here breast development and pubic hair development both are seen.
- Cyclical vaginal bleeding is also seen.
- M/C cause is idiopathic
- DOC= GnRH analogues (continuous)

→ **Peripheral/Pseudo precocious puberty**
- It is due to excessive sex steroid secretion from either adrenal gland or gonads and is independent of activation of HPO axis. Pubertal changes occur due to independent production of sex steroids, e.g., ovarian tumor producing estrogen
- It can lead to breast development, sexual hair development but not to cyclical bleeding as menarche requires not only production of estrogen but also its withdrawal
- Management – treat the cause.

Causes (See Flowchart 6.2)

Flowchart 6.2

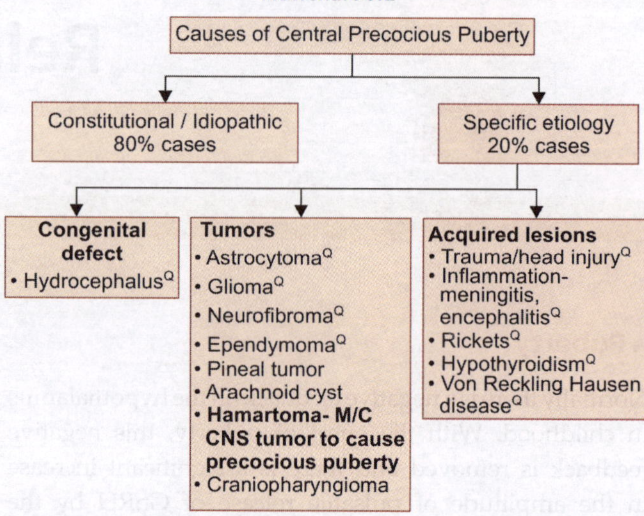

- The pathophysiology of central precocious puberty is unclear but most lesions are associated with increased intracranial pressure and are located in the region of hypothalamus.

Note: Up to 90% of children with central precocious puberty have no identifiable cause. However the disorder can be associated with a variety of central nervous system lesions including tumors, (like hamartoma astrocytoma, irradiation, hydrocephalus, cyst etc. Consequently head MRI is indicated even when there are no neurological signs or symptoms seen in all patients of Precocious puberty.

Peripheral Precocious Puberty

Causes (See Table 6.2)

Table 6.2: Causes of peripheral precocious puberty

Here hypothalamic pituitary ovarian axis is intact

Isosexual

A. Ovarian causes
- Granulosa cell Tm[Q]
- Theca cell Tm[Q]

B. Adrenal cause
- Feminizing adrenal neoplasia[Q] (generally adrenal causes lead to heterosexual puberty)

C. Ectopic Gonadotropin production
- Dysgerminoma[Q]
- Choriocarcinoma[Q]
- Hepatoblastoma[Q]

} Secrete hCG

D. Exogenous estrogen
- In the form of OCP's
- Corticosteroid intake

E. McCune-Albright syndrome

Contd...

Contd...

Heterosexual
- Congenital adrenal hyperplasia[Q]
- Ovarian/adrenal testosterone[Q] secreting tumors[Q]:
  - Androblastoma[Q]
  - Hilus cell Tm[Q]
  - Gynandroblastoma[Q]
  - Lipoid cell tumors[Q]
- Exogenous androgen[Q]

Note: Mc cause Albright syndrome is a rare disorder characterised by precocious puberty, cafe au lait skin spots and polyostotic fibrous dysplasia of bone caused by a somatic mutation of the alpha subunit of the G Protein.

Delayed Puberty

Delayed puberty is said to occur when there is **no breast development by the age of 13 years and no menarche by the age of 16 years.** *(Willams gynae 3/e p329)*

Note: In boys: Delayed puberty means no testicular growth by 14 years.

Causes of Delayed Puberty

1. **Constitutional delay** (M/c cause of delayed puberty in boys and overall M/c cause of delayed puberty).
2. **Hypogonadotropic hypogonadism:** Defect is at the level of hypothalamus or pituitary. Levels of FSH and LH are low (< 10 m IU/mL). Levels of estrogen are decreased (*See* Flowchart 6.3).

Flowchart 6.3

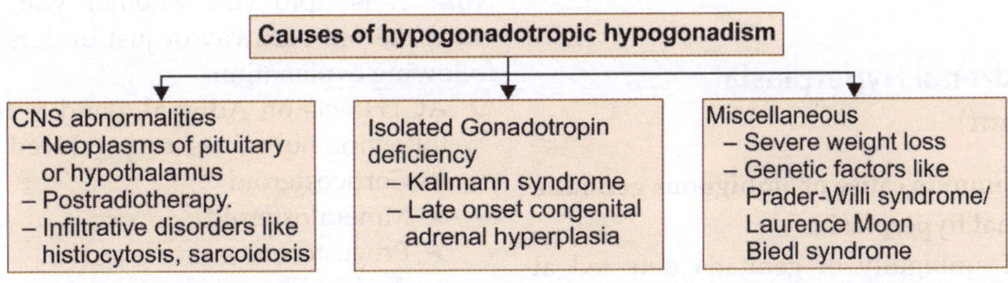

DOC for treating **hypogonadotropic** hypogonadism = Oestrogen/(ethinyl estradiol) in order to promote breast development and somatic growth.

3. **Hypergonadotropic hypogonadism**

- Defect lies at the level of ovary.
- There is sexual infantilism and FSH levels are elevated (as the negative feedback on FSH by estrogen decreases). Levels of FSH > 30 m IU/ml.

Causes:

- Turner syndrome (45 XO)
- Pure gonadal dysgenesis 46 XX, 46 XY
- Ovarian failure
  - Infections like mumps or tuberculosis of ovary
  - Iatrogenic (post-surgery/radiotherapy)
  - Swyer syndrome
  - Primary ovarian failure

M/c cause of primary amenorrhea and delayed puberty in females – Turner Syndrome
Other cause of delayed puberty is Kallmann Syndrome

Ambiguous Genitalia

Males	Females
Ambiguous genitalia in males is due to androgen insensitivity or decreased androgen levels.	Ambiguous genitalia is due to exposure to an increased androgen levels in intrauterine life.
E.g. • **M/c cause**: Testicular feminisation syndrome • 5-alpha reductase deficiency • Congenital lipoid adrenal hyperplasia.	**M/c cause**: Congenital adrenal hyperplasia • Cushing's disease • Maternal ovarian androgen secreting tumours • Aromatase deficiency • Maternal drug intake (Testosterone, Danazol)

True Hermaphroditism[Q]

Individuals with this disorder have both ovarian and testicular tissue, most commonly as composite ovotestes but occasionally with an ovary on one side and testis on the other.

Pseudohermaphroditism[Q]

The genetic sex indicates one sex whereas the external genitalia has characteristics of the other.

Female Pseudohermaphroditism

Genotype: Females external genetalia look like males. Genetic females (gonads ovaries) with masculinized external genitalia manifesting as – clitoral hypertrophy[Q] and some degrees of fusion of urogenital or labioscrotal folds.

Male Pseudohermaphroditism

Genetic males (Gonads testis) with feminized external genitalia manifesting as hypospadiasis, or incomplete fusion of the urogenital or labioscrotal folds, M/C cause of male pseudohermaphroditism is Testicular feminizing syndrome.

Congenital Adrenal Hyperplasia (Very Important)

In a female most common cause of ambiguous genitalia is congenital adrenal hyperplasia.

- Infact cases of ambiguity of genitalia detected at birth are due to adrenogenital syndrome (congenital adrenal hyperplasia) unless proved otherwise.
- It is an autosomal recessive[Q] disorder (if any couple has had one affected child, subsequent baby has 1 in 4 chance of having the same disability).

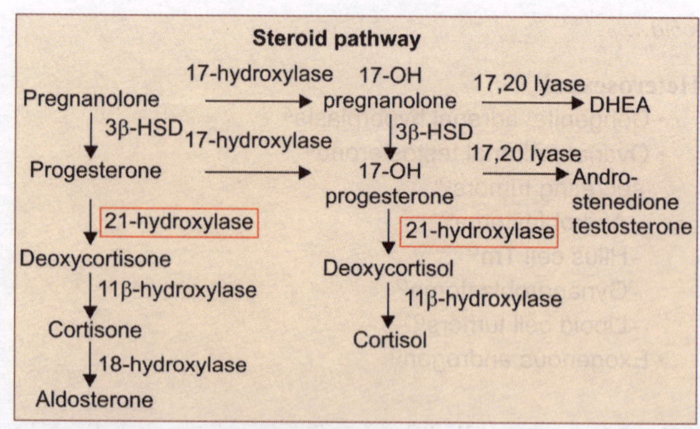

Fig. 6.2: Steroid pathway

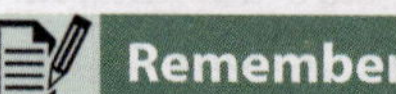

Remember

(3β 21 11β 18) for enzymes coming vertically.
The M/c enzyme deficiency in CAH is 21 hydroxylase enzyme deficiency.

Note: It is upto you whether you want to rug up entire steroid pathway or just understand CAH by the following explanation.

- ACTH acts on Adrenal gland & from the adrenals following hormones are produced
  - Corticosteroid
  - Mineralosteroid
  - Progesterone
  - Androgens
- As you can see from steroid pathway (Fig. 6.2) if 21 hydroxylase is deficient it will result in decreased corticosteroid & mineralosteroid production. But for production of progesterone and Androgens, 21 hydroxylase is not needed.

Flowchart 6.4: Congenital adrenal hyperplasia with 21 hydroxylase deficiency

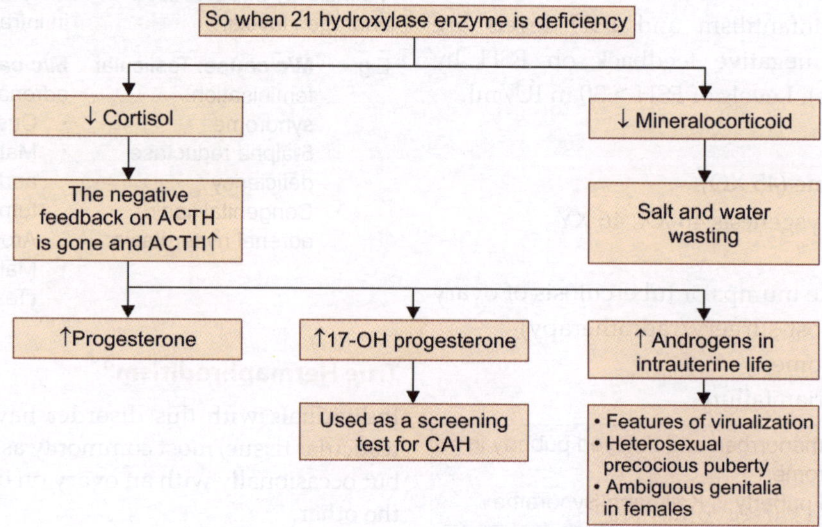

A point worth nothing is that development of the internal genitalia (i.e. Mullerian duct and its derivatives) is normal in females with classical CAH because the excess androgen is derived from adrenals and the ovaries are normal so they produce neither anti Mullerian hormone nor significant amount of androgen to promote Wolffian duct development.

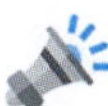

Important One Liners

Congenital adrenal hyperplasia is the M/c cause of ambiguous genitalia in females.
M/c enzyme deficiency in CAH is 21 hydroxylase deficiency.
Least common Enzyme deficiency = 3β HSD i.e. Hydroxysteroid dehydrogenase.

Physical Characteristics in Females

- Genotype = 46XX[Q].
- Gonads = ovaries[Q].
- Uterus and vagina are present, as Mullerian duct develops normally, but remain infantile therefore failure to menstruate[Q].
- Vulva and introitus are affected. There is clitoromegaly[Q] and the genital folds fuse to form penile urethra rather than labia minora.[Q] Labia majora are fused which appears like scrotum.
- **Heterosexual precocious puberty[Q]:** Pubic hair and axillary hair appear and voice deepens by the age of 2-4 years[Q]. (since these characteristics are dependent on androgen).
- Associated metabolic abnormalities (d/t decreased aldosterone): Hyponatremia[Q], hyperkalemia[Q] and hypotension[Q].
- Have high chances of short stature as adults.

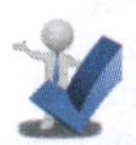

KEY POINTS

Nonclassical or late onset CAH–
There is no genital ambiguity at birth and usual presentation is androgen excess at puberty and hence it is a differential diagnosis of PCOD.

Investigation

- **USG:** shows presence of uterus, vagina, fallopian tubes and ovaries[Q]. (Thus, all patients are potentially fertile)
- **Sex chromatin study:** shows positive Barr body[Q]. (*Note*: Whenever a child presents with ambiguous genitalia always do karyotyping)

Screening Test for CAH

Flowchart 6.5: Screening test of CAH

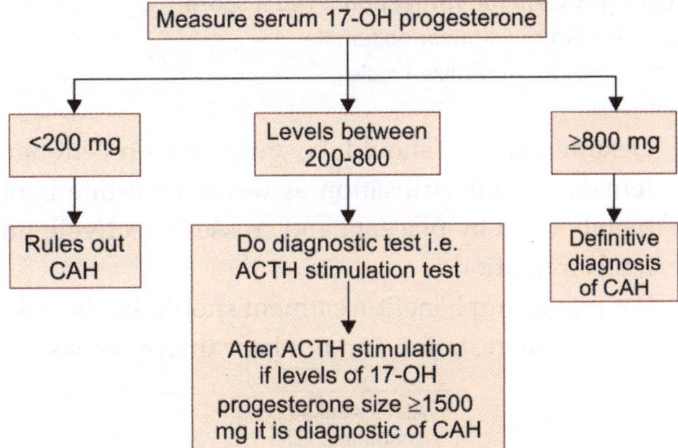

Treatment of CAH

Flowchart 6.6: Treatment of CAH

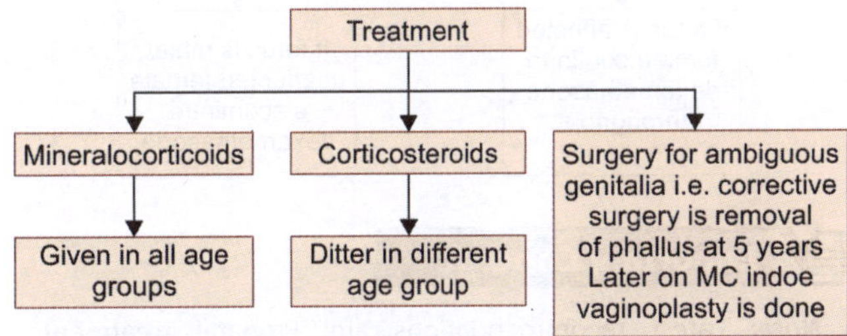

Choice of Corticosteroids in Treating CAH

Age	Corticosteroid of Choice
In neonate, childhood and uptil puberty (before closure of epiphyses)	Short acting corticosteroid i.e. Hydro cortisone (long acting can adversely affect the growth)
After closure of epiphysis	Long acting corticosteroid either Dexamethasone/ prednisolone
At reproductive age In these females fertility is decreased but they can conceive	
• Non pregnant female with CAH • Pregnant female with CAH who is carrying a male fetus or an unaffected female fetus	DOC = Hydrocortisone as it does not cross the placenta
• Pregnant female with CAH with an affected female fetus	DOC = Dexamethasone as it crosses the placenta

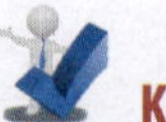

KEY POINTS

Scoring system for virilization: Prader score

Score 0 = Normal appearing female

Score 5 = Normal, virilized male

- Dexamethasone should be given to prevent fetal female genital virilisation as dexamethasone is not metabolized by placenta and crosses effectively into fetal circulation.
- For maximum benefit-treatment should begin at 4 to 5 weeks of gestation and not later than 8 weeks.

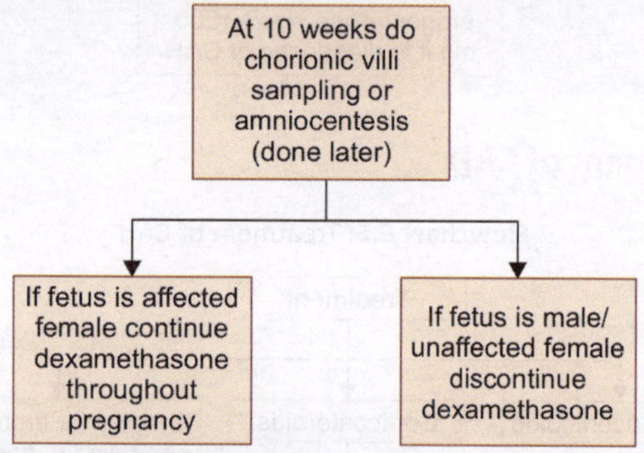

Important Concept

Note: Latest recommendations are: Prenatal treatment poses risks like postnatal failure to thrive and psychomotor developmental delay, hence best approach is early prenatal diagnosis by chorionic villi sampling with rapid sex determination (FISH for the X and Y chromosome) and Genotyping. Treatment should be given to only those mothers with an affected female child.

Androgen Insensitivity Syndrome

It consists of a spectrum of conditions ranging from complete insensitivity to less insensitivity towards testosterone

Complete Androgen Insensitivity	Incomplete Androgen Insensitivity	Reifenstein Syndrome

Complete Androgen Insensitivity Syndrome Testicular Feminizing Syndrome

Inherited as X linked Recessive disorders

Genotype = 46XY

Pathophysiology: See Flowcharts 6.7 and 6.8.

Flowchart 6.7: Androgen insensitivity syndrome at birth

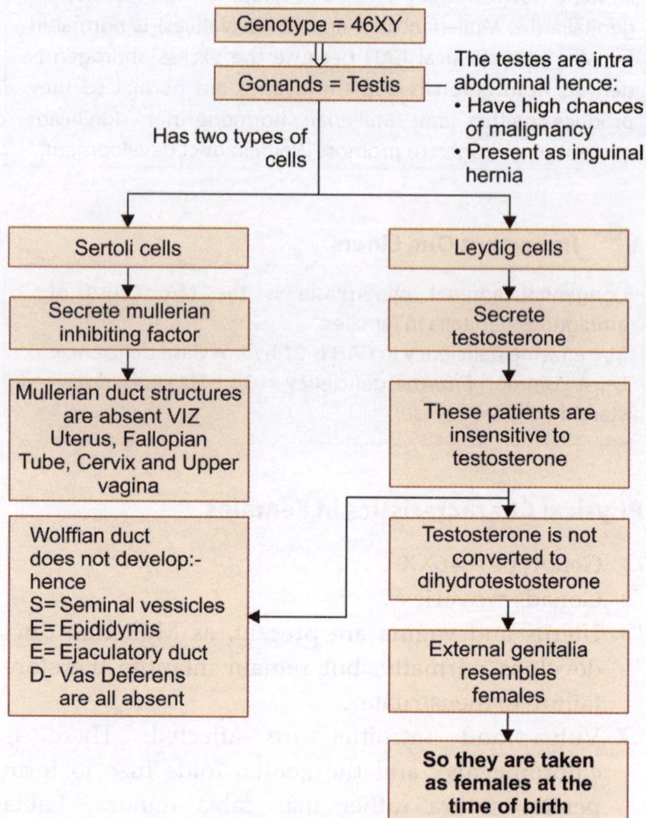

Flowchart 6.8: Androgen insensitivity syndrome at puberty

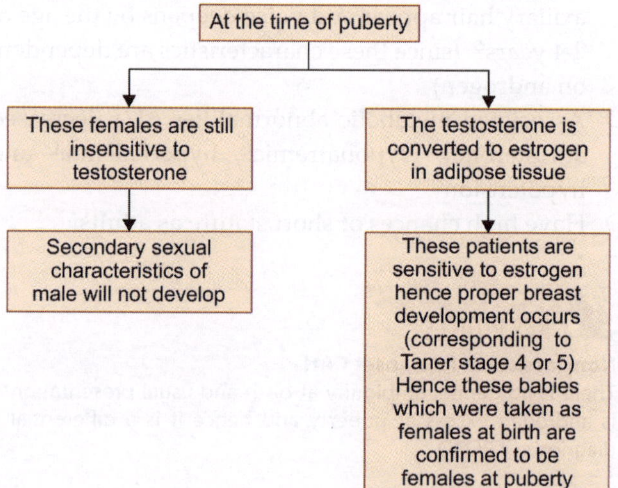

Note: In these females also, the hormone needed for pubic hair and axillary hair is androgen, that is why these females will not have proper pubic hair and Axillary hair (corresponding to Tanner Stage 1 or 2)

- Now since they are taken as females, they are expected to menstruate. Since uterus is absent, they cannot menstruate and hence they will complain of primary amenorrhea.

- ➤ D/D= Mullerian agenesis
- ➤ IOC to distinguish between the two is Karyotyping.

Management

Let them be Females

- The testis should be removed after puberty[Q] (16-18 years) as they have a high potential for malignant change, specially gonadoblastoma and dysgerminoma.[Q]
- Bilateral laparoscopic gonadectomy is the preferred procedure for removal of intra-abdominal testes.[Q]
- Estrogen therapy is desirable to prevent osteoporosis.[Q] since when testis are removed the source of testosterone and in turn estrogen is also gone.

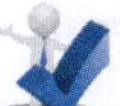

KEY POINTS

In Testicular feminizing syndrome patients, uterus is absent and hence no risk of developing endometrial cancer thus with oestrogen there is no need to add progestin.

- Vaginoplasty should be done just before or after marriage.[Q]

Incomplete Androgen Insensitivity Syndrome

- X linked recessive disorder
- Less severe than complete insensitivity (i.e. there is little responsiveness to Testosterone)
- Genotype = 46XY
- See Flowchart 6.9 for Pathophysiology

Flowchart 6.9: Pathophysiology in incomplete androgen insensitivity

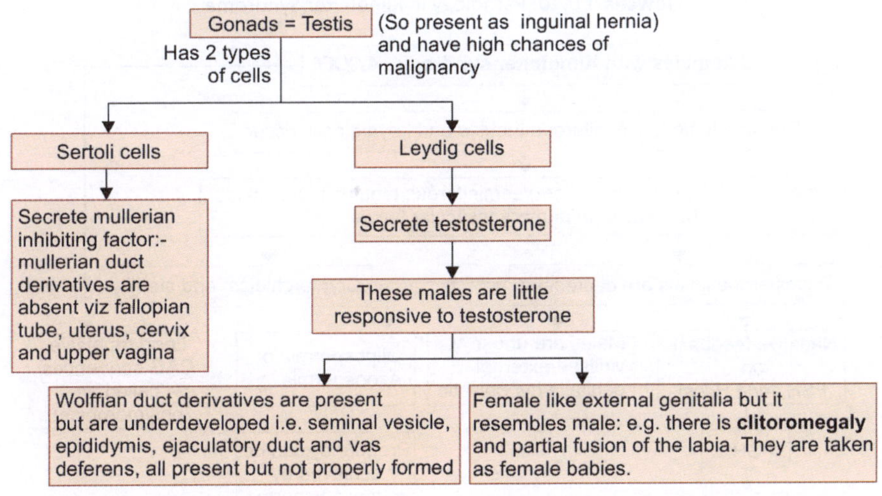

At the time of puberty

Again these children who are actually males but brought up like females: are partially sensitive to testosterone

These females will show virilizing features

Have proper breast development as testosterone gets converted to estrogen

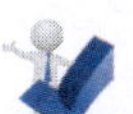

KEY POINTS

In Questions:

- If there is a female who complains of 1° amenorrhea with breast development corresponding to Taner Stage 4 or 5, but pubic hair absent, Bilateral Inguinal Hernia present: Always diagnosis is Complete Androgen Insensitivity Syndrome

Contd...

Contd...

- If there is a female who C/o 1° amenorrhea with proper breast development, inguinal hernia and clitoromegaly—then diagnosis is Incomplete AIS.

Reifenstein Syndrome

- Here patients are males but the males are undervirilised
- They have male genitalia but with bifid scrotum and hypospadias
- Male internal genitalia are present but are less developed.
- Patients complain of infertility
- Phenotypically also they are males but have gynecomastia.
- It is not inherited as X linked disorders.

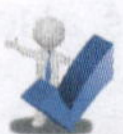

KEY POINTS

Testicular Feminization syndrome and Müllerian agenesis are differential diagnosis of each other.

- In both these conditions – a female (phenotypically) presents with:
  - Primary amenorrhoea
  - Normal breast development
  - Absent uterus.

The best test to differentiate between them is: Karyotyping

In Mullerian agenesis:

- Karyotype = 46 XX
- Barr body = Present
- Testosterone levels = N

In Testicular Feminization Syndrome:

- Karyotype = 46 XY
- Barr body = Absent
- Testosterone levels: Increased (as compared to females)

Klinefelter Syndrome (47XXY)

Pathophysiology

- The classic form of Klinefelter syndrome (47XXY) occurs following meiotic nondysjunction of the sex chromosomes during gametogenesis (40% during spermatogenesis, 60% during oogenesis).

Clinical Features

- Klinefelter syndrome (KS) is the **M/C cause of primary testicular failure** affecting 1 in 1000 males
- Pathology – See Flowchart 6.12.

Flowchart 6.10: Pathology in Klinefelter Syndrome

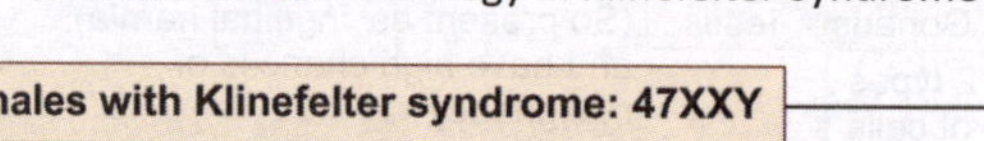

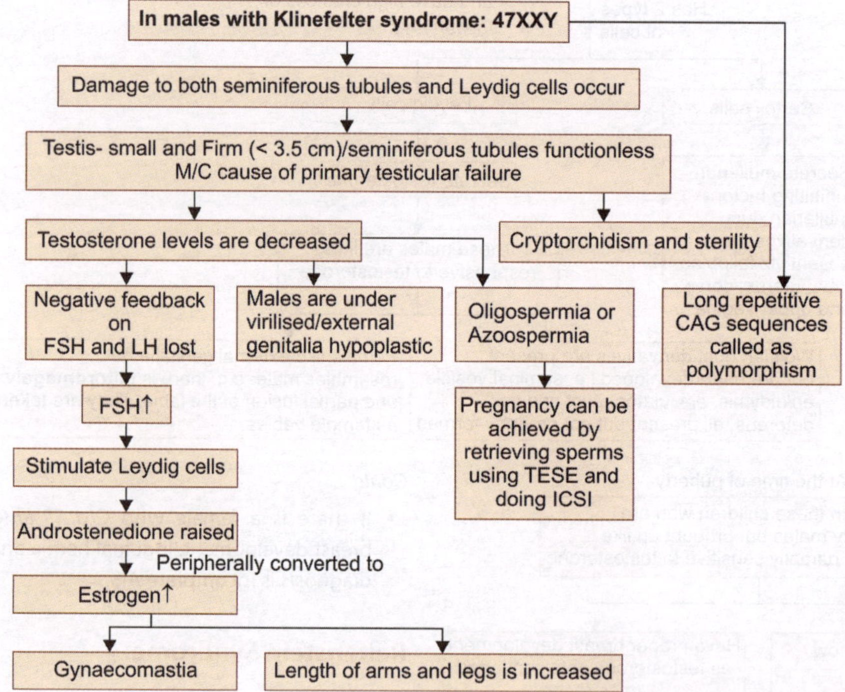

In addition to these, men with Klinefelter exhibit a number of psychosocial abnormalities like:

- Lack of insight
- Poor judgement
- Difficulty with complex speech
- Decreased attention span

In adult life, such males have increased risk of:

- Pulmonary diseases
- Breast CA
- Mediastinal germ cell tumor
- Varicose legs
- SLE
- Diabetes mellitus
- Antisocial mental disorder

Management

Give testosterone.

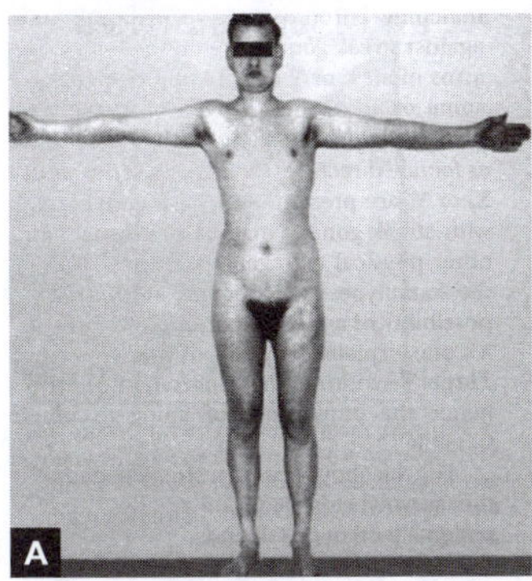
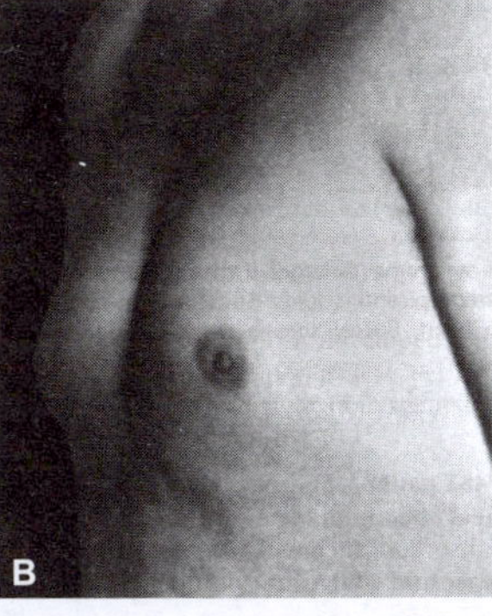

Figs. 6.3A and B: Klinefelter syndrome. Man aged 28 years, married but infertile and complaining of gynaecomastia. Chromosomes 47XXY (Professor Sir Cyril Clarke's case). (A) An apparently normal male but tall. The scrotum is small and contains very hypoplastic testes; (B) Slight gynaecomastia.

Diagnosis

Testicular biopsy shows hyalinised seminiferous tubules and hyperplastic Leydig cells.
Pituitary hormones (FSH, LH) are increased and testosterone levels are reduced.

Gonadal Dysgenesis

Gonadal dysgenesis: is a term where there is incomplete or defective formation of gonads which could be due to:

i. Disturbance in germ cell migration
ii. Chromosomal abnormality
iii. Defective formation of urogenital ridge.

It can be of following varieties:

i. Turner syndrome : 45XO
ii. Pure gonadal dysgenesis: 46XX
iii. Swyers syndrome 46XY

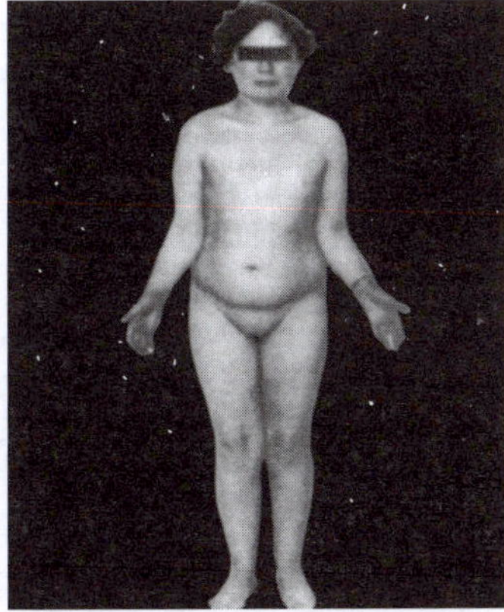

Fig. 6.4: Turner syndrome

Turner Syndrome

- **Genotype:** ***Most common*** **= 45XO**[Q] (loss of one X chromosome is due to Non- dysjunction during meiosis[Q], the X chromosome retained is ***maternal in origin***[Q] in most cases).
  - **Mosaics:** 45XO/46XX or 45XO/46XY

Note: In all **patients of Turners syndrome karyotype should be done because if they are Mosaic = 45XO/46XY then due to Y chromosome, gonads have high chances of developing gonadoblastoma**[Q]**.**

- **Pathophysiology (see Flowchart 6.11)**
- In Turner Syndrome–because estrogen levels are suboptimal. Therefore epiphyseal closure would occur late and hence height of the patient ideally should be more. But they are short statured due to-mutation in SHOX (short stature home box) containing gene.
- The clinical diagnosis of Turners is confirmed by the finding of **45 XO karyotype** (at least 30 cells should be examined due to possibility of mosaicism).
- **Gonads:** ***B/L Streak Gonads.***[Q] (since one single X chromosome is present, so ovaries are not properly formed).
- **Additional features of Turner syndrome**
  - Webbing of neck
  - Low posterior hair line
  - Widely spaced nipple (as breast is absent)
  - Shield shaped chest
  - Short 4th metacarpal
  - Cubitus valgus
  - CVS anomalies: M/C-Bicuspid aortic value (coarctation of aorta)
  - M/C Renal anomaly–Horse shoe shaped kidney
  - Increased risk of autoimmune diseases-diabetes/ Hashimoto thyroiditis.
  - IQ: Normal
- **Hormone levels:** LH: and FSH are increased

Flowchart 6.11: Pathophysiology of Turner Syndrome

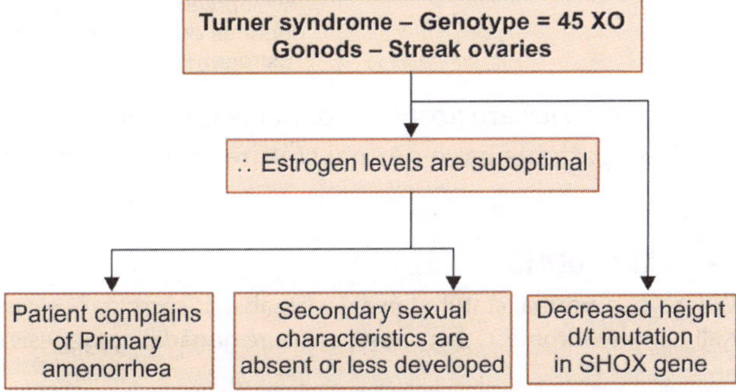

Management: Includes initially low dose estrogen to promote breast development; given at 12 years of age or at the time of diagnosis followed 1 year later by cyclical estrogen and progesterone.

Pure Gonadal Dysgenesis (46XX)

- In this condition although both X chromosomes are present but still ovaries are streak.
- The Gonads, i.e. ovaries are streak, so there is less estrogen and hence delayed puberty and 1° amenorrhea

This condition is similar to Turner syndrome except for following two conditions:

(i) Height of female is normal (in contrast to Turner Syndrome where height is short)
(ii) All the addition features of Turner syndrome are absent.

Swyers Syndrome (46XY)

In this condition: Gonads are testis. The testis are dysgenetic. In 85% cases, the cause is unknown but in 15% cases, it is due to mutation in SRY gene.

See Flowchart 6.12 for more details.

Flowchart 6.12: Pathophysiology of Swyer syndrome

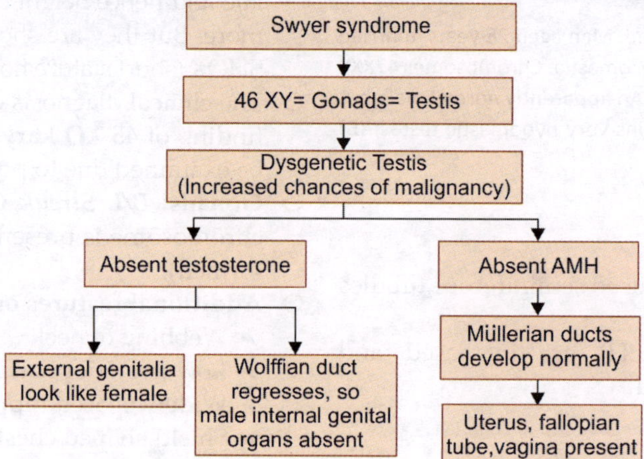

So although they are males, **they are taken as females.**

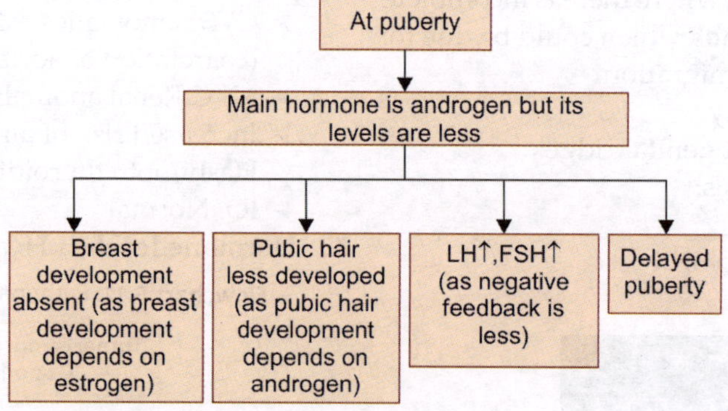

- Since ovaries are absent ∴ patients C/O primary amenorrhea.
- These patients have normal stature and present with primary amenorrhea.

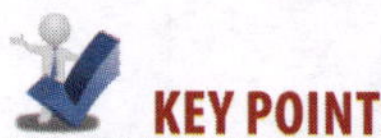

KEY POINTS

Wherever a normal stature female with absent secondary sexual characteristics presents with primary amenorrhea = M/c cause is Kallmann syndrome. Other causes are pure gonadal dysgenesis or Swyers syndrome or gonadal agenesis.

NEW PATTERN QUESTIONS

N1. Precocious puberty may be seen in all of the following conditions *except*:
a. Granulosa - cell tumour
b. Head - injury
c. Corticosteroid intake
d. Hyperthyroidism

N2. Precocious puberty associated with bony dysplasia and café au lait spots in skin is seen in:
a. Frohlichs syndrome
b. Alports syndrome
c. McCune-Albright syndrome
d. Laurence-Moon-Biedl syndrome

N3. An infant is found to have clitoral enlargement and some degree of labial fusion.
What is the first step in arriving at a diagnosis?
a. Perform a karyotype
b. Perform an ultrasound scan
c. Perform blood 17-hydroxyprogesterone levels
d. Perform serum testosterone levels

N4. An infant is found to have clitoral enlargement and some degree of labial fusion. The karyotype is XX.
What is the next step in arriving at a diagnosis?
a. Perform 5a-reductase levels
b. Perform an ultrasound scan
c. Perform serum cortisol levels
d. Perform blood 17-hydroxyprogesterone levels

N5. A 2-year-old child is found to have hirsutism clitoral enlargement and some degree of labial fusion. The karyotype is XX. Serum 17-hydroxyprogesterone levels are high.
What is the most appropriate first step in the management?
a. Commence treatment with cortisol after puberty
b. Commence treatment with glucocorticoids
c. Give a high salt diet
d. Perform surgery to remove the tumour

N6. A 13-year-old child, who is reared as female presents with primary karyotype XY. On examination, there is hirsutism, partial fusion of labia and clitoromegaly. Gonads can be felt in inguinal area. What is the most appropriate first step in management?
a. Rear the child as male
b. Treat with estrogen and progesterone
c. Treat with estrogen alone
d. Gonadectomy

N7. In testicular feminisation syndrome:
a. Buccal smear is chromatin positive
b. Normal breast size is observed
c. Menstruation is scanty and infrequent
d. Streak gonads seen

N8. All are true *except*, for Klinefelter syndrome:
a. M/C chromosomal cause of male infertility
b. Associated with gynecomastia
c. Associated with increased risk of breast cancer
d. Associated with short life span

N9. Normal size but non-functioning uterus is usually associated with:
a. Stenosis of the external os
b. Uterine synechiae
c. Partial agenesis of the vagina
d. Complete absence of vagina

N10. Exposure of a female fetus to androgen in early embryogenesis may arrest differentiation of:
a. Müllerian ducts
b. Ovary
c. Urogenital sinus
d. Mesonephric ducts

N11. Scoring system for virilization in females:
a. Ferriman–Gallwey score
b. Prader score
c. Nugent score
d. Dutchman score

N12. Main gene induced in 24 hydroxylase deficiency CAH:
a. Cyp 21 A2
b. Cyp 18
c. K ras
d. P ten

N13. Fate of Mullerian duct is determined by:
a. X chromosome
b. Y chromosome
c. Both
d. None

N14. Gonads are bipotential till:
a. End of 5 weeks
b. End of 6 weeks
c. End of 7 weeks
d. End of 8 weeks *Largman Embryology 13/e pg 261, 270*

N15. Delayed puberty is defined if menstruation does not occur by:
a. 13 years
b. 14 years
c. 15 years
d. 16 years

N16. Premature adrenarche is:
a. Development of pubic & axillary hair by 8 years
b. Development of pubic & axillary hair by 6 years
c. Pubic hair & axillary hair by 10 years
d. Pubic hair & axillary hair by 12 years

PREVIOUS YEAR QUESTIONS

1. **The sequence of development of puberty in girls is:** *(AI 00)*
   a. Thelarche, Pubarche, Menarche
   b. Pubarche, Thelarche, Menarche
   c. Pubarche, Menarche, Thelarche
   d. Menarche, Thelarche, Pubarche
2. **The first sign of puberty in girls is:** *(AI 08)*
   a. Breast budding
   b. Peak height velocity
   c. Menarche
   d. Pubic and axillary hair growth
3. **What is the first sign of puberty in a girl?** *(AIIMS Nov 2015)*
   a. Thelarche
   b. Menarche
   c. Adrenarche
   d. Pubarche
4. **Which of the following pubertal events in girls is not estrogen dependent?**
   a. Menstruation b. Vaginal cornification
   c. Height spurt d. Hair growth
5. **Which of the following is responsible for pubertal growth in females?** *(AIIMS May 2014)*
   a. Decreased level of adrenal androgens at puberty
   b. High level of estrogen at puberty
   c. Pulsatile release of GnRH during sleep
   d. Increased sensitivity of HPO axis to estrogen
6. **One of the following forms the basis for sex chromatin testing:** *(AIIMS May 2014)*
   a. Barr body
   b. Testosterone receptors
   c. Hormone levels
   d. Phenotypic features
7. **A 9-year-old girl presents with menarche. History reveals thelarche at the age of 7 years and adrenarche at the age of 8 years- the M/C cause of this condition in girls is:**
   a. Idiopathic
   b. Gonadal tumor
   c. McCune Albright syndrome
   d. Hypothyroidism
8. **What is the drug of choice for precocious puberty in girls?** *(AIIMS Nov 2016)*
   a. GnRH analogues
   b. Cyproterone acetate
   c. Danazol
   d. Medroxyprogesterone acetate
9. **Medication used in treatment of idiopathic central precocious puberty is:**
   a. Exogenous gonadotrophins
   b. Ethinyl estradiol
   c. GnRH analogues
   d. Ethinyl estradiol
10. **Gynaecomastia is seen in:** *(PGI June 07, Dec. 02)*
    a. Secondary syphilis
    b. Lepromatous leprosy
    c. HIV
    d. Klinefelter's syndrome
11. **Gynaecomastia is seen in all of the following conditions *except*:** *(AI 2012)*
    a. Prolactinoma
    b. TSH secreting adenoma
    c. HCG secreting tumor
    d. Estrogen secreting tumor
12. **During sexual differentiation in males:** *(Karnataka 05)*
    a. Leydig cells produce Mullerian Inhibiting Substance
    b. Primitive Gonads differentiate into testis due to the presence of SRY gene
    c. Androgen binding protein is responsible for the development of male external Genitalia
    d. Wolffian duct regresses
13. **Most common cause of ambiguous genitalia in a female child is:** *(AI 2011)*
    a. Placenta steroid sulfatase deficiency
    b. Fetal aromatase deficiency
    c. Wnt4 mutation
    d. Congenital adrenal hyperplasia
14. **Most common cause of female pseudohermaphroditism is:** *(AI 02)*
    a. Virlizing ovarian tumor
    b. Ovarian dysgenesis
    c. Exogenous androgen
    d. Congenital adrenal hyperplasia
15. **Female pseudohermaphroditism true is:** *(PGI Dec 04)*
    a. 46XX chromosomal pattern
    b. Absent ovary c. Absent uterus
    d. Presence of testis e. Clitoromegaly
16. **The treatment for a case of virilizing adrenal hyperplasia is:** *(AI 06)*
    a. Estrogens
    b. Antiandrogens
    c. ACTh
    d. Cortisone
17. **Best prenatal treatment for CAH is:** *(AIIMS Nov 2011)*
    a. Dexamethasone b. Betamethasone
    c. Prednisolone d. Hydrocortisone
18. **A newborn with 46XX has external genitalia of male. All the following are the possible causes *except*:**
    a. Placental aromatase deficiency
    b. Maternal androgen adrenal tumor
    c. Anti-Mullerian hormone deficiency
    d. Wnt 4 mutation
19. **A 15-year-old female presents with primary amenorrhea. Her breasts are Tanner 4 but she has no axillary or pubic hair. The most likely diagnosis is:** *(AI 06)*
    a. Turner's syndrome
    b. Mullerian agenesis
    c. Testicular feminization syndrome
    d. Premature ovarian failure

20. Androgen insensitivity syndrome true is: *(AIIMS May 08)*
a. Phenotype may be completely female
b. Predominantly ovarian component in gonads
c. Always in female
d. Testes formed abnormally and receptors are normal

21. Which of the following statement is/are true regarding androgen insensitivity syndrome? *(PGI Nov 2012)*
a. Absent vagina
b. Karyotype is XX
c. Karyotype is XY
d. Pubic hair is normally present
e. Breast development is normal

22. Regarding androgen insensitivity syndrome, which statement is/are true: *(PGI May 2013)*
a. Genotype is 46 XX
b. Scanty pubic hair
c. Well developed female external genitalia
d. Uterus absent
e. Breast development is adequate

23. All are seen in testicular feminization syndrome *except*: *(PGI June 99)*
a. 46XY
b. Primary amenorrhea
c. Short stature
d. Vagina may be present

24. A girl presents with; primary amenorrhea; grade V thelarche, grade II pubarche; no axillary hair; likely diagnosis is: *(AI 01)*
a. Testicular feminisation syndrome
b. Mullerian agenesis
c. Turners syndrome
d. Gonadal dysgenesis

25. All of the following statements about Androgen Insensitivity Syndrome are true *except*: *(AI 08)*
a. Patients have an XY genotype
b. Pubic hair are abundant
c. Short vagina may be present
d. Ovaries are absent

26. 16-year-old female presents with primary amenorrhoea with B/L inguinal hernia. She has normal sexual development with no pubic hair. USG shows no uterus and ovaries and a blind vagina. Diagnosis is: *(AIIMS May 07)*
a. Turner's syndrome
b. Mullerian agenesis
c. STAR syndrome
d. Androgen insensitivity syndrome

27. A young female presented to you with primary amenorrhea. Examination reveals normal breast development and absent axillary hairs. Pelvic examination shows a normally developed vagina with clitoromegaly. On ultrasound, gonads are visible in the inguinal region. What is the most likely diagnosis? *(AIIMS Nov 2016)*
a. Complete androgen insensitivity syndrome
b. Partial androgen insensitivity syndrome
c. Mayer Rokitansky Kuster Hauser syndrome
d. Gonadal dysgenesis

28. Among the following which is a feature of testicular feminization syndrome: *(PGI June 99)*
a. XX pattern
b. Commonly reared as male
c. Well formed female internal genitalia
d. High testosterone levels

29. In Testicular Feminization syndrome Gonadectomy is indicated: *(UPSC 04)*
a. As soon as it is diagnosed
b. At puberty
c. Only when malignancy develops in it
d. When hirsutism is evident

30. A 16-year-old female presents with Primary Amenorrhea. Examination shows a Short Blind Vagina, with absent Uterus. The Next Investigation of choice is: *(AI 00)*
a. Karyotyping
b. IVP
c. Gonadotrophin levels
d. Serum prolactin

31. True about Klinefelter syndrome: *(PGI May 2010)*
a. XXY
b. XO
c. Male hypogonadism
d. Female hypogonadism
e. FSH

32. A patient of 47 XXY karyotype presents with features of hypogonadism; likely diagnosis is: *(AI 01)*
a. Turners syndrome
b. Klinefelters syndrome
c. Edwards syndrome
d. Down syndrome

33. True about Klinefelter syndrome: *(PGI May 2015)*
a. Leg are more in length than trunk
b. Intrauterine fertilization can not be successful even with TESA and ICSI
c. Gynecomastia
d. FSH and luteinizing hormone (LH) are decreased

34. Young male presents with delayed puberty with decreased FSH, LH, and testosterone. Which of the following is NOT possible? *(AI 2012)*
a. Kallmann syndrome
b. Klinefelter's syndrome
c. Constitutional delay
d. DAX-1 gene mutation

35. In which of the following conditions do the ovaries functions normally? *(AIIMS Nov 2011)*
a. Turner's syndrome
b. Rokitansky-Kuster-Hauser syndrome
c. Androgen insensitivity syndrome
d. Swyer's syndrome

36. Which of the following statements is true about Swyer syndrome?
a. Can be fertile with surrogacy
b. Can be fertile with ovum donation
c. Presents with primary fertility
d. Gonadectomy is indicated for all patients

37. A mother brings her 19 years old daughter to your clinic with complaint that she has not started having menses. General examination reveals normally developed breasts and pubic hair. On pelvic examination, vaginal ending is blind and uterus is not palpable. Which of the following do you suspect? *(AIIMS May 2016)*

a. Mullerian agenesis
b. Asherman syndrome
c. Gonadal dysgenesis
d. Turner syndrome

38. True regarding testicular feminization syndrome:

a. Phenotype that of female
b. Phenotype and genotype of male
c. Genotype, phenotype and gonads of male
d. Gnods and genotype that of female

39. Which of the following is/are true regarding androgen insensitivity syndrome:

a. Absent vagina
b. Karotype is XX
c. Karyotype is XY
d. Pubic hair normally present
e. Breast development adequate

40. True about precocious puberty in girls: *(PGI May 2011)*

a. Secondary sexual characteristics before 8 years
b. Increase in testis size – earliest sign of puberty in boy
c. Commonest cause is Idiopathic
d. Hypothalamic hamartoma is least of central cause
e. MRI brain is a mandatory investigation

41. Least common cause of ambiguous genitalia in female is: *(JIPMER May 2017)*

a. 17 alpha hydroxylase
b. 21 hydroxylase
c. 3β steroid dehydrogenase
d. 11β hydroxylase

42. Young female history spontaneous abortion and secondary amenorrhea since then. FSH 6 IU/mL. What is the most probable cause of amenorrhea? *(AIIMS Nov 2018)*

a. Ovarian failure
b. Pituitary failure
c. Fresh pregnancy
d. Uterine synechiae

43. Which of the following can cause Precocious puberty? *(PGI MAY 2019)*

a. Congenital adrenal hyperplasia
b. McCune Albright syndrome
c. Granulosa cell tumor
d. Leydig cell tumor
e. Theca cell tumor

44. All are features of Turner's syndrome *except*: *(PGI December 2018)*

a. Karyotype is 46 XO
b. Normal breast
c. Underdeveloped uterus
d. Normal secondary sexual characters
e. Primary amenorrhoea

ANSWERS TO NEW PATTERN QUESTIONS

N1. Ans. is d, i.e. Hyperthyroidism *Ref: Jeffcoate 7th/ed, p116-118*

- Friend for the details on causes of precocious puberty kindly see the preceding text.
- Remember hypothyroidism and not hyperthyroidism causes precocious puberty.

Reason:

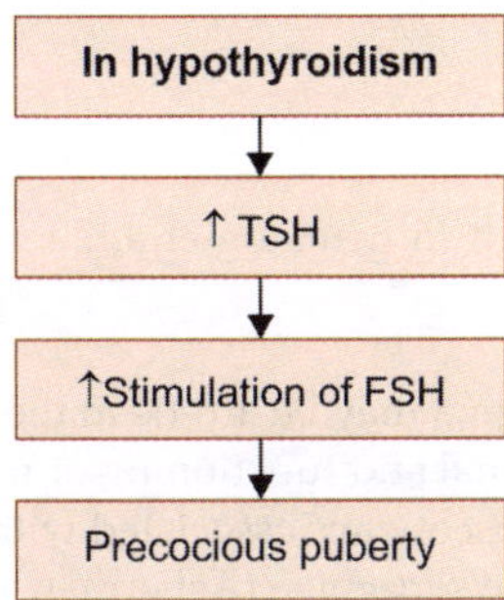

If precocious puberty is associated with delayed bone age it suggests primary hypothyroidism.Q

N2. Ans. is c, i.e. McCune-Albright syndrome *Ref: Novak 15th/ed, p1023*

Precocious puberty with bony dysplasia and cafe au lait spots points towards incure in McCune-Albright syndrome as the diagnosis.

> McCune-Albright Syndrome is characterised by the classic triad of polyostotic fibrous dysplasia of bone, irregular café au lait spots on skin and GnRH independent sexual precocity

- The precocious puberty is the result of secretion of estrogen from functioning ovarian cysts.
- The café au lait spots are usually large, do not cross the midline and have irregular "coast of maine" margins.
- They are located on the same side as the bony lesion

Laurence-Moon-Biedl syndrome is hypothalamic amenorrhea + mental retardation + polydactyl + retinitis pigmentosa.
Frohlich Syndrome is hypogonadotropic hypogonadism + obesity + genital hypoplasia
Both these are causes of delayed puberty and not precocious puberty

N3. Ans. is a, i.e. Perform a karyotype

A child born with ambiguous external genitalia could be a female who has been exposed to androgens, such as in the case of congenital adrenal hyperplasia, or a true hermaphrodite, or an under masculinised male. Such a male could have 5α-reductase deficiency, or abnormal androgen receptors, or Müllerian inhibitor deficiency. Therefore, the first step in the diagnosis is to perform a karyotype, to diagnose whether the child is a male or a female, because further investigations would depend on the genetic sex. However, a true hermaphrodite could be XX or XY.

N4. Ans. is d, i.e. Perform blood 17-hydroxyprogesterone levels

As the karyotype is XX the child is a female. The child has been exposed to androgens *in utero* from the mother or the child has congenital adrenal hyperplasia. The rare possibility of a true hermaphrodite with a XX karyotype should also be considered. The next step is to perform blood 17-hydroxyprogesterone levels, to confirm/exclude congenital adrenal hyperplasia, which is a treatable condition. An ultrasound scan should be performed next, because the uterus ovaries and vagina are present in congenial adrenal hyperplasia.

N5. Ans. is b, i.e. Commence treatment with glucocorticoids

A diagnosis of congenital adrenal hyperplasia can be made because the karyotype is XX and there is hirsutism, labial fusion and elevation of 17-hydroxyprogesterone. The first step in the management is to commence treatment with a large dose of corticosteroids to suppress the adrenal function. Treatment should be commenced immediately to prevent the harmful effects of excessive adrenal function. All female functions will be restored in due course. Cosmetic treatment will be required for hirsutism and clitoromegaly. Salt loss should be prevented.

N6. Ans. is d, i.e. Gonadectomy

The first step is to remove the gonads to prevent further secretion of androgens and malignant transformation. Corrective surgery and cosmetic therapy should be done for virilisation. Female secondary sexual characteristics can be induced with oestrogen alone as the uterus is absent so no chances of endometrial cancer. The cloacal vagina may be sufficient for sexual intercourse or a vagina can be reconstructed by vaginoplasty, just before or after marriage. Fertility and menstruation cannot be restored.

N7. Ans. is b, i.e. Normal breast size is observed *Ref: Dutta Gynae 6th/ed, p443*

In testicular feminization syndrome:

Genotype = 46 XY

- Hence Barr body is absent i.e. chromatin negative (i.e., option a is incorrect)
- Here gonads are testis and are not streak (option d is incorrect)
- There is primary amenorrhea (option c is incorrect)

(i.e. option d is correct).

Rest all options you know.

N8. Ans. is d, i.e. Associated with short life span

See the for explanation.

N9. Ans. is b, i.e. Uterine synechiae

Lets have a look at each option:

Option a: Stenosis of external os would result in hematometra, i.e. uterus would be large and non-functioning (hence ruled out).

Option c: Partial agenesis of vagina *Ref: Dutta Gynae 6th/ed, p43*

In partial agenesis of vagina a segment of vagina may be atretic in the upper-third. It is often associated with hypoplasia or even absence of cervix. Uterus may be normal and functioning or malformed.

Option d: Complete absence of vagina is almost always associated with absence of uterus. *Ref: Dutta Gynae 6th/ed, p44*

Hence by exclusion our answer is b i.e. uterine synechiae (Asherman syndrome)

In Uterine synechiae–the uterus does not function normally due to presence of adhesions size of uterus is normal.

N10. Ans. is c, i.e. Urogenital sinus *Ref: Read below*

This is common sense. We have discussed so many times that in females exposure of androgens in early embryogenesis results in ambiguous external genitalia.

The external genitalia are formed by urogenital sinus (so it is our answer of choice)

N11. Ans. is b, i.e. Prader score

Prader score is for scoring of virilization

Ferriman–Gallwey score is for hirsutism

N12. Ans. is a, i.e. Cyp 21 A2

The main gene involved in 21 hydrogxylase deficiency type of CAH is cyp 21 A2.

N13. Ans. is b, i.e. Y chromosome

Mullerian duct fate is determined by Y chromosome. If Y chromosome is present, then gonads are testis & testes have Sertoli & Leydig cells.

The Sertoli cells secrete mullerian inhibiting factor in males & that is the reason for regressing of mullerian duct in males.

N14. Ans. is b, i.e. End of 6 weeks *Ref: Langman Embryology 13th/ed, p261, 270*

N15. Ans. is d, i.e. 16 years *Ref: Williams gynae 3rd/ed, p329*

This is a controversial question *Williams gynae 3rd/ed, p329 says*

"Puberty is considered delayed if no secondary sexual characteristics are noted by age 13 or if menses have not commenced by age 16"

Williams gynae 3rd/ed, p329

As per Medicine uptodate – delayed puberty is if menstruation does not begin by 15 years of age

But I am going with Williams Gynae.

N16. Ans. is a, i.e. Development of pubic hair and axillary hair by 8 years of age *Williams gynae 3rd/ed, p329*

"Adrenarche is onset of DHEA and DHEA-S production from adrenal zona reticularis which can be detected around 6 years of age. This phenotypic result of adrenarche is axillary and pubic hair development termed pubarche which begins in girls at age 8 years. Premature adrenarche is defined therefore as growth of pubic hair prior to age 8, but other signs of estrogenization or virilization are absent."

ANSWERS TO PREVIOUS YEAR QUESTIONS

1. **Ans. is a, i.e. Thelarche, Pubarche, Menarche**
2. **Ans. is a, i.e. Breast budding**
3. **Ans. is a, i.e. Thelarche** *Ref: Ghai Essential Pediatrics 8th/ed, p531-535*

   The first sign of puberty in girls is Growth spurt. The first visible sign of puberty in girls is: Thelarche (appearance of breast budding).
4. **Ans. is d, i.e. Hair growth** *Ref: Williams Gynae 1st/ed, p315; Novak 14th/ed, p992, 15th/ed, p993*

   In girls the sequence of development of puberty is (Mnemonic: GTPH in males).Q
   G = **G**rowth spurt
   T = **B**reast development (**T**helarche)Q
   P = **P**ubic hair development (Pubarche)Q
   H = **He**ight increases; peak growth velocityQ attained
   in males = Menstruation starts (Menarche)Q
   (Axillary hair develop after menstruation starts)Q

   - The main hormone responsible for secondary sexual characteristics in females is estrogen
   - Estrogen leads to
     - Breast development
     - Growth spurt, i.e. height attained
     - Production of cervical mucus
     - Cornification of vaginal cells
     - Menstruation (menstruation occurs due to withdrawal of progesterone in an oestrogen primed uterus)
   - Estrogen leads to
   - As far as hair growth is concerned - in females also the hormone responsible is Androgens (produced by adrenals and ovary)
5. **Ans. is c, i.e. Pulsatile release of GnRH during sleep**

   Ref: Nelson 19th/ed, p1886; M.Fritz and L. Speroff's 'Clinical Gynecologic Endocrinology and Infertility' 8th/ed, p407

   Pulsatile release of GnRH during sleep is responsible for pubertal growth in females.

   "After a decade of quiescence, pulsatile secretion of GnRH increases and the hypothalamic-pituitary gonadal axis is reactivated (gonadarche), probably in response to metabolic signals from the periphery. FSH and LH levels rise moderately before age 10, followed by a gradual increase in estradiol concentrations, which stimulate breast development (thelarche). The increase in pulsatile gonadotrophin secretion occurs first at night, during sleep, but gradually extends throughout the day."

   - M. Fritz and L. Speroff's 'Clinical Gynecologic Endocrinology and Infertility' 8/e pe p407
6. **Ans. a, i.e. Barr body** *Ref: Gamong 24th/ed, p392-393*

   Barr body forms the basis for sex chromatin testing.

   Barr Body
   When two X chromosomes are present in a cell (as in a normal female) one of them becomes inactivated and condensed on the nuclear membrane and is called the 'Barr body'. This process is termed as X chromosome lyonization (inactivation)
   Presence or absence of Barr bodies helps in ascertaining the sex of an individuals
   - Absence of Barr body indicates that the patient has only one X chromosome (e.g. Normal male XY or Turner's syndrome (XO)
   - Nuclei of cells in females (XX) contain a darkly staining Barr body that is not present in the nuclei of cells in males.
   - Barr bodies are most easily seen in a smear of squamous epithelial cells obtained by scraping the buccal mucosaQ
   - Barr bodies react differently to histological stains and are best seen as dark staining bodies within the nucleus of non-dividing interphase cells.
7. **Ans. is a, i.e. Idiopathic**
8. **Ans. is a, i.e. GnRH analogue**
9. **Ans. is c, i.e. GnRH analogues** *Ref: Novaks 15th/ed, p1017,1020; Textbook of Gynae Shielabalakrishnan 1st/ed, p67-8*

   In question no. 7 female has developed both breast and axillary hair and she has cyclical vaginal bleeding, these findings favour central precocious puberty which is most commonly idiopathic.

   DOC for managing central precocious puberty is GnRH analogue –(Leuprolide)

   Principle → Continuous administration of GnRH agonist, downregulates and desensitizes GnRH receptor of pituitary, decreasing gonadotropin release leading to decreased estrogen production.

   Note: In these females GnRH should be withdrawn at the age of normal puberty.

10. Ans. is b, c and d, i.e. Lepromatous leprosy; HIV; Klinefelter's syndrome

11. Ans. is a, i.e. Prolactinoma *Ref: Harrisons 18th/ed, p2889, Schwartz 7th/ed, p541; Schwartz 7th/ed, p541; Behl 9th/ed, p223*

Gynaecomastia implies presence of female type mammary glands in male.

It can be:

Physiological	[Q]Pathological[Q]				
Neonatal period[Q] Systemic[Q]	Adolescence[Q] excess	Senescence[Q] androgens[Q]	D/t Estrogen[Q] intake diseases	D/t decreased	Drugs[Q]
• Occurs b/w 12 and 15 years[Q] • Unilateral[Q]	• Occurs b/w 50 and 70 years[Q] • Bilateral[Q]				

Causes of Gynaecomastia:

I. Estrogen excess states:

A. Gonadal origin:

1. True hermaphroditism
2. Gonadal stromal (Nongerminal) neoplasm of testis:
   - Leydig cell (interstitial)[Q]
   - Sertoli cell[Q]
   - Granulosa-theca[Q]
3. Germ cell tumours:
   - Choriocarcinoma[Q]
   - Seminoma, teratoma[Q]
   - Embryonal carcinoma[Q]

B. Nontesticular tumours:

1. Skin-nevus
2. Adrenal cortical Neoplasms[Q]
3. Lung carcinoma[Q]
4. Hepatocellular carcinoma[Q]

C. Endocrine disorders:

1. Hypothyroidism[Q]
2. Hyperthyroidism[Q]

D. Disease of the liver – Non-alcoholic and alcoholic cirrhosis

E. Nutrition alteration states: Starvation (As pituitary adrenal axis is suppressed)

II. Androgen deficiency states:

A. Senescent causes with aging

B. Hypoandrogen state (hypogonadism)

1. *Primary testicular failure*
   a. Klienfelter syndrome (XXY)[Q]
   b. Reifenstein syndrome, (XY)[Q]
   c. Rosewater, Gwinup, Hamwi familial gynecomastia (XY)
   d. Kallmann syndrome[Q]
   e. Kennedy disease with associated gynaecomastia[Q]
   f. Eunuchoidal males (Congenital anorchia)[Q]
   g. Hereditary defects of androgen biosynthesis
   h. ACTH deficiency
2. *Secondary testicular failure:*
   a. Trauma[Q]
   b. Orchitis: due to mumps and leprosy[Q]
   c. Crytorchidism[Q]
   d. Irradiation[Q]
   e. Hydrocele[Q]
   f. Varicocele[Q]
   g. Spermatocele

C. Renal failure

III. Drug related conditions that initiate gynaecomastia

1. Estrogen[Q]
2. Digitalis[Q]
3. Spironolactone[Q]
4. Methyldopa[Q]
5. Captopril[Q]
6. Calcium Channel blocker[Q]
7. Cimetidine (high doses)[Q]
8. Ketoconazole[Q]
9. Tricyclic Antidepressant[Q]
10. Diazepam[Q]

IV. Systemic disease 'with' idiopathic mechanisms

A. Non-neoplastic disease of the lung

B. Trauma (chest wall)

C. CNS - related causes from anxiety and stress

D. AIDS (Acquired Immunodeficiency Syndrome)

12. Ans. is b, i.e. Primitive Gonads differentiate into testis due to the presence of SRY gene

Ref: Dutta Gynae 5th/ed, p420, 6th/ed, p439; Williams Gynae 1st/ed, p403-404; Harrison 17th/ed, p2339-2340

As discussed earlier:

In males

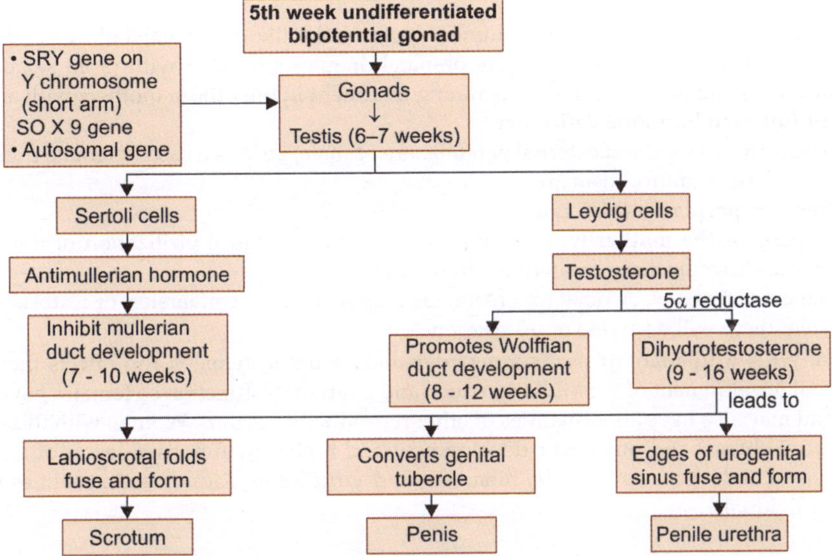

In males—masculinization of external genitals begin at 9–10 weeks and is completed by 12–14 weeks of gestation.

- Thereafter the only change is in the growth and length of penis.
- Since in males, mainly masculinization is due to testosterone/dihydrotestosterone, therefore if it is deficient it will lead to undermasculanization of external genitalia, i.e. males will have small phallus, hypospadias or scrotal defect, i.e. ambiguous genitalia.

13. Ans. is d, i.e. Congenital adrenal hyperplasia *Ref Leon Speroff 8th/ed, p349; Dutta Gyne 6th/ed, p440*

"CAH due to 21 hydroxylase deficiency is the most frequent cause of sexual ambiguity and the M/C endocrine cause of neonatal death." *Ref: Leon Speroff 8th/ed, p349*

Ambiguity of sex at birth—"Cases of ambiguity of sex detected at birth are due to adrenogenital syndrome unless proved otherwise". *Ref: Dutta Gynae 6th/ed, p404*

14. Ans. is d, i.e. Congenital adrenal hyperplasia

Ref: Dutta Gynae 4th/ed, p404; Williams Gynae 1st/ed, p409; Novak 14th/ed, p102

Most common cause of female Pseudohermaphroditism is Congenital adrenal hyperplasia

15. Ans. is a, and e, i.e. 46XX chromosomal pattern; and Clitoromegaly

Ref: Dutta Gynae 6th/ed, p440; William Gynae 1st/ed, p409; Shaw 15th/ed, p113

In a female most common cause of ambiguous sex is congenital adrenal hyperplasia.

As discussed in preceeding text in case of congenital adrenal hyperplasia:

Genotype: 46XX

Gonads: Ovary

Internal genital organs: Normal (i.e. uterus, vagina)

External genital organs: There is clitoromegaly and genital folds fused to form penile urethra rather than labia minora. Labia majora are fused which appears like scrotum

16. Ans. is d, i.e. Cortisone

17. Ans. is a, i. e. Dexamethasone *Ref: Shaw 15th/ed, p114; CGDT 10th/ed, p120; Leon Speroff 8th/ed, p355*

Treatment of CAH is aimed at providing sufficient amounts of the deficient hormone, cortisol, to reduce excessive ACTH secretion and to prevent consequences of excessive androgen production.

Thus in patients of CAH: Hydrocortisone 10–20 mg/m^2 body surface area is given per day.

Once the neonate is stable reconstruction surgery-clitoroplasty (by 5 years) and vaginoplasty are done

Prenatal Cases:
DOC is dexamethasone as dexamethasone is not metabolized by placenta and crosses effectively into fetal circulation. For maximum benefit-treatment should begin at 4 to 5 weeks of gestation and not later than 8 weeks

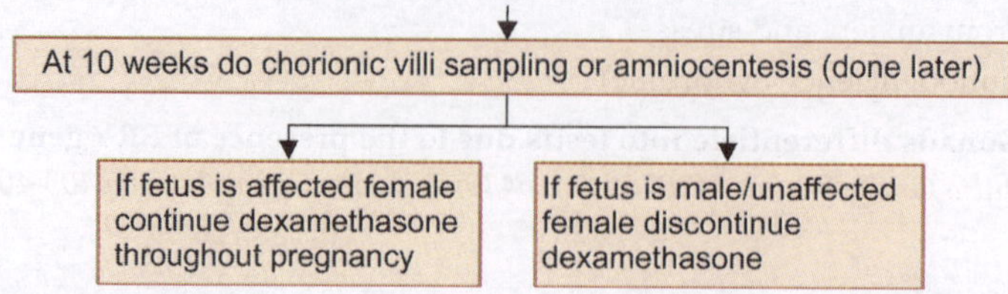

Note: Latest recommendations are prenatal treatment poses risks like postnatal failure to thrive and psychomotor developmental delay, hence best approach is early prenatal diagnosis by CVS with rapid sex determination (FISH for the X and Y chromosome) and genotyping and beginning treatment in only those mothers with an affected female child.

18. Ans. is c, i.e. Anti-Mullerian hormone deficiency *Ref: Leon speroff 7th/ed, p329,344*

The karyotype of the baby is 46 XX and external genitalia are of male, i.e. it is a case of female pseudohermaphroditism. Causes of female pseudohermaphroditism are:

- **Congenital adrenal hyperplasia. (M/C cause)**
- **Increased androgens in the mother** which cross the placenta and cause virilization of the external genitalia. Like maternal intake of androgenic drugs, maternal adrenal tumor, etc.
- **Placental aromatase deficiency.** Aromatase enzyme is responsible for conversion of testosterone to estradiol. If this enzyme is deficient there will be excess of testosterone.
- **Wnt4 mutation.** Wnt4 Mullerian aplasia is a disorder that occurs in females and affects their reproductive system. There is abnormal development of the Mullerian duct, and ovarian dysfunction so females have an underdeveloped or absent uterus and may also have abnormalities of other reproductive organs. Women with this condition have primary amenorrhea, normal breast and pubic hair development and higher than normal levels of androgens in their blood. These high levels of androgens cause acne, hirsutism and virilisation. Kidney abnormalities may also be present in some affected individuals.

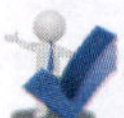

KEY POINTS

AMH Deficiency/ Uterine Hernia Syndrome/Persistent Mullerian duct syndrome

- It is seen in males
- It is an autosomal recessive congenital disorder.

Karyotype = 46 XY
Gonads = testis
Hormone = Testosterone
Thus, external genitalia are normal since levels of testosterone are normal. The problem is there is persistent Mullerian duct so uterus and other Mullerian duct derivatives are seen in a male.
Typical features: Include cryptorchidism and the presence of a small, underdeveloped uterus in a male infant or adult.
Here since both Mullerian duct and Wolffian duct both are seen in males so the tissue are often intertwined, resulting in obstruction or non patency of the vas deferens or other parts of the male excretory ducts. This can result in infertility.
The condition can come to attention because of a bulge in the inguinal canal of a male infant due to herniation of the uterus.
There is no ambiguity or malformation of the external genitalia. They look like a normal male.

19. Ans. is c, i.e. Testicular feminization syndrome *Ref: Novak 14th/ed, p1037-1038*

When a female comes with complain of primary amenorrhea the first thing to do is see her secondary sexual characteristics:

- *In Turner's Syndrome all secondary sexual characteristics are absent where as in the question the female has proper breast development with absent axillary and pubic hair (therefore option 'a' ruled out).*
- *In Mullerian agenesis – Patient presents with primary amenorrhea with well developed secondary sexual characteristics (both breast and pubic hair), i.e. option b ruled out.*
- *In option d, i.e. premature ovarian failure – patient will have no secondary sexual characteristic be it breast or pubic hair, i.e. this option is also incorrect.*
- *In testicular feminization syndrome as discussed in the preceeding text – Genotype is 46 XY, i.e. they are males but with testosterone resistance. Male secondary sexual characteristics do not develop. This testosterone is converted to estrogen and thus these males have well developed breasts (Tanner stage 4 or 5) and since development of pubic and axillary hair is dependent on testosterone, these are not developed or under developed (Tanner stage 1 or 2)*

20. Ans. is a, i.e. Phenotype may be completely female *Ref: Shaw 15th/ed, p111-112; Williams Gynae 1st/ed, p410*

21. Ans. is a, c and e, i.e. Absent vagina; Karyotype is XY; and Breast development is normal

- Testicular feminization syndrome is the most common form of male intersex
- The individual presents with female phenotype, but genotype is 46XY.
- Gonads are testis and ovary is absent.
- A short blind vagina is usually seen.

The etiology of testicular feminisation involves either *Ref: Williams Gynae 1st/ed, p410*

- Testicular enzyme defects in the biosynthesis of testosterone
- Peripheral enzyme defect
- Abnormalities in the androgen receptor

Thus testis are abnormal functionally & not anatomically

22. Ans. is b, d and e, i.e. Scanty pubic hair; Uterus absent; and Breast development is adequate
Ref: Shaw Gynae 15th/ed, p111-2; Dutta Gyane 6th/ed, p424

Androgen insensitivity syndrome/Testicular Feminizing syndrome:

- Genotype: 46 XY
- They are males who are resistant to testosterone
- Internal genitalia and external genitalia of males are present hence (no uterus).

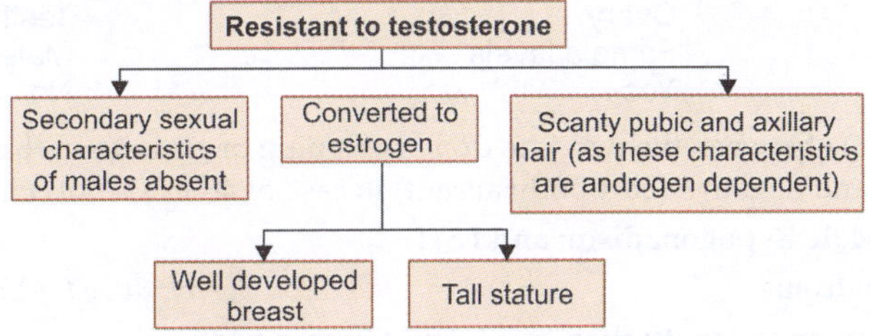

23. Ans. is c, i.e. Short stature

24. Ans. is a, i.e. Testicular feminisation syndrome

25. Ans. is b, i.e. Pubic hair are abundant

All options have been explained in detail in the preceeding text, I do not think there is any need to repeat them. Here I want to point out that in these patients testis are intra-abdominal which can present in the form of bilateral inguinal hernia and since the entire testosterone is converted to estrogen hence these patients are tall.

26. Ans. is d, i.e. Androgen insensitivity syndrome *Ref: Leon Speroff 7th/ed, p330; Shaw 15th/ed, p111-112; Novak 14th/ed, p1047; Harrison 17th/ed, p2344; Williams Gynae 1st/ed, p410*

Patient is presenting with primary amenorrhea + B/L inguinal hernia + Normal secondary sexual characteristic (i.e. breast) + No pubic hair & USG shows no uterus and ovaries.

All this points towards androgen insensitivity syndrome.

27. Ans. is b, i.e. Partial insensitivity syndrome

There is clitoromegaly which indicates partial androgen insensitivity.

28. Ans. is d, i.e. High testosterone levels *Ref: Harrison 17th/ed, p2344; Dutta Gynae 6th/ed, p443*

In Testicular Feminization Syndrome

- Genotype– 46XY
- Gonads – Testis (intraabdominal)
- Phenotype – Female

Internal Genitalia – Is of males (except a short vagina may be present)

They are reared as female.

Lab investigation:

- Testosterone levels may be normal/high/low depending on the degree of androgen resistance and the contribution of estradiol to feedback inhibition of the hypothalamus pituitary axis. *Ref: Harrison 17th/ed, p2344*

"Laboratory evaluation demonstrates elevated LH levels, normal or slightly elevated testosterone levels, and a 46XY Karyotype."
Ref: Williams Gynae 1st/ed, p410

- LH levels are high (due to insensitivity of pituitary and hypothalamus to testosterone) but FSH levels are Normal.

29. Ans. is b, i.e. At puberty *Ref: Novak 14th/ed, p1051, 15th/ed, p1050*

Patients of Testicular Feminization syndrome (Androgen insensitivity) are genotypically males (Karyotype 46XY) but phenotypically females (i.e. male pseudohermaphroditism). Due to the presence of Y chromosome gonads are testis which remain intra-abdominal and have a malignant potential (Most common = Gonadoblastoma, Dysgerminoma). Therefore testis should be removed in such patients. B/L Laparoscopic Gonadectomy is the preferred procedure[Q]. As far as timing of Gonadectomy is concerned:

"In patient with complete androgen insensitivity, the testis should be removed after pubertal development is complete to prevent malignant degeneration." *Ref: Novak 14th/ed, p1051, 15th/ed, p1050*

Whereas in cases other than Testicular Feminization syndrome, if patient has XY Karyotype and she develops virilization, the testes should be removed immediately to preserve the female phenotype and to promote female gender identity.

Extra Edge:

In case specific age at which Gonads should be removed in Testicular Feminization is asked go for 16-18 years.

Ref: Leon Speroff 7th/ed, p340

30. Ans. is a, i.e. Karyotyping *Ref: Jeffcoate 7th/ed, p198; CGDT 10th/ed, p931 Fig. 56-2*

A female presenting with absent uterus and short blind vagina:

Friend what are the D/D's which come to your mind.

I can think of only 2: Mullerian dysgenesis and Testicular feminizing syndrome (or male pseudohermaphroditism).

Presentation	Mullerian Agenesis	Androgen Insensitivity
Inheritance pattern	Sporadic	X-linked recessive
Karyotype	46XX	46XY
Breast development	Yes	Yes
Axillary and pubic hair	Yes	No
Uterus	No	No
Gonad	Ovary	Testis
Testosterone	Female levels	Male levels
Associated anomalies	Yes	No

So, the best way to differentiate between the two is to do karyotyping or chromatin/barr body test, which comes positive (barr body present) in 46XX and negative (barr body absent) in case of 46XY Genotype.

31. Ans. is a, c and e, i.e. XXY; Male hypogonadism; and FSH

32. Ans. is b, i.e. Klinefelter syndrome *Ref: Leon Speroff 8th/ed, p1261-1262; Harrison 17th/ed, p2340-42*

33. Ans. is a and c, i.e. Legs are more in length than trunk and Gynecomastia

Klinefelter Syndrome

Genotype – 47XXY

Clinical features

- Klinefelter syndrome (KS) is the M/C cause of primary testicular failure, i.e. male hypogonadism affecting 1 in 1000 males

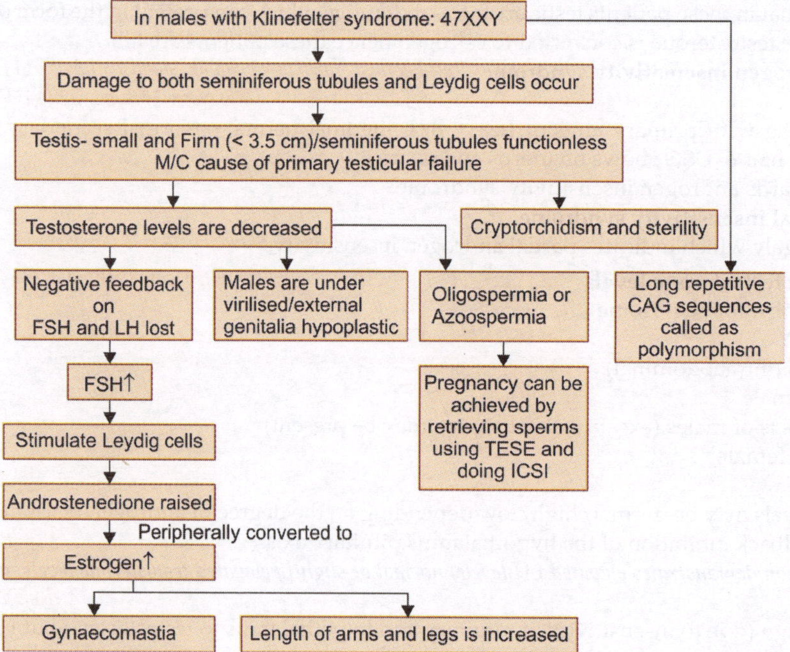

34. Ans. is b, i.e Klinefelter's syndrome *Ref: Leon Speroff 7th/ed, p404-407*

- Decrease in serum follicle-stimulating hormone (FSH), luteinizing hormone (LH), and testosterone indicates that this is a case of hypogonadotropic hypogonadism.
- Hypogonadism resulting from hypothalamic or pituitary defects is called as hypogonadotropic hypogonadism or central hypogonadism. Examples of hypothalamic defects include Kallmann syndrome. Examples of pituitary defects include hypopituitarism. DAX-1 (dosage-sensitive sex reversal, adrenal hypoplasia critical region, on chromosome X,

gene 1) is a nuclear receptor protein. Mutations in this gene result in both X-linked congenital adrenal hypoplasia and hypogonadotropic hypogonadism.

- Hypogonadism which results from defects of the gonads is called as primary hypogonadism/hypergonadotropic hypogonadism. Examples include Klinefelter syndrome, mumps, varicocele, etc.

In Klinefelters = Testosterone is decreased, which results in increase in LH and FSH.

35. Ans. is b, i.e. Rokitansky-Kuster-Hauser syndrome *Ref: Jeffcoates 7th/ed, p197-198; Shaw 14th/ed, p82; COGDT 10th/ed, p549*

- Ovaries develop from genital ridge, whereas fallopian tubes, uterus, cervix and upper part of vagina are formed by Mullerian duct.
- In Mullerian agenesis which is also called as Mayer-Rokintansky-Kuster-Hauser syndrome, fallopian tube, uterus, cervix and upper part of vagina are absent and not ovaries.
- Ovaries are normally functioning.

36. Ans. is b i.e. Can be fertile with ovum donation *Ref: Shaw's Textbook of Gynecology 15th/ed, p145*

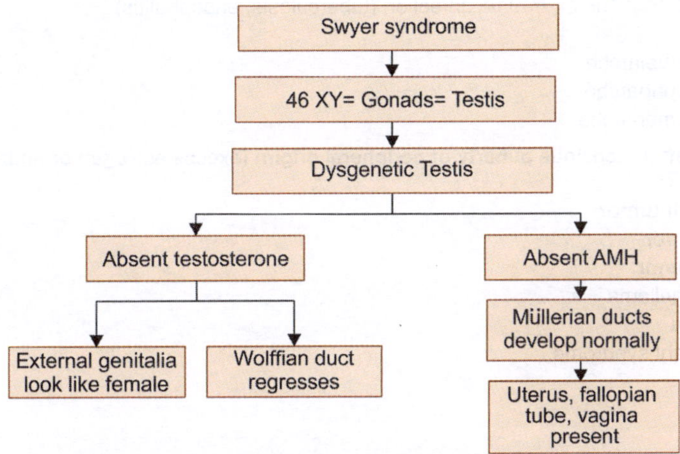

- Mgt: Estrogen and progesterone therapy for breast development and menstruation
- Gonadectomy: As intra-abdominal testis have risk of germ cell tumor
- Females can become pregnant by doing IVF with donor oocyte

37. Ans. is a, i.e. Mullerian agenesis

In the question - 19 year old c/o primary amenorrhea with -

(i) Normal secondary sexual characteristics (breast and pubic hair)
(ii) Uterus is absent
(iii) Short vagina is present

All these favor the diagnosis of Mullerian agenesis. As far as Ashermann Syndrome is concerned, uterus should be palpable. In Gonadal dysgenesis and Turner Syndrome, secondary sexual characteristics are absent.

38. Ans. is a, i.e. Phenotype that of female

In Testicular feminizing syndrome:
Genotype = 46 (XY) = male
Phenotype = Female (well developed breast)
Gonads = Testes.

39. Ans. is a, c and e, i.e. Absent vagina; Karyotype is XY and Breast development is adequate

See the text for explanation.

40. Ans. is a, b, c and e, i.e. Secondary sexual characteristic before 8 years; Increase in testis size earliest sign of puberty in boy; Commonest cause is idiopathic and MRI brain is a mandatory investigation.

See the text for explanation

41. Ans. is c, i.e. 3 Beta steroid dehydrogenase deficiency

As you can see, all the options given in the question are enzymes of steroid Pathway

- CAH which is the M/C cause of ambiguous genitalia in females is most commonly due to deficiency in enzyme 21 hydroxylase
- The least common cause is deficiency of 3 β hydroxysteroid dehydrogenase.

42. Ans. is d i.e. Uterine synechiae

- Since the lady in the question is having secondary amenorrhea following an abortion, uterine synechiae is the most likely cause. Here FSH levels are normal

- (Normal serum FSH value in adult woman is 5–20 lU/mL).
- In case of ovarian failure—FSH should be high (as no negative feedback from estrogen).
- In case of pituitary failure—levels of FSH are low.

43. Ans. is a, b, c and d, i.e. Congenital adrenal hyperplasia, McCune Albright syndrome, Granulosa cell tumor, and Leydig cell tumor

Precocious puberty: It is defined as appearance of any of the secondary sexual characteristics before the age of 8 years or occurrence of menarche before the age of 10 years *– Shaw's Gynae 17th/ed, p83*

Causes of precocious puberty.

GnRH dependent-80% (complete, central, isosexual or true)
- Constitutional—most common
- Juvenile primary hypothyroidism
- CNS lesions (30%): Tumor, trauma, infection (tuberculosis, encephalitis)
- Incomplete
  - Premature thelarche
  - Premature pubarche
  - Premature menarche

GnRH independent (precocious puberty of peripheral origin) (excess estrogen or androgen)

Ovary
- **Granulosa cell tumor**
- **Theca cell tumor**
- **Leydig cell tumor**
- Chorionic epithelioma
- Androblastoma
- McCune-Albright syndrome

Adrenal
- Hyperplasia
- Tumor

Liver

Hepatoblastoma

Iatrogenic

Estrogen or androgen intake

Aetiological classification of precocious puberty.	*Shaw's Gynae 17th/ed p83*
• Complete precocious puberty	• Idiopathic, familial or sporadic, genetic (75%) • Congenital lesions of the *hypothalamus-pituitary* • Acquired lesions—trauma, infection, neoplasm—tuberculosis (TB) meningitis in childhood • Part of a specific syndrome—***McCune-Albright*** (5%), von Recklinghausen's neurofibromatosis • Other causes—endocrine/metabolic disorders
• Incomplete precocious puberty:	• Premature thelarche • Premature adrenarche • Premature menarche
• Pseudoprecocious puberty: (GnRH independent)	• Feminizing ovarian tumors (10%) (hormone secreting) • **Adrenal hyperplasia** neoplasm – 20% • Hypothyroidism • Hepatoblastoma producing gonadotropins • Iatrogenic–estrogen administration

44. Ans. is b and d, i.e. Normal breast, and Normal secondary sexual characters

Ref: Robbin's 9th/ed, p166-67; Dutta's Gynae 6th/ed, p422-25; Shaw's Gynae 15th/ed p128-110-11

Explained in detail in book

CHAPTER 7

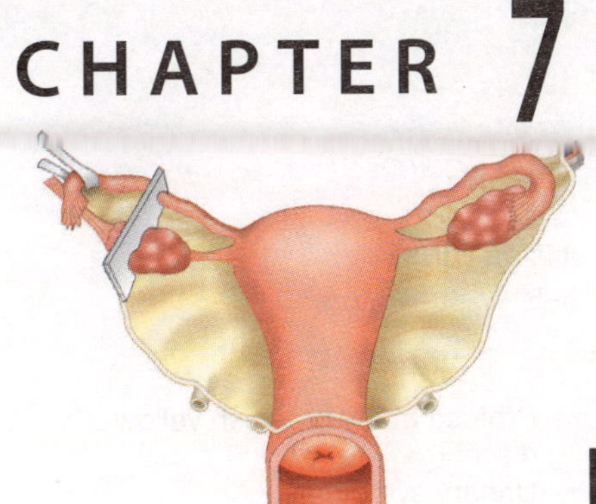

Infections of the Genital Tract

Vagina – Characteristics

- In adult females, vagina is lined by stratified squamous epithelium. In newborn females, it is lined by transitional epithelium.
- Squamous epithelium is resistant to gonoccocal and chlamydial infection. Thus, gonoccocal or chlamydial vaginitis cannot occur in young/adult females.

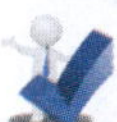

KEY POINTS

Theoratically gonoccocal vaginitis can occur in newborn females as their vagina is lined by transitional epithelium.
M/c site for gonoccocal infection in young females is endocervix since endocervix is lined by columnar epithelium and not squamous epithelium.

Vagina has local inhabitant bacteria called as *Doderlein's bacillus* (lactobacilli) which breaks down the glycogen present in vaginal epithelium into lactic acid resulting in acidic pH (Avg, 4.5; Range, 4–5.5) of vagina. The acidic pH of vagina acts as a barrier for external organisms.

Physiological Discharge

- Clear, white, and flocculent odorless discharge which becomes yellow on contact with air due to oxidation
- Smear contains epithelial cells and lactobacilli (which are normal in number)
- pH ranges from 3.8 to 4.2
- Increases with increased estrogen conditions: pregnancy, OCP, mid-cycle, PCOS, or premenarchal
- If increased in perimenopausal woman, investigate for other effects of excess estrogen (e.g. endometrial cancer).

Vulvovaginitis

Postmenopausal Vaginitis/Atrophic/Senile Vaginitis

Vaginitis in postmenopausal females is called as atrophic or senile vaginitis.

Etiology

Due to decreased estrogen in postmenopausal females which leads to vaginal dryness.

Clinical Features

- Discomfort, dryness, soreness in the vulva
- Dyspareunia.

Investigations

Diagnosis is usually a visual one – thinning of tissues, erythema, dryness

- Rule out malignancy.

Treatment

- Local estrogen cream is ideal – (Premarin cream)
- Oral or transdermal hormone replacement therapy (if treatment for systemic symptoms is desired).

Infectious Vulvovaginitis *(See Table 7.1)*

Table 7.1: Infectious vulvovaginitis

	Bacterial vaginosis	Candidiasis	Trichomonas vaginitis
Organism	Alteration of vaginal flora; lactobacilli decrease whereas coccobacilli and Gardnerella increase	*Candida albicans* > *Candida glabrata* > *Candida tropicalis*	*Trichomonas vaginalis* (flagellated protozoa) (Figs. 7.1A and B)
M/C	Most common vaginitis (overall)	M/C vaginitis in: • Pregnancy, diabetes • Immunocompromised people • OCP users, steroid users, antibiotic users	

Contd...

Contd...

STD	Not an STD	Usually not an STD	It is an STD
pH of discharge	> 4.5	< 4.5 (so it is the M/C vaginitis in acidic media) or during pregnancy	5–6
M/C complaint	Foul smelling dirty white discharge **No inflammation-hence no itching**	• Intense pruritis • Curdy white discharge (or cottage cheese like discharge) • **Splash dysuria**	• Profuse frothy greenish yellow discharge • Urinary symptoms • Dysuria • Dyspareunia
Signs	–	Examination reveals erythema and edema of labia and vulvar skin (Fig. 7.2A)	Strawberry vagina or angry looking vagina (Fig. 7.3)
IOC	**Saline microscopy** 'Clue cells', i.e. vaginal epithelial cells to which bacteria are adhered seen (Fig. 7.4)	**Saline microscopy** pseudohyphae seen (Fig. 7.2B)	**Saline microscopy** Typical motile flagellated trichomonas seen or some kind of motility seen Tricomonas may be seen on pap smear. If pap smear shows Trichomonas, doa saline microscopy to further confirm the diagnose before initiating treatment
Gold standard investigation	**Gram stain** On gram staining **Nugent scoring** is done-The Nugent score is calculated by assessing the presence of lactobacillus (Gram +ve rods-scored as 0 to 4), *Gardnerella vaginalis* (scored as 0 to 4) and mobiluncus (Gram variable rods-scored as 0-2) A score of ≥ 7 is consistent with bacterial vaginosis	Culture on Sabouraud's medium or Nickerson medium	Culture on—**Feinberg-Whittington media or Diamond media**
Amine test/Whiff test, i.e. 10% KOH added to discharge	Positive, i.e. on adding 10% KOH to discharge, fishy odour or amine like odour obtained.	Negative	May be positive/or negative due to its association with Bacterial vaginosis
T/t = Nonpregnant females	Metronidazole (500 mg BD × 7 days) or clindamycin Cream 2%, one full application (5 g) intravaginal at bedtime for 7 days or clindamycin 300 mg BID × 7 days	Azole group of antifungals like fluconazole/miconazole which can be applied topically or given orally (150 mg, single dose)	Metronidazole (2 gm single dose oral) or 500 mg BD × 7 day)
Pregnancy = DOC	Metronidazole (250 mg TDS x 7 days) To be avoided in first trimester	Topical azole antifungals to be avoided in first trimester	Metronidazole (250 mg TDS x 7 days)
Simultaneous treatment of male partner	Not needed as BV is not an STD	If partner has symptoms then treatment needed	Always done as *Trichomonas vaginalis* is an STD

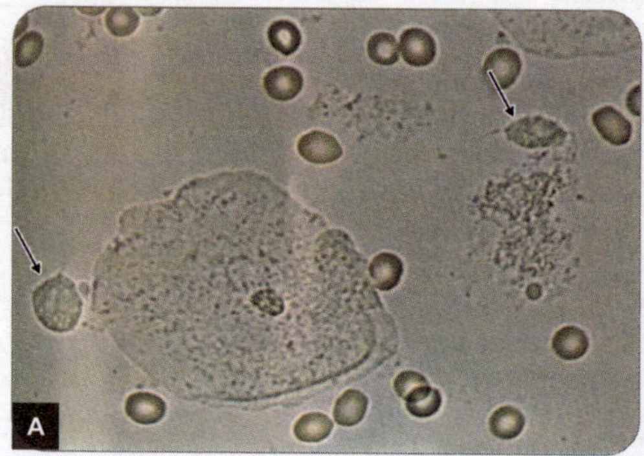

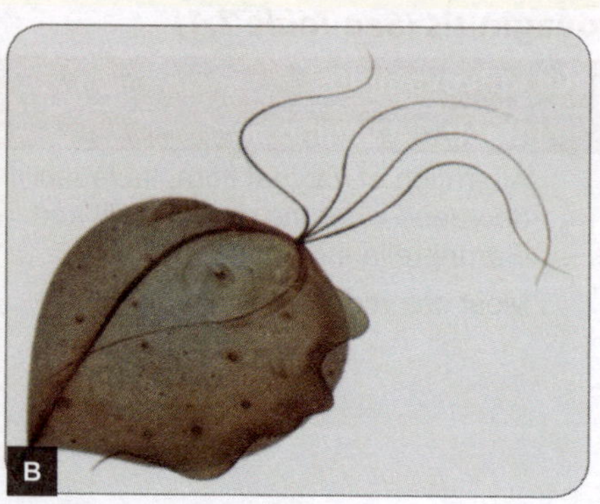

Figs. 7.1A and B: Trichomonas: (A) Saline preparation; (B) Showing depicting anatomic features of Trichomonas

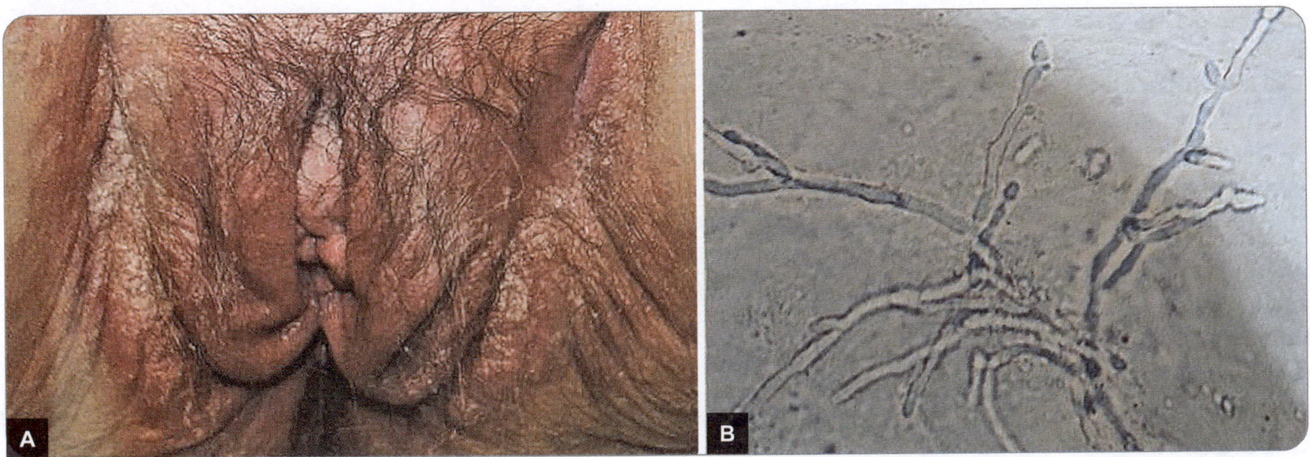

Figs. 7.2A and B: Candida infection: (A) Thick white discharge, labial erythema, (B) Candida albicans in KOH preparation, Pseudohyphae seen

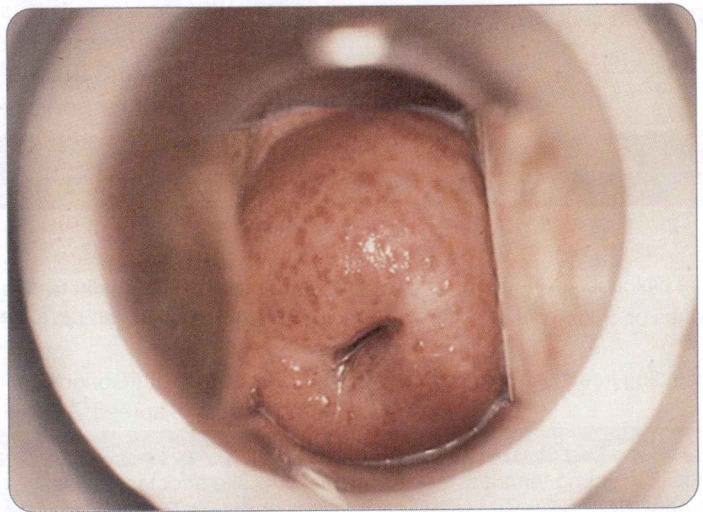

Fig. 7.3: Strawberry vagina

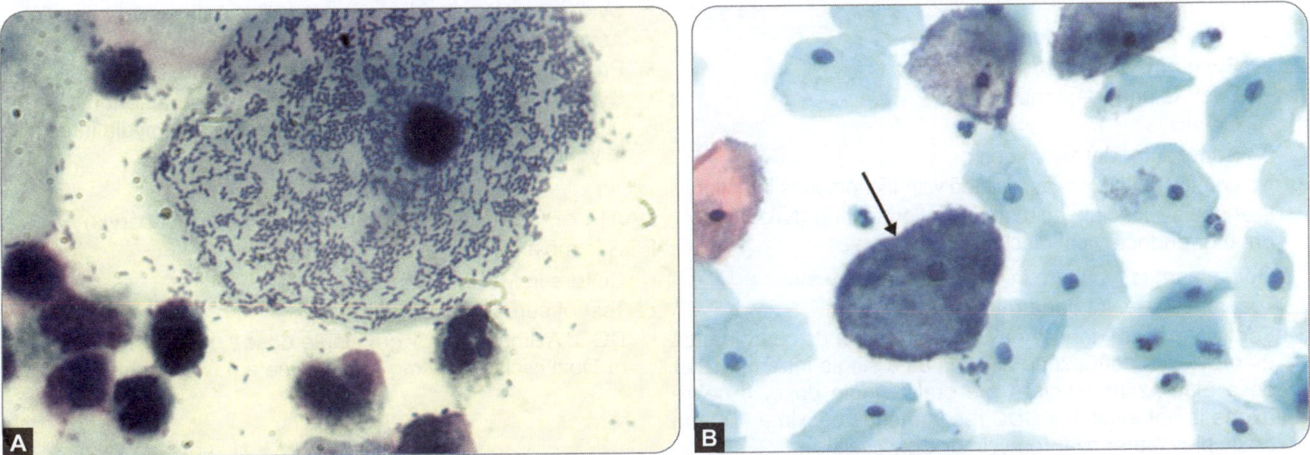

Figs. 7.4A and B: (A): Clue cells; (B): Pap smear showing clue cells with normal vaginal epithelial cells

Bacterial Vaginosis

Bacterial vaginosis is not considered by CDC to be an STD but an increased risk of BV is associated with sexual contact with multiple partners & new male & female partners condom use lowers its risk.

Risk factors for Bacterial vaginosis:

- Oral sex
- **Douching**
- Cigarette smoking
- **Sex during menses**
- Intrauterine device
- **Early age of sexual intercourse**
- New partner/multiple partners
- **Sexual activity with other women.**

Hazards of Bacterial Vaginosis

Women with BV are at increased risk for:

- PID
- Post abortal PID
- Postoperative cuff infections after hysterectomy
- Abnormal cervical cytology.

Pregnant women with BV are at risk for:

- PROM
- Preterm delivery
- Chorioamnionitis
- Post caesarean endometritis

Candidiasis:

CDC classifies vulvovaginal candidiasis into uncomplicated and complicated.

Uncomplicated: is sporadic, mild to moderate in severity, likely to be caused by Candida albicans & involves unimunocompromised females.

Complicated: is a recurrent disease, severe, caused by non albican species & M/c immunocompromised females. Longer treatment duration for 7-14 days needed in this case.

Recurrent vulvo vaginal candidiasis:

It is defined as **4 or more episodes of candidiasis in a year.**

- **Management**-Fluconazole 150 mg every 3 days for 3 doses (day 1, day 4, day 7) followed by 150 mg weekly for 6 months as a maintenance therapy.
- For Non albican recurrent infection = boric acid gelatin capsule intravaginally daily for 2 weeks as they are not responsive to azole treatment.

Table 7.2	
Gonorrhea	**Chlamydia**
• 2nd M/C cause of PID	Most common cause of PID M/C age group < 25 years
• Caused by Gram negative diplococcus N. gonorrhoeae • Associated with trichomonas or chlamydia infection in 60% cases	• Caused by chlamydia trachomatis (D-K serotype) an obligate intracellular parasite
• M/C route of spread: Ascending infection along with sperms	• Associated with Gonorrhea infection • M/C route of spread: Ascending infection along with sperms
Gonorrhea	**Chlamydia**
• M/C site affected: endocervix in young females, the urethra and Bartholin's gland	• M/C site affected-endocervix, urethra and Bartholin's gland: Like Gonococcus—stratified squamous epithelium is resistant to chlamydia also.
• Symptoms: – The PID which is non-commonly – **Purulent vaginal discharge** – Dysuria and frequency – Cervicitis – Adnexal tenderness seen • No pruritus unless it is associated with trichomonas infection	• Symptoms: It is insidious in onset & mostly asymptomatic • Asymptomatic in 80% cases • Presents with **clear mulcoid nonoffensive discharge** • Dysuria and frequency of micturition with bacteriuria < 10^5 organisms/ml of urine is pathognomic of chlamydia infection in young sexually active females.
• Diagnosis—Nucleic acid amplification testing **(NAAT)** of urine or endocervical discharge.	NAAT or PCR (Specimen: to be taken from endocervix) PCR is most reliable test
• Gold standard—culture in Thayer Martin media.	• Culture in McCoy lines
• Test for cure—Not done routinely.	• Test of cure not done routinely
• For treatment of gonorrhea CDC recommends combination therapy: with ceftriaxone 250 mg as a single intramuscular dose plus azithromycin 1 gm orally single dose. If ceftriaxone is not available CDC recommends cefixime 400 mg orally plus either azithromycin or Doxycycline. For gonorrhea if, cettriazone is not used in treatment than test of cure should be done after 1 week **(this is an important change in CDC guidelines).**	• DOC: Azithromycin 1 gm single dose or Doxycycline 100 mg orally twice a day × 7 days

Contd...

Contd...

Sex partners should be treated especially those exposed within 2 weeks prior to onset of symptoms or 4 weeks prior to diagnosis in an asymptomatic patient	
• DOC in pregnancy—Injection Ceftriaxone 250 mg single dose and azithromycin 1g orally single dose	DOC in pregnancy—Azithromycin 1 gm single dose or amoxicillin 500 mg TDS x 7 days or erythromycin 500 mg orally four times a day × 7 days. Test of cure for C. trachomatis is not routinely indicated. Repeat testing done 3 weeks after treatment is recommended for pregnant women only.

Condyloma Acuminata (Genital Warts)

- Most common viral sexually transmitted infection
- **Causative agent:** HPV (human papilloma virus)
- More than 200 subtypes HPV are known of which mostly are genital subtypes
- HPV types 6 and 11 are classically associated with anogenital warts/Condylomata Acuminata
- HPV types of 16 and 18 are the most oncogenic (classically associated with CIN and Ca cervix)
- Anatomical distribution of anogenital HPV infection is: cervix 70%, vulva 25%, vagina 10% and anus 20%.

Clinical Features

- Soft, multiple warts on any dermal or mucosal surface. Mostly seen on the posterior introitus, the labia majora and minora.
- Genital warts can be diagnosed by gross inspection. Colposcopic examination may help to rule out other cervical/vaginal lesions.

Treatment

- **Patient applied:**
  - Podofilox 0.5% solution or gel (Pregnancy category C)
  - Imiquimod 5% cream (Pregnancy category C).
- **Provider administered:**
  - Cryotherapy with liquid nitrogen (safe in pregnancy)
  - Podophyllin resin in tincture of benzoin (pregnancy category C)
  - Trichloroacetic acid (TCA) or bichloroacetic acid weekly (80–90%) (safe in pregnancy)
  - Surgical removal/laser
  - Intralesional interferon (not approved by FDA).

Prevention

- HPV types 6, 11, 16 and 18 are preventable with Gardasil (quadrivalent HPV recombinant) vaccine. Details of vaccine are given in chapter on Cancer Cervix (Chapter 14B) of the book.

Note: HPV cannot be prevented by using condoms.

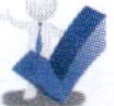

KEY POINTS

Genital Warts during Pregnancy

- Condylomata tend to get larger in pregnancy and should be treated early (consider excision)
- Cesarean section is done only if there is obstruction of birth canal or risk of extensive bleeding
- Do not use imiquimod, podophyllin, or podofilox in pregnancy
- Vertical transmission can occur during pregnancy leading to juvenile laryngeal papillomatosis in the neonate

Genital Ulcers

The M/c causes of genital ulcers in young, sexual active women are:

- Herpes simplex virus (HSV)
- *Treponema pallidum* (syphilis)
- *Haemophilus ducreyi* (chancroid).

Herpes Simplex Virus

SUPERFICIAL KNOWLEDGE

- It is the M/C cause of genital ulcers
- **Etiology**—90% cases are due to HSV-2; 10% cases are due to HSV-1

Classically

- HSV-1—causes disease above the belt (i.e. oral lesions)
- HSV-2—causes disease below the belt (i.e. genital lesion)
- Lesion first appears as erythematous plaque which later forms vessicles and then small ulcers with an erythematous halo and yellow base. Ulcers are extremely tender and inguinal lymph nodes are enlarged (Fig 7.5)
- **IOC:** Electron microscopy
- **DOC**: Acyclovir (200 mg 5 times a day × 7 days or 400 mg 3 times day for 7 days
- **Gold standard for diagnosis**: Tissue culture (William's Gynecology 3rd ed., p. 56).

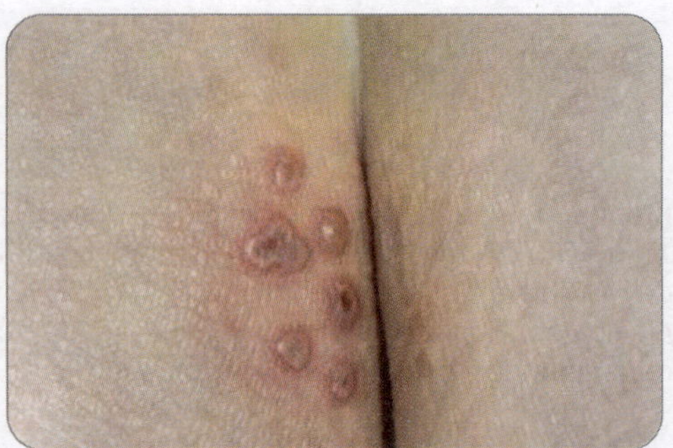

Fig. 7.5: Genital: Herpetic ulcers—vesicles prior to ulcer

Syphilis

- **Etiologic agent – *Treponema pallidum***
- **Primary syphilis** presents as a single hard, painless, solitary chancre (Fig. 7.6) on the vulva, vagina or cervix, although non-genital lesions may also be present. Non-tender inguinal lymphodenopathy is present. Primary chancre resolves spontaneously within 2–6 weeks
- **Screening test:** VDRL test (IM, 2.4 million IU).
- **Confirmatory test:** Fluorescent treponemal antibody test
- **DOC – Benzathine penicillin.**

Note: Tubes are not affected in 1° syphilis and infertility does not occur in syphilis.

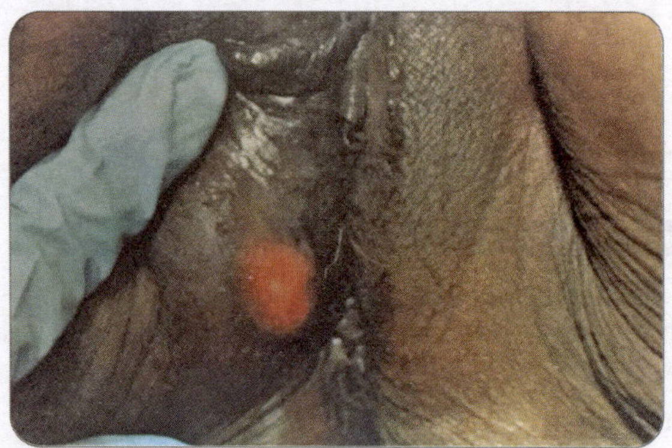

Fig. 7.6: Vulva syphilitic chancre

KEY POINTS

Manifestations of syphilis in genital tract:

Stage of syphilis	Lesion seen
Primary	Chancre/ulcer
Secondary	Condyloma lata-coarse flat topped moist necrotic lesion
Tertiary syphilis	Gumma-punched ulcer with rolled out margins.

Molluscum Contagiosum (Fig. 7.7)

- Caused by Pox virus
- M/c in developing countries
- **M/c route of spread:** Skin contact (sexual/non sexual)

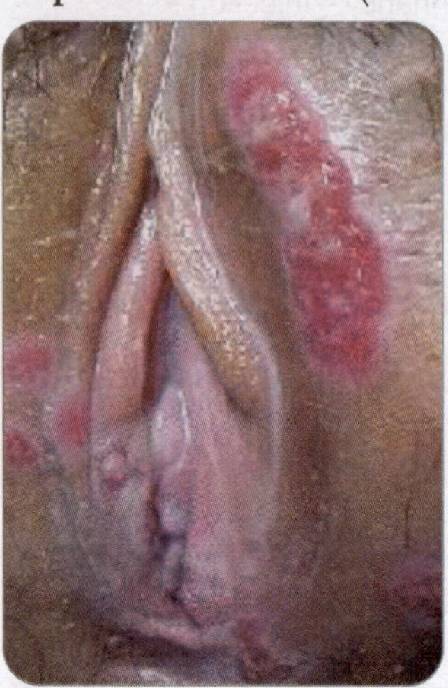

Fig. 7.7: Lesions of molluscum contagiosum

- Characteristic lesion: Multiple dome-shaped papules with central umblication. Edges of these painful ulcer are regular with erythematous non-indurated margins. Ulcer base is red and granular (Fig. 7.7)
- Diagnosis: Bygross inspection
- Management: Self-limiting condition
- If required: Cryofreezing/curettage of core material should be done

Note: For clinical features of genital ulcers *see* Annexure 7.

Pelvic Inflammatory Disease (PID)

Definition

- Infection or inflammation of the upper genital tract involving fallopian tube, ovaries and uterus

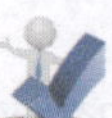

KEY POINTS

Note: Cervicitis and vaginitis are not included in PID

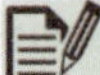

Important Concept

- M/C route of spread of PID–ascending infection along with sperms.
- The only PID which does not spread this way is genital TB. It has hematogenous spread.
- M/c symptom of PID: Dysmenorrhea (Abdominal pain rarely ever occur in PID)
- **IOC** for diagnosis of PID: Laparoscopy
- **Surest sign of salpingitis** is pus extruding from fimbrial end of tube.
- **Violin string like adhesions** in the pelvis and around liver suggests chlamydial infection.

Organisms Causing PID

Primary	Secondary
Chlamydia (M/C)	*E. coli* (M/C in postmenopausal females)
Gonorrhea	Group B *Streptococcus*
Mycoplasma genitalium	*Klebsiella*
	Anaerobes

- M/C cause of PID: Chlamydia
- M/C cause of acute PID/Symptomatic PID: Gonorrhea
- M/C PID due to IUCD: Actinomyces
- M/C route of spread of PID: Ascending infection along with a the sperms (STD) except genital TB
- M/C PID in virgin females: Genital TB
- M/C PID in postmenopausal females = E. coli (Williams)

Risk Factors:

- Multiple sex partners
- Low socioeconomic status
- Young age of intercourse (10-19 years)
- Douching
- H/O instrumentation
- Sexual partner with urethritis or gonorrhea
- Not using mechanical or chemical contraceptive barrier.

Protective Factor

- Use of barrier contraceptive
- OCP
- Pregnancy
- Menopause

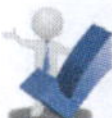

KEY POINTS

- As discussed earlier, squamous epithelium is resistant to Gonococcal & chlamydial infection and the M/C route of infection is ascending infection along with sperms.
- Hence, M/C site of asymptomatic carriage of Gonococcal infection in females: Endocervix (as it is lined by columnar epithelium) other sites are – Urethra, Bartholin's gland.
- Gonococcal vaginitis can never be seen in young females as their vagina is lined by squamous epithelium in all females except in newborns.
- Hence theoretically speaking gonococcal vaginitis can be seen in newborn females.
- The gonococcal/chlamydia from the Endocervix in young females ascends up & leads to PID.
- Then from fallopian tube, it spreads to peritoneum leading to abdominal tenderness. When it heals, **some fine Violin string adhesions** are formed (Fig. 7.8) between liver capsule and parietal peritoneum (Fig. 7.8).
- In women with PID and peritonitis, usually only lower abdomen is involved. However, inflammation of the liver capsule, may lead to right upper quadrant pain – condition called as **Fitz-High-Curtis syndrome** (sequelae of PID)
- Classically, symptoms of this perihepatitis include sharp, pleuritic upper quadrant pain that accompanies pelvic pain.

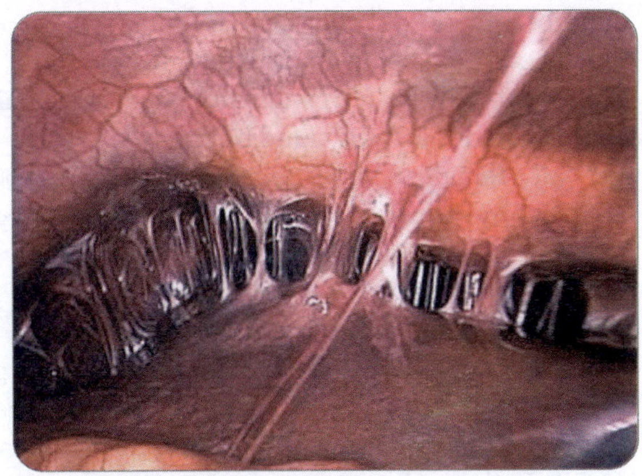

Fig. 7.8: Violin string adhesion seen in PID

Syndromic Approach

These days focus has shifted on **syndromic approach** for diagnosis of PID. This involves treatment based on signs and symptoms rather than laboratory tests.

The current CDC recommendations are that empirical treatment of PID should be initiated in sexually active young females and other females at risk for STD if they **experience pelvic or lower abdomen pain,** if no other cause can be identified and if **one or more of the minimum criteria specified below are present on pelvic examination.**

CDC 2006 Criteria for the Diagnosis of PID

Minimum Criteria

- Lower abdominal tenderness or
- Adnexal tenderness
- Cervical motion tenderness.

Additional Criteria

- Oral temperature more than 38.3°C (101.6°F)
- Abnormal cervical or vaginal mucopurulent discharge
- Presence of abundant WBC on saline mount of vaginal secretions
- ESR >15 mm/hours
- Elevated C-reactive protein
- Laboratory documentation of cervical infection with *Neisseria gonorrhoeae* or *Chlamydia trachomatis.*

Note: IOC in Gonorrhea = Nuclei and amplification test Gold standard = creatine in Thayer Nation media IOC for chlamydia - NAAT gold standard = creatine in McCoy cells.

Definitive Criteria

1. **Gold standard for diagnosis of PID is Laparoscopy.**

Findings on laparoscopy consistent with PID:
- i. Dilated hyperemic tube
- ii. Pyosalpinx
- iii. Tubo ovarian mass

Laparoscopy offers following advantages:

i. Biopsy can be taken from fallopian tube

ii. Prognostic scoring for conception, i.e. **Boer Maisel score** can be done at the same time.

But all females in whom PID is suspected, laparoscopy should not be done. Also by laparoscopy endometritis cannot be diagnosed.

2. **Endometrial Biopsy:**

   It is done to detect Endometritis:

   - **Acute Endometritis is** diagnosed by polymorpho nuclear leukocytes on the Endometrial surface. Chronic Endometritis is diagnosed by plasma cells in the endometrium.

3. **Sonography:**

   - Normal fallopian tubes are usually not visible on ultrasound
   - However with acute tubal inflammation, the tube swells, its lumen occludes distally, it distends & its walls and endosalpingeal folds thicken.

Findings on USG in Tubal Inflammation

1. Distended ovoid-shaped tube filled with anechoic on echogenic fluid.
2. Fallopian tube wall thickening
3. Incomplete internal septa.

Signs on USG in Tubal inflammation

1. **Bead on string appearance/cog wheel appearance** when inflamed tubes are imaged in cross section cogwheel appearance is seen due to endosalpingeal fold (Figs. 7.9A and B)
2. **Waist sign:** On longitudinal reaction, diametrically opposite indentations seen (Fig. 7.10)

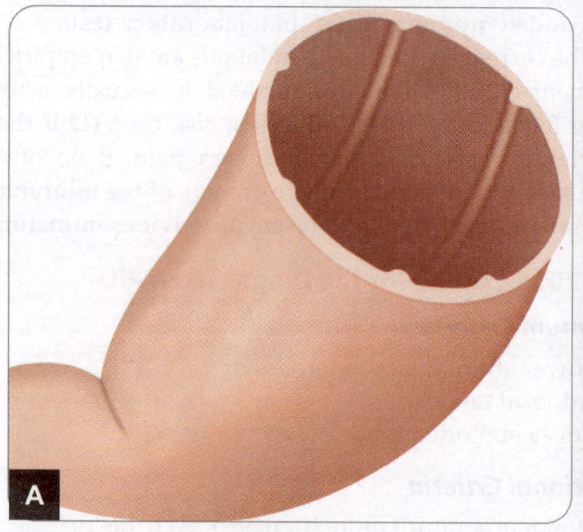

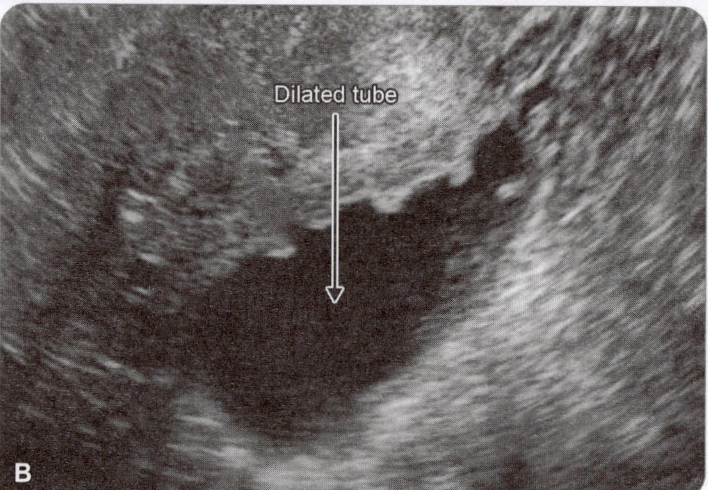

Figs. 7.9A and B: Cogwheal sign of PID

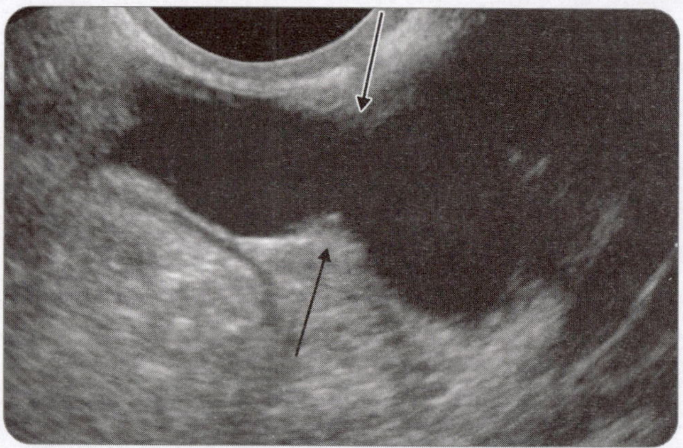

Fig. 7.10: Waist sign of PID

CDC Guidelines 2015 for treatment of PID

Dutta Gynae 6th/ed, p128

Principles for Managing PID

- The management of PID is antibiotics to cover Gonorrhea infection, Chlamydia infection and for anaerobic infection
- The management of PID is started based on symptoms without waiting for test reports.
- The sooner the treatment is initiated, lesser are the chances of sequale.
- In most cases PID is treated on OPD basis with oral antibiotics. If patient does not respond to oral antibiotics within 72 hours then parenteral antibiotics are given:

Indications for Hospitalisation in PID are:

1. Pregnancy
2. **Drug addicts/Adolescent**
3. Surgical emergency cannot be ruled out like appendicitis

4. Tubo ovarian abscess.
5. Failed oral treatment (No Response to oral antibiotics in 72 hours)
6. Patient not able to take oral drugs due to Nausea/Vomiting/high fever (> 38.3 °C).
7. WBC count > 15,000/nm^3
8. Poor compliance of patient

- Patient should have oral therapy for 14 days
- **Regimen A**
  - Ceftriaxone 250 mg IM single dose
    PLUS
  - Doxycycline 100 mg PO BID for 14 days with or without
    Metronidazole 500 mg PO BID
- **Regimen B:** Replace ceftriaxone with cefoxiler 2 gm 1/m with 1 g probenecid single dose
- Broad spectrum antibiotic coverage (cefotaxime/cefoxitin) is indicated as most PIDs are polymicrobial (Gram-negative and positive aerobes as well as anaerobic rods and cocci)

Inpatient Regimen/Parenteral Treatment

Regimen 1: CEFOTETAN 2g I/V every 12 hours. + Doxycycline 100 mg orally on I/V 12 hourly.
Regimen 2: Cefoxitin 2g I/V every 6 hours
+ Doxycycline 100 mg orally on I/V every 12 hours.
Regimen 3: Clindamycin 900 mg I/V every 8 hours. + Gentamicin Loading dose I/V or I/M – 2 mg 1 kg
Followed by maintenance dose 1.5 mg 1 kg every 8 hours

Note: The I/V Regimen should be continued for 24 hours after patient clinically improves and then shifted to oral forms of the drug.

Indications for surgery in PID:
Minimal invasive surgery is done by laparoscopic drainage of Tubo ovarian abscess or posterior colpotomy if:
- Size of abscess > 10 cm.
- Abscess ruptures
- Abscess fails to respond to antibiotic in 48-72 hrs

Remember

In Gonorrhea cervicitis:
- **Females C/O profuse, odorless, non-irritating & white-yellowish discharge or mucopurulent discharge.**
- Patients may have intermenstrual bleeding or post coital bleeding.
- **IOC: NAAT test**

Sample: For those with a cervix:-Vaginal swab specimen are as sensitive and specific as cervical swab specimen.
- For women without a cervix following hysterectomy first void urine samples are collected
- Gold standard = Culture

Single dose T/t of Gonococcal infection
Regimen A (Recommended) – Ceftriaxone 250 mg IM+ Azithromycin 1 g orally once
Regimen B (Alternative)–Cefixime 400 mg orally once Azithromycin 1g orally once.

Chlamydia: Mostly asymptomatic patient complaint of- **mucoid discharge** Due to urethritis, dysuria is prominent

IOC = NAAT or PCR
Gold standard = Culture

Treatment of Chlamydia
Recommended = Azithromycin 1g once *Or*
Doxycycline 100 mg twice daily for 7 day

Extra Edge

- **If PID occurs in females with Intrauterine device:** (Williams Gynae 3/ed, p69)
- Highest Risk of PID is during first 3 weeks after device insertion. After this time, there has to be some other reason.
- Theoretically, it is believed that on IUCD may worsen the infection or delay resolution
- Evidence supports leaving an IUCD during treatment in those with mild or moderate PID. Severe disease warrants removal or if patients symptoms fail to improve within 48 to 72 hours, then device is removed

Sequelae of PID

- Infertility – seen in 6–60% patients
- Ectopic pregnancy
- Chronic pelvic pain, dyspareunia
- **Fitz-Hugh-Curtis syndrome:** It is the development of perihepatic adhesions which lead to right upper quadrant pain. It is seen in PID due to chlamydia and gonorrhea.

Genital Tuberculosis

- Genital tuberculosis is almost always a secondary infection, with M/c primary sites being (in that order) Lungs > lymph nodes > abdomen
- Route of spread – Hematogenous (so it is the M/c PID in virgin females)
- **M/c site** for genital TB is Fallopian tubes (Bilateral involvement)
  - In Fallopian tubes – M/c affected part is Ampulla and M/c encountered pathology is endosalpingitis

Sites of Genital TB	% involvement
Tubes	90–100%
Uterus	50–60%
Ovaries	20–30%
Vagina and Vulva	1–2%

- **M/c age group:** 20–30 years (28 years specifically)
- **M/c symptom:** Infertility

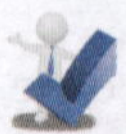

KEY POINTS

Infertility results from tubal as well as endometrial disease. The tubes may be patent on HSG but there is functional loss.

- If patient conceives spontaneously, ectopic pregnancy is the most likely outcome.
- **IInd M/c site of involvement: uterus**
- Cornu of the uterus is most commonly affected as it is in continuation with the fallopian tube and infection descends from the tubes. Thus B/L cornual block is seen.
- Uterine TB can manifest in the form of
  - Asherman's syndrome, i.e. destruction of the endometrial lining of uterine cavity with the formation of intrauterine synechiae or adhesions
  - Pyometra, i.e. pus-filled uterine cavity.

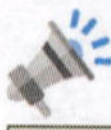

Important One Liners

- M/c cause of B/L cornual block on HSG is physiological spasm
- M/C pathological cause of B/L cornual block is Genital TB
- M/c cause of pyometra is senile endometritis
- M/c cancer causing pyometra is cancer cervix > cancer endometrium
- What % of TB patients are infertile – 70%
- What % of infertile patients have TB
- Worldwide: 10%
- India: 17%

Important Concept

Asherman syndrome

- M/c cause – dilatation and curettage done in post-partum period followed by D&C done for missed abortion
- Presentation:
  - **Hypomenorrhea** (Typical presentation)
  - Amenorrhea
  - Infertility
- IOC – Hysteroscopy as it is diagnostic and therapeutic.
- Hysterosalpingography shows honeycomb appearance
- Management – Hysteroscopic adhesiolysis followed by insertion of balloon catheter to prevent adhesion formation and a combination of estrogen & progesterone given to rebuild endometrium.

- **Menstrual problems occurring in TB patients:**

M/C menstrual complain: Oligomenorrhea/ Amenorrhea
1st menstrual complain: Menorrhagia (due to Endometritis in acute phase)
Pelvic examination: M/C finding = Normal pelvic examination
2nd M/C finding: Tenderness
M/C finding in genital TB in adolescent girls: B/L Adnexal mass

Hysterosalpingography in TB

HSG is contraindicated in patients of genital TB as it can lead to reactivation or spreading of disease. But, if unknowingly HSG is done in patients of TB, some typical characteristic findings seen are:

- **Lead pipe appearance of tube** (Fig. 7.11)
- **Beaded appearance of tube**
- Hydrosalpinx (*See* Fig. 7.13)
- B/L Cornual block
- **Golf club stick like appearance of tube**
- **Tobacco pouch like appearance of the fimbrial end of tube** (Fig. 7.12)
- Uterus – honeycomb appearance due to Asherman syndrome

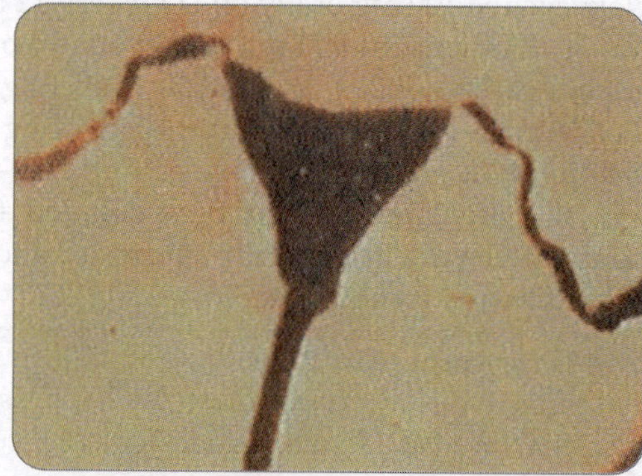

Fig. 7.11: HSG showing rigid pipe line tubes of genital tuberculosis

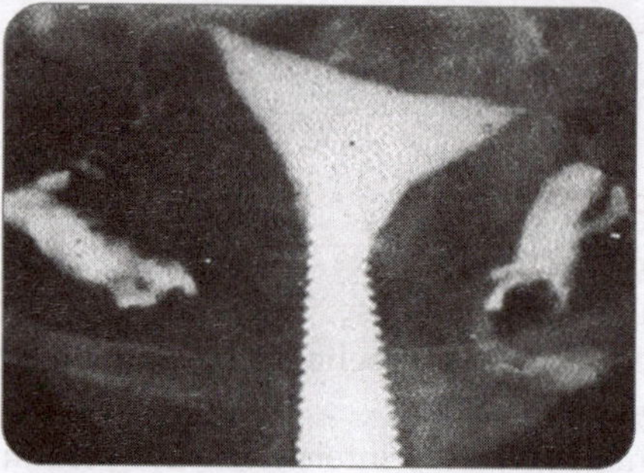

Fig. 7.12: HSG showing bilateral tobacco pouch appearance of genital tuberculosis

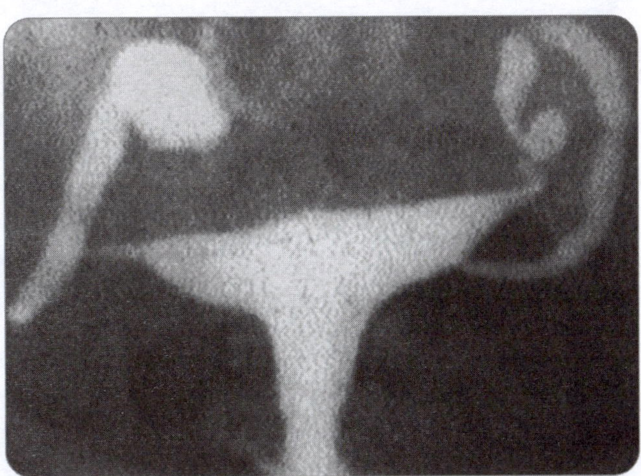

Fig. 7.13: HSG showing bilateral hydrosalpinx in Genital TB patient

Diagnosis

- **Endometrial biopsy:** Best time to do biopsy is 1–2 days before or 12 hours after onset of menses. In unmarried girls - menstrual blood can be collected within 12 hours of onset of menstruation for endometrial biopsy.
- PCR done on endometrium or menstrual blood is more sensitive than microscopy and bacteriological culture.
- Menstrual blood/curettings should be divided into 3 portions

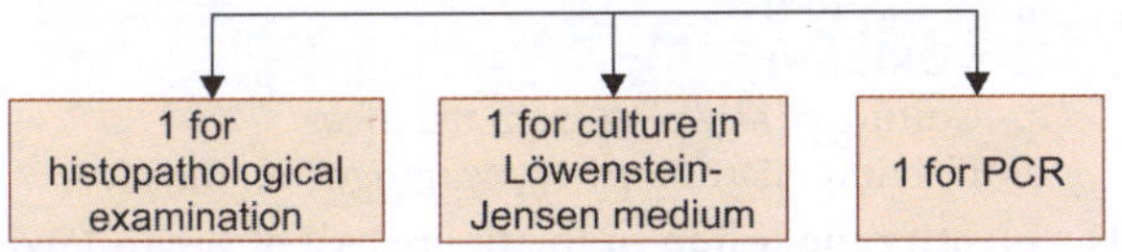

Treatment

- Genital tuberculosis falls in category 1. The treatment is for 6 months
- 4-drug AKT (isoniazid, ethambutol, pyrazinamide, and rifampicin) is given for 2 months, and 2 drugs (INH and rifampicin) are given for remaining 4 months. If a female conceives on ATT, continue ATT & continue her pregnancy.
- Surgery for restoration of fertility (corrective tuboplasty) is contraindicated in genital TB
- If a female conceives on ATT, continue ATT & continue here pregnancy
- IVF after completion of AKT is the treatment for infertility.

Note: The text of this chapter has been referenced and updated from CDC guidelines 2015.

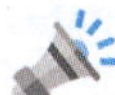

Important Common

- M/c cause of genital ulcers – Herpes
- M/c vaginitis in pregnant women – Candidiasis
- M/c vaginitis in young females – Trichomonas vaginitis
- M/c organism causing candidiasis – Candida albicans
- M/c cause of acute cervicitis and acute salpingitis – Gonorrhea
- M/c site for asymptomatic Gonorrhea in young females – Endocervix
- M/c cause of PID in virgin females – Tuberculosis
- Strawberry vagina seen in Trichomonas vaginitis
- Curdy white discharge/cottage cheese like discharge – Candidiasis
- Whiff test positive/clue cells/Amsel's criteria – Bacterial vaginosis
- Genital warts are caused by HPV 6 and 11 (Condyloma acuminata)
- Chancroid caused by Haemophilus ducreyi
- IOC for PID – Laparoscopy
- IOC for Chlamydia – NAAT > Polymerase chain reaction.

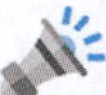

Important Percentages

- 50% of patients of gonorrhea are asymptomatic.
- 80% of patients of *Chlamydia* are asymptomatic.
- After treatment of Genital TB of the patients who conceive 50% have tubal pregnancy, 20–30% abort and 2% have live birth.

NEW PATTERN QUESTIONS

N1. The following are the primary sites of acute gonococcal infection *except*:
a. Urethra
b. Bartholin's gland
c. Skene's gland (paraurethral glands)
d. Exocervix

N2. M/C gynaecological problem in prepubertal females is:
a. Congenital prolapse b. Endometriosis
c. Vulvo vaginitis d. Polyp

N3. A 37-year-old female, on oral contraceptives presents with whitish vaginal discharge. She does not have soreness or itching. The discharge causes yellowish stains in her underwear. pH of discharge is acidic. Microscopy shows normal number of lactobacilli. Most appropriate diagnosis is:
a. Bacterial vaginosis
b. Leucorrhea
c. Chlamydial infection
d. Vaginal candidiasis

N4. Regarding bacterial vaginosis, all are true *except*:
a. Homogeneous vaginal discharge with pH 5.0 to 6.0
b. Positive KOH – With fishy odour
c. Positive clue cells in 100% of cases
d. It is due to Gardnerella vaginalis

N5. Criteria for diagnosis of gardenella vaginosis includes all *except*:
a. pH < 4-5
b. White discharge
c. Fishy odour when 10% KOH is added
d. Presence of clue cells

N6. A woman complains of an offensive fishy smelling yellowish discharge without pruritus. pH of discharge is > 4.5. Gram stained vaginal smear shows a reduced number of lactobacilli with large number of Gardnerella vaginalis. What is the best treatment option for this patient?
a. Clindamycine 300 mg twice daily × 7 days
b. Metronidazole 500 mg twice daily × 7 days
c. Metronidazole 2 gm as a single dose
d. Metronidazole vaginal gel once a day × 7 days

N7. Identify the infection shown in following Pap smear:

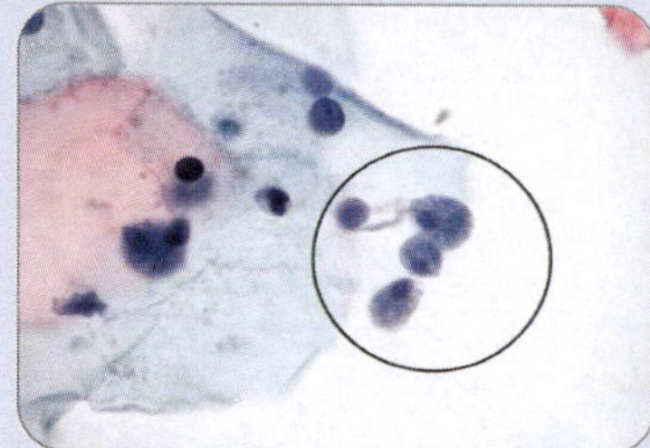

a. Cervical dysplasia
b. *Trichomonas vaginalis*
c. Bacterial vaginosis
d. Candidal infection

N8. A woman complains of clear, mucoid, non-offensive vaginal discharge without pruritis or soreness. The cervix appears inflamed on speculum examination and an endocervical swab is taken. What is the most appropriate test to confirm the diagnosis?
a. Perform ELISA test
b. Perform a culture
c. Perform a DNA amplification (PCR) test
d. Perform a direct fluorescent antibody test

N9. Ulceration of the vulva is commonly seen in all *except*:
a. Bacterial vaginosis
b. Syphilis
c. Chancroid
d. Behçet's disease

N10. A 30-year-old multiparous female complains of a painless ulcer in vulva. She has several sexual partners. Her previous pregnancy has ended in a still birth at 24 weeks. What is the first test, which should be performed in this case:
a. ELISA for HIV
b. VDRL Test
c. Culture of scraping from the ulcer
d. Election microscopy of scraping from the ulcer

N11. Identify the lesion in the figure. All of the following drugs can be used in this condition *except*:
a. Imiquimod b. Podophyllin
c. Methotrexate d. Trichlorocacetic acid

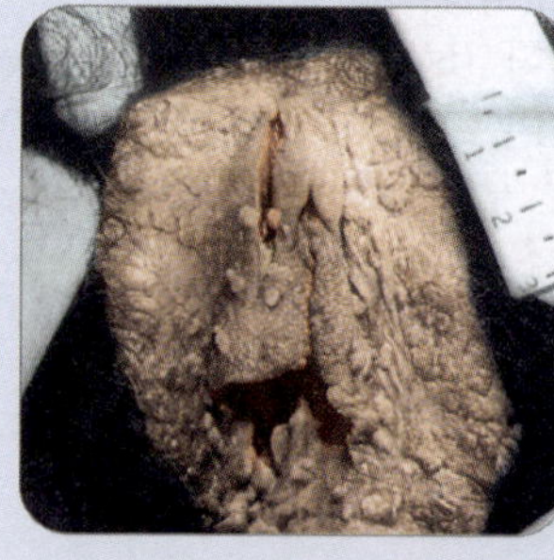

N12. A 32-year-old female complains of multiple small painful ulcers of the vulva of 2 days duration. She had a previous episode which healed spontaneously. What is the most likely diagnosis?
a. Chancroid
b. Genital herpes
c. Granuloma inguinale
d. Lymphogranuloma venereum
e. Primary syphilis

N13. In QN12 what is the best test to diagnose the infection?

a. Culture of scrapings from the ulcer
b. Electron microscopy of scraping from the ulcer
c. ELISA test
d. PCR of scrapings from the ulcer

N14. The risk factors of acute pelvic inflammatory disease (PID) are the following *except*:

a. Menstruating teenagers who have multiple sex partners
b. IUD users
c. Women with monogamous partner who had vasectomy
d. Previous history of acute PID

N15. A 30-year-old female complains of lower abdominal pain and purulent vaginal discharge.

Her pulse rate = 98/min
Temp = 101°F
WBC count and ESR are raised
P/V examination reveals lower abdominal tenderness and cervical motion tenderness. What is the best treatment option for her?

a. Single IM injection of ceftriaxone with oral doxycycline and oral metronidazole for 14 days
b. Single dose of cetotriaxone injectin with oral azithromycin for 14 days
c Oral metronidazole for 14 days
d. Oral ofloxacin and oral metronidazole for 14 days

N16. M/c organism causing PID in postmenopausal females:

a. *Chlamydia*
b. *E. coli*
c. *Klebsiella*
d. *Staphylococcus*

N17. M/c cause of B/L cornual block seen on HSG:

a. TB
b. Endometriosis
c. Physiological spasm
d. PID

N18. Which of the following is true with regards to genital tuberculosis?

a. Ovarian involvement can occur without tubal affection
b. Infertility is mainly due to anovulation
c. Acid fast bacilli is identified in 100% cases of tubercular endometritis
d. A negative Mantoux test reasonably excludes tuberculosis

N19. The following statements are related to tubercular salpingitis *except*:

a. The abdominal ostium may be patent with eversion of fimbriae
b. The early lesion may be confused with adenocarcinoma on histology
c. Genital tuberculosis is always secondary and the tubes are invariably the primary sites
d. Salpingitis isthmica nodosa is the exclusive pathology to tuberculosis

N20. True statement about female genital tuberculosis:

a. Genital tract involvement results from lymphatic spread
b. Premenstrual histopathological examination is diagnostic
c. Polymerase chain reaction (PCR) techniques have got higher sensitivity in detection
d. Reproductive outcome following antituberculous chemotherapy is satisfactory

N21. HSG findings in tubercular salpingitis are all *except*:

a. Tobacco pouch appearance
b. Powder burn appearance
c. Lead pipe appearance
d. Golf stick appearance

N22. Extensive endometrial TB presents with:

a. Menorrhagia
b. Amenorrhea
c. Polymenorrhea
d. Metrorrhagia

N23. Figure shows phthirus pubis. The pathogen was seen in pubic hair of a pregnant female complaining of genital itching.

DOC for pubic lice in pregnant females is:

a. Premetharin cream 1%
b. Malathion 0.5%
c. Overnectin
d. Petroleum jelly

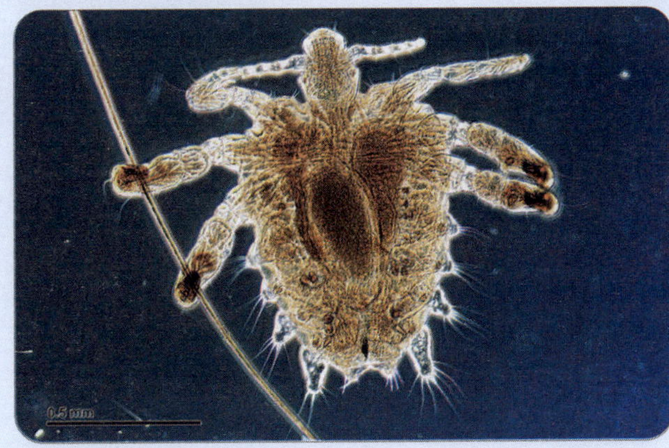

N24. M/C cause of PID is:

a. Chlamydia
b. Gonorrhea
c. TB
d. Salmonella

N25. All of the following screening test are recommended by CDC in pregnant female *except*:

a. ELISA for HIV
b. HBs Ag
c. NAAT for chlamydia and gonorrhea
d. Saline microscopy for bacterial vaginosis

N26. A 35 year old female complains of clear mucoid non offensive vaginal discharge without pruritus. She is infected due to tubal damage. The cervix appears inflamed on per speculum examination. What is the most likely cause?

a. Bacterial vaginosis
b. Chlamydia
c. Gonorrhea
d. Trichomonas

N27. A P3 woman complains of an offensive fishy smelling yellowish discharge without pruritus. Her previous pregnancy ended in preterm delivery. Best way to confirm the diagnosis is:
a. Culture of discharge
b. Microscopic examination of wet mount
c. Test vaginal pH
d. Do a NAAT

N28. M/c cause of vaginal discharge among reproductive age females
a. Trichomonas b. Candida
c. Bacterial vaginosis d. Gonorrhea

N29. All of the following are risk factors for bacterial vagnosis *except:*
a. Oral sex
b. Cigarette smoking
c. Sex during ....
d. Use of condoms during sex

N30. Following is STD *except*:
a. Trichomonas
b. Bacterial vaginosis
c. Gonorrhea
d. Candida infection

N31. Most sensitive diagnostic technique for Trichomonas infection
a. Culture in Diamond media
b. Culture in Thayer Martin media
c. Pap Smear
d. NAAT

N32. Whiff test is positive in:
a. Candidians b. Chlamydial infection
c. Trichomonas vaginitis
d. HSV infection

N33. Foul smelling fishy odour is seen on:
a. Trichomonas b. Gardnerella
c. Chlamydia d. Candidiasis

N34. All of the following are related to Bacterial vaginosis *except*:
a. Amsels criteria
b. Nugent score
c. Strawberry vagina
d. Whiff test

N35. All are correctly matched *except*
a. Trichomonas: Greenish discharge
b. Bacterial vaginosis: Foul smelling dirty white discharge
c. Chlamydia: Cottage cheese like discharge
d. Gonorrhea – Yellowish white discharge

N36. A 30-year-old female complains of pain in lower abdomen and vaginal discharge. O/E:- cervical movements are tender. Gram smear of discharge shows abundant pus cells but no bacteria. The best possible approach in this case is:
a. Culture on Diamond media
b. Culture on Thayer martin medium
c. Culture on MCoy cells
d. Culture on LJ media.

N37. All are true regarding treatment of PID *except*:
a. Prompt treatment is the key to successful patient outcome
b. If patient doesn't respond to oral therapy within 72 hours, parenteral therapy is initiated
c. Remove any IUCD in the patient, as soon as PID is diagnosed
d. Remove IUCD if patient fails to improve within 48 to 72 hours.

PREVIOUS YEAR QUESTIONS

1. **Which of the following is not sexually transmitted?** *(AIIMS June)*
   a. Echinococcus
   b. Candida
   c. Molluscum contagiosum
   d. Group B. Streptococcus
2. **A patient with discharge per vagina was evaluated and on endocervical biopsy Chlamydia was found. Treatment to be given in this case is:** *(AIIMS June)*
   a. Azithromycin and contact tracing
   b. Metronidazole only
   c. Doxycycline and metronidazole
   d. Azithromycin
3. **Strawberry vagina is seen in:** *(AIIMS June 98)*
   a. Candida albicans
   b. H. vaginalis
   c. Syphilis
   d. Trichomonas vaginalis
4. **All are risk factors for vaginal candidiasis *except*:** *(AIIMS Nov 10)*
   a. HIV
   b. Hypertension
   c. Pregnancy
   d. Diabetes mellitus
5. **Clue cells are seen in:** *(AIIMS May 08)*
   a. Bacterial vaginosis
   b. Candidasis
   c. Trichomoniasis
   d. Gonorrhoea
6. **A 40-year-old woman presented to the gynecologist with complaints of profuse vaginal discharge. There was no discharge from the cervix on the speculum examination. The diagnosis of bacterial vaginosis was made based upon all of the following findings on microscopy *except*:** *(AIIMS 06)*
   a. Abundance of gram variable coccobacilli
   b. Absence of lactobacilli
   c. Abundance of polymorphs
   d. Present of clue cells
7. **In hysterosalpingography, fallopian tubes are seen beaded in appearance with clubbing of fimbrial end and ampulla. Most likely cause is:** *(AIIMS June)*
   a. Tuberculosis
   b. Candidiasis
   c. Chlamydia
   d. Gonococcus
8. **What is the most likely cause for beaded appearance of fallopian tubes with clubbed ends of fimbriae on HSG?** *(AIIMS Nov 2015)*
   a. Genital tuberculosis
   b. Chlamydia
   c. Nisseria gonorrhoea
   d. Endometriosis
9. **A lady approaches a physician for contraceptive advice. On examination, there were two symmetrical ulcers on vulva, which were well-defined with firm base. Which of the following is the most likely cause?** *(AIIMS Nov)*
   a. Chancre b. Herpes
   c. Syphilis d. Malignancy
10. **A 25-year-old female with history of multiple contacts presenting with growth on vulva, the probable diagnosis is:** *(AIIMS June 98)*
    a. Condyloma accuminata
    b. Verruca plana
    c. Verruca vulgaris
    d. Condyloma lata
11. **A young lady presents to your office with complain of copious vaginal discharge, but there is no cervical discharge on per speculum examination. Which of the following should be given for the management?** *(AIIMS Nov 2012)*
    a. Metronidazole and fluconazole
    b. Metronidazole and azithromycin
    c. Metronidazole and doxycycline
    d. Fluconazole only
12. **Cervicitis is caused by:** *(PGI June 03)*
    a. Pseudomonus
    b. Staphylococcus
    c. Chlamydia
    d. Trichomonas
    e. N. gonorrhoea
13. **Minimum criteria to diagnose PID include(s):** *(PGI May 2013)*
    a. Lower abdominal tenderness
    b. Fever
    c. Cervical motion tenderness
    d. Adnexal tenderness
    e. Leucocytosis
14. **Acute PID is treated by:** *(PGI June 03)*
    a. IV antibiotics (broad spectrum)
    b. Drainage of TO mass
    c. Abdominal hysterectomy
    d. Laparoscopic exploration
15. **Nongonococcal urethritis is caused by:** *(PGI Dec 99)*
    a. Chlamydia
    b. LGV
    c. Syphilis
    d. Gardnerella vaginalis
16. **Which of the following statements about clinical features in a female suffering from Gonorrhoea is correct?**
    a. 50% patients are asymptomatic
    b. Excessive vaginal discharge is seen
    c. Vaginal discharge is purulent
    d. Features of perihepatitis present
    e. All of the above statements are correct

17. True about Trichomonas vaginalis: *(PGI June 05)*
a. Flagellated parasite
b. Fungal infection
c. Curdy white discharge
d. Pruritus
e. Sexually transmitted disease

18. Trichomonas—which of the following true is?
a. Foul smelling vaginal discharge *(PGI June 08)*
b. Vaginal pH is 4
c. Strawberry vagina
d. Infertility
e. Abortion

19. True about bacterial vaginosis: *(PGI June 05)*
a. Itching
b. Gray discharge
c. Clue cells found
d. Fishy odor discharge
e. Caused by *Gardnerella vaginalis*

20. True about bacterial vaginosis: *(PGI Dec 04)*
a. Intense pruritis
b. Gray and white discharge
c. Associated with vaginal pH >4.5
d. Commonly associated with intensive mucosal inflammation
e. Oral metronidazole is the drug of choice

21. Not true about bacterial vaginosis: *(PGI Nov 2012)*
a. Clue cells present
b. With KOH gives amine smell
c. pH <4.5
d. Yellow green discharge
e. Whiff test positive

22. In a patient with pelvic inflammatory disease due to tuberculosis, which of the following statements is true? *(PGI Dec 01)*
a. Mycobacterium can be grown from menstrual blood
b. Associated with infertility
c. Ectopic pregnancy is common
d. Dysmenorrhea is a common presentation

23. All are clinical features of PID *except*:
a. Temp > 38°C
b. WBC count of 15,000
c. ESR – 10 mm/hour
d. Tenderness on movement of cervix

24. During laparoscopy, the preferred site for obtaining cultures in a patient with acute PID is:
a. Endocervix
b. Endometrium
c. Pouch of Douglas
d. Fallopian tubes

25. Asymptomatic carriage of gonococcal infection in female is commonly seen in: *(AI 97)*
a. Endocervix b. Vagina
c. Urethra d. Fornix

26. Gonococcal vaginitis occurs in: *(TN 2007)*
a. Adults b. Children
c. Infants d. Adolescents

27. Which of the following cannot be detected by wet film? *(Delhi 08)*
a. Candida
b. Trichomonas
c. Chlamydia
d. Bacterial vaginosis

28. The most sensitive method for detecting cervical chlamydia trachomatis infection is: *(AI 04)*
a. Direct fluorescent antibody test
b. Enzyme immunoassay
c. Polymerase chain reaction
d. Culture on irradiated McConkey cells

29. A 45-year-old female complains of lower abdominal pain and vaginal discharge. On examination, there is cervicitis along with a mucopurulent cervical discharge. The Gram smear of the discharge shows presence of abundant pus cells, but no bacteria. The best approach to isolate the possible causative agent would be:
a. Culture on chocholate agar supplemented with hemin *(AI 05)*
b. Culture on McCoy cells
c. Culture on a bilayer human blood agar
d. Culture on Vero cell lines

30. Drug of choice for Chlamydia in pregnancy: *(AI 10)*
a. Doxycycline
b. Tetracycline
c. Erythromycin
d. Penicillin

31. A woman presents with a thick curdy-white vaginal discharge. The best treatment for her is: *(AI 00)*
a. Miconazole b. Metronidazole
c. Nystatin d. Doxycycline

32. Creamy fishy odor is caused by: *(AI 09)*
a. Trichomonas b. Gardnerella
c. Candida d. Chlamydia

33. A lady presented with creamy white vaginal discharge with fishy odor, drug of choice is: *(AIIMS May 09)*
a. Doxycycline b. Ofloxacine
c. Metronidazole d. Clindamycin

34. Most common site for genital tuberculosis is: *(AI 98)*
a. Ovary b. Uterus
c. Cervix d. Fallopian tube

35. Most common route of transmission of endometrial tuberculosis is: *(AIIMS June 98)*
a. Direct local spread b. Lymphatic spread
c. Retrograde spread d. Hematogenous

36. Salpingitis/Endosalpingitis is best confirmed by:
a. Hysteroscopy and laparoscopy *(AI 08)*
b. X-ray
c. Hysterosalpingography
d. Sonosalpingography

37. A 19-year-old girl with painless ulcer in labia majora with everted margins: *(AIIMS May 2013)*
a. Treponema pallidum
b. Chlamydia
c. Gonorrhoea
d. Herpes genital ulcer disease

38. True about Trichomonas vaginitis: *(PGI Nov 2014)*
a. Important cause of recurrent abortion
b. T. vaginalis is a flagellated protozoa
c. Metronidazole is used for treatment
d. Strawberry cervix
e. Curdy discharge

39. A milky white discharge with fishy odour with minimal itching is due to: *(JIPMER May 2017)*
a. Bacterial vaginosis b. Gonorrhea
c. Trichomonas d. Candida

40. True about bacterial vaginosis: *(JIPMER May 2016)*
a. pH > 6 and whitish discharge
b. pH > 4.5 and fishy odour on KOH mount
c. Caused by Trichomonas vaginalis
d. Predominance of lacto bacilli

41. A pregnant lady with gonorrhoea with white discharge TOC is:
a. Ceftriaxone single dose 1/m + metronidazole for 14 days
b. Ceftriaxone plus azithromycin single dose
c. Ceftriaxone plus doxy cycline 100 mg for 7 days + Metronidazole for 14 days.
d. Ceftriaxone single dose 1/m

42. Risk factor for acute PID includes: *(PGI May 2012)*
a. Advanced age
b. OCP use
c. IUCD use
d. Previous H/O PID
e. Increase number of sexual partners

43. Which of the following can be diagnosed on vaginal wet mount smear: *(PGI NOV 2008)*
a. Trichomonas vaginalis
b. Candida albicans
c. Herpes simplex
d. N. Gonorrhea
e. Atrophic vaginitis

44. True statement about bacterial vaginosis:
a. Metronidazole is the DOC
b. Dose of metrozole is 500 mg twice a day for 7 days
c. Intravaginal clindamycin is used
d. Male partner is also treated in all cases
e. Clotrimazole 2% clean is used intravaginally.

45. DOC for pregnant women with chlamydia Trachomatis infection: *(JIPMER Nov 2014)*
a. Clindamycin
b. Metronidazole
c. Amoxicillin
d. Cephazolin

46. A 16-year-old girl presented with pruritis & vaginal discharge. She has been previously treated for UT9 what is the diagnosis: *(JIPMER Nov 2014)*
a. Chlamydia
b. Candida
c. Trichomonas
d. Gardnerella vaginalis

47. Whiff test is used in the diagnosis of: *(JIPMER May 2014)*
a. Trichomonas
b. Bacterial vaginosis
c. Candida
d. PID

48. A female presents with 3 cms painless ulcer with raised edges on Labia majora M/c cause is: *(JIPMER May 2017)*
a. Syphilis
b. Gonorrhea
c. Herpes
d. Chlamydia

49. True about Trichomonas vaginitis: *(PGI Nov 2014)*
a. Important cause of recurrent abortion
b. T vaginalis is a flagellated protozoa
c. Metronidazole is used for treatment
d. Strawberry cervix
e. Curdy discharge

ANSWERS TO NEW PATTERN QUESTIONS

N1. Ans. is d, i.e. Exocervix *Ref: Dutta Gynae 6th/ed, p147*

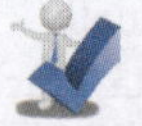

KEY POINTS

Ectocervix or exocervix is covered by squamous epithelium and squamous epithelium is resistant to Gonococcal infection

Primary genital sites of involvement of gonorrhea

- Endocervix
- Urethra
- Skene's gland
- Bartholin's gland

N2. Ans. is c, i.e. Vulvo vaginitis

N3. Ans. is b, i.e. Leucorrhea

The patient is having leucorrhea because she has white vaginal discharge without pruritus or soreness and normal number of lactobacilli are present. Chlamydia will cause a similar discharge, but the number of lactobacilli will be reduced, as it is an infection.

N4. Ans. is c, i.e. Positive clue cells in 100% cases *Ref: Dutta Gynae 6th/ed, p152*

We have discussed bacterial vaginosis in detail.

Clue cells are diagnostic but about 40% patients may not have clue cells.

N5. Ans. is a, i.e. pH < 4.5

The clinical criteria for bacterial vaginosis is **Amsel's criteria in** which out of the following 4 any 3 criteria should be positive:

a. Homogenous thin, grey discharge that thinly coats the vaginal walls
b. Clue cells (i.e. vaginal epithelial cells to which bacteria are adhered) should be present ≥ 20%
c. pH of vaginal fluid ≥ 4.5 (usually 4.7 to 5.7)
d. A fishy odour of discharge after adding 10% KOH (called as **Whiff test positive**)

N6. Ans. is b, i.e. Metronidazole 500 mg twice daily × 7 days

This patient has bacterial vaginosis based on following findings:

- Offensive fishy smelling vaginal discharge
- No pruritis
- pH > 4.5
- Reduced number of lactobacilli
- Increased number of Gardnerella

Mgt = Non pregnant females = 500 mg metronidazole twice daily × 7 days.

Pregnancy–250 mg twice a day × 7 days.

N7. Ans. is c, i.e. Trichomonas vaginalis

The papsmear shows motile flagellated trichomonas.

N8. Ans. is c, i.e. perform a DNA amplification (PCR) test

This patient is presenting with clear mucoid offensive discharge without pruritus or soreness, there is cervicitis. This points towards chlamydia as the diagnosis as in Gonorrhea the discharge is purulent.

IOC for chlamydia = PCR of endocervical swab.

N9. Ans. is a, i.e. Bacterial vaginosis *Ref: Dutta Gynae 6th/ed, p262*

Vulval ulcers

Vulval ulcers are predominantly due to sexually transmitted diseases. Rarely, it may be due to non-specific causes. Malignant ulcer is also rare. The various etiological factors related to vulval ulcers are given in the below Table.

Ulcers of the Vulva

STD related	Idiopathic	Tuberculosis	Malignancy	Systemic disease related or dermatoses
• Syphilis • Herpes genitalis • Chancroid • Granuloma inguinale • Lymphogranuloma venereum	• Behçet's disease • Aphthous ulcers • Lipschutz ulcers	Tubercular	**Primary** • Squamous cell carcinoma • Malignant melanoma • Basal cell carcinoma **Secondary** • Leukemia • Choriocarcinoma	• Lupus erythematosus • Crohn's disease • Lichen planus • Lichen sclerosus • Sjogren's syndrome

Note: **Lipschutz ulcer:** The lesion affects mainly the labia minora and introitus. In acute state, there may be constitutional upset with lymphadenopathy. The causative agent may be Epstein-Barr virus. Treatment is with antiseptic lotions and ointment.

N10. Ans is b, i.e. VDRL Test *Ref: Dutta Gynae 6th/ed, p262*

The female is presenting with a single painless ulcer, she has multiple sex partners and her pregnancy resulted in still birth at 24 weeks. All this points towards syphilis as the diagnosis.

The first test to be performed in this case is VDRL test (screening test).

Confirmatory test = specific treponemal test like Treponema haemaggluteration test or fluorescent treponemal antibody test.

Infection	Diagnosis
Chlamydia	NAAT or PCR
Gonorrhea	NAAT
Chancroid	Culture of scrapings from ulcer
Genital herpes	Electron microscopy of scrapings from ulcer
LGV	ELISA test

N11. Ans. is c, i.e. Methotrexate *Ref: Current diagnosis and treatment sexually transmitted diseases, p94, 95*

The condition shown in the figure is vulvar warts.

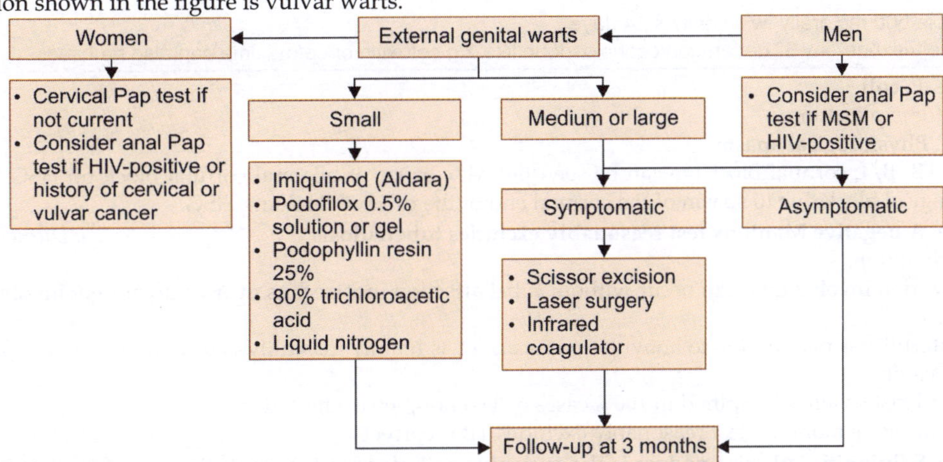

N12. Ans. is b, i.e. Genital herpes

The diagnosis is genital herpes as the patient has multiple small painful ulcers along with history of a previous episode in past. This is not a case of chancroid because in chancroid there is long history (here history is of 2 days) and it leads to enlarged lymph nodes although in chancroid also, multiple painless ulcers are seen.

In LGV, a small shallow ulcer with LN enlargement is present.

Syphilis leads to single painless ulcer. Granuloma inguinale leads to papules and ulcers with lymphedema.

N13. Ans is b, i.e. Electron microscopy of scrapings from the ulcer *Ref: Dutta Gynae 6th/ed, p128*

See N10 for explanation.

N14. Ans. is c, i.e. Women with monogamous partner who had vasectomy *Ref: Dutta Gynae 6th/ed, p128*

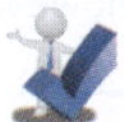

KEY POINTS

Women with monogamous partner who had vasectomy is a protective factor for PID and not risk factor

Risk factors of PID	Protective factors of PID
• Menstruating teenagers. • Multiple sexual partners. • Absence of contraceptive pill use. • Previous history of acute PID. • IUD users. • Area with high prevalence of sexually transmitted diseases	**Contraceptive practice** • Barrier methods, specially condom, diaphragm with spermicides • Oral steroidal contraceptives have got two preventive aspects. – Produce thick mucus plug preventing ascent of sperm and bacterial penetration – Decrease in duration of menstruation, creates a shorter interval of bacterial colonization of the upper tract. • Monogamy or having a partner who had vasectomy. **Others** • Pregnancy • Menopause • Vaccines: Hepatitis B, HPV

N15. Ans. is a, i.e. single IM injection of ceftriaxone with oral doxycycline and oral metronidazole for 14 days

This patient has PID. Any sexually active female who complains of lower abdominal pain and has at least 1 minimum criteria of PID–is taken as a case of PID.

Minimum criteria

1. Lower abdominal tenderness
2. Cervical movement tenderness
3. Adnexal tenderness

In this patient cervical motion tenderness is present so she is a case of PID.

As per 2015 CDC guidelines.

> **Best Treatment for OPD management of PID is:**
> Inj ceftriaxone 250 mg IM single dose
> +
> Doxycycline 100 mg orally twice daily × 14 days
> +/–
> Metronidazole 500 mg orally twice daily × 14 days
> Instead of ceftriaxone-any 3° generation cephalosporin like 2 g cefoxitin or cefotaxime can also be used.

N16. Ans. is b, i.e. E. coli

See the text for explanation.

N17. Ans. is c, i.e. Physiological spasm

On HSG in TB: B/L cornual blockage can be seen but M/c cause of bilateral cornual block on HSG is not genital TB. It is physiological block due to spasm of the cornual end of the tube while doing HSG.

N18. Ans. is d, i.e. A negative Mantoux test reasonably excludes tuberculosis *Ref: Dutta Gynae 6th/ed, p140*

Let's see each option.

Option a: Ovarian involvement can occur without tubal affection incorrect as ovaries do not get involved without tubes being affected

Option b: Infertility is mainly due to anovulation incorrect as mainly infertility is due to tubal blockage or adhesions in endometrial cavity

Option c: Acid fast basilli is identified in 100% cases of TB endometritis incorrect

Option d: A negative montoux test reasonably excludes TB is correct *Ref: Dutta Gynae 6th/ed, p140*

N19. Ans. is d, i.e. Salpingitis isthmica nodosa is the exclusive pathology to tuberculosis *Ref: Dutta Gynae 6th/ed, p138*

- In genital TB abdominal ostium may be patent with eversion of fimbrial end called as tobacco pouch appearance. Thus option 'a' is correct
- The early lesion may be confused with adenocarcinoma (i.e. option b is correct)
- Genital TB is always secondary and tubes are invariably the primary sites (i.e. c is correct)
- Salpingitis isthmica nodosa is the exclusive pathology of the TB incorrect (as it may be seen in endometriosis also)

In some cases of genital TB, nodules are present in the tuber first size in the isthmic part near the uterine cornu, it is called as salpingitis isthmic nodosa

> **Salpingitis isthmica nodosa** is the nodular thickening of the tube due to proliferation of tubal epithelium within the hypertrophied myosalpinx (muscle layer). Exact aetiology is unknown. It is diagnosed radiologically as a small diverticulum. It is however not specific to tubercular infection only. It is also observed in pelvic endometriosis.

N20. Ans. is c, i.e. PCR techniques have got higher sensitivity in detection *Ref: Dutta Gynae 6th/ed, p140*

Genital tuberculosis is usually secondary to primary infection (lungs, bones, lymph nodes).

It spreads by hematogenous route (not lymphatic route) leading to endosalpingitis.

Caseous granulomatous lesions with giant cells on pathological examination are suggestive of TB but is not diagnostic as it can be seen in fungal infection and sarcoidosis.

PCR is more sensitive (85–95%) than microscopy and bacteriological culture. This method can detect fewer than 10 organisms in clinical specimens compared to 10,000 necessary for smear positivity.

Reproductive outcome even after treatment is poor. Pregnancy rate is about 20%, live birth rate is only 7%. Risk of miscarriage and ectopic pregnancy are high.

N21. Ans. is b, i.e. Powder burn appearance

Powder burn appearance is seen in endometriosis and not genital TB.

N22. Ans is b, i.e. Amenorrhea

Extensive TB presents with amenorrhea due to Asherman syndrome.

N23. Ans. is a, i.e. Premetharin cream 1% *Ref: Current diagnosis and treatment sexually transmitted diseases, p227*

Pubic lice, a common condition is caused by the crab louse, Phthirus pubis.

The pubic louse is 0.8–1.2 mm in length and can be seen with the naked eye.

The louse primarily infests pubic hair but may attach to adjacent hair of the chest, abdomen, legs, and buttocks. Eyelashes may also become infested.

Phthirus pubis lives for approximately 2 weeks, during which females produce about 25 ova.

The nits incubate for 1 week, and the nymphs mature to adults over pruritus results from hypersensitivity to louse saliva, it may be 2 or more weeks before symptoms develop following initial infestation.

Bluish-gray macular lesions secondary to deep dermal hemosiderin deposition from the bites of the louse, known as maculae cerulean, may be noted in patients with established infestation.

Crab lice and nits may be seen with the naked eye; therefore, the presence of one or both of these forms in the hair is diagnostic.

Treatment

- Premetharin 1% cream rinse and pyrethrins with piperonyl butoxide are the primary agents recommended for the treatment of pubic lice and are the drugs of choice for pregnant or lactating women. These agents should be applied to the affected areas and washed off after 10 minutes.
- Malathion 0.5% lotion is in alternative when treatment failure is thought to be secondary to drug resistance. The agent should be applied to the affected area for 8–12 hours and rinsed off.
- Ivermectin (200 mcg/kg as a single dose, repeated in 2 weeks), provides an oral alternative for therapy.

Note: Pubic lice are primarily spread through sexual contact. Therefore, all partners with whom the patient has had sexual contact within the previous 30 days should be evaluated and treated, and sexual contact should be avoided until all partners have successfully completed treatment and are thought to be cured.

N24. Ans. is a, i.e. Chlamydia

M/c cause of PID–Chlamydia > Gonorrhea

M/c cause of PID in virgin females–Genital TB

N25. Ans. is d, i.e. Saline microscopy for bacterial vaginosis

Tests recommended by CDC–to be done at 1st antenatal visit for STD.
- ELISA for HIV
- HBs Ag for hepatitis B
- VDRL test for syphilis
- NAAT for chlamydia and gonorrhea (in pregnant females <25 years and older women).
- HCV antibodies testing for hepatitis C virus (most important basic factor being past or current drug use)
- Pap test.

No routine screening done for:
- Bacterial vaginosis (even in those females who are at high risk for preterm labor)
- Trichomonas vaginalis
- HSV-2.

N26. Ans. is b, i.e. chlamydia

In the question patient is complaining of vaginal discharge without pruritus. The cervix is also inflamed, i.e. cervicitis is also present and she has a tubal cause of infertility, which means the organism is leading to PID (i.e rules out Trichomonas and Bacterial Vaginosis).

Now we have 2 options - Gonorrhea and chlamydia.

In Gonorrhea, the discharge is purulent. Clear mucoid nonoffensive discharge means it is chlamydia.

N27. Ans. is b, i.e. Microscopic examination of a wet mount of vaginal discharge.

The patient is having Bacterial vaginosis as she presents with offensive, fishy smelling yellowish discharge, without pruritus. Her previous pregnancy had ended in a preterm delivery.

The IOC in Bacterial vaginosis is microscopic examination of the discharge mixed with saline. Clue cells will be visible.

N28. Ans. is c, i.e. Bacterial vaginosis *Ref: William Gynae 3rd/ed, p51*

"Bacterial vaginosis is the most common cause of vaginal discharge among reproductive age women."

Ref: Williams Gynae 3rd/ed, p51.

N29. Ans. is d, i.e. Use of condoms during sex *Ref: Williams Gynae 3rd/ed, p51*

Risk factors For Bacterial vaginosis
- Oral sex
- Douching
- Black race
- Cigarette smoking
- Sex during menses
- Intrauterine device
- Early age of sexual intercourse
- New or multiple sex partners
- Sexual activity with other women

N30. Ans. is b,, i.e. Bacterial vaginosis

Trichomonas:

"This protozoan infection is the most prevalent non viral STD in united states. Unlike other STD's its incidence appears to increase with patients age" *Ref: Williams Gynae 3rd/ed, p63*

- Undoubtedly Gonorrhea & chlamydia are STDs
- **Now for candida**

"It can be sexually transmitted and several studies have reported an association between candidians and arogenital sex." *Ref: Williams Gynae 3rd/ed, p51*

- **Bacterial vaginosis:**

"This condition is not considered by CDC to be sexually transmitted disease CSTD." *Ref: Williams Gynae 3rd/ed pg 51*

N31. Ans. is a, i.e. Culture in Diamond media: *Ref: Williams Gynae 3rd/ed, p63*

"The most sensitive diagnostic techniques is culture which is impractical because special media (Diamond media) is required."

N32. Ans. is c, i.e. Trichomonas infection *Ref: Williams Gynae 3rd/ed, p52*

- Whiff Test:

Vaginal discharge + 10% KOH gives a Fishy odour.

This test is characteristic of BV with vaginal pH > 4.5 and this stems from diminished acid production by bacteria. Similarly Trichomonas vaginals infection is also associated with anaerobic overgrowth & resultant elaborated lamines. Thus women diagnosed with bacterial vaginosis should have no microscopic evidence of trichomoniasis

N33. Ans. is b, i.e. Gardenerella:

Gardnerella is one of the organism responsible for bacterial vaginosis hence to the correct answer here

N34. Ans. is c, i.e. Strawberry vagina strawberry vagina is seen in Trichomonas vaginitis

N35. Ans. is c, i.e. Chlamydia: Cottage cheese like discharge

Cottage cheese like discharge is seen in candidiasis

N36. Ans. is c, i.e. Culture on McCoy cells.

In the clinical case – the female has- pain in lower abdomen vaginal discharge clinical movements are tender Gram smear shows abundant pus cells, all these indicate PID

Now since no bacteria are seen, hence it could be that the organism causing PID is intracellular i.e , chlamydia trachomatis. **Hence culture on McCoy cells for definitive diagnosis.**

N37. Ans. is c, i.e. Remove any IUCD in the patient as soon as PID is diagnosed. *(Ref: Williams Gynae 3rd/ed, p6a)*

See the text for explanation.

ANSWERS TO PREVIOUS YEAR QUESTIONS

1. **Ans. is a, i.e. Echinococcus** *Ref: Park 19th/ed, p278, 20th/ed, p289*

Classification of sexually transmitted disease

Bacterial	Viral	Protozoa	Fungal	Ectoparasites
• Neisseria gonorrhea • Chlamydia trachomatis • Treponema pallidum • Haemophilus ducreyi • Mycoplasma hominis • Ureaplasma urealyticum • Calymmatobacterium granulomatis • Shigella species • Group B streptococcus • Bacterial vaginosis • Campylobacter spp.	Herpes 1 – 2 Hepatitis B HPV HIV *Molluscum contagiosum*	*Entamoeba histolytica* *Giardia* *Trichomonas*	*Candida*	*Phthirus pubis* *Sarcoptes scabiei*

2. **Ans. is a, i.e. Azithromycin and contact tracing** *Ref: Harrison 18th/ed, p1426; William's Gynae 1st/ed, p66; Current diagnosis and treatment of sexually transmitted diseases p 81*

Management of Chlamydia

Uncomplicated chlamydia can be treated with Tetracycline (500 mg 4 times daily), Doxycycline (1000 mg twice daily), Erythromycin (500 mg 4 times daily), Fluoroquinolone -ofloxacin 300 mg twice daily, or Azithromycin -single dose – 1 g Drug of choice is Azithromycin 1g single dose.

Advantages of Azithromycin are

- Single dose regimen – 1 g stat dose (It is as effective as 7 days of doxycycline treatment).
- Better patient compliance.
- Fewer gastrointestinal side effects.

Disadvantage:

- High cost of azithromycin.

Contact tracing:

- Patients with asymptomatic infection and their sex partners form a major burden of chlamydial infection so, contact tracing should always be done (wherever possible).
  Alternative to azithromycin is doxycycline 100 mg orally twice a day for 7 days.

3. **Ans. is d, i.e. Trichomonas vaginalis** *Ref: Shaw 15th/ed, p146; Williams Gynae 1st/ed, p64,65; Jeffcoates 7th/ed, p340-342*

Strawberry vagina or angry-looking vagina is seen in case of Trichomonas infection.

4. **Ans. is b, i.e. Hypertension** *Ref: Shaw 15th/ed, p146*

Risk factors for Candidal (Monilla) Vaginitis

- Promiscuity
- **Immunosuppression** (like HIV)
- **Pregnancy**
- Steroid therapy
- Following long-term broad spectrum antibiotic therapy
- Oral contraception pills
- **Diabetes mellitus**
- Poor personal hygiene
- Obesity

5. **Ans. is a, i.e. Bacterial vaginosis** *Ref: Shaw 15th/ed, p131,132; CGDT 10th/ed, p670; William's Gynae 1st/ed, p51,63*
6. **Ans. is c, i.e. Abundance of polymorphs** *Ref: Shaw 15th/ed, p131,132; CGDT 10th/ed, p670; William's Gynae 1st/ed, pp 51,63*

"Clue cells are the most reliable indicator of bacterial vaginosis. The positive predictive value of this test for the presence of BV is 95%." *Ref: Williams Gynae 1st/ed, p51*

Microscopy in Bacterial vaginosis shows:

- Clue cells[Q] seen in wet mount
- ↑ number of Gardnerella vaginalis[Q]
- ↓ number of lactobacilli[Q]
- ↓ leukocytes (conspicuously absent)[Q]/polymorphs absent

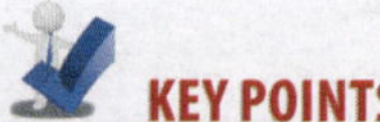

KEY POINTS

Clue cells are vaginal epithelial cells to which bacteria are adhered.

7. **Ans. is a, i.e. Tuberculosis** *Ref: Shaw 15th/ed, p157; Dutta Gynae 5th/ed, p137-38*
8. **Ans. is a, i.e. Genital tuberculosis**

HSG showing *'Bead-like fallopian tube and clubbing of ampulla are suggestive of genital tuberculosis'.*

9. **Ans. is a, i.e. Chancre** *Ref: Harrison 17th/ed, p1040; William's Gynae 1st/ed, p58-9*
Current diagnosis and treatment of STD's p21

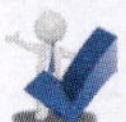

KEY POINTS

Painless well-defined ulcers with firm base should raise the suspicion of chancre.

(The lesion in the question is thought to be painless as the lady in the question is not coming because of ulcer, but for contraceptive advice. Presence of ulcer is an incidental finding).

Chancre is the primary lesion of primary syphilis.

- It is most commonly found on the labium majus, labium minus, fourchette, clitoris, urethral orifice or cervix but can be found anywhere on the lower genital tract.
- In 10% cases more than one primary lesion is present.
- The first manifestation is a small papule which breaks to form an ulcer.
- Ulcer **is firm, painless with raised edges and granulomatous base.**
- In fact any sort of discrete relatively painless ulceration on the vulva may be primary syphilitic lesion.
- Inguinal glands enlarge when the primary is on the vulva or lower vagina.
- Lymph nodes **are hard, shotty, painless, and do not suppurate.**

10. **Ans. is a, i.e. Condyloma accuminata** *Ref: Shaw 15th/ed, p138, 139; Current diagnosis and treatment of sexually transmitted diseases, p92-93*

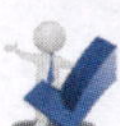

KEY POINTS

- History of sexual exposure and growths on vulva is consistent with condyloma accuminata.

- Condyloma accuminata:
  - It is a *sexually transmitted disease*[Q] caused by HPV 6[Q], 16,[Q] and 18.[Q]
  - Warts are seen on the vulval area.[Q]
  - Warts are common in the regions affected most directly by coitus[Q] i.e. posterior fourchette[Q] and lateral areas of vulva. These verrucous growths may coalesce to form large cauliflower growths.[Q]
  - Condyloma is associated with vulval,[Q] vaginal,[Q] and cervical cancers.[Q]
  - Diagnosis is by colposcopy which shows raised patches of aceto-white epithelium with speckled appearance.[Q]

Lets also rule out other options.

- **Verrucous plana:**
  - Hands and face are the most common site[Q], warts are not seen in genital area.
  - It is usually seen in children.[Q]
  - Sometimes, it can also occur in young women, but then face is the most common site involved.[Q]
- **Verruca vulgaris:**
  - Here also the site of warts is different; usually affected areas are exposed parts of the bodyQ, handQ, feetQ, nails, arms, and legs, face, and scalp.
- **Condyloma lata:**
  - Is the growth seen on genitalia in secondary syphilis.Q
  - The presence of these lesions without any other features of syphilis is very unlikely.

11. **Ans. is a, i.e. Metronidazole and fluconazole**
Ref: Dutta Gynae 6th/ed, p176; Internet search–www. naconlinr.org/upload/publication/ste

Syndromic management of sexually transmitted infections (WHO 1991)

Principle: Treatment of STDs should be initiated at the patient's first visit to a clinic. At the same time the couple is counseled about the importance of condom use and prevention of STD transmission.

Syndromic managements are based on epidemiological studies all over the world. Syndromic diagnosis and laboratory assisted diagnosis have been found similar in terms of accuracy.

Identifying Syndromes

Syndrome	Most common cause
Vaginal discharge	Vaginitis (Trichomonas, candidiasis, bacterial vaginosis) cervicitis (gonorrhea/ chlamydia)
Urethral discharge	Gonorrhea/chlamydia
Genital ulcers	Syphilis, Chancroid, Herpes
Lower abdominal pain	Gonorrhea/Chlamydia/mixed anaerobes

Now since in the question, it is specifically mentioned, patient does not have any cervicitis so we will treat her for vaginitis, i.e. for Trichomonas and bacterial vaginosis give her Metronidazole and for candidiasis give her fluconazole.

12. Ans. is b, c and e, i.e. Staphylococcus; Chlamydia; and N. gonorrhoea *Ref: Dutta Gynae 5th/ed, p163*

Cervicitis refers to infection of the endocervix including the glands and stroma.

Organisms causing cervicitis

- Streptococcus
- Staphylococcus
- Gonococcus
- E. coli
- Chlamydia

Trichomonas, Candida and Herpes simplex virus cause inflammation of the ectocervix (vaginitis) and not of endocervix.

13. Ans. is a, c and d, i.e. Lower abdominal tenderness, Cervical motion tenderness, and Adnexal tenderness.

Ref: Shaw 15th/ed, p449-50; Dutta's Gynae 6th/ed, p130; Johns Hopkins Manual of Gynecology and Obstetrics, The, 3rd/ed; William's Gynae 1st/ed, p73

CDC criteria for Diagnosis of PID has been discussed in detail earlier.

14. Ans. is a, b and d, i.e. IV antibiotics, Drainage of TO mass, and Laparoscopic exploration

Ref: Textbook of Gynae, Sheila Balakrishnan 1st/ed, p217-18; Novak 15th/ed, p565-66

Management of PID

- Broad-spectrum antibiotics (oral or IV)
- If tubo-ovarian mass/abscess is present – it should be treated medically but, if there is no response drainage should be done.
- Drainage of a pelvic abscess by colpotomy may occasionally be needed

Place of surgery in acute PID: Surgery can range from laparoscopy to laparotomy.

Indications

- No response to treatment and worsening of condition
- Ruptured tubo-ovarian abscess
- Drainage of a pelvic abscess
- Doubtful diagnosis

15. Ans. is a, i.e. Chlamydia *Ref: Harrison 17th/ed, p823; Current diagnosis and treatment of STI p15*

Non gonococcal urethritis is caused by: Rare Cases

- *Chlamydia trachomatis* (30 – 40%)
- *Ureaplasma urealyteum*
- *Mycoplasma genitalium*
- *E coli*
- *Ureaplasma urealyticum*
- Anaerobic bacteria
- *Trichomonas vaginalis*
- Adenovirus
- Herpes simplex virus

Management:

Azithromycin 1 g orally in a single dose or doxycycline 100 mg orally twice a day × 7 days

Alternative = Erythromycine 500 mg four times a day × 7 days

16. Ans. is e, i.e. All of the above statements are correct

Ref: Dutta Gynae 5th/ed, p143; CGDT 10th/ed, p671; William's Gynae 2nd/ed, p86,87

- Gonorrhea infection is caused by *Neisseria gonorrhoeae*—a gram-negative diplococci.
- Incubation period = 3–7 days[Q]

Clinical features in adults

- **50 percent** of patients with Gonorrhoea are asymptomatic[Q]
- Asymptomatic gonorrhoea in females is due to infection of endocervix.[Q]

In symptomatic cases, **M/c symptom is usually excessive vaginal discharge,** lower abdominal pain, and dysuria.

"In exceptional cases gonococcal septicemia is described and may be manifested by pyrexia and even vesicular or pustular dermatitis" Ref: Jeffcoate's 7th/ed, p313

Signs:

- ***Labia are swollen and look inflammed.***Q
- ***Cervicitis with a mucopurulent cervical discharge.***
- *Bartholin glands are enlarged and tender.*Q
- *On squeezing the ducts: purulent exudate escapes.*Q

Complications-PID, Fitz-Hugh-Curtis syndrome and septicemia.Q

17. Ans. is a, d and e, i.e. Flagellated parasite, Pruritus, and Sexually transmitted disease

Ref: Shaw 15th/ed, p146; William's Gynae 1st/ed, p64-5; Jeffcoate's 7th/ed, p340-42

Trichomonas vaginalis

- Is a flagellated protozoa which leads to trichomonas vaginitis.
- Patients complain of profuse frothy creamy/Slightly greenish discharge and pruritis

O/E = Multiple small punctate strawberry spots are seen on vaginal walls and portio vaginalis of cervix called as strawberry vagina.

- It is sexually transmitted.

18. Ans. is a and c, i.e. Foul smelling vaginal discharge; and Strawberry vagina *Ref: John Hopkins Manual of Gynecology and Obstetrics 4th/ed, p430; Shaw 15th/ed, p145; Novak 14th/ed, p544; Leon Speroff 7th/ed, p1090*

- There is no doubt that trichomonas infection cause foul smelling discharge and strawberry vagina.
- Vaginal pH favoring trichomonas infection is higher than 5 *(Novak 15/e p560)*

Trichomonas vaginalis has not been associated with infertility.

Infact *Jeffcoates 7th/ed, p702* says – *"Clinical observations show that many women with chronic cervicitis and Trichomonas vaginalis conceive repeatedly without difficulty."*

Common infections associated with infertility are:

- *Chlamydia trachomatis*
- N. gonorrhoea
- *Ureaplasma urealyticum*
- *Genital TB*

Ref: Shaw 14th/ed, p189

Infections and Infertility

"Infections of the female and male genital tracts have been implicated as causes of infertility. Chlamydia infection and gonorrhea are the major pathogens and should be treated appropriately. Ureoplasma urealyticum and Mycoplasma hominis have also been implicated and if positively identified by culture, they should be treated with oral doxycycline, 100 mg twice daily for 7 days. This has been shown to increase the pregnancy rate in patients with primary infertility."

Ref: John Hopkin's Manual of Gynecology and Obstetrics 4th/ed, p430

Effect of Trichomonas on Pregnancy Outcome –

"Pregnant women with trichomonas vaginitis are at increased risk for premature rupture of membranes and preterm delivery." *Ref: Novak 14th/ed, p544*

As far as abortions is concerned –

Organisms which have been associated with sporadic abortions are:

- *Chlamydia trachomatis*
- *Mycoplasma homins*
- *Listeria monocytogenes*
- Herpes virus
- *Ureaplasma urealyticum*
- *Toxoplasma gondii*
- *Campylobacter*
- Cytomegalovirus

Ref: Leon Speroff 7th/ed, p1090

19. Ans. is b, c, d and e, i.e. Gray discharge; Clue cells found; Fishy odor discharge; and caused by *Gardnerella vaginalis*

20. Ans. is b, c and e, i.e. Gray and white discharge; Associated with vaginal pH > 4.5; and Oral metronidazole is the drug of choice *Ref: Shaw 15th/ed, p131-32; CGDT 10th/ed, p670; William's Gynae 1st/ed, p50,51*

All the options we have discussed earlier.

KEY POINTS

Remember: There is no inflammation in bacterial vaginosis and hence pruritus is not seen in bacterial vaginosis

21. Ans. is c and d, i.e. pH < 4.5, and Yellow green discharge *Ref: Shaw 15th/ed, p131; Dutta Gynae 6th/ed, p152*

Bacterial vaginosis is characterised by homogeneous, greyish white discharge adherent to vaginal wall.

Yellowish green discharge is seen in case of trichomonas infection and not bacterial vaginosis.

22. Ans. is a, b and c, i.e. Mycobacterium can be grown from menstrual blood, Associated with infertility, and Ectopic pregnancy is common *Ref: Shaw 15th/ed, p156-58; Jeffcoate 7th/ed, p327*

Amongst the given option there is no doubt that TB leads to infertility and ectopic pregnancy rather M/C symptom of TB is infertility (i.e. options b and c are correct).

Mycobacterium can be grown from menstrual blood is again correct (i.e. option a). Now coming to option d, i.e. dysmenorrhea is a common presentation.

- ***Pain*** is uncommon and is a result of subacute PID.
- ***"Dysmenorrhea rarely ever occurs"***. *Ref: Jeffcoates 7th/ed, p327*

23. Ans. is c, i.e. ESR - 10 mm/hour *Ref: Textbook of Gynae Shiela Balakrishnan 1st/ed, p216; Novak 15th/ed, p565*

- Temp >38°C (100.4° F)
- WBC count >15,000 are all criteria for diagnosing PID
- Tenderness on movement of cervix

ESR ≥ 15 mm/hr is the criteria and not ESR ≥ 10 mm/hr.

For details of the criteria, kindly see the preceding text.

24. Ans. is d, i.e. Fallopian tubes *Ref: Telinde Operative Gynae 9th/ed, p678, 679; Dutta Gynecology 6th/ed, p126*

According to: *Dutta Gynae 6th/ed, p130*

For identification of organisms in PID the materials are collected from the following available sources:

- Discharge from urethra or Bartholin's gland
- Cervical canal
- Collected pus from the fallopian tubes during laparoscopy or laparotomy.

The material so collected is subjected to Gram's stain and culture (aerobic/anaerobic). The findings of Gram-negative diplococci is very much suggestive of gonococcal infection.

25. Ans. is a, i.e. Endocervix

26. Ans. is c, i.e. Infants *Ref: Dutta Gynae 5th/ed, p143, 6th/ed, p147; COGDT 10th/ed, p671,672*

There are 2 important points which we should be remembered about gonorrhoea infection.

- Squamous epithelium is resistant to gonococci infection
- Gonorrhoea is an STD (i.e. it is transmitted by ascending infection along with sperms)

Now, since squamous epithelium is resistant to gonococcal infection, in vagina and ectocervix gonococcal infection cannot occur (as both are lined by squamous epithelium). So from there, gonoccal infection will travel along with sperms and reach endo cervix which is lined by columnar epithelium.

∴ *M/C site for gonoccal infection in young females is endocervix.*

Other sites are

- Bartholin's gland (Bartholin cyst is caused by gonoccal infection)[Q]
- Skene glands
- Urethra

Note: In newborn females vagina is lined by transitional epithelium so theoretically gonococcal vaginitis can occur in them

27. Ans. is c, i.e. Chlamydia

28. Ans. is c, i.e. Polymerase chain reaction *Ref: Shaw 15th/ed, p145; Harrison 18th/ed, p1426; Dutta Gynae 6th/ed, p 126*

Chlamydia Infections

"Except in highly sophisticated centres, the detection of Cl. trachomatis is difficult by wet film". *Ref: Dutta Gynae 6th/ed, p126*

- "Polymerase and ligase chain reactions are fast highly sensitive and specific (96%) and now considered gold standard in the laboratory diagnosis. *Ref: Shaw 14th/ed, p131; 15th/ed, p145*

Note: *Ref: Harrison 18th/ed, p1426*

- ***The current diagnostic technique of choice for chlamydial infections is NAAT—Nucleic acid amplification tests.***
- *Choice of specimen*—Specimen can be urine or vaginal swabs.
- For screening asymptomatic women—CDC recommends—Self-collected vaginal swabs
- In symptomatic females—cervical swab sample
- In males—urine sample is the specimen of choice

29. Ans. is b, i.e. Culture on McCoy cells *Ref: Harrion 18th/ed, p1426*

Patient is complaining of abdominal pain and vaginal discharge. On examination, cervicitis and mucopurulent discharge is seen—which indicates she is having PID. The presence of pus cells in absence of organism indicates chlamydial infection (most common STD today). It is an intracellular organism that grows only on McCoy or HeLa cell cultures. It cannot be grown on other media and hence, often goes unnoticed, later leading to infertility.

Culture in Mc Coy cells is 100% specific for chlamydia but is inexpensive, technically difficult and takes 3-7 days to obtain the result.

30. Ans. is c, i.e. Erythromycin *Ref: Williams Obs 23th/ed, p124; Harrison 18th/ed, p1426*

In non pregnant females – DOC for *Chlamydia* = Azithromycin or Doxycycline

But Doxycycline is contraindicated during pregnancy.

Treatment of *chlamydia* infection during pregnancy

Regimen	Drug and Dosage
Preferred choice	Azithromycin (1 g) as a single dose Alternatives are: Amoxicillin 500 mg TDS × 7 days Erythromycin base 500 mg QID ×7 days Erythromycin ethylsuccinate 800 mg QID × 7 days

"Azithromycin is the first-line treatment and has been found to be safe and efficacious in pregnancy."

Ref: Williams Obs 23rd/ed, p1241

But since azithromycin is not given in the options, so the next best option is Erythromycin.

31. Ans is a, i.e. Miconazole *Ref: Shaw 15th/ed, p146 147; CGDT 10th/ed, p599-601*

Thick curdy discharge indicates the causative white organism is candida which is treated by Azole group of antifungals e.g. Fluconazole/Miconazole given orally or applied topically.

Management of Vulvovaginal Candidiasis in Pregnancy:

- 1st trimester: Nystatin vaginal tablets
- 2nd trimester: Topical azole antifungal

Management of Recurrent Vulvovaginal Candidiasis:

- Recurrent vulvovaginal candidiasis is defined as four or more episodes of vulvovaginal candidiasis in a year. It might be caused by *Candida tropicalis*[Q] or *Candida glabrata.*[Q]
- Antibiotic treatment needs to be prolonged (Fluconazole 150 mg weekly x 6 months or ketoconazole/Itraconazole 100 mg daily x 6 months).
- Simultaneous treatment of male partner.[Q]
- Patients on prolonged therapy should have their LFT monitored.

32. Ans. is b, i.e. Gardnerella

33. Ans. is c, i.e. Metronidazole *Ref: Shaw 15th/ed, p131; CGDT 10th/ed, p670; William's Gynae 1st/ed, p51*

Creamy white discharge with fishy odor is characteristic of bacterial vaginosis (M/C cause Gardnerella)

Drug of choice for management of bacterial vaginosis/Gardnerella vaginitis is–

Metronidazole:

Dose – 500 mg oral metronidazole is given twice daily for 7 days

Alternatively, metronidazole gel (can be applied once daily for 5 days or clindamycin cream (2%) at bedtime for 5 days.

Note: Treatment of male sexual partner is not required in bacterial vaginosis.[Q]

In pregnancy:

- Bacterial vaginosis is associated with preterm birth and premature rupture of membranes.
- Treatment is reserved for symptomatic women who usually complain of fishy odor.
- DOC – Metronidazole (oral) in the 2nd and the 3rd trimester.

Unfortunately, treatment does not reduce preterm birth and routine screening is not recommended.

34. Ans. is d, i.e. Fallopian tube

35. Ans. is a, Direct local spread *Ref: Shaw 15th/ed, p154*

- M/c Route of spread of Genital TB: Henatoze
- M/c Route of spread of Endometrial TB: Direct local spread
- Tubercular endometritis causes infertility due to uterine scarring resulting in destruction of endometrium[Q]
- Genital tuberculosis is almost always a secondary infection, with primary sites being lungs, lymph nodes, abdomen, etc.
- Hematogenous route is the most common mode of spread from the primary site.

36. Ans. is a, i.e. Hysteroscopy and laparoscopy *Ref: Shaw 15th/ed, p451; William's Gynae 1st/ed, p74; Gynecology by Ostrzenski (Lippincott Williams 2001/282); Dutta Gynae 6th/ed, p130*

Laparoscopy is considered the "gold standard". While it is the most reliable aid to support the clinical diagnosis but it may not be feasible to do in all cases. It is reserved only in those cases in which differential diagnosis includes salpingitis, appendicitis or ectopic pregnancy. Nonresponding pelvic mass needs laparoscopic clarification.

Hysteroscopy may also provide confirmatory evidence for salpingitis.

"Fallopian tube culture can be obtained laparoscopically and recently the hysteroscopic approach has been introduced. The specimen is obtained during hysteroscopy with a cytobrush." *Ref: Gynecology by Ostrzenski (Lippincott Williams) (2001)/282*

Also Know

Since laparoscopy is an invasive procedure for diagnosis of salpingitis/PID, diagnosis should first be made clinically.

37. **Ans. is a, i.e. Treponema pallidum**

The M/c causes of genital ulcers in young, sexual active women are:
- Herpes simplex virus (HSV)
- Treponema pallidum (syphilis)
- Haemophilus ducreyi (chancroid).

In this case, painless ulcer with everted margin leave no doubt that the cause of the ulcer is syphilis (treponema pallidum).

Clinical features of genital ulcers

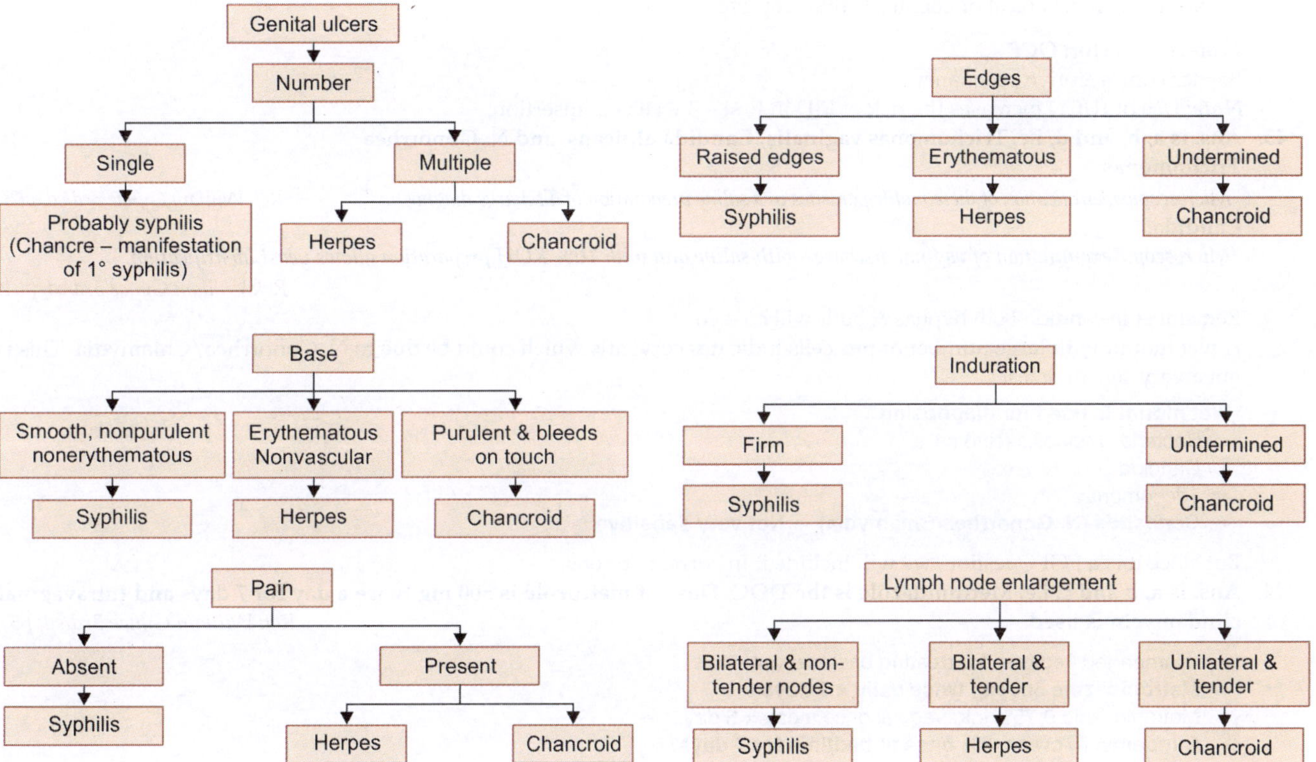

38. **Ans. is b, c and d, i.e T. vaginals is a flagellated protozoa, Metronidazole is used for treatment, and Strawberry cervix**
Ref: Dutta Obs 7th/ed, p167

Infection in genital tract may be responsible for sporadic abortion but its relation to recurrent abortion is inconclusive. Rest all options- have been explained earlier in the chapter.

39. **Ans. is a, i.e. Bacterial vaginosis**

(*See* the text for explanation)

40. **Ans. is b, i.e. pH > 4.5 fishy odour on KOH mount**

(*See* the text for explanation)

Note: In bacterial vaginosis, the number of lactobacilli disease

41. **Ans is b, i.e. Ceftriaxone plus azithromycin, single dose**

DOC for Gonorrhea in pregnancy:

Ceftriaxone 250 mg single dose and azithromycin 1g orally single dose

DOC for Chlamydia in pregnancy:

Preferred Regimen:

Azithromycin 1 gm single dose

Or

Amoxicillin 500 mg TDS × 7 days.

Or

Erythromycin 500 mg oral 4 times a day × 7 days.

42. Ans. is c, d and e, i.e. IUCD user, Previous H/O PID, Increase number of sexual partners

Ref: Table 3-11, Williams Gynae 3rd/ed, p66

Risk factors for PID

- Douching
- Single status
- Substance abuse
- **Multiple sexual partners**
- Lower socioecomomic status
- Recent new sexual partners
- **Younger age (10 to 19 years)**
- Sexual partner with urethritis or Gonorrhea
- **Previous diagnosis of PID**
- Not using mechanical or chemical contraceptive

Protective factor: OCP

Barrier contraceptive pregnancy

Note: Use of IUCD increases the risk of PID in first - 3 weeks of insertion.

43. Ans. is a, b, and d, i.e. Trichomonas vaginalis, Candida albicans, and N. Gonorrhea

Trichomonas:

"Microscopic identification of these motile parasites in a saline preparation of discharge diagnostic." *Ref: William Gynae 3rd/ed, p63.*

Candida:

"Microscopic examination of vaginal discharge with saline and with 10% KOH preparation allows yeast identification."

Ref: William Gynae 3rd/ed, p61.

Remember in candida-both hyphae & buds will be seen

A wet mount with large number of pus cells indicates cervicitis which could be due to N. Gonorrhea/Chlamydia. This is not a very sensitive test

Wet mount is used for diagnosing

- Bacterial vaginosis (clue cells)
- Candida
- Trichomonas
- **Cervicites (N. Gonorrhea/Chlamydia) → Not very sensitive**

But since it is a PGI Question, we will include it in correct options.

44. Ans. is a, b and c, i.e. Metronidazole is the DOC, Dose of metrozole is 500 mg twice a day for 7 days and Intravaginal clindamycin is used

Ref: William Gynae 3rd/ed, p52

Recommended Regimen for treating bacterial vaginosis

- **Metronidazole 500 mg twice daily × 7 days**
- Metronidazole 0.75% intravaginal once a day × 5 days
- **Clindamycin cream 2% once at bedtime for 7 days.**

Note: Treatment of male partner is not done in BV.

Clotrimazole cream is used for Candida infection.

45. Ans. is c, i.e. Amoxicillin

(See Q 41 for explanation)

46. Ans. is b, i.e. Candida

H/O use of antibiotics, UTI & vaginal discharge with itching all indicate towards Candidal vaginosis.

47. Ans. is b, i.e. Bacterial vaginosis

(*See* the text for explanation)

48. Ans. is a, i.e. Syphilis

Ref: Williams Gynae 3rd/ed, p56

"With pregnancy syphilis, the hallmark lesion is the chancre, in which spirochetes are abundant classically, it is an isolated non tender ulcer with raised sounded borders and an uninfected base."

Ref: Williams Gynae 3rd/ed, p56

49. Ans. is b, c, d, i.e. T vaginalis is a flagellated protozoa; Metronidazole is used for treatment; Strawberry cervix

Now no explanation is needed for any other option except its role in Abortions.

"Infection in genital tract may be responsible for sporadic spontaneous abortion but its relation to recurrent abortion is in conclusive."

Ref: Dutta Obs 7th/ed, p167

REVIEW/PRACTICE QUESTIONS

1. **Not included in PID:**
   a. Salpingitis b. Endometritis
   c. Cervicitis d. Oophoritis
2. **All of the following are risk factors for PID *except*:**
   a. LSES
   b. Substance abuse
   c. Pregnancy
   d. Not using barrier contraceptive
3. **Clue cells are seen in:**
   a. Bacterial vaginosis
   b. Trichomonas
   c. Candida
   d. Central TB
4. **M/C cause of PID in IUCD users:**
   a. Chlamydia b. E. coli
   c. Actinomyces d. Staphylococcus
5. **An acute inflammation of tube can be a result of:**
   a. Gonorrhea
   b. E. coli
   c. Enterococcus faecalis
   d. Chlamydia
6. **M/c symptom of PID:**
   a. Vaginal discharge
   b. Abdominal pain
   c. Bleeding per vagina
   d. Fever
7. **Gold standard for diagnosing PID:**
   a. USG b. MRI
   c. Culdocentesis d. Laparoscopy
8. **Risk factor for candidians are all *except*:**
   a. HIV b. Pregnancy
   c. Diabetes d. All of above
9. **Organism which flourishes in acidic medium:**
   a. Candida
   b. Trichomonas
   c. Bacterial vaginosis
   d. Monoliasis
10. **Frei test and Grove sign are seen in:**
   a. Primary syphilis
   b. Granuloma inguinale
   c. Lymphogranuloma venereum
   d. Herpes
11. **Prognostic scoring system in PID is:**
   a. Prader scoring
   b. Bear-Miesel
   c. Insler score
   d. Nugent score
12. **Staging of PID given by:**
   a. Boer misl score b. Gainesville
   c. Insler d. Nugent
13. **Mode of spread of TB to endometrium:**
   a. Hematogenous b. Local spread
   c. Lymphatic d. Retrograde
14. **DOC for Bacteria vaginosis in a pregnant female:** *(AIIMS Nov 2019)*
   a. Clindamycin
   b. Metronidazole
   c. Erythromycin
   d. Fluconazole
15. **A 40 years patient c/o foul smelling greyish white discharge, diagnosed to be *Gardnerella* vaginalis infection. Microscopic findings are suggestive of:** *(AIIMS Nov 2019)*

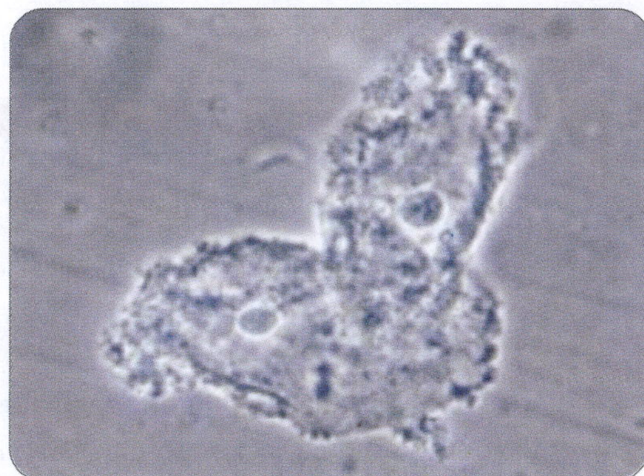

   a. Group of bacilli arranged in chain forms
   b. Bacteria found to be engulfed by macrophages
   c. Bacteria adherent to lining vaginal epithelial cells
   d. Bacteria arranged in cluster forms
16. **Which is/are NOT true about Asherman's syndrome?** *(PGI May 2019)*
   a. Can be caused by genital TB
   b. Progesterone challenge test +ve
   c. Elevated serum prolactin level and normal FSH/LH ratio
   d. Causes secondary amenorrhea
   e. May result from uterine curettage
17. **All are true regarding Asherman syndrome *except*:** *(PGI December 2018)*
   a. Can occur due to tubercular pathology
   b. Causes primary amenorrhea
   c. Can occur due to curettage and drainage
   d. Can be viewed by hysteroscope
   e. All of the above

REVIEW/PRACTICE ANSWERS

1. **Ans. c, i.e. Cervicitis** *Ref: Shaw 16th/ed, p177*
2. **Ans. c, i.e. Pregnancy** *Ref: Williams Gynae 3rd/ed, p66*
3. **Ans. a, i.e. Bacterial vaginosis**
4. **Ans. c, i.e.Actinomyces** *Ref: Shaw 16th/ed, p178*
5. **Ans. is a, i.e.Gonorrhea** *Ref: William Gynae 3rd/ed, p66*

Gonococcus can cause direct damage to fallopian tube. However chlamydia does not have any direct affect nor it leads to acute inflammation. The cell mediated immune reaction can later on result in scarring of tubes.

6. **Ans. b, i.e. Abdominal pain** *Ref: Shaw 16th/ed, p181*
7. **Ans. d, i.e. Laparoscopy** *Ref: William Gynae 3rd/ed, p67*
8. **Ans. d, i.e. All of above**
9. **Ans. a, i.e. Candida**
10. **Ans. c, i.e. Lymphogranuloma venereum**
11. **Ans. b, i.e. Bear-Miesel**
12. **Ans. b, i.e. Gainesville**
13. **Ans. b, i.e. Local spread**
14. **Ans. is b, i.e. Metronidazole**

- Metronidazole, tinidazole and clindamycin are preferred antibiotics for treatment of bacterial vaginosis; however the single best drug of choice is metronidazole.

First line	Second line
• Metronidazole (DOC) 500 mg orally BD for 7 days	• Tinidazole 2 gm orally OD for 2 days
• Metronidazole gel 0.75% 5 gm intravaginally once a day for 5 days	• Tinidazole 1 gm orally OD for 5 days
• Clindamycin cream 2% 5 gm intravaginally once a day for 7 days	• Clindamycin 300 mg orally BD for 7 days
	• Clindamycin ovules 100 mg OD intravaginally for 3 days

15. **Ans. is c, i.e. Bacteria adherent to lining vaginal epithelial cells** *Ref: William's Gynecology 3rd/ed, p51-52*

- The microscopic finding is vaginal epithelial cells with bacteria attached to them called as "*clue cells*".
- Clue cells are the most reliable indicator of bacterial vaginosis.
- These vaginal epithelial cells contain may attached bacteria, which create a poorly defined stippled border
- Saline microscopy with >20% of clue cells is diagnostic of bacterial vaginosis and is one of the 4 criteria described in Amsel's criteria.

Amsel Criteria: Diagnostic Criteria for Bacterial Vaginosis
- Abnormal gray discharge
- Vaginal pH ≥4.5
- Positive amine/whiff test (release of fishy, amine-like odor when vaginal fluid is alkalinized with KOH)
    - ≥ 20% of the epithelial cells are clue cells.

16. **Ans. is b, and c, i.e. Progesterone challenge test +ve, and Elevated serum prolactin level and normal FSH/LH ratio**

We have dealt with Asherman syndrome in detail in chapter on Genital TB and Amenorrhea:

- Asherman syndrome is mainly caused due to uterine curettage (i.e., option c is correct) and in developing countries, it may be due to TB and schistosomiasis (i.e. option a is correct)
- It leads to secondary amenorrhea (i.e. option d is true)
- Progesterone challenge test is negative in Asherman syndrome (i.e. option b is incorrect)
- Serum prolactin, LH and FSH are all normal in Asherman as in Asherman the pathology lies in the endometrium of uterus (i.e. option c is incorrect).

17. **Ans. is b, i.e. Causes primary amenorrhea** *Ref: Shaw's Gynae 16th/ed, p430-34; Dutta's Gynae 6th/ed, p438-441*

- ***Asherman syndrome causes secondary amenorrhea.***
- ***Asherman syndrome occurs primarily after a dilation and curettage.***
- In the developing world, ***it may also occur due to infections from schistosomiasis or tuberculosis.***
- *Hysteroscopy is the gold standard for diagnosis.*

Details on Asherman syndrome have been covered in chapter on TB of Genital Tract and Amenorrhea.

CHAPTER 8

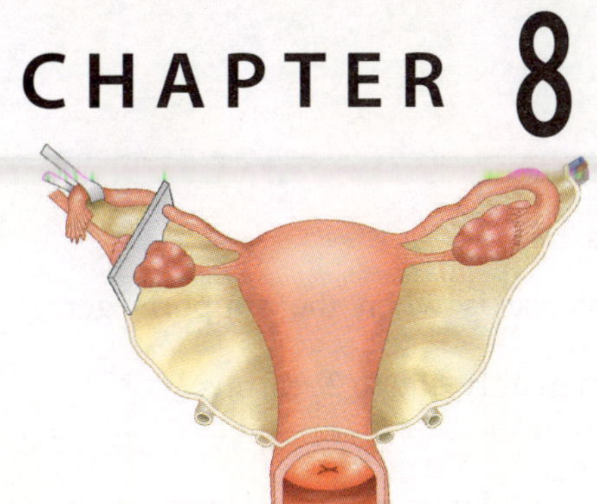

Prolapse/Fistulas and SUI

Pelvic Relaxation/Prolapse

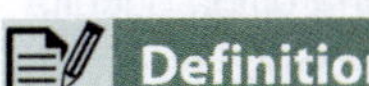

Definition

Pelvic Relaxation/Prolapse

Protrusion of pelvic organs into or out of the vaginal canal is called as **prolapse**. External Os lies at level of ischeal spine and internal Os at upper border of pubic symphysis. Hence any descent of uterus from these levels is a case of prolapse.

Prolapse Could be

i. Uterocervical prolapse
ii. Vaginal prolapse

Supports of Uterus

Supports of uterus are categorized as:

1. Mechanical supports of uterus
2. Ligaments supporting the uterus
3. Muscles supporting the uterus

1. Mechanical Supports of Uterus

- **Angle of arteversion**: Angle between vagina and cervix, i.e. 90°
- Angle of arteflexion Angle between cervix and uterus i.e. 120° Normally uterus is in arteverted and arteflexed position (Fig. 8.1)
- 1st step in prolapse is Retroversion of uterus.

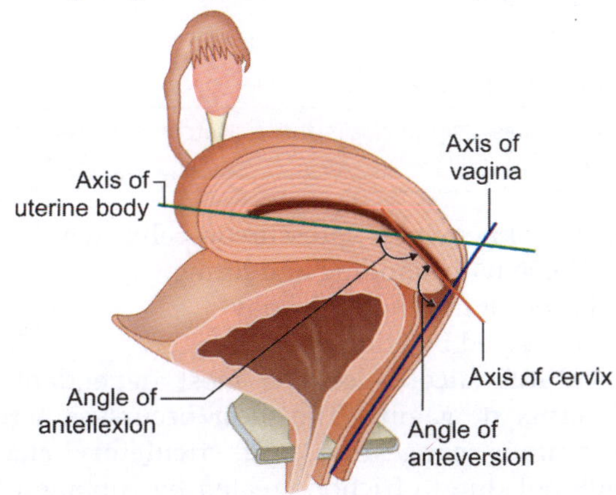

Fig. 8.1: Angle of anteversion and angle of anteflexion

2. Ligaments Supporting the Uterus

Primary supports	Secondary support	No support
1. Cardinal ligament (Main support) 2. Uterosacral ligament (2 main ligament) 3. Pubocervical ligament Together these are called as Triradiate ligament (Fig. 8.2)	Round ligament	Broad ligament

- **Round ligament of uterus** originates from the cornua of uterus, in the parametrium. It enters the pelvis via the deep inguinal ring, passes through the inguinal canal and continues on to the labia majora.
  - It helps to keep the uterus in anteverted position (therefore indirectly supports the uterus)
  - It develops from the gubernaculum
  - It is supplied by the artery of Sampson which is a branch of uterine artery.

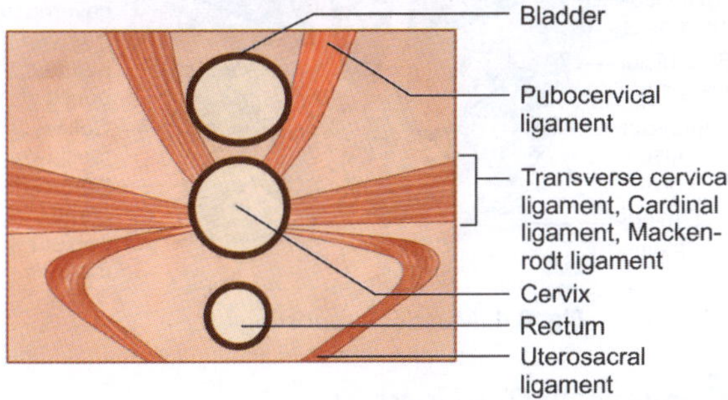

Fig. 8.2: Supports of uterus showing triradiate ligament

3. Muscles Supporting the Uterus

The muscles which support the uterus are:

1. Levator ani muscle which forms the pelvic diaphragm
2. Superficial and Deep Transverse perineal muscles which form the urogenital diaphragm
3. Bulbospongiosus muscle
4. External anal sphincter
5. External urethral sphincter muscle fibers.

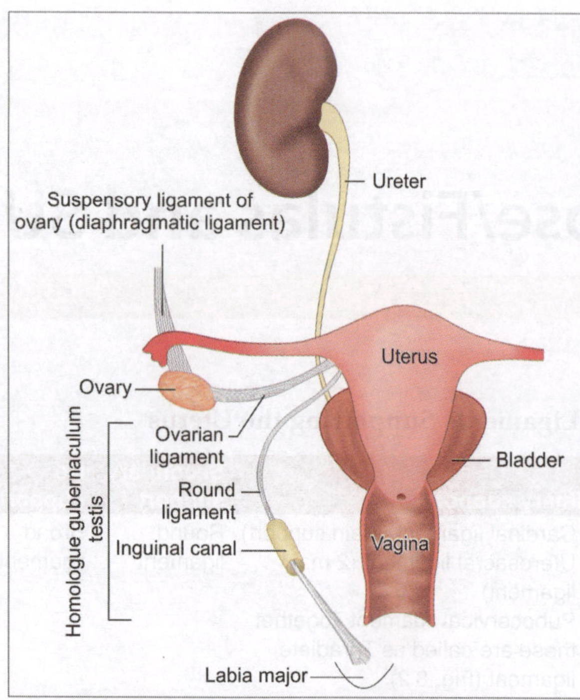

Fig. 8.3: Round ligament

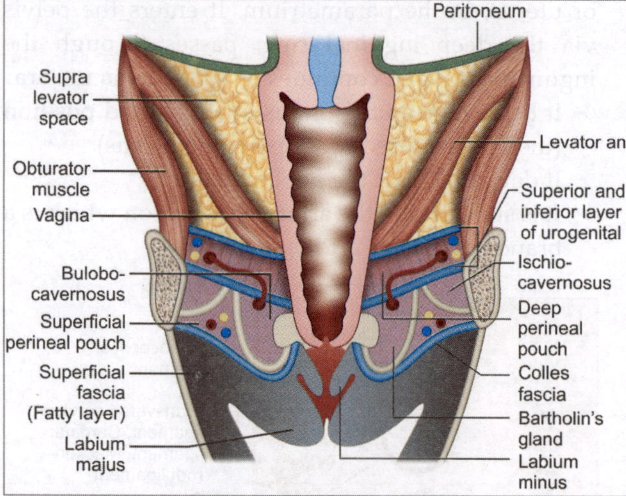

Fig. 8.4: Muscles supporting uterus

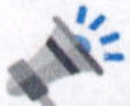

Important One Liners

- Normally uterus remains in anteverted and anteflexed position. Retroversion is the first step in prolapse. Therefore, whenever given a case of prolapse – in viva. You can safely say the females uterus is retroverted even without examining.
- Main ligament responsible for anteflexion and anteversion: Round Ligament
- Ligament preventing retroversion: Uterosacral ligament
- Broad ligament (fold of peritoneum) does not support the uterus at all.
- Most important overall uterine support is Levator ani muscle.

Etiology of Prolapse

- The cause of prolapse is when the supports get weakened.
  This could happen mainly due to 2 reasons:
  1. Repeated child birth
  2. Menopause

  This is the reason, prolapse is more common in elderly multiparous females.

The list of causes leading to prolapse are given in Table 8.1.

Table 8.1: Causes of prolapse.

Acquired Causes		Congenital Causes
• **Menopause** • **Repeated child birth**	} **2 main causes**	• Spina bifida occulta • Neurological disorders viz Ehler Danlos syndrome, Marfans syndrome
• Traumatic deliveries • Faulty birth practices • Precipitate labor • Iatrogenic trauma like in case of vaginal hysterectomy, vulvectomy • Increased intra-abdominal pressure like in COPD, constipation, obesity		

Note: If prolapse occurs in young, Nulliparous female, it is called as congenital prolapse.

Congenital Prolapse

Risk factors are:

1. Osteogenesis imperfecta
2. Ehler Danlos syndrome
3. Spina bifida
   - Cystocele is not seen in congenital prolapse
   - It is managed by sling surgeries/Cervicopexy

Symptoms of Prolapse

- Due to protusion of cervix and uterus into vagina, **patient feels something coming down or out.**
- **Groin/back pain** (due to stretching of **uterosacral ligaments)**[Q].

Important One Liners

Backache in case of prolapse is due to stretching of uterosacral ligaments.

- Feeling of heaviness/pressure in pelvis which is
  - Worse with standing and lifting
  - Worse at the end of the day
  - Is relieved by lying down
- **Decubitus ulcer** – on the most dependant part of cervix or vagina. The ulcer occurs as a **result of venous congestion and circulatory changes and**[Q] not due to friction created by rubbing of the prolapsed parts with the thigh.[Q]

Note: Infection and bleeding can occur if surgery is performed in presence of decubitus ulcers.

- **Treatment of decubitus ulcer:** Reduction of the prolapse part into the vagina and **daily packing with glycerine and acriflavine.[Q] Acriflavine is an antiseptic agent while glycerine is a hygroscopic agent.**
- **Urinary symptoms:** Incontinence, frequency or urgency.
- Cancer of cervix or vagina is rarely seen[Q], even in untreated cases of prolapse.

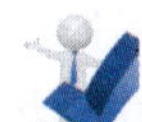

KEY POINTS

- Best Method to prevent prolapse-
- Perineal exercise/Kegels exercise x 3 to 4 times a day.

Classification of Uterine Prolapse

Uterine prolapse

Shaw's classification (old classification):

- 1^0 – descent of the cervix to the vagina
- 2^0 – descent of the cervix to the introitus
- 3^0 – descent of the cervix outside the introitus.
- Procidentia: All of the uterus outside the introitus.

Management of Uterine Prolapse

Uterine Prolapse

Management depends on age and parity of the female, (Flowchart 8.1):

Flowchart 8.1

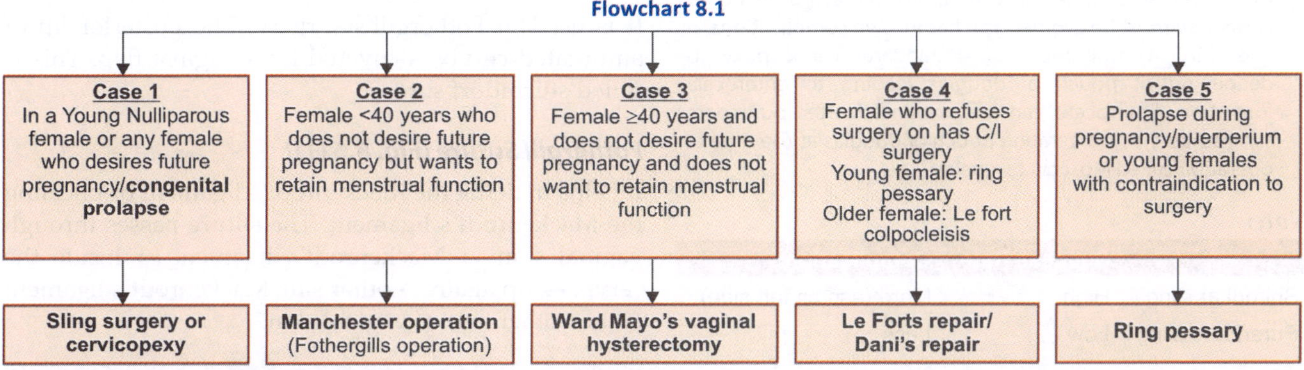

Details of Prolapse Surgeries

Abdominal Sling Surgeries–Management of Choice in Young Females with Prolapse Who are Desirous of Future Child Bearing

Purandare Sling/cervicopexy	Shirodkar Sling	Composite/Virkud Sling
• Sling made of fascia lata is used • It is an example of anterior sling • It is type of **dynamic/open sling** where central part of the sling is fixed anteriorly to the exposed part of **isthmus** and the two ends of the tape are attached to **posterior rectus sheath.** ***Note:*** It should be performed only in those females who have a good abdominal tone. • **Drawback:** It leads to retroversion of uterus, deepening of pouch of douglas and enterocele formation. ***Note***: Purandare sling has lesser complications as compared to Shirodkar but has lesser success rate also.	• It is type of **static sling** which aims at strenthening the uterosacrals. i.e. it is type of posterior sling. • Mersilene tape is attached anteriorly to posterior surface of cervix and posteriorly to **anterior longitudinal ligament** in front of Sacral promontory. • This surgery has drawback mainly **on left side** because tape has to pass below the mesentry of sigmoid colon to reach the sacral promontory. • In order to avoid it a hook of psoas muscle is made. **Drawback:** • Injury to sigmoid colon (left side) • Intestinal obstruction • Injury to ureter • Haemorrhage from mesenteric vessels • Injury to genitofemoral nerve present in psoas muscle. ***Note***: Shirodkar has more complications and that too on left side. It has better results as compared to Purandare	• In this surgery on the **Right side - shirodkar** sling is performed i.e. tape is attached to sacral promontory and on the **Left side purandare sling is performed** (as main drawback of Shirodkar sling is on left side).

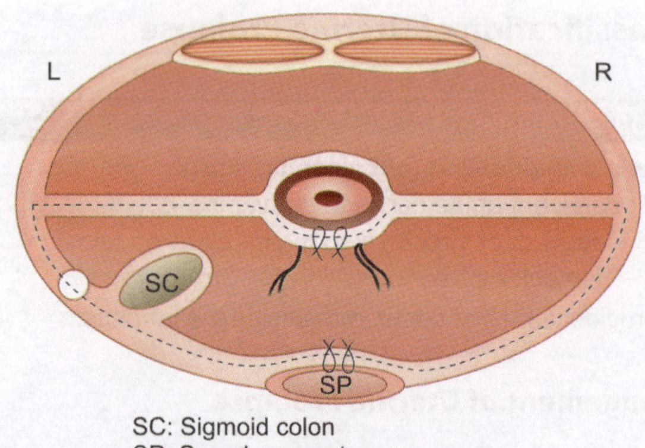

Fig. 8.5: Shirodkar sling surgery

KEY POINTS

- Goal of prolapse surgery is relief of prolapse symptoms-Over correction must be avoided as it has its own complications.
- The M/C complication of Purandare cervicopexy is deepening of pouch of douglas leading to enterocele formation. Enterocele can be prevented after purandare sling surgery by obliterating pouch of douglas at the time of operation called Moscowitz repair.

Note:

	Success Rate	Complication
Shirodkar sling	High	More (esp on left side)
Purandare sling	Low	Less

Fothergill's Repair/Manchester Operation

It is suitable for women under 40 years of age, who are desirous of retaining their menstrual function but do not desire future pregnancy.

Steps of Fothergill

1. Preliminary D and C
2. Amputation of cervix (can injure internal os or cervical stenosis)
3. Strengthening the cervix by suturing cut end of Mackenrodt ligament in front of cervix (plication of cardinal ligament)
4. Anterior Colporrhaphy
5. Colpoperineorrhaphy.

The most important steps are step 2 and 3, because of amputation of cervix. This surgery cannot be done in females who want future pregnancy.

Note: In Fothergill's surgery, the posterior lip of the amputated cervix is covered by a vaginal flap using **sturmdorf suture or by Bonney's method.**

Complications

- Cervical amputation leads to:
  - Incompetent os
  - Habitual abortion (second trimester abortions)
  - Preterm deliveries
  - Premature rupture of membranes (PROM)

  – Dutta Obs 6th/ed, p317
  - Decreased cervical fertility
- Excessive fibrosis causes stenosis leading to dystocia during labour
- Hematometra *(Very rare)*
- Recurrence of prolapse.

Note: Since all these complications of Fothergills are mainly due to amputation of cervix-**Shirodkars modification of Fothergills operation** (also called as Shirodkars uterosacral ligament advancement surgery), is done where amputation of cervix is not done, rest all steps are same as Fothergill's repair.

Sturmdorf Suture [Fig. 8.6 (2)]

It is used in Fothergill's surgery. The posterior lip of amputated cervix is covered by a vaginal flap. This is called sturmdorf suture.

Fothergill Suture [Fig. 8.6 (1)]

It helps in tieing the Mackenrodt's ligament or plicaling the Mackenrodt's ligament. The suture passes through vaginal skin → Mackenrodt's ligament → inside the cervix → up again → other side Mackenrodt's ligament & then other side of vaginal skin.

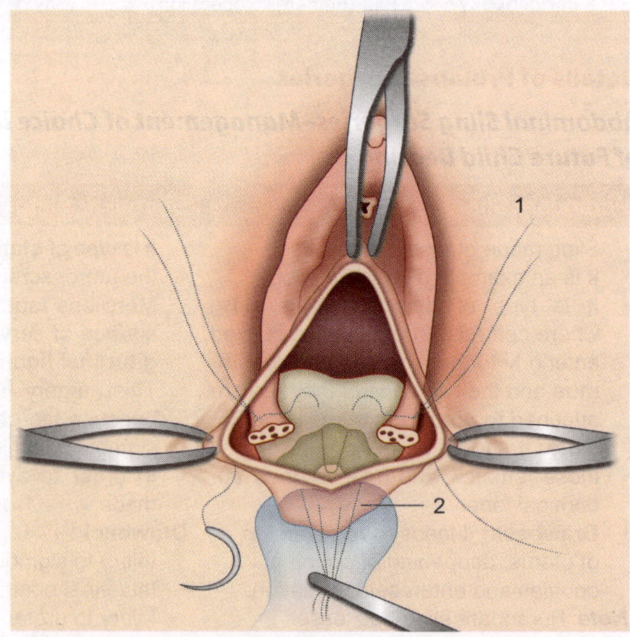

Fig. 8.6: Sturmdoff and Fothergill suture

Also Know

Apart from prolapse, the other indication for Fothergills surgery is elongation of cervix.

Ring Pessary

Pessaries are of 2 basic varieties:

- Supportive variety, e.g. ring pessary
- Space occupying variety e.g. Gellhorn pessary.

Indications for Using Pessary in Prolapse

- Prolapse during pregnancy.
- In puerperium—to facilitate involution
- Patient unfit or unwilling for surgery
- Women who have undergone atleast one previous attempt at surgical intervention without relief
  Diagnostic: It may be placed diagnostically to identify which women are at risk for urinary incontinence after prolapse correcting surgery.

Problems Associated with Pessary

- It is never curative and is only palliative
- Can cause vaginitis
- Has to be changed every 3 months
- Forgotten pessary can cause vaginal ulcerations, erosions, and fistula formation.
- May cause dyspareunia
- It does not cure stress incontinence.

Contraindication of Pessary

- Acute genital tract infections
- Adherent retroposition of uterus.

Note: For types of pessary.

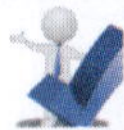

KEY POINTS

Management of 3° prolapse in pregnancy

In early months of pregnancy

(uptil 18 weeks as after that spontaneous correction occurs)

If Cervix can be replaced inside the vagina

- Cervix is to be kept inside the vagina with the help of ring pessary.
- Patients should lie with footend elevated.
- To decrease edema & congestion of the prolapsed mass-gauze soaked with acriflavine & glycerine is to be applied.

If Cervix is incarcerated & cannot be reposited

- Termination of pregnancy

In late months of pregnancy

Admit the patient at 36 weeks for safe confinement

Management of prolapse after childbirth

- Perineal exercise/Kegel's exercises
- Ring pessary
- Never do surgery within 6 months[Q] of delivery as there is always the possibility of recurrence of prolapse.[Q]

Le Forts Repair/Colpocleisis

- In females more than 60 years of age, who have medical complications like previous history of MI, hypertension and diabetes, vaginal hysterectomy is not possible as the anesthesist will not agree to give anesthesia.
- In such patients, procidentia or 3° prolapse can be managed by Le forts colpocleisis:
- In Le forts repair/colpocleisis: The vaginal epithelium is removed followed by suturing of the anterior and posterior walls of denuded vagina, thereby completely obliterating the vagina.
- The procedure is done under local anesthesia.
- Before performing this procedure, PAP smear and pelvic USG should be done to rule out cancers and pelvic pathology.
- *Note:* Le forts repair cannot be performed in young females because:
  - Their coital function will be hampered
  - Menstrual blood doesnot get way to come out after Le forts repair so blood will keep on collecting in uterine cavity leading to hematometra.

Note: In older females if sexual function is desired partial colpocleisis called as **Goodell Powel Surgery** can be done.

Vault Prolapse

- Refers to prolapse of the vaginal stump left behind after performing hysterectomy.
- Vault is the site where anterior and posterior vaginal walls are sutured. Incidence = 1–10%. It is usually accompanied by enterocele (70%.)

Degrees of vault prolapse:

- **First Degree**: The vaginal apex is visible at introitus
- **Second Degree**: The vault protrudes through introitus
- **Third Degree**: The entire vagina is outside the introitus.

Management of Vault Prolapse

Patient is fit for abdominal surgery	In obese, elderly patients, not fit for abdominal surgery
• **Transabdominal sacral colpopexy, i.e. uterosacral suspension** (Mesh is attached to the vault and sacral promontory). • It is the **Gold Standard Surgery for vault prolapse**	**Transvaginal sacrospinous ligament fixation/colpopexy** can be done. A special instrument: Miya Hook is used for the surgery. Recurrence rate—3%.

Important One Liners

- Suspension of the vault by sacrospinous colpopexy at the time of primary surgery can prevent vault prolapse.
- Uterosacral suspension is the surgery for vault prolapse but colposuspension is the surgery for stress urinary incontinenece

Extra Edge

Kegel's Exercise

Kegel's exercise are pelvic floor exercises which consists of contracting and relaxing the muscles that form part of the pelvic floor.

The aim of Kegel's exercises is to improve muscle tone by strengthening the muscles of the pelvic floor. They are good for treating first degree vaginal prolapse, preventing uterine prolapse, and to aid with child birth in females and for treating prostate pain and swelling resulting from benign prostatic hyperplasia (BPH) and prostatitis in males. These exercises reduce premature ejaculatory occurrences in men as well as increase the size and intensity of erections.

Kegel's exercises may be beneficial in treating urinary incontinence in both men and women. The treatment effect might be greater in middle aged women in their 40s and 50s with stress urinary incontinence alone.

Time for initiating Kegel's exercise in pregnant females

- In 1st trimester
- Following vaginal delivery-after 24 hours
- Following cesarean section-after 24 hours

Limitations of Kegel's exercises

—Jeffcoates 7th/ed, p286

- Kegel's exercise has a limited effect as it affects mainly voluntary muscles viz bulbocavernous, levator ani, and superficial and deep transverse perineal muscles and not the main fascial supporting tissues.

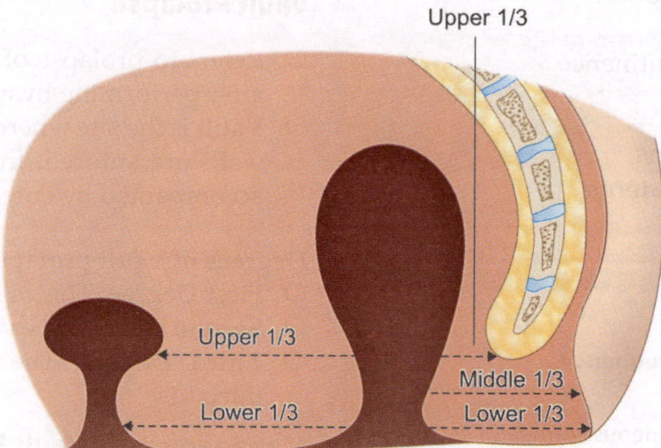

Fig. 8.7: Relationship of walls of vagina

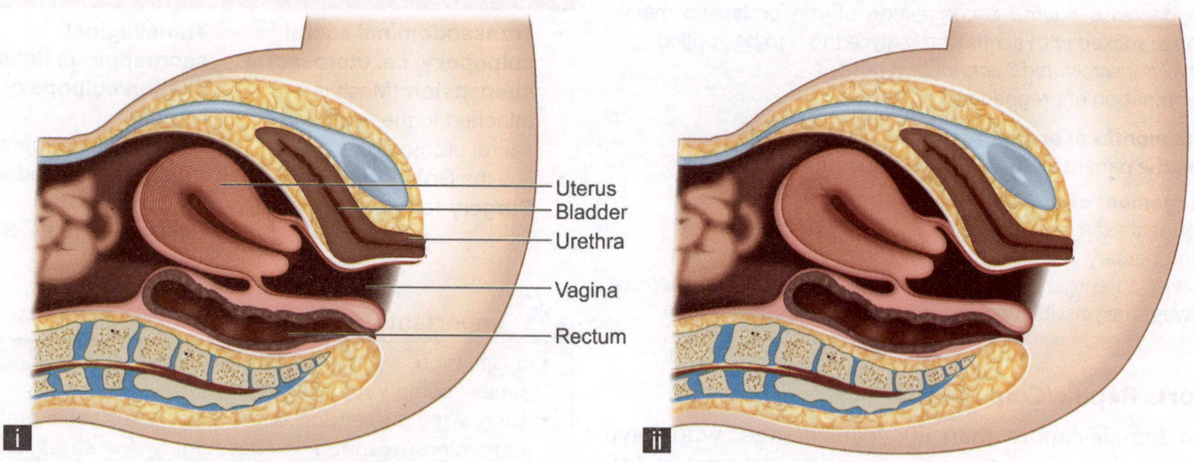

Figs. 8.8(i and ii): (i) Anterior vaginal wall prolapse; (ii) Distal posterior wall prolapse

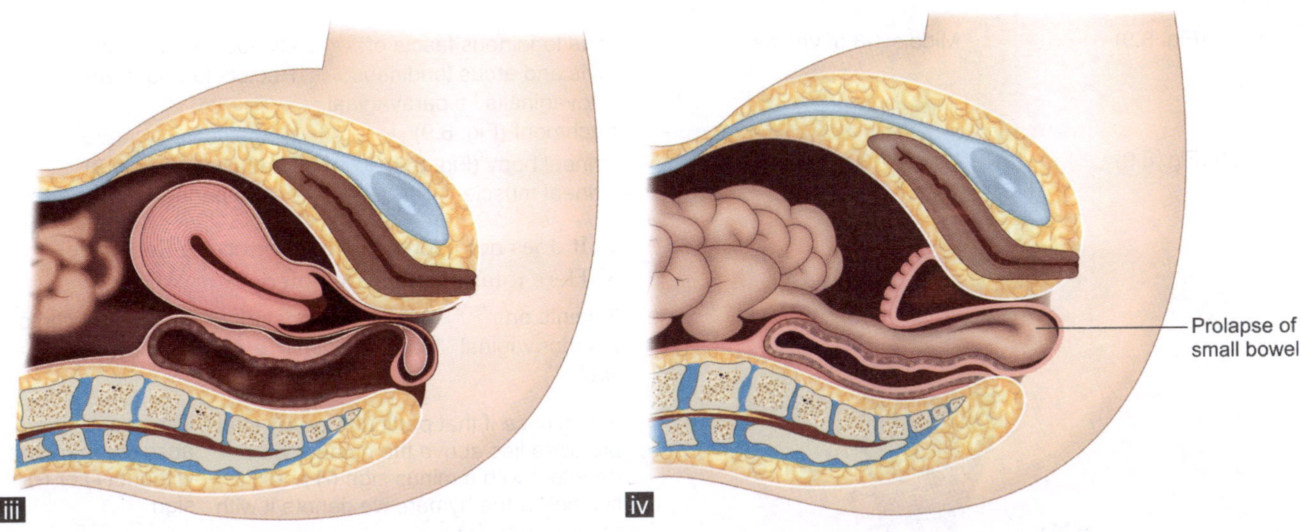

Figs. 8.8(iii and iv): (iii) Apical posterior wall prolapse; (iv) Prolapse of small bowel

Vaginal Prolapse

- Vaginal prolapse occurs basically due to defect in Endopelvic fascia

Classification of Vaginal Prolapse

Vaginal prolapse	(Figs. 8.8i to iii)
A. Anterior vaginal wall: • Upper two thirds prolapse, it is called as cystocoele/cytourethrocoele • Lower one third is called as urethrocoele	**B. Posterior vaginal wall :** • Upper one third is called enterocoele (pouch of Douglas herniates) • Middle one third is called rectocele. • Lower one third is called Laxed perineum

Management of Vaginal Prolapse

- **Management of vaginal prolapse is not dependent on age & parity of patient** (Flowchart 8.2).

Flowchart 8.2: Management of vaginal prolapse

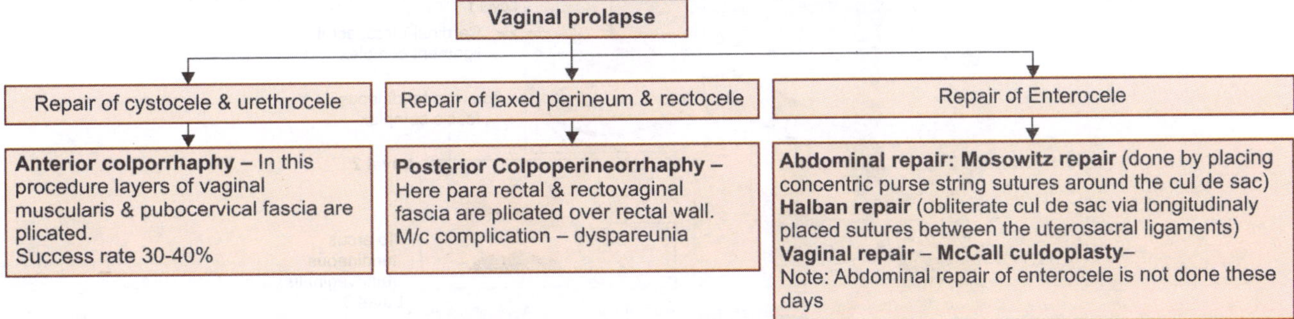

Support of Vagina – Delancey's Levels of Support (See Fig. 8.9)

Levels	Part which it is supporting	Structures supporting	Leads to
Level 1 (Fig. 8.9)	Apex of vagina/cervix	Cardinal ligament Uterosacral ligament (Fig. 8.10)	Vault prolapse Apical prolapse Elongation of cervix Enterocele (Fig. 8.9)

Contd...

Contd...

Level 2 (Fig. 8.9)	Middle 1/3 of vagina	Arcus tendineus fascia of pelvis and arcus tendineus rectovaginalis i.e paravaginal attachment (Fig. 8.9)	Cystocele (Fig. 8.8) Rectocele (Fig. 8.8)
Level 3 (Fig. 8.9)	Lower 1/3 of vagina	Perineal body (Fig. 8.9) Perineal muscle	Urethocele (Fig. 8.8) Laxed perineum (Fig. 8.8)

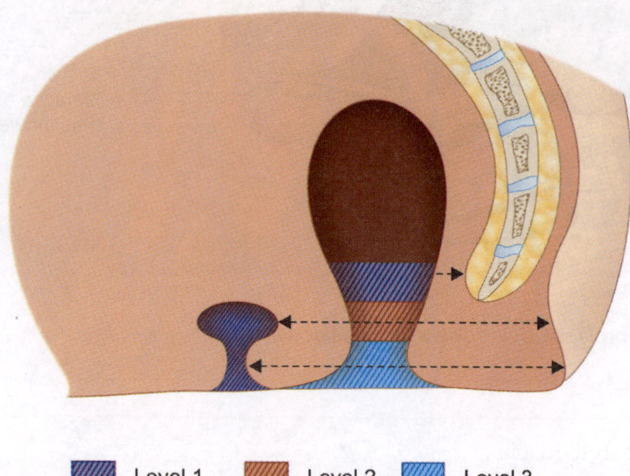

Fig. 8.9: Diagrammatic representation of Delancey's levels of defects caused by it

POP – Q Classification of Prolapse

- In this classification i.e. pelvic organ prolapse quantification (POP-Q) Classification, the reference point is **Hymen**
- It was accepted in 1996.
- It does not use terms like cystocele/Rectocele
- Here total 9 things are noted

3 points on anterior vaginal wall	3 points on posterior vaginal wall	3 measurements are noted
In this case if that particular point after prolapse lies above the hymen, we denote it with a minus sign (-) and if it lies below the hymen, we denote it with positive sign (+).		These are absolute numbers without (+) or (-) sign

Description of Points

- **Aa**: 3 cm above external urethral meatus on anterior wall of vagina. Range – 3 to +3.
- **Ba** = Most dependent part of anterior vaginal wall between Aa and anterior fornix. Range -3 to TVL.
- **C** = Cervix or vaginal cuff (after hysterectomy)
- **Ap** = 3 cm above hymen on posterior vaginal wall. Range -3 to +3 (Fig. 8.11)
- **Bp** = Most dependent part of posterior vaginal wall between Ap and posterior fornix. Range -3 to TVL. (Fig. 8.11)
- **D** = Posterior fornix (In patients of TAH, point D is removed) (Fig. 8.11)

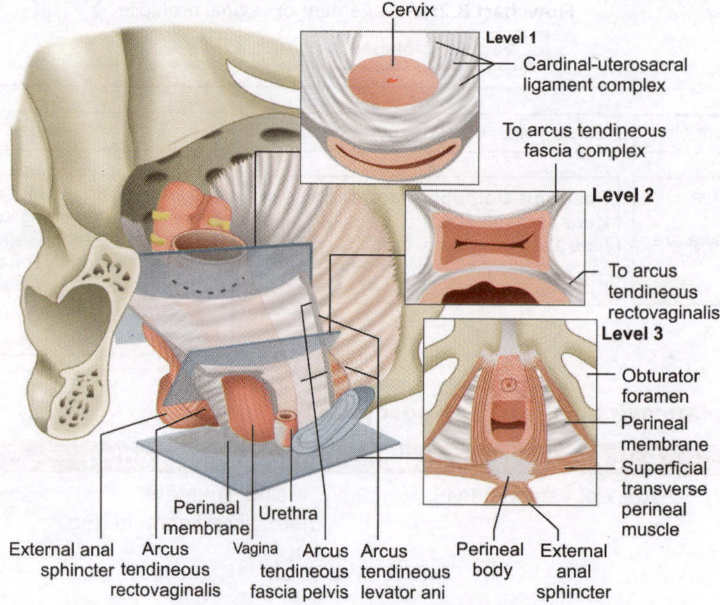

Fig. 8.10: Delancey's level of support

Three Measurements

- **Genital Hiatus (GH) measurement** from Middle of external urinary meatus to middle of Hymen (Fig. 8.12)
- Perineal Body Measurement from Middle of hymen to middle of anal opening (Fig. 8.12)
- Total vaginal length

Now these measurements are plotted on a 3 x 3 grid

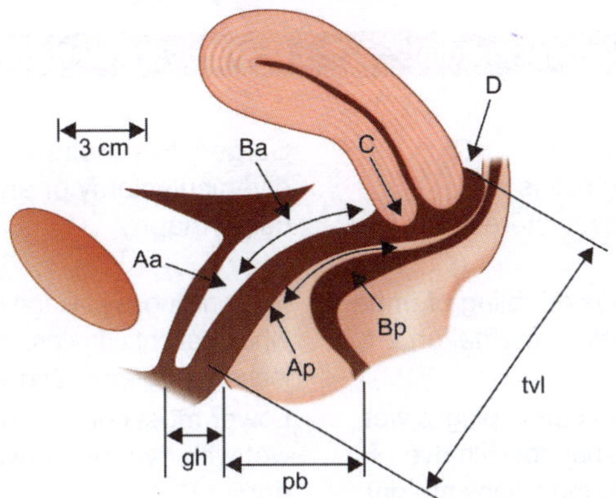

Fig. 8.11: Delancey level of support

Aa	Ba	C
GH	PB	TVL
AP	Bp	D

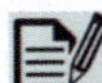

Remember

All the parts and measurements are measured with patient in dorsolithotomy position (Fig. 8.13) with patient performing Valsalva maneuver except total vaginal length where patient should be relaxed.

Note:

- Part Aa and Ba are Marker of anterior vaginal wall prolapse
- Part Ap and Bp are marker of posterior Vaginal wall prolapse
- C is a marker of uterine prolapse
- D is a marker of enterocele

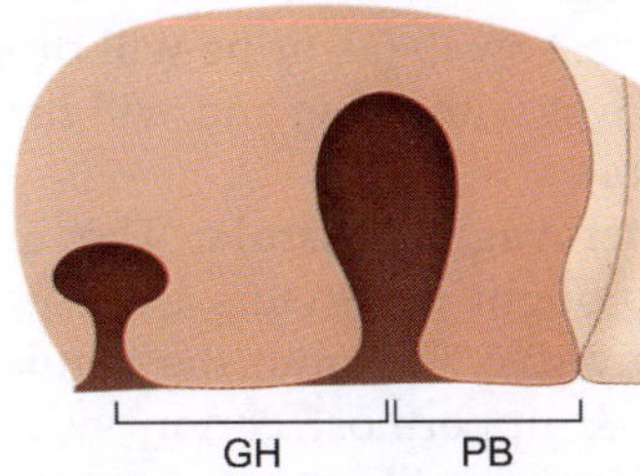

Fig. 8.12: Measurements done in POP-Q classification, GH: Genital hiatus; PB: Perineal body

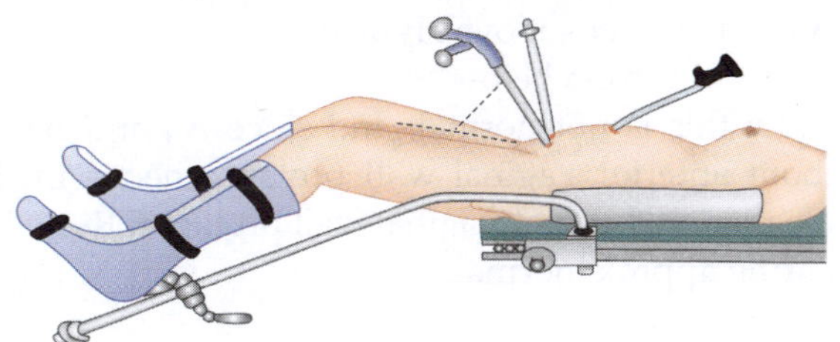

Fig. 8.13: Dorsolithotomy position

The leading parts of prolapse is noticed & staged as follows:

Staging of Prolapse

- **Stage 1**: Prolapsed part is > 1 cm above the hymen
- **Stage 2**: Prolapsed part is 1 cm on either side of Hymen
- **Stage 3**: Prolapsed part is > 1 cm below the hymen
- **Stage 4**: Procidentia i.e. complete prolapse.

Now to understand this – lets see a few examples:

Case 1

Aa –3	Ba –3	C –8
GH –2	PB –3	TVL 10
Ap –3	Bp –3	D –10

It Means

- Aa is –3 i.e. 3 cms above Hymen in this patient – which is normal (as by definition Aa is taken 3 cm above ext urethral meatus).
- Ba is = -3 = Normal
- C = is – 8 = 8 cms above Hymen is cervix
- TVL = 10 = Total vaginal length is 10 cms in this patient i.e Normal again
- Ap = -3 = Normal
- Bp = -3 = Normal
- D = -10 = i.e. posterior fornix is 10 cm

Now TVL = 10 cms & D = 10 cm i.e. everything is normal.

- Also note part C is 8 cm which again shows normal findings as normally also anterior vaginal wall is shorter than posterior vaginal wall.
- Thus this is a normal Grid i.e. Normal patient. No prolapse.

Case 2

Aa -1	Ba + 5	C -6
G1 + 4	PB 1	TVL 10
Ap -3	Bp -3	D -8

- Aa = -1 i.e. 1 cm above Hymen
- Ba = +5 i.e. 5 cm below.

Now this is not normal, and since Aa and Ba tell us about anterior vaginal wall prolapse hence in this female there is anterior vaginal wall prolapse. Rest all is appearing approx. normal.

Now in order to stage the prolapse → The leading point is seen, here since it is point B, which has prolapsed maximum we will take it as the leading point. Part B = +5 i.e. 5 cm below the hymen i.e. stage 3. So this is a case of stage 3 anterior wall prolapse.

Urinary Fistulas

	Vesicovaginal Fistula	Ureterovaginal Fistula	Urethrovaginal Fistula
M/C	VVF is the m/c urinary fistula		
Etiology	In developing countries – Obstructed labor. It is due to ischemic necrosis, so develops 3–5days after delivery. In Developed countries – hysterectomy	Hysterectomy Maximum risk is with Wertheims hysterectomy	Surgery like-urethral diverticulectomy or anterior colporrhaphy
Chief Complain	Continuous dribbling of urine from vagina + no normal urge for urination	Continuous dribbling of urine from vagina + normal urge for urination	No continuous leakage but when patient urinates, urine leaks from urethra and vagina.
Methylene blue 3 swab test (M oirs test)	Middle cotton plug is wet with dye and urine (blue in colour)	Uppermost cotton plug is wet with urine but not with dye. Other 2 cotton swabs are dry	Lower most cotton plug is wet with dye, other two are dry.
Investigation of choice	Cystoscopy	Dye test with indigo carmine demonstrates urinary extravasation and identifies the location of injury + Cystoscopy	
Management of Choice—Surgery	**Technique: Layer technique/Latzko repair** (for post-hysterectomy VVF repair) **Chassar Moir technique** **Time of repair: If it is due to obstructed labor** repair should be done **after 6 weeks.** (so that infection and inflammation subside)– *William Gynae 3/e pg 581* **If it is due to surgery:** • And is recognised within 24 hours—Immediate repair. • If recognised later—repair after **6 weeks** **Radiation fistulas** are repaired after 12 months	**Technique: Boari Flap technique** Time of repair: As early as possible	

Methylene Blue 3 Swab Test

The three swab test helps to differentiate between vesicovaginal, uretero vaginal and urethrovaginal fistula.

Procedure of 3 swab test:

- A red rubber catheter is introduced into the bladder through the urethra.
- Methylene blue dye is instilled into the bladder through catheter.
- 3 cotton swabs are placed in the vagina as follows:
  - One at vault,
  - One at the middle
  - One just above the introitus and removed after some time of instillation of dye

In case of

- **Urethrovaginal fistula:** The lower most cotton swab will get wet and will be blue in colour (as evident from Fig. 8.14).
- **Vesicovaginal fistula:** The middle swab and lower most swab (as urine will drop down) both will be wet with urine and will have blue colour (Fig. 8.14).
- **In ureterovaginal fistula:** The urine which is being brought by ureters is clear, i.e. does not have any dye. Through the fistula it will reach vagina' & uppermost cotton swab will be wet with urine but will not have any colour. (as dye is in bladder and not ureter) (Fig. 8.14).

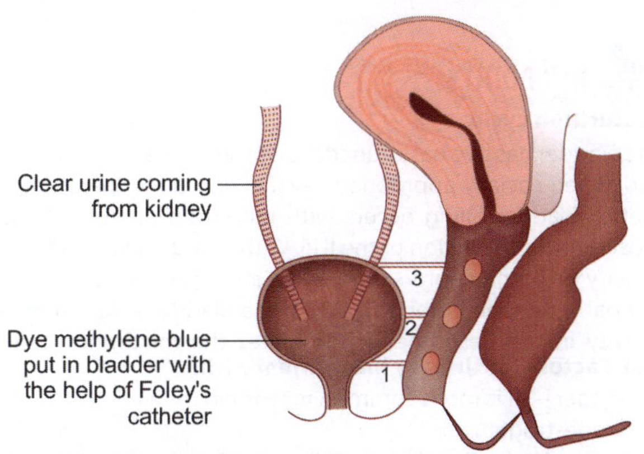

Fig. 8.14: Urinary fistulas: 1. Urethrovaginal fistula; 2. Vesicovaginal fistula; 3. Ureterovaginal fistula

Observation	Interpretation
Upper most swab soaked with urine but unstained with dye	Ureterovaginal fistula[Q]
Upper and lower swab remain dry but the middle swab soaked with dye	Vesicovaginal fistula[Q]
The upper two swab remain dry but lower one soaked with dye	Urethrovaginal fistula[Q]

Most Common in Fistulae

MC urinary fistula	Vesicovaginal[Q]
MC cause of VVF in India	Obstructed labour[Q]
MC cause of Uretero Vaginal Fistula	Injury to ureter after gynecological operation[Q] especially Wertheim' hysterectomy[Q]
MC cause of Vesico Uterine fistula	Cesarean section[Q]
MC cause of Recto Vaginal fistula	Cesarean perineal tear[Q]

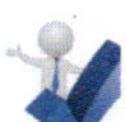

KEY POINTS

Sims Triad: For repair of VVF: **James** Sims described a method for closing very small fistula's called saucerization (where the margins of fistula are closed with interrupted sutures using silver wire without separating bladder from vagina. It is done is **SIMS position** using **SIMS speculum** so called as **SIMS triad**

New classification of Genitourinary fistulas

In this classification the Genitourinary fistulas are devided into 4 main types depending on distance of the fistulas distal edge from Ext. urinary meatus

- **Type 1**: Distal edge of fistula > 3.5 cms from Ext urinary meatus
- **Type 2**: Distal edge 2.5 – 3.5 cms from Ext urinary meatus

Contd...

Contd...

- **Type 3**: Distal edge 1.5 to < 2.5 cm from Ext urinary meatus
- **Type 4**: Distal edge < 1.5 cm from Ext urinary meatus.

Each type is further subdivided into 3 categories depending on size of fistula

- a = Size < 1.5 cm in diameter
- b = Size 1.5-3 cm in diameter
- c = Size > 3 cm in diameter

HOT TOPIC

Menouria

- It is seen in uterovesical fistulae[Q], i.e. fistula connecting uterus to bladder
- Usually follows cesarean section[Q]
- The patient complains of hematuria/passage of menstrual discharge via urethra at the time of menstruation. Patient does not have urinary incontinence.[Q]
- The fistula is between bladder and uterus– and the uterus lies at a higher level than bladder, so urine cannot go upwards against gravity, hence no urine incontinence. Rather at the time of mensturation, blood flows down and menouria is seen.
- The presence of the fistula can be demonstrated by hysterography (but not by cystography) and cystoscopy.[Q]
- Treatment is by abdominal repair.[Q]

Important One Liners

Another important cause of cyclical hematuria is endometriosis[Q] of bladder.

Rectovaginal Fistula

- **MC cause**—Complete tear of perineum repaired improperly
- **Other causes**—TB/Lymphogranuloma inguinale/ carcinoma acervix advanced stage or when RT is given in cancer cervix (takes 3 months to several years to develop)
- **Rare causes**—Congenital RV fistula; Diverticulitis rectal abscess and direct trauma.
- **Management**—Convert the fistula into complete perineal tear, repair
  - Fistula due to cancer cervix/rectum Exenteration surgery
  - Fistula due to radiation—Colpocleisis
- **Mode of delivery**—after repair of rectovaginal fistula is caesarean section.

Urine Incontinence

According to International continence society, **"incontinence" is defined as the complaints of any involuntary leakage of urine which is a social and hygienic problem to the patient.**

Physiology of Micturition

Bladder Supply

Sympathetic	Parasympathetic
Via T10 – L 2/ L3 Neurotransmitter – Norepinephrine that acts on 2 types of receptors • α receptor – located on urethra (close urethra and ↑ urine storage and continence) • β receptor- located mainly on bladder (↓ tone of bladder and urethra and promote storage of urine). (The somatic supply to bladder is mainly by pudendal nerves.)	Via S2 – S4 Neurotransmitter-acetyl choline that acts via muscarinic receptors in bladder. It promotes bladder emptying: • Contracts detrusor muscle • Relaxes urethra

KEY POINTS

Micturition cycle

The bladder has two basic functions: storing urine (sympathetic) and, when socially appropriate, evacuating urine (parasympathetic). Bladder filling occurs with relaxation of the detrusor muscle and contraction of the IUS. With bladder filling, afferent activity via baroreceptors triggers the storage reflex to maintain sympathetic tone in the IUS. When the bladder is full, afferent activity in the pelvic nerve stimulates the micturition reflex

Risk Factors for Urinary Incontinence (UI)

- Gender – UI is more common in women than men
- Hypoestrogenism
- Parity – Higher incidence of UI in multiparous females
- Repeated child birth
- Underlying medical conditions like diabetes, obesity parkinsonism, and multiple sclerosis
- Previous pelvic surgery with resultant scar formation
- Pharmacological agents like diuretics, caffeine, and anticholinergics
- Chronically increased intra- abdominal pressure as in COPD

Types of Urinary Incontinence

Stress urinary incontinence	Urge urinary incontinence	Mixed incontinence	Functional incontinence	Bypass incontinence
It is involuntary escape of urine when intra-abdominal pressure is increased as in sneezing or coughing or laughing.	Involuntary leakage accompanied by or immediately preceeded by the urge to void.	Both SUI and urge incontinence together	It is associated with cognitive, psychological or physical impairment that makes it difficult to reach the toilet.	May be caused by urogenital fistula or any congenital abnormality
It is the most common variety of urinary incontinence.	Involuntary detrusor muscle contractions are typically the cause of urge incontinence.		A useful mnemonic for functional incontinence is DIAPERS D = Delirum I = Infection A = Atrophy P = Pharmacological drugs E = Endourinopathy R = Restricted mobility S = Stool impaction	

Stress Urinary Incontinence (SUI)

- M/C type of urine incontinence in women accounting for 50–70% of cases.

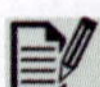

Definition

Defined as involuntary escape of urine when intra-abdominal pressure is increased as in sneezing or coughing or laughing.

SUI Can Be Due To

Bladder Neck Descent (Including urethral hypermobility) (75–80%)	Intrinsic Sphincter Defect (20–25%)
It occurs due to loss of integrity of the fibromuscular tissue that supports the bladder neck & urethra	It is diagnosed when the sphincter mechanism is compromised and fails to close the urethrovesical junction. These patients are severely incontinent.

Test for Detecting Stress Incontinence—Which Aim at Evaluating Urethral Support

- **Bonney's test:** In this test the patient is asked to insert 2 fingers, in the paraurethral region causing lifting of the bladder neck and then the patient is asked to cough. If SUI gets corrected, then it is due to bladder neck descent. If SUI persists, it is due to sphincter defect.

- **Marchetti test:** is same as Bonney's test, except that instead of fingers, two Allis forceps are used.
- **Q tip test:** A sterile cotton swab is introduced into the level of bladder neck. Then the patient is asked to strain. Marked upward elevation of cotton tip (>30°) indicates urethra hypermobility. Goniometer is used to measure the urethero - vesicle angle.

Management

- **1st line of mgt:** Pelvic floor exercise i.e. Kegel's exercises.
- **Definitive management:** Surgical management.

Earlier concept:

i. For bladder neck descent (urethral hypermobility): Surgery done was **colposuspension**.
ii. For intrinsic sphincter defect: Surgery done was pubovaginal sling surgery, e.g. aldridge, McGuire sling.

Colposuspension: See Flowchart 8.3

Flowchart 8.3

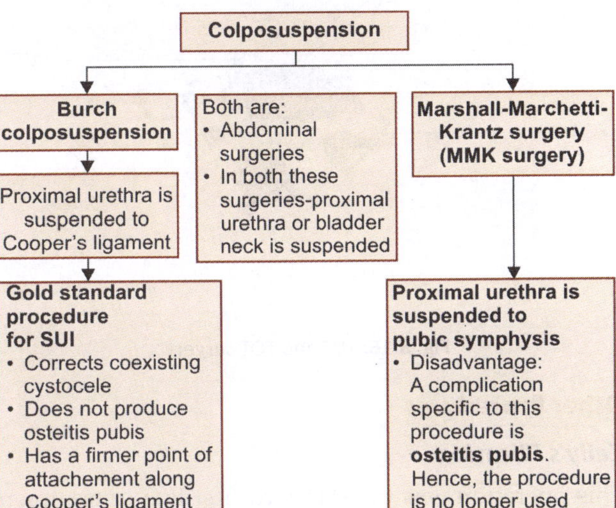

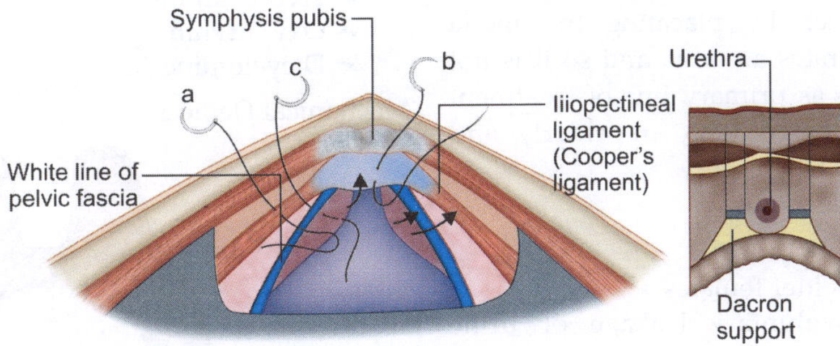

Fig. 8.15: Colposuspension surgeries

Important One Liners

Specific complication of Marshall Marchetti Krantz procedure for treating SUI is Osteitis Pubis

Current principle: These days—these surgeries have been replaced by minimally invasive synthetic midurethral slings—TVT and TOT.

Tension Free Slings (8.16)

TVT	TOT
(Tension-free vaginal tape)	**(Tension-free obturator tape)**
Common points of TVT and TOT • Both are vaginal surgeries • Both are day care surgeries • In both surgeries, midurethra is suspended	

TVT	TOT
• Devised by Nelson in 1998	• Devised by Delorne in 2001

Cont...

Cont...

TVT	TOT
• A mersilene tape is passed vaginally in a U-shaped manner under midurethra to either sides	• A multifilament polypropylene tape is passed through obturator foramen
• Retropubic space of retzius is entered, chances of bladder injury present	• Retropubic space is not entered: ∴ Less complications
• Cystoscopy should be done at the end of procedure	• It is the preferred method
• Complications: – Injury to bladder – Retropubic hematoma – Sling erosion – Overactive bladder	

Remember

Best surgery for SUI is TOT > TVT > Burch colposuspension

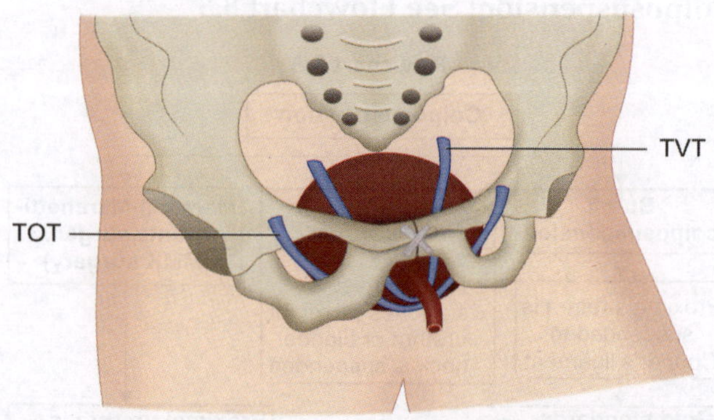

Fig. 8.16: TVT and TOT surgery

Other Procedures

Kelly's Plication

This operation was the standard first line of treatment previously. The principle was supposed to be elevation of bladder neck by placating the fascia under the urethra. Cure rates are low, and so it is not recommended nowadays as primary line of treatment but recommended in women who are elderly and medically unfit for prolonged surgery.

Urge Incontinence

- It is more common in older females.
- Characterized by involuntary leakage of urine accompanied by urgency

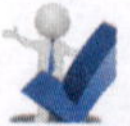

KEY POINTS

It is can be mainly due to detrusor over activity which can be

- Idiopathic (in 90% cases)
- Due to neurogenic causes like:
  - Cerebrovascular accidents
  - Alzheimer's disease
  - Multiple sclerosis
  - Parkinsonism
  - Diabetes
- Cystitis/UTI
- Bladder stones/Cancer
- Urethral obstruction

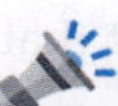

Important One Liners

Must rule out neurological cause for urge incontinence

- Multiple sclerosis
- Slipped disc
- Diabetes mellitus

Investigations

- Urine culture (to rule out infection)
- Cystourethroscopy (to rule out causes like bladder tumor/calculus)
- **Cystometry**

Management

Urge incontinence is best treated by behavioural therapy and anti-cholinergic drugs (to decrease detrusor contractions).

- **Anti-cholinergic drugs** used are:
  - Tolterodine
  - Hyoscyamine
  - Oxybutynin
  - Dicyclomine

Mechanical Devices

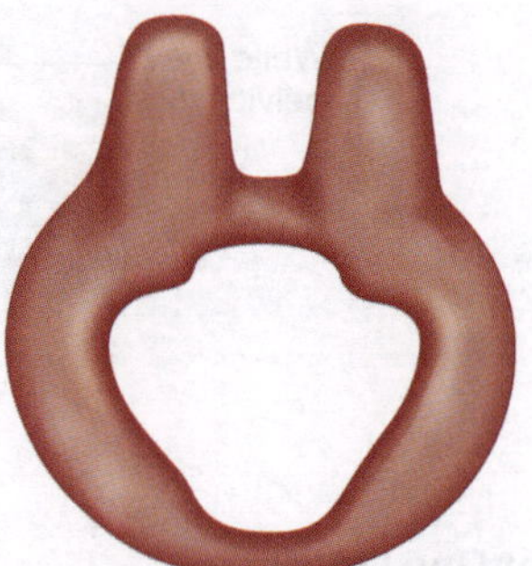

Fig. 8.17: Intriol

Vaginal: Intriol (Fig. 8.17) and continence guard (Fig. 8.18)

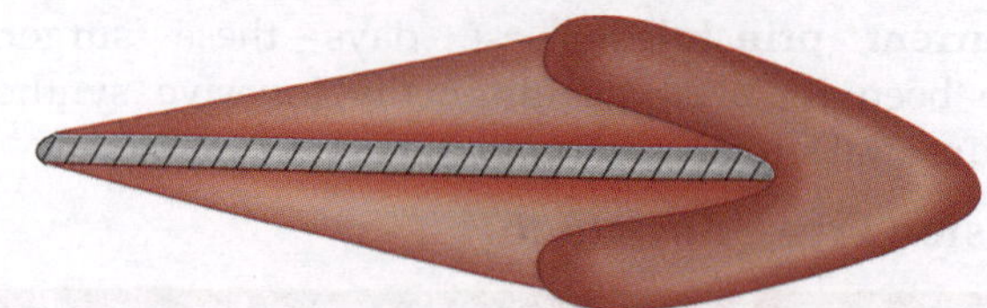

Fig. 8.18: Continence guard.

NEW PATTERN QUESTIONS

N1. The most important support of pelvic viscera is:
a. Levator ani muscle
b. Suspensory ligaments
c. Uterosacral ligament
d. Cardinal ligament

N2. All of the following support the uterus *except*:
a. Cardinal ligament b. Broad ligament
c. Pubocervical ligament d. Round ligament

N3. All of the following support uterus *except*:
a. Cardinal ligament
b. Round ligament
c. Pubocervical ligament
d. Mackenrodt's ligament

N4. Birth trauma is a risk factor for:
a. Endometriosis b. Prolapse
c. Abortion d. PID

N5. Childbirth trauma leading to urine incontinence is seen least in females with:
a. Android pelvis b. Anthropoid pelvis
c. Gynecoid pelvis d. Platypelloid pelvis

N6. In Baden Walker halfway system of classification of prolapse, the reference point is:
a. Hymen b. Introitus
c. Internal os d. External os

N7. Urinary symptoms of procidentia:
a. Frequency of micturition
b. Retention of urine
c. Stress incontinence
d. All of the above

N8. All of following are Type of urinary fistula *except*:
a. Ureterovaginal b. Vesicovaginal
c. Ureterouterine d. Urethro uterine

N9. In anterior colporrhaphy, the best method of suture apposing the vaginal flaps is:
a. Interrupted b. Continuous
c. Interlocking d. Interrupted mattress

N10. Enterocele formation is a common complication of:
a. Shirodkar sling b. Purandare sling
c. Virkud sling d. Khanna sling

N11. All of the following surgeries are done in vault prolapse *except*:
a. Uterosacral suspension
b. Colposuspension
c. Sacral colpopexy
d. Sacrospinous ligament fixation

N12. All of the following pairs are correctly matched *except*:
a. Uterine prolapse – Vaginal hysterectomy
b. Rectocele – Posterior colporrhaphy
c. Cystocele – Colposuspension
d. Vault prolapse – Sacrospinous fixation

N13. Latzko operation is done for:
a. VVF b. Ureterovaginal fistula
c. Urethrovaginal fistula d. All of the above

N14. The following are recognised surgical treatments for SUI *except*:
a. Laparoscopic colposuspension
b. Periurethral injection of collagen
c. TOT
d. Posterior colporrhaphy

N15. All of the following surgeries are done in SUI *except*:
a. Shirodkar sling
b. Aldridge sling
c. Kellys stitch
d. Marshall Marchetti Krantz

N16. Regarding the sling procedure for Urodynamic Stress Incontinence (USI):
a. Tension-free vaginal tape (TVT) elevates the bladder neck to a retropubic position
b. TVT is an autologous sling material
c. Intrinsic sphincter deficiency is an indication
d. Success rate of TVT is low than other retropubic procedures

N17. Complications of sling procedures (TVT) for USI are all *except*:
a. Injury to bladder and wound haematoma
b. Sling erosion particularly with polytetrafluoroethylene (Goretex)
c. Overactive bladder in about 7% cases
d. Obturator nerve injury is about 10%

N18. Baldy Webster operation is done in case of:
a. Congenital prolapse
b. Retroversion of uterus
c. Inversion of uterus
d. Prolapse in females <40 yrs of age

N19. A 26-year-old nulliparous female with third degree uterine prolapse but no cystocele and no rectocele is best treated by:
a. Abdominal sling surgery
b. Le fort colpocleisis
c. Fothergills repair d. Amputation of cervix

N20. The instrument shown in figure is used to measure:

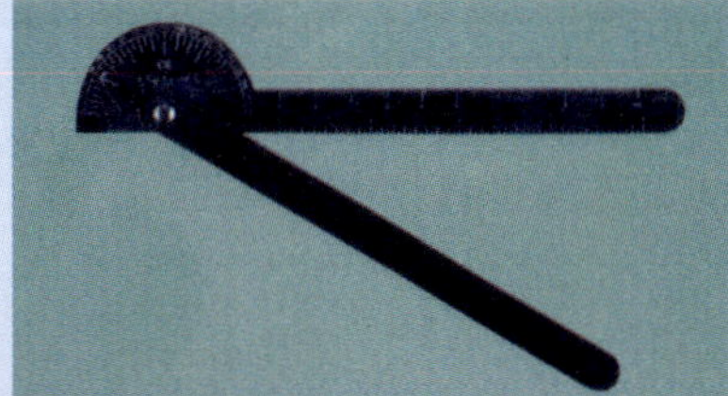

a. Urethrovesical angle b. Angle of arteflexion
c. Angle of Anteversion
d. Angle of vagina with horizontal

N21. The instrument shown in figure is used for:

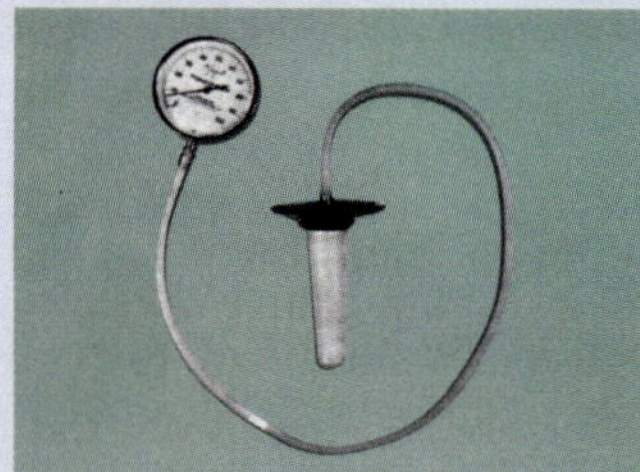

a. Kegel's exercise
b. Retroversion
c. Prolapse
d. Measuring rectal pressure

N22. The pessary shown in Figure is used for:

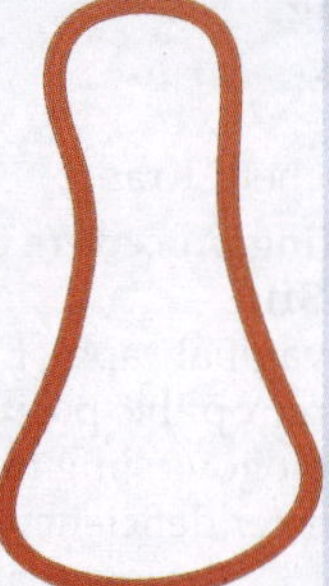

a. Prolapse of uterus
b. Stress urinary incontinence
c. Retroversion of uterus
d. Inversion of uterus

N23: A 65-year-old female has 3rd degree UV prolapse with a large decubitus ulcer. She gives history of urinary retention several times. What is the next step in management?

a. Manchester repair
b. Le fort repair
c. Insertion of ring pessary and application of estrogen cream
d. Vaginal hysterectomy

N24. All of the following are done in case of VVF *except*:

a. Methylene blue 3 swab test
b. Urine culture
c. Cystoscopy
d. MRI

N25. A VVF with leading point 2 cm from Ext urinary meatus is classified as:

a. Type 1
b. Type 2
c. Type 3
d. Type 4

PREVIOUS YEAR QUESTIONS

1. **A 30-year-old multipara has uterine prolapse, the management of choice is:** *(AIIMS Nov 99)*
   a. Fothergill's repair
   b. Fothergill's repair with tubal ligation
   c. Sling operation
   d. Vaginal hysterectomy
2. **A 28-year-old female P3, has IInd degree of utero-vaginal prolapse. The management of choice is:** *(AIIMS Dec 97)*
   a. Fothergill's repair
   b. Wertheim's hysterectomy
   c. Perineal exercises x 3 month
   d. Vaginal hysterectomy with vault repair
3. **A lady with prolapsed uterus after Fothergill's repair will complain of following *except*:** *(AIIMS Nov 00)*
   a. First trimester abortion
   b. Cervical dystocia
   c. Premature labour
   d. Premature rupture of membrane
4. **Fourteen weeks pregnancy with third degree prolapse. Best management will be:** *(AIIMS Dec 98)*
   a. Sling surgery b. Foot end elevation
   c. Ring pessary d. No treatment
5. **Most common cause of vesicovaginal fistula in India is:** *(AIIMS Nov 02)*
   a. Gynae surgery b. Irradiation
   c. Obstructed labour d. Trauma
6. **Kamla, a 48-year-old lady underwent hysterectomy. On the seventh day, she developed fever, burning micturation and continuous urinary dribbling. She can also pass urine voluntarily. The diagnosis is:** *(AIIMS May 01)*
   a. Vesicovaginal fistula b. Urge incontinence
   c. Stress incontinence d. Ureterovaginal fistula
7. **Postpartum VVF is best repaired after:** *(AIIMS 87)*
   a. 6 weeks b. 8 weeks
   c. 3 months d. 6 months
8. **Ureter is identified at operation by:** *(AIIMS 96)*
   a. Rich arterial plexus b. Peristaltic movement
   c. Relation to lumber plexus
   d. Accompanied by renal vein
9. **Most important structure preventing uterine prolapse is:**
   a. Round ligament b. Broad ligament
   c. Cardinal ligament d. Uterosacral ligament
10. **Cause of decubitus ulcer in uterine prolapse is:** *(PGI Dec 99)*
    a. Friction b. Venous congestion
    c. Intercourse d. Trauma
11. **Indication of Manchester operation in prolapse:** *(PGI Dec 03)*
    a. Nulliparous
    b. Women of < 35 years age
    c. Patient who wants child bearing function
    d. Congenital elongation of cervix
12. **Most common site of obstetric injury leading to uretero vaginal fistula:** *(PGI 96)*
    a. Infundibulo pelvic ligament
    b. Vaginal vault
    c. Ureteric tunnel
    d. Below cardinal ligament where uterine artery crosses
13. **Treatment of genuine stress incontinence:** *(PGI Dec 04)*
    a. Anterior colporrhaphy
    b. Posterior colporrhaphy
    c. Colposuspension
    d. Pelvic floor exercise
    e. Sling operation
14. **Cause(s) of retention of urine in reproductive age group:** *(PGI Dec 00)*
    a. Cervical fibroid
    b. Retroverted gravid uterus
    c. Unilateral hydronephrosis
    d. Severe UTI
    e. Posterior urethral valve
15. **Which is true regarding retroverted uterus?** *(PGI Dec 01)*
    a. May present congenitally
    b. Associated with endometriosis
    c. It is a cause of infertility
    d. Causes menorrhagia
    e. Associated with PID
16. **Most common genital prolapse is:** *(AI 02)*
    a. Cystocoele b. Procidentia
    c. Rectocoele d. Enterocoele
17. **Shirodkar sling operation may be associated with all complications *except*:**
    a. Enterocele
    b. Subacute intestinal obstruction
    c. Ureteral injury
    d. Paraesthesia over inner aspect
18. **Kegel's exercise should begin:**
    a. Immediately after delivery
    b. 24 hrs after delivery
    c. 3 weeks after delivery
    d. 6 weeks after delivery
19. **A 65-year-old P3+0 female complains of procidentia. She has past history significant of MI and is diabetic and hypertensive. Ideal management of prolapse in the patient is:**
    a. Cervicopexy b. Vaginal hysterectomy
    c. Wait and watch d. Le Fort's repair
20. **Best management of vault prolapse is:**
    a. Sacral colpopexy
    b. Sacrospinous ligament fixation
    c. Le forts repair
    d. Anterior colporrhaphy

21. The most appropriate method for collecting urine for culture in case of vesicovaginal fistula is: *(AI 04)*
a. Suprapubic needle aspiration
b. Midstream clean catch
c. Foley's catheterisation d. Sterile speculum

22. Most useful investigation for VVF is: *(AI 10)*
a. Three swab test b. Cystoscopy
c. Urine culture d. IVP

23. Chassar Moir technique is used in: *(AMU 05)*
a. VVF b. Stress incontinence
c. Urethrocoele d. Enterocoele

24. In a case of incontinence of urine, dye filled into the urinary bladder does not stain the pad in the vagina, yet the pad is soaked with clear urine. Most likely diagnosis is: *(UPSC 00)*
a. VVF b. Ureterovaginal fistula
c. Urinary stress incontinence
d. Urethero - vaginal fistula

25. A case of obstructed labor which was delivered by Cesarean section complains of cyclical passage of menstrual blood in urine. Which is the most likely site of fistula? *(AI 04)*
a. Uretherovaginal b. Vesico-vaginal
c. Vesico-uterine d. Uretero-uterine

26. Multipara with LSCS, presents With Cyclical Hematuria, Diagnosis can be: *(PGI Dec 08)*
a. VVF b. UVF
c. Bladder endometriosis d. Ca. Cervix

27. The recommended non surgical treatment of stress incontinence is: *(AI 09)*
a. Pelvic floor muscle exercises
b. Bladder training
c. Electrical stimulation d. Vaginal cone/weights

28. Kelly's plication operation is done in: *(PGI June 05)*
a. Stress incontinence b. Vault prolapse
c. Rectal prolapse d. Uterine prolapse
e. Cervical incontinence

29. Bonney's test demonstrates:
a. Stress urinary incontinence
b. Urge incontinence
c. Overflow d. All of the above

30. Which of the following surgeries for stress incontinence has highest success rate? *(AI 2011)*
a. Bursch colposuspension
b. Pereyra sling
c. Kelly's stitch
d. Tension free vaginal tape (TVT)

31. Among the surgeries to correct SUI, the long-term success rate is maximum with: *(AI 2002, 2011)*
a. Burch's colposuspension
b. Stamey's repair
c. Kelly's stitch d. Aldridge surgery

32. Site of placement of tension free vaginal tapes in stress urinary incontinence: *(PGI May 2013)*
a. At ureterovaginal junction
b. At urethrovaginal junction
c. At upper part of urethra
d. At middle part of urethra
e. At lower part of urethra

33. The disadvantage of Marshall Marchetti Krantz procedure compared with other surgical alternatives for treatment of stress urinary incontinence includes:
a. Urinary retention
b. Increased incidence of urinary tract infections
c. High failure rate
d. Osteitis pubis

34. A woman treated for infertility, presents with 6 week amenorrhea with urinary retention. The most likely etiology is: *(AI 00)*
a. Retroverted uterus b. Pelvic hematocele
c. Impacted cervical fibroid
d. Carcinoma cervix

35. Which of these is not a support of the uterus?
a. Urogenital diaphragm *(AIIMS May 2015)*
b. Pelvic diaphragm
c. Perineal body d. Rectovaginal septum

36. A lady underwent vaginal hysterectomy for Carcinoma cervix. Following the surgery after her urethral catheter was removed, she complained of urinary incontinence. On examination she has normal voiding as well as continuous incontinence. Methylene blue dye was instilled in her bladder through her urethra and she was given oral Phenazopyridine dye. After some time her pads were checked and it showed yellow staining at the top most pad, while the middle or bottom pads were unstained. She is likely to have:
a. Ureterovaginal fistula b. Vesicovaginal fistula
c. Urethrovaginal fistula d. Vesicouterine fistula

37 All of the following are SLING operation for uterine prolapse *except*:
a. Khanna b. Shirodkar
c. Abdomino cervicopexy
d. Manchester

38 Urinary incontinence in females is best investigated by: *(JIPMER May 2015)*
a. Cystometry b. Colonoscopy
c. Colposcopy d. Cystoscopy

39. Symptoms suggestive of Genuine Stress Incontinence is caused by:
a. Iliohypogastric nerve b. Inferior gluteal nerve
c. Pudendal nerve d. Genito Femoral nerve

40. Vaginal prolapse following abdominal hysterectomy is/are caused by damage of: *(PGI May 2017)*
a. Level I support b. Level II support
c. Level III support d. Urogenital diaphragm

41. Anterior colporrhaphy and colpoperineorrhaphy is know as: *(JIPMER 2012)*
a. Ward Mayo surgery b. Shirodkar repair
c. Manchester repair d. Pelvic floor repair

42. Main support of uterus is by: *(JIPMER 2011)*
a. Mackenrodt's ligament b. Broad ligament
c. Uterosacral ligament d. Round ligament

ANSWERS TO NEW PATTERN QUESTIONS

N1. **Ans. is a, i.e. Levator ani muscle**

N2. **Ans. is b, i.e. Broad ligament**

N3. **Ans. is b, i.e. Round ligament**

Remember

- Most important support of uterus is levator ani muscle
- Most important ligament supporting the uterus—Cardinal ligament/Mackenrodt's ligament
- Round ligament is a secondary support of the uterus as it does not support it directly but helps to keep it in anteverted position
- Broad ligament is a fold of peritoneum and does not support the uterus at all.

Note: Hence answer to question no. N2 is 'Broad Ligament' and question no. N3 where all other supports are primary supports, the answer is 'round ligament' which is only a secondary support.

N4. **Ans. is b, i.e. Prolapse**

N5. **Ans. is a, i.e. Android pelvis** *Ref: Dutta Gynae 6th/ed, p399*

Childbirth trauma causes damage of the pelvic floor and pubocervical fascia leading to urinary continence. The injury is more common in gynecoid and least in android pevis.

N6. **Ans. is a, i.e. Hymen** *Ref: Jeffcoates 8th/ed, p253*

Bader Walker Halfway's system of grading of prolapse is similar to Shaw's classification but uses the hymen as a reference point.

N7. **Ans. is d, i.e. All of the above** *Ref: Dutta Gyane 6th/ed, p208*

All the urinary symptoms given in the options can occur in case of prolapse.

"Retention of urine may rarely occur." *Ref: Dutta Gyane 6th/ed, p208*

N8. **Ans. is d, i.e. Urethro uterine**

Come on! You don't want me to explain that why urethro uterine fistula is not possible anatomically.

N9. **Ans. is a, i.e. Interrupted** *Ref: Dutta Gynae 6th/ed, p213*

The cut margins of the vagina are repaired by interrupted sutures.

N10. **Ans. is b, i.e. Purandare sling** *Ref: Dutta Gynae 6th/ed, p404*

Enterocele formation occurs with Purandare sling.

N11. **Ans. is b, i.e. Colposuspension**

Colposuspension i.e. Bursh colposuspension is done in SUI.

N12. **Ans. is c, i.e. Cystocele–Colposuspension**

Colposuspension (Burch colposuspension) is not a surgery for vault prolapse. It is done in SUI. Rest all surgeries are done in vault prolapse. Surgery for cystocele is Anterior colporrhaphy.

N13. **Ans. is a, i.e. VVF.**

Latzko repair/Chassar Moir technique/ Layer technique are all for repairing VVF.

N14. **Ans. is d, i.e. Posterior colporrhaphy**

Posterior colporrhaphy is done for managing rectocele.

N15. **Ans. is a, i.e. Shirodkar sling**

Surgeries done for SUI—Earlier

- Aldridge sling
- McGuire sling
- Kelly's stitch
- Marshall Marchetti Krantz surgery

Surgeries done for SUI—Now-a-days

Best – TOT
2nd Best – TVT
3rd Best – Burch colposuspension

N16. Ans. is c, i.e. Intrinsic sphincter deficiency is an indication

Lets see each option:

TVT acts by increasing urethral coaptation, kinking the urethra with the rise in abdominal pressure and not by elevating bladder neck hence option a is incorrect.

TVT is made from polypropylene (marlex) or polytetrafluoroethylene (Goretex) and not autologous sling material. Autologus sling material refers to natural sling materials made from rectus fascia or porcine dermis. These are less Antigenic; hence option b is incorrect.

TVT is done in case of intrinsic sphincter deficiency, i.e option c is correct.

Success rate of sling procedure are over 80%, i.e option d is incorrect

N17. Ans. is d, i.e. Obturator nerve injury is about 10% *Ref: Ieffwates 8th/ed, p803*

Complications of TVT are:

a. Injury to bladder
b. Retropubic hematoma
c. Sling erosion
d. Overactive bladder.

N18. Ans. is b, i.e. Retroversion of uterus *Ref: Jeffcoates 8th/ed, p274*

Surgeries for Retroversion:

- Baldy Webster operation
- Modified Gilliam's operation
- Laparoscopic ventrosuppression

Since round ligament helps to keep uterus in anteverted position in all these surgeries, round ligaments are tightened.

N19. Ans. is a, i.e. Abdominal sling surgery

Best surgery for prolapse when a female wants to conceive in future is – Abdominal sling surgery.

N20. Ans. is a, Urethrovesical angle *Ref: Novak Gynaecology 8th/ed, p918*

The instrument shown is a goniometer, which is used to measure baseline urethral angle and maximum strain angle of the urethra with a cotton tip swap in place.

N21. Ans. is a, Kegel's exercise *Ref: Jeffcoates 8th/ed, p883*

The instrument shown in the figure is a Kegel Perineometer used for pelvic floor exercise, i.e. –Kegel exercises.

It consists of a vaginal obturator with an air-containing sleeve connected to a manometer which measures the strength of vaginal muscle.

N22. Ans. is c, Retroversion of uterus *Ref: Jeffcoates 8th/ed, p882–883*

The pessary shown in is **Hodge pessary**. Hodge pessary is used for treating retroversion.

Indications of Hodge Pessary in Retroverted uterus:

1. Mobile retroversion of uterus (pessary is of no use in fixed retroversion)
2. Pessary test
3. During pregnancy.

N23. Ans. is c, i.e. Insertion of ring pessary and application of estrogen cream

Since this female has a decubitus ulcer, we cannot perform surgery immediately so we will insert ring pessary and apply estrogen cream and wait for decubitus ulcer to heal.

N24. Ans. is d, i.e. MRI *Ref: Shaw 16th/ed, p221 & 222*

The Investigation done in VVF are:

- **Urine culture**
- USG
- IVP
- Cystoscopy
- Methylene blue 3 swab test

N25. Ans. is c, i.e. Type 3 *Ref: William gynae 3/e p578*

See the text for explanation.

ANSWERS TO PREVIOUS YEAR QUESTIONS

1. **Ans. is b, i.e. Fothergill's repair with tubal ligation** *Ref: Shaw 15th/ed, p339; Jeffocate 7th/ed, p289*
2. **Ans. is a, i.e. Fothergill's repair** *Ref: Shaw 15th/ed, p339; Jeffocate 7th/ed, p289*

   Fothergill's operation (Manchester Repair) is done in women below 40 years, who want to retain their menstrual function.

   In both questions 1 and 2 patients are less than 40 years and multiparous so, Fothergill's repair is the ideal management for them.

   Fothergill's repair causes complications of pregnancy like incompetent os, habitual abortion and cervical dystocia therefore in a multipara who have completed their family we can do tubal ligation to prevent pregnancy.

   "If the family is completed, vaginal sterlization is to be done." *Ref: Dutta Gynae 6th/ed, p216*

   Thus in question 1 answer is Fothergill's repair with tubal ligation
3. **Ans. is a, i.e. First trimester abortion** *Ref: Shaw 15th/ed, p339-340; Dutta Obs 6th/ed, p169-170, 317*

   In Fothergills repair cervical amputation is done which leads to
   - Incompetent os
     - Habitual abortion (second trimester abortion and not first trimester, as incompetent os leads to second trimester abortion) *Ref: Dutta Obs 6th/ed, p169-170*
     - Preterm deliveries
     - Premature rupture of membranes *Ref: Dutta Obs 6th/ed, p317*
     - Other complications are decreased cervical fertility
   - Excessive fibrosis causes stenosis leading to dystocia during labour.
   - Hematometra (Very rare)
   - Recurrence of prolapse

   Note: Since all these complications of Fothergill's are mainly due to amputation of cervix-**Shirodkar's modification of Fothergills operation** (also called as Shirodkar's uterosacral ligament advancement surgery), is being done where amputation of cervix is not done, rest all steps are same as Fothergills repair.
4. **Ans. is c, i.e. Ring pessary**

   Ref: Dutta Obs 6th/ed, p312-3; Shaw 15th/ed, p337-8; Williams Gynae 1st/ed, p545-7 (for details of pessaries)

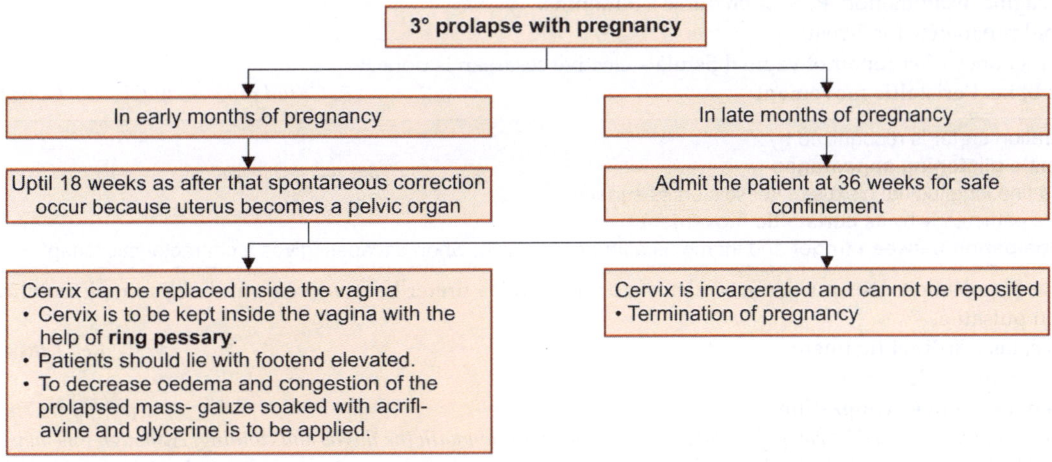

5. **Ans. is c, i.e. Obstructed labour** *Ref: Shaw 15th/ed, p184; William Gynae 1st/ed, p573*

   "In developing countries, 90% of genitourinary fistulas arise from obstetric trauma, specifically from prolonged or obstructed labor." *Ref: William Gynae 1st/ed, p573*

   Most common Genital Fistula is vesico vaginal fistula and so above statement holds good for VVF also.

   The fistula resulting from pressure during long and difficult labour always involve the trigone of the bladder.[Q]

   Whereas – "In developed countries, latrogenic injury during pelvic surgery is responsible for 90% of VVF. In industrialized countries, hysterectomy is the most common surgical cause of VVF, accounting for approximately 75% of fistula cases. Laparoscopic hysterectomies were associated with the greatest incidence followed be abdominal and vaginal." *Ref: Williams Gynae 1st/ed, p573*
6. **Ans. is d, i.e. Ureterovaginal fistula** *Ref: Jeffcoate 7th/ed, p263,265*
   - Continuous dribbling of urine following hysterectomy points towards urinary fistulas as the diagnosis.

- In case of urinary fistulas, if the patient never needs to void as there is continuous dribbling it signifies that the fistula communicates with the bladder. If, there is filling and emptying of bladder along with the fistula, it suggests fistula opening into one ureter i.e. Ureterovaginal fistula.[Q]
- As far as urethral fistula are concerned, they give little trouble because the urethra is normally empty of urine. However during micturition urine passes through the fistula and may then fill the vagina to dribble during body movements for a short time afterwards.

This patient is developing symptoms on the ***seventh day*** *can be explained by : "Fistulas resulting from accidental, surgical and obstetrical trauma are produced in two ways. They can be caused by* ***direct injury*** *such as cuts and then they* ***manifest themselves immediately*** *by hematuria and incontinence. Alternatively, if they are the outcome of* ***pressure necrosis*** *or of* ***ischemia,*** *in such a case urinary incontinence, fever and burning micturition develops 7-14 days after the accident."* *Ref: Jeffcoate 7th/ed, p263*

Before concluding let's rule out other options as well:
- In stress incontinence, dribbling of urine occurs only when intra-abdominal pressure is raised.
- In urge in continence, the patient has urge to void urine at a moment's notice and she is unable to control her bladder and passes urine instantly.

7. **Ans. is c, i.e. 3 months** *Ref: Shaw 15th/ed, p187; TB of Gynecology shiela Balakrishnan 335*

Management of VVF is: Surgical management:

Timing of surgery—
- Small urinary fistulas sometimes heal spontaneously during the first few weeks.
- However, in a case of established fistula – it is better to wait for about 3 months[Q] for all tissue inflammation to subside. If one attempt fails to heal fistula, second attempt is done after 3 months.[Q]
- In fistulas following surgery, if it is recognized within 24 hrs-repair immediately but if not then waiting period is 3–6 months.
- In fistulas following radiation – 2 years time can be taken before inflammation subsides.

Techniques of Repair
- Layer technique
- Latzko procedure (for fistulas following hysterectomy)
- Chassar Moir technique.[Q]

Post-operative Management—
- Continuous bladder drainage for 14 days.[Q]
- Antibiotic coverage.
- No vaginal examination, P/S, intercourse x 3 months.
- Avoid pregnancy for 2 years.
- In pregnancy after repair of vaginal fistula – elective cesarean is done.[Q]

8. **Ans. is b, i.e. Peristaltic movement** *Ref: Stud progress in Obs and Gynae Vol 16, p306*

At operation ureter is recognized by:
- Its **pale glistening appearance**
- By a fine longitudinal plexus of vessels on its surface
- More particularly by its **peristaltic movement**
- **By palpation between finger** and thumb as a firm cord which, when escapes, gives a characteristic 'snap'.

Absence of pulsation does not serve to identify a structure as ureter because veins and obliterated umbilical artery are also non pulsatile.

9. **Ans. is c, i.e. Cardinal ligament** *Ref: Jeffcoate 7th/ed, p46*

See the text for explanation.

10. **Ans. is b, i.e. Venous congestion** *Ref: Jeffcoate 7th/ed, p279-280*

"Ulceration of the prolapsed tissue is often said to be caused by friction with the thighs and clothing. Although this may be partly true, it is notable that the ulcer is nearly always on the most dependant part of the cervix or vagina and not at the sides where friction is greatest. It is to be regarded, therefore more as a result of circulatory and nutritional changes than of trauma."

Treatment of decubitus ulcer: Reduction of the prolapse into the vagina and daily packing with glycerine and acriflavine. Acryflavin is an antiseptic agent while glycerine is a hygroscopic agent.

Also know: Other important points to remember in symptoms of prolapse
- Backache in patents of prolapse is due to the stretching of uterosacral ligaments.
- Genuine stress incontinence is seen in patients of prolapse
- Cancer of cervix or vagina is rarely seen, even in untreated cases of prolapse.

11. **Ans. is b, i.e. Women of < 35 years age**

Ref: Shaw 15th/ed, p339; Principles and Practice of Obs & Gynae for PG's Pankaj Desai 3rd/ed, p559

Fothergill's repair/Manchester operation

"It is suitable for women under 40 years who are desirous of retaining their menstrual and reproductive function."

Ref: Shaw 14th/ed, p305; 15th/ed, p339

This means options b and c both are correct. But though this operation was initially advocated for young women desirous of child bearing, now the view has changed:

"Cervical amputation may adversely affect subsequent conception (infertility, cervical stenosis) and/or pregnancy outcome (repeated IInd trimester abortion, preterm labor, cervical dystocia). For these reasons, this repair is not considered as an operation of the choice in India" (for child bearing function). *– Principles and Practice of Obs & Gynae for PG's Pankaj Desai 3rd/ed, p559*

So I am not including **option "c"** in the answer.

In congenital elongation of cervix management is amputation of cervix which is just a part of Fothergill's repair, it does not require all components of this operation therefore, should not be considered amongst the correct options.

12. Ans. is d, i.e. Below cardinal ligament where uterine artery crosses

The crossing of the uterine vessels and ureter is at the level of internal os. Over here the ureter runs below the uterine vessels (water below the bridge) and the distance between the ureter and uterine vessels is only 1.5–2 cm.

The ureter can get injured at all the sites mentioned in the question but during gynaecological surgeries the commonest site of injury to ureter is where it crosses below the uterine arteries.

The next common site of injury is behind the infundibulopelvic ligament at the pelvic brim.

Close anatomical association between ureter and genital organs may lead to ureteric injury during gynecological surgery.

Incidence: 0.5–1% of all pelvic operations.

The sites of ureteric injuries are shown in Figure.

- At or below the pelvic brim (I)
- Along the course of ureter on lateral pelvic wall above the uterosacral ligaments (II)
- In the base of broad ligament where the ureter passes beneath the uterine vessels, about 1.5 cm lateral to cervix at the level of internal orifice (III)
- Beyond the uterine vessels as the ureter passes in the tunnel in Mackenrodt's ligament and turns anteriorly and medially to enter the bladder (IV)
- In the intramural portion of bladder (V).

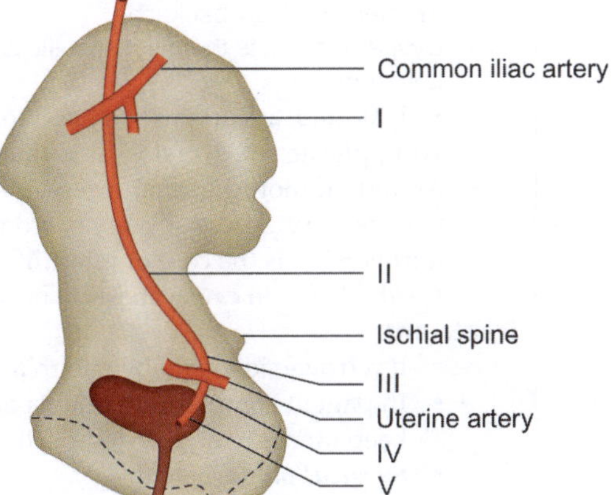

13. Ans. is c, d and e, i.e. Colposuspension; Pelvic floor excercises; and Sling operation *Ref: Shaw 14th/ed, p174; Dutta gynae 5th/ed, p387-9; Textbook of Gynae, shielaBalakrishnan 1st/ed, p329-330*

As explained in preceeding text:

- Pelvic floor exercises
- Sling operation
- Colposuspension (Burch) are all done for management of SUI.

14. Ans. is a, b, and d, i.e. Cervical fibroid; Retroverted gravid uterus; and Severe UTI

Ref: Jeffcoate 7th/ed, p855; Dutta Gynae 6th/ed, p410

Important gynecological causes of acute retention:

Period of life	Associated disorders	Provisional diagnosis
Postmenarchal	**Primary amenorrhea**	**Primary amenorrhea**
Childbearing period	• Short period of secondary amenorrhea • Menorrhagia • No menstrual abnormality • Irregular bleeding with pain • Irregular bleeding with fever	• Retroverted gravid uterus • Uterine fibroid impacted in POD • Impacted ovarian tumor, cervical or broad ligament fibroid • Pelvic hematocele • Pelvic abscess

Besides the above causes *Jeffcoate 6th/ed, pp 855-858* gives an exhaustive list of other causes of urinary retention- in which urethritis causing spasm of voluntary external urethral sphincter and acute urinary retention is given.

15. Ans. is b, c, d and e, i.e. Associated with endometriosis; It is a cause of infertility; Causes menorrhagia; and Associated with PID *Ref: Shaw 15th/ed, p345-7; Jeffcoate 7th/ed, p295-7*

The usual position of the uterus is one of ***anteversion*** and ***anteflexion***, in which the body of the uterus is bent forward at its junction with cervix.

Retroversion

Retroversion is a condition in which axis of cervix is directed upward and backward (instead of forward).

Causes		
Developmental	**Acquired**	
	Mobile retroversion	**Fixed retroversion**
• Seen in 20% of patients • Retroversion can never be congenital (it is always developmental) malformation as the uterus is without version and flexion at birth.	• Prolapse • Puerperium • Fibroid • Ovarian cyst (pushes uterus backward)	• **PID** • Pelvic tumors • Chocolate cyst of ovary • ***Pelvic endometriosis***

Symptoms:

- Mobile retroversion is usually symptomless, main disadvantage being increased risk of perforation of the uterus at the time of instrumentation.

Symptoms which can be seen are:

- Spasmodic dysmenorrhea[Q]
- Pelvic congestion syndrome causing:
  - Congestive dysmenorrhea
  - Polymenorrhagia
  - Premenstrual low backache
  - Dyspareunia (it is the most specific and genuine complain in case of retroversion)
  - Leucorrhoea
- *Infertility:* as cervix is directed forward away from the seminal pool.

  To implicate retroversion as a cause of infertility, it is necessary to perform Sims-Huhner test (postcoital test). Abundant motile sperms are seen in the vaginal pool but their failure to show up in the cervical canal indicates that the cervical canal is away from the seminal pool and is not accessible to the motile sperms. In such a case, retroversion is the case of infertility. Surgical correction of the retroversion should result in conception.
- *Abortion:* can cause abortion between 10th to 14th week.

Treatment:

- If retroversion is mobile no treatment is required.
- In patient complaining of dyspareunia and backache with retroverted uterus : Hodge pessary may be used to keep uterus in anteverted position.
- ***Surgical management:***
  - Modified Gilliams operation
  - Plication of round ligament[Q]
  - Baldy webster operation[Q]

16. Ans. is a, i.e. Cystocoele *Ref: Dutta Gynae 4th/ed, p193; Novak 14th/ed, p898*

Genital prolapse refers to protusion of the pelvic organ into or out of the vaginal wall.

Classification of prolapse:

The answer is further confirmed by following lines from Novak.

"Data from Women's Health Initiative revealed anterior pelvic organ prolapse in 34.3%, posterior wall prolapse in 18.6% and uterine prolapse in 14.3% of women in the study." *Ref: Novak 14th/ed, p898*

Anterior organ prolapse is cystocele

17. Ans. is a, i.e. Enterocele

As discussed in preceeding text enterocele is a long term complication of purandare sling surgery and not of Shirodkar's.

18. Ans. is b, i.e. 24 hrs after delivery *Ref: Internet search*

Kegel's exercise are pelvic floor exercises which consists of contracting and relaxing the muscles that form part of the pelvic floor.

The aim of Kegel exercises is to improve muscle tone by strengthening the pubococcygeus muscles of the pelvic floor. Kegel exercises are good for treating vaginal prolapse, preventing uterine prolapse and to aid with child birth in females.

Kegel's exercises: Time for initiating Kegel's exercise:

- Pregnancy 1st trimester
- After vaginal delivery after 24 hours
- After cesarean section after 24 hours.

19. Ans. is d, i.e. Le Fort's repair *Ref: Dutta Gynae 5th/ed, p197-205; Shaw 15th*

In females more than 60 years of age, who have medical complications like, in this patient previous H/O MI, hypertension and diabetes, Vaginal hysterectomy is not possible as the anesthetist will not agree to give anesthesia.

In such patients procidentia/3° degree prolapse can be managed by Le forts colpocleisis.

20. **Ans. is a, i.e. Sacral colpopexy** *Ref: Telende's 9th/ed, p1003, 1011; Text book of Gynae, Sheila Balakrishnan 1st/ed, p321-3*

Best management is sacral colpopexy.

21. **Ans. is c, i.e. Foley's catheterisation** *Ref: Shaw 15th/ed, p185; Dutta Gynae 5th/ed, p404*

"Urine culture is mandatory before surgery and infection should be treated. The urine is collected by Catheterization." *Ref: Shaw 14th/ed, p167*

In VVF

"Preoperative collection is best to be done through ureteric catheterization." *Ref: Dutta 5th/ed, p404*

So friends undoubtedly ureteric catheterization. (Don't get confused – it is not Foley's catheterization) is the best method for collecting urine for culture in a case of VVF. This option is not given, so, we will have to look for next best option.

- "Urine collected through a sterile vaginal speculum will not serve the purpose because of contamination. *Ref: Dutta Gynae 5th/ed, p405 (Option "d")*
- Midstream clean catch sample is also contaminated in vesicovaginal fistulas. (**Option "b"**)
- Suprapubic aspiration done after proper cleansing and draping the patient with full bladder, is easy and next best method of urine collection after ureteric catheterization. But the only prerequisite for this method of collection is 'A full bladder' which cannot be fulfilled in a case of VVF as urine continuously dribbles from the vagina and therefore, bladder is never full. (Ruling out **Option "a"**)

By exclusion our answer is Foley's catheterization, although chances of contamination are present in Foley's catheterization but they can be reduced if proper vaginal douching is done prior to collection of urine.

22. **Ans. is b, i.e. Cystoscopy** *Ref: Principles & Practice of Obs & Gynae Vol. II for PG's 3rd/ed by Pankaj Desai, Narendra Malhotra p613, Telinde 9th/ed, p1104*

The most useful investigation in case of VVF is cystoscopy as it helps to confirm the size, position and number of fistulas

23. **Ans. is a, i.e. VVF** *Ref: Shaw 15th/ed, p186-7; Dutta Gynae 6th/ed, p421,423*

Techniques for repairing VVF:

- Layer Technique
- Latzko procedure (for fistulas following hysterectomy)
- Chassar Moir technique

24. **Ans. is b, i.e. Ureterovaginal fistula** *Ref: Dutta Gynae 6th/ed, p420; Shaw 15th/ed, p186*

In the question : In methylene blue swab test, dye filled in the bladder does not stain the pad in vagina but it is soaked with clear urine which means it is a uretero vaginal fistula (for details see preceeding text).

Observation	Interpretation
1. Upper most swab soaked with urine but unstained with dye	Ureterovaginal fistula[Q]
2. Upper and lower swab remain dry but the middle swab soaked with dye	Vesicovaginal fistula[Q]
3. The upper two swab remain dry but lower one soaked with dye	Urethrovaginal fistula[Q]

25. **Ans. is c, i.e. Vesico-uterine** *Ref: Shaw 15th/ed, p188; Jeffcoate 7th/ed, p266*

26. **Ans. is b and c, i.e. UVF; and Bladder endometriosis** *Ref: Shaw 15th/ed, p188*

The condition of cyclical passage of menstrual blood in urine is called as **menouria.** *Ref: Jeffcoate 7th/ed, p266*

Menouria:

- *It is seen in uterovesical fistulae*[Q]
- *Usually follows cesarean section*[Q]
- The patient complains of hematuria/passage of menstrual discharge via urethra at the time of menstruation. Patient does not have urinary incontinence.[Q]
- Menouria is seen when uterovesical fistula opens into the uterus above the isthmus.[Q]
- The presence of the fistula can be demonstrated by hysterography (but not by cystography) and cystoscopy.[Q]
- Treatment is by abdominal repair.[Q]
- *Another Important cause of cyclical hematuria is endometriosis*[Q] *of bladder.*

27. **Ans. is a, i.e. Pelvic floor muscle exercises** *Ref: Dutta Gynae 5th/ed, p586; Novak 14th/ed, p875; Williams Gynae 1st/ed, p525-6; Textbook of Gynae Sheila Balakrishnan 1st/ed, p328*

The most recommended non surgical treatment for stress incontinence is pelvic floor muscle exercise.

"Pelvic floor muscle training should be offered as first line conservative management for stress incontinence." *Ref: Novak's 14th/ed, p875; Dewhurst 10th/ed, p486*

"Pelvic floor exercises are the mainstay of conservative therapy for stress incontinence." *– Urinary incontinence in primary care' (2000)/73*

28. **Ans. is a, i.e. Stress incontinence** *Ref: Shaw 14th/ed, p174; Textbook of Gynae Shiela Balakrishnan 1st/ed, p330*

Kelly's plication/Kelley's stitch was the standard first line of treatment for SUI previously but due to low cure rates, it is not being done these days. 5-year failure rate for Kelly's plication is approximately 50%.

29. Ans. is a, i.e. Stress urinary incontinence *Ref: Telinde 9th/ed, p1035-37*

Bonney's test is performed in the clinical evaluation of SUI. In the Bonney's test, two fingers are placed in the vagina at the UV junction on either side of the urethra and the bladder neck is elevated.

On straining or coughing, leakage of urine indicates of positive test. A positive test indicates that the SUI is due to bladder neck descent and urethral hypermobility and can be corrected by bladder neck suspension surgeries.

A negative test i.e. leakage of urine-means SUI is due to intrinsic urethral sphincteric deficiency and results of performing bladder neck suspension surgery will not be good.

Note: Marchetti test is same as Bonney's test, but two Allis forceps are used instead of fingers.

30. Ans. is d, i.e. Tension free vaginal taping (TVT)

31. Ans. is a, i.e. Burch's colposuspension *Ref: Telinde 9th/ed, p1052-6*

Evidence Based Urology' (Wiley Blackwell) 2010/193 'Pelvic Floor Dysfunction. A multidisciplinary Approach' (Springer) 2006/117: Hernia Repair Sequalae (Springer) 2010/440; Assessing and Managing A cutely Ill Adult Surgery Patient' (John Wiley and Sons) 2007/182

As discussed in preceding text SUI is managed basically by performing either of the two surgeries viz-

1. Burch colposuspension
2. Tension free vaginal tapes/tension free obturator tapes.

The rates of success of these two surgeries are comparable, so if either of them is given in options, we will chose it.

So in Q31-Answer is Burch colposuspension *Ref: Telinde 9th/ed, p1050-6*

Procedure	Long-term success rate (%)
• Burch's colposuspension	• 89.5
• Stamey's repair	• 85
• Kelly's repair	• 50–60
• Aldridge Repair	• 85

Now suppose both Burch colposuspension and TOT and TVT tape is given (like in Q30), then remember-

Tension Free Vaginal Tape (TVT) and TOT have emerged as the treatment of choice for genuine stress incontinence in recent years

Tension Free Vaginal Tape (TVT) and Tension Free Obturator Tape (TOT) are a simple procedures that may be performed under local anesthesia and have decreased operative and recovery time, and is as effective as 'Burch colposuspension' which was earlier considered the procedure of choice.

"A number of surgical procedures have been developed to treat genuine stress incontinence and most aim to elevate and support the bladder neck. Burch colposuspension was the procedure of choice, but in recent years this has been superseded by the 'Tension free Vaginal Tape' which is showing comparable results and is less invasive'"

Ref: Assessing and managing Acutely III Adult Surgery Patient' (John Wiley and Sonsd) 2007/440

Between TVT and TOT, TOT is better as it has less complications

∴ Best is TOT > TVT > Burch colposuspension.

32. Ans. is d, i.e. At middle part of urethra *Ref: Shaw 15th/ed, p193-194; Dutta gynae 6th/ed, p404*

Read the text for explanation.

33. Ans. is d, i.e. Osteitis pubis *Ref: Telinde 9th/ed, p1057-8; Textbook of Gynae, Sheila Balakrishnan 1st/ed, p329*

Marshall-Marchetti-Krantz (MMK) procedure, involves the attachment of the periurethral tissue to the symphysis pubis. In approximately, 3% of patients undergoing the procedure, osteitis pubis develops.

34. Ans. is c, i.e. Impacted cervical fibroid *Ref: Read below*

The patient in the question:

- Was being treated for infertility.
- Now has H/O 6 weeks of amenorrhea.
- Presents with urinary retention.

The first diagnosis which comes in our mind is *retroverted gravid uterus*.

Points which favour the diagnosis are: The woman is pregnant and has complain of urinary retention.

But friends, here it is important to understand that retroverted gravid uterus causes urinary retention at 14–15 weeks of gestation (not 6 weeks). *Ref: Jeffcoate 7th/ed, p299*

So **Option "a"** is ruled out

Option "b" Pelvic hematocele

"Pelvic hematocele is formed in a patient complaining of 6 weeks amenorrhea in case of ectopic pregnancy."
Ref: Jeffcoate 6th/ed, p212

Though pelvic hematocele causes urine retention but then other symptoms (pain) and signs of ectopic pregnancy should be present.

Option "c" Impacted cervical fibroid

"A cervical fibroid impacted in pouch of Douglas can cause retention of urine. The onset of retention is acute and usually occurs immediately before menstruation, when the uterus is further enlarged by congestion or during early pregnancy." *Ref: Jeffcoate 7th/ed, p493*

Fibroid is associated with infertility.

Thus, an impacted cervical fibroid can explain all features seen this woman and is our option of choice.

35. **Ans. is d, i.e. Rectovaginal septum** *Ref: Shaw's Textbook of Gynecology 15th/ed, p331*

For details see the text.

36. **Ans. is a, i.e. Ureterovaginal fistula** *Ref: Shaw's Textbook of Gynecology 15th/ed, p186*

The site of the fistula can be determined by the complaint and also by Methylene Blue 3 Swab test.

Complaint	Urogenital fistula
• H/O normal voiding + Continuous dribbling of urine from vagina	Ureterovaginal fistula
• Continuous dribbling of urine from vagina but no normal voiding	Vesicovaginal fistula
• No continuous leakage but when patient urinates, urine comes out from urethra and vagina	Urethrovaginal fistula

For details of methylene blue 3 swab test-Refer chapter 8 of the guide.

Observation	Interpretation
Upper most swab soared with urine (yellow) but not with dye. Remaining 2 swabs unstained	Ureterovaginal fistula
Upper and lower remain dry but middle swab soaked with dye. The upper two swabs remain dry but lower soared with dye	Vesicovaginal fistula

In the question, the lady is having normal voiding as well as continuous in continence and on methylene blue 3 swab test, she has yellow staining on upper most pad while other two pads are unstained.

This means she is having ureterovaginal fistula.

37. **Ans. is d, i.e. Manchester**

Manchester surgery is the other name for Fothergill surgery

38. **Ans. is a, i.e. Cystometry** *(Ref: William Gynae 3rd/ed, p526)*

Diagnostic procedures in urinary continence include-

- **Urinalysis and culture to rule out infection**
- Post voidal residual volume
- Urodynamic studies done by cystometry.

39. **Ans. is c, i.e. Pudendal nerve** *(Ref: Shaw's 15/e)*

40. **Ans. is a, b, c and d i.e Level I support, Level II support, Level III support and Urogenital diaphragm**

Disruption of level I support may lead to prolapse of the uterus or vaginal vault, while damage to level II and III supports predispose to anterior and posterior vaginal prolapse. All levels of defective support should be repaired during reconstructive surgery.

There are three levels of vaginal support as described by DeLancey.

- **Level I** support consists of paracolpium that suspends the apical portion of the vagina and is comprised of the cardinal-uterosacral ligament complex.
- **Level II** support comprises the paracolpium that is attached to the vagina laterally via the arcus tendineus fasciae pelvis and superior fascia of the levator ani.
- **Level III** support consists of the distal vaginal attachments: anteriorly, via fusion of the urethra to the vagina, laterally, to the levator ani, and posteriorly, with the perineal body.

41. **Ans. is d, i.e. Pelvic floor repair**

Anterior colporrhaphy and colpoperineorrhaphy together is called as pelvic floor repair

42. **Ans. is a, i.e. Mackenrodt's ligament**

Cardinal ligament also called as Mackenrodt's ligament is the main support of uterus.

REVIEW/PRACTICE QUESTIONS

1. **Best time to do surgery after VVF:**
   a. Immediately b. After 3 weeks
   c. After 1 month d. After 6 weeks
2. **Best time to repair an old perineal tear:**
   a. After 3-6 weeks
   b. After 3 months
   c. After 1 month
   d. After 12 months
3. **All of the following surgeries are done in vault prolapse *except*:**
   a. Colposuspension
   b. Uterosacral suspension
   c. Sacral colpopexy
   d. Sacral spinous ligament fixation
4. **All of the following surgeries are done in stress urinary incontinence *except*:**
   a. Marshall Marchetti Krantz & surgery
   b. Aldridge surgery
   c. Latzko repair
   d. Pereyra surgery
5. **The reference part in POP –Q classification is:**
   a. Hymen b. Internal os
   c. Introitus d. External os
6. **Strumdorf suture is applied in:**
   a. Fothergills repair
   b. Ward Mayo Hysterectomy
   c. Le fort colpocleisis
   d. Latzko repair
7. **In Baden Walker Halfway system of classification of prolapse, the reference point is:**
   a. Hymen b. Ext os
   c. Int os d. Introitus
8. **Enterocele is repaired by:**
   a. Shirodkar repair b. Sacropexy
   c. Colpopexy d. Moskowitz repair
9. **Investigation of choice for vesicovaginal fistula is:** *(AIIMS Nov 2018)*
   a. IVP b. Cystoscopy
   c. 3-swab test d. X-ray
10. **While performing Burch operation there was significant bleeding and pooling of blood in the space of Retzius. The source of bleeding cannot be visualized. What is the next step in the management?** *(AIIMS May 2018)*
   a. Call vascular surgeon
   b. Give a generalized suture in bleeding area
   c. Lift endopelvic fascia by putting fingers in vagina
   d. Placing surgical drain

REVIEW/PRACTICE ANSWERS

1. **Ans. is d, i.e. After 6 weeks** *Ref: Ahow 16th/ed, p231-233.*
2. **Ans. is b, i.e. After 3 months** *Ref: Shaw 16th/ed, p202*
3. **Ans. is a, i.e. Colposuspension**
4. **Ans. is c, i.e. Latzko repair** *Ref: Shaw 16th/ed, p231-233*
5. **Ans. is a, i.e. Hymen** *Ref: Jeffcoate 7th/ed, p46; CGDT 10th/ed, p49*
6. **Ans. is a, i.e. Fothergills repair** *Ref: Shaw 15th/ed, p5*
7. **Ans. is a, i.e. Hymen**
8. **Ans. is d, i.e. Moskowitz repair**
9. **Ans. is b i.e. Cystoscopy**
   See explanation of Q. 22 of chapter 8 of book
10. **Ans. is c i.e. Lift endopelvic fascia by putting fingers in vagina** *Ref: Te Linde's Operative Gynecology, 11th/ed*
   In Bursch operation, space of Retzius is assessed. If there is any bleeding from space of Retzius, first step is to lift the endopelvic fascia by putting fingers in 12 vagina.

CHAPTER 9

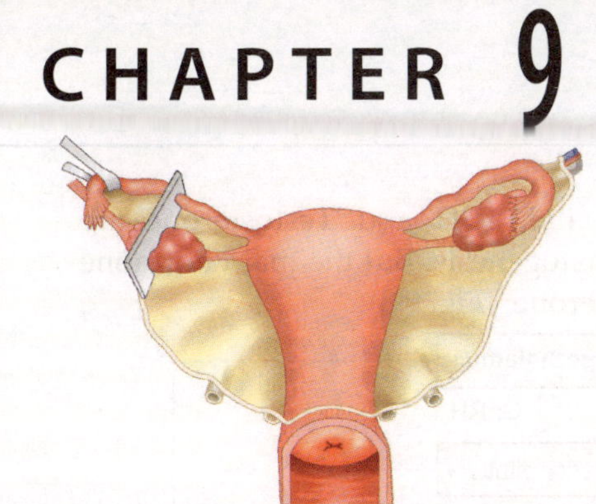

Infertility

Definitions

- **Infertility:** Failure of a couple of reproductive age to conceive even after at least 1 year of regular coitus without contraception.
  - **Primary infertility:** Infertility in a woman who has never been pregnant.
  - **Secondary infertility:** Infertility in a woman who has had one or more previous pregnancies but is now unable to conceive. Incidence is 10–15%.
- **Fecundability:** Probability of achieving pregnancy within one menstrual cycle. For a normal couple, this is approximately 25%.
- **Fecundity:** Ability to achieve a live birth within one menstrual cycle.

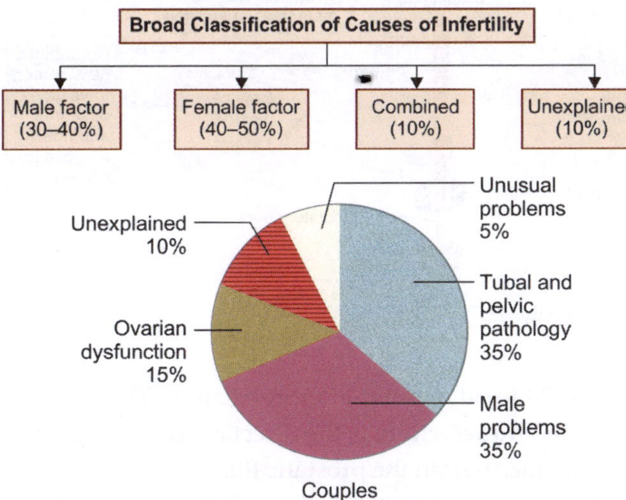

Fig. 9.1: Couples: Causes of infertility

Causes of Female Infertility

The main causes of female infertility include

- **Ovarian cause:** (i) Decreased ovarian reserve (ii) Anovulation.
- **Decreased ovarian reserve**
- **Tubal factor**
- **Uterine factor**
- **Pelvic factor**
- **Unexplained**

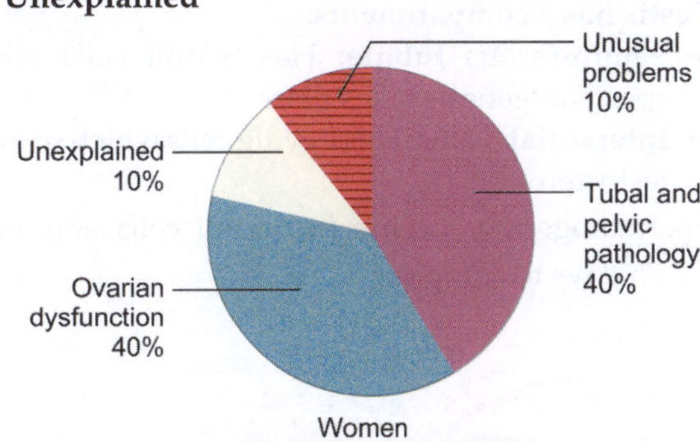

Fig. 9.2: Females: Causes of infertility

Evaluation

- Evaluation is indicated for women who fail to conceive after one or more years of regular, unprotected intercourse.
- Women over the age of 35 should be evaluated sooner (i.e., after 6 months of regular, unprotected intercourse).
- No woman should be denied her request for infertility services or counseling, regardless of duration.
- Successful reproduction requires proper structure and function of the entire reproductive axis, including hypothalamus, pituitary gland, ovaries, fallopian tube, uterus, cervix, and vagina.

> - **Infertility evaluation** comprises eight major elements:
>   - History and physical examination
>   - Semen analysis (first investigation)
>   - Sperm–cervical mucus interaction [postcoital testing (PCT)]–for select patients
>   - Assessment of ovarian reserve
>   - Tests for occurrence of ovulation
>   - Evaluation of tubal potency
>   - Detection of uterine abnormalities

- With proper coordination, the evaluation can be completed within one menstrual cycle. No abnormality or cause of infertility can be identified in 10% to 15% of couples. This group comprises a category known as "unexplained infertility."

Male Infertility

Male factor is the only cause of infertility in about 20% of infertile couples but it a contributing cause in 50% case.

Physiology of Sperm Formation in Males

- **Testis has 2 compartments:**
  - **Seminiferous tubule:** Has Sertoli cells where spermatogenesis takes place
  - **Interstitial tissue:** Has Leydig cells which secretes testosterone
- Spermatogenesis occurs in Sertoli cells and takes 74–75 days to complete.
- All 3 hormones LH, FSH and Testosterone are needed for spermatogenesis. But the main hormone needed is Testosterone. (Fig. 9.3)

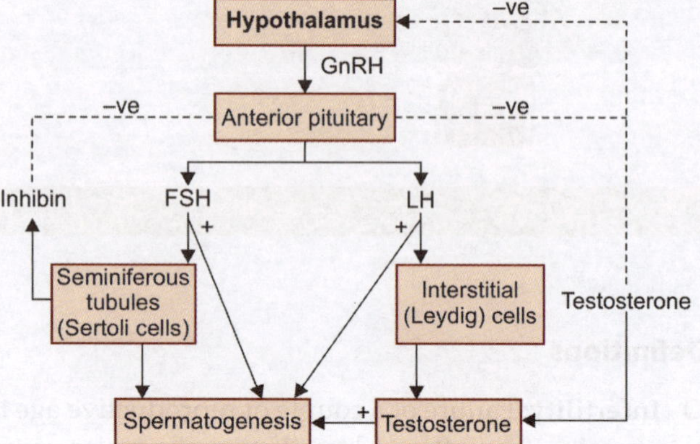

Fig. 9.3: Hypothalamus pituitary testis axis in males

- The resultant spermotozoa are released into the seminiferous tubule lumen and then enter the epididymis where they mature and become motile. They take 7–10 days to transverse this tortous structure and reach the vas deferens.

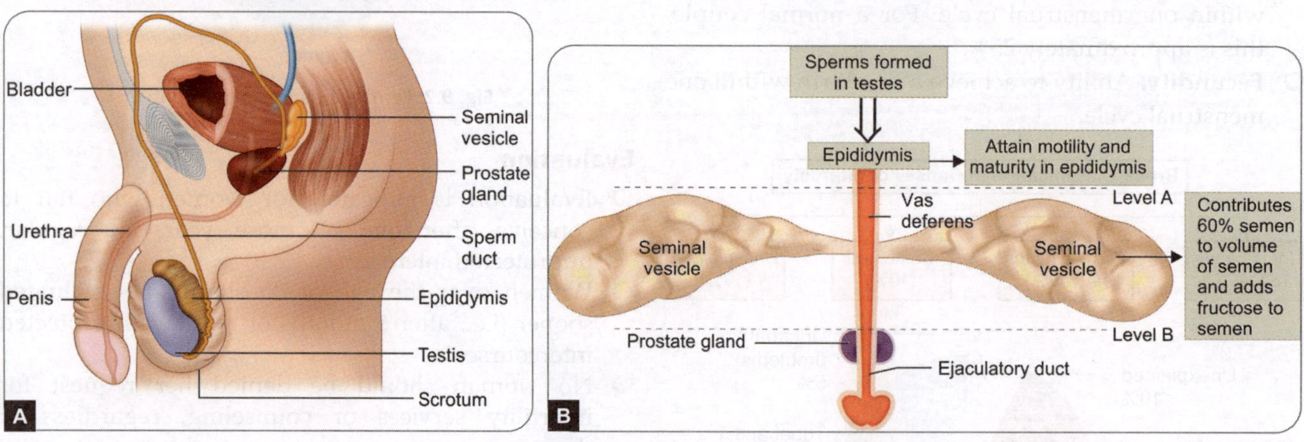

Figs. 9.4A and B: Sperm pathway

- The fluid from seminal vesicle **fluid contributes 60% of the semen volume. Seminal vesicle fluid contains large amount of fructose, which is used by the sperm mitochondria to generate ATP to allow movement through female** genital tract.
- Now after this prostate Gland adds its secretion to the semen and then at the time of ejaculation, bulbourethral gland gives its secretion. The sperms and semen pass into ejaculation duct is ejaculate out.
- The released semen is a gelatinous mixture of spermatozoa and seminal plasma: However, it thins out 20 to 30 minutes after ejaculation. This process, called **liquefaction, is the** direct result of proteolytic enzymes within the prostatic fluid.
- Following ejaculation, the released spermatozoa must undergo capacitation to become competent to fertilize the oocyte.
- Capacitation starts in the cervix and most importantly occurs in fallopian tube.
- Sperm transport from the posterior vaginal fornix to the fallopian tubes occurs within 2 minutes during the follicular phase of the menstrual cycle.

Also Know

The sertoli cells are supporting cells also called as **sustentacular cells** and they surround all stages of the developing sperm cells (Fig. 9.5).

The tight junction between these sertoli cells create the **blood testis barrier** which keeps the blood borne toxins from reaching the germ cells and at the same time keeps surface antigens on the developing germ cells from escaping into the bloodstream and prompting an autoimmune response.

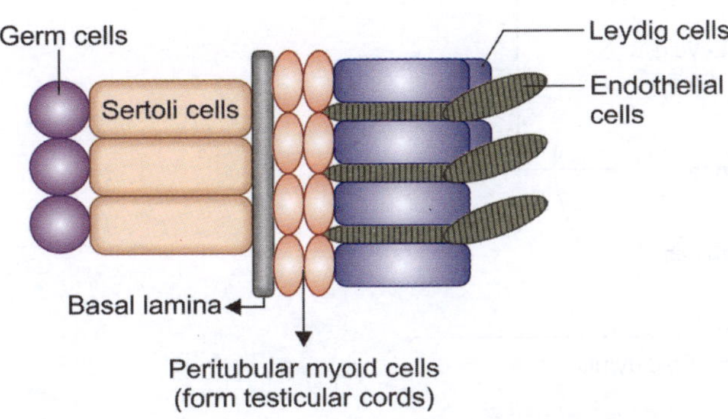

Fig. 9.5: Blood testis barrier

Investigation of male infertility

Semen Analysis

It is the first investigation to be done when a couple comes with the complaint of infertility. Abstinence of 3 days is needed

Normal parameters of semen Analysis (WHO–2010)

Normal parameters of semen analysis (WHO–2010)	
Semen analysis	**Minimum (Normal values)**
Volume	≥1.5 mL
pH	7.2–7.8
Viscosity	<3 (scale 0–4)
Sperm concentration	≥15 million/mL
Total sperm count	39 million/ejaculate
Motility	Progressive motility : 32%
	Total motility ≥40
Morphology	Normal forms 4%
Viability	Living 58%
Leucocytes	Less than 1 million/mL
Round cells	< 5 million/mL
Sperm agglutination	< 10% spermatozoa with adherent particles

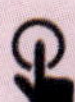

Most important criteria in semen analysis is sperm morphology > sperm motility > sperm concentration

Other Important Values in Semen Analysis

- pH = > 7.2 (between 7.2 and 7.8)
- Round cells (including WBC + epithelial cells + immature cells) = < 5 million/mL.
- Sperm agglutination = <2

Extra Edge

- When no motile sperms are observed a **sperm viability** test differentiates viable or non motile sperms from dead sperms.
- Round cells in semen analysis includes epithelial cells, prostate cells, immature sperms (spermatogonia, round spermatids, spermatocytes) and leucocytes. If total round cells is > 5 million/mL it is abnormal. True leukocytospermia means > 1 million leukocytes/mL and requires semen culture for Mycoplasma hominis, Ureaplasma urealyticum and Chlamydia.
- Lymphocytes can be distinguished from other cells by immunoperoxide staining **"Endtz Test".**

Terminology related to semen analysis

Normospermia	All semen parameters normal
Oligozoospermia[Q] / oligospermia	Decreased sperm number < 20 million/mL
Asthenozoospermia[Q] / asthenospermia	Decreased sperm motility[Q]
Teratozoospermia[Q]	Increased abnormal forms of sperm[Q]
Oligoasthenoterato-zoospermia	All sperm variables abnormal[Q]
Azoospermia[Q]	No sperm in semen[Q]
Aspermia	No ejaculate (ejaculation failure)
Leucocytospermia[Q]	Increased white cells in semen[Q]
Necrozoospermia[Q]	All sperms non-viable or non-motile[Q]

Note: If no spermatozoa are observed in wet preparation, WHO recommends an examination of centrifuged sample (3000 × g or greater for 15 minutes). If no sperms are observed in the centrifuged sample, the semen analysis should be repeated. The presence of a small number of sperms in either of centrifuged sample is defined as **cryptozoospermia** and complete absence is called as **azoospermia.**

Causes of Male Infertility

All causes of male infertility can be classified as:

1. **Pre-testicular cause** i.e. involving Hypothalamus or Pituitary
2. **Testicular cause** i.e. involving testis
3. **Post-testicular cause** i.e. below level of testis (Flowchart 9.1)

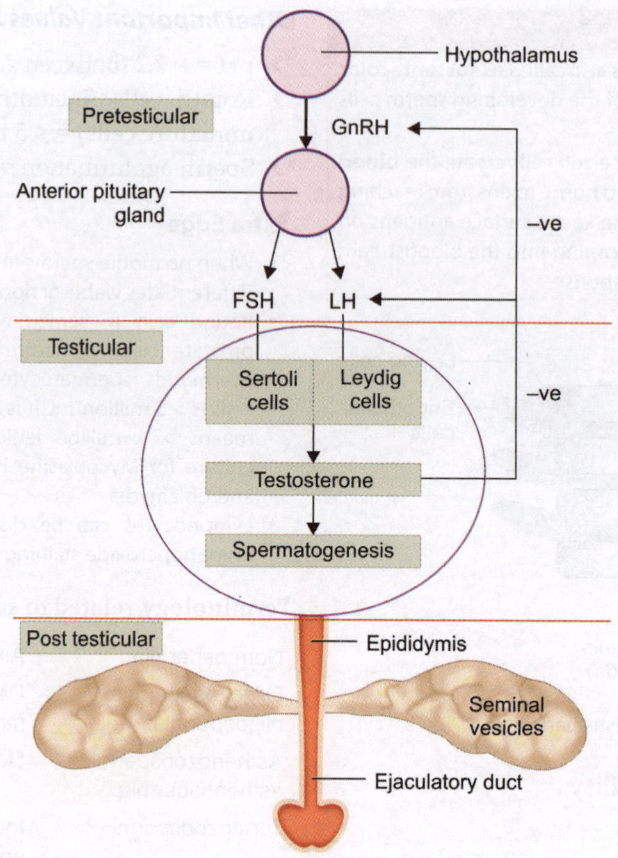

Fig. 9.6: Causes of male infertility.

Flowchart 9.1: Causes of male infertility

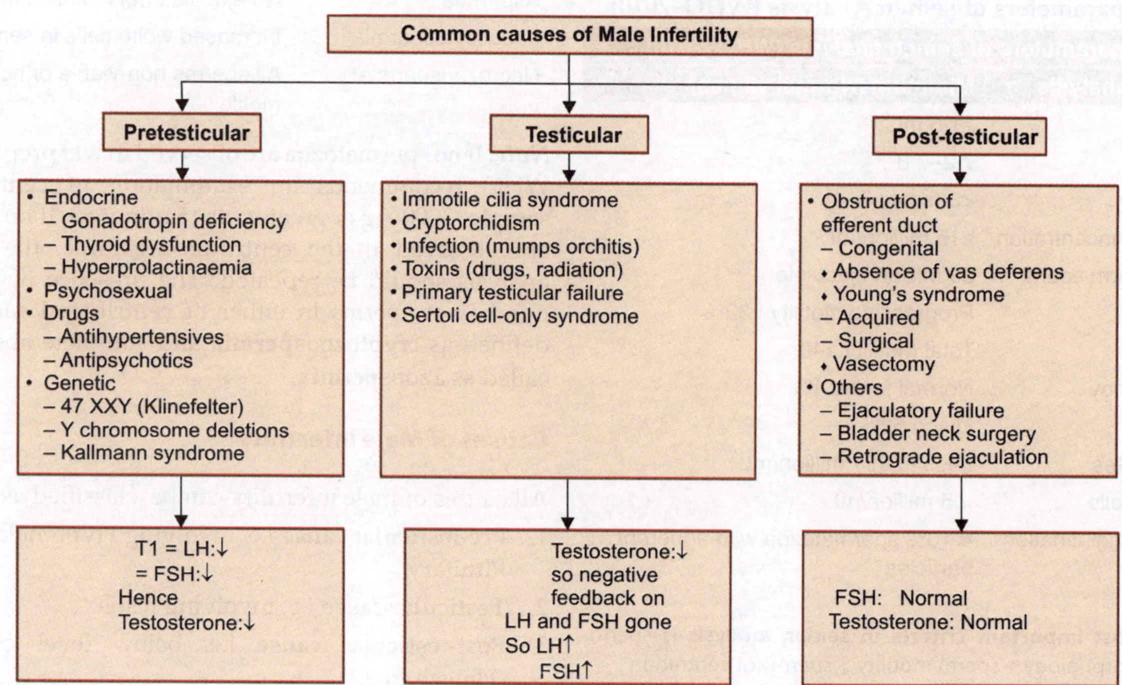

Azoospermia

In patient with azoospermia workup as shown in Flowchart 9.2 is done.

Flowchart 9.2

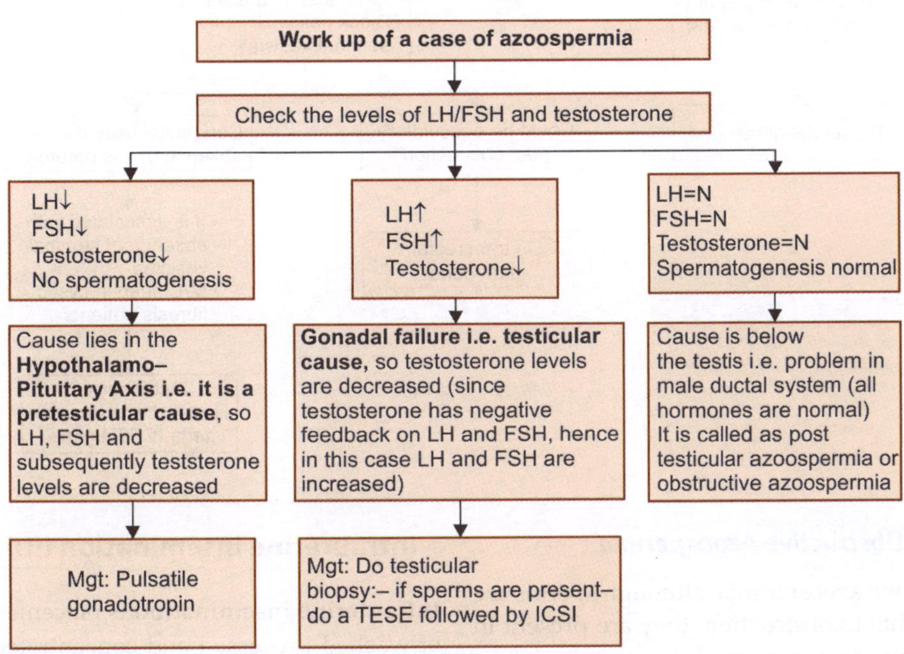

Note: Always in men who have low semen volume rule out Retrograde ejaculation.
In case of obstructive azoospermia, spermatogenesis occurs normally so it will have the best prognosis.

Important Concept

A very important question and very frequently asked in all exams is to find out the site of block in case of azoospermia.
Now for all questions like these:
Check the levels of FSH and testosterone.

Hormone Levels	Site of Problem
FSH ↓ Testosterone ↓	Hypothalamus or Pituitary
FSH ↑ Testosterone ↓	Testis
FSH N Testosterone N	Problem is below the testis called as **obstructive azoospermia**

In case of obstructive azoospermia:

- The site of block can be determined by seeing whether Fructose is present or absent in semen
- As seen in Fig. 9.4B seminal vesicles add fluid (which accounts for 60% of semen) and fructose to it
  - (i) **So if block is below the level of seminal vessicles (Level B shown in Fig. 9.4B): There will be**
    Then when the man will ejaculate its semen will have fluid from bulbourethral Gland and prostate Gland.
    It will not have fluid from seminal vesicle, hence fructose will be absent and semen will be low in volume. It will not have sperms (i.e. azoospermia).
  - (ii) **If block is above the level of seminal vesicle (Level A) shown in Fig. 9.4B):**
    Then when the male ejaculates his semen will have:
    Fluid from seminal vessicle hence it will be of good volume and fructose will be present
    Fluid from prostate Gland
    Fluid from bulbourethral Gland the semen **will not** have—sperms (i.e. azoospermia).

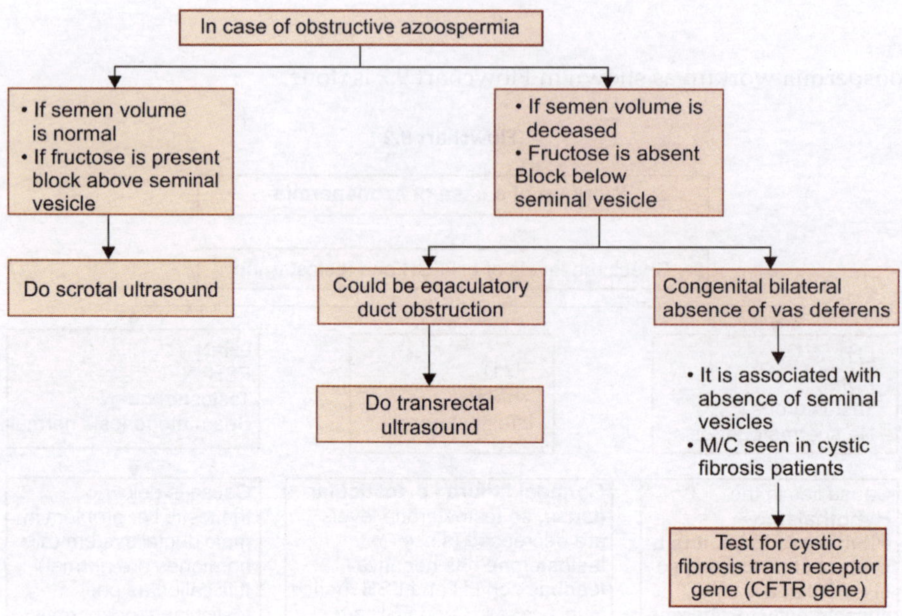

Management of Obstructive Azoospermia

In case of obstructive azoospermia, although sperms are absent in semen due to obstruction, they are present in the testis as in testis spermatogenesis is normal.

Sperms can be retrieved from testis or epididymis by following surgical techniques:

TESA	Percutaneous testicular sperm aspiration
TESE	Testicular sperm extraction
MESA	Microsurgical epididymal sperm aspiration
PESA	Percutaneous epididymal sperm aspiration

The recovered sperms are then injected into the **oocyte by ICSI** (explained latter).

Note: Repeat retrieval should be done after 3–6 months.

In case of Testicular azoospermia—there are slight chances of pregnancies; if sperms can be retrieved from the testis using retrieval method followed by ICSI.

Epididymal aspiration is not an option in them.

Management Options in Decreased Sperm Count in Males

Sperm count	Management
Oligospermia = Sperm count 10–15 million/mL	IUI
Sperm count = **5–10 million/mL**	IVF
In case of **severe oligospermia (< 5 million/mL)**	ICSI

Intrauterine Insemination (IUI)

Intrauterine insemination is placement of 0.3 to 0.5 mL of washed processed and concentrated sperms (devoid of seminal plasma/semen) into the intrauterine cavity **by transcervical catheterization.**

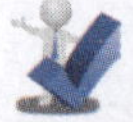

KEY POINTS

Prerequisite for IUI:
- Fallopian tube of the female should be patent so IUI cannot be done in tubal infertility in females
- Total number of motile sperms should be more than 10 million and 14% of sperms should have normal morphology

Methods of processing the sperm:
1. Swim up technique (Most commonly used)
2. Swim down technique
3. Density centrifugation technique (Best)

The purpose of IUI is to bypass endocervical canal and to place increased number of motile sperms close to fallopian tube.

Components of the ejaculate removed in IUI include seminal fluid, excess debris, leukocytes and morphologically abnormal sperms. Best results are achieved when the final specimen contains 10 million total motile sperms.

IUI done with husband sperm is IUI-H and with donor sperm is IUI-D.

Indications

Intrauterine insemination is done in **males** with:

- Severe hypospadias, epispadias
- Retrograde ejaculation (Immediate postcoital urine is taken and sperms are extracted from it.)
- Neurogenic impotence
- Sexual dysfunction
- Oligospermia with sperm count 10–15 million/mL.
- Low ejaculate volume (IUI + clomiphene × 2 cycles).

In female infertility IUI is useful in:

- Cervical infertility-Antisperm antibodies are present in cervix
- Vaginismus (involuntary contraction of perineal muscles during intercourse)
- Unexplained infertility. (IUI + clomiphene × 3 cycles).

Procedure

Patient is laid in supine position and an insemination catheter is inserted in cervical canal and is advanced slowly in the uterine cavity. 0.5 mL of semen is slowly introduced and patient is then asked to lay supine for 15 minutes.

Timing for IUI

- In natural and clomiphene stimulated cycles, urinary LH monitoring should be started 3 days before expected ovulation and insemination done on the day after midcycle urinary LH surge or IUI is done on 5 and 7 days after completion of clomiphene.
- If ovulation is triggered by exogenous hCG, IUI is performed 36 hours later.

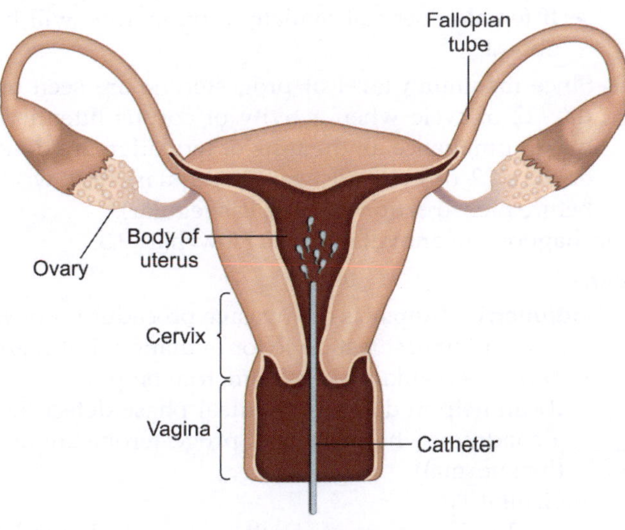

Fig. 9.7: IUI

IVF (In Vitro Fertilization)

Indications

In females:

- Tubal disease best is for distal tube obstruction
- Endometriosis leading to infertility
- In case of decreased ovarian reserve using donor oocyte
- In Mullerian agenesis – using IVF followed by surrogacy
- If female has a risk of transferring a genetic disease then IVF with pre- implantation genetic diagnosis is done

In males:

- For oligospermia (sperm count 5–15 million/mL)
- Unexplained infertility

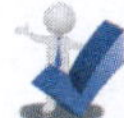

KEY POINTS

- **Most important parameter for IVF**-Motility of sperms.
- **Most important parameter for ICSI**- Morphology of sperms

ICSI: Intracytoplasmic Sperm Injection

Indications

- Female indications same like IVF

Male:

- For severe oligospermia sperm count < 5 million/mL
- Motility of sperms < 5%
- Whenever sperms are retrieved surgically using techniques of MESA/PESA/TESA/TESE
- In case of IVF failure

Procedure: Common for IVF and ICSI

- Semen is collected, washed processed like in IUI and incubated in media for 3-4 hours to promote sperm capacitation and acrosome reaction.
- **To the female partner:** Ovulation inducing drugs like clomiphene or gonadotropins are given so that she hyperovulates. This is followed by follicular monitoring from D10 onwards. When at least 2 follicles are 17–18 mm in size or larger (but not more than 24 mm) and endometrial thickness is 8 mm or more, injection hCG is given as **ovulation trigger.** This is because hCG and LH are functionally similar.
- Oocyte retrieval is done via TVS under general anesthesia. Prophylactic antibiotics are recommended at the time of retrieval oocyte. Retrieval should be done 36 hrs after hCG injection.

In IVF

- Now **50,000 to 1,50,000** motile sperm are inseminated for each oocyte in a small droplet of media under oil.

In ICSI (Figs. 9.8A to C)

- Here the aspirated oocyte is stipped off its follicular cells, followed by insertion of a single sperm into the cytoplasm of the mature metaphase II egg.
- Hence in ICSI for 1 oocyte, only 1 sperm is needed. That is why this procedure can be done in severe oligospermia or in azoospermia when sperms are surgically retrieved from testes.

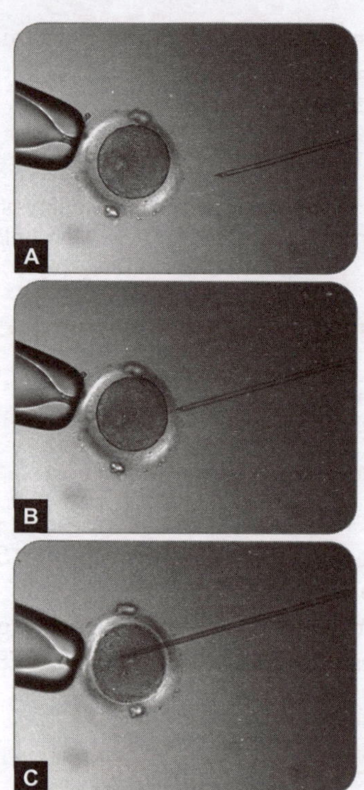

Figs. 9.8A to C: Intracytoplasmic sperm injection (ICSI) procedure: (A) The holding (left) and the injecting (right) pipettes are seen; (B) The oolemma is penetrated; (C) The injection pipette has reached nearly the center of the oocyte

Common Steps for Both IVF & ICSI Continued

- Once the fertilization occurs, either by IVF or by ICSI, it is known by presence of 2 pronuclei and extrusion of second polar body. The embryos are cultured. Embryos are incubated in atmosphere of ≤ 5% CO_2 and 37°C temperature. Various culture media are used.
- The embryo transfer can be done at **cleavage stage or 8 cell stage** i.e. day 3 or **at blastocyst stage** (i.e. day 5). Blastocyst transfer is associated with lower implantation failure, higher pregnancy rate and 7% higher live birth.
- It is done transcervically using TAS to ensure that embryos are **transferred 1.5 to 2 cm below the fundus of uterus. (As this is the site for implantation)**
- Success rate with single embryo = 30%
- Cumulative success rate = 40–50%

FEMALE INFERTILITY

A–Ovarian Cause (40% Cases)

The 2 major causes of ovarian infertility in females are:

1. Anovulation e.g. PCOS.
2. Decreased ovarian reserve e.g. premature menopause

WHO classifications of ovarian causes of infertility

Class I (10%):	Hypothalamic pituitary failure (Hypogonadotrophic hypogonadism) e.g. Kallman syndrome
Class II (85%):	Hypothalamic pituitary ovarian dysfunction e.g. PCOS (Anovulation) (Most easily treatable form of infertility) hyperprolactinaemia
Class III (5%):	Ovarian failure (premature menopause).

1. Anovulation

It is the most easily reversible and treatable cause of female infertility.

Diagnosis

- This is based on the fact that:
  - It female ovulates: Progesterone will be present
  - If female does not ovulate: Progesterone will be absent
- Since maximum level of progesterone are seen on day 22 of cycle when activity of corpus luteum is maximum, hence all the tests of ovulation are done on day 22 of cycle (if cycle is regular) or 1 week before menstruation (if cycle is irregular).

For diagnosis of anovulation see Flowchart 9.3.

Note:

1. **Endometrial Biopsy** is an invasive procedure & now a days not the best test done for ovulation. But there are certain advantages of endometrial biopsy:
   i. It can help in diagnosing luteal phase defect (i.e. a condition where levels of progesterone are less than normal)
   ii. Genital TB
   - The first sign of ovulation on endometrial biopsy is subnuclear vacuoles.

Flowchart 9.3

Diagnosis of Ovulation

- Indirect
- Direct → Laparoscopy
- Conclusive → Pregnancy

Basal Body Temperature
In ovulatory cycle, there is biphasic[Q] pattern of temperature variation. At the time of ovulation BBT is raised to 0.5 to 1°F. The rise sustains throughout the 2nd half of the cycle and falls two days prior to next period - called biphasic pattern. In anovulatory cycle - No Rise of temperature throughout the cycle.[Q]

Cervical Mucus Study
Under the influence of oestrogen cervical mucus shows ferning[Q] or stretchability (spinnbarkeit)[Q]. After ovulation progesterone causes loss of ferning and stretchability[Q]. Persistence of ferning/spinnbarkeit beyond 22nd days means anovulation.[Q]

Vaginal Cytology
Maturation index shifts to left[Q] under the effect of progesterone after ovulation i.e. there is predominance of intermediate cells.

Hormonal Estimation
- **S. progesterone: done on 8 th[Q] and 22nd[Q] day of cycle.**
  An increase in value from <1 mg/ml to >3–6 mg/ml suggests ovulation
- **Serum LH or Urine LH**
  estimation daily can indicate LH surge and LH peak. Ovulation occurs 10–12 hrs after LH peak.[Q]
- Best time test for LH is in late afternoon i.e. between 4 pm–10 pm
  Once the test is positive intercourse s/b advised
  Best time is 24 hours after test positive
- The female remains tertile till 45 hours after test is positive

Endometrial Biopsy
It should be in premenstrual phase day of regular cycle. In case of irregular cycles it is done within 24 hours of the period 2 samples should be taken one for HPE and other for means ovulation has occurred.
Secretory endometrium with coiled (cork screw glands) means ovulatory cycle. Proliferative endometrium with simple cystic tubular glands means anovulatory cycle.

USG
Serial sonography can precisely measure the size of Graffian follicle, and thus the exact time of ovulation. Features[Q] of recent ovulation[Q] are – collapsed follicle and some fluid in pouch of Douglas.

Note: Apart from all the Indirect evidences of ovulation discussed above, if a female has dysmenorrhea that also indicates ovulatory cycle. Pain is absent in anovulatory cycles.

2. **Best investigation for anovulation:** Hormone estimation
   i. If one wants to know only that whether a female has ovulated or not then, S. progesterone level estimation is done.
   ii. If one wants to know the time at which ovulation occurs - serum LH estimation is done
3. M/C done test for ovulation - Follicular monitoring on TVS.

Signs of Ovulation on USG

- Size of follicle increases by 2-3 mm everyday till it becomes 18-20 mm in size and then it suddenly decreases.
- Some fluid is seen in pouch of Douglas
- Endometrium appears triple layered/TRILAMINAR appearance (Fig. 9.9)

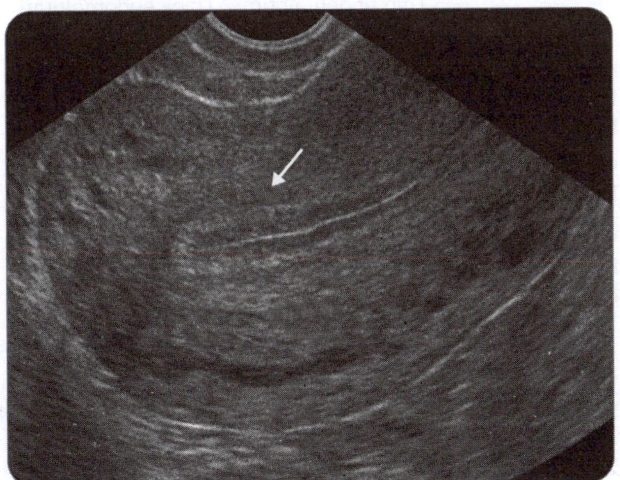

Fig. 9.9: Ultrasound showing triple layered appearance of endometrium

Management

Management of Anovulation is by ovulation induction. Ovulation induction aims at the release of one egg per cycle in a woman who has not been ovulating regularly.

Ovulation Inducing Agents

1st line drugs for anovulation
(i) Letrozole (Best)
(ii) Clomiphene citrate (2nd best):
- Nowadays the DOC for anovulation is Letrozole.
- Earlier there was a ban on use of letrozole but now it has been removed & letrozole is considered as DOC for PCOD/PCOS.
- The first step in all patients with PCOD/ anovulation is to advise them weight reduction.
- Weight reduction in itself restores ovulation in some cases.
- Weight reduction can be achieved by:
  - Diet modification
  - Physical exercise
  - Bariatric surgery
- The ideal time to conceive after bariatric surgery is after 12-18 months.
- If patient has insulin resistance, then along with clomiphene citrate or letrozole, add metformin.
- If patient has hyperprolactinemia, then along with clomiphene citrate or letrozole, add cabergoline.

Comparative analysis of Letrozole and Clomiphene

	Clomiphene	Letrozole
Mechanism of action	SERM	Aromatase inhibitor
Half life	Long 5–7 days	Short 45 hrs
Anti-estrogenic effects	Clomiphene has anti-estrogenic effects Thin endometrium and altered cervical mucus	Letrozole does not have anti-estrogenic effects Thick endometrium and favourable cervical mucus
Uterine blood flow	↓	↑
Ovulation rate Pregnancy rate	60–85% 10–12% per cycle	70–80% 10–15% per cycle
Multiple pregnancy rate	High	Low
OHSS	High	Low

Hence, first choice drug for ovulation induction is Letrozole (as per ACOG guidelines)

Note: If Letrozole is not given in options then mark clomiphene.

Dose of Letrozole = 2.5 mg/day
Maximum dose = 7.5 mg/day
To be given from D3-D7

Clomiphene Citrate

Clomiphene Citrate: It is a racemic mixture of enclomiphene and zuclomiphene. Enclomiphene is a more potent isomer responsible for its ovulation-inducing action.

- **Dose** = 50–250 mg. The US FDA-approved maximum dose for clomiphene citrate is 100 mg. **Maximum approved time** = 1 year
  Initial dose = 50 mg × 5 days (either from D2 to D6 or D5 to D9)
- Clomiphene blocks "Estrogen" receptors, so negative feedback on FSH gone so levels of FSH → increase from pituitary, which leads to growth of multiple follicles hence multiple pregnancy.
- Thus it can be used **only in patients with intact hypothalamic -pituitary ovarian axis**
- From D10 follicular monitoring is done and as the follicles reach 18–20 mm size, **hCG injection is given as ovulation trigger.**

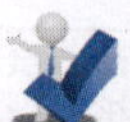

KEY POINTS

hCG is functionally and structurally similar to LH hence giving hCG injection creates LH surge like condition.

- Ovulation occurs in 80% cases
- After 32 to 36 hours of inj hCG, IUI is done.

Side Effects of Clomiphene

- Multiple pregnancy: Rate 5–8% (< 10%)
- Menopausal symptoms–like vasomotor symptoms (Hot flashes)–(M/C side effect).
- Risk of ovarian hyperstimulation syndrome (< 1%)
- Ovarian cyst formation
- Visual symptoms—**If visual symptoms occur, its use should be immediately discontinued**
- As it leads to hyperovulation, it increases chances of ovarian cancer.

KEY POINTS

- Clomiphene is not teratogenic but it is classified as category X drug by FDA and is C/I in suspected pregnancy.
- Clomiphene doesn't increase the risk of ectopic pregnancy.

2nd Line Drug for Anovulation

Gonadotropins: HMG (Human Menopausal Gonadotropin) is obtained from the urine of the menopausal women.

- Menopausal women have high FSH and LH levels in their blood and urine, and HMG is extracted from urine of menopausal females.
- Dose of HMG = 130–300 IU daily
- Maximum dose = 450 IU for superovulation
- With HMG the chances of multiple pregnancy are 30% and OHSS are 5%.

3rd Line Drug

GnRH: Synthetic GnRH can be given in a pulsatile manner for ovulation induction and as treatment for delayed puberty. GnRH agonist can be given for maximum 6 months, because they cause significant osteoporosis. If it has to be continued for more than 6 months, then add back therapy should be given.

Ovarian Hyperstimulation Syndrome

Background

All ovulation inducing drugs, directly or indirectly increase FSH which in turn stimulates a number of follicles. The granulosa cells of the follicles secrete Estrogen.

Estrogen (E2) secreted per follicle = 150-200 pg/mL

Hence if the number of follicles increase, the levels of E2 increase.

- If estrogen ≥ 3500 pg/mL, the chances of OHSS are 1.5%.
- If estrogen ≥ 6000 pg/mL, the chances of OHSS are 38%.

What is OHSS

This is a clinical symptom complex associated with ovarian enlargement resulting from exogenous gonadotropin therapy.

Pathophysiology

The increased estrogen levels increase vascular endothelial growth factor (VEGF) which increases vascular permeability and loss of fluid, protein and electrolytes into the peritoneal cavity which leads to hemoconcentration.

- Another factor involved is Angiotensin II.
- There is also associated electrolyte imbalance.
- Due to hemoconcentration, hematocrit increases & there are increased chances of thromboembolic events.
- As the size of ovary increases due to enlarged follicles, there are chances of torsion, rupture and haemorrhage of ovary.

Risk Factors for OHSS

- Young female
- Female has PCOS
- Injection hCG – it triggers OHSS.

Symptoms

Abdominal pain is the most prominent symptom caused by ovarian enlargement and accumulation of peritoneal fluid.

Due to leakage of fluid to third space, it can lead to ascites, pleural effusion, edema, etc. Due to decreased intravascular volume there can be decreased urinary output, hypovolemic and renal failure.

Grading

Grade 1:	Abdominal distension
Grade 2:	Abdominal distension + Nausea/vomiting or diarrhea Size of ovary = 6–12 cms
Grade 3:	Ascites present on ultrasound
Grade 4:	Clinical evidence of ascites/hydrothorax/ difficult breathing
Grade 5:	Findings of grade 4 with evidence of hemoconcentration, coagulation abnormalities and decreased renal perfusion.

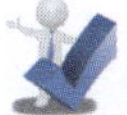

KEY POINTS

In all cases of ovulation induction, injection hCG is given as an ovulation trigger.

Ideal condition for injection hCG

- E2 levels = 450–1000 pg/mL
- 1–2 follicles ≥ 16 mm in size
- Endometrial thickness = 8 mm

BUT

Injection hCG also triggers OHSS if Estrogen levels are very high

E2 ≥ 3500 pg/mL -> chances of OHSS are 1.5%

E2 ≥ 6000 pg/mL -> chances of OHSS are 30%

Hence to prevent OHSS

- Delay hCG injection
- Withhold hCG injection (if E2 ≥ 5000 pg/mL or if follicles are ≥ 13 in number)
- Decrease the dose of hCG from 10,000 IU to 5000 IU.
- Cancel the cycle (in grade 3, 4, 5 of OHSS)
- Give cabergoline as it decreases VEGF.

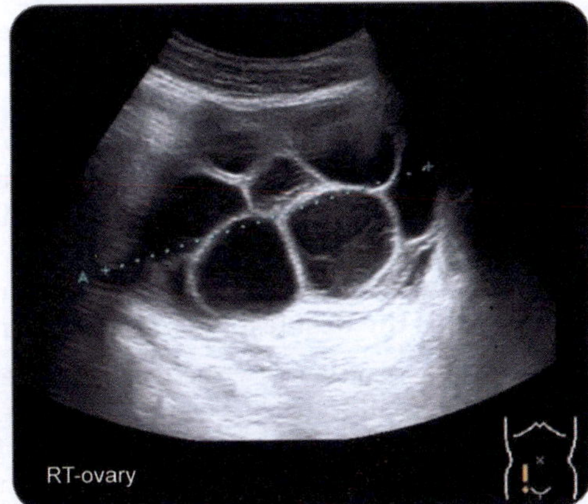

Fig. 9.10: USG of OHSS

Management

- Admit the patient
- 1st line treatment - correction of hypovolemia by IV fluids or colloids
- In case of tense ascites – Paracentesis is done
- Prophylactic heparin to reduce the risk of thromboembolism.

2. Decreased Ovarian Reserve

Decreased ovarian reserve, i.e. less number of follicles in the ovary is the second ovarian cause of female infertility.

Ovarian reserve tests are to assess the quantity as well as the quality of primordial follicles present in the women's ovary. These tests are done to determine how the ovaries will respond to therapy (ovulation induction). In other words it is the assessment of the reproductive potential of the woman.

Tests for Ovarian Reserve

1. **Serum Day 3 FSH levels**
   Basis of Test: As the number of follicles decrease serum estrogen decreases so negative feedback on FSH is lost, hence serum FSH levels increase.

> **FSH levels**
> - Normal = 0–10 IU
> - Borderline = 10–15 IU
> - Poor ovarian reserve = ≥ 15 IU
> - Suggestive of premature ovarian failure = ≥ 20 IU
> - Diagnostic of premature ovarian failure = ≥ 40 IU

2. **Serum Inhibin B levels:**
   In poor ovarian reserve patients, levels of Inhibin B on Day 3 are less than 45 pg/mL as Inhibin is secreted by granulosa cells of the follicle
3. **Clomiphene citrate challenge test:**
   In this case FSH levels are measured on Day 3 of the cycle and again on Day 10 after administering clomiphene citrate (100 mg orally each day) from Day 5 to Day 9.
   The Day 3 levels of FSH are increased in patients of poor ovarian reserve and further increase on Day 10 after clomiphene
4. **Serum antimüllerian hormone (AMH)**: Levels of serum AMH is a good predictor of ovarian stimulation response. Levels of AMH (< 0.5 ng/mL) decline with age and with poor ovarian reserve. Levels of AMH can be measured any time in the menstrual cycle, hence it is **the best test for ovarian reserve.**

> **AMH**: AMH is produced by the granulosa cells of the preantral small follicles. Serum levels of estradiol and inhibin B depend on pituitary FSH feedback mechanism. Level of AMH is not dependent on feedback mechanism.
>
> This is one of the reasons for which AMH is a better predictor of ovarian reserve compared to estradiol and inhibin B. Levels of AMH can be measured at anytime in the menstrual cycle.

5. **Antral Follicle Count (AFC)** is done by using TVS in early follicular phase in both the ovaries. AFC reflects qualitative the primordial follicular pool in the ovary. It is done between D2–D4 of cycle.
   - AFC more than 6 in each ovary (2–10 mm size) reflects adequate ovarian follicular reserve.
   - AFC, less than 4, indicates poor ovarian reserve and poor response to ovarian stimulation during IVF.
   - In both ovaries if follicles are <10, it reflects poor ovarian reserve.

- AFC decreases with age.

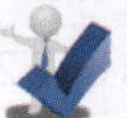

KEY POINTS

AFC is the best quantitative marker of ovarian reserve.
AMH is the best overall marker of ovarian reserve.

6. **Serum estradiol levels:** Per se it does carry any significance. But if the levels are correlated along with FSH levels then it has significance.

Management

In poor ovarian reserve cases the female will not have her own eggs so she can become pregnant by using donor oocytes followed by IVF.

Tubal Factors

Tubal factors leading to infertility include endometriosis, pelvic adhesion disease or previous bilateral tubal ligation. These conditions lead to blockage of tube.

The block could be at the level of:

- Proximal block
- Mid segmental block
- Distal block

The problem is if only both the tubes are blocked. Unilateral block does not need treatment.

Tests for Detecting Tubal Potency

Investigation of Choice—Hysterosalpingography (HSG)

- **Hysterosalpingogram (HSG)** assesses uterine and fallopian tube contour and tubal patency. It shows Mullerian anomalies as well as most endometrial polyps, synechiae and submucosal fibroids.
  - Performed in the early follicular phase, D 10 of the cycle to minimize chances of interrupting a possible pregnancy.

- It is an OPD procedure and does not need any anesthesia.
- The procedure is performed by injecting a radiopaque dye using **Leech-Wilkinsion cannula (Fig. 9.11)** through the cervix. As more dye is injected, the dye normally passes through the uterine cavity into the fallopian tubes and then spills into the peritoneal cavity.
- X-ray films are taken under fluoroscopy to evaluate tubal patency (Fig. 9.12).
- Nonsteroidal anti-inflammatory drugs may be given to prevent cramping.

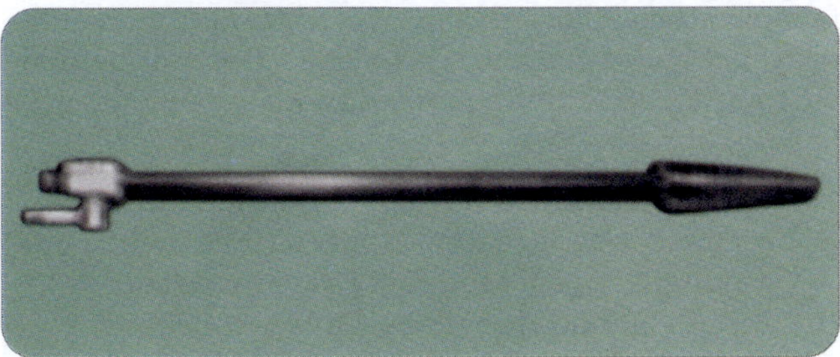

Fig. 9.11: Leech-Wilkinsion cannula

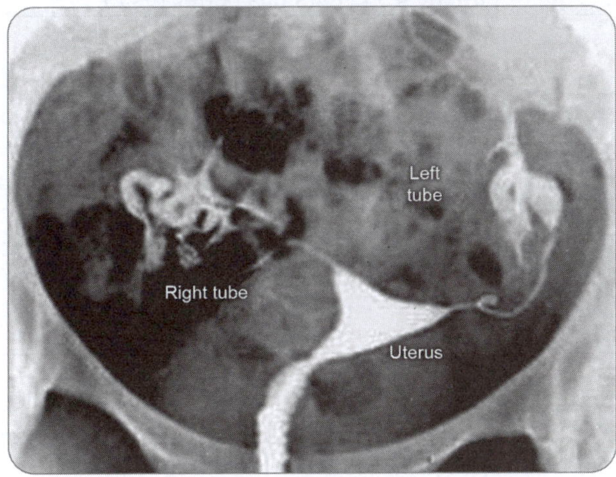

Fig. 9.12: Normal HSG

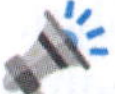

Important One Liners

- First test to assess tubal patency – HSG.
- HSG is not the best test because in some patients while doing HSG cornual spasm occurs which leads to bilateral cornual block. HSG cannot differentiate between cornual spasm and cornual block and it cannot visualise the exterior of the tube.
- Obsolete test for tubal patency – Rubins test/CO_2 insufflation test
- Best test or Gold standard test for tubal patency is – Laparoscopic chromopertubation.

- **Saline infusion ultrasonography** [Sonohysterography (SHG)]
  - SHG involves transvaginal ultrasound after the introduction of sterile water or saline into the uterine cavity.
  - Useful in assessment of uterine cavity abnormalities such as polyps or submucosal fibroids. But it does not provide information regarding fallopian tubes on its patency.
- **Laparoscopic Chromopertubation**
  - This is the most definitive and **gold standard test** for tubal patency.
  - It can assess both the tubal patency and exterior of tube, that is why it is the gold standard test.

Chromopertubation means: Dye (usually a dilute solution of indigo carmine) is instilled through the fallopian tubes and seen by laparoscopy to document tubal patency.

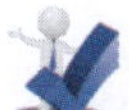

KEY POINTS

Laparoscopy with chromopertubation is the best investigation for confirming tubal patency.

It is both diagnostic and therapeutic as any pathology can simultaneously be corrected with operative laparoscopy.

As it requires general anaesthesia and admission, so it is not the first line investigation for tubal patency, hence first line of investigation is HSG.

Management of Tubal Factor Infertility

Tubal Blocks

Tubal factor infertility means that their is tubal blockage.

Tubal Blocks can be at 3 levels viz:

a. Proximal block, i.e. cornual block (Fig. 9.13)
b. Midsegmental block
c. Distal block (Fig. 9.14).

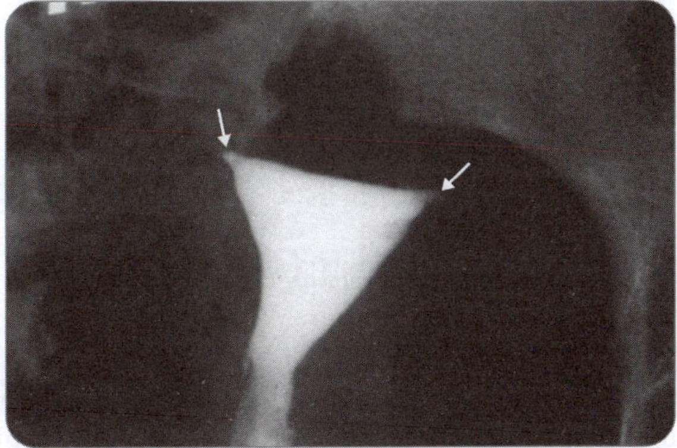

Fig. 9.13: HSG showing B/L Cornual Block

a. Proximal Block i.e. B/L Cornual Block *(Fig. 9.13)*

Mostly it is due to cornual spasm at the time of HSG.

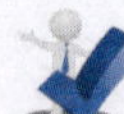

KEY POINTS

M/C cause of B/L cornual block on HSG is physiological (due to cornual spasm)

Management in this Case

- **Tubal cannulation or catheterization** i.e. passage of a soft catheter into the tubal ostia under hysteroscopic guidance or USG guidance. This is followed by laparoscopic chromopertubation. So a very oftenly asked question is the management of bilateral cornual spasm, which would be hysteroscopic cannulation followed by laparoscopic chromopertubation.
- If the blockage is **unrelieved, then it is a pathological block and M/C cause of B/L pathological cornual block** is **Genital Tuberculosis**. In this case management is IVF.

So the initial management of B/L cornual block is laparoscopy and hysteroscopy but best management is IVF.

b. Distal Block *(Fig. 9.14)*

Distal tubal disease and occlusion are causal in 85% of all tubal infertility and can be secondary to a variety of inflammatory conditions including infection (gonococcal), endometriosis or prior abdominal or pelvic surgery.

- **Management of mild distal block** – fimbrioplasty
- **Management of severe distal block** – IVF.

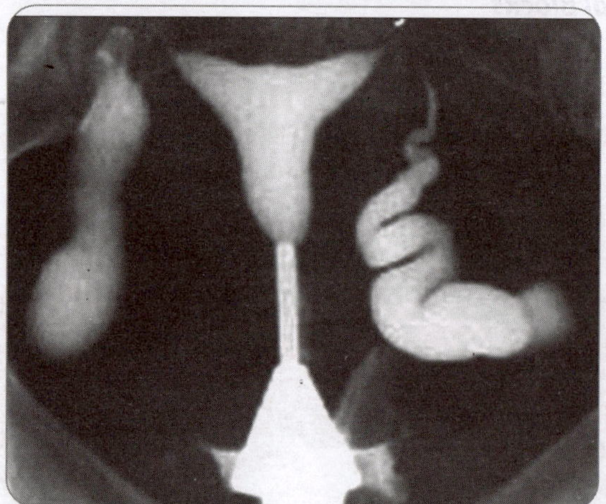

Fig. 9.14: HSG showing Distal Block

c. Midsegmental Block *(See Fig. 9.15)*

This is seen in those cases who had tubectomy done earlier, regret their decision (20% cases) and require reversal of sterilization procedure (5%)

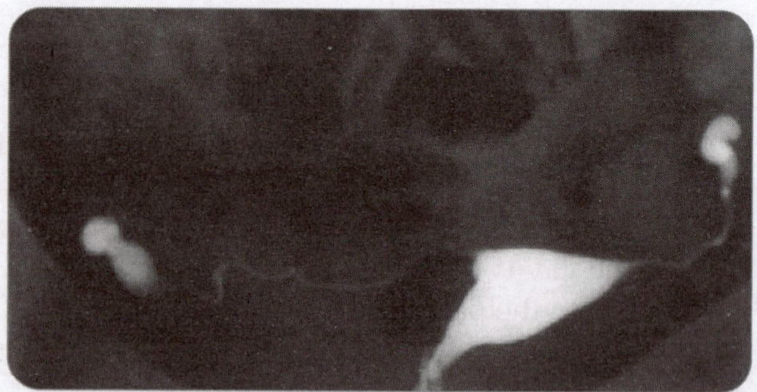

Fig. 9.15: HSG showing midsegmental block

The technique for sterilization reversal involves microsurgical dissection of the occluded ends of the fallopian tube followed by a layered reapposition of the proximal end distal tubal segments. This can be done by mini laparotomy, laparoscopy on robotic asserted laparoscopy.

Success of Recanalization depends on certain factors.

a. Method of sterilization – Reversal is best **with clips > fallope rings > Modified Pomeroy > cautery.**
b. Length of final anastomised tube – ≥ 4 cm
c. Type of anastomosis – best result seen with Isthmo-Isthmic anastomosis
d. Age of patient < 35 years has better result.

Cervical Factor

Cervical factor infertility can be due to abnormal or deficient mucus in cases of:

i. Infection
ii. Prior cervical surgery
iii. Use of antiestrogens (e.g. clomiphene citrate) for ovulation induction
iv. Presence of Antisperm antibodies

The treatment of cervical factor depends on the cause

- If it is due to chronic cervicitis/infection - Treatment of infection by antibiotics is the cure.
- If is due to decreased mucus volume - Treatment includes short-term supplementation with exogenous estrogen like ethinyl estradiol and use of mucolytic expectorant like guaifenesin. However, their value has not been confirmed.
- If it is due to antisperm antibodies -Investigation done to detect antibodies is postcoital test.

Postcoital Test (Sims or Huhner's Test)

It is designed to assess:

- *The quality of cervical mucus.*
- Presence and number of motile sperms in the female reproductive tract after coitus.
- Interaction between cervical mucus and sperms.

- *It gives an approximate idea of sperm count: (normally 10–50 motile sperms are seen per high power field in cervical mucus, if count is < 10 sperms/HPF it indicates the need for complete semen analysis).*

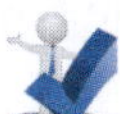

KEY POINTS

Prerequisites for the post-coital test:
- Abstinence of 2 days.[Q]
- Intercourse to be performed 2 – 8 hours before the test.[Q]
- No use of lubricant.[Q]

Time of test:
- It should be performed in D10–D12 of cycle

Method: The couple is advised to have intercourse and present to the doctor within 2-12 hours of intercourse. The cervical mucus of the female partner is collected and examined under microscope.

Note: Normally sperms show slow forward motility but in case of Antisperm antibodies, sperm show rotatory motion.

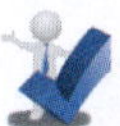

KEY POINTS

Postcoital test is only a screening test for detecting antisperm antibodies.
Confirmatory tests for detecting antisperm
- Sperm agglutination test
- MAR (mixed agglutination reaction) test
- Immunobead test

- **Treatment options include:**
  - Use of *condom or diaphragm as a barrier method for 3 months.* During this period, the antibodies will disappear and conception may occur then.
  - ***Corticosteroids*** given to female partner can also help in getting rid of these antibodies.
  - IUI is the best method for treating cervical factor infertility and unexplained infertility. So many clinicians forgo cervical mucus testing and proceed directly to IUI treatment in absence of tubal disease.

Also Know

Tests for studying sperm function
- Sperm Penetration assay
- Miller kurzrok test[Q]

(Tests for studying sperm penetration[Q])

Hypoosmotic swelling test[Q]: Test for studying tail function.
Hemizona Test: Test for studying the ability of sperm to bind to human zona pellucida.
Scoring system for permeability of cervical mucus is Insler score (A score of 10–12 is considered good score).

Uterine Factors

Uterine factors, such as leiomyomas, intrauterine synechiae (Asherman's syndrome), and uterine deformities or septa, cause approximately 2% of infertility. The mainstay of treatment for these conditions is surgical correction, frequently via a hysteroscopic approach.

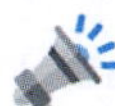

Important One Liners

M/c fibroid leading to abortions and infertility is submucous fibroid.
M/C congenital malformation of uterus leading to infertility : septate uterus

Luteal Phase Defect

During normal luteal phase when their is adequate progesterone secretion by the corpus luteum, adequate development of secretory endometrium occurs for blastocyst implantation. **Luteal phase defect refers to a condition when production of progesterone is suboptimal by corpus luteum.**

Inadequate progesterone secretion could be due to:
- Inadequate follicular development
- Inadequate FSH or LH secretion
- Hyperprolactinemia

It is an inevitable phenomenon in all ART cycles.

LPD may cause implantation failure and is thought to account for 4% of infertility.

Diagnosis of LPD is not based on uniform criteria:
- Low levels of midluteal serum progesterone (<10 ng/mL)
- Endometrial histology done on 25th-27th day of cycle shows endometrium more than 2 day out of phase
- A shortened luteal phase <14 days, are considered for the diagnosis.

Management – Micronized Progesterone

Unexplained Infertility

Management: Clomiphene citrate and IUI for 3-4 cycles. If it is not successful then IVF or ICSI.

Preimplantation Genetic Diagnosis (PGD)

- Preimplantation genetic diagnosis describes a number of techniques for preconceptional genetic evaluation of the embryos resulting from IVF
- It can be used to detect:

- Numerical aneuploidy
- Structural chromosomal anomalies (like translocation, inversion)
- To identify single gene disorders like cystic fibrosis, thallasemia, hemophilia, sickle cell disease
- To determine gender

- The technique requires one or two cells that may be obtained from:
  - Blastomere of cleavage stage hence also called cleavage stage embryo biopsy
  - Polar body
  - Trophoectoderm tissue from a blastocyst stage (day 5 embryo).

Method of cleavage stage embryo biopsy: Laser or a dilute solution of acid Tyrode solution is used to create a small hole in the zona pellucida and one or two cells are aspirated, typically on the third day after oocyte retrieval and fertilization when embryos are at the 6-8 cell stage.

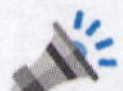

Important One Liners

For Preimplantation genetics (PGD) how many blastomeres are needed = 1 or 2

Polar bodies are not preferred for PGD as it cannot detect paternal defects

NEW PATTERN QUESTIONS

N1. The secretion of FSH in a male is inhibited by negative feedback effect of:
a. Inhibin secreted by Sertoli cells
b. Inhibin secreted by Leydig cells
c. Testosterone secreted by Sertoli cells
d. Testosterone secreted by Leydig cells

N2. Sperms attain maturity in:
a. Vas deferens
b. Ejaculatory duct
c. Epididymis
d. Seminal vesicle

N3. Liquefaction time of semen is:
a. 30 mins b. 60 mins
c. 50 mins d. 10 minutes

N4. Time taken by the sperms to reach fallopian tube
a. 2 mins b. 5 mins
c. 10 minutes d. 30 seconds

N5. Time taken for capacitation is:
a. 2 hrs b. 3 hrs
c. 5 hrs d. 7 hrs

N6. The cells which lie outside blood testis barrier:
a. Sertoli cells b. Spermatocyte
c. Spermatid d. Leydig cells

N7. The axial filament of sperm tail has following arrangement of filaments:
a. 1 + 5
b. 3 + 5
c. 7 + 5
d. 9 + 2

N8. The major contribution to the human seminal fluid is from:
a. Testes
b. Seminal vesicles
c. Prostate
d. Bulbourethral and urethral glands

N9. True about normal sperm count:
a. 60–100 lakh/mm^3
b. 4–5 million/mm^3
c. 60–120 lakh/mm^3
d. 60–120 million/mL

N10. Absent fructose content in the seminal fluid suggests:
a. Congenital absence of seminal vesicle
b. Ejaculatory duct obstruction
c. None
d. Both

N11. Semen analysis of a male of an infertile couple, shows absence of spermatozoa but presence of fructose. The most probable diagnosis is:
a. Prostatic infection
b. Mumps orchitis
c. Block in efferent duct system
d. All of the above

N12. Indications of intrauterine insemination (IUI) are all *except*:
a. Hostile cervical mucus
b. Unexplained infertility
c. Oligoasthenospermia
d. Luteal phase defect

N13. In which case homologous artificial insemination is used in females:
a. Hormonal disturbance
b. Tubal block
c. Cervical factor
d. All of the above

N14. Artificial insemination with husband's semen is indicated in all the following situations, *except*:
a. Oligospermia
b. Impotency
c. Antisperm antibodies in the cervical mucous
d. Azoospermia

N15. Indications for ICSI are all *except*:
a. Motility of sperms < 5%
b. Sperm count < 5 million/mL
c. Obstructive azoospermia
d. Morphologically normal sperm < 2%

N16. M/C time for embryo transfer after IVF is:
a. 2 days
b. 3 days
c. 4 days
d. 5 days

N17. A couple semen analysis report shows oligospermia. Which of the following can be given to increase sperm count?
a. FSH
b. LH
c. Estrogen
d. Progesterone

N18. Which of the following is suggestive of ovulation?
a. Oligomenorrhea
b. Regular cycle with dysmenorrhea
c. Day 21 estrogen levels increased
d. Drop in basal body temperative by 0.5°C in second half of cycle
e. Day 8 progesterone elevated

N19. Ovulation can be diagnosed by all *except*:
a. Measuring day 14 serum progesterone
b. Rise in basal body temperature in the second half of cycle
c. Study of cervical mucus
d. Endometrial histology

N20. Pulsatile GnRH is used for treating:
a. Precocious puberty
b. Anovulation
c. Size of fibroid
d. Pain in endometriosis

N21. IOC for tubal patency:
a. HSG
b. Laparoscopic chromopertubation
c. Saline infusion ultrasonography
d. USG

N22. Identify the instrument shown:

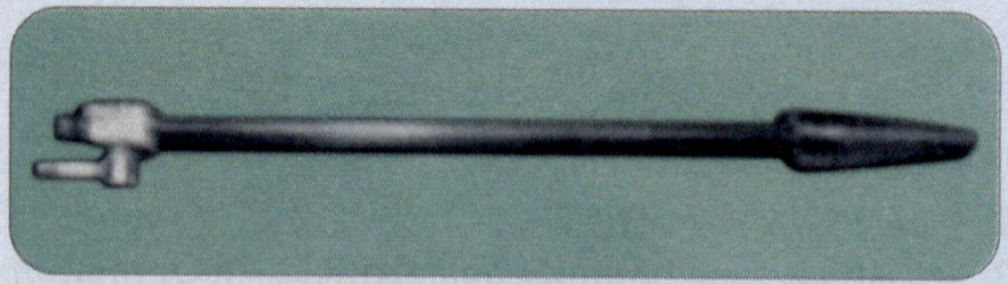

a. Hegars dilators
b. Drew smiths cather
c. Leech Wilkinson cannula
d. Uterine manupulators

N23. What is the M/C cause of condition shown in figure?

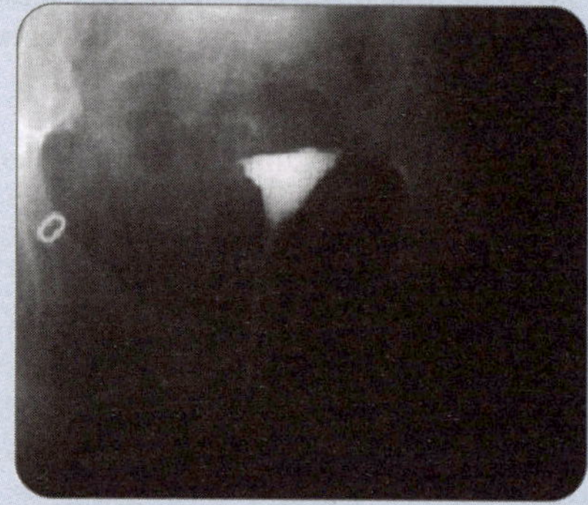

a. Genital TB
b. Gonococcal salpingitis
c. Clomydial salpingitis
d. Physiological

N24. Reversal of sterilization is best with:
a. Fallope rings
b. Clips
c. Modified Pomeroy technique
d. Uchida technique

N25. Which is not an assisted reproduction technique?
a. GIFT b. ZIFT
c. IVF and ET d. Artificial insemination

N26. In semen banks, semen is preserved at low temperature using:
a. Dry ice b. Deep freeze
c. Liquid nitrogen d. Liquid air

N27. Cytokine involved in ovarian hyperstimulation syndrome:
a. IL-2 b. VEGF
c. TNF-alpha d. Endothelin

N28. Which testicular cells are located outside the blood testis barrier:
a. Spermatogonia
b. Sertoli cells
c. Leydig cells
d. Primary spermatocyte

N29. For oil-based dye used in HSG all are true *except*:
a. Higher pregnancy rates
b. Better image quality
c. Higher chances of granuloma formation
d. Less Patient discomfort

N30. All of the following risks are increased in pregnancy achieved by IVF in comparison to normal pregnancy *except*:
a. Multiple gestation
b. Ectopic pregnancy
c. Heterotopic pregnancy
d. Chromosomal anomaly in fetus

N31. Reversal of sterilization is best with:
a. Falope ring
b. Cauterization
c. Pomeroy method
d. Irving method

N32. Best type of anastomosis for reversal of sterilization:
a. Isthmo-isthmic anastomosis
b. Isthmo-ampullary anastomosis
c. Ampullary-ampullar anastomosis
d. Interstitial-Isthmic anastomosis

PREVIOUS YEAR QUESTIONS

General Infertility

1. **In the perspective of the busy life schedule in the modern society, the accepted minimum period of sexual cohabitation resulting in no offspring for a couple to be declared infertile is:** *(AIIMS May 05)*
   a. One year
   b. One- and- a- half year
   c. Two years
   d. Three years
2. **Infertility is defined as** *(PGI May 2014)*
   a. If a couple fail to conceive after 18 months of unprotected regular intercourse
   b. If a couple fail to conceive after 15 months of unprotected regular intercourse
   c. If a couple fail to conceive after 12 months of unprotected regular intercourse
   d. Termed primary if conception has never occurred
   e. Termed secondary if conception has never occurred
3. **Infertility is seen in:** *(PGI Dec 02)*
   a. Fibroid uterus
   b. Endometriosis
   c. Adenomyosis
   d. PID
4. **Common causes of infertility are:** *(PGI Dec 00)*
   a. Chlamydia b. Gonorrhea
   c. Mycoplasma d. Pneumococcus
5. **Best prognosis in infertile women is seen in/most reversible form of infertility is:** *(PGI June 98, Dec 97)*
   a. Tubal block b. Anovulation
   c. Oligospermia d. Endometritis
6. **TB endometritis causes infertility by:** *(PGI Dec 98)*
   a. Causing anovulation
   b. Destroying endometrium
   c. Tubal blockage
   d. Ciliary dysmotility
7. **Kamla, a 30 yrs old lady examined for infertility by hysterosalpingography, reveals 'Bead-like' fallopian tube and clubbing of ampulla. Most likely cause is:** *(AI 02)*
   a. Gonococcus
   b. Mycoplasma
   c. Chlamydia
   d. Mycobacterium tuberculosis
8. **The risk of Asherman syndrome is the highest if Dilatation and Curettage (D and C) is done for the following condition:** *(AIIMS May 06)*
   a. Medical termination of pregnancy
   b. Missed abortion
   c. Dysfunctional uterine bleeding
   d. Postpartum hemorrhage
9. **What is the cause for luteal phase defect?** *(PGI Dec 05)*
   a. Progesterone is inadequately secreted
   b. Excess estrogen is secreted
   c. Excess progesterone is secreted

Female Infertility: Ovarian Cause

10. **Smita is a case of infertility. What is the right time in her menstrual cycle to do endometrial biopsy:**
    a. 12–14 days b. 17–19 days *(AIIMS Nov 00)*
    c. 20–22 days d. 3–5 days
11. **Fern test is due to:** *(SGPGI 05)*
    a. Presence of NaCl under progesterone effect
    b. Presence of NaCl under estrogenic effect
    c. LH/FSH
    d. Mucus secretion by Glands
12. **Drugs used for ovulation induction are:** *(PGI Nov 10)*
    a. GnRH
    b. Clomiphene citrate
    c. Gonadotropins
    d. Letrozole
    e. Danazol
13. **Antihormonal substance used to induce ovulation:** *(AI 07)*
    a. Mifepristone
    b. Clomiphene citrate
    c. Tamoxifen
    d. Raloxifen
14. **A patient treated for infertility with clomiphence citrate presents with sudden onset of abdominal pain and distension with ascites, the probable cause is:** *(AIIMS May 01)*
    a. Uterine rupture
    b. Ectopic pregnancy rupture
    c. Multifetal pregnancy
    d. Hyperstimulation syndrome

Female Infertility: Tubal Cause

15. **Fallopian tube dysmotility is seen:** *(AIIMS Nov 09, 08)*
    a. Noonan syndrome
    b. Turner syndrome
    c. Kartagener syndrome
    d. Marfan syndrome
16. **Best Investigation to assess tubal patency:** *(TN 95)*
    a. Rubin's test
    b. HSG
    c. Laparotomy
    d. Laparoscopic chromotubation
17. **Fallopian tube patency is checked by:** *(PGI Dec 02)*
    a. Hysterosalpingography
    b. Laparoscopy
    c. Hysteroscopy
    d. USG
    e. CT scan
18. **Lady with infertility with bilateral tubal block at cornual best method of management is:** *(AIIMS Nov 06)*
    a. Laparoscopy and hysteroscopy
    b. Hydrotubation
    c. IVF
    d. Tuboplasty

19. **An infertile women has bilateral tubal block at cornua diagnosed on hysterosalpingography. Next step in treatment is:** *(AIIMS Nov 2011)*
   a. IVF
   b. Laparoscopy and hysteroscopy
   c. Tuboplasty
   d. Hydrotubation
20. **Tubal patency is checked by all *except*:** *(PGI Nov 2010)*
   a. HSG
   b. Laparoscopy
   c. Falloscopy
   d. Celphorcopy
   e. Sonosalpingography

Female Infertility: Cervical Cause

21. **Postcoital test detects all of the following *except*:** *(AIIMS May 01)*
   a. Fallopian tube block
   b. Cervical factor abnormality
   c. Sperm count
   d. Sperm abnormality
22. **Cervical hostility is tested by following *except*:**
   a. Spinnbarkeit
   b. Postcoital test
   c. Miller kuzrole test
   d. Keller test *(PGI Dec 97)*
23. **Postcoital test showing non motile sperms in the cervical smear and Motile sperms from the posterior fornix suggests:** *(UPSC 97)*
   a. Faulty coital practice
   b. Immunological defect
   c. Hypospadias
   d. Azoospermia
24. **Treatment for Cervical infertility can be all *except*:** *(Delhi 99)*
   a. Condom for 3 month
   b. IUI
   c. Gamete Intrafallopian transfer
   d. Clomiphene citrate
25. **If the life style factor that is causing infertility in a young male is identified. Which of the following life style modification will have no effect?** *(AIIMS Nov 2014)*
   a. Weight gain b. Less exercise
   c. Vegetarian diet d. Weight loss

Male Infertility

26. **According to WHO criteria, the minimum normal sperm count is:** *(AIIMS)*
   a. 10 million/mL b. 15 million/mL
   c. 40 million/mL d. 60 million/mL
27. **Which is a not an essential criteria according to WHO for normal semen analysis?** *(AIIMS)*
   a. Sperm count >15 million/mL
   b. Volume >1 mL
   c. Sperm with normal morphology (strict criteria) > 4%
   d. Motility >32% with rapidly progressive motility
28. **According to the 2010 WHO criteria what are the characteristics of normal semen analysis.** *(AIIMS May 2015)*
   a. Volume 1.5 ml, count 15 million, morphology 4% progressive motility 32%
   b. Volume 2.0 mL, count 20 million, morphology 4% progressive motility 32%
   c. Volume 1.5 ml, count 20 million, morphology 4% progressive motility 32%
   d. Volume 2.0 ml, count 15 million, morphology 40% progressive motility 32%
29. **Aspermia is the term used to describe:** *(AI 05)*
   a. Absence of semen
   b. Absence of sperm in ejaculate
   c. Absence of sperm motility
   d. Occurrence of abnormal sperm
30. **Which of the following is true about obstructive azoospermia?** *(AI 09)*
   a. ↑ FSH and ↑ LH
   b. Normal FSH and normal LH
   c. ↑ LH, Normal FSH
   d. ↑ FSH, Normal LH
31. **A male with azoospermia. On examination size of testis normal FSH normal testosterone normal. Most probable cause is:** *(AIIMS Nov 09)*
   a. MAL descended testis
   b. Klinefelter's syndrome
   c. Kallmann's syndrome
   d. VAS obstruction
32. **Not found in seminal fluid:** *(PGI May 2013)*
   a. Fructose b. PG's
   c. Spermine d. Citric acid
   e. Inositol
33. **Sertoli cells secrete:** *(JIPMER 2012)*
   a. FSH
   b. LH
   c. Testosterone
   d. Androgen binding protein
34. **A couple having unprotected intercourse for one year and not able to conceive presents to infertility clinic. Woman has normal menstrual cycle. Semen analysis shows abnormal sperm morphology, low count and normal volume. Best next step would be:** *(JIPMER May 2016)*
   a. Perform HSG in woman
   b. Check LH, FSH levels
   c. Repeat test
   d. Get a scrotal USG done
35. **In azoospermia, the diagnostic test which can distinguish between testicular failure and obstruction of Vas deferens is:** *(UPSC 04)*
   a. Estimation of FSH level
   b. Estimation of testosterone level
   c. Karyotyping
   d. FNAC of testes
36. **A couple complains of primary infertility in spite of staying together for 4 year and having unprotected intercourse, all tests in wife are normal. Semen analysis shows a volume of 0.8 mL/sperm count is 0, fructose is absent what is done next?** *(AIIMS Nov 2013)*
   a. Testicular FNAC
   b. Ultrasound for obstruction
   c. Local palpation of vas
   d. Karyotyping

IUI

37. Intrauterine insemination means implantation of: *(PGI June 05)*
a. Semen
b. Washed semen
c. Million of sperm
d. Fertilized ova

38. IUI is indicated in all *except*: *(PGI Nov 2010/June 09/PGI Nov 15)*
a. Unexplained infertility
b. Endometriosis
c. Male infertility
d. PCOD
e. Tubal factor infertility

IVF

39. In vitro fertilization is indicated in: *(AIIMS Dec 97)*
a. Tubal pathology
b. Uterine dysfunction
c. Ovarian pathology
d. Azoospermia

40. Aspiration of sperms from testis is done in: *(AI 07)*
a. TESA
b. MESA
c. ZIFT
d. GIFT

41. A 25 years old female comes to your clinic for evaluation of infertility. A hysterosalpingogram reveals Asherman's syndrome. What symptoms will the patient have? *(AIIMS May 2016)*
a. Menorrhagia
b. Oligomenorrhea
c. Polymenorrhea
d. Hypomenorrhea

42. Indications for in-vitro fertilization (IVF): *(PGI Nov 2016)*
a. Bilateral tube blockage
b. Normal male factor
c. Hostile cervical factor
d. Proximal tubal block
e. Premature ovarian insufficiency

43. ICSI is/are useful in: *(PGI Nov 2015)*
a. Mullerian agenesis
b. Unexplained infertility
c. Hostile cervical mucus
d. Oligospermia
e. Presence of sperm antibodies

44. In Kartagener syndrome cause of infertility is: *(AIIMS May 2018)*
a. Oligospermia
b. Asthenospermia
c. Undescended testis
d. Epididymis obstruction

45. Which of the following is the important marker of male infertility in semen analysis? *(AIIMS May 2018)*
a. Motility
b. Concentration
c. Volume
d. Sperm Count

46. A 25-year-old women underwent induced clomiphene ovulation. On USG, ovary showed 8 follicles. Hypo-stimulation Serum estradiol level was 808 pg/mL. What is the next step in the management of this patient? *(AIIMS May 2018)*
a. Retrieve follicles
b. Give cabergoline
c. Cancel cycle
d. Withhold hCG

47. A young lady presents to the gynecology OPD with complaints of primary infertility, excessive weight gain and hirsutism. Laparoscopy shows the following finding. What is the most likely diagnosis? *(AIIMS May 2019)*

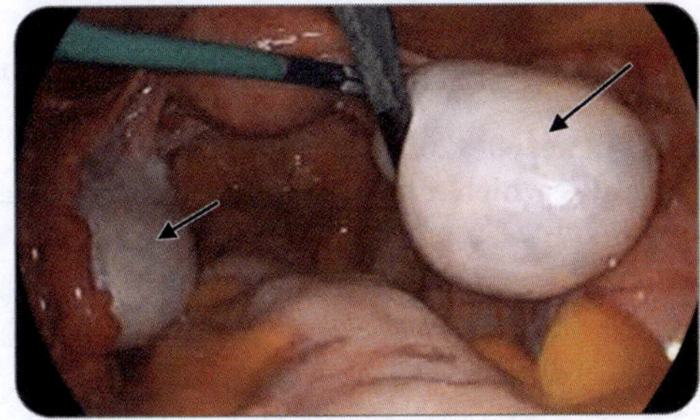

a. Turner's syndrome
b. Pituitary adenoma
c. PCOS
d. Bilateral dysgerminoma

48. Which is/are not true about lower reference range for semen analysis according to WHO recommendation? *(PGI May 2019)*
a. Sperm concentration–55 million spermatozoa per mL
b. Total sperm count–39 million per ejaculate
c. Sperm volume–1.5 mL
d. Morphology–4% normal
e. Progressive motility–62%

ANSWERS TO NEW PATTERN QUESTIONS

N1. Ans. is a, i.e. Inhibin secreted by Sertoli cells

See the text for explanation

N2. Ans. is c, i.e. Epididymis

Sperms attain motility and maturity in **caudal part of epididymis**

N3. Ans. is a, i.e. 30 mins

N4. Ans. is a, i.e. 2 mins

N5. Ans. is d, i.e. 7 hrs

Process	Time taken
• Liquefaction time	• 20–30 minutes
• Time taken by sperms to reach fallopian tube	• 2 minutes
• Capacitation time	• 7 hours

N6. Ans. is d, i.e. Leydig cells

Blood testis barrier is formed by Sertoli cells which keeps the growing germ cells (its all stages) separated from blood.

N7. Ans. is d, i.e. 9 + 2 arrangement

The tail of the sperm has 2 main parts:

- The principal piece which has a central core made of axial filaments with a 9 + 2 arrangement.
- The end piece is the small tapering part of tail.

N8. Ans. is b, i.e. Seminal vesicles

Major contribution to semen is by seminal vesicle, followed by prostatic fluid followed by secretion of bulbourethral glands.

N9. Ans. is d, i.e. 60–120 million/mL.

The values which are given in the text are normal minimum values.

Normal values are:

Volume 2–6 mL
pH = Alkaline = 7.2–7.8
Liquefaction within half an hour
Count: 15–200 million per mL
Mobility and motility 60% progressive forward motility
Morphology 60% normal forms

N10. Ans. is d, i.e. Both

Fructose is added to seminal fluid, by seminal vessicle and hence would be absent in case of both congenital absence of seminal vesicle (seen in case of **Congenital Bilateral Absence of Vas Deferens**) and ejaculatory duct obstruction.

N11. Ans. is c, i.e. Block in efferent duct system

See explanation of precious question

N12. Ans. is d, i.e. Luteal phase defect

IUI is done in case of:

- Hostile cervical mucus
- Unexplained infertility
- Oligoasthenospermia.

But it is not the treatment for Luteal phase defect. Treatment for LPD is progesterone.

N13. Ans. is c, i.e. Cervical factor

Homologous artificial insemination means husbands semen used for IUI.

N14. Ans. is d, i.e. Azoospermia

For IUI, minimum number of motile sperms needed are 10 million. It cannot be used in azoospermia.
Management in Azoospermia: superficial sperm retrieval from testis followed by ICSI.

N15. Ans. is d, i.e. Morphologically normal sperms < 2%

ICSI can be done

- When sperm count is < 5 million/mL
- Motile sperms are < 5%
- Morphologically normal sperms < 4% (not < 2%)
- In obstructive azoospermia when sperms are surgically retrieved
- In case of repeated IVF failure

N16. Ans. is b, i.e. 3 days

M/C time of embryo transfer = Day 3 (8 called Blastomere stage). Best result obtained with Day 5 transfer (Blastocyst transfer)

N17. Ans. is a, i.e. FSH *Ref: Novaks p1143*

In males with oligospermia, pregnancy rates have been improved by administering exogenous FSH. Clomiphene citrate can also benefit to some extent but not as much as FSH.

N18. Ans. is b, i.e. Regular cycle with dysmenorrhea

Lets see each option one by one:

Option a – Oligomenorrhea → means ovulatory dysfunction or anovulation

Option b – Regular cycles with dysmenorrhea – only ovulatory cycles are painful: So if in a female dysmenorrhea is present, it suggests ovulation.

Option c – Day 21 oestrogen levels increased; this suggests that female has not ovulated, as if she would have ovulated, on Day 21, levels of progesterone would have increased and not estrogen.

Option d – If a female ovulates, basal body temperature increases and does not decrease, due to the thermogenic effect of progesterone

Option e – On Day 8 main hormone is oestrogen and not progesterone in ovulatory cycles.

N19. Ans. is a, i.e. Measuring day 14 serum progesterone *Ref: Dutta Gynae 6th/ed, p240*

Serum progesterone is measured on D8 and D21 to show the rise and not on D14.

N20. Ans. is b, i.e. Anovulation

Pulsatile GnRH therapy is used for treating –

- Anovulation
- Delayed puberty

Rest everywhere continuous GnRH is used so as to decrease the levels of estrogen in hyperestrogenism conditions like–Precocious puberty, fibroid, endometriosis.

N21. Ans. is a, i.e. HSG

IOC for Tubal patency – HSG
Gold standard – Laparoscopic chromopertubation.

N22. Ans. is c, i.e. Leech Wilkinson cannula.

The figure shows Leech Wilkinson cannula which is used to insert dye into the uterus during HSG.

N23. Ans. is d, i.e. Physiological

- The HSG shows B/L cornual block which is most commonly physiological due to cornual spasm
- M/C pathological cause of cornual block: Genital TB
- M/C cause of distal block of fallopian tube: Gonococcus

N24. Ans. is b, i.e. Clips

See the text for explanation

N25. Ans. is d, i.e. Artificial insemination *Ref: Novak 14th/ed, p1237; Williams Gynae 1st/ed, p462*

All methods of ART, by definition, involve interventions to retrieve oocytes. These techniques includes IVF, ICSI, GIFT, ZIFT, Cryopreserved embryo transfers, and the use of donor oocytes.

Different methods of ART

IVF - ET	In vitro fertilization and embryo transfer
GIFT	Gamete intra-fallopian transfer
ZIFT	Zygote intra-fallopian transfer
POST	Peritoneal oocyte and sperm transfer
SUZI	Subzonal insemination
ICSI	Intra-cytoplasmic sperm injection

N26. Ans. is c, i.e. Liquid nitrogen *Ref: Jeffcoate 7th/ed, p723*

Cryopreservation of semen:

Involves cooling of embryos in the pronucleate stage or early cleavage stage to very low temperature in the presence of cryoprotectants such as:

- I_2 - Propanediol (Iodine)
- Glycerol
- Dimethyl sulphoxide (DMSO) with sucrose.
- They are then stored in liquid nitrogen till required.[Q]
- Over half the embryos survive thawing process.

N27. Ans. is b, i.e. VEGF

Cytokine involved in ovarian hyperstimulation syndrome is VEGF.

N28. Ans. is c, i.e. Leydig cells

See the text for explanation

N29. Ans. is d, i.e. Less patient discomfort *Ref: COGDT 10/e pg884*

Comparison of oil-based versus water-based dye used in the hysterosalpingogram	
Fertility enhancement	Oil: Higher pregnancy rates
Patient discomfort	Water: less cramping
Image quality	Water: rugae seen Oil: better image
Embolization	Minimal risk with either dye
Granuloma	Greater risk for retained oil

N30. Ans. is d, i.e. Chromosomal anomaly is fetus *Ref: COGDT 10/e p924*

In pregnancies achieved by IVF:

1. Multiple gestation—Likelihood of twins is increased by 20–30%

Multiple pregnancy:
- With clomiphene = < 10%
- With HMG = 30%
- With IUI = 10–20%

2. Ectopic pregnancy = chances are twice with IVF as compared to normal pregnancy
3. Heterotopic pregnancy (Twin pregnancy with 1 intrauterine and other ectopic) otherwise is rare but with IVF chances are increased.
4. Chances of preterm and low birth weight baby are higher in patients undergoing IVF

Chances of miscarriage
Chances of chromosomal anomaly] Same in IVF and normal pregnancy

N31. Ans. is a, i.e. Falope ring

- Chances of reversal are best when tubectomy was done with: Laparoscopic clips > Laparoscopic falope rings
- Chances of Reversal are least with: Cauterization.

N32. Ans. is a, i.e. Isthmo-isthmic anastomosis

See the text for explanation.

ANSWERS TO PREVIOUS YEAR QUESTIONS

General Infertility

1. **Ans. is a, i.e. One year** *Ref: Shaw 15th/ed, p200*
2. **Ans. is c, i.e. If a couple fail to conceive after 12 months of unprotected regular intercourse**

   If a couple fails to achieve pregnancy after one year of "unprotected" and regular intercourse, it is an indication to investigate the couple for infertility. *Ref: Novak 13th/ed, p973*

   - **Infertility:**
     - *Primary :* When no previous pregnancies have occurred.
     - *Secondary :* When a prior pregnancy although not necessary although not necessary a live birth, has occurred.
3. **Ans. is a, b, c and d, i.e. Fibroid uterus; Endometriosis; Adenomyosis; and PID**

   Ref: Dutta Gynae 5th/ed, p222-223; Novak 15th/ed, p1160, 1157; Williams Gynae 1th/ed, p427; Jeffcoates 7th/ed, p701-703

Common causes of female Infertility are:

a. Decreased ovarian reserve

b. Ovarian Factor

It is the most easily diagnosed and most treatable cause of infertility[Q]. It includes:

Anovulation / Dysovulation:

- Like in case of hypothalamic dysfunction[Q], Kallmann syndrome
- Hyperprolactinemia (due to drugs, pituitary adenoma[Q])
- Primary hypothyroidism[Q]
- PCOS[Q]
- Subclinical adrenal failure
- Diabetes mellitus

Luteinized unruptured follicle
Luteal phase defect

c. **Tubal Factors:** Partial or complete bilateral tubal obstruction resulting from previous salpingitis/PID. It could be: Postabortal[Q]
   - Gonococcal[Q]
   - Chlamydial[Q]
   - Tuberculous[Q]

- Tubal inflammation related to endometriosis
- Following Inflammatory bowel disease
- Following surgical trauma

d. **Peritoneal Factors:**
   - Pelvic adhesions
   - Endometriosis

e. **Uterine Factors:**
   - Uterine absence, atrophy
   - Congenital malformations (Among all congenital uterine abnormalities, septate uterus is the M/C and most highly associated with reproductive failure and obstetrics complications).

- Intrauterine adhesions (Asherman's syndrome)[Q]
- Endometrial polyps
- Leiomyomas (most common with sub mucous variety)[Q]
- Chronic endometritis (TB)[Q]
- Exposure to DES in utero

f. **Cervical Factors:**
   - Impenetrable cervical mucus or poorly penetrable cervical mucus due to presence of local sperm antibodies.
   - Loss of mucus due to amputation of cervix, cone biopsy or over enthusiastic cervical diathermy.
   - Faulty direction of cervix as seen in retroversion or severe prolapse.
   - Cervical stenosis.

g. **Others:** Anxiety/apprehension use of contraceptives; anorexia nervosa.

As such adenomyosis is not given as a cause of infertility but if you go through the chapter of adenomyosis: *Jeffcoate 7th/ed, p382 says* (In chapter on Adenomyosis): **"The patient may also complain of infertility".**

So, I am including it in the correct options.

4. **Ans. is a, b and c, i.e. Chlamydia; Gonorrhea; and Mycoplasma** *Ref: Williams Gynae 1st/ed, p434; Novak 14th/ed, p1227*

PID resulting in salpingitis is an important cause of infertility.

Infertility from PID can occur due to following organisms:

a. Chlamydia
b. Gonorrhea
c. Tuberculosis } *Ref: Williams Gynae 1st/ed, p434*
d. Mycoplasma (Specifically ureoplasma) *Ref: Novak 14th/ed, p1227*

Certain Infections cause Intrauterine synechiae or asherman syndrome thus leading to infertility like:

e. Schistosoma

5. **Ans. is b, i.e. Anovulation** *Ref: Kistner's Gynecology 6th/ed, p279; Novak 14th/ed, p1206*

"Disorders of ovulation account for about 30–40% of all cases of female infertility. These disorders are generally among the most easily diagnosed and most easily treatable causes of infertility." *Ref: Novak 14th/ed, p1206*

- In couples with infertility ovulatory disorder have the best prognosis. Relatively poor prognosis is observed in male factor infertility and tubal factor infertility.
- Prognosis can be arranged as below in descending order on the basis of cumulative pregnancy.

Ovulatory factor > unexplained > Male factors > Endometriosis > Tubal factors.

6. **Ans. is b and c, i.e. Destroying endometrium; and Tubal blockage** *Ref: Shaw 15th/ed, p154-156; Williams Gynae 1st/ed, p423*

- Most common site for genital TB is fallopian tube (90% cases).

- Uterus is involved in 70% cases of genital tuberculosis.
- The infection to uterus descends from the tube, i.e. if TB endometritis is present, invariably tubes are involved.
- Most common symptom of Genital TB: Infertility (35–60%). Infertility[Q] is either due to blockage of fallopian tube[Q] or due to loss of tubal function even if tubes are patent.[Q]

Tubercular endometritis causes uterine scarring which destroys the endometrium leading to synechia formation (Asherman syndrome) and infertility.

"In developing countries, genital TB may account for 3% or more of patients with infertility. In these cases tubal damage and endometrial adhesions are the underlying cause." *Ref: Williams Gynae 1st/ed, p423*

7. **Ans. is d, i.e. Mycobacterium tuberculosis** *Ref: Shaw 15th/ed, p157*

The following findings on hysterosalpingogram strongly suggest tubercular salpingitis:

- A rigid nonperistaltic pipe like tube, called ***lead pipe appearance***[Q]
- ***Beading and variation in filling density***[Q]
- ***Calcification of the tube***[Q]
- ***Cornual block***[Q]
- A jagged fluffiness of the tubal outline[Q]
- Vascular or lymphatic intravasation of the dye[Q]
- Tobacco-pouch appearance seen on naked eye examination.

Also Note:

- In a proven case of genital tuberculosis, hysterosalpingography is contraindicated as it may spread the infection.
- In TB Endometritis on HSG: The uterine cavity is shrivelled and obliterated by adhesions giving honeycomb appearance.
- On USG: Incomplete septation of the tubal wall "Cogwheel sign" is a marker for acute disease. Thin wall and beaded string appearance is a marker for chronic disease.

8. **Ans. is d, i.e. Postpartum hemorrhage**

Ref: Clinical Gynecologic Endocrinology & Infertility, Leon Speroff 7th/ed, p1045, Net search www.asherman syndrome.com

Asherman syndrome

Asherman syndrome is the presence of intrauterine adhesions.

Pathophysiology: It is the result of scanty or poorly vascularized and dysfunctional endometrium resulting from trauma. Any insult severe enough to remove or destroy endometrium can cause adhesions.

Etiology:

Asherman syndrome: ***"Generally is the result of an overzealous postpartum curettage resulting in intrauterine scarification."*** *... Leon Speroff 7th/ed, p 417*

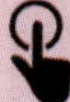

Most common etiology is: D and C done for postpartum haemorrhage.

Other Etiologies:

D and C done:

- After previous elective pregnancy termination.[Q]
- For missed abortion[Q]
- For hydatidiform mole[Q]
- After cesarean section[Q]

As a postoperative complication of:

- Abdominal/hysteroscopic myomectomy[Q]
- Metroplasty[Q]
- Septoplasty[Q]
- Uterine artery embolisation for the treatment of uterine fibroids
- Chronic infection-like genital tuberculosis[Q] and Schistosomiasis[Q] or infection due to IUCD's for 1-2 weeks.

Symptoms:

- Menstrual disorders like (hypomenorrhea, amenorrhea, dysmenorrhea).
- Hypomenorrhea is the typical symptom of Asherman syndrome.
- Infertility (it results due to absence of viable endometrium for implantation as well as from obstruction of fallopian tubes).
- Recurrent miscarriage (due to insufficient normal endometrial surface)
- If patients of asherman syndrome conceives, pregnancy is complicated by preterm labour, placenta accreta, placenta previa and/or PPH.

Diagnosis:
- Hysterosalpingography: (X-ray dye test) and saline hysterosalpingogram (fluid ultrasound) demonstrate filling defect.
- Hysteroscopy is both is the method of choice for diagnosis and treatment.[Q]

Treatment:
- Hysteroscopic lysis of adhesions is the preferred surgical treatment.
- Following surgery some method is used to keep the walls of the uterus apart in the immediate postoperative period to minimize the chances of recurrence. This is can be done by the use of balloon catheter or nonmedicated IUCD's for 1–2 weeks.
- Antibiotics are administered prior to the procedure and continued for approximately 10 days after the surgery.
- Postoperative treatment with exogenous estrogens 2.5 mg daily overlapping with progestin is given to promote rapid reepithelialization and reduce the risk of recurrent adhesion.

9. **Ans. is a, i.e. Progesterone is inadequately secreted** *Ref: Novak 14th/ed, p1225, 15th/ed, p1161*
Read the preceding text for explanation

Female Infertility: Ovarian Cause

10. **Ans. is c, i.e. 20–22 days** *Ref: Shaw 15th/ed, p215; Duta Gynae 5th/ed, p229*
See the text for explanation.

11. **Ans. is b, i.e. Presence of NaCl under estrogenic effect** *Ref: Shaw 15th/ed, p215*
- Fern test is for documenting ovulation.
- **Procedure:** A specimen of cervical mucus is obtained and is spread on a clean glass slide and allowed to dry. It is then viewed under the low power microscope.
- **Result and interpretation:** Under the influence of estrogen on Day12-Day 14 cervical mucus shows characteristic pattern of fern formation. *The ferning is due to the presence of sodium chloride in the mucus secreted under estrogen effect.*
- After ovulation on Day 21–23, ferning disappears because protein content increases and Sodium chloride decreases under the effect of progesterone.
- Disappearance of ferning after ovulation and if previously present is presumptive evidence of corpus luteum activity.

12. **Ans. is b, c and d, i.e. Clomiphene citrate; Gonadotropins; and Letrozole**
Ref: Williams Gynae 1st/ed, p450-452; Novak 14th/ed, p1210-1213

Most commonly used drugs for ovulation induction:
1. Clomiphene citrate (CC)
2. Letrozole
3. Gonadotropins

13. **Ans. is b, i.e. Clomiphene citrate** *Ref: Shaw 15th/ed, p217; Williams Gynae 1st/ed, p450-451*
See the text for Explanation

14. **Ans. is d, i.e. Hyperstimulation syndrome** *Ref: Shaw 15th/ed, p 315; Novak 14th/ed, p 1225; Recent Advances in Obstetrics & Gynecology no 21, p123 Onwards; Williams Gynae 1st/ed, p452-455*
History of clomiphene citrate and presence of ascites, abdominal pain and distension strongly suggest ovarian hyperstimulation syndrome.

Female Infertility: Tubal Cause

15. **Ans. is c, i.e. Kartagener syndrome** *Ref: Leon Speroff 7th/ed, p239; www.emedicine.com*
- **Primary ciliary dyskinesia (PCD)**, also known as immotile ciliary syndrome or Kartagener syndrome (KS), is a rare autosomal recessive genetic disorder in which there is a congenital absence of dynein arms (a protein structure associated with motility) in all body cilia.
- It can lead to male factor infertility due to diminished sperm motility in males. As far as female infertility is concerned–*patients with kartageners can conceive because motility of the cilia of fallopian tube is distorted and not totally absent.*

16. **Ans. is d, i.e. Laparoscopic chromotubation** *Ref: Shaw 15th/ed, p213; Leon Speroff 7th/ed, p1048*
17. **Ans. is a, b and d, i.e. HSG; Laparoscopy; and USG.**

The gold standard/best investigation to assess tubal patency is laparoscopic chromotubation.

Contraindication of tubal Patency tests.
- HSG should not be performed during and immediately before menstruation and in the post ovulatory period.
- HSG should not be performed after curettage.
- In recently active salphingitis.

- In suspected tuberculosis of genital tract.
- In infection of the lower genital tract.

18. Ans. is a, i.e. Laparoscopy and hysteroscopy *Ref: Leon Speroff 8th/ed, p1184-1185; Jeffcoates 7th/ed, p720; Advanced Infertility Management – Mehroo Hansotia p10*

19. Ans. b, i.e. Laparoscopy and hysteroscopy *Ref: Leon speroff 8th/ed, p1184-1185*

As discussed in text, M/C cause of B/L cornual block is physiological sperm hence it should be managed by cannulation under hysteroscopic guidance followed by Laparoscopic Chromopertubation to see whether the dye is coming out or not.

"In general, success rates achieved with surgery have been extremely poor and IVF represents the best treatment option"

Ref: Leonsperoff 8th/ed, p1184

"Hysteroscopic transcervical cannulation of the tubes has been used in case of proximal tube obstruction. This method has been successful in cases where there is no significant pathology but if there is endosalpingiosis or infection, this method cannot be curative." *... Jeffcoate 7th/ed, p720*

Hysteroscopic cannulation:

"Considering the simplicity of the procedure hysteroscopic cannulation should be tried as the first procedure for proximal tubal block. If the procedure is not successful or pregnancy is not achieved IVF is recommended."

... Advanced Infertility Management – Mehroo Hansotia p10

Management of Bipolar tubal obstruction, i.e. both proximal and distal tubal obstruction. Best is IVF

20. Ans. is a, b and c, i.e. HSG, Laparoscopy & Falloscopy

HSG & Laparoscopy (Laparoscopic chromopertubation) are used for assessing patency of tube. The other investigations which can be useful are:

Salpingoscopy: It is used to complement laparoscopy to assess the mucosa of infundibulum and ampulla

Falloscopy: It is microendoscopy of oviductal lumen from the utero-tubal ostium to the fimbriae by a transcervical approach.

As far as: Sonosalpingoscopy is considered – It is infusion of saline into endometrial cavity during sonography performed during follicular phase

But:

"The primary limitation of SIS is that it does not provide information about fallopian tube although rapid loss of saline into pelvis is certainly consistent with at least unilateral patency. **It is preferred if information about patency is not required.**"

Williams gynae 3rd/ed, p440

Female Infertility: Cervical Cause

21. Ans. is a, i.e. Fallopian tube block *Ref: Shaw 15th/ed, p204*

See the text for explanation.

22. Ans. is d, i.e. Keller test *Ref: Shaw 15th/ed, p20*

Post coital test and miller kurzrok test can detect cervical hostility as noted by rotatory/shaky movement of the sperm in post coital test, or < 3 cm of penetration of cervical mucus in 30 minutes in miller kurzrok test.

Spinbarkeit is basically a test for assessing ovulation: At the time of ovulation, the cervical mucus is thin and so profuse that the patient may notice a clear discharge *(called Normal ovulatory cascade)*. This ovulatory mucus has the property of great elasticity and will withstand stretching up to a distance of over 10 cm. This phenomenon is called spinbarkeit, or thread test for oestrogen activity. Under the influence of progesterone after ovulation mucus becomes thick and opaque and breaks on stretching i.e. hostile for sperms

Therefore, indirectly Spinbarkeit test can also detect cervical hostility.

23. Ans. is b, i.e. Immunological defect *Ref: Shaw 15th/ed, p204; Jeffcoate 7th/ed, p714*

Postcoital test showing non motile sperms in the cervical smear and motile sperms in the posterior forix suggest that the sperms are normal and motile when they reach fornix. After that in cervix they become immotile, i.e. antisperm artibodies are present in the cervix, i.e. immunological defect is seen.

24. Ans. is d, i.e. Clomiphene citrate *Ref: Dutta Gyane 5th/ed, p 241; Williams Gynae 1st/ed, p460*

Cervical factor infertility can be due to abnormal or deficient mucus *... William Gynae 1st/ed, p60*

i. Infection
ii. Prior cervical surgery
iii. Use of antiestrogens (e.g. clomiphene citrate) for ovulation induction (so clomiphene is a cause of cervical factor infertility rather than management)
iv. Sperm antibodies

The treatment of cervical factor thus depends on the cause:

- If it is due to chronic cervicitis/infection - Treatment of infection by antibiotics is the cure.
- If it is due to decreased mucus volume - Treatment includes short term supplementation with exogenous estrogen like ethinyl estradiol and use of mucolytic expectorant like guaifenesin. However, their value has not been confirmed.
- If it is due to antisperm antibodies. Treatment options include:

- Use of *condom or diaphragm as a barrier method for 3 months.* During this period, the antibodies will disappear and conception may occur then.
- ***Corticosteroids*** given to female partner can also help in getting rid of these antibodies.
- ***Intrauterine insemination*** at the time of ovulation (most acceptable method for cervical factor infertility) or *GIFT (Gamete intrafallopian transfer)* are very useful techniques in such cases.

• **IUI is the best method for treating cervical factor infertility and unexplained** infertility. So many clinicians forgo cervical mucus testing and proceed directly to IUI treatment in absence of tubal disease.

25. Ans. c, i.e. Vegetarian diet *Ref: http://www.cincinnatifertility.com/holistic-treatment/fertility-diet; http://www.baby-hopes.com/articles/exercise-fertility.html*

Vegetarian diet will have minimal or no effect on fertility.

"Weight definitely matters when it comes to fertility. Women who are overweight- or underweight-tend to have a more difficult time conceiving. The same goes for men, but more about that later." *- http://www.early-pregnancy-tests.com/weight-fertility.html*

"Exercise can affect fertility in several ways. Over-exercising is one of the bigger causes of infertility for women. *If a woman exercises too much, she is at a risk of losing too much of her body fat. Body fat plays an essential role in the production of estrogen; without enough estrogen, a woman who over-exercises might not ovulate. The technical term for not ovulating is oligomenorrhea, and is a major cause of fertility problems.* ***Women who don't get enough exercise can impact their fertility negatively as well. By not getting enough exercise, a woman runs the risk of becoming overweight or obese. An overweight or obese woman,*** *because she has more fat cells, can actually have too much estrogen. This overproduction of estrogen can negatively impact ovulation and conception. In addition,* ***being overweight puts you at risk for insulin resistance, which can ultimately keep you from ovulating."*** *-http://www.babyhopes.com/articles/exercise-fertility.html*

Male Infertility

26. Ans. is b, i.e. 15 million/mL

27. Ans. is b, i.e. Volume > 1 mL *Ref: Novak 14th/ed, p 1193; 15th/ed, p 1141; Leon Speroff 7th/ed, p1144*

Normal seminal fluid analysis:

Semen analysis - WHO

Parameter	2010 Guidelines
Volume	> 1.5 mL
Sperm concentration	> 15 million/mL
Sperm motility	> 32% progressive or > 25% rapidly progressive
Morphology (Strict Criteria) WBC	> 4% normal forms
Immunobead or mixed anti globulin reaction test	< 1 million/mL
	< 50%

28. Ans. is a, i.e. Volume 1.5 mL, count 15 million/mL morphology 4% and progressive motility 32%

Ref: Dutta Gynae 4th/ed, p218

29. Ans. is a, i.e. Absence of semen

Aspermia refers to failure of formation or emission of semen.

The absence of spermatozoa in semen is *known as* ***Azoospermia.***

For other terminologies related to semen analysis – refer preceding text

30. Ans. is b, i.e. Normal FSH and normal LH

In obstructive azoospermia, there is some obstruction due to which the sperms are absent in semen. Now since pituitary is normal hence LH, FSH levels will be normal, and since testis is normal so testosterone will be normal.

31. Ans. is d, i.e. VAS obstruction

Since all FSH, LH and Testosterone are normal therefore, it has to be an obstructive cause. Amongst the option, VAS obstruction is the only obstructive cause and hence our answer.

Ref Ganong

32. Ans. is e, i.e. Inositol

Composition of Semen

Organ	Contributes % of Semen	Feature
Testis/Epididymis	5%	Spermatozoa
Seminal vesicle	50-65%	Fructose, phosphorylcholine, ergothioneine, ascorbic acid, prostaglandins, flavins, Bicarbonate

Contd...

Contd...

Organ	Contributes % of Semen	Feature
Prostate	20-30%	Prostate Spermine Citric acid Cholesterol Phospholipids Zinc acid Fibrinolysin Phosphatase
Bulbourethral glands	<5%	Clean mucus

33. **Ans. is d, i.e. Androgen binding protein**

First of all by exclusion our answer is – Androgen Binding protein.

FSH stimulates Sertoli cells to produce Androgen binding protein which may serve to increase the accumulation of androgen in the seminiferous tubular epithelium & make it available for binding by intracellular androgen receptors.

34. **Ans. is c, i.e. Repeat test** *Williams Gynae 3rd/ed, fig 19.11, p445*

If a semen analysis report comes abnormal then a repeat semen analysis should be done at 1 month interval. If that also comes abnormal then other investigations should be done.

35. **Ans. is a, i.e. Estimation of FSH level** *Ref: Shaw 13th/ed, p203*

As discussed above

In Pretesticular cause e.g. Kallmann syndrome	LH decreased FSH decreased Testosterone decreased
In Testicular cause (orchitis, trauma, torsion, varicocele)	Testosterone decreased so LH↑ FSH↑
Post-testicular cause (obstruction, congenital B/L absence of vas deferens)	Testosterone Normal LH Normal FSH Normal

36. **Ans. is b, i.e. Ultrasound for obstruction** *Ref: Reproductive medicine secrets by Peter Chan 1st/ed, p33*

Absent fructose in semen means block is below the level of seminal vesicles which is not allowing sperms from testis and seminal fluid with fructose from seminal vesicle to be present in the semen. This means there is an obstructive pathology. The best way to detect obstruction is to perform a Transrectal Ultrasound.

Also Know

- **Role of Transrectal ultrasound in male infertility: Transrectal ultrasound (TRUS):** is done to visualize the seminal vesicles, prostate and ejaculatory ducts obstruction. Indications of TRUS are: (i) Azoospermia or severe oligospermia with a normal testicular volume, (ii) Abnormal digital rectal examination, (iii) Ejaculatory duct abnormality (cysts, dilatation or calcification), (iv) Genital abnormality (hypospadias).

IUI

37. **Ans. is b, i.e. Washed semen**

Intrauterine insemination is placement of 0.3 mL of **washed processed** (maxm = 0.5 mL) and concentrated sperms (devoid of seminal plasma)/semen into the intrauterine cavity by transcervical catheterization.

38. **Ans. is b, d and e, i.e. Endometriosis, PCOD and Tubal factor infertility**

In PCOD – Management is ovulation inducing drugs.

Endometriosis and Tubal factor infertility – Management is IVF.

IVF

39. **Ans. is a, i.e. Tubal pathology** *Ref: Shaw 15th/ed, p214; Clinical Endocrinology & Infertility by Leon Speroff 7th/ed, p1216, John Hopkins Manual of Obs and Gynae 4th/ed, p432*

IVF was first developed as a means to overcome infertility resulting from irreparable tubal disease as fertilization takes place in fallopian tube.

Now the spectrum of IVF has broadened and is indicated in number of conditions - as discussed in text.

40. Ans. is a, i.e. TESA *Ref: Novak 14th/ed, p1201*

Friends, we have studied in detail IVF and IUI but either of them cannot be performed if appropriate methods for sperm recovery are not available in cases of male infertility.

Sperm retrieval or recovery can be done by:

- Microsurgical epididymal sperm aspiration : **MESA**[Q]
- Percutaneous epididymal sperm aspiration : **PESA**[Q]
- Testicular sperm extraction : **TESE**[Q]
- Percutaneous testicular sperm fine needle aspiration : **TESA**[Q]

- The choice of the method depends on:
  - i. The underlying diagnosis,
  - ii. Whether goal of the procedure is diagnostic or therapeutic
  - iii. Whether, isolated sperm will be used immediately or cryopreserved.

For further details refer to the preceding text.

Note: GIFT: (Gamete Intra Fallopian Transfer)/ZIFT: (Zygote Intra Fallopian Transfer)

They are alternatives to IVF in which oocytes and sperm (in GIFT) or zygote (in ZIFT) are transferred to fallopian tube instead of uterus via laparoscopy. Once commonly used, as they offered high success rates to women with normal tube anatomy (whereas IVF is mainly used in cases where tubal pathology is present), both procedures are relatively rare now.

41. Ans. is d, i.e. Hypomenorrhea

The typical presenting symptom in adenomyosis is hypomenorrhea, i.e. less blood loss during menstruation.

42. Ans. is a, d and e, i.e Bilateral tube blockage, Proximal tubal block and Premature ovarian insufficiency

43. Ans. is a, b and d, i.e. Mullerian agenesis; Unexplained infertility and Oligospermia

ICSI can be done in all these conditions where IVF is done hence their is no doubt about Mullerian agenesis and oligospermia.

In cases of unexplained infertility—if IUI fails, it is followed by IVF/ICSI.

Indications of IVF

1. Tubal factor infertility
   a. In distal tubal obstruction- IVF is treatment of choice for severe distal disease
   b. In proximal tubal obstruction as discussed in chapter on infertility, M/C causes physiological spasm hence management is tubal cannulation under hysteroscopic guidance followed by Laparoscopic chromopertubation. If it persists then IVF is done
2. Endometriosis
3. Preimplantation genetics diagnosis
4. Premature ovarian failure- using donor eggs.
5. Mullerian agenesis = IVF followed by surrogacy.
6. Male factor infertility with sperm concentration 5-15 million/mL
7. Fertility preservation in case female is having cancer and needs chemotherary. In these cases eggs are cryopreserved

Indications of ICSI: ICSI can be used in all cases where IVF is used and also:

- Male factor infertility with sperm court < 5 million/mL
- Asthenospermia (<5% progressive motility)
- Terato spermia (<4% normal forms)
- Or in surgical retrieved sperms from testis in case of obstructive 9200 Azoospermia
- For preimplantation genetic diagnosis
- Repeated IVF failure

Note: In the question- for hostile cervile factor i.e antisperm antibodies, IUI is done

44. Ans. is b i.e. Asthenospermia *Ref: Clinical Gynecologic endocrinology and infertility, Leon speroff*

- Kartagener syndrome is also known as **primary ciliary dyskinesia**.
- It is identified as a cause of male infertility as it affect ciliary structure and function and thus causes oligo-asthenospermia (poor sperm motility). It is primarily a disorder of sperm transport so if one option is to be chosen, asthenospermia is the answer of choice.
- Affected individuals also have chrome respiratory infections as cilia of respiratory tract are also affected.

45. Ans. is b i.e. Concentration *Ref: Clinical Gynecologic Endocrinology Infertility 8th/ed*

See Chapter 10 of book.

46. Ans. is d i.e. Withhold hCG *Ref: Berek and Novak's Gynaecology*

Now lets first understand a few concepts before jumping at the answer

1. For hCG trigger: at least 2 follicles measuring 17-18 mm should be present.

2. Per follicle 150-200 pg/mL of estrogen is adequate.
- Now in this patient: Number of follicles shown on USG are: 8 follicles
- Since day on which USG is done is not mentioned we presume it to be Day (2) i.e. the usual time.
- Now on day (2) = 8 follicles are seen on USG.
- Levels of estradiol are 800 pg/mL.
- This means: Out of the 8 follicles approx. 4 are mature & rest are immature.
- Now comes the TRICK:
- If question would have said we are doing IVF and since age of patient is 25 years, I would have cancelled the cycle as this is too less an estrogen and less follicles (mature) to go ahead with retrieving of follicles.
  Now the question is saying simply Induced ovulation i.e. either we are using clomiphene or letrozole.
- Now in this case 800 pg/mL or 4 follicles are good enough. I will not give hCG otherwise patient will land into OHSS. So answer as per me should be withhold hCG (best answer) or cancel cycle (2nd best answer).

47. Ans. is c, i.e. PCOS

- The Laparoscopic image shows bilaterally enlarged ovaries.
- Patient has H/O weight gain, primary infertility and hirsutism.

Now amongst the given options:

- *In Turner's syndrome*: Patient will have streak gonads (ovaries will not be enlarged, so it is ruled out)
- *In Pituitary Adenoma*: They are pituitary tumors which may be functional (have more secreting) or non-functional. Mostly pituitary tumors are functional prolactin secreting lactotroph or non-functional. In a prolactin secreting lactotroph, due to increased levels of prolactin, the levels of LH and FSH decrease. Hence the size of ovary is never increased. Only in rare cases of Gonadotroph secreting pituitary tumors, the levels of LH and FSH are high and hence the size of ovary is increased due to hyperstimulation. But then it is a rare case of enlarged ovaries.
- *In B/L dysgerminoma*: Which is a germ cell tumor of ovary. There will be B/L enlarged ovaries but then patient will be cachexic and will have weight loss. The tumor is grows rapidly and leads to pain in abdomen. Patient will not present as weight gain, hirsutism and primary infertility.

All these symptoms along with by laterally enlarged ovaries are constant with PCOS.

48. Ans. is a and e, i.e. Sperm concentration—55 million spermatozoa per mL, Progressive motility—62%

Semen analysis (WHO-2010).

Semen analysis	***Normal reference value***	***Lower reference limit***
Volume	2.0 mL or more	1.5 mL
pH	7.2–7.8	
Viscosity	<3 (scale 0–4)	
Sperm concentration	20 million/mL	**15 million/mL**
Total sperm count	>40 million/ejaculate	**39** million/ejaculate
Motility	>50% progressive forward motility	**Progressive motility = 32%**
Morphology	>14% normal form	**4%**
Viability	75% or more living	58%
Leukocytes	Less than 1 million/mL	
Round cells	<5 million/mL	
Sperm agglutination	<10% spermatozoa with adherent particles	

Latest WHO recommendations for normal semen analysis reference values.

- Volume: ***1.5***-5.0 mL
- pH: >7.2
- Viscosity: <3 (scale 0-4)
- **Sperm concentration: >15 million/mL**
- **Total sperm number: >39 million/ejaculate**
- **Per cent motility: >32%**
- Forward progression: >2 (scale 0-4)
- **Normal morphology: >4%**
- Round cells: <1 million/mL
- Sperm agglutination: <2 (scale 0-3)

CHAPTER 10

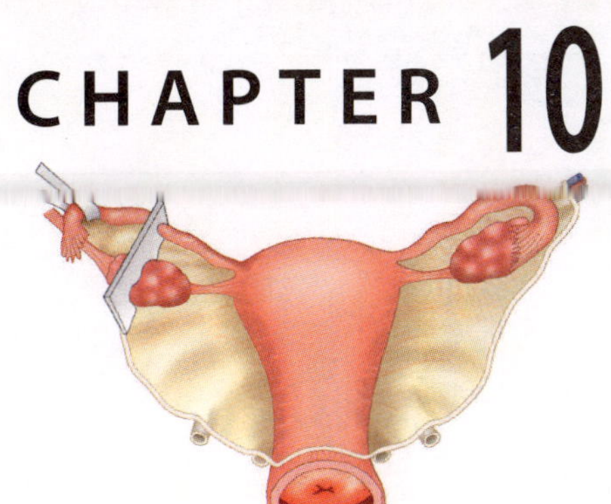

Contraception

Flowchart 10.1

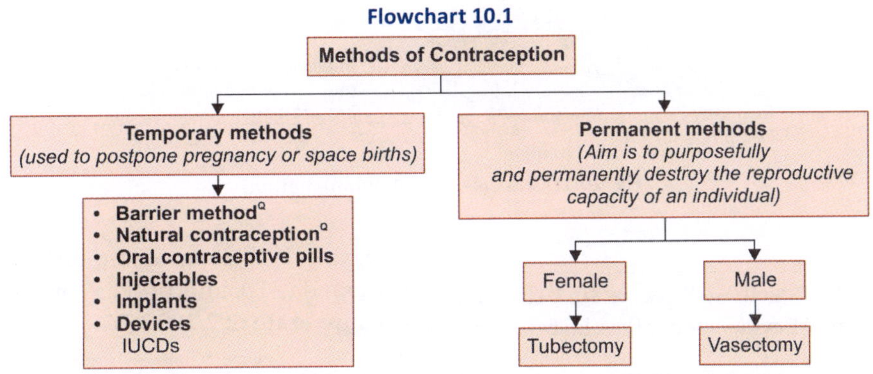

Contraceptive methods are classified as:

- **Top Tier:** Method - Most effective & easy to use. They include = IUCD/Implants/Male and Female sterilization methods.
- Second Tier: Include OCP's, injections, transdermal patches and transvaginal rings.
- Failure Rates - 3–9/100 users
- **Third tier** = Include Barrier methods. Failures rates: 10–100/100 users.
- Fourth tier includes spermicidal preparations.
- Failure Rates - 21–30/100 users.

Natural Family Planning Method

It is the method of planning family without using any drugs or contraceptives.

Flowchart 10.2

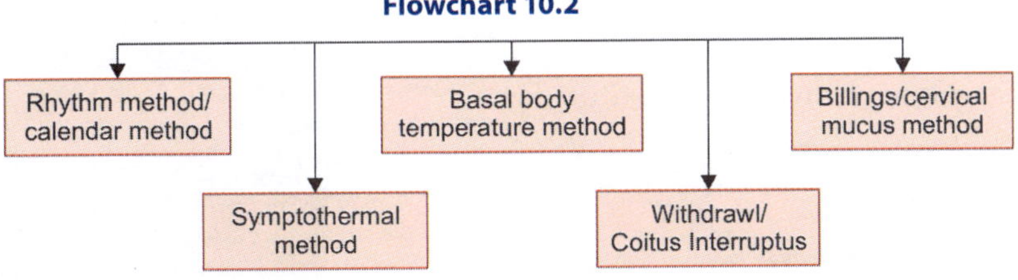

Basis: These methods aim at avoiding sexual intercourse around ovulation.

The timing of ovulation can be judged on calendar basis and symptom basis.

1. Rhythm method/calendar method: It is based on Ogino-Knaus theory which states ovulation occurs on day 14 ± 2 in a female with a regular 28 days cycle (i.e. avoid sex between 12th and 16th day)

But fertilizable span of sperm is 48 – 72 hours and ova is 12 – 24 hours.

Therefore, unsafe period = 8–18 day (Failure rate = 25 – 35%)
Failure rate can be reduced if sex is avoided from 7–21 day if (failure rate = 10%)

Thus sex is safe only in the first and last 7 days of a menstrual cycle *(park 20/e, p436)* (Fig. 10.1)

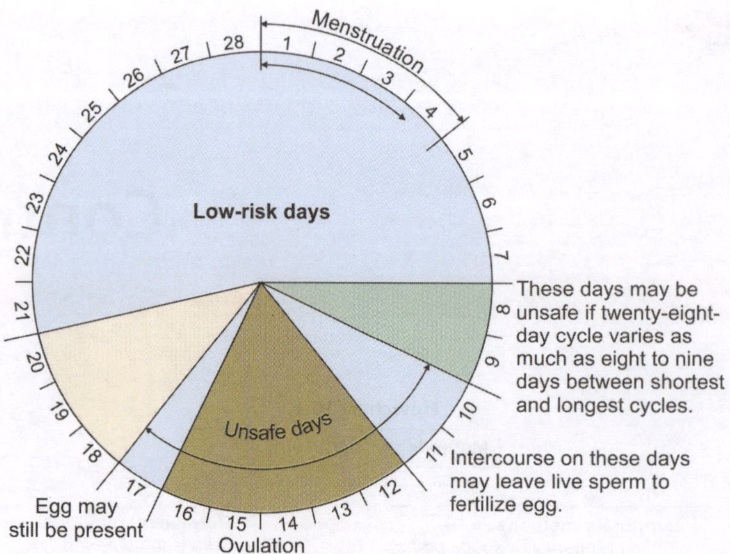

Fig. 10.1: The Calendar (Rhythm) method

In irregular cycle:

Safe period is = shortest cycle - 18 (gives first day of the fertile period) longest cycle - 11 (gives last day of the fertile period).

Advantage: Low cost and lack of side effects

- **Drawback:** Difficult to predict safe period if cycles are irregular
- Can only be used by educated and responsible couples with a high degree of motivation and cooperation.
- Compulsory abstinence of sexual intercourse for nearly half month called as programmed sex.
- Not applicable during postnatal period.
- High failure rate -9/100 WY.

Standard Days Method (In India called as Tirumala Method)

- Developed by Georgetown University's Institute for Reproductive Health.
- It has a simpler rule set and is *more effective than the rhythm* method.
- A product, called ***Cyclebeads,*** was developed alongside the method to help the user keep track of estimated high and low fertility points during her menstrual cycle.
- The Standard Days Method can only be used by women whose cycles are always between 26 and 32 days in length.

In this system:

- Days 1–7 of a woman's menstrual cycle are considered infertile.
- Days 8–19 are considered fertile.
- From day 20, infertility is considered to resume.
- Failure rate of **2/100 WY**.

Cervical Mucus Method (Billings Method) (Figs. 10.2 and 10.3)

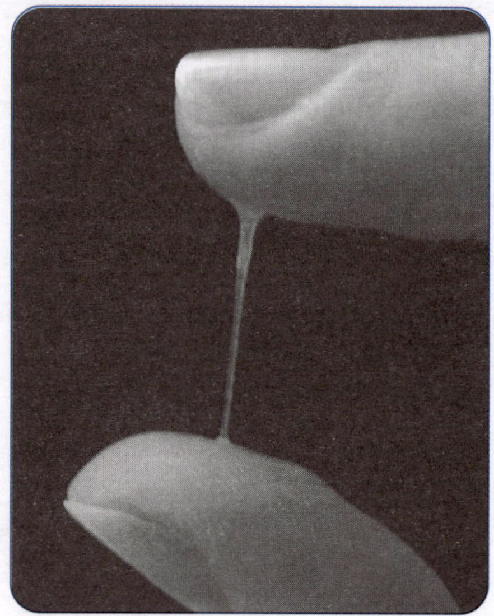

Fig. 10.2: Cervical mucus method

- This method is based on the observation of changes in the characteristics of cervical mucus.
- At the time of ovulation: Cervical mucus is watery, clear (resembling raw eggs white), smooth, slippery and profuse. After ovulation, under the influence of progesterone, the mucus thickens and lessens in quantity.

- It is recommended that women use tissue paper to wipe inside the vagina to assess the quantity and character of mucus.
- Intercourse is considered to be safe during the dry days immediately after the menses and till the mucus is detected. Thereafter the couple must abstain until the fourth day after the peek day.
- To practice this method, the women should be able to distinguish between the different types of mucus. This requires a high degree of motivation.

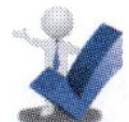

KEY POINTS

Cervical mucus method (Billings method) is based on the principle that under the influence of estrogen, cervical mucus is thin, watery, profuse and elastic (it can be stretched between fingers called Spinnbarkeit). Whereas after ovulation under the influence of progesterone it becomes thick, scanty and loses its elastic nature and breaks on stretching called as Tack.

Basal Body Temperature Method

A woman's basal body temperature (BBT) drops briefly and then rises half a degree following ovulation, due to thermogenic effect of ping progesterone and remains elevated in the secretory phase. Normal BBT is between 96 and 98 degrees, and after ovulation rises to 97 – 98 degrees fahrenheit or rises by 0.2–0.5°C. A rise in temperature that persists for at least 3 days indicates that ovulation has occurred. ***The safe period begins from the fourth day (first day being the day of ovulation) to the last day of the next period.*** For this method to be effective, a chart of daily temperature reading needs to be kept.

Symptothermic Method

This method makes use of at least two indicators to identify the fertile period. Usually the cervical mucus method and the BBT methods are combined.

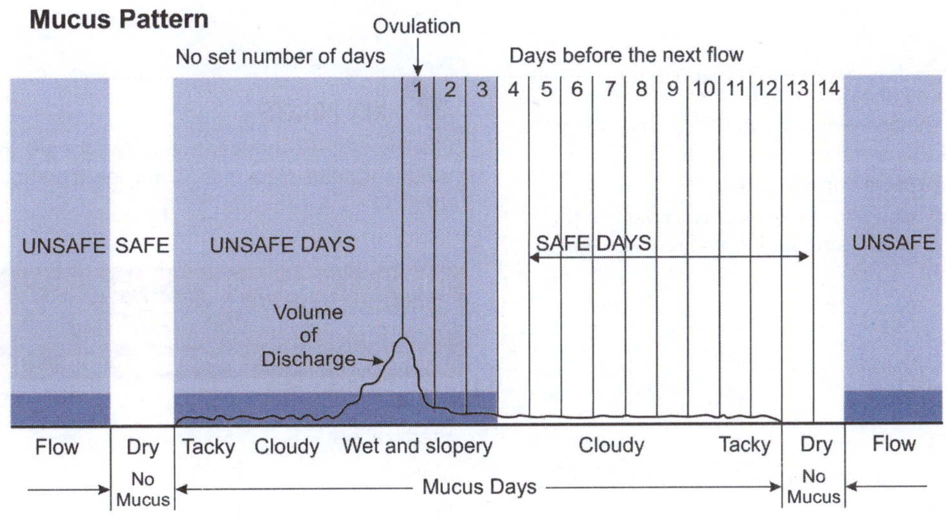

Fig. 10.3: Billings method

Lactational Amenorrhea Method (LAM)

Basis

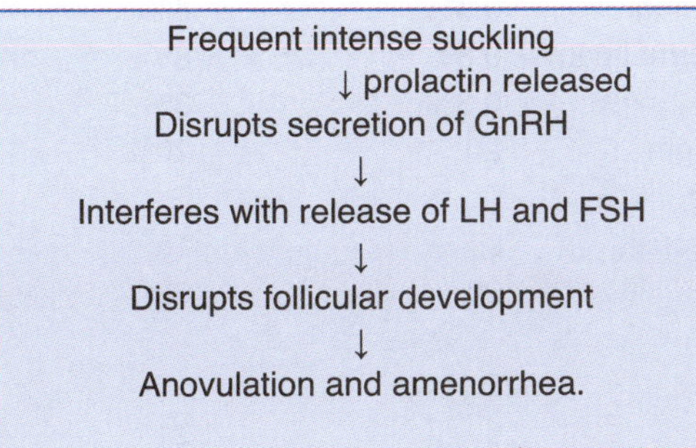

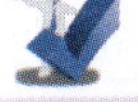

KEY POINTS

The 3 prerequisites for lactational amenorrhea to ensure effective contraception

1. Exclusive breast feeding
2. Baby <6 months of age
3. There is amenorrhea (menses should not have resumed after delivery)

Failure rate = 5/HWY.

Recent Advances

Special digital thermometers and use of the ovumeter to note changes in cervical mucus are under experiment.

Another device called PERSONA (unipath) consists of dipsticks to detect urinary estrone 3- glucuronide (which indicates the onset of the fertile period) and LH (which indicates ovulation).

Natural Family Planning Methods are not Suitable for Women

- With irregular cycles, cycles shorter than 21 days
- During adolescence, lactation, and premenopausal
- Who have had cervical surgery (cautery and conization)
- With vaginal infection (until cure)
- Who have sexually transmitted disease (STD) or pelvic inflammatory disease (PID) in the last 3 months
- Who had abortion recently
- Noncooperative husbands and couples who have casual sex.

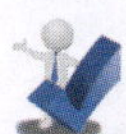

KEY POINTS

The typical failure rate of natural family planning method is 20 per 100 women in the first year of use but it can be reduced to 1–9 % with correct usage and practice.

Characteristic of an Ideal Contraceptive

An ideal is safe, effective, inexpensive, reversible, simple to use, independent of coitus, long lasting and requires minimal medical supervision.

Pearl Index

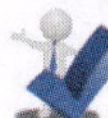

KEY POINTS

Pearl index indicates the effectiveness of a contraceptive or is an index of contraception failure.

- It is expressed in terms of *"failure rate per hundred women - years of exposure (HWY)"*.
- Failure rate per HWY =

$$\frac{\text{Total accidental pregnancies} \times 1200\ (12 \times 100)}{\text{No. of patients observed} \times \text{Months of use}}$$

- In applying the above formula the following points must be kept in mind:
  a. The total accidental pregnancies shown in the numerator must include every known conception, whatever its outcome.
  b. The factor 1200 is the number of months in 100 years.
  c. The total months of exposure in the denominator is obtained by deducing from the period under review of 10 months for a full term pregnancy and 4 months for an abortion.

Lets understand this by an example.

Suppose 100 couples have used a method for a period of 3 years and have resulted in 24 pregnancies, the pearl index is $\frac{24 \times 1200}{100 \times 36} = 8$

WHO Eligibility Criteria for Contraceptives

WHO divides the contraceptive methods into 4 categories in a particular condition:

WHO category 1: Means that there is no contraindication for the use of the contraceptive. There is no restriction for its use. These methods can be used freely.

WHO category 2: The contraceptives should be used with caution in these conditions.

WHO category 3: The proven risks of the contraceptives in these conditions outweigh the advantages. Avoid these methods.

WHO category 4: There are absolute contraindications for the use of a particular contraceptive. Never use the method.

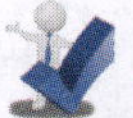

KEY POINTS

Efficiency of a contraceptive is considered to be high if the pregnancy rate is less than 10 and low if pregnancy rate is more than 20.

Table 10.1: Pearl Index

User Independent		
Contraception	**Perfect use rate**	**Typical use**
Implants	.05	.05
Sterilization		
Male	0.1%	0.15%
Female	0.5%	0.5%
IUCD		
Mirena	0.2%	0.2%
CuT 380 A	0.6%	0.8%
User Dependant		
OCP's	0.3%	8%
Vaginal ring	0.3%	8%
Transdermal path	0.3%	8%
DMPA	0.3%	3%
Diaphragm	20	20%
Sponge		
Nullliparous	9	16
Parous	20	32
Condom		
Male	2	15
Female	5	21

Note: Least failure rate is with perfect use. If in question nothing is mentioned take it as Typical use.

Barrier Methods

Males	Females
• Condoms	• Female condoms (Femshield) • Today contraceptive/vaginal sponge • Vaginal diaphragm/cervical cap

Note: Spermicidal agents like nonoxynol octoxynol and menfegol are added to any of the above barrier methods to increase its effectiveness.

Male Condoms/French Letters

- **Types:**
  - Latex
  - Vylex
  - Natural membrane condoms
  - Polyurethane
  - Polyisoprene

Note:

Polyurethane condoms have a longer shelf life and can be used with oil based lubricants (latex condoms get damaged when oil based lubricant is used).

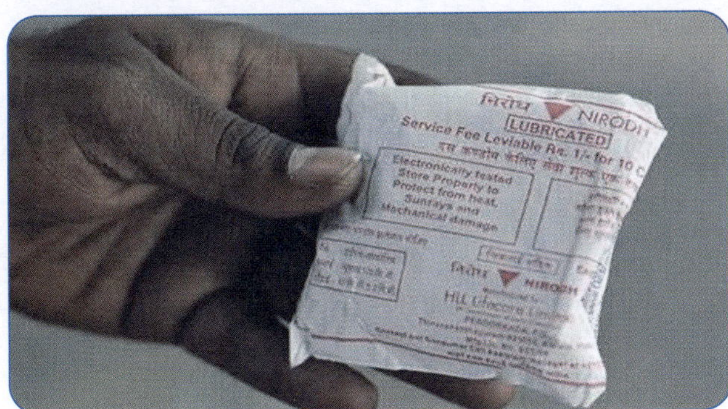

Fig. 10.4: Nirodh is available free of cost at government hospitals

Directions for Use

- The condom should be put on by unrolling it over the erect penis after pulling back the foreskin, before there is any contact between the male and female organs. An airfree space should be left by squeezing the tip and holding it up till it is unrolled fully for better collection of semen.
- It should be used only once.
- It should not be inflated for testing.
- Vaseline oils, skin lotions, cold creams, i.e. oil based lubricant should not be used as they increase the chance of rupture. If lubrication is needed, water based lubricant K-Y jelly or spermicidal jelly can be used.
- Soon after discharge, the male should withdraw the penis holding the condom firmly against his body
- To increase the effectiveness, a dose of spermicidal jelly or foam tablet may be used at the same time. In case of breakage, slippage, or defective use, women should report or use emergency contraceptive within 72 hours and a spermicidal agent should be quickly inserted into the vagina.

Condoms: Prevent PID
Prevent ectopic pregnancy

Advantages

- Condoms gives very good protection against STDs. These include syphilis gonorrhea, trichomoniasis, moniliasis, nongonococcal urethritis, and infection with chlamydia and herpes virus.
- They are the only contraceptives to protect against HIV and against sexually transmitted hepatitis B Virus.
- Condoms reduce the chances of developing cervical dysplasia and cancer cervix (by preventing HPV infection).

Non-contraceptive Uses

- After vasectomy to be used till semen analysis confirms azoospermia.
- As condoms catheter in males
- After vaginoplasty
- As condom tamponade for managing atonic PPH
- In patients with antisperm antibodies present in cervical mucus.

Disadvantages

It can lead to contact dermatitis in female partners.

Female Condom (Reality Condom/Femshield) (Fig. 10.5)

- Consist of Polyurethane/sac about 15 cm long and 7 cm in diameter with 2 flexible rings.
- The ring at closed end covers the cervix internally like a diaphragm and rug at open end covers the vulva.
- It is pre lubricated with silicon based lubricant (dimethicone)
- The condom is to be inserted like a tampon before intercourse and removed soon after intercourse.
- Sexual intercourse takes place within the cavity of the device.
- The advantage of female condom is its use depends on the will of the female partner and does not require male cooperation. **It prevents STDs and HIV.**

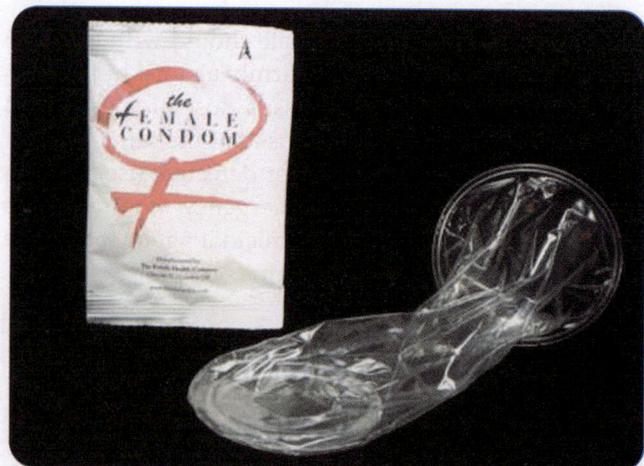

Fig. 10.5: Female condom

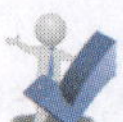

KEY POINTS

Female condoms

FC-1 = made of polyurethane is not used now

FC-2 = Nitrile based female condom, socially marketed free of cost by Govt. of India to female sex workers.

FC-3 = Made of latex.

Important One Liners

Female condoms protect against STDs and HIV.

Disadvantages of female condom

- High failure rate = 5–20%
- Small risk of Toxic shock syndrome
- Increased risk of UTI
- Interferes with sexual pleasure
- Unsuitable for women with uterine prolapse, cystocele, rectocele or retroverted uterus

Occlusive Caps (Vaginal Diaphragm and Cervical Caps) (Figs. 10.6 and 10.7)

- Occlusive caps do not act as sperm proof mechanical barriers like condoms but are used as a means to retain spermicides in contact with cervical os, so spermicides must be used along with these devices.
- After intercourse, the vaginal diaphragm and vault cap should not be removed before 6-8 h of the last act and should not be kept for more than 24 h.
- The best time to introduce it is, from a few minutes to 2 h before the sexual act.
- Like condoms, diaphragms and cervical caps prevent the spread of STDs, but AIDS is not prevented by them.

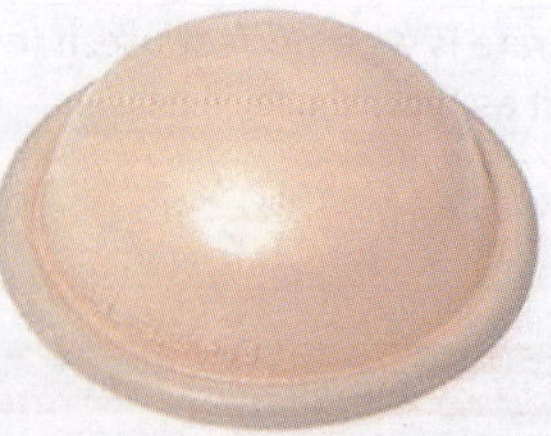

Fig. 10.6: Vaginal diaphragm

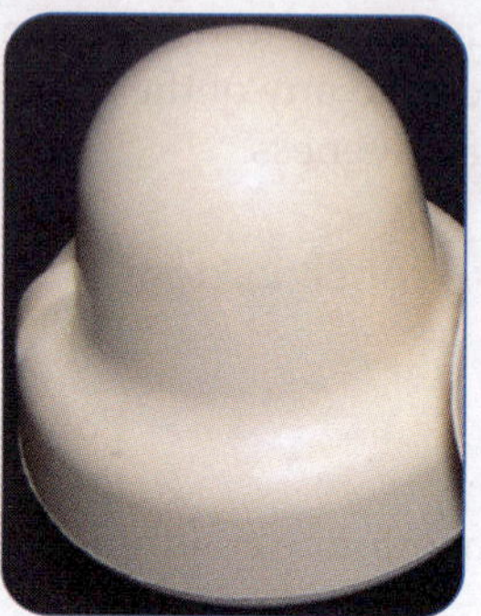

Fig. 10.7: Cervical cap

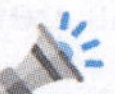

Important One Liners

Contraindications to the use of diaphragm—

a. Prolapse, cystocele, rectocele
b. Retroversion
c. Vesico Vaginal Fistula/Rectovaginal Fistula
d. Badly eroded or lacerated cervix
e. Recurrent UTI

Multiple sex partners is not a contraindication for the use of diaphragms, rather barrier contraceptives protect against STD's so these are contraception of choice in them.

Disadvantages

- Diaphragms increase the chance of UTI and cervical erosion
- They do not protect against HIV
- Not suitable for women with uterine prolapse

Spermicides

- *Spermicidal agents are chemical agents with kill the sperms before it enters to the cervical canal. They are available as foam tablets, soluble pessaries, creams, jellies or as films.*
- Contents are:
  - **Nonoxynol - 9 (N - 9)**
  - Menfegol
  - Benzalkonium chloride.
  - Octoxynol
  - Enzyme inhibiting agents

– Jeffcoates 7th/ed, p794

- **The main mechanism by which spermicidal jelly acts is by disruption of sperm cell membrane.**
- Failure rate is 20–25 per 100 WY, when used alone. When used in conjunction with a mechanical barrier, they give a reliable contraceptive effect.

Recent Advances

Recent evidences indicate spermicides are not effective in preventing cervical gonorrhea, Chlamydia, or HIV infection. In addition, frequent use of spermicides containing N-9 has been associated with an increased risk of HIV transmission. *– CGDT 10th/ed, p581*

- Advantage 24 is a new contraceptive gel which contains nonoxynol.

Today/Vaginal Sponge (Fig. 10.8)

- It is mushroom shaped polyurethane disposable sponge.
- It is contains 1 gm of NONOXYNOL - 9 and is provided with a loop for easy removal.
- It is a barrier contraceptive which prevents entry of sperm into the cervical canal and contains a spermicidal agent.
- It should be placed high up in the vagina with concave side covering the cervix & should be kept for 6 hrs in vagina after intercourse (maximum wean time is 30 hrs)
- It remains effective for 24 hours regardless of the frequency of coitus and should be kept for 6 hrs in vagina after intercourse (maximum wear time is 30 hrs)
- It is to be used only once.
- It should be left in vagina and removed 6 hrs after sexual intercourse.

Side Effects

- Allergic reactions
- Vaginal dryness, soreness, or itching
- It can lead to genital lesions which may damage the vaginal mucosa and enhance HIV transmission.

> ***Note:***
> Different books have a different say on role of Today in preventing STD's and toxic shock syndrome. But *Leon Speroff* is the most authentic book for this issue. It says – *(Leon Speroff 7th/ed, p 1003)*
> - There is no risk of toxic shock syndrome, infact nonoxynol 9 retards staphylococcal replication and toxin production.
> - It decreases the risk of infection with gonorrhea, Trichomonas, and Chlamydia.

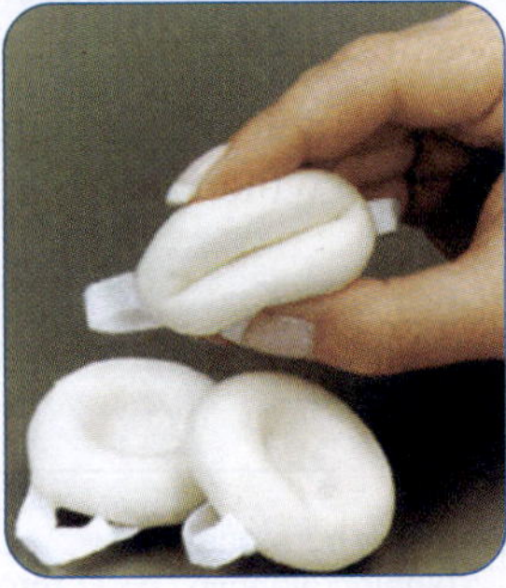

Fig. 10.8: Vaginal contrceptive sponge (Today)

Oral Contraceptives

Mechanism of Action

Prevention of ovulation[Q]	Prevention of fertilization[Q]	Interference with Implantation[Q]
• Progestin reduces frequency of LH secretory pulses, while estrogen primarily reduces FSH secretion. • Both synergise each other to inhibit GnRH • As a result, follicles fail to develop and rupture and ovulation does not occur.	• Thick cervical mucus, hostile to sperms may inhibit fertilization. • Uterine and tubal contractions may be modified to disfavor fertilization.	• Endometrium is rendered either hyperproliferative, hypersecretory, or atrophic and out of phase with fertilization and not suitable for nidation Thus, even if ovulation and fertilization occur, implantation does not occur normally.

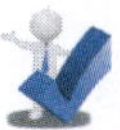

KEY POINTS

- Standard dose pills have = Estrogen 50 mcg
- Lose dose pills have = Estrogen < 50 mcg (M/C = 35 mcg).
- Very low dose < 20 mcg
- Minimum effective doses of Estrogen in OCP's = 10 mcg.
- Minimum effective doses of estrogen in OCP = 10 mcg.

In 2011, FDA approved the first pill containing only 10 mcg of ethinyl standard LO-Loestrin FE.

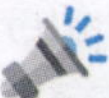

Important One Liners

- Main mechanism of action of combined pills is prevention of ovulation.
- Combined pills act by decreasing both LH and FSH
- They do not interfere with placental functioning.
- When taken daily for 3 out of 4 weeks, they provide virtually absolute protection against conception.

Progesterones in OCPs

Generation	Progesterone	Comments
Ist generation: (Estranes derived from Testosterone)	Norethisterone, Norethindrone, Norethynodrel, lynestrenol	Used in pills with ≥50 mcg of EE
2nd generation	Levonorgestrel Norgestrel	Levonorgestrel is the M/c used progesterone in OCPs E.g. = Mala N, Mala D
3rd generation (Gonanes)	Desogestrel (active from 3-keto DSG), Gestodene, Norgestimate	Pills with 3rd generation progesterones are very beneficial (see flowchart 10.3) e.g. of pills are femilon, Loette, Novelon
4th generation	Drospirenone Dienogest, nomegestrol	Useful in women with hirsutism, acne, and those who have fluid retention after taking OCP and in treating PMS, PMDD

Note: The fourth generation pill used in India contains Ethinylestradiol and drospirenone — Yasmin (Fig. 10.11). Another is Diane 35 which has cyproterone a acetate 2 mg.

Flowchart 10.3: Benefit of 3rd generation Progesterone

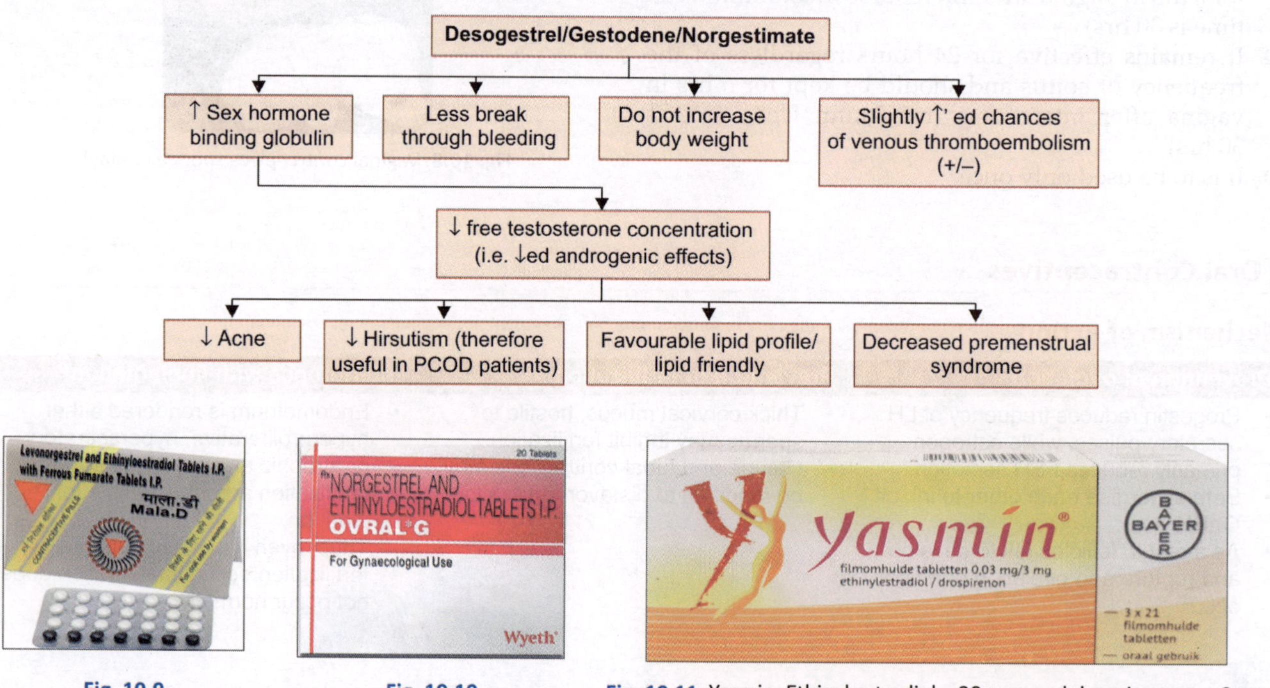

Fig. 10.9

Fig. 10.10

Fig. 10.11: Yasmin: Ethinyl estradiol = 30 mcg and drospirenone = 3 mg

Some important OCPs and their Composition

- **Mala D (Fig. 10.9) and Mala N** both have ethinyl estradiol–30 mcg and levonorgestrel–0.15 mg. Mala D available at ₹ 2 and Mala N free of cost. Both have 21 hormonal tablet and **7 ferrous fumarate tablets**.
- **Yasmin (Fig. 10.11:** Ethinyl estradiol 30 mcg Drospirenone = 3 mg

Non-contraceptive Benefits of OCPs-Oral Contraceptive Pills (OCPs) are Beneficial in

Cancers/Cysts

- Uterine cancer (endometrial CA)
- Ovarian cancers[Q]
- Fibroid uterus (Progesterone only pills)
- Ovarian cysts[Q]
- Colorectal cancer
- Choriocarcinoma

Benign Disease of Genital Tract

- Benign breast diseases[Q]
- Endometriosis (if used continuously)
- **PID**[Q] (but incidence of chlamydia and candida is ↑)
- Ectopic pregnancy (as it decreases incidence of PID)

They decrease ovulation thus are helpful in

- Dysmenorrhea, premenstrual tension, and mittelschmerz syndrome.
- **By decreasing blood loss they are helpful in menorrhagia and polymenorrhea.**
- Acne and hirsutism (especially those containing desogestrel)
- Rheumatoid arthritis

OCPs are also Beneficial in: *– Leon Speroff 7th/ed, p914*

- Dysfunctional uterine bleedings (DUB)
- Hormone therapy for hypothalamic amenorrhea
- Prevention of menstrual porphyria.

Note: OCPs are protective against benign breast diseases but as far as carcinoma breast is concerned, their role is controversial OCPs are being considered in the etiology of Ca breast. The progestogen component of pills is attributable to the Ca breast as the risk is same in users of OCPs 2 progestin only pills.

M/C side effect of OCPs-Break through bleeding

KEY POINTS

In OCPs users there is

- Increased risk of depression. Vit B_{16} helps in curing depression after OC use.

Tumors and OCPs—

Tumors associated with OCP use

1. Cervical cancer (adeno CA)
2. Hepatic cancer/Hepatic focal nodular Hyperplasia & benign hepatic adenoma
3. Pituitary adenoma
4. Breast cancer *William Gynae 3rd/ed, pg126*

OCPs provide protection against

1. Ovarian tumors/cysts
2. Uterine tumors and fibroid
3. Benign breast disease
4. Colon CA

Failure Rate of OCPs-0.1

Table 10.2: Some Benefit of Combination Estrogen plus Progestin Oral Contraceptives

Increased bone density
Reduced menstrual blood loss and anemia
Decreased risk of ectopic pregnancy
Improved dysmenorrhea from endometriosis
Fewer premenstrual complaints
Decreased risk of endometrial and ovarian cancer
Reduction in various benign breast diseases
Inhibition of hirsutism progression
Acne improvement
Prevention of atherogesis
Decreased incidence and severity of acute salpingitis
Decreased activity of rheumatoid arthritis

Contraindications of OCPs

Absolute Contraindications-WHO Category 4

KNOW IN-DEPTH

Mnemonic

- **Banks** Known or suspected **B**reast cancer
- **Have** Severe **H**ypertriglyceridemia/**H**ypercholesterolemia
- **Various** (Undiagnosed abnormal) **V**aginal bleeding
- **Schemes** **S**mokers over the age of 35 years
- **To** **T**hrombophlebitis/**T**hromboembolic disorders, (present H/O, past H/O, family H/O) Cerebral and Cardiac disease
- **Provide** **P**regnancy
- **Home** **H**ypertension (Moderate to severe) (> 160/110 mm of Hg)
- **Loans** Impaired **L**iver function/infective hepatitis
- **During**-**D**iabetes mellitus with vascular disease
- **May**-**M**igraine with aura

Relative Contraindications

KNOW SUPERFICIALLY

- Migraine without Aura
- Diabetes mellitus/Gestational diabetes
- Hypertension (mild)
- Smoking < 35 years of age
- Uterine leiomyoma
- Elective surgery (OCP should be stopped 4 weeks before any scheduled surgery)
- Seizure disorders
- Obstructive jaundice in pregnancy
- Sickle cell disease
- Gallbladder disease
- SLE
- Mitral valve prolapse
- Hyperlipidemia
- Hepatic disease.

OCP's are desirous in following class of patients:

- Molar pregnancy after evacuation
- Young adolescents in unstable relationship.
- Recently married couple
- In women wanting to space their pregnancy
- Women with:
  - Acne
  - Endometriosis
  - Dysmenorrhea
  - Menorrhagia
  - Family H/O ovarian cancer

Important Practical Applications

- **When to begin a pill–**
  In menstruating females: Between day 1 - of menstrual cycle (no backup contraceptive required). If she begins after day 5, backup contraceptive should be used for 7 days.
- After Medical Termination of Pregnancy (MTP)/ abortion: Can begin immediately (no backup required) after first trimester abortion and one week after 2nd trimester abortion.
- After delivery: 6 to 8 weeks.

In the event of missing a pill:

(See Flowchart 10.4)

According to Williams Gyne 3/ed, p122

During COCs use, if one dose is missed, conception is unlikely with higher-dose monophasic COCs. When this is recognized, taking that day's pill plus the missed pill will minimize breakthrough bleeding. The remainder of the pill pack is then completed with one pill taken daily.

It several dose are missed, or if a dose is missed with the lower-dose pills, then two pills are taken but an effective barrier technique is added for the subsequent 7 days. The remainder of the pack if completed with one pill taken daily. Alternatively, a new pack can be started and a barrier method added as additional contraception for a week. With any scenario of missed pills, the pills are continued, but the women should seek medical attention to exclude pregnancy. Fortunately, CHC are not teratogenic if taken accidentally during early pregnancy (Lammer, 1986).

KEY POINTS

1. Ovulation returns within 3 months of with drawl of the drug in 90% cases
2. If OCPs are taken in early pregnancy the risk of congenital malformations is 2–3% same like general population.

Flowchart 10.4

Most recent missed pill immediately, use condoms for 7 days and continue the packet

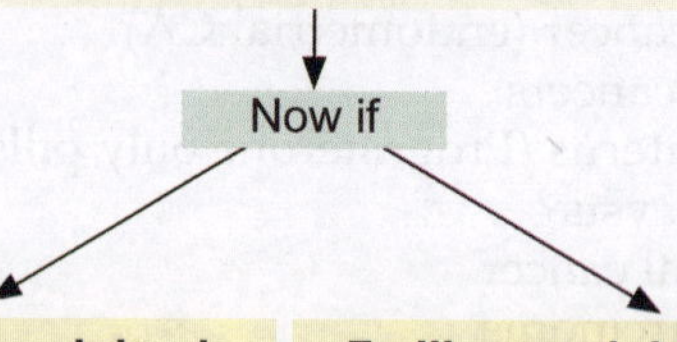

≥ 7 pills are remaining in packet	**< 7 pills remaining in packet**
Finish the remaining tablets and start the new packet after 7 days gap	Finish the remaining pills and start the new packet next day without a 7 days gap

Combined Hormonal Contraception and Medical Disorders

Obese and Overweight Women. In general, OCPs are highly effective in obese women. However, obesity may result in altered pharmacokinetics of some Combined Harmonal Contraceptive (CHC) methods. That said, data regarding overweight women are conflicting from lowered bioavailability.

Excessive weight gain is a concern with use of any hormonal contraceptive. Gallo and associates (2014) again concluded in their review that available evidence was insufficient to determine the influence of CHCs on weight gain, although no large effect was obvious.

Diabetes Mellitus. Higher-dose COCs were associated with insulin antagonistic properties, particularly those medicated by progestins. However, with current low-dose. CHCs, these concerns have been mitigated. In healthy women, large long term prospective studies have found that OCP's do not appear to increase the risk for diabetes. Moreover, these agents do not appear to increase the risk for overt diabetes in women with prior gestational diabetes. Use of these contraceptives in approved for nonsmoking diabetic women who are younger than 35 years and who have no associated vascular disease (American College of Obstetricians and Gynecologists, 2013d).

Cardiovascular Disease. In general, sever cardio-vascular disorders limit the use of CHCs. For less severe disorders, however, current formulations do not increase associated risks.

First, low-dose CHCs do not appreciably increase the absolute risk of clinical significant hypertension (Chasan-Taber 1996). However, it is common practice for patients to return 8 to 12 weeks following CHC initiation for evaluation of blood pressure and other symptoms. For those with already established chronic hypertension,

CHC use is permissible in those with well-controlled, otherwise, uncomplicated hypertension (American College of Obstetricians and Gynecologists, 2013d). Severe forms of hypertension, especially those with end-organ involvement, usually preclude CHC use.

Women who have had a documented *myocardial infarction* should not be given CHCs.

Cerebrovascular Disorders. Women who have had either an *ischemic* or *hemorrhagic stroke* should not use CHCs. But the incidence of strokes in nonsmoking young women is low and use of CHCs does not increase the risk for either type of stroke.

Migraine headaches may be a risk factor for strokes in some young women Curtis had coworkers (2002) reported that women using COCs who had *migraine headaches with aura* had a two- to fourfold increased risk for stroke compared with nonusers. Because of this, the WHO (2010) recommends against CHC use in this subset of migraineurs. Alternatively, the American College of Obstetricians and Gynecologists (2013d), because the absolute risk is low, has concluded that CHCs may be considered for young nonsmoking women who have migraine headaches without focal neurologic changes. For many of these women, an intrauterine contraceptive method or a progestin only pill may be more appropriate (World Health Organization, 2010).

Venous Thromboembolism. Early in CHC history, it was apparent that *deep-vein thrombosis* and *pulmonary embolism* risk were significantly increased in women who used these contraceptives (Realini, 1985). These risks were found to be estrogen dose related and have been appreciably lowered with evolution of low-dose formulations that contain only 10 to 35 μg of ethinyl estradiol.

Seizure Disorders. One mechanism with several antiepileptic drugs is potent induction of cytochrome P450 system enzymes. In turn, this increased contraceptive steroid metabolism, and serum levels of these decrease by as much as half (American College of Obstetricians and Gynecologists, 2013d; Zupanc, 2006).

These metabolic interactions usually do not result in increased seizure activity. One possible exception is combined use of CHCs and monotherapy with the anticonvulsant lamotrigine. Serum anticonvulsant levels are decreased by up to 50 percent, which may increase seizure risks (Gaffield, 2011).

Evidence-based guidelines for use of contraceptives by women with epilepsy are listed in the US MEC. Use of CHCs in epileptic women is rated as category 3, that is, theoretical or proven risks usually outweigh the method advantages. CHCs used concurrently with anticonvulsants may reduce contraceptive or anticonvulsant effectiveness. Thus, epileptic women using cytochrome P450 enhancing aniconvulsants are counseled regarding alternate contraceptive methods if feasible. If not, a COC containing at least 30 μg of ethinyl estradiol should be used. For those using lamotrigine monotherapy, CHCs are not recommended.

Other Combined (E + P) Contraceptives

Transdermal patch called as ortho EVRA	**Vaginal ring called as Nuva ring** (Launched in India in November 2009) (Fig. 10.12A and B)
P = Norelgestromin (eluted 150 mcg/day) EVRA Estrogen = Ethinyl estradiol (eluted = 20 mcg/day)	P = Etonorgestrel (active metabolite of desogestrel) E = Ethinyl estradiol (Releases 15 μg EE and 120 mcg etonogestrel[Q])
• Applied weekly to any body location but not breast, for 3 weeks followed by 1 week patch free withdrawal bleeding week	• Placed in vagina for 3 weeks and removed for 1 week • Made of diethyl polysiloxane
Advantages • Better compliance • Avoids first pass hepatic metabolism and maintains a steady hormone level. **Disadvantages** • Less effective in obese women (>90 kg) • Not yet available in India • Increased risk of thrombosis as compared to COC's.	**Advantages** • Increased compliance and satisfaction • Decreases incidence of vaginal yeast and bacterial infections • All systemic side effects of OCPs are absent **Disadvantages** • ↑ Leucorrhea • Failure rate 0.3%

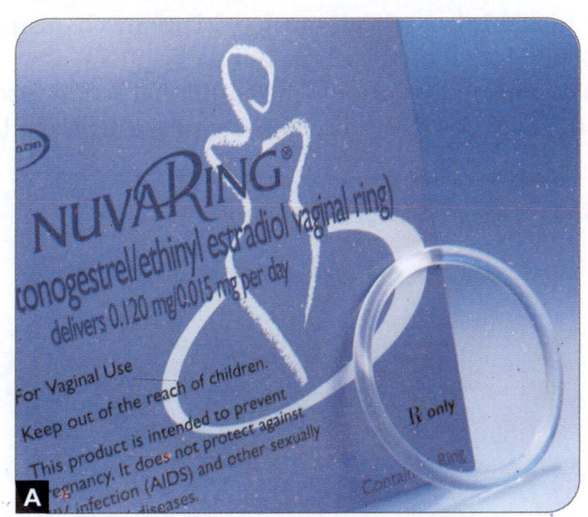

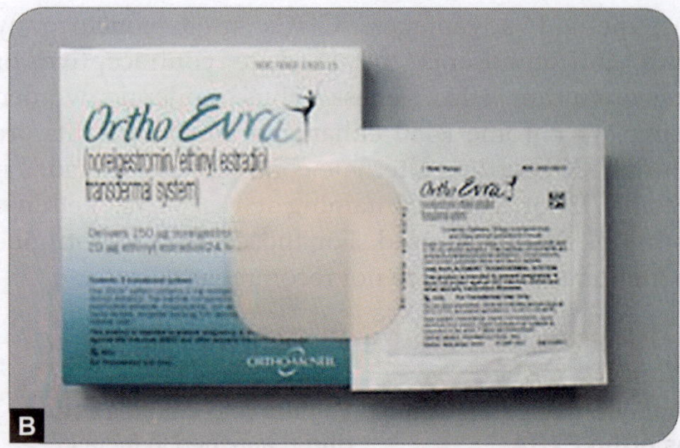

Figs. 10.12A and B: A: Vaginal ring, B: Ortho Evra patch

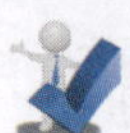

KEY POINTS

Other Rings

- Silastic vaginal rings (SVR) containing levonorgestrel and releasing 20 mcg of LNG daily.
- Nestorone –150 mcg progesterone + 15 mcg EE_2

Recent Advance

Continuous use pill: 'Seasonale' available in western countries. It contains 0.15 mg LNG and 30 mcg EE. Women take a pill every day for 84 days and then take a 7 day hormone free interval. This causes withdrawal bleeding four tenes in an year & not 12 time.

Progestin-only Pills (POP)

They contain very low doses of a progestin and no estrogen, and so can be used throughout breastfeeding and by women who cannot use methods with estrogen like in smokers, with past H/O uterine fibroid,

Progestin only pills (POPs) are also called "minipills".

Mechanism of Action

- **Thickening cervical mucus:** Main mechanism of action for all progesterone pills.
- **Preventing ovulation:** This additional action is seen in newer desogestrel containing progesterone pill.

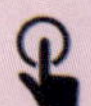

Minipill available in India = Cerazette (Fig. 10.13) containing—Desogestrel (75 mcg)

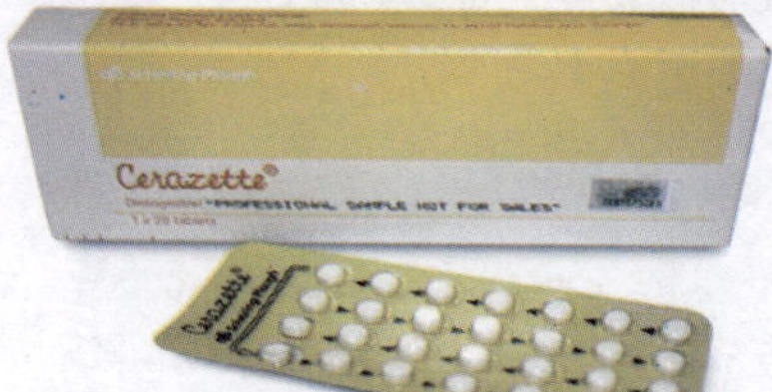

Fig. 10.13: Cerazette

How to Use

In regular cycles	Amenorrhea	During lactation
• Recent WHO recommendations suggest POP should be started **within 1st five days of menstrual cycle without need of additional contraception (preferably 1st day).**	• Start **any time after being sure that there is no pregnancy** (Additional protection or abstinence from sex being advised for the first 48 hours)	• *As per CDC guidelines it can be stated any time after delivery according to WHO it is started after 6 weeks*

- Traditional progesterone only pill should be taken every day without break and **at the same time.**[Q] Safety margin (3 hrs). If delay was for > 3 hrs - back method should be used.
- For newer desogestrel containing pill, **a delay of ~12 hours** can be accepted.

POPs have minimal if any effect on carbohydrate metabolism and coagulation factors. They do not cause or exacerbate hypertension and thus may be ideal for some women at increased risk for other cardiovascular complications. Such women include those with a history of thrombosis or migraine headaches or smokers older than 35 years. Because they do not impair milk production, POPs are suitable for lactating women. When used in combination with breast feeding, POPs are virtually 100-percent effective for up to 6 month.

Side Effects

- **Menstrual disturbances:** Most common reason for discontinuation of POP's is irregular bleeding pattern.
- **Other side effects:** Headache, acne, breast pain, nausea, vaginitis, and dysmenorrhea.

KEY POINTS

Failure rate of POPs

Breast feeding women

- Typical use: 1/HMY
- Perfect use: 0.3/HMY

Nonbreast feeding women

- Typical use: 3-10/HMY
- Perfect use: 0.3/HMY

Progesterone Injections

DMPA	Net En
150 mg DMPA	200 mg of norethindrone enanthate
Given i/m	Given i/m
To be repeated every 3 months	To repeated every 2 months
Pt can wait upto 4 weeks late for next injection	Pt can wait uptil 2 weeks late

Mode of action–inhibit ovulation

Advantages:

1. Raises the threshold for seizures in epilepsy pts
2. Reduces sickling of anemia
3. Should be used if female wants to delay pregnancy for at least 1 year

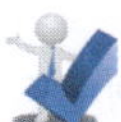

KEY POINTS

DMPA is suited ideally for—

- Lactating women
- Sickle cell anemia (best contraceptive)
- Seizure disorder (raises seizure threshold)

Disadvantages:

1. Decreases bone mass
2. Delayed return of fertility–avg 12 months, maxm–18 months
3. DMPA use is commonly associated with weight gain and patients develop diabetes mellitus

M/C side effect: Irregular vaginal bleeding Others-weight gain, breast tenderness and depression.

Contraindication: Absolute: Pregnancy unexplained genital bleeding, severe coagulation disorder, Previous sex steroid induced adenoma.

Relative Contraindication: Liver disease, depression, CVS disease, Rapid return of fertility desired.

Note: Subcutaneous DMPA called as Depo sub Q provera available these days with 104 mg of DMPA. Repeat injection–3 months.

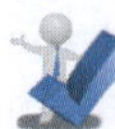

KEY POINTS

Injection - cyclofem/cyclo-provera

DMPA = 25 mg

+

Estradiol cypionate 5 mg

Administered monthly **Mesigyna:**

Norethindrone = 50 mg Enanthate

+

Estradiol valerate (5 mg)

Administered-monthly

Progestin Only Implants

Subdermal Progesterone Implants Includes

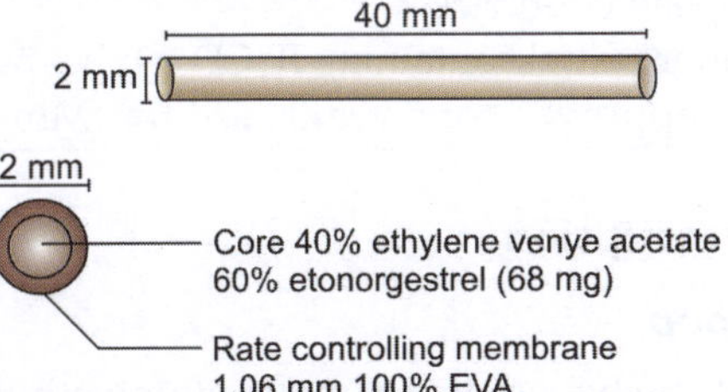

Diagrammatic representation of implanon

Implanon (Fig. 10.14A)

- It has a single rod **4 cms** in size containing **68 mg of 3 ketodesogestrel** (etonorgestrel). Released@67 mcg/day.
- Both removal & insertion are OPD procedures
- Most popular implant these days.[Q]
- Replaced after 3 years.[Q]
- Mechanism of action inhibition of ovulations like newer pills having desogestrel.

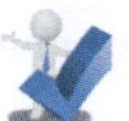

KEY POINTS

Note: Now implanon has been replaced by **Nexplanon (Fig. 10.14B)** which has same characteristic like implanon, only difference is, it is radiopaque.

Implants have the lowest failure rate-.05%

- M/C side effect; irregular vaginal bleeding

Site of Insertion

- Implants are inserted subcutaneously on the inner surface of the upper arm of non dominant arm (6–8 cm superior and lateral to medial epicondyle of humerus) using a 10 gauge trocar as an inserter, under local anesthesia.

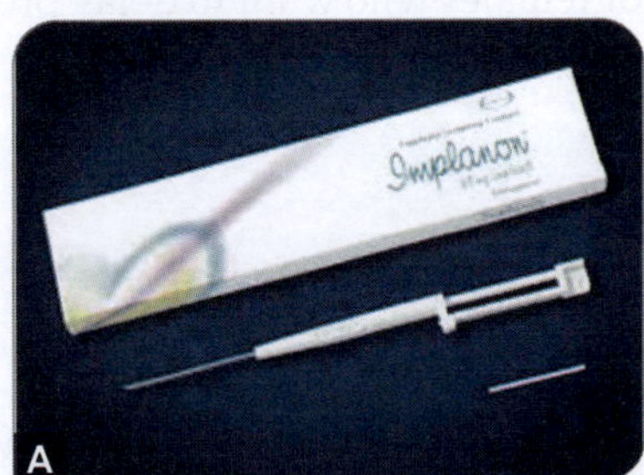

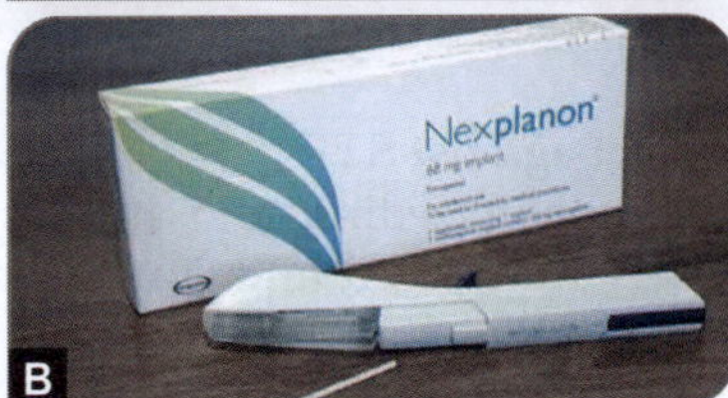

Figs. 10.14A and B: (A) Implanon (B) Nexplanon

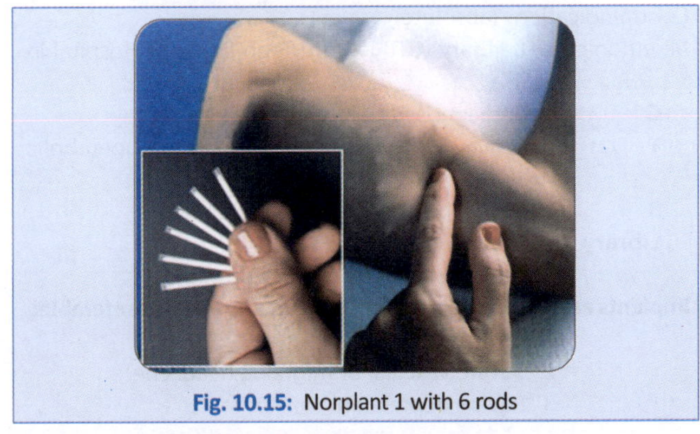

Fig. 10.15: Norplant 1 with 6 rods

- Each rod 3 cm long & has 36 mg each of LNG
- Effective for 5 years
- Not available in India now

- The implant should be inserted within day-5 of a menstrual cycle, immediately after abortion and 3 weeks after postpartum.

Advantages

- Should be used in females who need next pregnancy after 2–3 years.
- Can be used in females with contraindication for the use of estrogen containing contraceptives.
- Can be used immediately postpartum.[Q]
- Can be used by lactating females.[Q]
- Not associated with changes in carbohydrate or lipid metabolism.
- No adverse effect on bone density.
- No pregnancies have been reported so far with the use of implanon.

Indications

Best suited for females who want to delay pregnancy for 2–3 years.

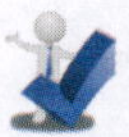

KEY POINTS

Return of fertility after removing implants—
- In 40% cases fertility returns by end of 3 months
- In 76% cases fertility by end of 2 years
- In 90% cases fertility by end of 3 years

Disadvantages

- **Do not protect against STD**
- Irregular vaginal bleeding and headache are the main reasons for discontinuation of implants by females

Mnemonic

Contraindications (absolute)

Mnemonic: GTB library (GTB is Guru Tegh Bahadur Hospital in Delhi).

G – Undiagnosed **G**enital bleeding
T – Active **T**hrombophlebitis or **T**hromboembolic disease
B – Known or suspected **B**reast cancer
Library – Acute **L**iver disease
– Benign or malignant **L**iver Tumours.

Implants are not contraindicated but other methods preferable:
1. Severe acne
2. Severe vascular or migraine headache
3. Severe depression

Intrauterine Contraceptive Devices (IUCDs)

The intrauterine devices are classified as follows:

Generation	Description
First generation IUDs	These are inert or non-medicated devices. e.g. Lippe's loop.
Second generation IUDs	It consists of copper or silver containing IUDs e.g. T Cu-220 C, T Cu 380- Ag, Nova T, Multiload Cu 250/375
Third generation IUDs	This consists of hormone releasing IUDs. e.g. Progestasert, Mirena.

Mechanism of Action of IUCD

Cu containing IUCD	Progestin releasing IUCD
• Elute copper which bring about enzymatic and metabolic changes in the endometrial tissue (aseptic inflammation) • They prevent implantation of fertilized ovium • Increase tubal motility • Impair sperm ascent	• They cause decidualization ***with atrophy of endometrial glands, therefore inhibit implantation*** • Alter cervical Mucus causing inhibition of sperm penetration and capacitation. • In 40% cases ovulation is also inhibited.

The contraceptive action of all IUCDs is mainly in the uterine cavity. Ovulation is not affected and the IUCD is not an abortifacient. It is currently believed that the mechanism of action for IUCDs is the production of an intrauterine environment that is spermicidal (Fig. 10.16).

Life Span of IUCD

Most of the IUCDs have an average life span of 3 years.

Exceptions are:

- Nova T/Multiload 375/Levonova – 5 years
- CuT 380 A (also known as Paragard) – 10 years – Distributed free of cost
- Progestasert – 1 years
- CuT200 B – 4 years, in US and 3 years in India and in European countries
- Levonorgestrel containing IUCD can be–7–10 years, but is approved for 5 years used for (Mirena)

IUCD's Description

Lippe's Loop

- Double S-shaped device made of polyethylene
- Available in 4 size A, B, C, D

- D is the largest
- Can be left in the uterus as long as desired
- Now not used.
- Method of insertion—Push out technique

CuT 200 (Gyne T)- Copper wire of 200 mm³ is wound around vertical stem. Earlier, it was M/C used by Indians. Now it is replaced by CuT 380A.

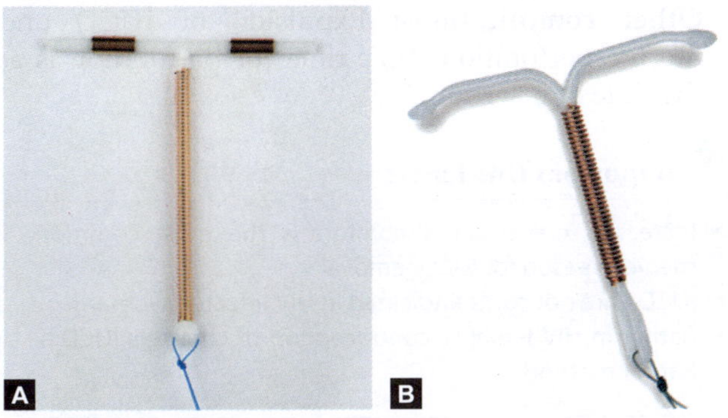

Figs. 10.16A and B: (A) Copper T380A (ParaGard) intrauterine device (B) Silver line Cu 380 Ag (M/C CuT used worldwide)

CuT380A: (Paraguard) (Fig. 10.16A)

- Named like this because it has copper wire (∴ Cu).
- The total area of copper wire = 380 mm²
- 'A' because copper wire is also found on arms.
- Note: 314 mm² copper wire is wrapped on vertical stem and 33 mm² on each aim.
- It is distributed free of cost by Government of India.
- It releases copper @ 50 mcg/day
- Method of insertion of CuT 380 is **withdrawal method. Using no touch technique**
- Used as emergency contraceptive also
- **It is the only CuT currently approved for use in India.**
- **Effective for 10 years**

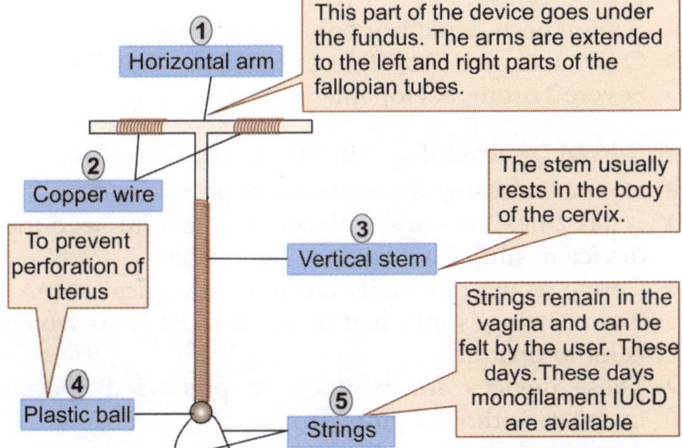

Diagramattic representation of CuT380A

Silver line Cu 380 Ag: (Fig. 10.16B)

It has flexible arms and, has a silver core and rest is similar to CuT 380A

It is the M/C CuT used worldwide

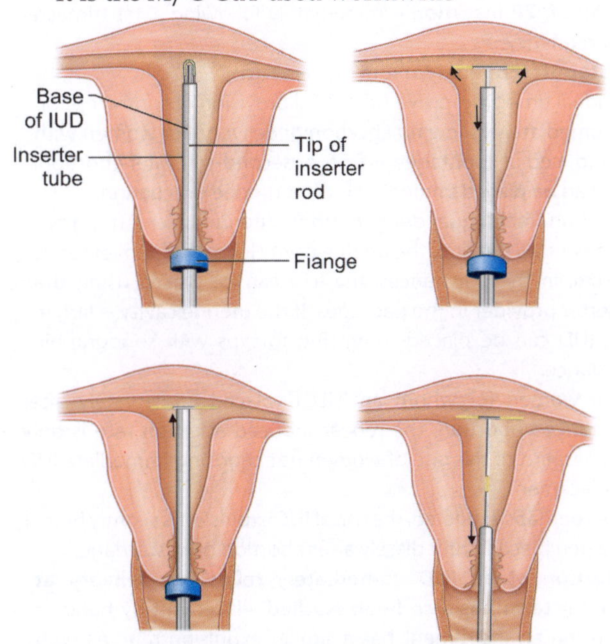

Figs. 10.17A to D: Insertion of ParaGard T 380A. The IUD is loaded into its inserter tube not more than 5 minutes before insertion. If longer, the malleable arms can retain "memory" of the inserter and remain bent inward. A blue plastic flange on the outside of the inserter tube is positioned from the IUD tip to reflect the uterine depth ascertained during sounding. The IUD arms should lie in the same plane as the flat portion of the blue flange; **A.** The inserter tube, with the IUD loaded, is passed into the endometrial cavity. When the blue flange abuts the cervix, insertion stops; **B.** To release the IUD arms, the solid white rod within the inserter tube is held steady while the inserter tube is withdrawn no more than 1 cm.; **C.** The inserter tube is then carefully moved upward toward the top of the uterus until slight resistance is felt; **D.** First, the solid white rod and then the inserter tube are withdrawn individually At completion, only the threads are visible protruding from the cervix. These are trimmed to allow 3 to 4 cm to extend into the vagina.

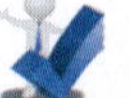

KEY POINTS

Method of insertion of IUCD—(Figs. 10.17A to D)

No touch technique and **withdrawal method.**

- Insertion of Lippes loop by pushout technique
- Insertion of Multiload
  - **Withdrawl technique without plunger**

Ideal time for insertion of Cu -T

- **Within 10 days of start of menstrual cycle.** It has the advantage that cervical canal is dilated, uterus is relaxed and chances of pregnancy are remote

Contd...

Contd...

- **Post-puerperal insertion immediately after delivery** (recommended by Govt. of India) or 6 weeks after delivery (Interval insertion)
- **Post-MTP insertion** - immediately following a 1st trimester pregnancy.

Postabortal or Postpartum Placement:

An ideal time to improve successful provision of contraception is immediately following abortion of delivery. For women with an induced or spontaneous first- or second-trimester abortion. IUC can be placed immediately after uterine evacuation.

Insertion technique depend upon uterine size. After first-trimester evacuation, the uterine cavity length seldom exceeds 12 cm. In these instances, the IUD can be placed using the inserter provider in the packages. If the uterine cavity is larger, the IUD can be placed using ring forceps with sonographic guidance.

- In women for whom an IUD is placed immediately after induced abortion, the repeat induced abortion rate is only one third of the rate of women not choosing immediate IUD placement.
- As perhaps expected, the risk of IUC expulsion is slightly higher when placed immediately after abortion or miscarriage.

Insertion of an IUD immediately following delivery at or near term has also been studied. Placement by hand or by using an instrument has a similar expulsion rate. As with postabortion insertion, expulsion rate by 6 months are higher than those in women whose IUD is placed after complete uterine involution. Even be beneficial because in some populations up to 40 percent of women do not return for a postpartum clinic visit.

Despite these findings, many chose to delay insertion for several weeks postpartum. Insertion at 2 weeks is quite satisfactory, and in most of the Clinics, is scheduled at 6 weeks postpartum to ensure complete uterine involution.

Ideal candidate for Cu-T insertion

- Should have had at least one child
- Are in mutually monogamous relationships; (IUDs do not protect against sexually transmitted diseases)
- Has no history of PID
- Choose not to use hormonal contraceptives.
- Previous ectopic pregnancy is not a C/I for IUCD insertion
- M/C infection seen with IUCD use is actinomyces

Complications of Copper IUCD

- **M/C complication:** Bleeding (increased blood loos of 80 mL/cycle).
- **2nd M/C complication:** Pain (M/c reason for removal of IUCD)
- **Expulsion rate of CuT:** 8 – 10%
- **Infection:** With current devices, IUCD incertain does not increased the risk of pelvic infection. There is no evidence that prophylactic antibiotic are necessary with insertion for women at lower risk for STD (ACOG 2014 guidances). **Most typical infection associated with Cu T use is actinomyces. Cut is associated with increased risk of PID in only first 20 days of use.**
- **Ectopic pregnancy:** As such it is seen that ectopic pregnancy is 50% less likely in women using IUCD than in women using no contraception. However. If pregnancy occurs count a centre female occurs her chances of ectopic are high.
- **Other complications:** Expulsion of IUCD and uterine perforation (M/c time for perforation is at the time of insertion).

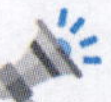

Important One Liners

- Increased menstrual discomfort is the most common medical reason for IUCD removal.
- IUCD's are not contraindicated in HIV infected women.
- Rather in HIV females, contraception of choice is IUCD + Barrier method

Absolute Contraindication for IUCD—Category 4 of WHO

Mnemonic

Please—peurperal sepsis, or postabortal sepsis
Postabortal/Postpartum endometritis in last 3 months
You → **U**terine distortion like fibroid causing it
Don't — **D**UB/unexplained vaginal bleeding
Try to — Gestational **t**rophoblastic neoplasia
Put — **Current P**ID/STD or within the past 3 months puerperal sepsis, known pelvic TB
Wet — **W**ilson disease
Condom — **C**ancer cervix
Cancer endometrium *(Novak 15th/ed, p 224)*
Mnemonic: Please You Don't Try to Put Wet Condom

Relative Contraindications of IUCD/WHO Category 3

Ref: JB Sharm Obstetrics p682

- Postpartum 48 hrs – 4 weeks
- Benign gestational trophoblastic disease
- Ovarian cancer (Absolute CI for LNG - IUCD)
- Severe Thrombocytopenia

Multiload Devices (Fig. 10.18)

- Copper releasing device made of polypropylene.
- It has 2 flexible arms with serrated fins (to keep the device in situ). The arms are radiolucent
- Copper is wrapped only around the vertical stem.
- Nylon string is attached to the vertical shaft which is radio-opaque
- These devices are available in preloaded special inserters without a plunger

  Multiload Cu 250 – life prespan = 3 years.

  Multiload Cu 375 – life span-5 years (Fig. 10.18).

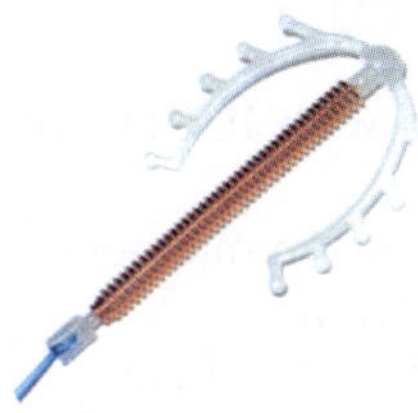

Fig. 10.18: Multiload 375 has 375 mm² of copper wire wound around its stem

Progesterone Containing IUCD MIRENA (Figs. 10.19 and 10.20)

- It has T shaped radio-opaque polyethylene frame on whose stem is present polydimethylsiloxane – Levonorgestreal.
- It contains **52 mg levonorgestrel**, eluting **20 μg daily**.
- It has 2 brown threads attached to stem
- **Life span** = 5 years
- Highly effective = failure rate = 1–3/1000 women (as effective as sterilization but easy reversible).
- **It cannot be used as an emergency contraception.**

Non Contraceptive uses of LNG Containing IUCD

- Decrease menstrual blood loss and are used for management of menorrhagia (can be used as an alternative to hysterectomy).
- Significant reduction in dysmenorrhea[Q]
- Decrease pelvic infection rates[Q].

–Williams Gyne 1st p119

- Can be used in treatment of endometrial hyperplasia, adenomyosis, uterine leiomyomas, and endometriosis. But in woman with uterine leiomyomas. Its placement is problamatic due to distorted cavity.
- It provides the benefits of hormone replacement therapy when used over the transition years of reproduction to perimenopause.

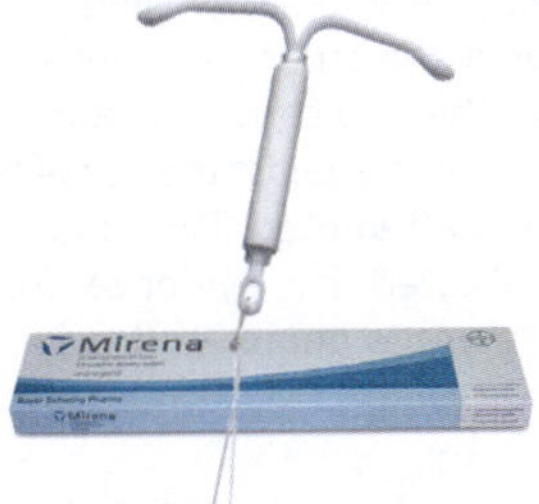

Fig. 10.19: Mirena

KEY POINTS

Advantages of 3rd generation IUCD (i.e. hormonal IUCD) over other IUCD's

- High efficacy with low pregnancy rates
- Longer duration of action
- Low expulsion rates
- Can be given to nursing mothers.

Drawback

- Irregular bleeding and oligomenorrhea which are common in first 3-4 months of use
- Amenorrhea (seen in 20–50% cases by 1 year of use).
- Not used as an emergency contraceptive
- Very costly = ₹ 7000.
- **Expulsion rate** = 5–6%
- Women who have had previous ectopic pregnancy may have increased risk for another because of diminished tubal motility from progesterone action.
- Contraindications: Apart from all the contraindications general to all IUCD progesterone IUCD cannot be used in breast cancer patients or any cancer responsive to progesterone & it cannot be used in liver disease

Progestasert

- It is a T shaped device
- Has a capsule containing 38 mg of progesterone
- Releases progesterone @ 65 mcg/day
- Life span: 1 year
- It is no Longer used these days and is replaced by mirena.

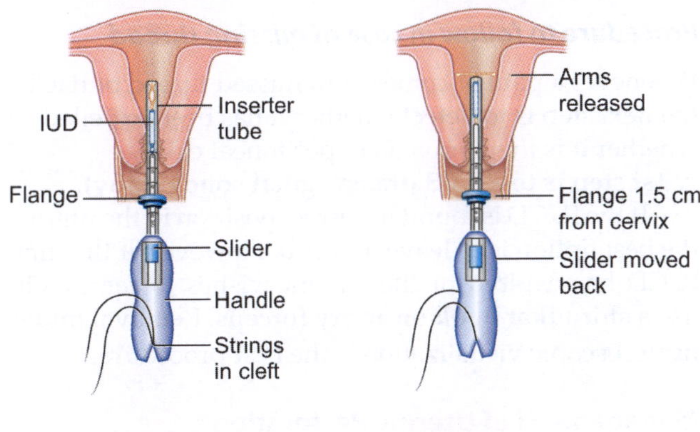

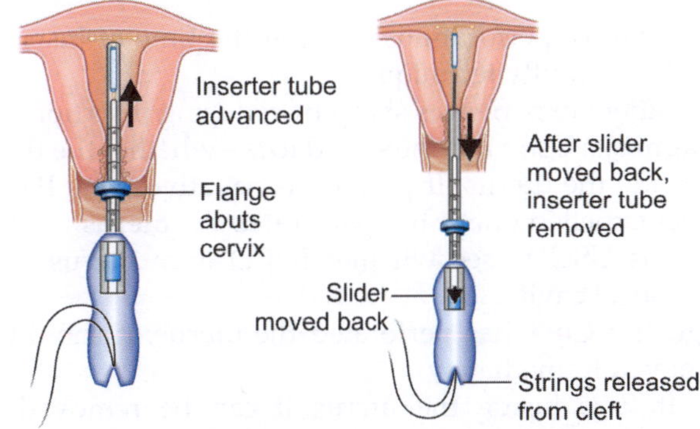

Figs. 10.20A to D: Insertion of Mirena intrauterine system. Threads from behind the slider are first released to hang freely. The teal-colored slider found on the handle should be positioned at the top of the handle nearest the device. The IUD arms are oriented horizontally. A. As tightly fixed into the handle's cleft. A flange on the outside of the inserter tube is positioned from the IUD tip to reflect the depth

Contd...

Contd...

found with uterine sounding; **B.** While inserting the Mirena device, the slider is held firmly in position at the top of the handle. Gentle traction is created by outward traction on the tenaculum to align the cervical canal with the uterine cavity. The inserter tube is gently threaded into the uterus until the flange lies 1.5 to 2 cm from the external cervical os to allow the arms to open. While holding the inserter steady, the IUD arms are released by pulling the slider back only to the raised horizontal line on the handle. This position is held for 15 to 20 seconds to allow the arms to fully open; **C.** The inserter is then gently guided into the uterine cavity until its flange touches the cervix; **D.** The device is released by holding the inserter firmly in position and pulling the slider back all the way. The threads will be released automatically. The inserter may then be removed. IUD strings are trimmed to leave approximately 3 cm visible outside the cervix.

Misplaced IUD (Missing Thread)

Causes

- Expulsion of IUD
- Curling of thread inside the uterus/breakage of thread
- Pregnancy
- Uterine perforation

Procedure to follow in case of missing thread

Whenever a patient comes with missed thread of IUCD, the next step is to detect whether it has been expelled or whether it is the uterus on in peritoneal cavity.

∴ **1st step is to a TVS (transvaginal sonography).**

If the IUCD is found in correct position in the uterus, the best option is to leave it in situ. However; if the time IUCD has expired or the patient wishes to remove it, use a **shirodkar hook on artery forceps**. Removal under hysteroscopic visualization is the best procedure.

Management of Uterine Perforation

- Majority perforations occur at the time of insertion due to faulty technique.
- Patient experiences sharp pain during insertion

Diagnosis: Use a uterine sound to see whether the IUCD is inside the uterus. If probing is negative, then IUD is either expelled out or has perforated the uterus.

IOC: is USG to see whether IUCD is in uterus or in peritoneal cavity.

Mgt: If a Cu T has perforated the uterus, it should be removed immediately.

If it is inside the uterus it can be removed by shirodkar hook or artery forceps under hysteroscopic guidance.

If Cu T is partly inside the uterus and partly in peritoneal cavity, removal by both hysteroscopy and laparoscopy is required.

If Cu T is inside peritoneal cavity, removal is by laparotomy or laparoscopy.

Pregnancy with IUCD

If pregnancy occurs with IUCD, around 30% cases are ectopic

There are 3 options in management

a. Therapeutic abortion
b. USG guided removal of IUD
c. Continuation of pregnancy with the device left in situ

If the patient wishes to continue the pregnancy, ultrasound evaluation of the location of the IUD should be considered. If the IUD is not in a fundal location, ultrasound-guided removal using small alligator forceps may be successful. If the location is fundal, the IUD should be left in place. When pregnancy continues with an IUD in place, the patient must be warned of the following complication.

- **Most common complication:** miscarriage/abortion
- Infection
- Preterm labor
- PROM
- IUGR

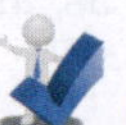

KEY POINTS *Williams Gyne 3rd/ed, p119–508*

Of special note, Vessey and associates (1979) had previously reported that fetal malformations were not increased in pregnancies in which the device was left in place. In the Ganer study, it is particularly worrisome that this rate was doubled compared with women in whom the device was removed. The distribution of malformations was notable in that 12 percent were skeletal malformations. In contrast, there were no chromosomal anomalies identified in fetuses born to women from the two IUD groups.

Because of these findings, if pregnancy continuation is desired, it is recommended that with early pregnancies with IUD be removed. However, if the strings are not visible, attempts of locate and remove the device may result in pregnancy loss. This risk must be weighed against the risk of leaving the device in place. It removal is attempted, TVS can be used. If attempts at removal are followed by evidence for infection, then antimicrobial treatment is begun and is followed by prompt uterine evacuation.

Emergency Contraception

It can be started up to five days (120 hours) after unprotected intercourse but **greatest protection occurs if it is given within 72 hours of unprotected sex.** Emergency contraception is also known as emergency birth control, backup birth control, and the morning after pill.

M/C method used = Levonorgestrel 1.5 mg single dose (Tablet = 0.75 mg 2 tablets together)

Note: The overall risk of having pregnancy after single unprotected intercourse is 8%.

Indications

- Breakage or slipping of condom
- Forgot to take OC pills or insert diaphragm or sponge
- Diaphragm slipped out of place
- Miscalculated "safe" days
- Failure to practice coitus interruptus
- Not using any birth control method
- Forced to have unprotected vaginal sex, or were raped.
- **Contraindications**: None

Mechanism of Action

- Delay ovulation-Hormonal methods
- Spermicidal-Nonhormonal methods
- Prevents implantation by affecting endometrial lining.

Note: E-pills are available free of cost by Govt. of India. It has Levonorgest.

M/C side effect: Nausea, vomiting

Important One Liners

- **Most effective method of emergency contraception** CuT IUCD
- **Most effective Hormonal method:** Ullipristal (best choice) followed by Levonorgestrel (2nd best choice)
- **M/C used method**–Levonorgestral
- **Not used as emergency contraceptives**
  - LNG-IUCD (mirena)
  - Progesterone only pills
  - Misoprost (abortifacient)

Methods and Dose

1. **Levonorgestrel** (progestin) 0.75 mg, two doses given at 12 hours interval at the earliest after unprotected coitus but within 72 hours. It may be given upto 120 hours (5 days), but efficacy will be much lower. It is very successful and without any side effects. A single dose of 1.5 mg (2 tablets) is equally effective. Failure rate is 1%. It is the method of choice for emergency contraception in current practice.
2. **Combined estrogen and progestogen pills (Yuzpe method**) is also effective. It consists of oral intake of 100 µgm ethinyl estradiol with 1 mg. levonorgestrel in two divided doses 12 hours apart starting within 72 hours of unprotected intercourse (total 4 tablets of ovral i.e. 2 tablets followed 12 hours later by 2 tablets each containing 50 µg of ethinylestradiol and 0.25 mg d-levonorgestrel. Alternately 4 tablets of low dose COCs followed 12 hours apart. By 4 more tablets very low dose pulls with 20 mcg of estogen should be taken 5 tablets as a single dose followed by 5 tablets later. Failure rate is 3.2%. Popular in past, its use is now superseded by LNG.)
3. **Conjugated equine estrogen** 15 mg. The drug is taken orally twice daily for 5 days, beginning soon after the exposure but not later than 72 hours.
4. **Mifepristone** 25 or 50 mg single dose is used. Failure rate is 0 to 1.6%. it is expensive (about 900 rupees).
5. Alternative to the above hormonal pills emergency contraception can be achieved by **insertion of an IUD** (not LNG-IUS) within 5 days of an unprotected intercourse which can be continued later. Failure rate is only 0 to 1% (15 times more effective than Yuzpe Regimen). It is useful for married women needing continued contraception.
6. **Centchroman:** 50 mg 12 hours apart
7. **New tablet: Ulipristal:** brand name **Ella** is available in US, which is selective Progesterone receptor antagonist.

   Dose: 30 mg single dose can be used uptil 120 hrs. Not available in India.

Table 10.3: Methods Available for Use as Emergency Contraception

Method	Formation	Pills per dose
Progestin-Only Pill		
Plan B[a]	0.75 mg levonorgestrel	1
Plan B One-Step[b]	150 mg levonorgestrel	1
SPRM Pill		
Ella[b]	30 mg ulipristal acetate	1
COC Pills[a,c]		
Ogestrel	0.05 mg ethinyl estradiol + 0.5 mg norgestrel[d]	2
Lo/Ovral, Cryselle	0.03 mg ethinyl estradiol + 0.3 mg norgestrel[d]	4
Trivora (pink), Enpress (orange)	0.03 mg ethinyl estradiol + 0.125 mg levonorgestrel	4
Aviane, Lessina	0.02 mg ethinyl estradiol + 0.1 mg levonogestrel	5

Contd...

Contd...

Copper-containing IUD
ParaGard T 380A

[a]Treatment consists of two doses taken 12 hours apart.
[b]Treatment consists of a single dose taken once.
[c] Use of an antiemetic agent before taking the medication will lessen the risk of nausea, which is a common side effect.
[d]Norgestrel contains two isomers, and only one of these isomers is bioactive, namely levonogestrel.
Thus, the amount of norgestrel needed for efficacy is twice that of the levonogestrel-based regiments.
COC = combination oral contraceptive; SPRM=selective progesterone-receptor modulator.

Permanent Method of Contraception

Female Sterilization

- First performed in 1823 in London by Dr J Blundell.
- Female sterilization is the most commonly used contraceptive method in the world
- **Child norm for sterilization in India: 1 child at least 1 year old**
- Husband concent for sterilization is not necessary.

Techniques

It can be done laparoscopically (procedure of choice these days) or by mini laparotomy (incision < 3 cms)

Methods of female sterilization

The basic fundamental principle in female sterilization is breaking the continuity of both fallopian tubes by removing a small segment of both tubes.

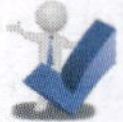

KEY POINTS

Site of Sterilization

Sterilization is done at the junction of proximal and middle third of tube – the loop formed consists mainly of isthmus and part of ampullary region.

- Best chances for reversibility is seen in—
Isthmo - isthmic type of anastomosis.

Prerequisites

A. Criteria for Eligibility

(Self-declaration by the client should be the basis of this information)

- Patient should be married.
- Female should be below the age of 49 years and above the age of 22 years.
- The couple should have at least one child whose age is above one year unless the sterilization is medically indicated.
- Female or her partners must not have undergone sterilization in the past (not applicable in cases of failure of previous sterilization).
- Clients must be in a sound state of mind so as to understand the full implications of sterilization.
- Mentally ill clients must be certified by a psychiatrist and a statement should be given by the legal guardian/spouse regarding the soundness of the client's state of mind.

1. Surgical Techniques by doing minilaparotomy (mini lap)

Important points to be kept in mind about surgical techniques are:

- The operating surgeon should identify each fallopain tube clearly by following it up to the fimbrial end.
- The site of the occlusion of the fallopain tube must always be within 2–3 cm from the uterine cornua in the isthmic portion (this will improve the possibility of reversal if required in the future).
- Excision of at least 1 cm of the tube should be done. Use of cautery and crushing of the tube should be avoided.

a. **Pomeroy technique (Figs. 10.21A and B):** (Most commonly done laparotomy method). The middle part of tube (3-4 cm away from fundus) is formed into a loop using **babcock forceps** which is tied at the base with catgut and excised. Site of ligation—Isthmus.
Failure Rate = 1 in 300/400 surgeries

b. **In Modified Pomeroy Technique:** The technique is similar to Pomeroy technique but here Double ligation of tube is done

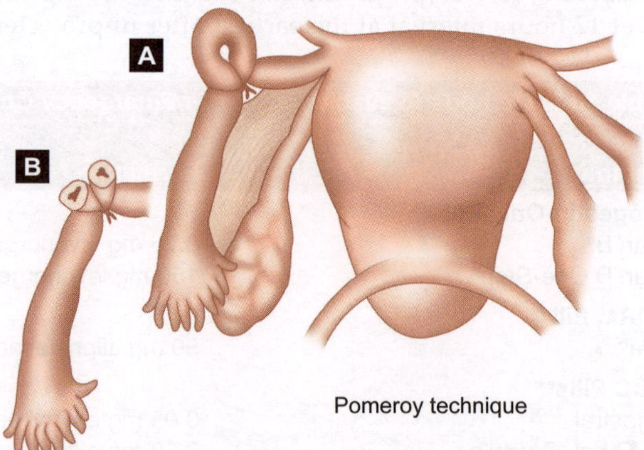

Figs. 10.21A and B: Pomeroy technique

- The Cut end of the tube is sent for histopathological examination to ensure, it is the tube which is cut.

This is because M/C cause of failure of female sterilization–is identification of wrong structure.

c. **Irving method–**Ligating and burying the proximal tubal end in serosa of posterior uterine wall.
   Failure Rate = 1 in 1000 surgeries.
d. **Uchida technique–**No Failure Rate in 19000 surgeries
e. **Fimbriectomy/kroeners technique–**Very high failure rate 2–3 in 100 surgeries
f. **Madlener technique–**High failure rate–0.3–2 in 100 surgeries
g. **Parkland technique–**Failure Rate 3 in 400 surgeries
   Note: Amongst the conventional methods - Uchida followed by Irwing has the least failure rate.

2. Laparoscopic ligation (Figs. 10.22A to C)

- Done using laparoscope.
  - It is a safe and effective method.
  - **It should not be done concurrently with 2nd trimester MTPs and in post-partum period.**

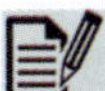

Remember

M/C method of female sterilisation is Laparoscopic sterilisation.
M/C method of postpartum sterilisation is: minilaparotomy.

- The patient is laid in lithotomy position and with a help of verses needle (introduced at an angle of 45°) pneumoperitoneum is created.
- **The gas used is CO_2** (M/C)
- **Intraabdominal pressure is maintained between 8-12 mm; max = 15 mm of Hg.**
  The procedure is done on an outpatient basis under sedation and local anaesthesia.
- **The methods of occlusion used during laparoscopy are (Flowchart 10.5)**

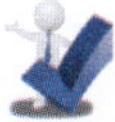

KEY POINTS

Timing for Female Sterilization

Per abdomen
- Post partum: within 48 hours uptil 7 days of delivery
- After MTP
- After cesarean section
- Interval sterilization: After a waiting period of 6 weeks after delivery

Laparoscopic sterilization
- With 1st trimester MTP
- As interval sterilisation

Note: Laparoscopic sterilization should not be performed along with second trimester MTP or in post partum period uptil 6 weeks after delivery, on D5-D11 of cycle avoid any pregnancy.

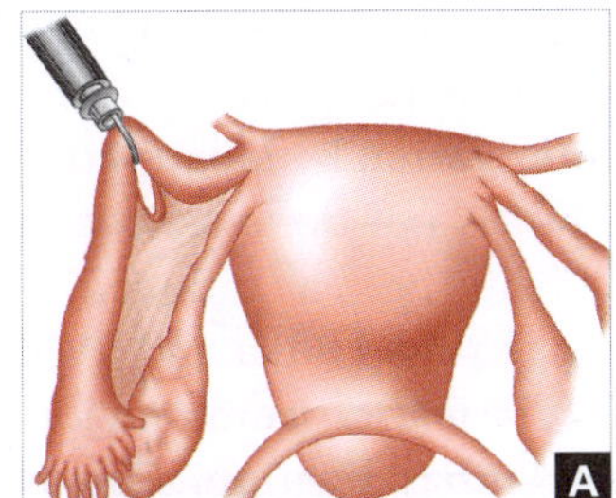

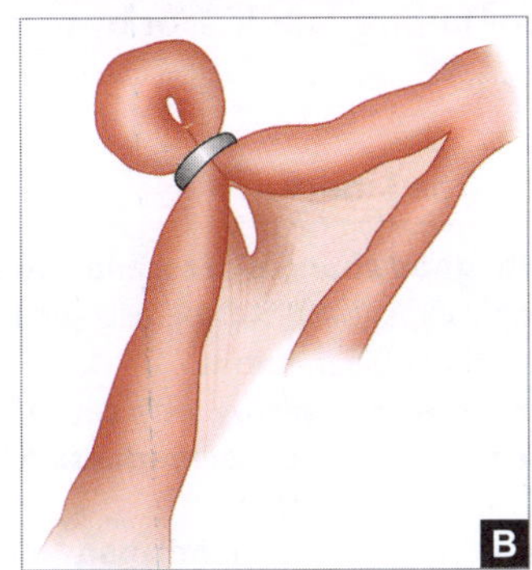

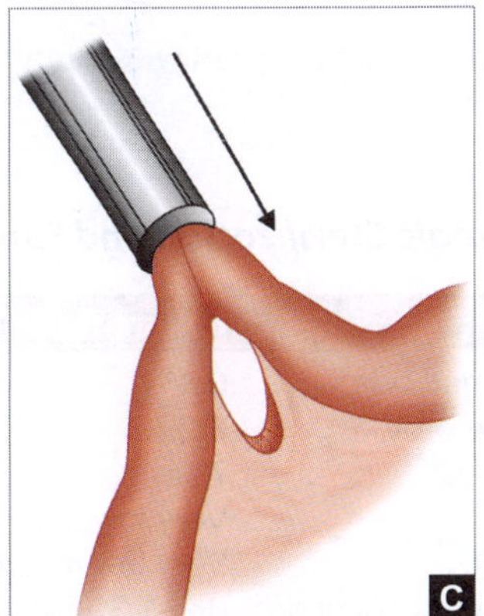

Figs. 10.22A to C: Laparoscopic sterilization

Flowchart 10.5

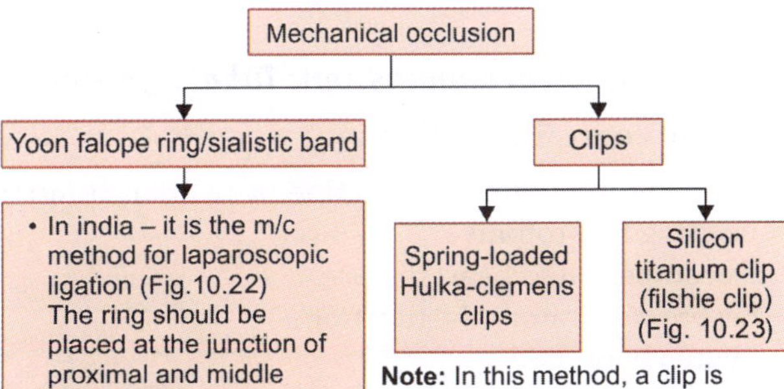

Note:
- Falope rings introduced by Yoon in 1974
- Clips cause least damage to tube = 4–5 mm

- With pomeroy technique damage is 3-4 cm. With Falope ring = damage is 3 cm

Unipolar cauterization by laparoscopy although has least failure but is not done as it leads to intestinal burns and has thus been abandoned.

Note: The falope ring, Hulka and filshie clips cannot be applied if tube is trick from previous salpingitis.

3. **Hysteroscopic tubal ligation:** Can be done using cauterization- failure rate 30% or by using sclerosants - failure rate, 15%

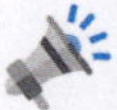

Important One Liners

- **Methods with good chances of recanalization:**
  - Laparoscopic clips (best) > Laparoscopic Falope ring > Pomeroy and Uchida methods.
- **Lowest chances of reversal are with cautery.**
- **Least failure rate with open techniques:** Uchida > irving > Modified Pomeroy > Pomeroy
- **M/C used method used in minilaparotomy:** Modified Pomeroy

Highest risk of ectopic pregnancy: Cautery > Madlenar > Modified pomeroy

Method of Female Sterilization and Failure Rates

Method	Failure Rate
• Pomeroy's method	0.4%[Q]
• Modified pomeroy	0.2%
• Madlener	7%
• Irwing	Very low failure rate
• Uchida	Very low failure rate
• Laparoscopic sterilization	0.2–1.3%
• Hysteroscopic tubal block	
– Cauterization	30%
– Sclerosants	15%

Contraindication of Laparoscopic Tubal Ligation

Absolute contraindications

- Large abdominal mass (uterine or ovarian tumors) needing laparotomy.
- Decompensated heart disease.
- Severe respiratory dysfunction.
- Hiatus hernia.
- Immediate post partum period

Relative contraindications

- Gross obesity with thick abdominal wall and
- Pelvic adhesion due to previous pelvic infection or operations. Laparoscopic sterilization should not be done soon after delivery or abortion of more than 12 weeks pregnancy.

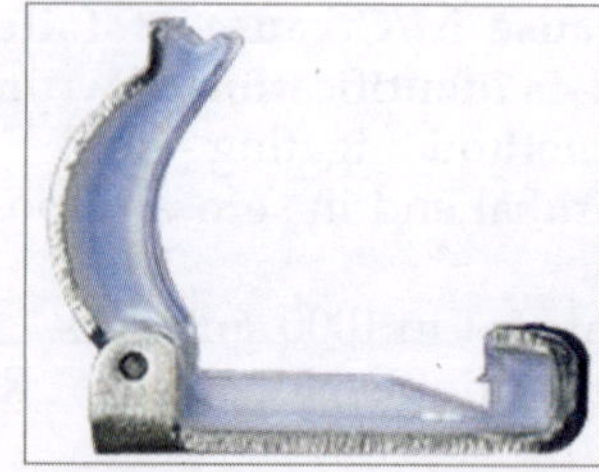

Fig. 10.23: Filshie clip for tubal sterilization

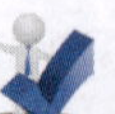

KEY POINTS

Post-ligation syndrome

Some patients after tubal ligation can experience post ligation syndrome characterized by:

- Menstrual irregularities like menorrhagia or irregular periods,
- Pelvic pain or congestive dysmenorrhea and
- Cystic ovaries.

It is vascular in origin and its incidence can be reduced if the blood vessels adjacent to the mesosalpinx are not unduly disturbed.

Reversal of Tubal Ligation

- The most important factor affecting successful reversal is length of the remaining tube
- For reversal the minimum length of reconstructed tube should be 4 cms (with ampullary part 2 cms)
- The chances of ectopic pregnancy after reversal are very high
- Reversal is best if site of sterilization is isthmus & anastomosis is isthmo-isthmic
- **Reversal depends on procedure adopted for sterilization.**
  It is best with clips > fallope ring > Modified pomeroy.
- **Reversal chances are least with cautery** (monopolar, followed by bipolar).

Male Sterilization

Vasectomy

- It is a simple, safe and effective surgical procedure that permanently ends a man's fertility.
- There are two methods by which the vasdeferens can be approached ***conventional vasectomy*** and ***no scalpel vasectomy***.
- Vasectomy consists of dividing and excising a part of vas deferens and disrupting the passage of sperms.
- It is done under local anesthesia.
- The first step in the vasectomy is to identify and immobilize the vas through the skin of the scrotum. The second step is to bring the vas into the open.
- Once the vas deferens is brought out into the open it is then occluded using a variety of methods viz:
  - Ligation and excision (most common method used in India)

- ➢ Electrocautery
- ➢ Thermal cautery
- ➢ Clips
- ➢ Open ended vasectomy

Conventional Vasectomy

- In the conventional incisional method of vasectomy, the surgeon uses a scalpel to make either one midline incision or two incisions in the scrotal skin, each usually 1.2 cm long and one overlying each vas deferens
- The incision +is routinely closed with sutures after the vasectomy has been completed
- In general, with conventional vasectomy, only the area around the skin entry site is anesthetized.

No-scalpel Vasectomy: Introduced in China by Dr Li Shuangjiang

- No-scalpel vasectomy *(also known as NSV)* is a unique method of gaining access to vas deferns
- Instead of a scalpel, two specialized instruments: *a ringed clamp* and a *dissecting forceps* (a sharp, curved hemostat) are used
- Because the scrotal skin puncture made with the dissecting forceps is so small, sutures are not needed.

Advantages of No-scalpel Vasectomy

- A smaller wound than conventional technique
- Earlier resumption of sexual activity after surgery (because it requires no scrotal incision)
- Neither conventional nor no-scalpel vasectomy is time-consuming, but it has been reported that the vasectomy procedure time is shorter when skilled providers use the no-scalpel technique
- Failure Rate = 0.1 - 0.15%
- Reversibility: Reversal is possible with microsurgery (vasovasotomy) giving 90% return of sperm and 70% pregnancy rate

Note: The longer the time interval between vasectomy and reversal, poorer the chances of reversal.

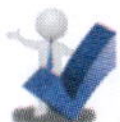

KEY POINTS

Sterility does not occur immediately after vasectomy.
Sperms remain in the semen for 15–20 ejaculation, requiring continued contraception for about 3 months. So, the couple is advised to use some form of contraception for the next 3 months or 15–20 ejaculates, generally. Before discontinuing contraceptive method, azoospermia should be confirmed by semen analysis (done either at 16 weeks or at 12 and 16 weeks)
Contraindications of vasectomy–

- Local skin infection
- Varicocele, hernia
- Undescended testis

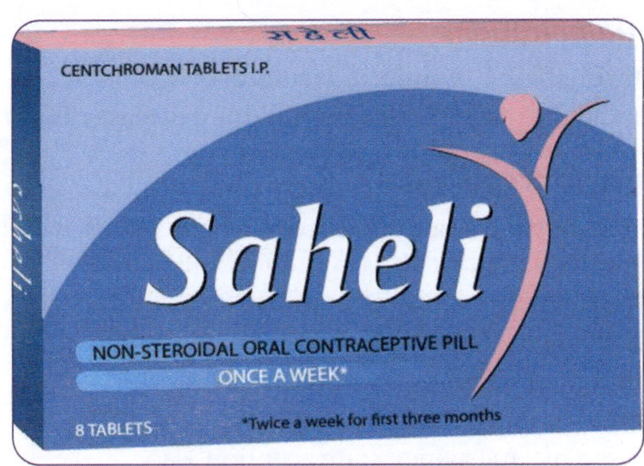

Fig. 10.24: Centchroman Saheli

Also Know

Gossypol

It has been discovered in China; an extract from cotton seed. It acts directly on the seminiferous tubules inhibiting spermatogenesis. The side effects are: fatigue, decreased libido and delayed recovery of sperm count. The serious side effects are hypokalemic paralysis and cardiac arrhythmias.

Centchroman (Fig. 10.24)

- It is a synthetic **non-steroidal** contraceptive.
- Active component– Ormeloxifene
- A tablet of 30 mg started on 1st day of menstruation and taken twice weekly for (12 weeks or 3 months), and weekly thereafter (t½ - 170 hours).

Mechanism of Action

- It prevents implantation through endometrial changes by making it out of phase and does not inhibit ovulation.
- Developed by CDRI, Lucknow and released in India by 2 trade names Saheli and Centron.
- Exhibits strong antiestrogenic and a weak estrogenic actions peripherally at receptor level.
- It is not teratogenic or carcinogenic
- It does not protect against STD.
- Pregnancy rate is (1–4)/100 WY.
- Return of fertility is within 6 months of stopping the drug.
- The drug can also be used as a post coital pill, given in 60 mg dose within 24 hours of coitus, 2 tablets repeated after 12 hours with a failure rate of 1%.

Side Effects

- Headache, nausea, vomiting, gain in weight, does not protect against HIV and STD, prolonged cycles (due to prolonged proliferative phase) and oligomenorrhea (in 8% cases). There is some delay in return of fertility.

Contraindications

a. During first 6 months of lactation
b. PCOD, hepatic dysfunction, kidney disease, TB, etc.

Non-contraceptive Use

Because of its potent antiestrogenic activity it is being tried in:

- DUB
- Endometrial hyperplasia
- Endometriosis
- Breast cancer

It is used as emergency contraception also.

Essure (Figs. 10.25A and B)

It is a spring-like device which is introduced via females vagina (with the help of a hysteroscope) into the fallopian tube. It blocks the fallopian tube and prevents sperms from reaching the ova. It has an outer coil of Nickel and Titanium and inner coil of stainless steel. It incites tissue reaction. Success rate 99%. Now available in India.

- For the first 3 months–back up method of contraception should be used.
- 3 months following device insertion, HSG required to confirm complete obstruction.

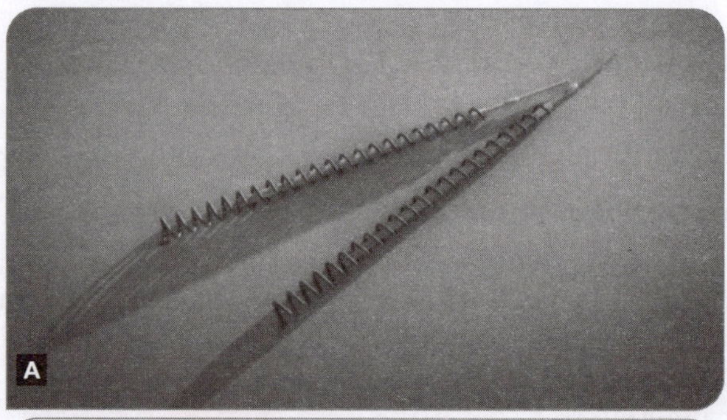

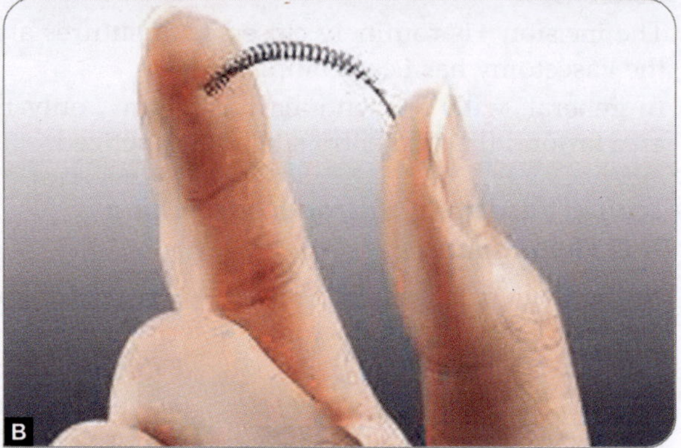

Figs. 10.25A and B: (A) Essure device for hysteroscopic sterilization. (B) Essure device with guide wire and handle

Lactation

- Among others, lactation is one factor addressed in the US MEC guidelines. **Approximately 20 percent of breast-feeding women will ovulate by 3 months postpartum. Ovulation often precedes menstruation, and these women are at risk for unplanned pregnancy.**
- For women who breast feed intermittently, effective contraception should begin as if they were not breast feeding. Moreover, contraception is essential after the first menses unless pregnancy planned.
- Of available methods, Cu-IUD in breast-feeding women has a category 1 or 2 rating.
- Women are counseled that effects of the etonogestrel-releasing contraceptive implant (Nexplanon) or LNG-IUS and breast feeding are not known, but studies have mostly shown no adverse association (Gurtcheff, 2011).
- Because POPs have little effect on lactation, they are also preferred by some for use up to 6 months in women who are exclusively breastfeeding.
- According to the Obstetricians and Gynecologists (2012), POPs and DMPA may be initiated prior to discharge regardless of breast-feeding status.
- For the etonogestrel implant, insertion is delayed until 4 weeks postpartum for those exclusively breast-feeding but can be inserted anytime for those not nursing.
- Combination hormone contraception may begin at 6 weeks following delivery, if breast feeding is well established and the infant's nutritional status is surveilled.

Table 10.4: U.S. Medical Eligibility Criteria for Use of Various Contraceptive Methods While Breastfeeding

Method	*Category*	*Comments*
CHCs[b]		Evidence limited. Guidelines based on theoretical concerns
Breastfeeding	3	
<1 month	2	
>1 month		

Contd...

Contd...

Method	Category	Comments
Non-breastfeeding		Theoretical concerns for thrombosis risks. Blood coagulation and fibrinolysis virtually normalized by 3 weeks pp
<21 days	4	
21–42 days, with risksc	3	
21–42 days, with no risks	2	
>42 days	1	
DMPA, POPs, Implants		Theoretical concerns that early use may diminish breast milk production are not supported by evidence. Limited studies
Breastfeeding		
<1 month	2	
>1 month	1	
Non-breastfeeding	1	Limited evidence suggests no adverse side effects
LNG-IUS		Theoretical risk of diminished breast milk production. Minimal evidence
Breastfeeding or not		
<10 mins	2	
10 mins to ≤4 wks	2	
≥4 wks	1	
Puerperal sepsis	4	IUD insertion could worsen condition
Cu-IUD		IUC placement <10 min pp is associated with lower expulsion rates compared with later IUD placement up to >72 hr pp. No comparative data for insertion >72 hr pp
Breastfeeding or not		At c-section, postplacental placement associated with lower expulsion rate than after vaginal delivery
<10 min	1	
10 min to <4 wks	2	No increased risk of infection or perforation associated with pp insertion
>4 wks	1	IUD insertion could worsen condition
Puerperal sepsis	4	

[a]Time reflects time from delivery.
[b]Combined hormonal contraceptive (CHC) group includes pills, vaginal ring, and patch.
[c]Associated risks that increase category score include: age >35, transfusion at delivery, BMI >30, postpartum hemorrhage cesarean delivery, smoking, I preeclampsia.
c-section = cesarean delivery; Cu-IUD = copper-beating intrauterine device; DMPA = depot medroxyprogesterone acetate; LNG-IUS - levonorgestrel-releasing intrauterine system; POPs - progestin-only pills, pp = postpartum.
Adapted with permission from Centers for Disease Control and Prevention, 2010, 2011. *Taken from Williams Gyne 3rd/ed, p108*

Important Points

- M/C method of contraception used by couples in India—Barrier method
- Best method for couples staying far—Barrier method
- Best method for newly married couples—OCPs
- Safest method of contraception—Barrier method
- In HIV patients best method—IUCD + Barrier method
- Female sterilization—Most commonly used method in Minilap Modified Pomeroy technique
- Most effective method—Modified Pomeroy technique
- Least effective Hulka Clip > Bipolar cautery
- Highest risk of ectopic pregnancy > Cautery > Madlener > modified Pomeroy
- Least failure rate in Minilap = Uchida > Irving > Modified Pomeroy
- Least failure rate in laparoscopy: Unipolar cautery > Ring.

PREVIOUS YEAR QUESTIONS

General

1. **Which of the following is correct for the calculation of pearl index?** *(AIIMS Nov 03)*
   a. $\frac{\text{No. of accidental pregnancies} \times 1200}{\text{No. of patient observed} \times \text{months of use}}$
   b. $\frac{\text{No. of accidental pregnancies} \times 1200}{\text{No. of patient observed} \times 2400}$
   c. $\frac{\text{No. of patients observed} \times \text{months of use}}{\text{No. of accidental pregnancies}}$
   d. $\frac{\text{No. of patient observed} \times 2400}{\text{No. of accidental pregnancies} \times 1200}$
2. **Pearl's index indicates:** *(PGI June 05)*
   a. Malnutrition b. Population
   c. Contraceptive failure d. LBW
   e. IUGR
3. **Reversible methods of contraception are:** *(PGI June 05)*
   a. Female sterilization b. OCP
   c. IUCD d. Barrier
   e. Depot injection
4. **Failure Rate of <2/100 women years is/are seen**
   a. Male condom b. Implanon
   c. COC d. vaginal diaphragm
   e. IUCD *(PGI Nov 2015)*

Barrier Methods

5. **Not a barrier contraceptive:** *(UP 2008)*
   a. Diaphragm b. Centchroman
   c. Condom d. Today
6. **Which one of the following is not a correct statement regarding the use of condom?** *(UPSC 07)*
   a. Air should be squeezed out of tip
   b. It should be tested by inflating
   c. It should be unrolled on erect penis
   d. K-Y jelly may be used for lubrication
7. **Which one of the following is the most common problem associated with the use of condom?** *(UPSC 02)*
   a. Increased monilial infection of vagina
   b. Premature ejaculation
   c. Contact dermatitis d. Retention of urine
8. **All are contraindications of diaphragm *except*:** *(UP 05)*
   a. Multiple sex partners b. Recurrent UTI
   c. Uterine prolapse d. Herpes vaginitis
9. **Contraceptive vaginal foam tablet "today "contains:**
   a. Nonoxynol 9 b. Octoxynol 9
   c. Menfegol d. None of the above
10. **True about Nonoxynol-9:** *(PGI May 2015)*
    a. Decrease risk of HIV
    b. Prevent STD infection
    c. Remain effective for 1–2 hours after application
    d. Spermicidal action
    e. Causes itching of vagina in female and itching of penis in male
11. **Spermicidal jelly acts through:** *(AIIMS Dec 98)*
    a. Acrosomal enzyme
    b. Cervical enzyme alteration
    c. Glucose uptake inhibition by sperms
    d. Disruption of cell membrane
12. **Spermicidal agents are:** *(PGI June 06)*
    a. Nonoxynol b. Menfegol
    c. Progestasert

OCPs

13. **All of the following mechanisms of action of oral contraceptive pills are true, *except*:** *(AI 06)*
    a. Inhibition of ovulation
    b. Prevention of fertilization
    c. Interference with implantation of fertilized ovum
    d. Interference with placental functioning

Composition

14. **Version I**
    Amount of estrogen in low dose oral contraceptive pills: *(AIIMS Nov 01)*
    a. 30 µg b. 40 µg
    c. 50 µg d. 20 µg
    Version II
    Minimum effective dose of ethinyl estradiol in combination oral pills is: *(AIIMS May 04)*
    a. 10 µg b. 35 µg
    c. 50 µg d. 75 µg
15. **Low dose OCP's contain:**
    a. Levonorgestrel b. Desogestrel
    c. Norgestrel d. Norethisterone
16. **Norgestimate OCP's have the following advantage *except*:**
    a. Reduces venous thrombosis
    b. Is cheaper than standard OCP's
    c. Reduces acne and hirsutism
    d. Useful in heart disease
17. **The progesterone component of OCP acts by:**
    a. Preventing ovulation
    b. Inhibiting implantation
    c. Bringing about alterations in cervical mucus
    d. All of the above
18. **Amount of estrogen in Mala D is:** *(UP 00)*
    a. 30 µg b. 50 µg
    c. 10 µg d. 80 µg
19. **Which of the following OCP's have the least amount of estrogen:**
    a. Mala N b. Triquilar
    c. Femilon d. Novelon

Benefits of OCPs

20. Which of the following is/are true about combined oral contraceptive pills: *(PGI Nov 2016)*
a. Reduces risk of venous thromboembolism
b. Reduces risk of benign breast disease
c. Protects against endometrial cancer
d. ↓ Bone density

21. Oral contraceptive pills decrease incidence of all of the following conditions *except*: *(AI 99)*
a. Salpingitis
b. Hepatic adenoma
c. Ovary CA
d. Fibroadenosis

22. Use of OCP's are known to protect against following malignancies *except*: *(AIIMS Nov 02)*
a. Ovarian carcinoma
b. Endometrial carcinoma
c. Uterine sarcoma
d. Carcinoma cervix

23. Use of oral contraceptives decreases the incidence of all of the following *except*: *(AIIMS May 05)*
a. Ectopic pregnancy
b. Epithelial ovarian malignancy
c. Hepatic adenoma
d. Pelvic inflammatory disease

24. OCP gives protection against following cancers: *(PGI June 06)*
a. Endometrial b. Ovary
c. Cervix d. Breast
e. Liver

25. Chronic use of combine oral contraceptive (COC) helps in all *except*: *(PGI Nov 2016*
a. Dysmenorrhea b. Breakthrough bleeding
c. Menorrhagia d. Migraine
e. Anaemia

Side Effects of OCPs

26. OCPs cause all *except*: *(AIIMS Dec 98)*
a. Dysmenorrhea b. Mastalgia
c. Nausea d. Chloasma

27. Adverse effects combined OCPs: *(PGI Dec 09)*
a. Liver disorders b. Increased size of PID
c. Weight gain d. Acne
e. Endometriosis

28. OCP's intake causes all *except*: *(AIIMS June 98)*
a. Decreased risk of ovarian tumour
b. Increased risk of fibroadenosis
c. Increased risk of liver adenoma
d. Increased risk of fibroadenoma

29. The use of combined OCPs is associated with an increased incidence of: *(AIIMS Nov 03)*
a. Bacterial vaginosis b. Chlamydial endocervicitis
c. Vaginal warts d. Genital herpes

Contraindications of OCPs

30. In a young female of reproductive age an absolute contraindication for prescribing OCP's is: *(AIIMS May 05)*
a. Diabetes b. Hypertension
c. Obesity d. Impaired liver function

31. Absolute contraindication of OCP's is: *(PGI June 02)*
a. Breast cancer b. Mentally ill
c. Migraine d. Fibroid
e. Hyperlipidemia

32. Contraindications to OC pills: *(PGI June 01)*
a. Heart disease b. Uterine malformations
c. Menorrhagia d. Liver failure
e. Epilepsy

33. OCPs is absolutely contraindicated in: *(PGI May 2014)*
a. Age >40 years with smoking
b. H/O Epilepsy
c. Cancer breast and genitalia
d. Thrombophlebitis
e. Hyperlipidemia

34. Contraindication of combined oral contraceptive (COC) include(s):
a. Severe hypertension
b. Ischemic heart disease
c. Pre-menstrual tension
d. Active liver disease

35. OCPs are contraindicated in all *except*: *(PGI Dec 99)*
a. Smoking 35 years
b. Coronary occlusion
c. Polycystic ovarian disease
d. Cerebrovascular disease

36. OCP's intake cause psychiatric symptoms, and abdominal pain. Diagnosis is: *(PGI Dec 98)*
a. Acute intermittent porphyria
b. Systemic lupus
c. Thrombosis
d. Anemia

Drug Interaction

37. A 20-years old nulliparous women is on oral contraceptives pills. She is currently diagnosed as having pulmonary tuberculosis. Which anti-tubercular drug decreases the effect of OCP: *(AIIMS May 01)*
a. INH b. Pyrazinamide
c. Ethambutol d. Rifampicin

38. OCP's efficiency is reduced by simultaneous use of: *(PGI Dec 98)*
a. Rifampicin b. Carbamazepine
c. Propranolol d. Tricyclic antidepressants

39. OCPs are C/I in pts receiving: *(AIIMS Nov 07)*
a. Rifampicin b. Ethambutol
c. Streptomycin d. Pyrazinamide

40. Hypokalemic paralysis is a side effect of:
a. Gossypol
b. DMPA
c. Testosterone enanthate
d. Cyproterone acetate

41. True about combined oral contraceptive:
a. Pelvic examination is mandatory before prescribing COC *(PGI May 2015)*
b. Pregnancy resumes soon after discontinuation of pill
c. Protect from endometrial cancer, & ovarian cancer
d. HIV antiviral drugs reduce effectiveness of COC
e. Pregnancy rate equal to non-hormonal contraceptive after discontinuation

Progesterone only Pills/Implants/Injections

42. Progestational contraceptives primarily act by: *(AIIMS May 03)*
a. Oviductal motility
b. Uterine endometrium
c. Altering cervix mucus
d. Inhibiting ovulation

43. True statement about Minipill is: *(AI 99)*
a. Irregular vaginal bleeding may be a side effect
b. Used in with combination with oral contraceptive pills
c. Cannot be used in lactation
d. Prevents ectopic pregnancy

44. True about progestogen only pili: *(PGI May 2015)*
a. Weight gain occurs
b. Cause irregular bleeding
c. It can be given to lactating mother
d. Should not be given to women over 35 years
e. Protect from breast cancer

45. True about MIRENA: *(PGI May 2015)*
a. Effective life is 5–10 years
b. Protects against HIV and STD
c. Contraindicated in suspected pregnancy
d. Contraindicated in breast cancer
e. Useful in controlling menorrhagia in fibroid

46. True about progestogen only pill (POP): *(PGI May 2016)*
a. It is taken daily on the same time
b. Higher failure rate than COC
c. Fertility return to normal after discontinuation without any delay
d. Suited for lactating women
e. Ectopic pregnancy risk are same as DOC

47. Use of Levo-norgestrel releasing, IUCD is helpful in all of the following conditions *except*: *(AIIMS Nov 02)*
a. Menorrhagia
b. Dysmenorrhea
c. Premenstrual symptoms
d. Pelvic inflammatory disease

48. Benefits of LNG IUCD: *(PGI Dec 09)*
a. Endometriosis
b. Fibroid uterus
c. PID
d. Contraception
e. Endometrial hyperplasia

49. Which of these is not a noncontraceptive use of levonorgestrel IUCD? *(AIIMS Nov 2015)*
a. Endometriosis
b. PreMenstrual Tension
c. Complex endometrial hyperplasia
d. Emergency contraception

50. All are true about LNG IUCD *except*: *(PGI Nov 2014)*
a. Cause Endometrial suppression
b. Can be used as emergency contraception
c. Cannot be given to lactating women
d. Devoid of estrogenic side-effects

51. True about Mirena: *(PGI Nov 2012)*
a. Progestrone containing IUCD
b. Contain desogestrel
c. Causes endometrial hyperplasia
d. Decreases menstural blood flow

52. Which of the following statements is incorrect regarding levonorgestrel releasing intrauterine contraceptive devices? *(AI 06)*
a. There is increased incidence of menorrhagia
b. This system can be used as hormone replacement therapy
c. This method is useful for the treatment of endometrial hyperplasia
d. Irregular uterine bleeding can be a problem initially

53. True about Mirena: *(PGI Nov 2014)*
a. Effective life is 2 year
b. LNG containing IUCD
c. Cause endometrial hyperplasia
d. Suppression of endometrium
e. No significant effect on ovaries

54. All of the following mechanisms might account for a reduce-risk of upper genital tract infection in users of progestin – releasing IUDs, *except*: *(AI 06)*
a. Reduced retrograde menstruation
b. Decreased ovulation
c. Thickened cervical mucus
d. Decidual changes in the endometrium

55. Contraceptive LNG–IUD (levonorgestrel intra–uterine device) has the cumulative pregnancy rate at 5 years of: *(AI 02)*
a. 0.5
b. 1.0
c. 1.5
d. 2.0

56. DMPA-True: *(PGI Dec 09)*
a. Failure @ 0.3/100 WY
b. 150 mg/3 monthly delivered
c. Weight gain
d. Glucose intolerance occur
e. Anemia improves

57. True regarding DMPA including the following *except*: *(AI 09)*
a. 3% failure rate
b. Does not have protective effect on Ca endometrium
c. Can be given in seizures
d. Useful in treatment of menorrhagia

58. Side effect of depot MPA are all, *except*: *(AI 00)*
a. Weight gain
b. Irregular bleeding
c. Amenorrhea
d. Hepatitis

59. To avoid contraception, DMPA is given: *(HP 05)*
a. Monthly
b. 3 Monthly
c. 6 Monthly
d. Yearly

60. Characteristic problem in females taking norethisterone is: *(AI 00)*
a. Irregular bleeding
b. Thromboembolism
c. Hirsutism
d. Weight gain

61. True about implanon: *(PGI May 2015)*
a. Releases > 76 mg/day of drug
b. Prevent STD
c. Life span is 3 years
d. Contains LNG
e. Has 6 implants

62. In a woman on subdermal progesterone implant, the menstrual abnormality seen is: *(AIIMS May 01)*
a. Menorrhagia
b. Metrorrhagia
c. Polymenorrhea
d. Amenorrhea

63. POPs carry a risk of: *(Jimper 2012)*
a. Hypertension
b. Embolism
c. Irregular bleeding
d. Ectopic pregnancy

IUCDs

64. **Characteristics of an ideal candidate for copper-T insertion include all of the following *except*:** (AIIMS May 05)
   a. Has born at least one child
   b. Is willing to check IUD tail
   c. Has a history of ectopic pregnancy
   d. Has normal menstrual periods

65. **Mechanism by which IUCD does not act:** (AIIMS Dec 98)
   a. Chronic endometrial inflammation
   b. Increase the motility of tubes
   c. Inducing endometrial atrophy
   d. Inhibition of ovulation

66. **Appropriate time of IUCD insertion is/are:** (PGI May 2015)
   a. Immediately after delivery
   b. 1 week after delivery
   c. Post-puerperal period
   d. Before menstruation
   e. Any time during lactation period

67. **All IUCDs are changed every 4–5 year *except*:** (AIIMS Dec 97)
   a. Cu 280
   b. Cu 320
   c. Multiload devices
   d. Progestasert

68. **Among the following IUCD's which has life span for 10 years?**
   a. CuT380A
   b. CuT200
   c. Nova T
   d. Multiload

69. **Composition of Nova - T:** (PGI June 05)
   a. Copper and silver
   b. Copper and aluminium
   c. Copper only
   d. Copper and selenium
   e. Copper and molybdenum

70. **A lady with IUCD becomes pregnant with tail of IUCD being seen, next course of action is:** (PGI Dec 98)
   a. MTP
   b. Remove the IUCD
   c. Continue the pregnancy
   d. Remove IUCD and terminate pregnancy

71. **An intrauterine pregnancy of approximately 10 weeks gestation is confirmed in a 30 year old, gravida 5, para 4 woman with an IUD in place. The patient expresses a strong desire for the pregnancy to be continued. On examination, the string of the IUD is noted to be protruding from the cervical os. The most appropriate course of action is to:**
   a. Leave the IUD in place without any other treatment
   b. Remove the IUD to decrease the risk of malformations
   c. Remove the IUD to decrease the risk of infection
   d. Terminate the pregnancy because of the high risk of malformations.

72. **A 28-year-old P1L1 had Cu T inserted 2 years back, on examination Cu T threads are not seen. USG shows Cu T partly in abdominal cavity. Method of removal is:**
   a. Hysteroscopy
   b. No need of removal (wait and watch)
   c. IUCD hook
   d. Laparoscopy

73. **Absolute contraindication for IUCD includes all of the following *except*:** (AI 97)
   a. Undiagnosed vaginal bleeding
   b. Suspected pregnancy
   c. Congenital malformation of uterus
   d. PID

74. **IUCD is absolutely contraindicated in:** (PGI Nov 2014)
   a. HIV positive women
   b. Previous ectopic tubal pregnancy
   c. Mild anaemia
   d. Undiagnosed vaginal bleeding

75. **Absolute contraindication of IUCD is:** (AIIMS Dec 97)
   a. Endometriosis
   b. Iron deficiency anemia
   c. Dysmenorrhea
   d. Pelvic tuberculosis

76. **Contraindications of IUCD:** (PGI June 09)
   a. Undiagnosed vaginal bleeding
   b. PID
   c. Smoking
   d. Obesity
   e. Diabetes

77. **Contraindications for IUCD:** (PGI May 2017)
   a. Postabortal sepsis more than 1 year ago
   b. Present cervicitis and vaginitis
   c. Past history of ectopic pregnancy
   d. Unknown cause of vaginal bleeding
   e. Severe dysmenorrhea

78. **Contraindication of IUCD:** (PGI Dec 04)
   a. Oligomenorrhea
   b. PID
   c. Uterine malformation
   d. Controlled diabetes
   e. Previous cesarean section

79. **Contraindication of IUCD:** (PGI Dec 04)
   a. Oligomenorrhea
   b. PID
   c. Uterine malformation
   d. Controlled diabetes
   e. Previous ectopic pregnancy

80. **The most common complication of IUCD is:** (AI 95)
   a. Ectopic pregnancy
   b. Bleeding
   c. Backache
   d. Cervical stenosis

81. **IUCD which may not be changed for 10 years:** (Jimper Dec 16)
   a. Cu T380A
   b. Cu 200
   c. NovaT
   d. MIRENA

82. **Best IUCD in a woman with menorrhagia** (Jimper 2011)
   a. Lipple Loop
   b. CuT 375
   c. CuT 200
   d. Levonorgestrel IUCD

Emergency Contraception

83. **Emergency contraception prevents pregnancy by all of the following mechanisms, *except*:** (AI 06)
   a. Delaying/inhibiting ovulation
   b. Inhibiting fertilization
   c. Preventing implantation of the fertilized egg
   d. Interrupting an early pregnancy

84. Emergency contraception is required in: *(AIIMS Nov 99)*
a. Partner not willing to use any contraceptive
b. In emergency, where sexual intercourse is done in camps in emergency like floods
c. Contraception failure
d. Unprotected sex

85. Drugs used in emergency contraception are all *except*: *(PGI Dec 06, PGI June 08)*
a. Levonorgestrel
b. Estrogen + progesterone
c. Danazol
d. Mifepristone
e. Misoprostol

86. All of these can be used for postcoital contraception *except*: *(AIIMS Nov 2015)*
a. Desogestrol b. Copper-T
c. Levonorgestrol d. OCP

87. Which is not an emergency contraceptive? *(PGI Nov 2012)*
a. Combined oral pills
b. Estrogen
c. Desogestrel
d. Levonorgestrel
e. Medroxyprogesterone acetate

88. Emergency contraceptive of choice is: *(PGI Dec 09)* *(Jimper Dec 16)*
a. OCP
b. Danazol
c. Levonorgestrel
d. Mifepristone

89. A 32-year-old P2L2 lady comes five days after unprotected sexual intercourse. What will be your advice for contraception in this lady? *(AIIMS May 2015)*
a. Levonorgestrol 0.75 mg
b. Copper IUD
c. Two tablets of high dose OCP, repeated after 24 hours
d. Laparoscopic tubectomy

90. Emergency contraceptives are effective if administered within following period after unprotected intercourse: *(AIIMS May 04)*
a. 24 hours
b. 48 hours
c. 72 hours
d. 120 hours

91. Antiprogester used for Emergency contraception: *(Jimper 2015)*
a. RU486 b. Misoprost
c. Methotrexate d. Estrogen

Permanent Method

92. A young lady can be counselled for sterilization operation in all *except*: *(PGI May 2015)*
a. A woman having no child may undergo sterilization
b. Women with HIV either taking or not ART can go for sterilization
c. Husband consent is present
d. Young lactating women more than 25 years can go for sterilization
e. If the couple has 3 or more living children, the lower limit of age of the husband or wife may be relaxed at the discretion of the operating surgeon

93. Permanent sterilization is all, *except*: *(PGI Dec 05)*
a. Electrocoagulation
b. Vasectomy
c. Clipping
d. Tube ligation
e. Medroxyprogesterone

94. Which of the following is not an abdominal laparoscopic technique for tubal ligation?
a. Pomeroy b. Parkland
c. Essure d. Irving

95. Method of sterilization which is least effective is: *(AIIMS Dec 98)*
a. Pomeroy's technique
b. Laparoscopy
c. Vaginal fimbriectomy
d. Hysteroscopic tubal occlusion

96. Sterilization procedure with maximum chances of reversal is: *(AIIMS May 02)*
a. Pomeroy's tubal ligation
b. Irwing's technique
c. Laparoscopic tubal ligation with silastic bands
d. Laparoscopic tubal ligation with clips

97. Sterilization is commonly performed at which site of fallopian tube: *(AI 07)*
a. Ampulla b. Infundibulum
c. Isthmus d. Cornua

98. Best prognosis for reversibility is seen in: *(AI 97)*
a. Isthmo – isthmic type
b. Isthmic – ampullary type
c. Ampullary – interstitial type
d. Ampullary – fimbrial type

99. Which of the following procedure is associated with maximum chance of recanalization during surgery for reversal of tubal ligation?
a. Isthmo-isthmic anastomosis
b. Isthumo-ampullary anastomosis
c. Ampullo-ampullary anastomosis
d. Cornual obstruction

100. Which of following is/are not fertility awareness based methods:
a. Withdrawal method
b. Rhythm method
c. Cervical mucus method
d. MTP pill
e. Sympto-thermal method

101. All of the following are features of post-tubal ligation syndrome *except*: *(PGI Nov 2016)*
a. Abnormal menstrual bleeding
b. Dysmenorrhea
c. Pelvic pain
d. Dysparaunia

102. Failure rate of vasectomy is:
a. 0.2% b. 0.1%
c. 3% d. 10%

103. **A couple is advised to use barrier methods after vasectomy till:**
 a. 3 months
 b. No sperms in ejaculate
 c. Next 15 ejaculations
 d. None of the above

Contraceptive of Choice

104. **PID occurs least common with:** *(AI 00)*
 a. OCPs b. Condom
 c. IUCD d. Diaphragm

105. **Ideal contraceptive for newly married couple is:**
 a. Barrier method *(AIIMS May 2011)*
 b. Combined OCP
 c. IUCD
 d. Progesterone only pill

106. **Ideal contraceptive for a couple living in different cities meeting only occasionally:** *(AIIMS May 2011)*
 a. Barrier method
 b. IUCD
 c. OCP
 d. DMPA

107. **Ideal contraceptive for lactating mother is:**
 a. Barrier method *(AIIMS May 2011)*
 b. Combined OCP
 c. Lactational amenorrhoea
 d. Progesterone only pill

108. **Peritoneum is opened in all of the following sterilization procedures *except*:** *(AP 97)*
 a. Mini lap
 b. Laparoscopy
 c. Vasectomy
 d. Transvaginal tubectomy

109. **Contraceptive to be avoided in epilepsy:**
 (AIIMS May 2011)
 a. OCPs b. Condom
 c. IUCD d. Mirena

110. **All of the following are reversible long acting contraceptives *except*:** *(AIIMS Nov 2018)*
 a. Copper T
 b. Laparoscopic tubal ligation
 c. LNG-IUS
 d. Implanon

111. **A female is on Mala N for contraception. After the end of the first strip, there was no withdrawal bleeding. What should be done?** *(AIIMS May 2018)*
 a. Start next cycle of tablets from 5th day
 b. Start next cycle from next day
 c. Urgent visit to hospital and check for pregnancy
 d. Take two pills after 12 hours

112. **A 30 years female is on warfarin for deep vein thrombosis. Which contraceptive should not be advised?**
 a. Progesterone only pills *(JIPMER May 2019)*
 b. Levonorgestrel
 c. IUCD
 d. Implanon

113. **Which can be used as emergency contraceptive?**
 a. Intrauterine copper device *(PGI May 2019)*
 b. Levonorgestrel (LNG)
 c. Estrogen plus progesterone
 d. Mifepristone
 e. Misoprostol

114. **Post-coital contraceptive which are used to prevent pregnancy include?** *(PGI December 2018)*
 a. Levonorgestrel
 b. Copper T up to 5 days before after the unprotected intercourse
 c. Progesterone only pill
 d. Progesterone and estrogen
 e. None of the above

115. **Mechanisms of action of depot MPA include all *except*:**
 a. Thinning of inner uterine layer *(PGI December 2018)*
 b. Thickening of cervical mucosa
 c. Immobilization of sperms
 d. Inhibition of ovulation
 e. Decreased entry of sperms in uterus

ANSWERS TO PREVIOUS YEAR QUESTIONS

General

1. **Ans. is a, i.e. No. of accidental pregnancies × 1200/No. of patients observed × months of use**
2. **Ans. is c, i.e. Contraceptive failure** *Ref: Dutta Obs 6th/ed, p531-532*

Pearl index indicates the effectiveness of a contraceptive or is an index of contraception failure.

- It is expressed in terms of "failure rate per hundred women - years of exposure (HWY)".
- Failure rate per HWY = $\frac{\text{Total accidental pregnancies} \times 1200\ (12 \times 100)}{\text{No. of patients observed} \times \text{months of use}}$
- In applying the above formula the following points must be kept in mind:
  a. The total accidental pregnancies shown in the numerator must include every known conception, whatever its outcome.
  b. The factor 1200 is the number of months in 100 years.
  c. The total months of exposure in the denominator is obtained by deducing from the period under review of 10 months for a full term pregnancy and 4 months for an abortion.

3. **Ans. is b, c, d and e, i.e. OCP; IUCD; Barrier, and Depot injection** *Ref: Dutta Obs 6th/ed, p532; Park 20th/ed, p424*

Methods of contraception (can be classified as)

Temporary methods
(used to postpone pregnancy or space births)
- *Barrier method*[Q]
- *Natural contraception*[Q]
- *Oral contraceptive pills*
- *Injectables*
- *Implants*
- *Devices like IUCD's*

Levonorgestrel IUCD's

Permanent methods
(Surgical methods arm is to purposefully and permanently destroy the Reproductive capacity of an individual)

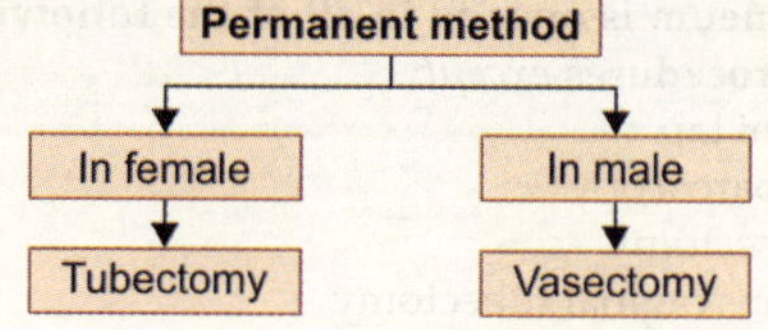

4. **Ans. is b and e, i.e. Implanon & IUCD**

Failure Rate <2/100 users means that it belongs to 1st tier method. Contraceptive methods included in First Tier method is IUCD/Implant/Sterilization methods.

Barrier Methods

5. **Ans. is b, i.e. Centchroman** *Ref: Shaw 15th/ed, p222*

Barrier Methods include:
- Condoms (for male use)
- Diaphragms (for female use) – Types
  1. Femshield (female condom)
  2. Today contraceptive/vaginal sponge
  3. Vaginal diaphragm/cervical cap

Besides these spermicidal agents like nonoxynol 9, octoxynol, and menfegol can be added to any of the above barrier contraceptive, to increase its effectiveness.

6. **Ans. is b, i.e. It should be tested by inflating**

Ref: Practice of Fertility Control S.K. Chaudhari 6th/ed, p82; Leon Speroff 7th/ed, p998

7. **Ans. is c, i.e. Contact dermatitis** *Ref: Shaw 14th/ed, p202*

See the text for explanation

8. **Ans. is a, i.e. Multiple sex partners** *Ref: Shaw 15th/ed, p225*

Occlusive caps (vaginal diaphragm and cervical cap):

Occlusive caps donot act as sperm proof mechanical barriers like condoms but are used as a means to retain spermicides in contact with cervical os, so spermicides must be used along with these devices.

Contraindications to the use of diaphragm
- Prolapse,cystocele, rectocele
- Retroversion
- VVF/RVF
- Badly eroded or lacerated cervix
- Recurrent UTI

Multiple sex partners is not a C/I for the use of diaphragms, rather barrier contraceptives protect against STD's so are contraception of choice in them.

9. **Ans. is a, i.e. Nonoxynol 9** *Ref: Shaw 14th/ed, p203*
   TODAY: It contains 1 gm of NONOX Y NOL–9
10. **Ans. is c, d and e i.e. Remain effective for 1–2 hrs after application, Spermicidal action and Causes itching of vagina in female and itching of penis in male** *Ref: Leon Speroff 8/e, p1129-1131*
    - Nonoxynol-9 is spermicidal agent
    - All spermicidal agents-have low efficiency with failure rate 20–25%
    - Effectiveness lasts for 1–2 hrs only.
    - They do not prevent HIV or STD infection(Rather HIV infection chances increases)
    - Only side effects in minor allergy in the form of itching
    - There is a possible association between spermicidal use and congenital abnormalities on spontaneous abortions, if pregnancy occurs.
11. **Ans. is d, i.e. Disruption of cell membrane** *Ref: Current Concepts in Contraception and Women Health by Jaypee Publication p32*
12. **Ans. is a and b, i.e. Nonoxynol, and Menfegol** *Ref: Shaw 15th/ed, p224*
    Spermicides
    "Spermicides are contraceptive chemical agents. They comprise,of a chemical capable of destroying sperm, incorporated into an inert base. The commonly used spermicidal agents contain nonionic surfactants which alter sperm surface membrane permeability, causing osmotic changes resulting in killing of sperm. Most of the spermicides contain nonoxynol-9 which is the best for this purpose."
    Ref: Current Concepts in Contraception and Women Health by Jaypee Publication p32
    - Spermicidal agents kill the sperms before it enters to the cervical canal. They are available as foam tablets, soluble pessaries, creams, jellies, or as films.
    - Contents are:
      - **Nonoxynol - 9 (N - 9)**
      - **Menfegol**
      - Benzalknonium chloride.
      - Octoxynol
      - Enzyme inhibiting agents

      – Jeffcoates 7th/ed, p794
    - Failure rate is 20–25 WY 100 woman years when used alone. When used in conjunction with a mechanical barrier, they give a reliable contraceptive effect.

    Note:
    - Recent evidences indicate spermicides are not effective in preventing cervical gonorrhoea, Chlamydia or HIV infection. In addition, frequent use of spermicides containing N-9 has been associated with an increased risk of HIV transmission. *– CGDT 10th/ed, p581*
    - Advantage 24 is a new contraceptive gel which contains nonoxynol.

OCPs

13. **Ans. is d, i.e. Interference with placental functioning** *Ref: KDT 6th/ed, p314-315*
    Friends, even if we don't know the mechanisms by which OCP's act, by sheer common sense we know that ***"Interference with placental functioning"*** is the incorrect option as if placenta is formed it means pregnancy is occuring which in itself is incorrect with regard to OCP's (as OCP's are used to prevent conception).
    The mechanism of action of OCP's has been discussed in detail in text.

In brief:
- Main mechanism of action of combined pills is - prevention of ovulation.
- Combined pills act by decreasing both LH and FSH
- They do not interfere with placental functioning.
- When taken daily for 3 out of 4 weeks, they provide virtually absolute protection against conception.

Composition

14. **Version I**
    Ans. is a, i.e. 30 μg *Ref: Dutta Obs 6th/ed, p543; Novak 14th/ed, p268,277*

Version II

Ans. is a, i.e. 10 µg *Ref: Dutta Obs. 6th/ed, p542; Shaw 15th/ed, p231*

Friends, I had a tough time in finding answers to these questions.

"Low dose pills have estrogen less than 50 mcg." *Ref: Dutta Obs 6th/ed, p543*

But it does not specify how much estrogen

"The low dose OCP (estrogen 30–35 mg EE) reduces the risk for a thromboembolic event when compared with higher dose (50 mg estrogen) OCs." *Ref: Novak 13th/ed, p251, 14th/ed, p268*

It further says *(Novak 14th/ed, p277)* *"For the average patient, the first choice of preparation for contraceptive purposes is a low estrogen OCP (20–35 µg EE) or a very low estrogen OC (20 µg EE)".*

So, from here it can be concluded that low dose OCP's are those pills with estrogen < 50 mcg (Normally 35 mcg). Very low dose OCPs are those pills with estrogen ≤ 20 µg EE.

My answer of choice for low dose OCPs is 30 µg.

Newer OCPs like femilon are a type of very low dose OCP's with estrogen = 20–30 or 35 µg of EE

Version II

"Intensive pharmacological research clinical trials conducted to minimise the adverse effects of estrogen without reducing the contraceptive efficacy, resulted in lowering the dose of oestrogen to a minimum of 20 µg or even 15 µg."

Thus, Remember: Low dose OCPs have estrogen = less than 50 mcg (30-35 mcg usually) *Ref: Dutta Obs 6th/ed, p542*

- Very low dose OCPs have estrogen = 20 mcg
- Minimum effective dose of Estrogen = 10 mcg

15. Ans. is b, i.e. Desogestrel *Ref: Reffcoate 7th/ed, p802, Dutta Gynae 6th/ed, p465; SK Chaudhary 7th/ed, p120-130*

Low dose OCPs on 3rd generation OCP have desogestrel.

16. Ans. is a, i.e. Reduces venous thrombosis *Ref: Lawrence 9th/ed, p723-725*

See the text for explanation

17. Ans. is d, i.e. All of the above *Ref: SK Chaudhary 7th/ed, p125-126,14*

Actions of the progesterone component of combined oral contraceptives:

- Suppresses ovulation by its inhibitory action on the pituitary and the hypothalamus. This is predominantly achieved by estrogens but even by progesterone.
- Causes atrophic changes in the endometrium and prevents nidation even if fertilization occurs.
- Acts on the cervical mucus, making it thick and tenacious and impenetrable by sperms.

The third-generation progestogens have a higher affinity for progesterone receptor and have a role in inhibiting ovulation. The main function of progestogens in combined pills is, to counteract the undesirable effects of estrogen such as endometrial hyperplasia and heavy withdrawal bleeding.

18. Ans. is a, i.e. 30 µg *Ref: Dutta Obs 6th/ed, p543*

19. Ans. is c, i.e. Femilon

Commercial name	Composition Progestin (mg)	Estrogen (µg)
1. Mala N (Distributed free of cost by govt. of India)	Levo norgestrel 0.15	Ethinyl estradiol 30
2. Mala D	D-levo Norgestrel 0.15	Ethinyl estradiol 30
3. Femilon	Desogestrel 0.15	Ethinyl estradiol 20
4. Loette	Levonorgestrel 0.1 mg	Ethinyl estradiol 20

- Eg's of very low dose OCP'S are femilon and Loette
- Triphasic//Triquilar

		Days ---->		
		1.6	7-11	12-21 day
Contain	EE	30 µg	40 µg	30 µg
	+			
	LNG	50 µg	70 µg	125 µg

Benefits of OCPs

20. Ans. is b and c. Reduces risk of benign breast diseases and Protects against endometrial cancer.

As discussed in chapter 10:

OCP's reduce risk benign breast disease and protect against endometrial cancer

- The estrogen component of pill increases clotting factors & hence OCP's are contraindicated in patient with history of thrombosis
- OCPs may have a role in decreasing osteoporosis by increasing bone mass.

Also Know:

Non contraceptive Benefits of OCPs

Table 10.7 Novak pa 236

Established benefits Menses related	Emerging benefits
• **Increased cycle regularly**	Increased bone mass
– Decreased blood loss	Reduced acne
– Decreased iron deficiency anemia	Reduced colorectal cancer
– Decreased dysmenorrhea	Reduced uterine leiomyomas
– Reduced symptom of premenstrual dysphoric disorder	Reduced rheumatoid arthritis
• Inhibition of ovulation	Treatment of bleeding disorder
– Few ovarian cysts	Treatment of Hyperandrogenic anovulation
– Few ectopic pregnancy	Treatment of endometriosis
Others	Treatment of perimenopausal changes
• Reduced fibroadenomas/fibrocystic breast changes	
• Reduced PID	
• Reduced Endometrial cancer	
• Reduced ovarian cancer	

21. Ans. is b, i.e. Hepatic adenoma *Ref: Shaw 15th/ed, p231-232; Dutta Obs 6th/ed, p545; Harrison 17th/ed, p563*

Friends, it is absolutely essential to mug up the benefits, side effects and contraindications of OCPs. Many questions are framed from these topics.

Here, I am repeating the list of Non-contraceptive benefits of OCPs:

Cancers/cysts

- Uterine cancer
- Ovarian cancers[Q]
- Fibroid uterus (Progesterone only pills)
- Ovarian cysts[Q]
- Benign breast diseases[Q]

Benign disease of genital tract

- Endometriosis (if used continuously)
- PID (here Salpingitis)[Q]
- Ectopic pregnancy (as it decreases incidence of PID)

They decrease ovulation thus, are helpful in

- Dysmenorrhea, premenstrual tension and Mittleschemerz syndrome.
- By decreasing blood loss they are helpful in menorrhagia and polymenorrhea.
- Acne and hirsutism (especially those containing desogesterel)

OCPs are also beneficial in: *Ref: Leon Speroff 7th/ed, p914*

- DUB
- Hormone therapy for hypothalamic amenorrhea
- Prevention of menstrual porphyria.

22. Ans. is d, i.e. Carcinoma cervix *Ref: Dutta Obs 6th/ed, p545; Shaw 14th/ed, p208; Harrison 17th/ed, p563*

23. Ans. is c, i.e. Hepatic adenoma

24. Ans. is a and b, i.e. Endometrial and Ovary

Friends, in the previous question I have given a list of conditions in which OCP's are beneficial. Here I would like to mention in brief.

OCPs	
Tumors associated	**Provides protection**
• Cervical cancer • Hepatic cancer • Pituitary adenoma • Breast cancer +/–	• Ovarian tumors/cysts • Uterine tumor • Benign breast disease

OCP's are protective against benign breast diseases, but as far as carcinoma breast is concerned their role is controversial. OCP's are considered in the etiology of Ca breast.

"The most credible metanalysis of oral contraceptive use suggest that these agents cause little if any increased risk of breast cancer. By contrast, oral contraceptives offer a substantial protective effect against ovarian epithelial tumors and endometrial cancer." – Harrison

25. Ans. is b and d, i.e. Breakthrough bleeding and Migraine *Ref: Novaks 15th/ed, p236*

Ref: Table (Novak's Gynae 15th/236): Established and Emerging Non-contraceptive Benefits of Oral Contraceptives

Side Effects of OCPs

26. Ans. is a, i.e. Dysmenorrhea *Ref: KDT 6th/ed, p315; Jeffcoate 7th/ed, p804*

27. Ans. is a and c, i.e. Liver disorders and Weight gain

28. Ans. is b and d, i.e. Increased risk of fibroadenosis and Increased risk of fibroadenoma

Ref: Dutta Obs 6th/ed, p545; Shaw 14th/ed, p208

OCP's have antiovulatory effect and by virtue of this property, relieve dysmenorrhea (rather than causing it), premenstrual tension and Mittleschmerz syndrome.

Side effects of OCPs are:

Nonserious side effects	Side effects which appear later	Serious side effects
• **Nausea,** vomiting • Headache (Migrane may be precipitated) • Break through bleeding[Q]/spotting[Q]/ amenorrhea • Breast discomfort/**Mastalgia**[Q]	• **Weight gain** • **Chloasma** • Pruritis vulva • Carbohydrate intolerance • Mood swing • Abdominal distension[Q] • Monilial Vaginitis[Q] • Corneal edema and irritation	• Leg vein/Pulmonary Thrombosis[Q] • Coronary Artery/[Q] • Cerebral Artery Thrombosis[Q] • Hypertension • Increased MI and stroke[Q] • Cholestatic Jaundice[Q] and Gall bladder stone[Q]

Cancers related to OCP use:

- Carcinoma cervix[Q]
- Hepatic adenoma[Q]
- Pituitary adenoma (+/–)[Q]
- Breast cancer (+/–)[Q]

Note:

- OCPs are protective against STDs
- OCPs are protective against PID

"The risk of hospitalization for PID is reduced by approximately 50–60% but atleast 12 months of use are necessary and the protection is limited to current use." *Ref: Leon Speroff 7th/ed, p905*

- At present time, no known association exist between oral contraception and viral sexually transmitted infections.

29. Ans. is b, i.e. Chlamydial endocervicitis *Ref: Novak 14th/ed, p275; CGDT 9th/ed, p727; Leon Speroff 7th/ed, p904-905*

This is a **tricky question** as some believe ***Option "b"*** i.e. chlamydial endocervicitis should be the answer while others believe Option "c" i.e. vaginal warts should be concerned. As far as candidial (monilial) vaginitis is concerned, OCP's use increase their incidence.

But for Chlamydial infections: *CGDT 9th/ed, p727 says:*

"Persons who use barrier contraception are less frequently infected by C. trachomatis than those who use no contraception, and women who use oral contraceptives may have a higher incidence of cervical infection than women not using oral contraceptives".

As if replying to CGDT *Novak 13th/ed, p259; 14th/ed, p275* says:

"Chlamydial colonization of the cervix appears more likely in OC users than in non users, but despite this, there is a 40–50% reduction in risk for Chlamydial PID"

I then had to confirm the answer from *Clinical gynaecologic endocrinology and Infertility 7th/ed by Leon Speroff* (It is the most authentic and reliable book for all problems related to Endocrinology, Contraception and Infertility)

"Fifteen of the Seventeen published studies reported a positive association of oral contraception with lower Genital tract infections caused by Chlamydial cervicitis. Because lower genital tract infection are on the rise (now the most prevalent STI in the US) and the rate of hospitalization for PID is also increased, it is worthwhile for both patients and clinicians to be alert for symptoms of cervicitis or salpingitis in women on oral contraceptives who are at high risk of sexually transmitted infections." *Ref: Leon Speroff 7th/ed, p905*

As far as HPV infection i.e. Vaginal warts is concerned

'The viral sexually transmitted infections (STI's) include HIV, human papilloma virus (HPV), herpes simplex virus (HSV) and hepatitis B (HBV). At the present time, no known associations exist between oral contraception and the viral STI'S'

Ref: Leon Speroff 7th/ed, p904

So, now we can be sure that the answer is Chlamydial endocervicitis.

Also Know

Infections and Oral contraception:

Use of OCP is associated with		
Increased risk of infection	Decreased risk of infection	No association with
• Candida (Moniliasis) • Chlamydia • Urinary tract infections	• Gonorrhea[Q] • Trichomonas[Q] • Bacterial vaginosis	• Viral STI's i.e. HIV[Q], HPV[Q] • Hepatitis B virus • Herpes simplex virus

Note:

- If question says PID and does not specify any organism—Then OCP'S overall not only decrease the incidence of PID but also risk of hospitalisation and severity of the disease is decreased.
- For protection against PID, at least 12 months of continuous use is necessary and this protection is limited only to current users.

Contraindications of OCPs

30. **Ans. is d, i.e. Impaired liver function** *Ref: Leon Speroff 7th/ed, p906*
31. **Ans. is a, i.e. Breast cancer**
32. **Ans. is a, d and e, i.e. Heart disease; Liver failure and Epilepsy**
33. **Ans. is a, b, c, and d, i.e. Age >40 years with smoking; H/O Epilepsy; Cancer breast and genitalia Thrombophlebitis Hyperlipidemia** *Ref: William Gynae 3rd/ed, p125*
    See the text for explanation. Only remember: Severe hyperlipidemia is an absolute C/I for OCP. Not just hyperlipidemia
34. **Ans. is a, b and d i.e. Severe hypertension, Ischemic heart disease, and Active liver disease** *Ref: Dutta Obs 8th/623; Shaw's Gynae 16th/273-75; Harrison 19th/2391; Katzung 10th/668- 670*
    See chapter text for explanation
35. **Ans. is c, i.e. Polycystic ovarian disease**
    Contraindications of OCPs:
    Absolute contraindications include:

Mnemonic

- Banks — Known or suspected Breast cancer
- Have — Severe Hypertriglyceridemia/Hypercholesteremia
- Various — (Undiagnosed Abnormal) Vaginal bleeding
- Schemes — Smokers over the age of 35 years
- To — Thrombophelebitis/Thromboembolic disorders, (present H/O, past H/O, family H/O) Cerebral and Cardiac disease
- Provide — Pregnancy
- Home — Hypertension (Moderate to severe)
- Loans — Markedly Impaired Liver function/infective hepatitis
- During — Diabetes mellitus with vascular disease
- May — Migraine disease with aura

For relative contraindications of OCP's: see the preceeding text

Epilepsy is a relative CI for the use of OCP's

36. **Ans. is a, i.e. Acute intermittent porphyria** *Ref: Harrison 17th/ed, p2439*
    Patient taking OCP's and presenting with abdominal pain and psychiatric problem, diagnosis is undoubtedly acute intermittent porphyria as OCP's can precipitate porphyria.

Some drugs which precipitate porphyria are:

- Barbiturates
- Sulfonamide antibiotics
- Meprobamate
- Phenytoin
- Valproic acid
- Griseofulvin
- Synthetic estrogen/progestogen (OCP)
- Alcohol
- Glutethimide
- Carbamazepine
- Pyrazolines
- Ergots
- Danazol
- Succinimide

Drug Interaction

37. Ans. is d, i.e. Rifampicin

38. Ans. is a and b, i.e. Rifampicin and Carbamazepine

39. Ans. is a, i.e. Rifampicin *Ref: KDT 6th/ed, p317; Novak 14th/ed, p276*

Interactions of OCP's with other Drugs.

Effect of other drugs on OCP's:

Drugs reducing the effectiveness of OCP		Drugs which increase the plasma level of steroids of OCP
• Rifampicin[Q] • Carbamazepine[Q] • Phenytoin • Antifungals like – Griseofulvin – Ketoconazole – Itraconazole	Induce synthesis of cytochrome P450 enzymes in liver.	• Ascorbic acid • Acetaminophen
• Ampicillin • Tetracycline	Kill gut bacteria and cause hydrolysis of steroid glucuronides in intestine.	

40. Ans. is a, i.e. Gossypol *Ref: Dutta obs 7th/ed, p561*

Gossypol

- It is a male contraceptive pill which contains–Disequilterpene aldehyde
- Discovered in China from an extract of cotton seed.
- Mechanism of action It inhibits spermatogenesis and decreases epididymal sperm motility
- Side effect: Hypokalemic paralysis in 1% patients

Other male hormonal contraceptives:

Testosterone enanthate injectable

Testosterone bucolate injectable

41. Ans. is b, d and e, i.e. Pregnancy resumes soon after discontinuation of pill, HIV antiviral drug reduce effectiveness of COC, Pregnancy rate equal to non hormonal contraception after discontinuation. *Ref: Leon Speroff, 8th/ed, p996-100*

- Many women can be prescribed hormonal contraception without clinical breast and pelvic examination (Thus, option 'a' is incorrect)

> Leon Speroff 8/e, page 1015 says—pelvic examination is not mandatory before prescribing CoCs in all women. Patients requiring further evaluation can be identified with careful medical history and measurement of BP. Subsequently, in view of the increased safety profile of low dose OCPs, for young healthy women with no risk factors, patients should be seen only after every 12 months for measurement of BP, urinalysis, breast examination, palpitation of liver and pelvic examination with pap smear.
>
> Women with risk factors should be seen every 6 months by trained personel. In females also, breast and pelvic examination is done yearly. Blood lipid profile and glucose levels should be checked only:
>
> i. Once in young women
> ii. Women > 35 years
> iii. Women with family H/O heart disease, diabetes, hypertension
> iv. Women with xanthesis
> v. Obese women
> vi. Diabetic women

- OCPs protect from endometrial and ovarian cancers but not cervical cancer (Therefore option 'c' is incorrect)
- HIV drugs reduce the effectiveness of OCPs i.e. option 'd' is incorrect.
- Reproduction after discontinuation of OCPs

> **According to Leon Speroff 8/e**
>
> It is unlikely that women discontinuing low-dose steroid contraception experience any significant delay in achieving pregnancy compared with the experience in general population.
>
> This is in contrast to the earlier findings that ovulation returns 3 months after stopping OCPs and to the finding that OCP users took 24 months, IUC users 14 months and diaphragm users 10 months to become pregnant.

Progesterone only Pills/Implants/Injections

42. Ans. is c, i.e. Altering cervix mucus *Ref: FOGSI Focus-Jan '06 issue-The Modern Pill, Chapter Estrogen Free Pills, p41; Current Concepts in Contraception and Women Health p49*

Major action of all POP's is alteration in cervical mucus and making it thick. The Newer POP's containing desogestrel also act by inhibiting ovulation.

43. Ans. is a, i.e. Irregular vaginal bleeding may be a side effect *Ref: Leon Speroff 7th/ed, p922*

I have already discussed minipil/progesterone only pill/lactation pill/Estrogen free pill in detail earlier and hence you know minipill can be used during lactation (i.e. ***option "c"*** is correct).

It is not used in combination with other pills therefore ***option "b"*** is incorrect.

Minipill

"Ectopic pregnancy is not prevented as effectively as intrauterine pregnancy. Although the overall incidence of ectopic pregnancy is not increased, When pregnancy occurs (with minipill use) the clinician must suspect that it is more likely to be ectopic. A previous ectopic pregnancy should not be regarded as a contraindication to the minipill." *Ref: Leon Speroff 7th/ed, p922*

So ***option "d"*** is incorrect

Main side effect of Minipill/progesterone only pill: Irregular bleeding and amenorrhea (i.e. ***option "a"*** is correct).

Pearl index-3%

44. Ans. is. a, b and c, i.e. Weight gain occurs, Cause irregular bleeding and It can be given to lactating mothers *Ref: JB Sharma Obs p694-695*

As discussed in the chapter, Minipills or Progesterone Only Pills are most effective means of contraception in lactating females.

- They should be taken everyday at the same time (hence, they are not good for unorganised females)
- Ectopic pregnancy is not prevented as effectively as intrauterine pregnancy. Although overall incidence of ectopic pregnancy is not increased
- Main side effect—breakthrough bleeding
- Other minor side effects—weight gain, acne and formation of follicular cysts in ovary
- Immediate return to fertility in lactating women with recent gestational diabetes
- Good choice for females in whom estrogen is C/I like smokers more than 35 years of age
- Can be used in females with previous episodes of vascular thrombosis
- It protects from endometrial and ovarian cancer

45. Ans. is Contraindicated in suspected pregnancy; Contraindicated in breast cancer; Useful in controlling menorrhagia in fibroid

Levonorgestrel-releasing Intrauterine System

Three levonorgestrel-releasing intrauterine contraceptive are which Food and Drug Administration (FDA)-approved in the United States Named Mirena, Skyla, and Liletta. These devices are T-shaped polyethylene structures with the stem encased by a cylinder containing polydimethylsiloxane and levonorgestrel. The cylinder has a permeable membrane that regulates continuous daily hormone release. The Mirena is currently approved for 5 years following insertion, but evidence supports use for 7 years (Thonneau, 2008). Liletta and Skyla are currently approved for 3 years. In addition to having a lower dose of progestin, Skyla is also marginally smaller in size. Mirena and Liletta have a length of 32 mm and width of 32 mm, but with Skyla, these same dimensions measure 28 mm.

There are several progestin-mediated mechanisms by which LNG-IUS may prevent pregnancy. The progestin renders the endometrium atrophic; it stimulates thick cervical mucus that blocks sperm penetration into the uterine cavity; and it may ectopic pregnancy may be at increased risk for another because of diminished tubal motility from progestin action. In women with uterine leiomyomas, placement of the LNG-IUS may be problematic if the uterine cavity is distored. In their metaanalysis, Zapata and associates (2010) reported the expulsion rate to be approximately 10 percent in women with coexistent liomyomas. However, in affected women women who retained the device, menstrual blood loss will be lessened in most.

Mirena, Liletta, and Skyla—Contraindication

Pregnancy or suspicion of pregnancy, Uterine abnormality with distorted uterine cavity
Use for postcoital contraception
Acute PID or history, of, unless there has been a subsequent intrauterine pregnancy.
Postpartum endometritis of infected abortion in the past 3 months.
Known or suspected uterine or cervical neoplasia
Uterine bleeding of unknown etiology
Untreated acute cervicitis or vaginitis or other lower genital tract infections
Acute liver disease or liver tumor (benign or malignant)
Increased susceptibility to pelvic infection
A previously placed IUD that has not been removed
Hypersensitivity to any component of the device
Known or suspected breast cancer or other progestinsensitive cancer

46. Ans. is b, c and d i.e. Higher failure rate than COC, Fertility return to normal after discontinuation without any delay and Suited for lactating women

See Text for explanation

47. **Ans. is c, i.e. Premenstrual symptoms**

48. **Ans. is a, b, c, d and e, i.e. Endometriosis, Fibroid uterus, PID, Contraception, and endometrial hyperplasia**

Ref: Shaw 15th/ed, p228

Mirena is a progesterone IUCD. It contains 52 mg levonorgesterel, eluting 20 μg daily.

Life span- 5 years

Failure rate = 0.2%

The biggest contraceptive advantage of progesterone IUCD's is–It can be given to nursing mothers.

For details see the text.

49. **Ans. is d, i.e. Emergency contraception**

LNG IUCD's cannot be used as emergency contraception

50. **Ans. is b, i.e. Can be used as emergency contraception**

51. **Ans. is a and d, i.e. Progesterone containing IUCD and Decreases menstrual blood now**

52. **Ans. is a, i.e. there is increased incidence of menorrhagia**

53. **Ans. is b, d and e, i.e. LNG containing IUCD, Suppression of endometrium and No significant effect on ovaries**

See the text for explanation

54. **Ans. is b, i.e. Decreased ovulation**

Ref: The Contraception Report' March 02, Vol. 13 No. 1

Several mechanisms account for a potential reduced risk of upper-genital-tract infection in users of progestin releasing IUDs.

- First, the local effect of progestin on cervical mucus make it thick and relatively impenetrable to bacteria.
- Since uterine bleeding is eventually greatly decreased in users of the LNG-IUD (progestin releasing IUD), any retrograde menstruation (which might seed the fallopian tubes with bacteria) should be reduced as well.
- In addition, decidual changes in the endometrium may make it less susceptible to infection.

In other words, progestin-releasing IUDs may mimic the protective effect of combined oral contraceptives and depot medroxyprogesterone acetate against upper-genital-tract infection.

Also Know

- PID is common in non hormonal IUCD.
- IUCD related bacterial infections are due to contamination of endometrial cavity at the time of insertion.
- Actinomycosis infection is related to IUCD use.
- Most common side effect of IUCD's is increased vaginal bleeding.
- Contraception of choice in patients with current recent or recurrent PID is hormonal or barrier method:

55. **Ans. is a, i.e. 0.5**

Ref: Leon Speroff 7th/ed, p981

LNG - IUD has a pregnancy rate of 0.2 100 women years (HWY) *(here nearest is 0.5 so that is the answer)*.

56. **Ans. is a, b, c and e, i.e. Failure @ 0.3/100 WY; 150 mg/3 monthly delivered; Weight gain and; Anemia improves**

57. **Ans. is b, i.e. Does not have protective effect on Ca endometrium**

58. **Ans. is d, i.e. Hepatitis**

59. **Ans. is b, i.e 3 monthly** *Ref: Jeffcoate 7th/ed, p812; Dutta Obs 6th/ed, p548; Park 20th/ed, p433-434; Leon Speroff 7th/ed, p962-963*

DMPA i.e. depot medroxyprogesterone acetate (depot provera) and Net en are progesterone only injectable contraceptives

DMPA is discussed in detail in preceeding text:

60. **Ans. is a, i.e. Irregular bleeding**

Ref: Dutta Obs 6th/ed, p548

Norethisterone acetate is commonly used as an injectable steroid - **'NET-EN'**

It is a progesterone based contraceptive like DMPA and its side effect are similar to those of DMPA.

The most frequent side effect is irregular bleeding.

NET-EN is given in doses of 200 mg at 2 monthly interval.

Extra Edge: Combined injectable contraceptive.

	Composition	Features
• Lunelle/cyclofem	25 mg DMPA + 5 mg estradiol cypionate	Monthly injection
• Mesigyna	50 mg NET-EN + 5 mg estradiol valerate	Monthly injection

61. **Ans. is c i.e. Life span is 3 years**

Ref: JB Sharma Obs, p696-697

- Implanon is a long-acting single rod subdermal implant
- Rod measures 4 cm in length
- It contains 68 mg of etonogestrel dispersed in ethylene vinyl acetate polymer
- Initial release rate is 60–70 mg/day and declines to 25–30 mcg at the end of third year
- Recommended use 3 years
- In UK, Nexplanon has now replaced implanon.

62. **Ans. is b, i.e. Metrorrhagia** *Ref: Novak 14th/ed, p283*
In progesterone only contraceptives whether injections/IUCDs/implants, the most common problem is–irregular vaginal bleeding, i.e. metrorrhagia.

63. **Ans. is d, i.e. Ectopic pregnancy** *Ref: William Gynae 3rd/ed, p127*
Irregular bleeding is a side effect of POPs. They carry an increased risk of ectopic pregnancy (if failure of method occurs)
Other drawbacks:
- Increased rate of failure as compared to OCPs
- Increased chances of developing functional ovarian cyst.

IUCDs

64. **Ans. is c, i.e. Has history of ectopic pregnancy** *Ref: Parks 20th/ed, p427*
The planned parenthood federation of America (PPFA) has described Ideal IUCD candidate as a woman.
- Who has no history of pelvic disease.
- Who has born at least one child
- Has normal menstrual periods
- Is willing to check IUCD tail
- Has access to follow up and treatment of potential problems
- Is in a monogamous relationship.

Extra Edge

Some important points from 'Leon Speroff' on patient selection for IUD.
- Age and parity are not critical factors in selection, the risk factors for STI's (sexually transmitted infection) are the most important considerations
- Patients with heavy menstrual periods should be cautioned regarding the increase in menstrual bleeding associated with copper IUD. Women who are anticoagulated or have bleeding disorder are obviously not good candidates for copper IUCD, but might benefit from progestin IUCD.
  - Women who have abnormalities of uterus like bicornuate uterus are not good candidates for IUD insertion.[Q]
  - Patients with Wilson's disease are not recommended, copper containing IUCD as contraceptive
  - Immunosuppressed individuals should not use IUCD.
- Patients at risk for endocarditis should be treated with prophylactic antibiotics at the insertion and removal of IUCD.
- According to Speroff: cervical dysplasias are not contraindication for use of IUCD'sQ but in patients with cervical stenosis it may be difficult to insert IUCD.
- No increase in adverse events has been observed with copper containing IUCD in women with either insulin dependent or non-insulin dependent diabetes. Infact Cu containing IUCD's can be the ideal choice for a woman with diabetes especially if vascular disease is present.

65. **Ans. is d, i.e. Inhibition of ovulation** *Ref: Shaw 15th/ed, p229; Leon Speroff 7th/ed, p980*

Remember
- Main action of OCPs = Inhibition of ovulation.
- Main action of IUCD = Prevent Implantation.

66. **Ans. is a, b, c, d and e Immediately after delivery, 1 week after delivery, Post puerperal period, Before menstruation and Anytime during lactation period.** *Ref: JB Sharma Obs- 680, Leon Speroff 8/e, p1113*

Timing of insertion:
1. Interval insertion- Insertion-6 weeks after parturition or MTP or abortion
2. Insertion immediately after delivery or 1st trimester(Abortion, spontaneous or induced)
3. Insertion at the time of caesarean section
4. Insertion immediately after menstruation (as cervix is more open-although insertion can be done at anytime of menstrual cycle after being sure patient is not pregnant)
5. After 2nd trimester abortion-Insertion should be done after uterine involution
6. Post cortal insertion-As an emergency contraceptive *Ref: JB Sharma, Obs, p680*

Insertion during lactation period- IUD can be safely inserted during lactational period after ruling our pregnancy, IUD does not affect lactation in any way. It is preferable to use smaller device during this period.
Immediate post partum insertion- IUD is inserted following delivery of the placenta both after normal delivery and caesarean section. Govt. of India is recommending it now. Large and long sponge holding forceps (Keely's forceps) have been devised to place the IUD near fundus. Expulsion rate is slightly high.

67. Ans. is d, i.e. Progestasert *Ref: Shaw 15th/ed, p227*

68. Ans. is a, i.e. CuT380A *Ref: Shaw 15th/ed, p227; Novak 14th/ed, p263*

Most of the IUCDs have an average life span of 3 years.

Exceptions are:

- Nova T/Multiload 375/Levonova – 5 years
- CuT 380 A (also known as Paragard) – 10 years – Distributed free of cost
- Progestasert – 1 years
- CuT200 B – 4 years, in US and 3 years in India and in European countries.
- Levonorgestrel containing IUCD can be used for: (Mirona) – 7–10 years, but is approved for 5 years

69. Ans. is a, i.e. Copper and silver *Ref: Shaw 15th/ed, p227*

Nova-T is nothing but Cu-T, where silver is added to the copper wire thereby increasing lifespan of Cu-T from 3 years to 5 years in Nova-T.

70. Ans. is b, i.e. Remove the IUCD

71. Ans. is c, i.e. Remove the IUD to decrease the risk of infection

Ref: Dutta Obs 6th/ed, p540; Novak 14th/ed, p263; Pretest Obs and Gynae Q. No. 426, SK Chaudhary 7th/ed, p110-111

A woman with an IUCD in place, with amenorrhea should have a pregnancy test and pelvic examination.

An intrauterine pregnancy can occur and continue successfully to term with an IUCD in place.

A. If an intrauterine pregnancy is diagnosed and IUCD strings are visible:

- IUCD should be removed as soon as possible in order to prevent septic abortion, premature rupture of membranes, and premature birth. Also do an USG to know whether it is intrauterine or ectopic pregnancy

B. If an intrauterine pregnancy is diagnosed and IUCD strings are not visible:

- An ultrasound examination should be performed to localize the IUCD and determine whether expulsion has occurred.
- If the IUCD is present there are 3 options for management.
  1. Therapeutic abortion
  2. If IUCD is not fundal in location: ultrasound guided intrauterine removal of IUCD.
  3. If IUCD is present in fundus of uterus: it should be left in place and pregnancy continued with the device left in place.

- If pregnancy continues with the device in place, the patient should be warned of the symptoms of intrauterine infection like fever or flue like symptoms, abdominal cramping or bleeding.
- At the earliest sign of infection, high dose intravenous antibiotic therapy should be given and the pregnancy evacuated promptly.

Note: Fetal malformations have not been reported to be increased with a device in place. *Ref: William Gynae 1st/ed, p120*

72. Ans. is d, i.e. Laparoscopy *Ref: SK Chaudhary 7th/ed, p114*

Copper can cause inflammatory reaction and can cause intestinal obstruction. Therefore, never wait and watch.

When Cu T is embedded within uterine cavity, hysteroscopic removal is the method of choice. It is preferred over IUCD hook. Hysteroscopy cannot visualize the Cu T that is in the abdominal cavity.

So when IUCD enters the abdominal cavity (partly or completely), laparoscopy is the preferred modality for retrieval.

Sometimes due to dense adhesions around the Cu T, a laparotomy may be required to remove it.

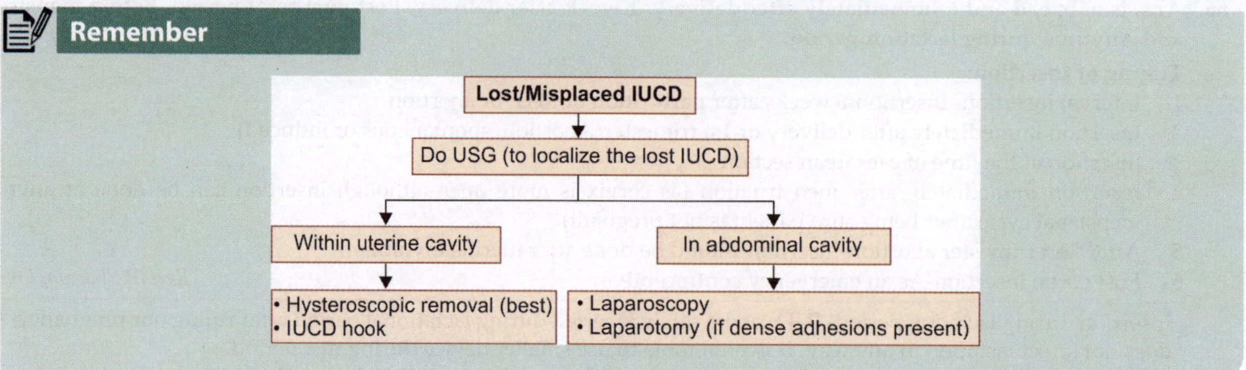

73. Ans. is c, i.e. Congenital malformation of uterus *Ref: Shaw 15th/ed, p228*

74. Ans. is d, i.e. Undiagnosed vaginal bleeding

75. **Ans. is d, i.e. Pelvic tuberculosis** *Ref: Shaw 15th/ed, p228*

76. **Ans. is a and b, i.e. Undiagnosed vaginal bleeding and PID** *Ref: Park 20th/ed, p427; Shaw 15th/ed, p228; Novak 15th/ed, p224*
See the text for explanation

77. **Ans. is b, d and e i.e Present cervicitis and vaginitis, Unknown cause of vaginal bleeding, and Severe dysmenorrhea**
Ref: Dutta Obs 8th/616; J B Sharma 1st/682; William's Obs 23rd/; Novak's Gyae 15th/224
"**Relative contraindication:** Purulent cervical discharge" *Ref: Park 24th/531*
WHO Category 4 for IUCD: Do not use (Absolute contraindications of IUDs in Gynecologic/Obstetric conditions)
Ref: J B Sharma 1st/682

- PID, current or within past 3 months
- Current STD or STD within past 3 months
- Known pelvic tuberculosis
- Unexplained or suspicious vaginal bleeding
- Malignant gestational trophoblastic disease
- Cervical and endometrial cancer
- Uterine/cervical abnormality incompatible with IUD insertion
- Uterine fibroids with distortion of uterine cavity.
- Puerperal or postabortal sepsis
- Suspected pregnancy

Contraindications for Insertion of IUCD *Ref: Dutta Obs 8th/616*
- Presence of pelvic infection, current or within 3 months
- Undiagnosed genital tract bleeding
- Suspected pregnancy
- Distortion of the shape of the uterine cavity as in fibroid or congenital uterine malformation;
- Severe dysmenorrhea
- Past history of ectopic pregnancy
- Within 6 weeks following cesarean section
- STIs—Current or recurrent
- Trophoblastic disease
- Significant immunosuppression.

Additionally for CuT are:
- Wilson disease and
- Copper allergy.
- For LNG-IUS are:
- Hepatic tumor or hepatocellular disease (active);
- Current breast cancer and (15) Severe arterial disease.

78. **Ans. is b, c and e, i.e. PID; Uterine malformation; and Previous cesarean section**

79. **Ans. is b, and c, i.e. PID; Uterine malformation** *Ref: Park 18th/ed, p364; Shaw 15th/ed, p228; Jeffcoate 7th/ed, p798-799*
Some books mention diabetes as a contraindication for IUCD but according to Leon Speroff Cu containing IUCDs can be the ideal choice for women with diabetes especially if there is associated vascular disease.
"No increase in adverse events has been observed with copper IUD use in women with either insulin dependent or non insulin dependent diabetes. Indeed, the IUCD can be an ideal choice for a woman with diabetes, especially if vascular disease is present."
Ref: Leon Speroff 7th/ed, p988

"IUCDs-They are the contraceptive method of choice in woman with either type I or type II diabetes."
– Current Concept in Contraception and Women Health, p95

Earlier it was believed IUCD's are contraindicated in patients of HIV but now it is not so - rather IUCD's are the method of choice in HIV infected women.
HIV and AIDS: *"IUD's are the method of choice in these women owing to their high efficacy, minimal maintenance and no drug interaction."* *– Current Concept in Contraception and Women Health, p97*
Leon Speroff 7th/ed, p985 also supports the use of IUCD's in HIV infected females.

80. **Ans. is b, i.e. Bleeding** *Ref: Park 20th/ed, p428*
Complication of IUCD
- M/C complication–Bleeding
- IInd M/C complication–Pain
- Infection–Doxycycline 200 mg/azithromycin 500 mg should be given 1 hour before insertion to reduce infection.
- Most typical infection associated with Cu T use is actinomyces.
- Ectopic pregnancy-It is seen that ectopic pregnancy is 50% less likely in women using IUCD than in women using no contraception.

81. Ans. is a, i.e. CuT380A *(see text for explanation)*

82. Ans. is d, i.e. Levonorgestrel IUCD *(see text for explanation)*

Emergency Contraception

83. Ans. is d, i.e. Interrupting an early pregnancy *Ref: Leon Speroff 7th/ed, p925-926*

Emergency Contraceptives are also called as **INTERCEPTIVES.**

It refers to a type of contraception that is used as an emergency to prevent pregnancy after an unprotected intercourse.

Mechanism of action

The mechanism of action is not known with certainty, but it is believed with justification that this treatment combines delay of ovulation (***Option 'a'***) with a local effect on endometrium (***Option "c"***) and prevention of fertilization (***Option "b"***).

As far as ***option 'd'*** is concerned

"How much a post fertilization effect (option d) contributes to efficacy is not known, but it is not believed to be the primary mechanism." *Ref: Leon Speroff 7th/ed, p925-926*

"Contrary to popular belief, it is not an abortifacient i.e. will not act after implantation has occurred." *—Current Concepts in Contraception and Womens Health p108*

Mechanism of action of emergency contraception versus medical method of MTP.

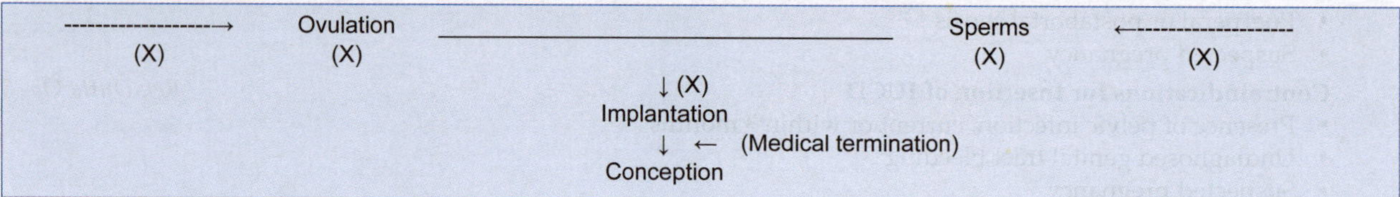

(X) steps inhibited by emergency contraception.

84. Ans. is c and d, i.e. Contraception failure; and Unprotected sex *Ref: Dutta Obs 6th/ed, p549; Leon Speroff 7th/ed, p925*

Sorry, friends I am not able to get you the exact answer. According to me both are correct.

Indications for emergency contraception *Ref: Dutta Obs 6th/ed, p549*

- Unprotected intercourse
- Condom rupture (Contraception failure)
- Missed pill (Contraception failure)
- Sexual assault/teenage assault
- Rape

Ref: Leon Speroff 7th/ed, p925

Emergency contraception

"It is an important option for patients and should be considered when condom break, sexual assault occurs, if diaphragms or cervical caps dislodge or with the lapsed use of any method."

85. Ans. is c and e, i.e. Danazol and misoprostol.

86. Ans. is a, i.e. Desogestrel

87. Ans. is c and e, i.e. Desogestrel and medroxyprogesterone acetate.

88. Ans. is c, i.e. Levonorgestrel. *Ref: Leon Speroff 7th/ed, p927; Novak 14th/ed, p283-285*

Drugs used for Emergency contraception:

1. OCP's (Morning after pill)
2. Levonorgestrel alone-Mostly used drug/progesterone for Emergency contraception
3. Copper Intrauterine device
4. Mifepristone/RU-486
5. Centchroman
6. Ulipristal

Note: LNG-IUCD cannot be used for emergency contraception

As far as Danazol is concerned, it was earlier used as an emergency contraceptive but not nowadays.

"The use of danazol for emergency contraception is not effective". *Ref: Leon Speroff 7th/ed, p927*

Also Know

- Emergency contraception should be initiated as soon as possible after exposure and the standard recommendation is that it should not be initiated later than 72 hours.
- Greatest protection occurs, if it is started within 12 hours of exposure.
- Emergency contraception will be ineffective in the presence of an established pregnancy.

89. Ans. is b, i.e. Copper IUD *Ref: Williams Obstetrics 24/ed, p714; JB Sharma Obs, p698*

Since the couple presented five days after unprotected sex and the family is complete, intrauterine devices are best for emergency contraception. Only copper containing IUD's can be used and not LNG-containing (like Mirena)
LNG tablet, can be given up till 120 hours. But its efficacy will be much less.

90. Ans. is d, i.e. 120 hours *Ref: Shaw 15th/ed, p237; Current Concepts in Contraception and Women Death, p105, Leon Speroff 8th/ed, p1042*

The standard recommendation is to start emergency contraceptive not later than 72 hours. The greatest protection is offered, if it is taken within 12 hours, as postponing the dose by 12 hours raises the chances of pregnancy by almost 50%. For this reason, the treatment should be initiated as soon as possible after sexual exposure.
Note: But here the question says - till how long are ECs effective or till how long can they be administered.

Ref: Shaw 14th/ed, p213 says

"The tables can be offered upto 120 hours, but its efficacy decreases with the longer coital - drug interval."
"Treatment should be initiated as soon after exposure as possible, and the standard recommendation is that it be no later than 120 h." *Ref: Leon Speroff 8th/ed, p1042 According to current concepts in contraceptions and women health also*
Emergency contraception can be given upto 5 days.
This is because
"Emergency contraception is not an abortifacient i.e. it will not act after implantation has occurred. This is also the basis for the window period of 5 days for use effectiveness of EC, as the whole process from deposition of sperms to implantation takes about 5 days."

Ref: Current Concepts in Contraception and Women Health p108

91. Ans. is a, i.e. RU486
RU486 is Mifeprestone which is a progesterone antagonist used as Emergency Contraceptive

Permanent Method

92. Ans. is a, i.e. A woman having no child/may undergo sterilization *Ref: Shaws Gynecology 16th/ed, p281-82*

Female sterilization

- Tubal ligation can be done at any convenient time to the patient. Postpartum ligation is done within the first week of delivery when the patient is already hospitalized. Interval sterilization is done when the woman is not pregnant or any time after 6 weeks of delivery. It can be combined with caesarean section
- Indications
  - Multiparity
  - Need of permanent method
  - Obstetrics- Three caesarean deliveries
  - Medical diseases at high risk of pregnancy
  - Psychiatric problems
  - Breast cancer
  - Eugenic conditions- repeat fetal malformations such as hemophilia, Rh incompatibility, Wilson's disease, Tay Sachs disease & Marfan syndrome
- Contraindication
  - Young women less than 25 years (as dictated by GOI)
  - Parity less than one child (as per the government rule)
  - Local infection
  - Prolapse- tubectomy can be done at the time of repair surgery

Government guidelines for sterilization *Park 23/ed, p508-09*

- The age of the husband should not ordinarily be less than 225 years nor should it be over 50 years
- The age of the wife should not be less than 20 years or more than 45 years
- The motivated couple must have 2 living children at the time of operation
- If the couple has 2 or more living children, the lower limit of age of the husband r wife may be relaxed at the discretion of the operating surgeon
- It is sufficient if the acceptor declares having obtained the consent of his/her spouse to undergo sterilization operation without outside pressure, inducement or coercion & he/she knows that for all practical purposes, the operation is irreversible, & also that the spouse has not been sterilized earlier

93. Ans. is e, i.e. Medroxyprogesterone *Ref: Dutta Obs 6th/ed, p532*

Methods of contraception (can be classified as)

Temporary methods *(used to postpone or space births)*	Permanent methods *(Surgical methods arm is to purposefully and permanently destroy the Reproductive capacity of an individual)*
• **Barrier method**[Q] • **Natural contraception**[Q] • Oral contraceptive pills • Injectables • Implants • Intrauterine devices like Copper T, Levonorgestrel IUCD's	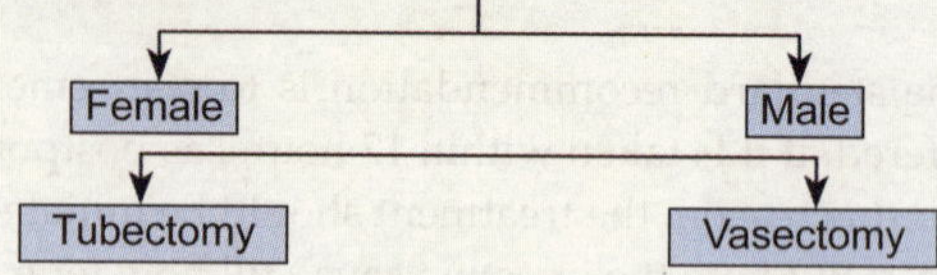

Electrocoagulation is using cauterization for the purpose of tubal ligation and clipping is done during laparoscopic tubal ligation, i.e. they are permanent methods.

Friends, here do not get confused by lines of *Shaws* which says some of these methods are reversible, it does not mean they are not permanent methods.

94. Ans. c, i.e. Essure *Ref: Williams 23/ed, p698-701*

Essure is a permanent intratubal implant inserted transcervically using hysteroscope, not an abdominal technique for tubal ligation.

95. Ans. is d, i.e. Hysteroscopic tubal occlusion *Ref: Shaw 15th/ed, p241*

Hysteroscopic tubal occlusion is done by 2 methods and both these methods have high failure rates.

Hysteroscopic tubal occlusion

Cauterization *(Failure rate 30%)*	**Sclerosants** *(Failure rate 15%)*
• Due to high failure rate these methods are obsolete now	

96. Ans. is d, i.e Laparoscopic tubal ligation with clips *Ref: Leon speroff 8th/ed, p935,929*

Most suitable for reversal is clips followed by ring, BUT most commonly used for laparoscopic tubal ligation is silastic ring followed by clips

Least suitable for reversal is monopolar cautery followed by bipolar cautery technique.

97. Ans. is c, i.e. Isthmus *Ref: Dutta Obs 6th/ed, p553*

98. Ans. is a, i.e. Isthmo-isthmic type

99. Ans. is a, i.e. Isthmo-isthmic anastomosis *Ref: Jeffcoate 7th/ed, p825; Novak 14th/ed, p294*

Read the following lines

"It is important to select the site of tubal ligation carefully which should ideally be done at the tubal isthmus. This is because in the event of the patient desiring a tubal recanalization procedure, the isthmo-isthmic anastomosis carries the best chances of success".

Ref: Jeffcoate 7th/ed, p825

100. Ans. is a and d, i.e. Withdrawal method and MTP pill.

In withdrawal method & MTP pill, patient need not be aware of safe period & day of ovulation. Rest all methods given in the option are based on fertility awareness

101. Ans. is d, i.e. Dyspareunia *Ref: Dutta obs 7th/ed, p 557*

Post ligation syndrome-

Some patients after tubal ligation can experience post-ligation syndrome characterized by menstrual irregularities like menorrhagia, or irregular periods along with pelvic pain or congestive dysmenorrhea and cystic ovaries.

It is vascular in origin and its incidence can be reduced if the blood vessels adjacent to the mesosalpix are not unduly disturbed.

102. Ans. is b, i.e. 0.1% *Ref: JB Sharma Obs 1st/ed, p672*

Read the text for explanation

103. Ans. is b, i.e. No sperms in ejaculate *Ref: Textbook of Gynae Sheila Balakrishnan 1st/ed, p373, Dutta Obs 7th/ed, p553*

Sterility does not occur immediately after vasectomy.

Sperms remain in the semen for 15–20 ejaculation, requiring continued contraception for about 3 months. So the couple is advised to use some form of contraception for the next 3 months or 15–20 ejaculates, but this can vary from person to person. So the best thing to do is to repeat the semen analysis and confirm that the male partner has become azoospermic. This is the reason why after vasectomy, 2 separate semen analysis should be done to confirm the absence of sperms in the ejaculate and then additional contraception discontinued.

Contraceptive of Choice

104. Ans. is b, i.e. Condom *Ref: Shaw 15th/ed, p231*

Barrier methods (especially condom) and OCP's both protect against PID, but the protection offered by OCP's is less than that by Barrier method.

"The incidence of pelvic inflammatory disease (PID) is reduced, though it does not reach the same low level as seen with the barrier methods." *Ref: Shaw 14th/ed, p208*

As far as diaphragm is concerned, it does not protect against HIV, whereas condom do. So I have chosen condom as the answer.

105. Ans. is b, i.e. Combined OCP

106. Ans. is a, i.e. Barrier method

107. Ans. is d, i.e. Progesterone only pill *Ref: Read below*

For newly married couples oral contraceptive pill is the method of choice provided there are no contraindications.
It has many noncontraceptive benefits along with effective contraception.
Barrier and Natural methods have high failure rate.
IUCD are not prescribed in nulliparous females due to increase risk of PID and infertility

In a couple who are living separately in two cities and meet only, occasionally contraception of choice is barrier method.

"Condom are suitable for use in old ager for couple who have infrequent coitus, during lactation, during holidays, subject who can not tolerate OCP, IUCD". *Ref: Practice of fertility control S.K. Chaudhuri 7th/ed, p71*

In Breastfeeding Females

For lactating mothers, contraceptive should be chosen in such a way that in addition to providing effective contraception, they do not adversely affect the success of lactation or the health of the infant. Barriers have a high failure rate of 4–14% and not reliable for long-term control.

As estrogens decrease the quality and quantity of milk, COC pills are absolutely contraindicated in lactating mothers.

Lactation Amenorrhea Method (LAM)

- Excessive secretion of prolactin, which controls lactation, inhibits the pituitary. Prolactin inhibits luteinizing hormone (LH) but has no effect on follicle-stimulating hormone (FSH). However, it partially inhibits ovarian response to both of these gonadotropins. As a result, while the prolactin level remains high, the ovary produces little estrogen and no progesterone. Hence, ovulation and menstruation are affected.
- LAM is effective only till 6 months postpartum. Beyond this, it is not a reliable method.
- Even for the 6 months, it is effective only if there is exclusive breastfeeding.
- It any time in the first 6 months the menses starts, then it cannot be used as birth control.
- POPs are safe with breastfeeding and very effective. They were mainly designed especially for lactating mothers.

108. Ans. is c, i.e. Vasectomy *Ref: Shaw 15th/ed, p238*

Vasectomy consists of dividing the vas deferens and disrupting the passage of sperms. It is done through a small incision in the scrotum under local anesthesia (LA). There is no need to open the peritoneum.

109. Ans. is a, i.e. OCPs *Ref: Leon speroff 8th/ed, p1026; text book of gynecology, Sheila Balakrishnan 1st/ed, p344,345*

In Epilepsy

"Consideration should be given to methods that neither affect antiepileptic drug metabolism nor the methods affected by drugs. These include intrauterine contraception with copper IUD, or levonorgestrel releasing IUD, long acting progestine only methods, barrier methods and sterilization." *Ref: Leon Speroff 8th/ed, p1026*

Epilepsy/seizure disorder is a relative contraindication for the use of OCP's as antiepileptic drugs like phenytoin, carbamazepine and phenobarbitone induce the synthesis of liver enzyme thereby reducing the plasma levels of ethinyl estradiol in women on combined pills, thereby increasing the chances of contraceptive failure.

So in epilepsy OCPs should be avoided.

110. Ans. is b i.e. Laparoscopic tubal ligation

- Laparoscopic tubal ligation is a surgical sterilization procedure in which a woman's fallopian tubes are either clamped and blocked or severed and sealed. Both methods prevent eggs from being fertilized. Tubal ligation is a permanent method of sterilization and not reversible for all practical purposes

111. Ans. is c i.e. Urgent visit to hospital and check for pregnancy *Ref: WHO guidelines; CDC guidelines, William Gynae 3/e, p122*

After ruling out pregnancy, next cycle of OCPs can be started

With any scenario of missed pills, if withdrawal bleeding does not occur during the placebo pills, the pills are continued but the woman should seek medical attention to exclude pregnancy. *William Gynae 3/e, p122*

112. Ans. is d, i.e. Implanon *Ref: DC Dutta's Textbook of Gynaecology, p509*

Since the patient has history of DVT and is on warfarin, hence we cannot give her—any contraceptive containing estrogen. Now in the option, none contains estrogen.

Amongst progesterone only containing contraceptives: POPs and progesterone injections are the only ones which can be given. As far as Implanon is concerned an absolute contraindication for its use is previous H/O DVT.

Note: As per Williams gynae 3rd/ed pg 127. Progesterone injections cannot be given to females with H/O thromboembolism. But the latest edition of Leon Speroff 9/e pg 930 says:

"DMPA can be considered for patients with congenital heart disease, sickle cell anemia, patients with previous H/O thromboembolism, women over 30 years who smoke or have other risk factors such as hypertension or diabetes mellitus."

113. Ans. is a, b, c and d, i.e. Intrauterine copper device, Levonorgestrel (LNG), Estrogen plus progesterone, and Mifepristone

"**Misoprostol** is used for medical termination of pregnancy **(MTP)**" *– Shaw's Gynae 17th/ed, p283*

It is not used as emergency contraceptive.

114. Ans. is a, b and d, i.e. Levonorgestrel, Copper T up to 5 days before after the unprotected intercourse, Progesterone and estrogen *Ref: Shaw's Gynae 16th/ed, p279-285; Dutta's gynae 6th/ed, p480-81, 500*

- As discussed in chapter on contraception, Levonorgestrel, cuIUCD and estrogen and progesterone are used as emergency contraception.
- Mirena (progesterone IUCD) and progesterone only pill (minipill) are not used as emergency contraceptives.

115. Ans. is c, i.e. Immobilization of sperms *Ref: Show's Gyne 15th/ed, p234; Dutta's Gyne 6th/ed, p471*

- High-dose progestogen-only contraceptives, such as DMPA, inhibit follicular development and prevent ovulation as their primary mechanism of action
- A secondary mechanism of action of all progestogen-containing contraceptives is inhibition of sperm penetration by changes in the cervical mucus. The cervical mucus remains thick and viscid.
- Inhibition of ovarian function during DMPA use causes the endometrium to become thin and atrophic.

Note: There is no medicinal contraceptive available which acts by immobilization of sperms.

CHAPTER 11

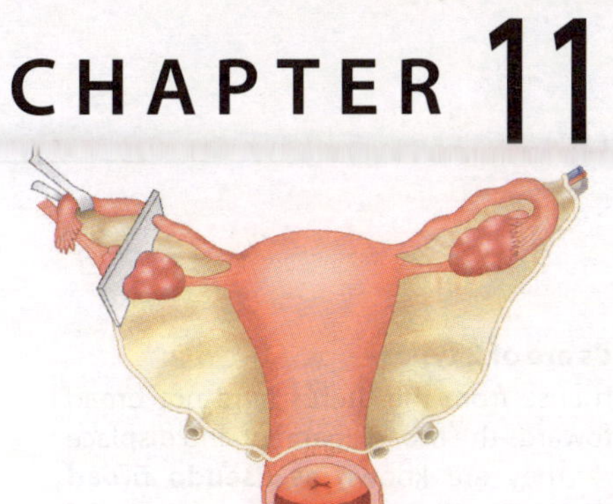

Uterine Fibroid

Fibroids

- Fibroids are the most common benign solid tumors in females.[Q]
- It is the most common pelvic tumor.[Q]
- **It is an estrogen and progesterone-dependant tumor**
- Most common age group affected is 35–45 years[Q]
- Fibroids are most commonly seen in nulliparous female.[Q]
- Locations of fibroid is described as follows (Fig. 11.1):

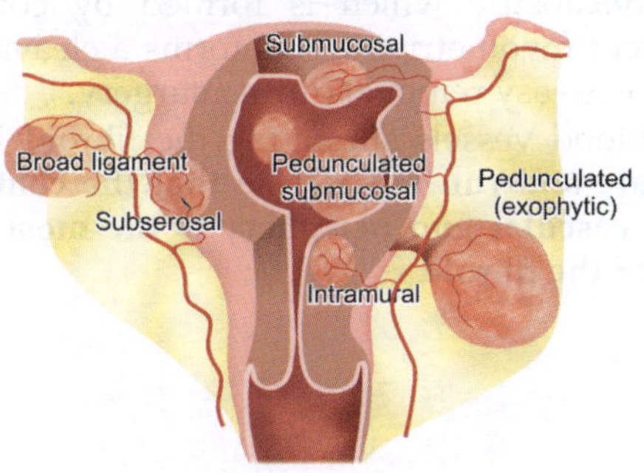

Fig. 11.1: Locations of fibroid

Flowchart 11.1

- **Fibroid**
  - Uterine
    - Intramural/Interstitial grow within the myometrial wall (M/C) 75%
    - Submucous grow toward the uterine cavity 15%
      - **Wansteker's classification: Hysteroscopically they are further divided into:** (Fig. 11.2)
        - **Type 0:** Fibroid totally in cavity
        - **Type 1:** ≥ 50% in cavity (i.e.< 50% in myometrium)
        - **Type 2:** < 50% in cavity (i.e.≥ 50% in myometrium)
    - Subserous grow outward toward the peritoneal surface 5%
  - Extrauterine
    - Most common is cervical fibroid[Q] followed by broad ligament fibroid (which could be anterior or posterior)

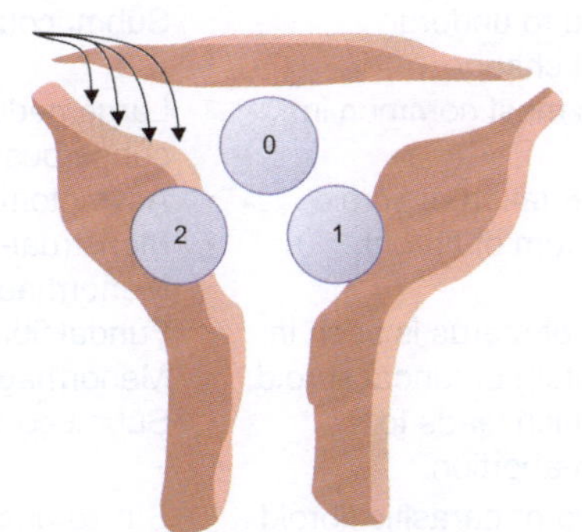

Fig. 11.2: Hysteroscopic classification of fibroid

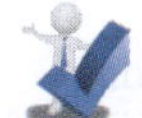

KEY POINTS

Diseases commonly associated with leiomyomas—
- Follicular cysts of ovary
- Endometrial hyperplasia
- Endometrial cancer
- Endometriosis

Etiology/Pathogenesis of Fibroids

- Fibroid is **monoclonal in origin.**[Q] i.e it is derived from a single progenitor myocyte.
- Multiple chromosomal abnormalities are detected in 40% of all fibroids—most common being translocation between the long arms of chromosomes 12 and 14 followed by deletion of chromosome 7.
- Gene mutations involved in origin of fibroid involved MED12 and HMGA2 gene.
- Similar to all hyperestrogenic conditions:
  - Fibroid is m/c in nulliparous females
  - It is m/c in obese females
  - M/C in females with Early menarche
  - Smoking, increased parity and exercise are **protective for leiomyomas.**
- There is no definite relationship between OCP and presence of fibroid.
- First degree relatives of women with fibroid have 2.5 times increased risk of developing fibroids.

- Risk of fibroid is more in African females.
- Most fibroids do not increase in size during pregnancy.

Most Common in Fibroid

• Most common (M/c) variety of fibroid	• Intramural/interstitial (75%) followed by submucous (15%) and subserous (10%)
• Fibroid with maximal symptoms	• Submucous fibroid
• To start with, all fibroids are	• Interstitial (Intramural)
• M/c fibroid to undergo malignant change	• Submucous
• Torsion is most common in	• Large pedunculated subserous fibroid
• M/c presentation of fibroid	• Asymptomatic
• M/c symptom of fibroid	• Menstrual-Menorrhagia
• Inversion of uterus is seen in	• Fundal fibroid
• M/c symptom of fundal fibroid	• Menorrhagia
• Fibroid which leads to maximum abortion	• Submucous fibroid
• Wandering or parasitic fibroid	• Subserous fibroid
• Lantern on dome of St Paul	• Peduculated cervical fibroid
• Pseudocervical fibroid	
• M/c fibroid to undergo calcareous degeneration	• Fibroid polyp • Subserous fibroid
• M/c fibroid to cause urinary symptoms	• Cervical fibroid
• Anterior cervical fibroid causes	• Urinary frequency
• Posterior cervical fibroid causes	• Urinary retention

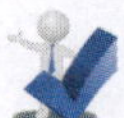

KEY POINTS

Broad ligament fibroids are of 2 types—

- Those fibroids which arise from the uterus (and not broad ligament) and grow towards the broad ligament and displace the ureter laterally – they are known as **Pseudo broad ligament fibroids** (Fig. 11.3A). **They are pedunculated and are covered by pseudocapsule similar to uterine fibroids.**
- Those fibroids which arise **de novo from broad ligament** and ureter is medial to this type of fibroid (i.e. ureter is between uterus and fibroid) are called as **True broad ligament fibroid** (Fig. 11.3B). **They are unpedunculated and never covered by a pseudo-capsule (unlike uterine fibroids).**
- Normally in uterine fibroids. M/C complain is heavy menstrual bleeding i.e., Menorrhagia. So patients have anemia ureter but in case of broad ligament fibroid, fibroid will press on ureter leading to hydroureter and hydronephrosis which increases erythropoietin levels & cause polycythemia.

Structure of Fibroids

- Grossly, Leiomyoma are round, rubbery tumors that when bisected display a whorled pattern.
- Fibroid is a well circumscribed tumor **with a pseudocapsule** which is formed by compressed adjacent myometrium. This forms a cleavage plane & allows easy removal during surgery.
- The blood vessels supplying the fibroid lie in the **capsule and run radially so that the center is the least vascular and periphery is the most vascular part of the fibroid**

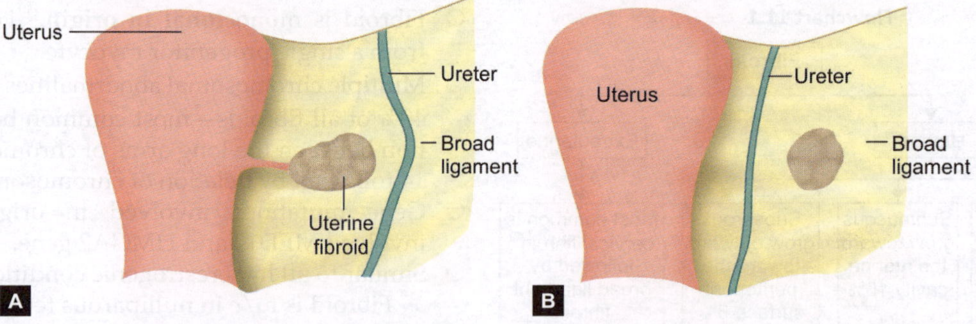

Figs. 11.3A and B: (A) Pseudo broad ligament fibroid; and (B) True broad ligament fibroid.

Thus, calcifications begin from the periphery of fibroid and degenerations begin from the center.[Q]

- Most fibroids are slow growing.
- Histologically, leiomyoma contain elongated smooth muscle cells aggregated in dense bundles
- Mitotic activity, however is rare and is a key point in differentiating it from malignant leiomyosarcoma.

Degenerations/Secondary Changes in a Fibroid

Mnemonic

Avoid	=	Atrophy
Red	=	Red degeneration
Hot	=	Hyaline degeneration (Most common degeneration)
Fatty	=	Fatty degeneration or calcification
Meat	=	Myxomatous degeneration
of **Chicken**	=	Cystic degeneration
Mnemonic:		*Avoid red hot fatty meat of chicken*

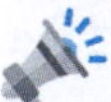

Important One Liners

- **M/c degeneration:** Hyaline degeneration
- Cystic degeneration is M/c in postmenopausal females and M/c in interstitial fibroid
- Calcareous degeneration is M/c in subserous fibroids
- Least common charge in fibroid is malignant transformation.

Red Degeneration of Fibroid (also called as Carneous Degeneration)

- **It is seen mostly during pregnancy, (but not exclusively) especially in mid pregnancy-2nd trimester**^Q
- It is an aseptic condition.^Q
- The myoma suddenly becomes acutely painful,^Q enlarged^Q and tender.^Q

Pathogenesis

- There is aseptic thrombosis in the blood vessels which supply the fibroid leading to subacute necrosis of fibroid

Clinical Features

- *Patient presents with:*
  - Acute abdominal pain^Q
  - Vomiting^Q
  - Malaise^Q
  - Slight fever^Q (This is not due to, infection but is reactionary)

Pathological Changes

- Fibroid becomes soft, necrotic or homogeneous especially in its center.
- It is stained **Salmon pink**^Q, or red (due to diffusion of blood pigments from the thrombosed vessels).
- It has a **fishy odor**^Q (due to secondary infection with coliform organisms)
- *Histologically:* There is evidence of thrombosis in some vessels.^Q
- Diagnosis is by ultrasound

Lab Investigations

- Although it is an aseptic condition, there is reactionary leukocytosis (due to fever)
- Raised ESR^Q

Management

- Conservative management^Q with analgesics antipyretics and antiemetics.

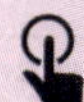

Steps Not Done for Management of Red Degeneration

- Do not give antibiotics
- Do not terminate pregnancy
- Do not do myomectomy

- The acute symptoms subside in 3–10 days^Q and pregnancy proceeds uneventfully.

Differential Diagnosis

- Appendicitis,^Q twisted ovarian cyst,^Q pyelitis^Q and accidental hemorrhage.^Q

Sarcomatous Change/Malignant Transformation of Fibroid

- **This is the least common change to be seen in fibroid.**^Q

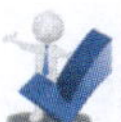

KEY POINTS

- Malignant change %: 0.2–0.5% (<0.5%)^Q
- M/c fibroid to become malignant: *Submucous fibroid*^Q
- M/c malignancy seen In fibroid: *Leiomyosarcoma*^Q
- Endometrial cancer is associated with fibroids in 3% cases

- Diagnosis is made by histological examination of the removed myoma.^Q

- **Macroscopic features suspicious for malignancy:**
  - *Loss of whorled pattern*
  - *Loss of capsule*
  - *Heterogeneity*
  - *Margins not well defined, blurred and irregular margins*
  - *Yellow, tan or gray color*
  - *Softer, less rubbery, less resilient (normally fibroid is firm).*

Sarcomas with malignant behavior have 10 or more mitosis per ten high power field.

- Development of sarcoma can be suspected clinically, when a leiomyoma (usually in a postmenopausal woman) becomes painful, tender, grows rapidly, and produces systematic upset and pyrexia.
- Overall 5 years survival rate in such patients = **20–30%.**

Symptoms of Fibroid

1. M/C presentation in a fibroid is asymptomatic
2. Most common symptom: Menstrual disturbances[Q]

- **Most common menstrual disturbance: Progressive menorrhagia**[Q] (seen in 30% cases). Cause: Due to increased estrogen, there is increased vascularity & due to increased surface area of uterus

Other Menstrual Symptoms:

- Metrorrhagia[Q] – (Irregular bleeding)[Q] – Normally a fibroid does not lead to metrorrhagia but if it does then it is a case of fibroid polyp.

Dysmenorrhea – congestive[Q] as well as spasmodic[Q] type seen.

3. **Pressure symptoms** (see Flowchart 11.2)

Flowchart 11.2

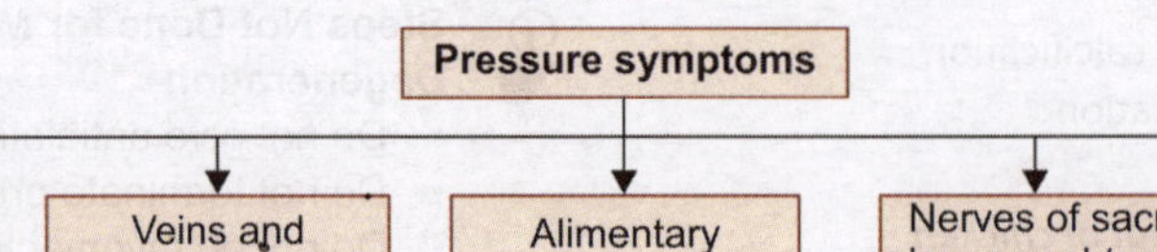
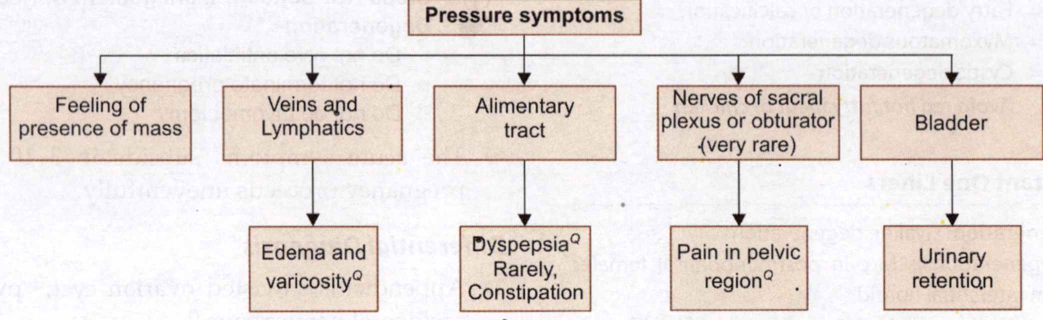

4. **Infertility:** As a sole cause, fibroid is responsible for < 3% cases of infertility.

Causes:

- Fibroid hinders with the ascent of the sperm.[Q]
- Interferes with implantation of fertilized ovum[Q] by distorting endometrium.
- Can cause associated disturbance in ovulation[Q]
- Lead to occlusion of tubal ostia.

> M/C fibroid to cause infertility and abortions is submucous fibroid

Note: Presence of submucous fibroids decrease fertility rates and removing them increases fertility rates.

- Subserous fibroids do not affect fertility rates but removing them increases fertility. Intramural fibroid slightly decreases fertility but removal does not increase fertility.

5. **Pain:** A fibroid usually does not cause pain in abdomen. If pain occurs it is due to:

> **Causes:**
> - Malignancy[Q]
> - It is being extruded from body as a polyp[Q]
> - Associated endometriosis[Q]
> - Torsion of a pedunculated fibroma[Q]
> - Degeneration[Q]

Mnemonic

My PET Dog.

5. **Other rare features of fibroid:**
   a. **Polycythemia:** (*Interesting as fibroids generally cause anemia due to blood loss. Polycythemia is seen in broad ligament fibroids*).[Q]
   b. **Hypoglycemia and hypokalemia.**
   c. Rarely it may lead to pseudo Pseudo-Meigs' syndrome
6. **Effect of fibroid on pregnancy**

   Fibroids lead to:
   - Infertility
   - Since fibroid is taken as a foreign body by uterus, so uterus tues to expel it out & hence contractility of uterus increases. This can lead to pertain labor
   - Fibroid can lead to malpresentation
   - It can lead to abruptio placenta
   - It can lead to PPH d/t increased surface area of uterus

Investigations

- M/C investigation done in fibroids or IOC is USG. (It is most readily available, least cost-effective but not as accurate as MRI at determining the precise location or size of fibroids especially in larger uteri or those with multiple fibroids)
- Best investigation to detect a small submucous fibroid – hysteroscopy.

Appearance of Leiomyoma on USG

- Uterus with a leiomyoma appears heterogenous in appearance.
- Focal myomas are usually heterogenous but mostly hypoechoic when compared with surrounding myometrium (Fig. 11.4).

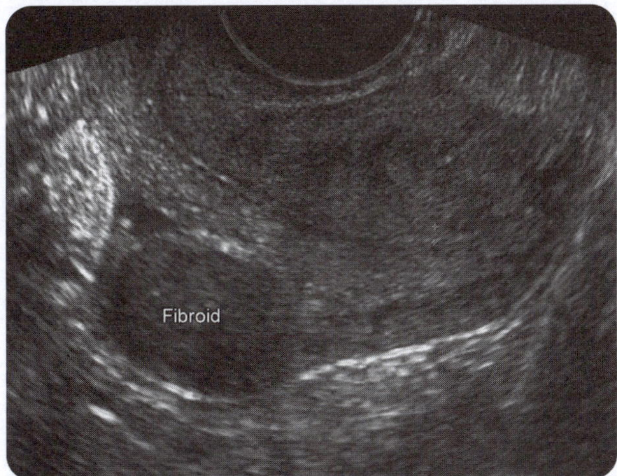

Fig. 11.4: USG of fibroid

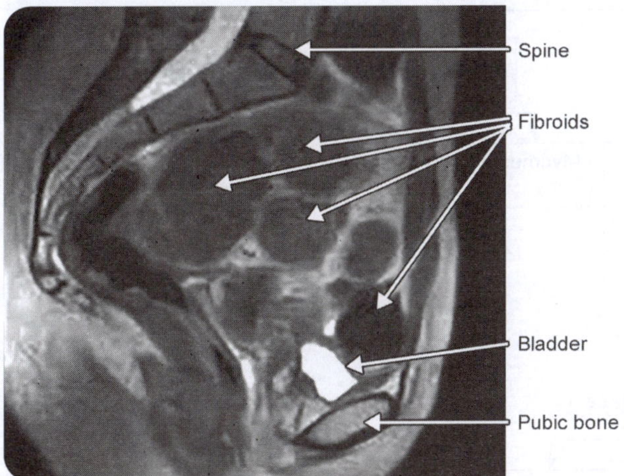

Fig. 11.5: MRI in fibroid

Differential diagnosis of fibroid is adenomyosis

Fibroid	Adenomyosis
Presenting symptom-menorrhagia	Menorrhagia and secondary dysmenorrhea
Irregular growth of uterus	Symmetrical growth of uterus
Non tender uterus	Uterus is tender to touch (called as **Halban sign**)
Uterine size = 16 to 20 weeks pregnancy sized uterus	10–12 weeks pregnancy sized uterus
IOC : USG	IOC : TVS > MRI. Gold standard–Histo-pathological examination

Management of Fibroids

See Flowchart 11.3: Asymptomatic fibroid

- **Asymptomatic fibroids** are managed expectantly i.e by observation
- Regardless of their size, asymptomonatic fibroids can be observed and surveilled with an annual pelvic examination.

Indications for surgical management of asymptomatic fibroid are:
- Pedunculated fibroid likely to undergo torsion.
- Suspecting malignancy.
- **Size of fibroid increasing rapidly**

The best management of symptomatic fibroids is surgical management

Indications of Medical Management[Q]

- To treat anemia and recover hemoglobin levels before surgery.[Q]
- To reduce the size of large fibroid and facilitate surgery.[Q]
- In women with medical contraindication to surgery or those who are postponing surgery.[Q]
- For preservation of fertility in women with large myomas before conservative surgery like myomectomy.[Q]

In the text, earlier we have read fibroid is an estrogen and progesterone dependent tumor.

∴ All those drugs which either decrease estrogen or progesterone will decrease the size of fibroid and in turn decrease blood loss.

Drugs which decrease estrogen are:

- Continuous GnRH agonist/GnRH antagonist
- Aromatase Inhibition: Lectrozole.
- Danazol: But it can lead to androgenic side effect like hirsutism in hence it should not be used in young females.
- Gestrinone

Drugs which decrease progesterone

- Progesterone antagonist: Mifepristone or RU 486.
- Selective Progesterone Receptor Modulator: Ulipristal.

Also Know

- Dose of Mifepristone = 2.5 mg to 10 mg
- Mifepristone given for 3-6 months daily can reduce volume of fibroid by 50%
- Mifepristone has 2 drawbacks:
  - Approximately 40% of treated common complain of vasometer symptoms
  - Due to its antiprogestational effects, endometrium is exposed to unopposed estrogen
- The efficacy of ulipristal is same like GnRH agonist (leuprolide) Dose is 5-10 mg oral daily doses.
- It controls bleeding in 90% cases of fibroid. But again concern of endometrial cancer limits its use solely to preoperative adjunct.

Flowchart 11.3: Management of Fibroid

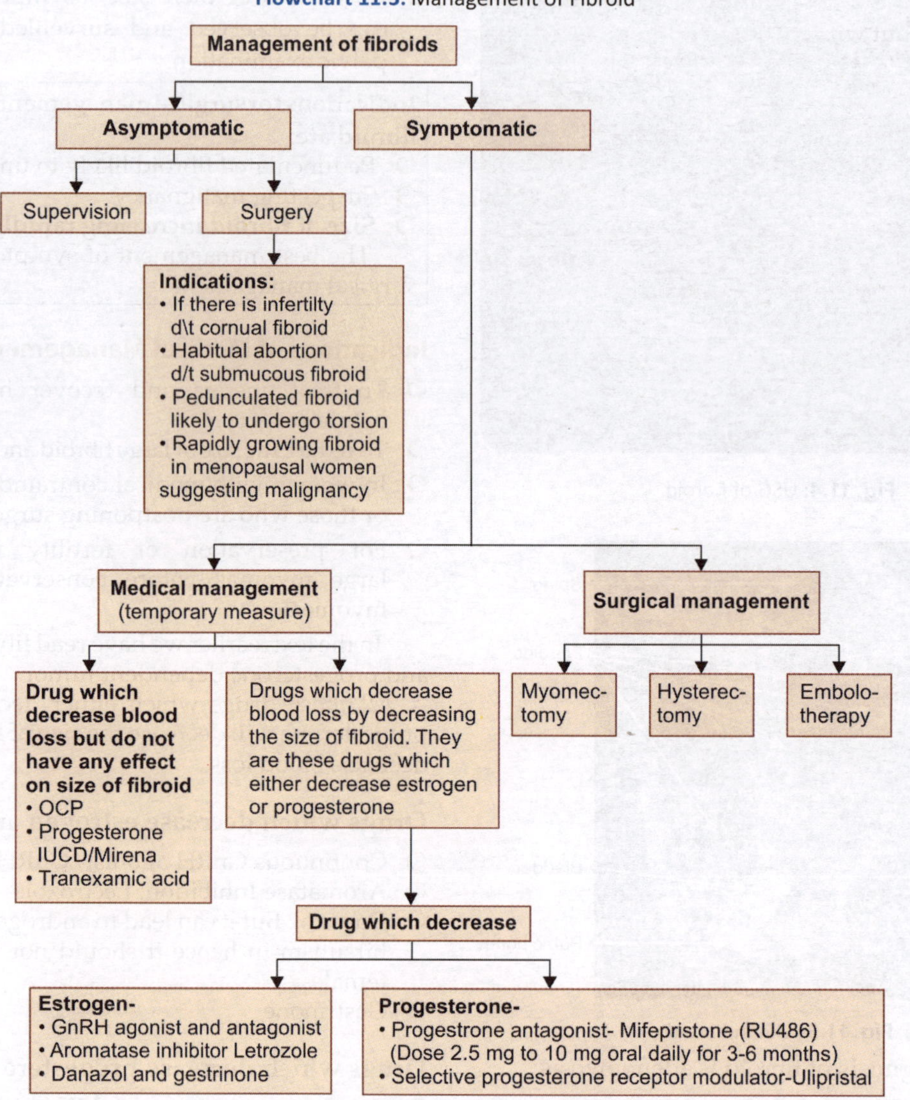

- **GnRH** agonist are synthetic derivatives of GnRH decapeptide. They are inactive orally but can be given intranasally, subcutaneously and intramuscularly. Leuprolide is FDA approved for fibroid treatment & is available as 3.75 mg monthly dose or 11.25 mg 3 monthly dose, both given 1. M. The other 3 GnRH agonist: Goserelin, Triptorelin and Nafarelin are not approved by FDA for fibroid treatment but are used off label.
- Size of fibroid decreases by 40-5% by use of GnRH.
- **Side effect of GnRH**: Decrease in estrogen leads to menopause like symptoms hot flashes and bone loss in 95% patients. *These drugs are not recommended for more than 6 months* (ACOG Recommendation) After starting GnRH agonist, add back therapy should be started after 1-3 months
- The GnRH agonist suppress leiomyoma cell proliferation & induce cell apoptosis at the fourth week of GnRH agonist therapy hence we say add back therapy should be given after 1-3 months. Add back therapy includes Estrogen & Progesterone
- According to ***Williams Gynae 3rd/ed,*** GnRH antagonist are also available. Two agents in this class **cetrorelix** and **ganirelix**, are currently FDA-approved for infertility use in women undergoing controlled ovarian hyperstimulation. A depot form of cetrorelix did not provide adequate or consistent suppression of estrogen production on leiomyoma growth.

On the other hand:

- **OCP's:** When given continuously can cause amenorrhea, but will not decrease the size of fibroid (as fibroid is Estrogen + Progesterone dependent).

- **Progesterone:** When given continuously will cause amenorrhea, but will not decrease the size of fibroid.
- The LNG-IUC's may be a reasonable treatment for women with fibroid associated Menorrhagia.
- **Tranexamic acid:** Will decrease blood loss but not affect the size of fibroid.
- As per ***Novaus* 15th/ed**, Ganirelix results in 29% reduction in fibroid volume.

Indications of Surgical Management[Q]

Fibroids causing any symptoms like

Flowchart 11.4

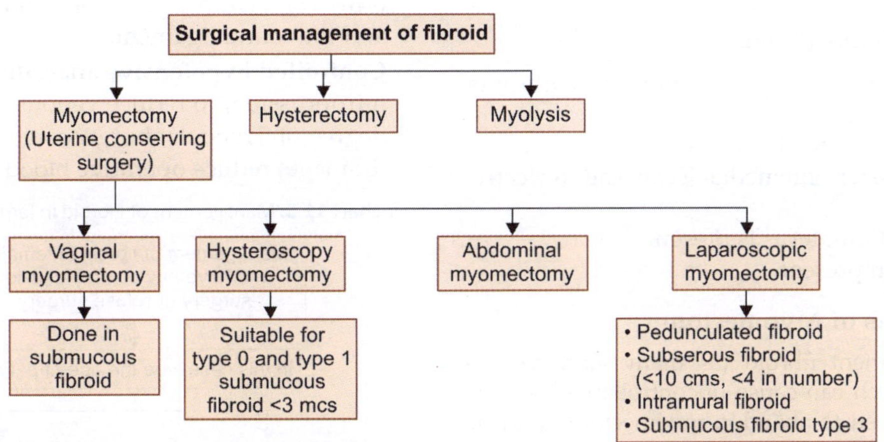

- Menorrhagia[Q] or pressure symptoms[Q] like urinary retention (by a cervical or broad ligament fibroid) or chronic pelvic pain with[Q] severe dysmenorrhea, acute pelvic pain as in torsion of a pedunculated fibroid, or prolapsing submucosal fibroid
- Unexplained infertility
- Recurrent abortions due to submucous fibroid
- Rapidly growing fibroid.

For details of surgical management see Flowchart 11.4.

Some Specific Indications for Hysterectomy

- In patients > 40 years of age.[Q]
- Multiparous women.[Q]
- If fibroid is associated with malignancy.[Q]
- During myomectomy, if their is uncontrolled hemorrhage or other surgical difficulty.[Q]

Hysterectomy for fibroids can be done by

- Abdominal route
- *Vaginal route*: It is done, if size of uterus is less than 12 weeks in size

Myomectomy

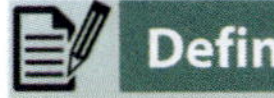 **Definition**

Myomectomy

Myomectomy is the enucleation of myomata from the uterus leaving behind a potentially functioning organ capable of future reproduction[Q]

- Myomectomy is specifically indicated in an infertile woman or woman desirous of bearing child and wishing to retain the uterus.[Q]

Prerequisites

- Anemia should be corrected.[Q]
- All other causes of infertility should be excluded.[Q]
- Male factor infertility should be ruled out.[Q] (husband semen analysis should be normal)
- Diagnostic D and C or hysteroscopy should be performed in case of irregular cycles, to detect any polyp and to rule out endometrial cancer[Q]
- Hysteroscopy or hysterosalpingography (HSG) should be done to detect a fibroid encroaching the uterine cavity or a polyp or tubal block.[Q]
- **Arrange for blood**
- In case of large fibroid decrease the size of fibroid by giving GnRH.

Time of Myomectomy

- It should be performed in immediate postmenstrual phase to reduce blood loss during surgery[Q]
- It should not be performed during pregnancy and at the time of cesarean section.[Q]

Route of Myomectomy

- Laparoscopic
- Abdominal
- Hysteroscopic

Laparoscopic Myomectomy

- Preferred as it needs less operative time

- Less blood loss
- Less postoperative stay
- Early ambulation
- It is done in subserosal (size < 10 cms and number < 4)/ intramural/type 2 submucosal fibroid (Fig. 11.2)
- **Disadvantage**–Earlier it was said it had **higher recurrence rate**, but now studies have proved it to be incorrect.

Hysteroscopic Myomectomy

- Done for type 0 and type 1 submucosal fibroids, < 5 cm in size (Fig. 11.2)
- Associated with more blood loss
- Due to saline distension media–it can lead to electrolyte imbalance
- Risk of perforation uterus is present
- Risk of infection present.

Contraindications of Myomectomy

- Big broad ligament fibroid (as many large vessels are present which can cause uncontrollable bleeding and thus the need to abandon myomectomy and do hysterectomy[Q])
- Multiple tiny fibroids scattered through the uterine wall.[Q]
- Infected fibroid
- Pelvic or endometrial TB
- During pregnancy of following cesarean section.

Results (Important)

- Pregnancy rate following myomectomy: 40–60%
- Recurrence rate: 40–50%
- Persisting menorrhagia: 1–5%[Q]

20–25% women subjected to myomectomy ultimately come for hysterectomy.

- Rupture of myomectomy scar during pregnancy is rare.
- Low-grade postoperative pyrexia is a rule and should not be treated by antibiotics (pyrexia is due to slight extravasation of blood in uterine wall or peritoneal cavity and settles spontaneously in 7–14 days).
- Myomectomy has higher chances of post operative intra-abdominal adhesions.

Measures to control blood loss during myomectomy

...*Dutta Gynae 6th/ed, p604*

- **Timing the surgery** in immediate **postmenstrual phase.**
- **Preoperative treatment with GnRH analogue** reduces the vascularity of the tumour and thereby reduces operative blood loss
- **Injection of vasoconstrictive** agents (commonly used is **vasopressin**) into the serosa overlying myoma.
- **Use of tourniquets:** To occlude the uterine vessels and also the ovarian vessels at the infundibulopelvic ligament.

  Note: If surgery duration is becoming ≥ 45 minutes, the tourniquets or clamp relieved intermittently.
- **Use of Victor Bonney's specially** designed clamp (Figs. 11.6A and B) to reduce uterine artery blood flow. This clamp is placed around the uterine vessels and the round ligament.
- **Controlled hypotensive anaesthesia** (using sodium nitroprusside) to reduce venous tone and moderate degree of Trendelenburg position (enhance venous drainage) reduce operative blood loss.

Flowchart 11.5: Management of Fibroid in females with C/I to surgery

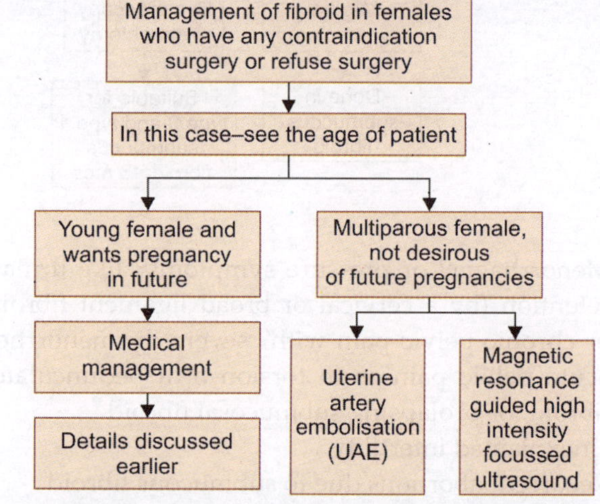

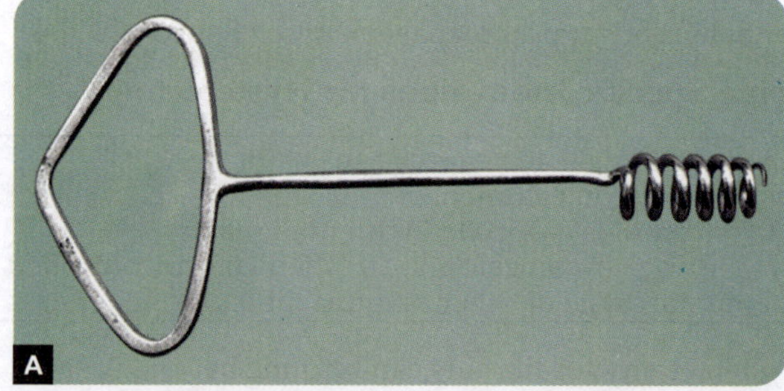

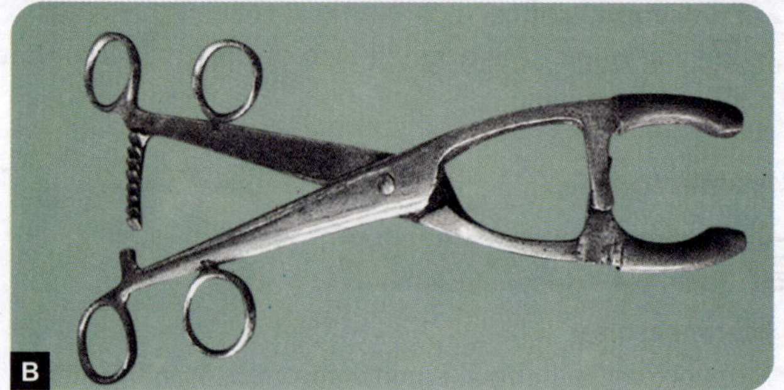

Figs. 11.6A and B: Important instruments used during myomectomy; (A) Bonneys myomectomy hook; (B) Bonneys myomectomy clamp

Embolotherapy/Uterine Artery Embolization

- **Uterine artery embolization** is done using **polyvinyl**[Q] **alcohol or gel foam**[Q]. It is performed by an ***interventional radiologists*** and involves catheterization of ***the femoral artery to gain*** access to the ***hypogastric arteries*** (Fig. 11.7). Under fluoroscopic guidance the uterine arteries are occluded using gel foam, polyvinyl alcohol, in patients not suited for or not desirous of surgical therapy.

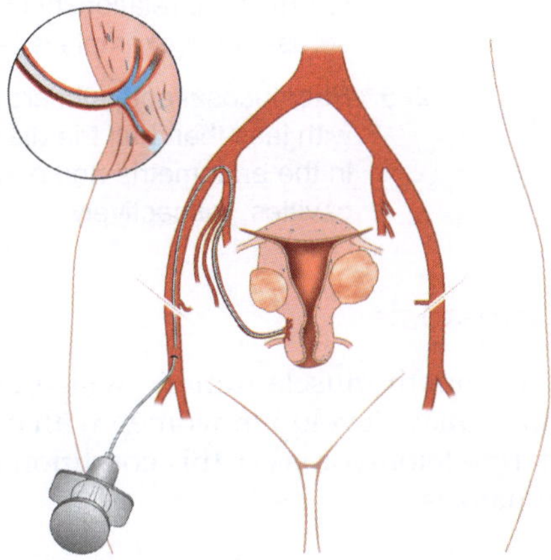

Fig. 11.7: UAE techniques. A catheter is threaded to the uterine arteries and embolic material injected to block off blood flow to the uterus

- In this manner, uterine blood flow is obstructed producing ischemia and necrosis.
- It shrinks the fibroid **volume by 40–50% in selective young women**[Q] **and menorrhagia resolves by 90% pressure symptoms in 40–70%. If patient is still symptomatic** after year then surgery should be considered.
- UAE is a management option for women with documented uterine leiomyoma despite medical management and who might otherwise be considered candidate for Hysterectomy or myomectomy

 **Remember**

Pedunculated submucous and subserous tumors are not suitable as these tumors can infarct and slough.

Investigations to be done before UAE:
- Cervical cancer screening
- Tests for *N. gonorrhoeae/Chlamydia*
- Endometrial Biopsy
- General investigation, CBC creatinine, prothrombin

Results

These patients experience:
- Lowered fertility rate[Q]
- Risk of placental insufficiency[Q]
- Uterine rupture in subsequent pregnancy[Q] because of interference with the blood supply and embolotherapy induced necrosis of the leiomyoma.
- Early ovarian failure, thus uterine artery embolization should not be done in females who desire future childbearing.
- Rate of reoperation is as high as 30% and reoperation rate is age-dependant, with higher likelihood in women over 40 years of age.
- Around 25% patients develop post embolization syndrome

- Post embolization syndrome lasts for 2 to 7 days and is marked by pelvic pain, nausea, low grade fever, mild WBC elevation and malaise.
- The syndrome is due to necrosis of fibroid after embolization, hence antibiotics have no role in it.
- Management: Conservative management and analgesics

- Other complications are:
  - Passage of necrotic tissue through vagina
  - Groin hematoma and vaginal discharge
  - Amenorrhea

Magnetic Resonance-guided High-intensity Focused Ultrasound (MR-HIFU) Surgery

It is used in managing fibroid. In MR-HIFU, fibroid tissue is heated and destroyed using targeted ultrasonic energy passing through the anterior abdominal wall.

- During MR-HIFU sessions lasting 2 to 3 hours, a patient lies prone within the MR imaging unit, & bladder is continuously drained.
- The normal uterine muscles, at a temperature of ≥ 57 °C remain intact following the procedure.
- Like UAE, 8-25% of patients who get MR-HIFU done their symptomatic relief waves with time and at ≥ 12 months they seek alternative procedure for their symptoms like Hysterectomy
- The fibroid does not disappear; however, it shrinks in size leading to a reduction in symptoms.

- **C/I to procedure (like normal MRI):**
  - Pregnancy
  - Energy path—obstruction like abdominal wall scars, bowel on foreign bodies.
- **Other exclusive C/I are:**
  - Desire for pregnancy in future
  - Current pelvic infection
  - Menopause
  - Myoma size > 10 cms
  - Uterine size > 24 weeks

Advantages

- Non invasive & requires only conscious sedation
- Associated with rapid recovery
- Well tolerated

Complications

- Skin burns
- Adjacent tissue energy
- Venous Thromboembolism

Extra Edge

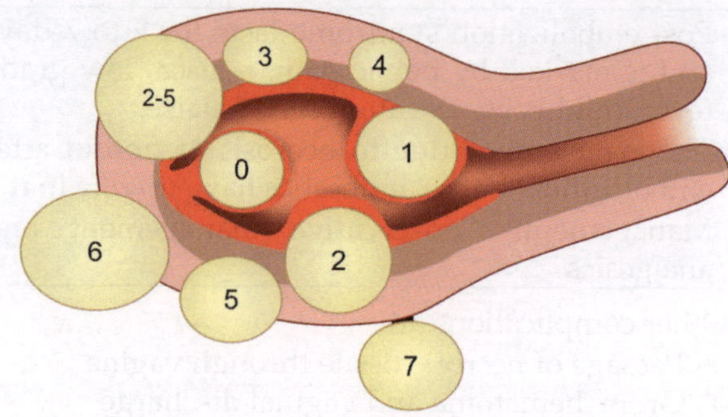

Fig. 11.8: FIGO classification of fibroids

FIGO Fibroid Classification

FIGO Leiomyoma Classification System		
SM-Submucosal	0	Pedunculated intracavitary
	1	< 50% intramural
	2	≥ 50% intramural
O-Other	3	Contacts endometrium; 100% intramural
	4	Intramural
	5	Subserosal ≥50% intramural
	6	Subserosal <50% intramural
	7	Subserosal pedunculated
	8	Other (specify e.g. cervical, broad ligament, parasitic)
Hybrid leiomyomas (impact both endometrium and serosa)		Two numbers are listed separated by a hyphen. By convention, the first refers to the relationship with the endometrium while the second refers to the relationship to the serosa. One example is below
	2–5	Submucosal and subserosal, each with less than half the diameter in the endometria and peritoneal cavities, respectively.

Leiomyomatosis

Extrauterine smooth muscle tumors, which are benign yet infiltrative, may develop in women with concurrent or prior uterine leiomyomas & this condition is termed as leiomyomatosis.

Intravenous Leiomyomatosis

- Invades into uterine veins such as pelvic veins, inferior vena cava.
- It is rare
- Female can C/O leiomyoma & right sided congestive cardiac symptoms.
- Benign & Recurrent

Disseminated Pentioneal Leomyomatosis (DPL)

- Multiple, benign small peritoneal nodules on abdominal cavity.
- M/C in Reproductive age & associated with pregnancy or OCPs use.

NEW PATTERN QUESTIONS

N1. Submucous fibroid protruding ≥ 50% in cavity is classified as:

a. Type 0 b. Type I
c. Type II d. Type III

N2. All of the followings are true with regards to fibroid *except*:

a. Fibroids are mostly asymptomatic
b. First degree relatives of females with fibroid have 2.5 times increased risk of developing fibroid
c. OCP's can increase the chances of fibroid in premenopausal females
d. Most fibroids do not increase in size during pregnancy

N3. Broad ligament fibroid is related to:

a. Ovaries
b. Fallopian tube
c. Ureter
d. Gartner's duct

N4. Most consistent symptom of fibroid:

a. Menorrhagia
b. Metrorrhagia
c. Dysmenorrhea
d. Urinary symptoms

N5. M/c degeneration in fibroid is:

a. Red degeneration
b. Hyaline degeneration
c. Calcific degeneration
d. Malignant transformation

N6. A 40-year-old female complains of heavy menstrual bleeding and dysmenorrhoea. On USG-an echogenic area of 20 weeks of pregnancy is seen in the uterus. Tenderness is present. Most likely diagnosis is:

a. Fibroid uterus b. Adenomyosis
c. Endometriosis d. PID

N7. All are complications of fibroid in pregnancy *except*:

a. Red degeneration
b. Obstructed labor
c. PPH
d. Placenta previa

N8. Regarding imaging of uterine fibroids all are correct *except*:

a. Ultrasound is ideal to confirm the diagnosis
b. Saline Infusion Sonography (SIS) is more sensitive to detect any submucous fibroid
c. MRI is superior to USG to identify the exact location of myoma
d. CT scanning is an alternative to MRI

N9. All of the following are the indications for myomectomy in a case of fibroid uterus *except*:

a. Associated infertility b. Recurrent pregnancy loss
c. Pressure symptoms d. Red degeneration

N10. All are prerequisites for myomectomy *except*:

a. Husbands semen analysis
b. D and C report
c. Hysterectomy consent
d. None of the above

N11. Identify the instrument:

a. Myoma clamp
b. Myoma screw
c. Uterine manipulator
d. IUCD removing hook

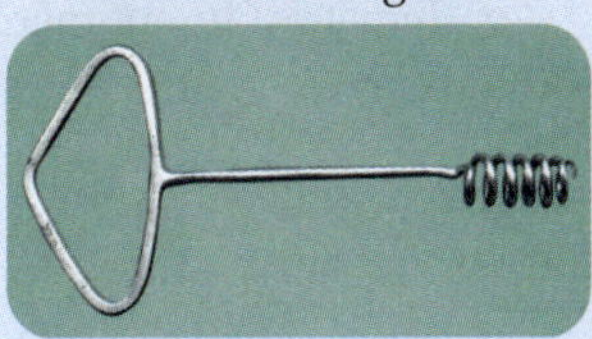

N12. Identify the instrument:

a. Bonneys myoma screw
b. Bonneys myoma clamp
c. Cervical occlusion clamp
d. Uterus holding forcep

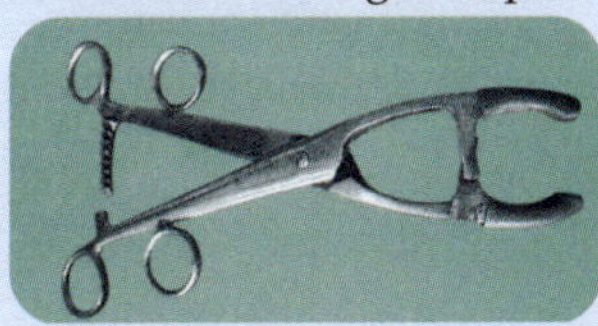

N13. All of the following measures reduce bleeding during myomectomy *except*: *(DNB 08)*

a. Preoperative correction of anemia
b. Preoperative oc pills
c. Ligation of pedicle
d. GNRH analogues
e. Local injection of vasoconstrictive agents

N14. A 36-year-old female presents with heavy menstrual bleeding. She has one child of 7 years. USG shows a single 3 × 3 cm submucosal fibroid. Hemoglobin is 10.5 gm/dl. What is the best treatment option for her?

a. GnRH injection
b. UAE
c. Hysteroscopic myomectomy
d. Laparoscopic myomectomy
e. TAH

N15. A 42-year-old female presents with heavy menstrual bleeding. She has one child (aged 7 years). Uterus is enlarged to 24 weeks with multiple fibroids. Her hemoglobin is 9 gm/dl. What is the best treatment option for her?

a. GnRH injection
b. Myomectomy
c. TAH + BSO followed by HRT
d. TAH

N16. Identify the fibroid based on FIGO classification:
a. Type 3 b. Type 4
c. Type 5 d. Type 7

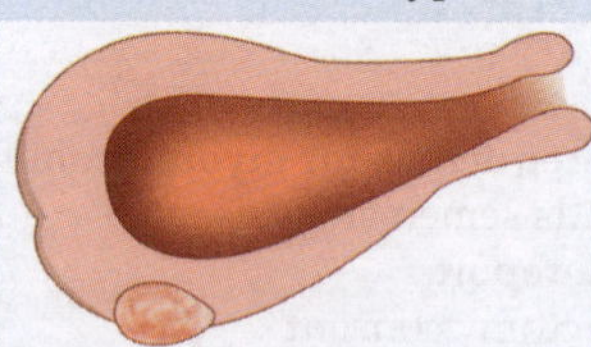

N17. Most common type of uterine polyp is:
a. Mucous polyp b. Fibroid
c. Placental polyp d. None

N18. Leiomyosarcoma is characterized by all *except*:
a. Presence of necrosis b. Vascular invasion > 50%
c. Mitosis ≥ 10 HPF d. Indistinct tumor margins

N19. All are true about fibroid *except*:
a. Monoclonal in origin
b. Both estrogen and progesterone dependent
c. Familial inheritance been
d. M/C in white females

N20. M/C gene nutation in fibroid.
a. MED-12 b. COL 4 A5-A6
c. FH d. None of above

N21. All of the following predispose to fibroid *except*:
a. Obesity b. Early menopause
c. Nulliparity d. African females

N22. Polycythemia or myomatous erythrocytosis syndrome is seen in______% cases:
a. 0.5% b. 5%
c. 10% d. 15%

N23. All of the following may be associated with fibroid *except*:
a. Pseudo-Meig's syndrome
b. Polycythemia
c. Amenorrhea
d. Dysmenorrhea

N24. All of the following are absolute C/I to uterine artery embolization *except*:
a. Pregnancy
b. Uterine infection
c. Endometrial cancer
d. Age of patient ≥ 50 years

N25. All of the following techniques are used for merging fibroid *except*:
a. UAE
b. MRg HIFU
c. TCRE
d. Myolysis

N26. GnRH approved by FDA for managing fibroid:
a. Leuprolide acetate = 1/m
b. Goserelin = 1/m
c. Nafarelin = 1/m
d. Triptorelin = nasal

N27. Broad ligament fibroid belongs to FIGO class___:
a. 5 b. 6
c. 7 d. 8

N28. Acute pain in fibroid is due to all *except*:
a. Torsion
b. Red degeneration
c. Hyaline degeneration
d. Sarcomatous change

PREVIOUS YEAR QUESTIONS

1. **All changes occur in fibroid uterus *except*:** *(AIIMS June 97)*
   a. Atrophy b. Squamous metaplasia
   c. Hyaline degeneration d. Calcification
2. **A pregnant woman with fibroid uterus develops acute pain in abdomen with low-grade fever and mild leukocytosis at 28 week. The most likely diagnosis is:**
   a. Preterm labor *(AIIMS Nov 03)*
   b. Torsion of fibroid
   c. Red degeneration of fibroid
   d. Infection in fibroid
3. **Not true about red degeneration of myomas is:** *(AIIMS May 02)*
   a. It occurs commonly during pregnancy
   b. Immediate surgical intervention is needed
   c. Due to interference with blood supply
   d. Treated with analgesics
4. **Red degeneration in uterine fibroid is most common in:** *(AI 99; AIIMS June 97)*
   a. Second trimester b. Third trimester
   c. Puerperium d. First trimester
5. **All are methods of managing fibroid uterus *except*:**
   a. Myomectomy *(AIIMS Nov 99)*
   b. Radiofrequency ablation
   c. Embolization of uterine artery
   d. Laser myomectomy
6. **Sucheta, a 29-year-old nulliparous women complains of severe menorrhagia and lower abdominal pain since 3 months. On examination there was a 14 weeks size uterus with fundal fibroid. The treatment of choice is:** *(AIIMS May 01)*
   a. Myomectomy b. GnRH analogs
   c. Hysterectomy d. Wait and watch
7. **To start with all fibroids are:** *(PGI Dec 98)*
   a. Interstitial b. Submucous
   c. Subserous d. Ovarian
8. **Calcareous degeneration occurs most commonly in which type of fibroids:** *(PGI 97)*
   a. Submucous b. Subserous
   c. Interstitial d. Cervical
9. **Uterine fibromyoma is associated with:** *(PGI June 02)*
   a. Endometriosis
   b. Pelvic inflammatory disease
   c. Ovarian Ca
   d. Amenorrhea
   e. Tamoxifen
10. **Treatment of red degeneration of fibroid during pregnancy:** *(PGI Dec 03)*
    a. Analgesics b. Laparotomy
    c. Termination of pregnancy
    d. Removal at cesarean section
11. **Submucosal fibroid is detected by:** *(PGI Dec 05, 02)*
    a. Hysteroscopy b. Hysterosalpingography
    c. USG (Transabdominal) d. Laparoscopy
12. **The drug which reduces the size of myoma includes:** *(PGI Dec 05)*
    a. GnRH agonist b. Danazol
    c. Progesterone d. Mifepristone
    e. Estrogen
13. **Drugs that reduce the size of fibroid are:** *(PGI June 03)*
    a. Danazol b. GnRH analog
    c. RU-486 d. Estrogen
    e. Progesterone
14. **Decreased vascularity of fibroid is seen with:**
    a. GnRH agonist b. Danazol *(PGI Dec 06)*
    c. Mifepristone d. Clomiphene citrate
15. **Management options in a 26-year-old women with 7 × 8 cm size fibroid:** *(PGI June 09)*
    a. Follow-up b. OCP
    c. Myomectomy d. Hysterectomy
    e. Danazol
16. **Malignant prevalence in fibroid is:** *(UP 99)*
    a. 0.5% b. 1%
    c. 5% d. 10%
17. **Least common complication of fibroid is:** *(AI 98)*
    a. Menstrual disorder b. Malignancy
    c. Urinary retention d. Degeneration
18. **In fibroid which is not seen:** *(AI 07)*
    a. Amenorrhea b. Pelvic mass
    c. Infertility d. Menstrual irregularity
19. **What is the earliest most common presenting feature of anterior cervical fibroid?**
    a. Frequency of urine b. Bleeding
    c. Acute abdomen d. Constipation
20. **HSG image below shows:** *(AIIMS Nov 2015)*
    a. Endometrial polyp b. Genital TB
    c. Fibroid uterus d. Asherman syndrome

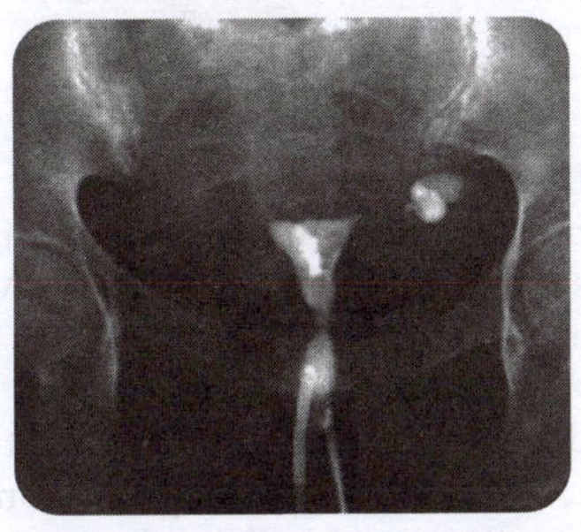

21. **Ulipristal acetate is a/an:** *(AIIMS Nov 2015)*
    a. GnRH agonist
    b. Androgen antagonist
    c. Selective estrogen receptor modulator
    d. Selective progesterone receptor modulator

22. Medical Treatment of myoma includes: *PGI Nov 2015.*
a. Tamoxifen
b. LNG IVCD
c. Mifepristone
d. GnRH agonist
e. GnRH antagonist

23. True statement regarding myoma of uterus:
a. Mostly asymptomatic *(PGI Nov 2011)*
b. Red degeneration decus
c. Sarcomatous change is common
d. Mifepristone is used for treatment

24. A uterine fibroid (7x8 cm) is seen in woman of age 26 years. Management options include: *(PGI June 2009)*
a. Follow-up
b. OCP
c. Myomectomy
d. Hysterectomy

25. Operative Haemorrhage during myomectomy can be minimised by prior administration:
a. GnRH analogue
b. OCP
c. Danazol
d. LH
e. Mifepristone

ANSWERS TO NEW PATTERN QUESTIONS

N1. Ans. is b, i.e. Type I
See the text for explanation.

N2. Ans. is c, i.e. OCP's can increase the chances of fibroid in premenopausal females *Ref: Novaks 15th/ed p438*
- **There is no definite relationship between oral contraceptives and the presence of fibroids.**

N3. Ans. is c, i.e. Ureter
If broad ligament fibroid lies medial to ureter. It is pseudo broad ligament fibroid and if it lies lateral to ureter it is true broad ligament fibroid.

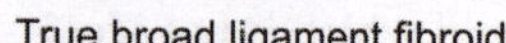

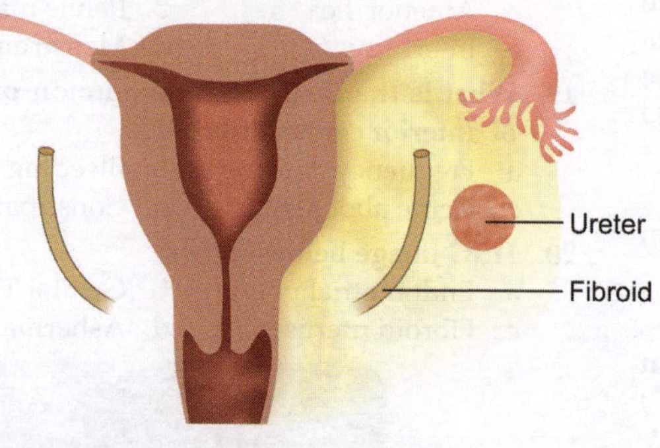

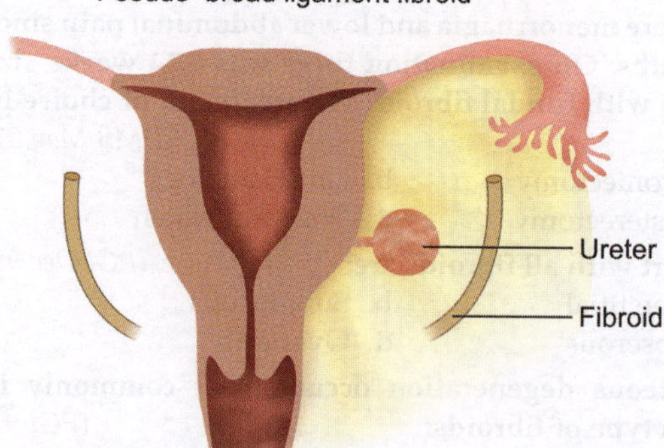

N4. Ans. is a, i.e. Menorrhagia
- M/c presentation of fibroid-asymptomatic
- M/c symptom-Menstrual symptom-Menorrhagia

Metrorrhagia is seen in fibroid polyp.

N5. Ans. is b, i.e. Hyaline degeneration
- M/c degeneration-Hyaline degeneration
- Least common change-Malignant transformation
- Degenerations become from the centre of fibroid
- M/c fibroid to undergo malignancy-Submucous fibroid

N6. Ans. is a, i.e. Fibroid uterus
In this case: point which favours the fibroid are
1. Size of growth = 20 weeks size

2. Menorrhagia and dysmenorrhea
3. Age of patient

The point which goes against it is tenderness seen in uterus. (This is seen in Adenomyosis, but in adenomyosis size of uterus is never more than 10–12 weeks pregnant uterus size).

Remember: In a big fibroid some tenderness can be seen due to necrosis of fibroid.

N7. Ans. is d, i.e. Placenta previa *Ref: Jeffcoate 7th/ed p493-4*

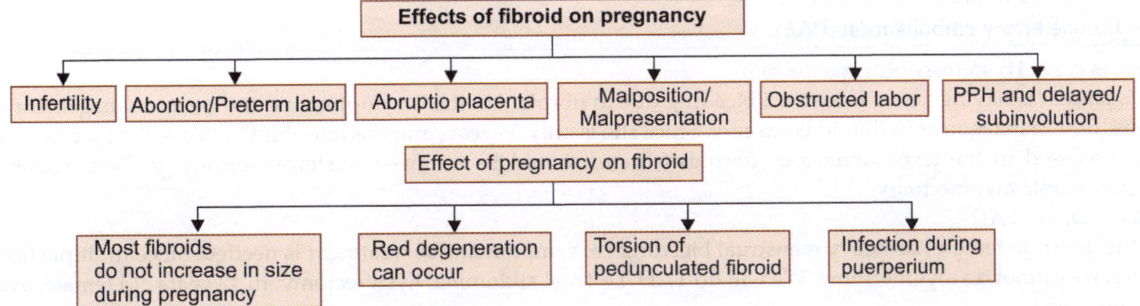

Thus, placenta previa is not a complication of fibroid → Abruptio placenta is a complication.

N8. Ans. is d, i.e. CT scanning is an alternative to MRI *Ref: Dutta Gynae 6th/ed p278-279*

The M/C investigation done to diagnose/detect fibroids is USG *"USG is an useful diagnostic tool to confirm its diagnosis".* *Ref: Dutta Gynae 6th/ed p278*

Three dimensional ultrasonography can locate fibroids accurately.

Although MRI are better (more accurate) than USG but is not routinely used as it is expensive and not widely available.

CT scan has got limited contrast resolution than MRI (i.e. option d is incorrect).

For submucous fibroid hysteroscopy or saline infusion semiography can be done.

N9. Ans. is d, i.e. Red degeneration *Ref: Shaw 15th/ed p360-2; Jeffcoat's 7th/ed p502*

From the given options the answer is quite obvious as red degeneration of fibroid is managed conservatively not by any surgery. But let us look at other options also.

Indication of myomectomy: Myomectomy is specifically indicated in an infertile woman, in recurrent abortions and patients with symptomatic fibroid but desirous of bearing child and wishing to retain the uterus.

Thus, option a and b are ruled out. As far as pressure symptoms are concerned, it means fibroid is symptomatic and all symptomatic fibroids need surgical management which could either be myomectomy or hysterectomy.

N10. Ans. is d, i.e. None of the above *Ref: Dutta Gynae 6th/ed p269*

Prerequisites for myomectomy: Anemia should be corrected.[Q]
- All other causes of infertility should be excluded.[Q]
- Male factor infertility should be ruled out.[Q] (husband semen analysis should be normal).
- Diagnostic D and Cor endometrial biopsy should be performed in case of irregular cycles, to detect any polyp and to rule out endometrial cancer.[Q]
- Hysteroscopy or HSG: To detect a fibroid encroaching the uterine cavity or a polyp or tubal block.[Q]

N11. Ans. is b, i.e. Myoma screw *Ref: Dutta Gyane 6th/ed p635*

It is a myoma screw:

Uses: To fix the myoma after the capsule is cut open to give traction while the myoma is enucleated of its bed (myomectomy) To give traction in a big uterus (multiple fibroids are requiring hysterectomy while the clamps are placed).

N12. Ans. is b, i.e. Bonneys myoma clamp *Ref: Dutta Gyane 6th/ed p635*

The Figure shows **Bonney myomectomy clamp.**

The clamp is used in myomectomy operation. It curtails the blood supply to the uterus temporarily, thereby minimizing the blood loss during operation. Simultaneous, bilateral clamping of the infundibulopelvic ligaments by rubber guarded sponge holding forceps may be employed.

The instrument is placed at the level of internal os with the concavity fitting with the convexity of the symphysis pubis. The round ligaments of both sides are included inside the clamp to prevent slipping of the instrument and preventing the uterus from falling back. The clamp is removed after suturing the myoma bed but before closing the peritoneal layers.

It is seldom used nowadays. Alternative methods are: Preoperative use of GnRH analogue, and/or intraoperative use of tourniquets, vasoconstrictive agents (vasopressin) and others.

N13. Ans. is b, i.e. Preoperative OC pills *Ref: Dutta Gynae 6th/ed p604*

Measures to control blood loss during myomectomy

- Preoperative **GnRH analogs**
- Moderate degree of **Trendelenburg position** to enhance venous return
- Timing the surgery in **immediate postmenstrual phase.**
- **Hypotensive anaesthesia** (using sodium nitroprusside)
- Use of **vasoconstrictive agents** mainly vasopressin **intraoperatively**
- Use of victor **Bonney's myomectomy clamp** around blood vessels and round ligament
- Use of **tourniquets** around blood vessels
- Uterine **artery embolisation (UAE)**

N14. Ans. is c, i.e. Hysteroscopic myomectomy

This patient is having heavy menstrual bleeding due to fibroid, i.e. she is symptomatic and hence management has to be done. Best management in fibroid is surgery. Since she is only 36 years and has one child ∴ We will go for myomectomy. As discussed in the text, submucous fibroid < 5 cm, should be removed hysteroscopically. ∴ Best management is hysteroscopic myomectomy.

N15. Ans. is d, i.e. TAH

In the question female has heavy menstrual bleeding i.e. symptomatic so treatment is needed. Since multiple fibroids are there, we cannot do myomectomy. We will do TAH, i.e Total abdominal hysterectomy. In 42 years old female, ovaries can be preserved.

N16. Ans. is c, i.e. Type 5 *Ref: Novaks Gynae 15th/ed p445*

The fibroid shown is the figure is subserosal formed with 50% intramural component. Hence it is type 5.

N17. Ans. is a, i.e. Mucous polyp[Q] *Ref: Jeffcoate 7th/ed p488*

- **M/C uterine polp is mucous (endometrial/adenoma) polyp**[Q].
- Polyps are mostly symptomless, if they become ulcerated, then features of menorrhagia/metrorrhagia are seen.
- M/C in postmenopausal females
- Predisposing factors: HRT, tamoxifen therapy and Increased patient age
- IOC = Hysteroscopy
- Management: Hysteroscopy-guided polypectomy.
- Rarely, polyps undergo malignant change (0.5%):
  - Endometrial polyp develops into adenocarcinoma
  - Fibroid polyp into sarcoma
  - Placental polyp into choriocarcinoma.

N18. Ans. is b, i.e. Vascular invasion > 50% *Ref: Robboy's Pathology of Female Repr tract 2nd/ed p474*

Parameter	Leiomyoma	Leiomyosarcoma
Age	30	50
Invasiveness	None	Present
Tumor margin	Distinct	Indistinct
Vascular invasion	None	33%
Size	< 5 cm	> 10 cm
Necrosis	None	tnt
Nuclear atypia	None	Marked
Mitosis	< 5	≥ 10
Abnormal mitosis	None	Frequent
p 16	10%	> 50%
Ki-67	Low (< 5%)	High (≥15%)

N19. Ans. is d, i.e. M/C in white females *(Ref: Jeffcoates 9th/ed, p583; Williams Gynae 3rd/ed, p203)*

We dealt with all the options given in question in the text.

The only option which needs more light- is option d – Fibroid is M/C in white females

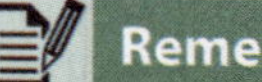

Remember

"The women of certain races, notably African, are especially prone to develop uterine leiomyomas."

– Jeffisates 9/c pg 583

N20. Ans. is a, i.e. MED-12 *(Ref: Williams Gynae 3rd/ed, p203)*

The 2 M/C gene mutations in fibroid are

- MED-12 mutation
- HMGA2 gene mutation

N21. Ans. is b, i.e. Early Menopause-

Fibroid is an estrogen and progesterone dependent tumor. Hence early menarche and late menopause predispose to fibroid and not the vice versa.

N22. Ans. is a, i.e. 0.5% *(Ref: Williams Gynae 3rd/ed, p205)*

"Less than 0.5% of women with leiomyoma develop myomatous erythrocytosis syndrome. This may result from excessive erythropoietin production by kidneys or by the leiomyoma themselves."

N23. Ans. is c, i.e. Amenorrhea *(Ref: Williams Gynae 3rd/ed, p206)*

There is absolutely no confusion now that fibroids can lead to polycythemia especially a broad ligament fibroid.

Fibroids can lead to 2° dysmenorrhea—

"Spasmodic dysmenorrhea is possible when a submucous tumor stimulates expulsive uterine contractions but is not common"

Jeffiorate 9th/ed, p586.

"Leiomyomas occasionally may cause pseudo- Merig syndrome." *–Williams Gynae 3rd/ed, p206.*

N24. Ans. is d, i.e. Age of patient ≥ 50 years *(Ref: Williams Gynae 3rd/ed, p210 Table 9-2)*

Absolute C/I to uterine artery embolization

- Pregnancy
- Active uterine or adnexal infection
- Suspected reproductive tracts malignancy.

Relative C/I:

- Coagulopathy
- Renal impairment
- Desire for future fertility
- Uterine size > 20-24 weeks
- Prior salpingectomy
- Prior pelvic radiation
- Large hydrosalpinx

N25. Ans. is c, i.e. TcRE

See the text for explanation

N26. Ans. is a, i.e. Leuprolide acetate = 1/m *Ref: Williams Gynae 3rd/ed, p208*

GnRH Receptor agents

"Leuprolide acetate is FDA approved for leiomyoma treatment and is available in a 3.75 mg monthly dose or 11.25 mg 3 month dose, both given 1/m" *Ref: Williams Gynae 3rd/ed, p208*

The other 3 GnRH agonist:

- Goserelin
- TRIPTORELIN
- NAFARELIN

Are not FDA approved but used as off label drugs in managing fibroid.

N27. Ans. is d, i.e. 8

See the text for explanation (Fig. 11.8)

N28. Ans. is c, i.e. Hyaline degeneration *Ref: Shaw 16/ed, p397*

Pain in a fibroid can be due to Torsion/Haemorrhage & Red degeneration. Hyaline degeneration is a painless condition.

ANSWERS TO PREVIOUS YEAR QUESTIONS

1. Ans. is b, i.e. Squamous metaplasia

Fibromyoma can have following complications and degenerative changes:

Complications	Changes/Degenerations	
• Torsion[Q]	• Avoid	= Atrophy
• Hemorrhage[Q]	• Red	= **Red** degeneration
• Infection[Q]	• Hot	= **H**yaline degeneration (MC)
• Ascites; pseudo-Meig's syndrome[Q] (Produced by pedunculated[Q] subserous fibroid)[Q]	• Fatty	= **Fatty** degeneration or calcification
	• Meat	= **M**yxomatous degeneration
	• Of chicken	= **C**ystic degeneration
• Malignant change[Q] (rarest)		
	***(Mnemonic:** Avoid Red hot fatty meat of chicken)*	

2. Ans. is c, i.e. Red degeneration of fibroid *Ref: Shaw 15th/ed p355; Dutta Obs 6th/ed p314; High Risk Pregnancy 2nd/ed p77*

Friends, the answer is quite obvious but let's see how other options can be ruled out.

Option "a" Preterm labor

Points in favor	Points against
• Patient is pregnant	• Preterm labor is diagnosed
• Pain in abdomen at 28 weeks (preterm labor is where labor starts before the 37th completed weeks. The lower limit is 28 weeks in developing countries and 20 weeks in developed countries	– When there are regular uterine contractions. (Not acute pain) With or without pain at least in every 10 minutes. – Dilatation of cervix is > 2 cm – Effacement of cervix = 80% – Length of cervix as measured by TVS < 2.5 cm and funneling of the internal OS. – Pelvic pressure backache, vaginal discharge, or bleeding. None of the above criteria are being fulfilled
	• Presence of leukocytosis and fever can also go against it as even if there is intra-amniotic infection causing preterm labor features like—fever, leukocytosis, uterine tenderness, and fetal tachycardia are absent. Rather, if these features are present it means a final stage of uterine infection has reached. And here our patient is having fever, leukocytosis without regular uterine contractions (off and on pair) but with acute pain in abdomen, so it can be ruled out

Option "b" Torsion of fibroid

Points in favor	Points against
• Patient has fibroid (Though no mention has been made whether it is pedunculated or not, Remember torsion is seen in subserous pedunculated myomas)[Q] • Patient is complaining of acute pain in abdomen	• Torsion is not associated with fever and leukocytosis

Option "d" Infection of fibroid

Points in favor	Points against
• Presence of fibroid (*Remember*: Infection is common in submucous fibroids)[Q] • Fever • Leukocytosis	• Acute pain in abdomen (Infection of fibroid will not cause acute pain in abdomen). • Infection of fibroid occurs following abortion or labor (Here patient is pregnant but there is no history of abortion or labor) • Infection causes blood stained discharge (Not seen in this patient)

So, from above discussion infection can be kept in ± status. If we have no better option, we can think about it.

Option "c" i.e. Red degeneration of fibroid is the diagnosis–let's have a look.

Red degeneration of fibroid

- It is seen mostly during pregnancy and mid pregnancy[Q]
- The myoma suddenly becomes acutely painful[Q], enlarged,[Q] and tender.[Q]
- **Patient presents with:**
  - Acute abdominal pain[Q]
  - Vomiting[Q]
  - Malaise[Q]
  - Slight fever[Q]

Lab investigations: Show moderate leukocytosis^Q and raised ESR^Q

Thus, all the features given in the question favor the diagnosis of red degeneration.

3. **Ans. is b, i.e. Immediate surgical intervention is needed** *Ref: Shaw 15th/ed p355; Jeffcoate 7th/ed p502*

   See the text for explanations.

4. **Ans. is a, i.e. Second trimester** *Ref: Jeffcoate 7th/ed p502*

   Friends, answer to this question was quite obvious as each one of us have mugged it up; but finding an appropriate reference was a difficult task.

   Read for yourself what *Ref: Dutta Obs. 6th/ed p309 has to say*

   "Red degeneration; It predominantly occurs in a large fibroid during the second half of pregnancy or puerperium."

   From the above statement answer could be second trimester, third trimester or puerperium.

   "Red degeneration; manifests typically about midpregnancy when the leiomyoma suddenly become acutely painful, enlarged and tender." *Ref: Jeffcoate 7th/ed p502*

   This clears the doubts and confirms our answer, i.e. red degeneration is most common during second trimester (mid pregnancy).

   Friends you should also keep in mind the following important points regarding-**Fibroids and pregnancy.**

   - Most fibroids do not increase in size during pregnancy.
   - Only 5% females with fibroid have degeneration during pregnancy.

5. **Ans. is b, i.e. Radiofrequency ablation** *Ref: Shaw 15th/ed p360-2; Jeffcoate 7th/ed p497-9; Dutta Gynae 5th/ed p269-73*

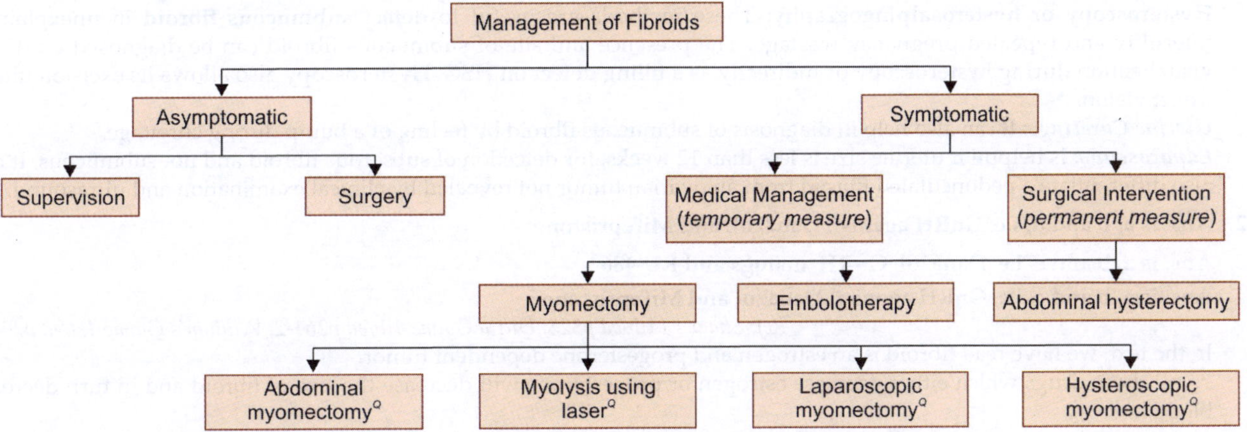

6. **Ans. is a, i.e. Myomectomy** *Ref: Shaw 15th/ed p 360; Jeffcoate 7th/ed p 496-8*

   First, let us see whether we would like to go for medical management or surgical intervention.

   The patient is presenting with:

   - Severe menorrhagia^Q
   - Chronic lower abdomen pain^Q

   These indications are strong enough for surgical intervention. Earlier size of fibroid >12 weeks was also an indication for surgery but nowadays it is not.

   Now comes the question – whether myomectomy or hysterectomy should be done.

   Indication of Myomectomy: Myomectomy is specifically indicated in an infertile woman or woman desirous of bearing child and wishing to retain her uterus.

   Since, our patient, Sucheta is just 29 years and nulliparous – Myomectomy should be done.

7. **Ans. is a, i.e. Interstitial** *Ref: Shaw 15th/ed p352*

   - Most common variety of fibroid is intramural/interstitial (75%) followed by submucous (15%) and subserous (10%).
   - To start with all fibroids are intramural/interstitial.^Q

8. **Ans. is b, i.e. Subserous** *Ref: Dutta Gynae 6th/ed p265*

   "Calcareous degeneration usually involves the subserous fibroids with small peduncle or myomas of postmenopausal women. It is usually preceded by fatty degeneration. There is precipitation of calcium carbonate or calcium phosphate within the tumor, when whole of the tumor is converted into a calcified mass it is termed as 'womb stone'" *Ref: Dutta Gynae 5th/ed p265*

9. **Ans. is a, i.e. Endometriosis** *Ref: Jeffcoate 7th/ed p490*

Diseases commonly associated with leiomyomas are:
a. *Follicular cysts of ovary*^Q
b. *Endometrial hyperplasia*^Q
c. *Endometrial cancer*^Q
d. *Endometriosis*^Q

- It is sometimes said salpingitis (i.e. pelvic inflammatory disease) is a common finding in patients of fibroid, but it is not true, the only possible link between the two is infertility (so **option "b"** is ruled out)
- Leiomyomas are associated with follicular cysts of ovaries (Not ovarian cancer-ruling out **option "c"**).
- Most common symptom of fibroid is menorrhagia and not amenorrhea (so obviously amenorrhea is not correct).

Now coming to the last option – Tamoxifen.

Tamoxifen causes Endometrial hyperplasia[Q] and Endometrial cancer, not Fibromyoma.

10. Ans. is a, i.e. Analgesics *Ref: Shaw 15th/ed p364; Dutta Obs 6th/ed p309; Jeffcoate 7th/ed p502*

Management of red degeneration of fibroid.

- Patient is managed conservatively using analgesics, antipyretics and antiemetics.[Q]

- **No need of**
  - Antibiotics
  - Myomectomy
  - Termination of pregnancy

11. Ans. is a, b and c, i.e. Hysteroscopy; Hysterosalpingography; and USG (Transabdominal)

Ref: John Hopkin's Manual of Obs and Gynae 4th/ed p449; William's Gynae 1st/ed p203; Dutta Gynae 6th/ed p278-9

USG: Ultrasound is the most readily available, least costly imaging technique to diagnose fibroid.[Q] It checks the number[Q], location[Q], and size[Q] of fibroids and helps to reduce overlooking small fibroids during surgery (which might lead to persistence or recurrence of symptoms).

Sonohysterography – is instillation of saline into endometrial cavity during TVS

Hysteroscopy or hysterosalpingography: These methods are useful to detect **submucous fibroid** in unexplained infertility and repeated pregnancy wastage. The presence and site of submucous fibroid can be diagnosed by direct visualization during hysteroscopy or indirectly as a filling defect on HSG. Hysteroscopy also allows its excision under direct vision.

Uterine Curettage: It can also help in diagnosis of submucous fibroid by feeling of a bump during curettage.[Q]

Laparoscopy: is helpful if uterine size is less than 12 weeks, for detection of subserous fibroid and not submucous. It can also differentiate a pedunculated fibroid from an ovarian tumor not revealed by clinical examination and ultrasound.

12. Ans. is a, b and d, i.e. GnRH against; Danazol; and Mifepristone

13. Ans. is a, b and c, i.e. Danazol; GnRH analogs and RU-486

14. Ans. is a, b and c, i.e. GnRH agonist, Danazol and Mifepristone

Ref: Shaw's 14th/ed p323; Dutta Gynae 4th/ed p261-2; William's Gynae 1st/ed p204-5

In the text, we have read fibroid is an estrogen and progesterone dependent tumor.

∴ All those drugs which either decrease estrogen or progesterone will decrease the size of fibroid and in turn decrease blood loss.

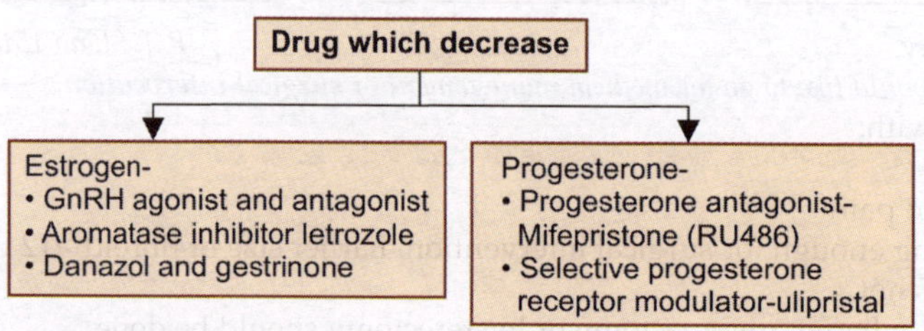

Mnemonic

Drugs which decrease size of fibroid and hence ↓ blood loss:

U:	Ulipristal
Are	Aromatase inhibitor–Letrozole
Gynae	GnRH agonist
	GnRH antagonist
M	Mifepristone
D	Danazol/Gestrinone

Drugs which decrease blood loss but will not have any effect on size of fibroid.

- **OCP's:** When given continuously can cause amenorrhea, but will not decrease the size of fibroid (as fibroid is Estrogen + Progesterone dependent).
- **Progesterone:** When given continuously will cause amenorrhea, but will not decrease the size of fibroid.
- **Tranexamic acid:** Will decrease blood loss but not affect the size of fibroid.

Mechanism of action:

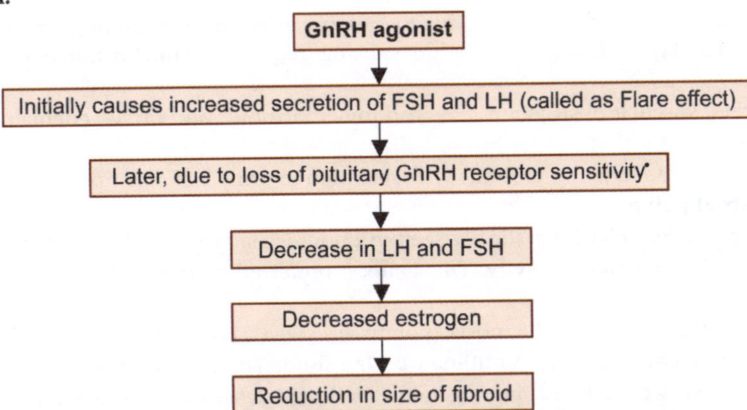

GnRH analogs cause reduction in size (50%) when used for a period of 6 months. But size comes back to previous state after the drug is withdrawn and the hypoestrogenic state induced by GnRH-agonists causes significant loss after 6 months of therapy.

"Because of these limitations of GnRH agonist therapy, The American College of Obstetricians and Gynaecologists currently recommends it only as a temporizing agent in women nearing menopause or as surgical pretreatment in selected women."

Ref: William's Gynae 1st/ed p205

GnRH analogs are used preoperatively:

- To decrease the vascularity and blood loss during surgery
- To induce amenorrhea - to build up hemoglobin in cases of anemia
- May facilitate laparoscopic or hysteroscopic surgery.

GnRH antagonist: They don't cause initial stimulatory effect and cause immediate suppression of pituitary and thus, decrease the size of fibroid.

15. **Ans. is a and c, i.e. Follow-up and Myomectomy** *Ref: Williams Gynae 1st/ed p205*

The question here does not specify whether the fibroid is asymptomatic or symptomatic.

In case of asymptomatic fibroid–

"Regardless of their size, asymptomatic leiomyomas usually can be managed expectantly by annual pelvic examination (ACOG 2001). If the assessment of the adnexa is hindered by uterine size or contour, some may choose to add annual sonographic surveillance."

Ref: Williams Gynae 1st/ed p203

So management of an asymptomatic fibroid is–simply follow-up

In case of symptomatic fibroid –

Medical management is a temporary measure and should be undertaken with the sole purpose of decreasing the size of fibroid or building hemoglobin levels, in females awaiting surgery.

Surgical management:

Between myomectomy and hysterectomy–

Myomectomy is preferred here because patient is too young (only 26 years) and may desire future pregnancy.

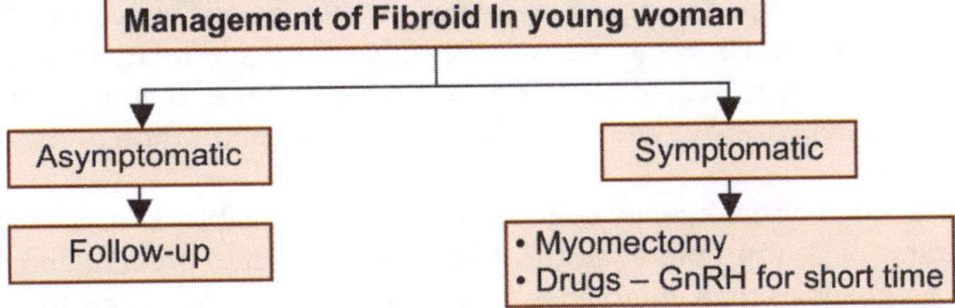

16. **Ans. is a, i.e. 0.5%**
17. **Ans. is b, i.e. Malignancy** *Ref: Shaw 15th/ed p353-5; Jeffcoate 7th/ed p500-2*
    - Sarcomatous change is seen in 0.2–0.5% of fibroids. It is the least common complication of fibroid.
    - Sarcomas with malignant behavior have ≥ 10 mitoses/high power field.
    - M/c fibroid to undergo malignancy is Submucous followed by Intramural.

Ref: Textbook of Gynae Sheila Balakrishnan 1st/ed p163

Ref: Shaw 15th/ed p356-7; Jeffcoate 7th/ed p492-3

18. **Ans. is a, i.e. Amenorrhea**

Fibroids do not lead to amenorrhea, they lead to menorrhagia/metrorrhagia

19. Ans. is a, i.e. Frequency of urine *Ref: Dutta Gynae 6th/ed p284*

Symptoms of cervical fibroid are predominantly due to pressure effect on surrounding structures.

Anterior cervical fibroid irritates the trigone of bladder causing frequency of micturition or even retention due to pressure effects.

In lateral cervical fibroid, vascular obstruction may lead to hemorrhoids and rarely, edema of legs. The ureter is pushed laterally and below the tumor.

Posterior cervical fibroid predominantly presents with retention of urine and constipation.

20. Ans. is a, i.e. Endometrial polyp *Ref: Shaw's Textbook of Gynecology 15th/ed p103*

The HSG shows a filling defect, characteristically seen in Endometrial polyps. Polyps may be seen as pedunculated or sessile-filling defects within the uterine cavity. This is not a preferred method for evaluation compared with the other modalities.

Although not always necessary for a diagnosis, polyps are well characterized on sonohysterography and appear as echogenic, smooth, intracavitary masses outlined by the fluid. The typical appearance of an endometrial polyp at sonohysterography is as a well-defined, homogenous, polypoid lesion that is isoechoic to the endometrium with preservation of the endometrial-myometrial interface. There is usually a well-defined vascular pedicle within the stalk.

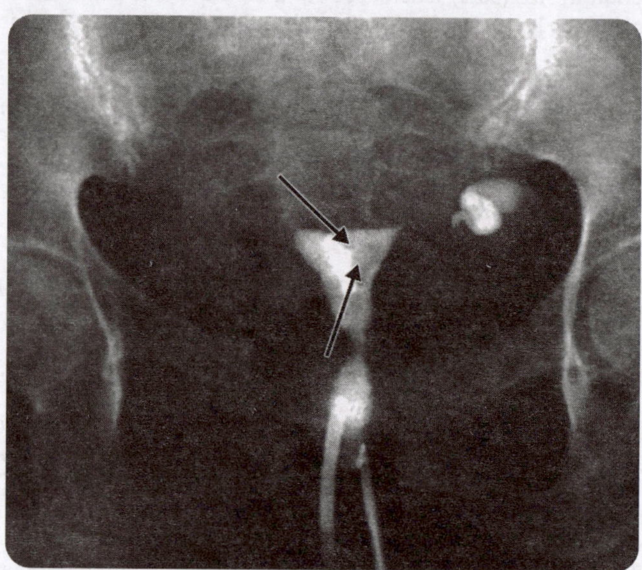

21. Ans. is d, i.e. Selective progesterone receptor modulator *Ref: Harrison's Principles of Internal medicine 19th/ed p2391*

Ulipristal acetate (trade name EllaOne in the European Union, Ella in the US for contraception, and Esmya for uterine fibroid) is a selective progesterone receptor modulator (SPRM).

1. **Pharmacodynamics**

   As an SPRM, ulipristal acetate has partial agonistic as well as antagonistic effects on the progesterone receptor. It also binds to the glucocorticoid receptor, but is only a weak antiglucocorticoid relative to mifepristone, and has no relevant affinity to the estrogen, androgen and mineralocorticoid receptors. Phase II clinical trials suggest that the mechanism might consist of blocking or delaying ovulation and of delaying the maturation of the endometrium.

2. **Medical Uses**
   - **Emergency contraception:** For emergency contraception, a 30 mg tablet is used within 120 hours (5 days) after an unprotected intercourse or contraceptive failure. It has been shown to prevent about 60% of expected pregnancies, and prevents more pregnancies than emergency contraception with levonorgestrel.
   - **Treatment of uterine fibroids:** Ulipristal acetate is used for preoperative treatment of moderate to severe symptoms of uterine fibroids in adult women of reproductive age in a daily dose of a 5 mg tablet. Treatment of uterine fibroids with ulipristal acetate for 13 weeks effectively controlled excessive bleeding due to uterine fibroids and reduced the size of the fibroids.

3. **Interactions**

   Ulipristal acetate is metabolized by CYP3A4 in vitro. Ulipristal acetate is likely to interact with substrates of CYP3A4, like rifampicin, phenytoin, St John's wort, carbamazepine or ritonavir. Therefore, concomitant use with these agents is not recommended. It might also interact with hormonal contraceptives and progestogens such as levonorgestrel and other substrates of the progesterone receptor, as well as with glucocorticoids.

4. **Adverse Effects**

   Common side effects include abdominal pain and temporary menstrual irregularity or disruption. Headache and nausea were observed under long-term administration (12 weeks), but not after a single dose.

5. **Contraindications**

   Ulipristal acetate should not be taken by women with severe liver diseases because of its CYP-mediated metabolism. It has not been studied in women under the age of 18.

   Pregnancy: Unlike levonorgestrel, and like mifepristone, ulipristal acetate is embryotoxic in animal studies. Before taking the drug, a pregnancy must be excluded.

22. Ans. is b, c, d, and e, i.e. LNG IUCD , Mifepristone, GnRH agonist and GnRH antagonist

Ref: Williams Gynae 15/ed p450

"The levonorgestrel releasing IUCD may be a reasonable treatment for selected women with fibroid associated menorrhagia."

Ref: Novaus 15/ed p450

"The immediate suppression of endogenous GnRH by daily subcutaneous injection of GnRH antagonist Ganirelix results in a 29%. reduction in fibroid volume within 3 weeks." *Ref: Novaus 15/ed p450*

"Treatment with GnRH – a decrease uterine volume, fibroid volume & bleeding." *Ref: Novaus 15/ed p449*

23. Ans. is a, b and d, i.e. Mostly asymptomatic, Red degeneration occurs and Mifepristone is used for treatment

See the text for explanation.

24. Ans. is a, b and c, i.e. Follow-up, OCP & Myomectomy

Since the female is young - 26 years, management options are:

(1) Follow-up - If fibroid is asymptomatic

(2) Myomectomy - If fibroid is symptomatic

(3) OCP i.e. medical management if patient refuses surgery or if surgery is contraindicated.

25. Ans. is a, i.e. GnRH analogue

See the text for explanation.

REVIEW/PRACTICE QUESTIONS

1. **All are true about uterine artery embolization:**
   a. Done by interventional radiologist using polyvinyl alcohol microspheres
   b. The angiographic catheter is placed in female artery
   c. Single uterine artery is embolized
   d. Both uterine arteries are embolized
2. **All of the following are not done in management of red degeneration of fibroid *except*:**
   a. Antibiotics
   b. Analgesics
   c. Myomectomy
   d. Termination of pregnancy.
3. **All of the following are true about sarcomatous changes in a fibroid *except*:**
   a. To Naked eye it appears yellowish grey in colour
   b. Soft and friable in consistency
   c. Non encapsulated
   d. Covered by a pseudocapsule
4. **Wombstone appearance of fibroid is seen in:-**
   a. Hyaline degeneration
   b. Red degeneration
   c. Calcareous degeneration
   d. Atrophy
5. **All of the following changes may be seen in fibroid *except*:**
   a. Degeneration
   b. Atrophy
   c. Squamous metaplasia
   d. Sarcomatous charge
6. **Acute pain in fibroid may be seen in all *except*:**
   a. Torsion
   b. Haemorrhage
   c. Red degeneration
   d. Calcareous degeneration
7. **A 25-year-old lady with submucosal fibroid was undergoing myomectomy. The surgeon was using 1.5% glycine as irrigating fluid for the cavity. During the surgery the nurse informs the surgeon that there is a 500 mL fluid deficit. What is the next step to be done?** *(AIIMS May 2018)*
   a. Stop the surgery
   b. Change the fluid to normal saline
   c. Continue the surgery with careful monitoring of fluid status
   d. Give furosemide to the patient and continue surgery
8. **A patient presents with heavy menstrual bleeding. Hysteroscopy was done, which revealed the following finding. What is the most likely diagnosis?**

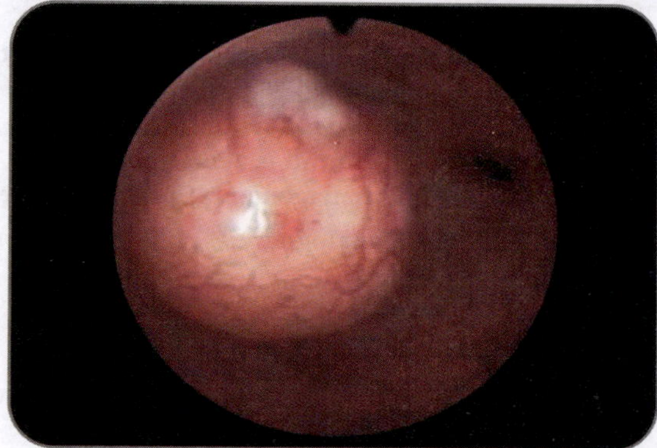

   a. Asherman syndrome
   b. Cervical carcinoma
   c. Endometrial carcinoma
   d. Submucosal fibroid
9. **Most common site for fibroids in uterus is:** *(JIPMER May 2019)*
   a. Subserous
   b. Intramural
   c. Subserous
   d. Cervical

REVIEW/PRACTICE ANSWERS

1. **Ans is c, i.e. Single uterine artery is embolized** *Ref: Williams gynae 3rd/ed, I p209.*
2. **Ans is b, i.e. Analgesics**
3. **Ans is d, i.e. Covered by a pseudocapsule** *Ref: Shaw gynae 15th/ed, p355*
4. **Ans is c, i.e. Calcareous degeneration** *Ref: Shaw 15th/ed, p354*
5. **Ans is c, i.e. Squamous metaplasia** *Ref: Shaw 15th/ed, p353-355.*
6. **Ans is d, i.e. Calcareous degeneration** *Ref: Shaw 15th/ed, p357*
7. **Ans. is c i.e. Continue the surgery with careful monitoring of fluid status**
   Ref: BSGE/ESGE guideline on management of fluid distension media in operative hysteroscopy/Williams Gaynae 3/e pg 903, 904
   - A fluid deficit of more than 1000 mL should be used as threshold to define fluid overload when using hypotonic solutions glycine 1.5%, sorbitol 3% in healthy women of reproductive age. A fluid deficit of 2500 mL should be used as threshold to define fluid overload when using isotonic solutions (Normal saline) in healthy women of reproductive age. Surgery is immediately stopped on reaching these limits. (ACOG 2013 Guidelines)

Distension Media

Because the anterior and posterior uterine walls lie in apposition, a distension medium is required to expand the endometrial cavity for viewing. Fluid media include saline, and low-viscous fluids, such as sorbitol, mannitol, and glycine solutions (Table 1). Historically, carbon dioxide was used for diagnostic hysteroscopy but is infrequently employed today. Each group has distinct advantages and properties. To expand the cavity, intrauterine pressures of these media must reach 45 to 80 mm Hg. Rarely is more than 100 mm Hg required. Moreover, because for most women, mean arterial pressure approximates 100 mm Hg, higher pressures can result in increased intravasation of media into the patient's circulation to create fluid volume overload.

Table 1: Hysteroscopic Media

Medium	Properties	Indications	Risks	Safety Measures
Gas				
Carbon dioxide	Colorless gas	Diagnostic	Gas embolism	Avoid Trendelenburg Keep flow <100 mL/min Intrauterine pressure <100 mm Hg
Electrolyte fluid				
0.9% saline	Isotonic 380 mOsm/kg H_2O	Diagnostic Operative w/bipolar tools	Volume overload	Plan to complete procedure at 750 mL deficit Stop procedure at 2.5 L deficit End earlier in patients with comorbidities or elderly
Lactated Ringer	Isotonic 273 mOsm/kg H_2O	Same as above	Volume overload	Same as above
Electrolyte-poor fluid				
Sorbitol 3%	Hypoosmolar 178 mOsm/kg H_2O	Operative w/ monopolar tools	Volume overload Hyponatremia Hypoosmolality Hyperglycemia	Plan to complete procedure at 750 mL deficit Stop procedure at 1-1.5L deficit End earlier in patients with comorbidities or elderly
Mannitol 5%	Isoosmolar 280 mOsm/kg H_2O	Operative w/ monopolar tools	Volume overload Hyponatremia	Same as above
Glycine 1.5%	Hypoosmolar 200 mOsm/kg H_2O	Operative w/ monopolar tools	Volume overload Hyponatremia Hypoosmolality Hyperammonemia	Same as above

Data from Cooper, 2000; American Association of Gynecologic Laparoscopists, 2013; American College of Obstetricians and Gynecologists, 2011.

Carbon Dioxide

This gasceous distension medium, when used under pressure, tends to flatten the endometrium and provides excellent visibility. A continuous flow is necessary to replace any gas lost through the tubes, and typically flow rates of 40 to 50 mL/min are adequate. Rates higher than 100 mL/min are associated with increased risks for gas embolism and therefore discouraged. Importantly, because *laparoscopic* insufflating machines can permit flow rates >1000 mL/min, these should not be used for hysteroscopy.

Disadvantages to CO_2 include its tendency, when mixed with blood or mucus, to form visually obstructive gas bubbles. Accordingly, prior to hysteroscope insertion, blood and mucus are carefully removed from the cervical os with a dry swab (Sutton, 2006). Similarly, use of CO_2 with thermal energy sources is avoided as smoke production prohibits adequate viewing. Because of these limitations, CO_2 is best used in cases in which minimal bleeding is anticipated, such as diagnostic hysteroscopy. The most serious complication associated with CO_2 use is venous gas embolism.

Fluid Media

Bleeding is common with operative hysteroscopy procedures. Thus rather than CO_2, fluid media are typically selected because of their optical clarity and ability to mix with blood. The main risk of fluid distension media, however, involves increased fluid absorption and circulatory fluid volume overload.

Fluid distension media can be divided according to their viscosity and electrolyte status. In general, low-viscosity fluids are used in modern hysteroscopy. An appropriate medium is selected based on its compatibility with electrosurgical instrumentation.

Low-viscosity Electrolyte Fluids

Normal saline and lactated Ringer solutions are isotonic, electrolyte fluids. They are readily available in the operating room and are frequently used for diagnostic hysteroscopy. However, these fluids cannot be used with monopolar electrosurgery. Specifically, these solutions conduct current; thus, dissipate the energy; and thereby render the instrument useless.

These electrolyte-containing, isotonic fluids have lower associated risks of hyponatremia compared with hypoosmolar fluids, described in the next section. Still, rapid absorption can lead to pulmonary edema. In general, when using isotonic medium in a healthy patient, a surgeon should consider terminating the procedure when the fluid deficit nears 2500 mL (American Association of Gynecologic Laparoscopists, 2013; American College of Obstetricians and Gynecologists, 2011).

Low-viscosity, Electrolyte-poor Fluids

Of other available media, 1.5-percent glycine, 3-percent sorbitol, and 5-percent mannitol are all low-viscosity, electrolyte-poor fluids. Because they are nonconducting, these media are used for electrosurgery involving monopolar instruments. Unfortunately, these fluids can create volume overload with con-current development of hyponatremia and hypoosmolality and the potential for cerebral edema and death (American College of Obstetricians and Gynecologists, 2011). Mechanistically, sorbitol is a six-carbon sugar and is metabolized following absorption. This effectively leaves free water in the intravascular space. Normal serum sodium levels are 135 to 145 mEq/L, and levels significantly below this may lead to seizure followed by respiratory arrest. In addition, hypokalemia and hypocalcemia can often develop concurrently. Five-percent mannitol, also a six-carbon sugar, is isoosmolar and so has diuretic properties but does not lead to serum osmolality changes (American Association of Gynecologic Laparoscopists, 2013).

In cases in which large fluid volume deficits are calculated, measurement of serum electrolyte levels is warranted. If a serum sodium level lower than 125 mEq/L is reached, postoperative care should be continued in a critical care setting. Treatment includes stimulation of diuresis with furosemide (Lasix), 20 to 40 mg given intravenously. Correction of hyponatremia is achieved with 3-percent sodium chloride, administered at a rate of 0.5 to 2 mL/kg/hr. In those with acute neurologic symptoms, 3-percent saline can instead be given in a 100 mL infusion over 30 minutes and repeated an additional two times. The goal of therapy is to reach a serum sodium level of 135 mEq/L within 24 hours. Overcorrection is avoided to prevent additional cerebral effects.

To assist with intraoperative fluid volume calculation, most operative hysteroscopes contain continuous flow systems that allow fluid deficits to be calculated. Calculation of deficits is performed every 15 minutes during procedures. If deficits of a hypotonic solution reach 1000 mL, a surgeon should consider procedure termination, measure electrolytes, and give diuretics as indicated (American Association of Gynecologic Laparoscopists, 2013). At the end of every hysteroscopic procedure, a final deficit is determined, and this value is recorded in the operative note.

8. **Ans. is d, i.e. Submucosal fibroid**

   The image shows a small tumor arising from uterus and coming inside the uterine cavity. It is a submucous fibroid.

9. **Ans. is b, i.e. Intramural** *Ref: Shaw's Textbook of Gynaecology, 15th/ed, p352*

   See the chapter on fibroid for explanation.

CHAPTER 12

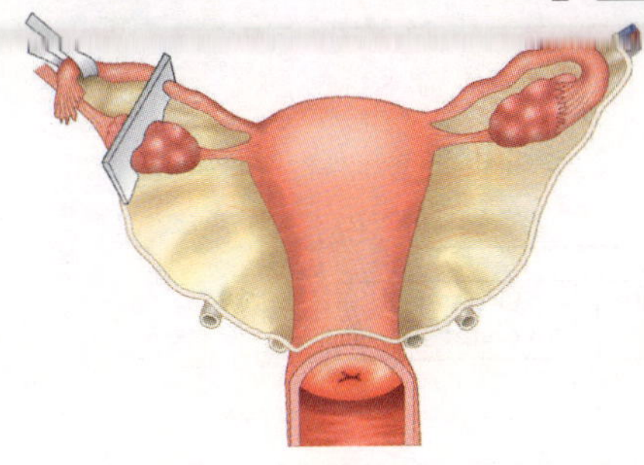

Endometriosis and Dysmenorrhea

Endometriosis

Definition

Endometriosis

The presence of endometrial tissue (glands and stroma) outside of the uterine cavity

Etiology

- Not fully understood
- Many theories have been proposed to explain endometriosis.

Theory	Proposed by	Mechanism
Implantation theory/ Theory of Retrograde menstruation	Sampson	Endometriosis occurs as a result of reflux of menstrual endometrium through the fallopian tubes and its subsequent implantation and growth on ovary, pelvic peritoneum and surrounding structures
Coelomic metaplasia	Meyer and Ivanoff	Endometriosis arises as a result of metaplastic changes in embryonal cell rests of embryonic mesothelium, which are capable of responding to hormone stimulation
Metastatic theory	Halban	Explains occurrence of endometriosis at less accessible sites like umbilicus, pelvic nodes, ureter, etc. The theory suggests embolization of menstrual fragments occurs through vascular or lymphatic channels. This leads to launching of endometriosis at distant sites

Contd...

Contd...

Theory	Proposed by	Mechanism
Histogenesis by induction		The theory proposes that an endogenous (undefined) biochemical factor can induce undifferentiated peritoneal cells to develop into endometrial tissue

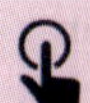

Endometriosis is an estrogen dependant condition
What happens to estrogen in endometriosis patients:
- In patients of endometriosis, both estrogen production and metabolism are altered in ways that promote the disease.
- Also in these women, substantial amounts of estrogen are synthesized locally.

- This estrogen augments PGE 2 production by stimulating Cox-2 enzyme & thus due to increased PGE 2 there is increased inflammation and pain

Risk Factors	Protective Factors
• Family history (7–10 fold increased risk if affected 1st degree relative) • Early menarche and late menopause • Heavy alcohol and caffeine consumption • Nulliparity • High socioeconomic status due to late marriage and late childbirth • *In utero* exposure to DES • Hormone – estrogen dependant condition • Mullerian agenesis leading to early onset of endometriosis @ puberty. • Food rich in fat/obesity	• Regular exercise • Smoking • Pregnancy • Multiparity

Epidemiology

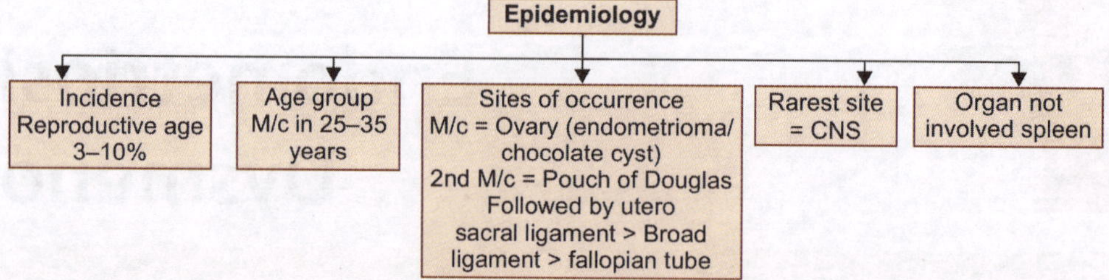

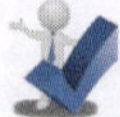

KEY POINTS

Endometriosis can occur anywhere in body including abdominal wall, lung, pleura, brain, and arm. It can also be seen in scars of certain surgeries, then it is called as scar endometriosis.

Scar Endometriosis is seen in

- Hysterotomy scar
- Classical cesarean section scar
- Myomectomy scar
- Ventrofixation scar
- Scar involving section of fallopian tube operation.
- Episiotomy scars.

Extrapelvic Endometriosis

- M/c site for extrapelvic endometriosis is GIT. (In GIT M/c site is sigmoid colon > Rectum).
- M/c site for urinary endometriosis: Bladder > lower ureter.
- Least common in urinary system: kidney.
- Overall the least common site or Rarest site is CNS.

Clinical Features

- May be asymptomatic

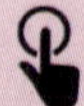

M/c symptom is pain: M/c pain: Secondary dysmenorrhea (commencing after 30 years and gradually increasing) > chronic pelvic pain > Dyspareunia > low backache

- Dyspareunia occurs when pouch of Douglas and rectovaginal septum are involved.

Important Concept

Reason for pain in endometriosis:

1. Direct and indirect effects of focal bleeding from endometriotic implants, as this endometriotic lesion is hormonally active.
2. Actions of inflammatory cytokines in the peritoneal cavity.
3. Invasion or direct infiltration of nerves in pelvic floor. This is the reason why pain coincides with depth of lesion.[Q]

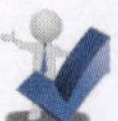

KEY POINTS

- Classic triad of endometriosis
  - Dysmenorrhea
  - Infertility
  - Dyspareunia
- M/c cause of secondary dysmenorrhea is Endometriosis followed by PID

- **2nd M/c presentation of endometriosis is infertility:** 30–40% of patients with endometriosis will be infertile
- 15–30% of those who are infertile will have endometriosis.

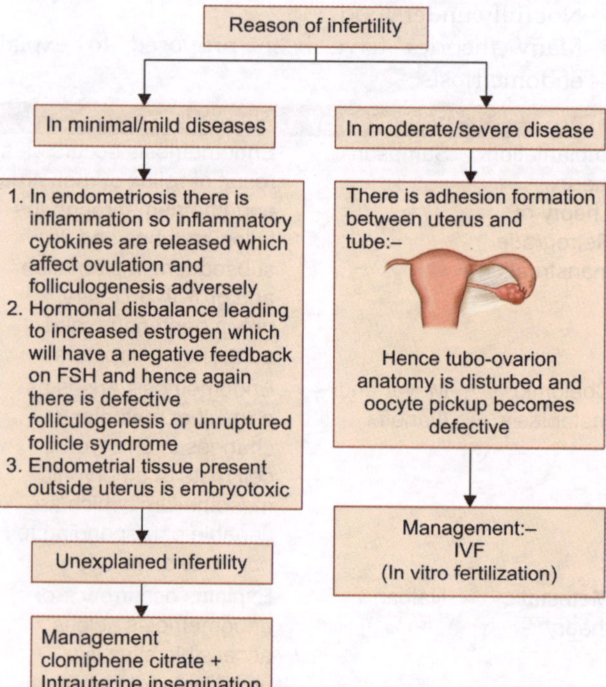

Important One Liners

M/c presentation in endometriosis — Pain
2nd M/c presentation in endometriosis — Infertility
3rd M/c presentation is ovarian mass i.e. Chocolate cyst
4th M/c presentation is menstrual symptoms like menorrhagia as due to excessive estrogen there is proliferation of endometrial tissue.

Examination Findings

- Fixed retroversion of uterus (due to adhesions)
- Firm fixed adnexal mass **(endometrioma)**
- Tender nodularity of uterosacral ligament **(cobble stone appearance)** and cul-de-sac felt on rectovaginal examination

Ovarian Endometriosis

- M/C site of Endometriosis is ovary
- Ovary is involved in 30-40% cases
- There is Bilateral involvement of ovary

Pathology:

- In Endometriosis, due to retrograde menstruation, blood & endometrial tissue shedding from tubes falls on ovary. This endometriotic implant inside ovary is hormonally active and like normal endometrial tissue it will proliferate and shed during menstruation.
- Thus a lot of blood starts collecting in ovary & organises to form a cyst. Now blood in cyst starts undergoing degradation & converts into bilirubin, biliverdin and hemosiderin (brown in colour). Thus this cyst in ovary appears brown in colour & is called as chocolate cyst/Endometrioma.

- Chocolate cyst will have tarry, thick viscous fluid having hemosiderin pigment (Fig. 12.1).

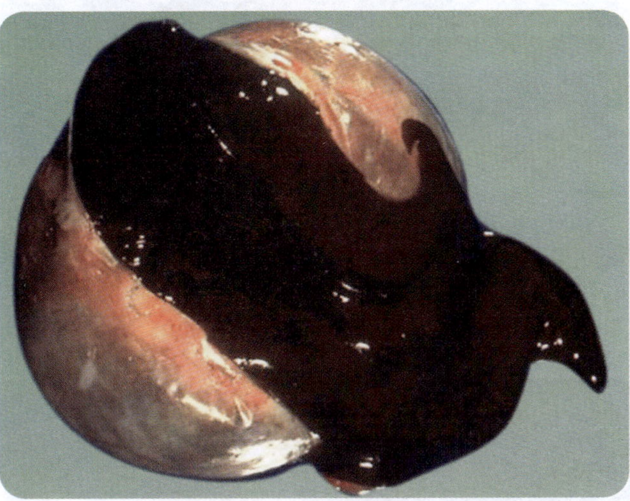

Fig. 12.1: Chocolate cyst with brown tarry liquid

Flowchart 12.1: Findings on Laparoscopy

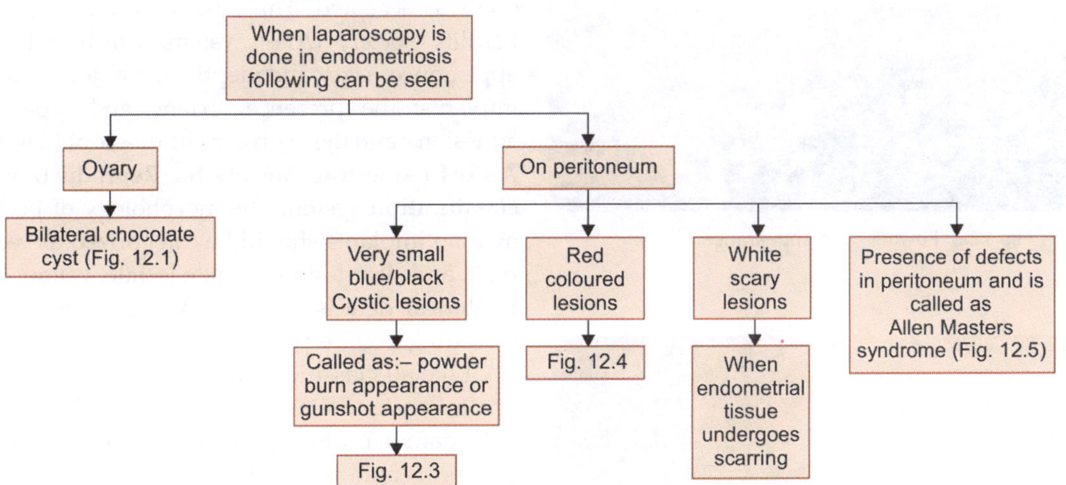

- This cyst is lined by granulation tissue or pseudo xanthoma cells
- Chocolate cyst are bilateral & size will be ≤ 12 cms.
- They may be unilocular (M/C) or multilocular (less common). M/C is menopausal females.
- Because this fluid, they may be contained in other conditions such as corpus luteum cysts ∴ biopsy and preferably removal of the ovarian cysts for histological confirmation are necessary for diagnosis. If this is not possible then following clinical criteria should be used for diagnosis.

- Cyst diameter < 12 cms
- Adhesion present till pelvic side wall or broad ligament
- Endometriosis on surface of ovary
- Tarry thick chocolate colored fluid content

Investigations

1st Investigation = TVS – on TVS chocolate cyst gives ground glass appearance (Fig. 12.2).

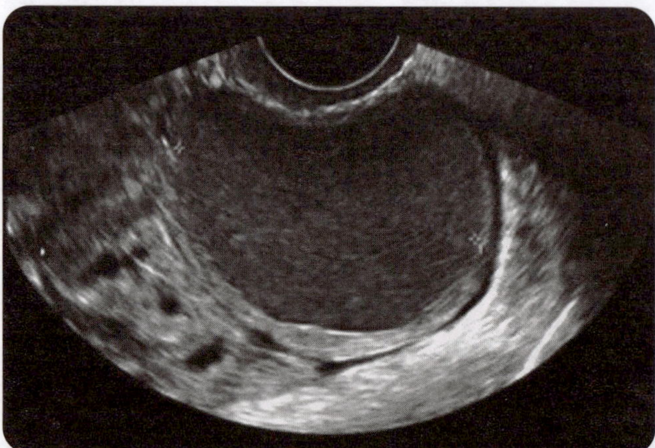

Fig. 12.2: Ground glass appearance in USG of chocolate cyst

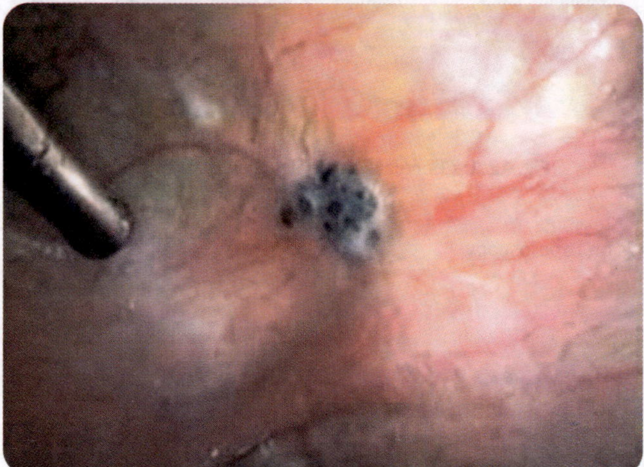

Fig. 12.3: Powder burn appearance

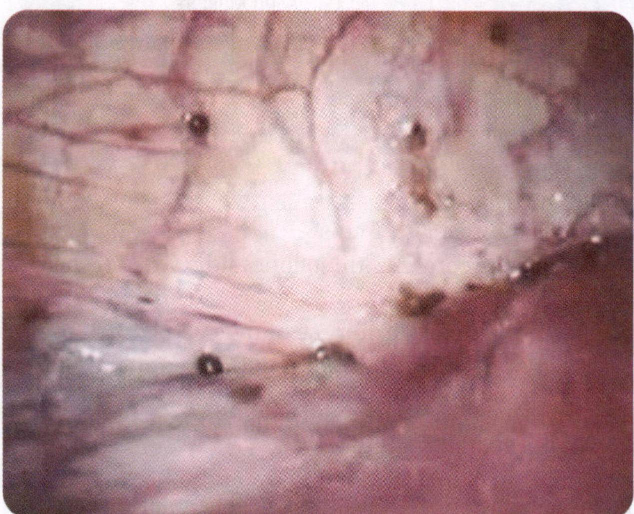

Fig. 12.4: Reddish of chocolate cyst lesions

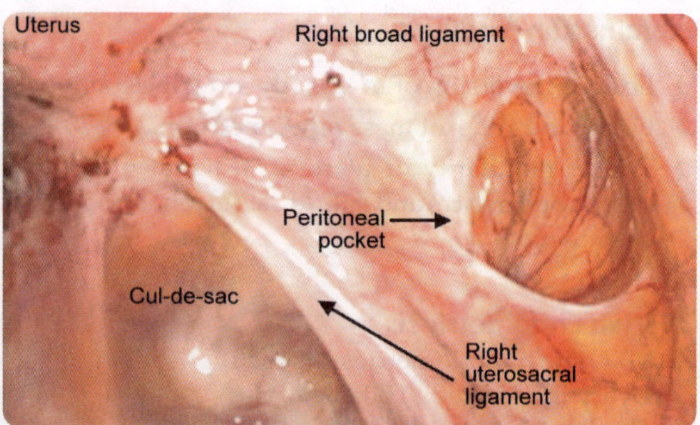

Fig. 12.5: Peritoneal defect: Allen Masters defect

- **IOC: laparoscopy:** Findings seen in laparoscopy. See Flowchart 12.1.
- **Gold standard:** Histopathological examination
- Others = **CA-125** levels are raised in endometriosis.
- Monocyte chemotatic protein (MCP–1) levels are rised in peritoneal fluid of women with endometriosis

Laparoscopic Classification

Many classification systems were proposed, but only one was accepted. This system is the revised American Fertility Society (AFS) system, which is based on the appearance, size, and depth of peritoneal and ovarian implants; the presence, extent, and type of adnexal adhesions; and the degree of cul-de-sac obliteration. **In this ASRM (American Society for Reproductive Medicine) classification system,** the morphology of peritoneal and ovarian implants should be categorized as red (red, red-pink, and clear lesions), white (white, yellow-brown, and peritoneal defects), and black (black and blue lesions), according to color photographs provided by ASRM.

Like all classification systems, the ASRM classification for endometriosis is subjective and correlates poorly with pain symptoms, but may be of value in infertility prognosis and management.

In 2009, a new staging system was proposed, called as **Endometriosis Fertility Index (EFI)**. The EFI score is given from 0 to 10, 0 has poorest and 10 best prognosis.

ASRM Classification of endometriosis:
Minimal: Isolated superficial disease on peritoneal surface.
Mild: Superficial multiple implants <5 cms with no significant adhesions.
Moderate: Multifocal disease, both superficial and invasive and associated with adhesions in tube and/or ovaries.
Severe: Multifocal disease like in moderate cases along with **large ovarian endometriomas** and **adhesions** in tube, ovaries, and **cul de sac**

Treatment

Treatment is justified in all patients regardless of clinical profile as endometriosis progresses in 30–60% patient's within an year of diagnosis.

Management of Endometriosis: consists of

A. Managing pain
B. Managing infertility

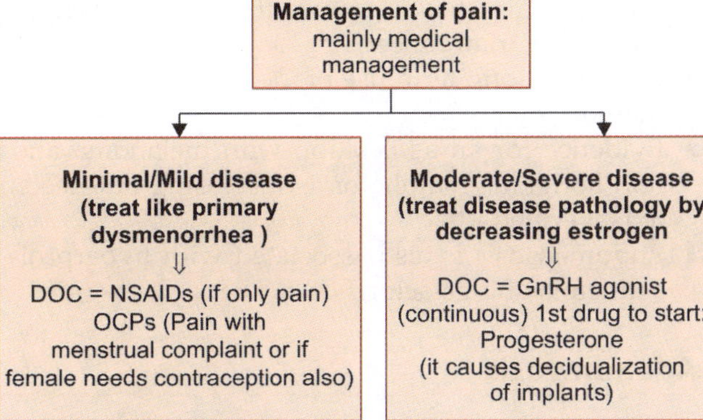

Drugs which can be used: In pain management of endometriosis are all these drugs which decrease estrogen

1. Continuous GnRH (DOC)
2. Progesterone
3. Letrozole (aromatase inhibitor)
4. Danazol
5. Gestrinone
6. Mifepristone

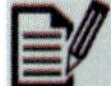

Important Concept

Mechanism of action of various drugs used in Endometriosis:

OCP's: Any low dose OCP (30–35 mcg EE) when given continuously creates pseudo pregnancy like state by inducing amenorrhea and endometrial decidualization. The drawback is:

1. Beakthrough bleeding episodes
2. Reactivation for disease after termination of treatment

Aromatase inhibition: Letrozole or anastrozole act by decreasing peripheral conversion of androgens to estrogens.

Anti progestins (Mifepristone/onapristone): action is based on their anti proliferative effect on endometrium

Dose: Mifepristone = 50–100 mg/day.

Progesterone: Inhibits the growth of endometrial tissue first inducing decidualization and then atrophy. According to Novak 15/e, pg 535, they are the first choice drugs for endometriosis.

- Medroxy progesterone acetate (orally 20–100 mg daily)
- DMPA injection
- LNG IUGD-is more value for females with deeply infiltrating rectovaginal endometriosis.

Contd...

Contd...

Dienogest: It is a semisynthetic progesterone with anti androgenic activity

- Orally active (Dose = 2 mg/day)
- Half-life: 10 hours
- It is as effective as GnRH in relieving pain associated with endometriosis. More trials are undergoing to prove its efficacy.

Remember: Although progestins are effective treatment of pain associated with endometriosis, their adverse effects on fertility limit its use in infertile women seeking pregnancy.

GnRH: Induces hypogonadal state (i.e. continuous GnRH leads to decrease in LHL PSH), which deprives existing disease of estogen and since it brings about amenorrhea, therefore prevents new peritoneal seedling. But its major side effects is decreased bone mineral density

Remember: Almost 75% females become hypogonadal by 4 weeks and 100% by 8 weeks

Example of GnRH: Leuprolide (IM), Goserelin (IM or SC), Triptorelin (IM) and Nafarelin (Nasal)

Danazol: Brings about high androgen and low estrogen environment that inhibits growth of endometriosis.

Dose = 400–800 mg OD for 3–6 months. But due to its androgenic side effects it is not used in young females.

Gestrinone: It has antiprogestational, anti-estrogenic and androgenic effect. Gestrinone unlike GnRH does not lower bone density, but decreased HDL.

Management of Infertility

- *In minimal/mild endometriosis the cause of infertility is unexplained.* Hence, management is superovulation with clomiphene followed by intrauterine insemination.
  This should be tried for 3 cycles and if patient does not conceive in 3 cycles, do IVF (or ICSI).
- *In moderate/severe endometriosis,* causes of infertility are both:

Ovarian (as discussed above) and tubal—there is distorted tubal anatomy and formation of dense adhesions in the tubes.

Management = IVF

Results of infertility management are better with advanced endometriosis as IVF is the management

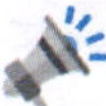

Important One Liners

- Best time to become pregnant in a patient of endometriosis is immediately after surgery
- Recurrence rate: After medical therapy = 30–50%. After conservative surgery = 4–14%

Surgical Management of Endometriosis

Indications:

1 Non responsive to medical management
2. Acute intolerable pain
3. Bowel/urinary tract involvement
4. Chocolate cyst.

Contd...

Contd...

Options:
1. Adhesiolysis
2. Fulguration of implants using laser or cryosurgery
3. Laparoscopic uterosacral nerve ablation if patient has excessive dysmenorrhea
4. Hysterectomy and B/L salpingo-oophorectomy-Reserved for patients with intractable pain who do not want future childbearing.

Note: Ovarian Remnant Syndrome: persistent a recurrent disease and pain associated with residual functional ovarian tissue even after surgery. This is seen more commonly when ovaries are enlarged or densely adhered to pelvic side walls and dissection is technically difficult.

Management of Endometrioma

Laparoscopic management of the endometrioma is the preferred management, i.e. it cannot be medically managed

Important Concept

The most common procedures for ovarian endometriomas are: *Ref: Novar 15th/ed, p527)*

i. **If cyst < 3 cms: Laparoscopic drainage and electrocoagulation**
ii. **If cyst > 3 cms: Laparoscopy cystectomy**
iii. In cases where excision is technically difficult without removing a large part of ovary:

Three steps procedure is done:
1. Marsupialization and rinsing
2. Hormonal treatement with GnRH.
3. Followed after 3 months by cyst wall electrocoagulation or laser vaporization.

Remember

Sites where endometriosis cannot be medically managed:
1. Ovary
2. Bowel
3. Urinary system

Also Know

Triad of symptoms: M/C seen in Endometriosis:

Intertility
Dyspareunia
2° dysmenorrhea

On P/V in Endometriosis:
- Fixed retroverted uterus
- Due to chocolate cyst-get adnexal mass
- Nodules may be palpated on uterosacral ligament called as **Cobblestone** appearance
- If endometriosis occurs in pubertal females always rule out mullerian malformations.

Recent Advances *Ref: Novak 15th/ed, p527*

- Latest edition of Novaks 15th/ed, p 506 and John Hopkins Manual of obs and gynae 4th/ed, p 459—mention increased risk of ovarian cancer (Endometroid and clear cell variety) in women with endometriosis.
- Definitive surgery to remove all visible evidence of endometriosis is not recommended as a prophylactic measure to reduce the risk of development of ovarian cancer.
- However, long term use of OCPs is the preferred method.
- Evidence for an association with melanoma and non hodgkins-lymphoma is increasing but needs to be verified.
- Endometriosis is also associated with hyperprolactinemia and galactorrhea.

Adenomyosis

Adenomyosis is a condition where there is ingrowth of endometrium (both gland + stroma) directly into the myometrium[Q] (Fig. 12.1). Earlier it was called **endometriosis interna.**

The most widely accepted theory regarding adenomyosis development describes the downward invagination of the endometrial basalis layer into the myometrium. The endometrial-myometrial interface is unique in that it lacks an intervening submucosa. Accordingly, even in normal uteri, the endometrium commonly invades the myometrium superficially.

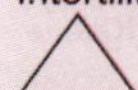

Remember

- Adenomyosis is associated with aromatase expression and higher tissue estrogen levels. Thus it is also a hyperestrogenic condition but unlike the other hyperestrogenic conditions it is not common in nulliparous females.
- Another fact worth noting is that it is M/C in females on SERM- Tamoxifen. Rather use of OCP's is not a risk factor for adenomyosis.

Age group : Mature reproductive patients > 40 years[Q]
Parity : Multiparous[Q]
Symptoms : Most common symptom: *Menorrhagia*[Q]
2nd most common symptom: *Dysmenorrhea*[Q]
Note: In adenomyosis intensity of pain correlates with number of lesions and depth of invasion
Presenting feature: Menorrhagia and secondary Dysmenorrhea

On per vaginal examination: Symmetrical enlargement of uterus[Q] (not more than 10–12 weeks of pregnancy, i.e. < 14 cms in size)[Q], mobility not restricted, (*Note:* In endometriosis uterus was fixed. Here in adenomyosis it is mobile) no associated adnexal pathology (whereas in endometriosis chocolate cyst were felt).

Halban's sign - ***tender, softened uterus*** on premenstrual bimanual examination.

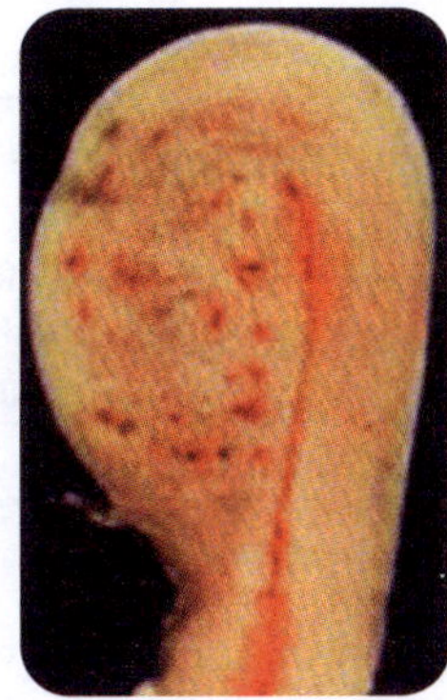

Fig. 12.6: Gross appearance of adenomyosis

The surface contour of uterus is smooth regular reddish and soft. It has focal areas of hemorrhage.

Diagnosis

- IOC - USG (TVS)

TVS Findings

- **Diffuse myometrial bulkiness typically of posterior uterine wall**
- Myometrium is heterogeneous with hyperechoic areas representing endometrial glands and hypoechoic areas showing muscle hypertrophy. This heterogeneous appearance is **called as salt and pepper appearance** (Fig. 12.7).
- Thickening of transition zone ≥ 12 mm thick
- **Myometrial cyst** (most specific sign) (Fig. 12.7).

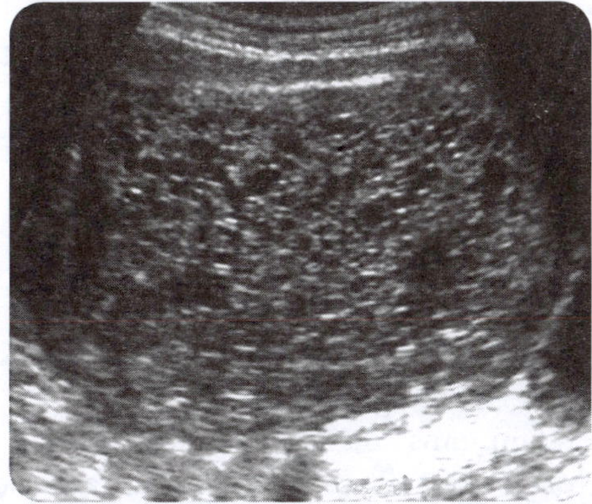

Fig. 12.7: Enlarged uterus with typical features of adenomyosis: Multiple bright ectogenic foci are seen throughout the myometrium (Salt and pepper appearance).

- **Subendometrial striations** called as **Venetian Blind appearance**.

MRI Findings (T2 weighted image): IOC

- Thickening of junctional zone ≥ 12 mm (normal is up to 5 mm)
- Diffusely enlarged uterus especially posterior part

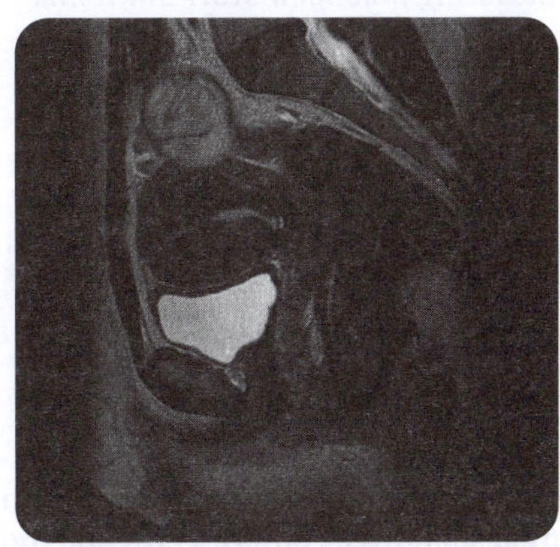

Fig. 12.8: MRI of adenomyosis

HPE Findings (Fig. 12.9)

- Endometrial glands are present in myometrium surrounded by stroma. These glands should be 2.5 mm deep to junctional zone
- Myometrial cells show hyperplasia and hypertrophy

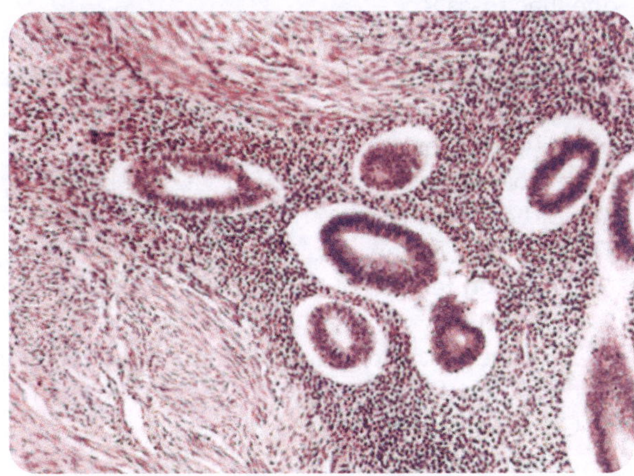

Fig. 12.9: HPE of for adenomyosis

Remember for Adenomyosis

- IOC – TVS
- Gold standard–histopathological examination after hysterectomy

IOC is TVS: as clear from following lines of Williams Gynae 3/e

"TAS does not consistently identify the often subtle myometrial changes of adenomyosis, thus imaging with TVS is preferred. In comparison, MR imaging may be equal or slightly superior to TVS. Thus, MR imaging may be appropriate when diagnosis is in conclusive, when further deliberation would affect patient management or when coexisting myoma distort anatomy."

Management

- TOC–Surgery (total hysterectomy)[Q] in most of the patient, as most of the patients are elderly.
- In younger women–progesterone pills, Levonorgestrel containing IUCDs, GnRH, or Aromatase Inhibitors can be given
- Recently uterine artery embolization is being tried.

Mittelschmerz/Ovular Pain

- **A female giving history of sharp pain in lower abdomen, every month, 2 weeks before menstruation suggests mittelschmerz as the diagnosis.**
- Mittelschmerz is synonymous to painful ovulation. Pain is associated with rupture of ovarian follicle at the time of ovulation

Characteristics

- It appears in the mid-menstrual period.[Q]
- Pain is usually situated in the hypogastrium or to one iliac fossa.[Q]
- Pain is usually located on one side and does not change side according to which ovary is ovulating.[Q]
- Nausea and vomiting is conspicuously absent.[Q]
- It rarely lasts for more than 12 hours.[Q]
- It may be associated with slight vaginal bleeding or mucoid discharge.[Q]
- The probable factors are:
  - Increased tension of Graafian follicle just prior to rupture.[Q]
  - Peritoneal irritation by follicular fluid following ovulation.[Q]
  - Contraction of tubes and uterus.[Q]

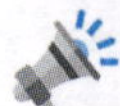

Important One Liners

Important one liner
A young female giving history of pain in lower abdomen, every month- two weeks before menstruation suggests **Mittleschmerz** as the diagnosis.

Management

- Assurance and analgesics
- In refractory cases, cycles are made anovular by giving OCPs.

Also Know

The phenomenon of ovulation bleeding or mucus tinged with blood at the time of ovulation is called as mittlebutt.[Q] This may be associated with ovulation pain, although each may occur independently.

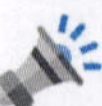

Important One Liners

Right ovarian vein syndrome: Right ovarian vein crosses the ureter at right angle. During premenstrual period, due to pelvic congestion or increased blood flow, there may be marked engorgement in the vein → pressure on ureter → stasis → infection → pyelonephritis → pain.

Premenstrual Disorders

- Frequently women of reproductive age experience symptoms during the late luteal phase of their menstrual cycle, and collectively these complaints are termed **premenstrual syndrome (PMS) or premenstrual dysphoric disorder (PMDD)**
- It is mostly seen in women aged to 30–45 years

Symptoms

The patients must have at least **five** of the following symptoms for most of the time during the premenstrual week, with symptoms remitting completely in the postmenstrual week (in order to make the diagnosis, the symptoms must be characteristic of PMS/PMDD, limited to luteal phase and not attributable to a general medical condition):

- Depressed mood, hopelessness, self-depreciation
- Anxiety tension
- Affective lability
- Anger, irritability, and interpersonal conflict
- Decreased interest in usual activities
- Difficulty in concentrating
- Decreased energy
- Appetite changes or cravings
- Changes in sleep
- Feeling overwhelmed or out of control
- Physical symptoms such as breast tenderness, headache, bloating

The symptoms markedly interfere with work, family, or academic responsibilities; are not only exacerbations of another existing disorder and are corroborated by at least 2 months of prospective daily ratings.

Pathophysiology of Premenstrual Syndromes (PMS)

The exact causes of premenstrual disorders are unknown, although several different biologic factors have been suggested. Of these, estrogen and progesterone, as well as the neurotransmitters, γ-amino butyric acid (GABA), and serotonin have been implicated.

Treatment of PMS

Conservative measures	Inhibition of ovulation	Medications directed at symptoms
• Elimination of caffeine from diet • Smoking cessation • Counselling, emotional support • Low-fat, high-fiber diet, and essential fatty acids in diet. • Regular exercise • Adequate sleep • Stress reduction	• Oral contraceptives (especially drospirenone containing) • GnRH agonist	• For fluid retention: diuretics • For pain: prostaglandin synthetase inhibitor • For mastalgia: evening primrose oil and pyridoxine • For anxiety/depression: SSRI like fluoxetine are preferred Tricyclic antidepressants can also be used.

NEW PATTERN QUESTIONS

N1. M/c accepted theory for endometriosis is:
a. Implantation theory
b. Coelomic metaplasia
c. Metastatic theory
d. Histogenesis theory

N2. All of the following protect against endometriosis *except*:
a. Pregnancy
b. Nulliparity
c. Exercise
d. Smoking

N3. Scar endometriosis can occur following:
a. Classical cesarean section
b. Hysterotomy
c. Episiotomy
d. All of the above

N4. A 30-year-old female complains of infertility for 2 years with dysmenorrhea and dyspareunia. On bimanual examination, her uterus is retroverted with limited mobility and tenderness in pouch of Douglas. What is the next step in management?
a. Perform a diagnostic laparoscopy
b. Perform an HSG
c. Perform TVS
d. Perform a laparotomy

N5. In same patient as in QN4-if TVS scan is normal and patient wishes to conceive soon. What is the next step in management:
a. Perform a diagnostic laparoscopy
b. Perform an HSG
c. Treat with medroxy progesterone acetate
d. Treat with GnRH analogues

N6. Best investigation to establish the diagnosis of endometriosis is:
a. Laparoscopy
b. USG
c. X-ray pelvis
d. CT Scan

N7. M/c site for extrapelvic endometriosis is:
a. Broad ligament
b. Sigmoid colon
c. Rectum
d. Ovary

N8. Which of the following drugs not used in endometriosis?
a. Danazol
b. Progestin
c. GnRH agonist
d. Misoprost

N9. A 40-year-old infertile woman suspected to be suffering from endometriosis is subjected to diagnostic laparoscopy. Findings indicate - uterus normal, both the ovaries show presence of chocolate cysts; endometriotic deposits are seen on the round ligament right side, both the fallopian tubes and the pouch of Douglas; moderately dense adhesions are present between the fallopian tubes and the pouch of Douglas. The treatment of choice in this case is:
a. Total hysterectomy with bilateral salpingo-oophorectomy
b. Danazol therapy
c. Progesterone therapy
d. Fulguration of endometriotic deposits

N10. A 36-year-old female, with two alive children complains of dysmenorrhea and dyspareunia. TVS shows a thin walled cyst 4 cm × 5 cm with echogenic fluid and no solid areas in left ovary. She doesn't wish to conceive. What is the first line of management?
a. Perform laparoscopic cystectomy
b. Treat with OCP's continuously
c. Treat with GnRH
d. Treat with medroxy progesterone acetate

N11. A 30-year-old-female complains of dysmenorrhea, dyspareunia and infertility. TVS shows a thin walled cyst 4 × 5 cm in diameter with echogenic fluid and no solid areas in left ovary. She wishes to conceive soon. What is the best treatment option?
a. Perform laparoscopic cystectomy
b. Treat with continuous OCP's
c. Treat with GnRH
d. Treat with injection DMPA

N12. True regarding adenomyosis is:
a. Most common in nullipara
b. Progestin are agents of choice for medical management
c. Presents with menorrhagia, dysmenorrhea, and an enlarged uterus
d. More common in young women

N13. All of the followings are presentations of adenomyosis *except*:
a. Menorrhagia
b. Infertility
c. Dysmenorrhea
d. Abdominal lump

N14. Gold standard for diagnosing adenomyosis:
a. MRI
b. USG
c. Histopathology
d. Saline infusion sonography

N15. A 28-year-old female patient presented with lower abdominal pain along with dysmenorrhea. The following finding was seen on laparoscopic examination. What is the likely diagnosis?
a. Krukenberg tumor
b. Polycystic ovaries
c. Endometriosis
d. Cystadenoma of ovary

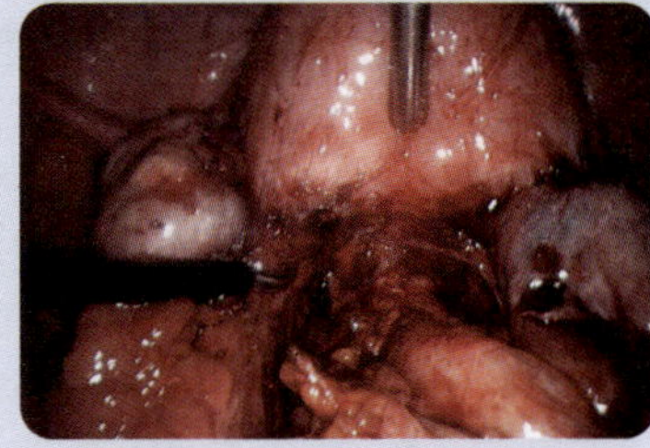

N16. Not true about Endometriosis:
a. Sampson gave implantation theory
b. Cause infertility
c. Laparoscopy is gold standard for diagnosis
d. Common in low socio-economic status

N17. All of the following are used in endometriosis *except*:
a. Progesterone
b. Danazol
c. GnRH agonist
d. Estrogen

N18. The organ NOT involved by endometriosis:
a. Liver
b. Lymph nodes
c. Brain
d. Spleen

PREVIOUS YEAR QUESTIONS

1. All are true regarding endometriosis, *except*:
a. Hormone dependent condition (*AIIMS Dec 94*)
b. Can involve lung, pleura
c. Contains clear fluid
d. Ovary is the most common site

2. True about endometriosis is/are: (*PGI June 06*)
a. MC in 3rd or 4th decade
b. Premenstrual spotting
c. Endometrial sarcoma is most common malignancy associated with it
d. True cyst
e. Ist degree relative seen

3. Endometriosis is commonly associated with:
a. B/L chocolate cyst of ovary (*PGI Dec 02*)
b. Adenomyosis
c. Fibroid
d. Luteal cyst
e. Endometritis

4. Pain in endometriosis correlates with: (*PGI June 00*)
a. Depth of invasion
b. Multiple sites
c. CA 125
d. Stage of disease

5. The M/C extrauterine site to be affected by endometriosis is: (*Delhi PG 09*)
a. Rectovaginal septum
b. Vagina
c. Sigmoid colon
d. Broad ligament (except tubes and ovaries)

6. A 35-year-old woman presents with infertility and palpable pelvic mass. Her CA-125 level is 90 mIU/mL diagnosis is: (*AIIMS May 2010*)
a. Ovarian Ca
b. Endometrioma
c. Tuberculosis
d. Borderline ovarian tumor

7. All are used in treatment of endometriosis *except*:
a. Medroxyprogesterone acetate (*AIIMS Dec 97*)
b. Tibolone
c. OCP
d. Danazol

8. Treatment of endometriosis include: (*PGI Dec 02*)
a. Estrogen b. Progesterone
c. OCP d. Danazol
e. GnRH

9. Drugs used in endometriosis are: (*PGI Dec 01*)
a. Testosterone b. Danazol
c. GnRH d. Progesterone
e. Estrogen

10. Treatment of endometriosis in infertile female: (*MAHE 05*)
a. GnRH b. Danazol
c. Clomiphene d. Progesterone

11. Not true about Endometriosis:
a. Sampson gave implantation theory
b. Cause infertility
c. Laparoscopy is gold standard for diagnosis
d. Common in low socio-economic group

12. A 45-years-old patient presented with complaints of pain in abdomen and menorrhagia. Endometrial biopsy was normal and sonogram of uterus showed diffusely enlarged uterus with no adnexal mass. What is the diagnosis? (*AIIMS May 2016*)
a. Fibroid uterus b. Endometritis
c. Endometriosis d. Adenomyosis

13. IOC for Endometriosis (*JIPMER Dec 2016*)
a. USG b. CA 125
c. Hysteroscopy d. Laparoscopy

14. Infertility in Endometriosis is due to: (*PGI May 12*)
a. Anovulation
b. Tubal obstruction
c. Implantation failure
d. Increased sperm phagocytosis
e. Altered tubal mobility

15. A 45-year-old woman presented with lower abdominal discomfort on examination uterus appears uniformly enlarged and adnexa is free. Biopsy taken shows endometrial glands inside the myometrium. The diagnosis is: (*JIPMER Dec 2016*)
a. Adenomyosis
b. Endometriosis
c. Leiomyoma
d. Endometrial Hyperplasia

16. True statement about primary dysmenorrhea: (*PGI May 2017*)
a. Pain starts 2–3 day before menstruation and stops after 1 day of menstruation
b. Pain begins a few hours before or just after the onset of a menstrual period and may last 48 to 72 hours
c. May be associated with psychological factors
d. GnRH antagonists are always used in 1st line treatment

17. True about endometriosis: (*PGI May 2016*)
a. Laparoscopy is gold standard for diagnosis
b. COC is used to relieve mild pain
c. GnRH antagonist is used to relive severe pain
d. Can be managed expectantly in asymptomatic cases

ANSWERS TO NEW PATTERN QUESTIONS

N1. Ans. is a, i.e. Implantation theory

See the text for explanation.

N2. Ans. is b, i.e. Nulliparity

As discussed in chapter 2, Endometriosis is a hyper estrogenic condition and is thus more common in Nulliparous females.

Protective factors are multiparity, pregnancy, smoking and exercise.

N3. Ans. is d, i.e. All of the above *Ref: Jeffcoate 7th/ed, p371*

Endometriosis sometimes occurs in abdominal wall scars following operations on uterus or tubes and is known as ***scar endometriosis.***

Operations most likely to be followed by scar endometriosis:
- Hysterotomy[Q]
- Classical cesarean section[Q]
- Myomectomy[Q]
- Ventrofixation[Q]
- Following operations for section of fallopian tube[Q]
- Following operations for removal of pelvic endometriosis[Q]
- Episiotomy[Q]

N4. Ans. is c, i.e. Perform TVS

Whenever a female comes with dysmenorrhea, dyspareunia and infertility, although we are suspecting endometriosis—we should not straight away do laparoscopy as it is invasive procedure. First do TVS to rule out fibroid or any other uterine pathology.

N5. Ans. is a, i.e. Perform a diagnostic laparoscopy

Now since here already TVS has been done and is normal, we will do IOC for endometriosis i.e. Laparoscopy.

Remember

	In Endometriosis	In Adenomyosis
1st Investigation	TVS	TVS
IOC	Laparoscopy	TVS
Gold standard	Histopathology	Histopathology

N6. Ans. is a, i.e. Laparoscopy

See the text for explanation.

N7. Ans. is b, i.e. Sigmoid colon

M/C site for extrapelvic endometriosis = GIT
In GIT M/C site is = sigmoid colon > Rectum
Overall M/C site of endometriosis = Ovary
Rarest site of endometriosis = CNS

N8. Ans. is d, i.e. Misoprost

Drugs used in the management of Endometriosis:
Proctor: Progesterone (oral/DMPA inj/Mirena IUCD)
And: Anti progestin (Mifepristone/onapristone)
Gamble: GnRH agonist
Always: Aromatase inhibitor (Letrozole/Anastrozole)
Offer: OCP's (continuous)
Good: Gestrinone
Deals: Danazol

N9. Ans. is d, i.e. Fulguration of endometriotic deposits *Ref: William's Gynae 1st/ed, p235; Bijoy Sree Sen Gupta 2nd/ed, p138*

In the question it is given, dense adhesions and chocolate cyst are present and patient is infertile. This cannot be treated by medical therapy and so, some form of surgery is required.

Main question is whether we would like to go for conservative surgery or radical surgery (i.e. TAH with BSO)

Remember: Mostly in endometriosis conservative surgery is done.

Conservative surgery: The clinical situations involving conservative surgery include ovarian endometrioma, pelvic adhesions, peritoneal implants and deep infiltrative rectovaginal septum disease. In addition, laser laparoscopy can be used in order to perform uterine nerve ablation. *Ref: Bijoy Sree Sen Gupta 2nd/ed, p138*

According to *William's Gynae 1st/ed, p239*

"Hysterectomy with bilateral oophorectomy should be reserved for women who have completed childbearing and recognise the risk of premature hypoestrogenism including possible osteoporosis and decrease libido."

N10. Ans. is d, i.e. Treat with medroxy progesterone acetate (MPA)

Friends: in the patient-

Lets see her age = 36 years old

And her chief complain = Pain

No desire to conceive

Treatment of pain = moderate/severe-as discussed is

1. 1st line = Progesterone—here inj Medroxy progesterone acetate
2. Best drug = GnRH

Since GnRH is costly, we initiate the treatment with progesterone.

Note: If this patient would have wanted to conceive, then we would not have given her progesterone as fertility is delayed with progesterone.

N11. Ans. is a, i.e Perform laparoscopic cystectomy

Here patient's age = 30 years

Main complain = Infertility

Management of chocolate cyst = Laparoscopic cystectomy.

N12. Ans. is c, i.e. Presents with menorrhagia, dysmenorrhea and an enlarged uterus

Ref: Shaw 15th/ed, p474-5; Novak 15th/ed, p484-5

As discussed in text-***adenomyosis is a condition where there is ingrowth of endometrium (both gland + stroma) directly into the myometrium.***[Q] ***Earlier it was called as Endometriosis interna***

It is more common in Multiparous[Q] *females (i.e. option a is correct).*

It is more common in elderly patients (> 40 years, i.e. option d is incorrect).

Mainly manifests as menorrhagia, dysmenorrhea and enlarged uterus (i.e. option c is correct).

N13. Ans. is b, i.e. Infertility

See the text for explanation.

N14. Ans. is c, i.e. Histopathology

See the text for explanation.

N15. Ans. is c, i.e. Endometriosis

Ref: Shaw's Textbook of Gynecology, 15/ed, p471

As seen in the figure, the cysts are showing blue gray color and small follicles of endometriosis are also visible. It is chocolate cyst seen in endometriosis.

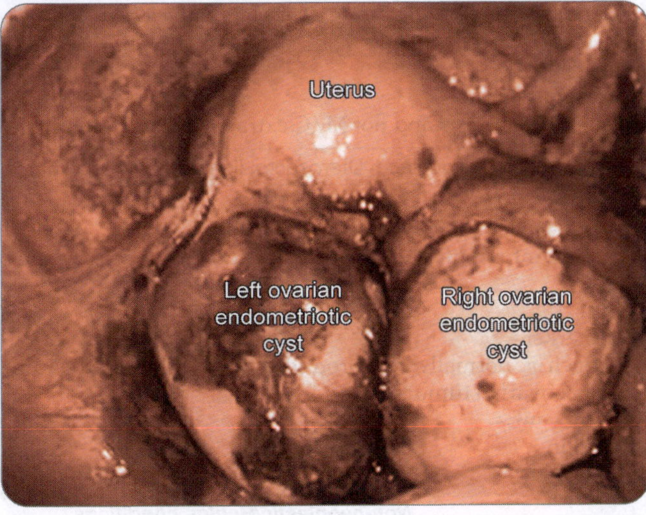

N16. Ans. is d, i.e. Common in low socio-economic status

Endometriosis is common in high socio-economic status. Rest all options are correct and have been discussed in the text.

N17. Ans. is d, i.e. Estrogen

As discussed Endometriosis is as hyperestrogenic condition so all drugs which directly or indirectly decreased estrogen are used in managing it, not estrogen itself.

N18. Ans. is d, i.e. Spleen

Ref: Williams Gynecology, 3/ed, p23

One pathological review revealed that endometriosis has been identified in all organs except spleen.

ANSWERS TO PREVIOUS YEAR QUESTIONS

1. **Ans. is c, i.e. Contains clear fluid**

Ref: Shaw 15th/ed, p466 for option a, 466-7 for option c; Jeffcoate 7th/ed, p370 for option 'd'; p372 for option 'b'

Endometriosis is occurrence of functioning endometrial tissue (glands + stroma) outside the uterine cavity.

Whatever the initial genesis of endometriosis its further development depends mainly on estrogen **(Option "a").** *Ref: Shaw 14th/ed, p420*

- It can occur anywhere in body, Most common site being ovary[Q] **(Option "d").** *Ref: Jeffcoate 7th/ed, p370*
- Can also involve lungs and pleura[Q] **(Option "b").** *Ref: Jeffcoate 7th/ed, p372*
- In endometriosis ovary contains tarry dark brown fluid (due to presence of blood pigments like hemosiderin) and cul de sac has yellow brown fluid.

Clear fluid is not seen anywhere, So, **Option "c"** is incorrect.

2. **Ans. is a, b, d and e, i.e. Most common in 3rd or 4th decade; Premenstrual spotting; True cyst; and 1st degree relative seen**

Ref: Shaw 15th/ed, p466-9; Jeffcoate 7th/ed, p368-70; CGDT 10th/ed, p715

As discussed in the preceeding text-

i. Endometriosis occurs most commonly in 3rd or 4th decade i.e "option a" is correct.
ii. If first degree relative is affected , there are 7-10 fold increased chances of a female having endometriosis i.e. option e is correct.
iii. Endometrioma/chocolate cyst is a true cyst–"option d" is correct.
iv. Premenstrual spotting is seen in endometriosis– thus proving "option b" is correct.
iv. Endometriosis is associated with granulosa cell tumors of ovary but not with endometrial sarcomas.

3. **Ans. is a, b and c, i.e. B/L chocolate cyst of ovary, Adenomyosis and Fibroid uterus**

Ref: Shaw 15th/ed, p466; Jeffcoate 7th/ed, p370; Novak 14th/ed, p1145,15th/ed, p517

As discussed in the text:

- B/L chocolate cysts are seen in ovary in patients of endometriosis (i.e. option a is correct)
  "Adenomyosis, endometriosis and uterine leiomyomas frequently coexist"..........Novaus 15/e, p484, i.e. Option b and c are also correct.
- **Luteal cysts:** These are seen in ovary in case of increased HCG for e.g.:
  - Pregnancy
  - H mole
  - Choriocarcinoma
  - Multiple pregnancy
  - hcg therapy

They donot have relation to endometriosis. Similarly endometritis and endometriosis are not related.

4. **Ans. is a, i.e. Depth of invasion** *Ref: Leon Speroff, 8/ed, p1230–1231*

"The intensity of pain associated with deeply infiltrating endometriosis relates to the depth of penetration and to the proximity or direct invasion of nerves". *Ref: Leon Speroff, 8th/ed, p1230*

"However there is no relationship between stage, site or the morphological characteristic of pelvic endometriosis and pain". *Ref: Leon Speroff, 8th/ed, p1231*

5. **Ans. is d, i.e. Broad ligament**

Guys: Read the question very carefully

It is asking M/C extrauterine site of metastasis and not M/C extrapelvic site.

- Sites of endometriosis = Ovary > Pouch of Douglas > Uterosacral ligament > Broad ligament > Fallopian tube

6. **Ans. is b, i.e. Endometrioma**

Ref: Novak Gynecology 14th/ed, p1466, 1146, 1147; William's Gynae 1st/ed, p232,210 Textbook of Gynae, Sheila Balakrishnan p185

In this question we have insufficient information to make any definite diagnosis. At the best we can try to make the most probable diagnosis.

CA-125

- This is a non-specific tumor marker
- CA-125 is a glycoprotein which is normally not produced by ovarian epithelium but may be produced by both malignant and benign epithelial ovarian tumors.
- Cut off level of CA-125 is < 35 U/mL.
- Levels of CA-125 can be raised in

↑ CA-125	
Neoplastic conditions	***Non-neoplastic/Benign conditions***
Gynecological • Ovarian cancer (nonmucinous) • Endometrial cancer • Tubal cancer *Non-gynecological* • Lung cancer • Breast cancer • Ca Pancreas • Colon cancer	• Endometriosis • Peritoneal inflammation, including PID • Tuberculosis • Hemorrhagic ovarian cysts • Liver disease • Leiomyoma • Pregnancy • Menstruation

- Thus, CA-125 levels, can be raised in all the four options, given in the question
- Palpable mass may also be present in all the four conditions.
- Infertility is a feature of endometriosis and tuberculosis. But for ovarian cancers, infertility (due to use of ovulation inducing drugs) is a risk factor, not a presenting symptom.
- Coming to Age: Patient is 35 years old.
- Age of 35 years favors endometrioma (endometriosis) the most.
- Peak incidence of invasive epithelial ovarian cancer (most common ovarian cancer) is at 56–60 years of age and for border line tumor average age is 46 years approximately *(Novak 14th/ed, p1466)*
- Patient with tuberculosis are in their twenties commonly, the maximum age incidence at diagnosis being 28 years.
- Also in tuberculosis, CA-125 has least significance as it is neither used for diagnosis nor for follow up
- Thus, based on age and infertility → the most probable diagnosis is endometrioma/endometriosis.
- Our answer is further supported by following lines from – *Textbook of gynae, Sheila Balakrishnan 1st/ed, p185*
- Serum CA 125 *"This is useful in post menopausal women when a high level may indicate malignancy. In the reproductive age group, the predictive value is not good as the marker may be raised in endometriosis".*

In young females if the value of CA-125 is >200 IU/mL, it is considered to indicate malignancy.

7. **Ans. is b, i.e. Tibolone** *Ref: Shaw 15th/ed, p472-3; Novak 14th/ed, p1164-9*
8. **Ans. is b, c, d and e, i.e. Progesterone, OCP, Danazol, and GnRH**
9. **Ans. is b, c and d, i.e. Danazol, GnRH, and Progesterone** *Ref: Shaw 15th/ed, p472-3; Novak 14th/ed, p1164-9*

Drugs used in the management of endometriosis

Hormone Therapy Empirical Therapy

Proctor–Progesterone-First line management → Oral progestins- continuous administration; → Injectable progestin-DMPA; → LNG-IUS
and–Antiprogestin = Mifepristone
Gamble–GnRH analogue (Best management)
Always–Aromatase inhibitor: Letrozole
Offer–OCP
Good–Gestrinone
Deals–Danazol

Mnemonic—Proctor and Gamble Always Offer Good Deals

10. **Ans. is c, i.e. Clomiphene**

As discussed in text:

> **For infertility: Mgt in mild cases Superovulation with clomiphene + IUI**
> **Mgt in moderate/severe cases–IVF**

11. **Ans. is d i.e. Common in low socio-economic group**

As discussed in text Endometriosis more common in high socio-economic status, not low.
Rest all options are correct and have been discussed earlier.

12. **Ans. is d i.e. Adenomyosis**

The patient is 45 years old and complaining of pain in abdomen and menorrhagia.
Her endometrial biopsy is normal and USG shows diffusely enlarged uterus.
This points towards Adenomyosis as the diagnosis.
"In adenomyosis-the uterus is typically diffusely enlarged, although less than 14 cm in size and is often soft and tender, particularly at the time of menses. Mobility of uterus is not restricted and there is no associated adnexal pathology"
Remember- Dysmenorrhea with diffuse uterine enlargement is attributed to adenomyosis *Novak 14th/ed, p484*

13. **Ans is d i.e. Laparoscopy.** *Ref: Williams 3rd/ed, p237*
14. **Ans. is a, c, d, and e, i.e. Anovulation; Implantation failure; Increased sperm phagocytosis; and Altered tubal mobility** *Ref: Jeffioates 9/ed, p442*

> **Causes of infertility: in Endometriosis** *Ref: Jefroates 9th/ed, p442*
> 1. Altered folliculogenesis
> 2. Poor oocyte quality
> 3. Ovarian dysfunction
> 4. Luteal phase defect
> 5. Reduced fertilisation
> 6. Abnormal embryogenesis
> 7. Reduced implantation (option C)
> 8. Altered granulosa rates cell kinetics
>
> *"The investigation of infertility, especially since the introduction of the laparoscope, has led to an increase in the diagnosis of endometriosis. Several possible mechanisms have been suggested for this association. The tubes are invariably open, but there may be pelvic adhesions, impaired ovum pick up; the alterations in prostaglandins, macrophases and cytokines mentioned above may lead to enhanced phagocytosis of sperm; hormonal disfunction may lead to anovulation, the lutenised unruptured follicle and lateral phase defect and there may be early pregnancy loss."* *Ref: Jefficoates 9th/ed, p441.*

15. Ans. is a, i.e. Adenomyosis

No doubt about diagnosis as biopsy says endometrium is inside the myometrium.

16. Ans. is b and c, i.e. Pain begins a few hours before or just after the onset of a menstrual period and may last 48 to 72 hours and May be associated with psychological factors

Ref: Shaw's 16th/ed, p471-73; Dutta Gynae 6th/ed, p178-80; Novak's Gyae 15th/ed, p481-83

Table (Novak's Gynae 15th/ed, p236)

Established and Emerging Noncontraceptive

- Benefits of Oral Contraceptives
- Established Benefits
- Menses-related
  - Increased menstrual cycle regularity
  - Reduced blood loss
  - Reduced iron-deficiency anemia
  - Reduced dysmenorrhea
  - Reduced symptoms of premenstrual dysphoric disorder
  - Inhibition of ovulation
  - Fewer ovarian cysts
  - Fewer ectopic pregnancies
- Other
  - Reduced fibroadenomas/fibrocystic breast changes
  - Reduced acute pelvic inflammatory disease
  - Reduced endometrial cancer
  - Reduced ovarian cancer
- Emerging Benefits
  - Increased bone mass
  - Reduced acnes
  - Reduced colorectal cancer
  - Reduced uterine leiomyomata
  - Reduced rheumatoid arthritis
  - Treatment of bleeding disorders
  - Treatment of hyperandrogenic anovulation
  - Treatment of endometriosis
  - Treatment of perimenopausal changes

Primary Dysmenorrhea

"The pain of primary dysmenorrhea usually begins a few hours before or just after the onset of a menstrual period and may last 48 to 72 hours" *Ref: Novak's Gyae15th/ed, p481*

i.e **"Option a"** is incorrect and option b correct

GnRH antagonists (Leuprolide, buserelin, nafarelin) are used for pelvic endometriosis (cause of secondary dysmenorrhea) and not primary dysmenorrhea i.e option d is incorrect

"Premenstrual syndrome is associated with psychological symptoms (like emotional liability, irritability, mood swing, depression)" *Ref: Shaw's 16th/ed, p471*

"Hormonal contraceptives are indicated for primary dysmenorrhea unresponsive to NSAIDs. If the patient does not respond to this regimen, hydrocodone or codeine may be added for 2 to 3 days per month; before addition of the narcotic medication, psychological factors should be evaluated, and diagnostic laparoscopy to rule out pathology should be considered." *Ref: Novak's Gynae 15th/ed, p481*

17. Ans. is a, b and d. Laparoscopy is gold standard for diagnosis, COC is used to relieve mild pain and can be managed expectantly in asymptomatic cases

As discussed in text

- Gold standard test for Endometriosis is Laparoscopy
- In case of mild pain due to Endometriosis i.e. mild dysmenorrhea-management is OCP's and in severe dysmenorrhea-management is GnRH agonist

"OCP's are a good choice for patients with minimal or mild pain" *Ref: COGDT 10th/ed, p916*

GnRH antagonist are not used these days hence option c is incorrect.

"In asymptomatic patients, those with mild discomfort or infertile woman with minimal or mild endometriosis, expectant management may be appropriate"

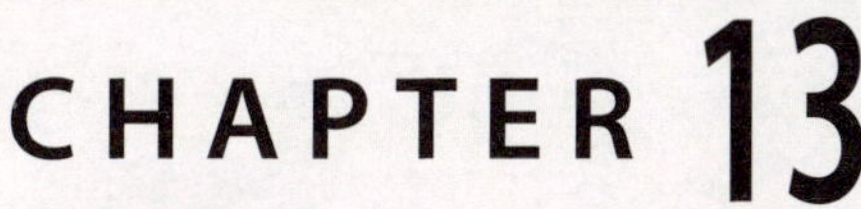

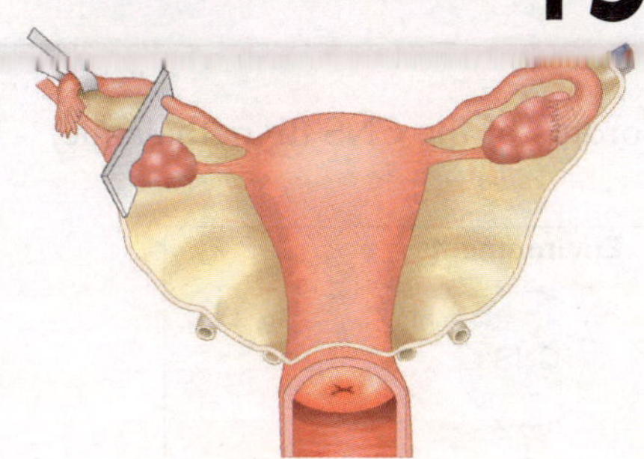

Disorders of Menstruation

Amenorrhea

Literally means absence of menstruation

Flowchart 13.1

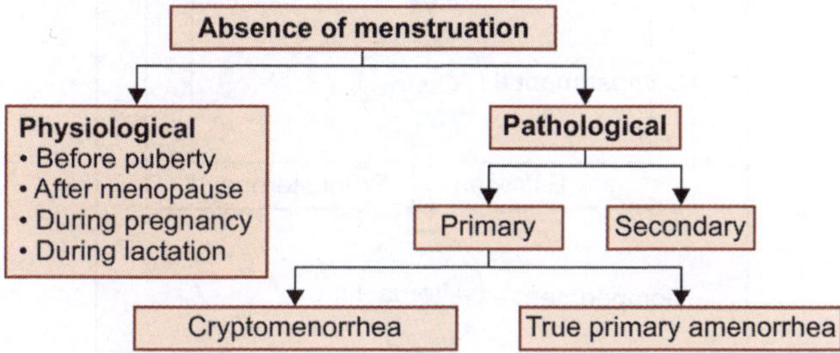

KEY POINTS

1° **Amenorrhea**—Condition where a female has not attained menarche by the **age of 13 years in the absence of development of secondary sexual characteristics** or no menarche by the age of **15 years regardless of the presence of normal growth and** development of secondary sexual characteristics.

2° **Amenorrhea**—Absence of menstruation for 3 months or oligomenorrhea in involving less than a cycles a year.

Recap of development in females

For normal development of Gonads (ovaries). Absence of Y chromosome & presence of XX (2X) chromosomes is required.

- Ovary
  ↓ secretes
  Estrogen
  (Required for normal development of secondary sexual characteristic in females)
- Absence of Y chromosome means
  ↓
  Absent testis i.e. absent sertoli cells
  ↓
  i.e. Müllerian inhibiting factor is absent
  ↓
  i.e. Müllerian duct grows normally and forms fallopian tubes, uterus, cervix, upper part of vagina.

Cryptomenorrhea

Definition: Occurrence of menstrual symptoms without external bleeding. Menstrual blood fails to come out from genital tract due to obstruction in the outflow passage.

Causes

Table 13.1

Congenital	Acquired
• Imperforate hymen (M/C cause) • Transverse vaginal septum	Cervical stenosis following: • Amputation • Cauterization • Conization

Pathology

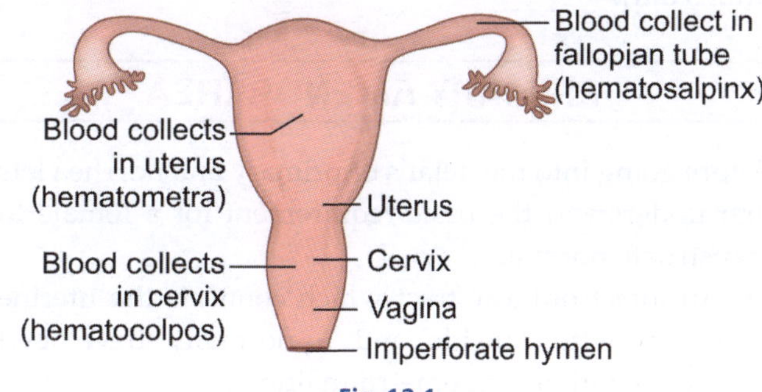

Fig. 13.1

Symptoms

Flowchart 13.2

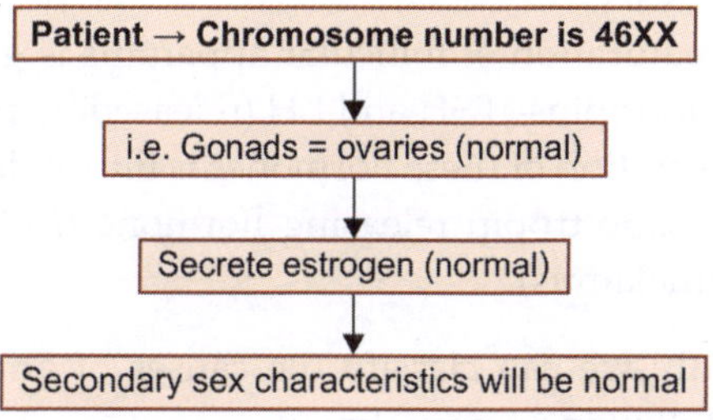

In Cryptomenorrhea

- A female with normal secondary sexual characteristics complains of primary amenorrhea
- H/o cyclical abdominal pain is present

- Patient may complain of urinary symptoms as hematocolpos can cause pressure symptoms.

O/E – A tumor, dull on percussion is found in lower abdomen (partly due to distended vagina & partly due to overfill bladder).

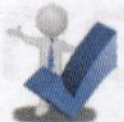

KEY POINTS

In a normal looking female, with normal secondary sexual characteristic always rule out cryptomenorrhea.

Local Examination

On separating labia, bluish bulging hymen is seen. Per Rectal examination shows uterus is present.

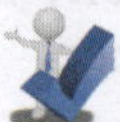

KEY POINTS

Never do P/V examination in a virgin females. To know whether uterus is present/absent and to assess the size of the uterus – do a Per Rectal examination, never Per vaginal examination.

Management

Urgent surgical management by giving a cruciate incision on the hymen (the collected blood automatically drains out).

PRIMARY AMENORRHEA

Before going into the details of primary amenorrhea lets first understand the basic requirement for a female to menstruate normally.

- An intact outflow tract which connects the uterine cavity with outside and a normally developed uterus with its endometrium lining.
- Proper quantity and sequence of steroid hormones i.e. estrogen and progesterone which inturn originate from ovary.
- The maturation of follicular apparatus is guided by gonadotropins– FSH and LH (released by pituitary).
- The secretion of these hormones is inturn dependent on gonado-tropin releasing hormone (re-leased by hypothalamus).

So, broadly we can classify the causes of amenorrhea into the following compartments.

Compartment I Disorders of the out flow tract or uterine target organs.

Compartment II Disorders of the Ovary

Compartment III Disorders of the Pituitary

Compartment IV Disorders of the CNS (hypothalamic) factors.

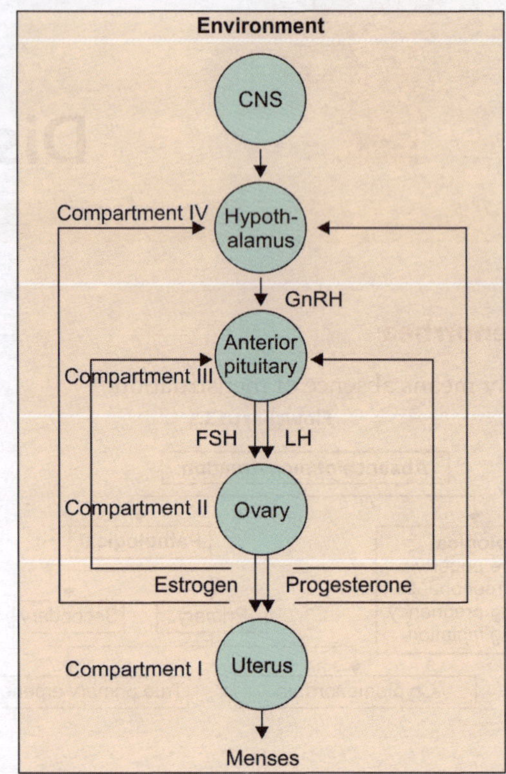

Fig. 13.2: Hormonal control of menstruation

Major Causes of Primary Amenorrhea (Compartment Wise)

Table 13.2

Compartment I (Disorders of outflow tract/ uterus)	*Mullerian Anomalies*[Q] *(2nd M/c cause of primary amenorrhea)* Androgen insensitivity syndrome (Testicular feminization syndrome)[Q]
Compartment II (Disorders of Ovary)	*Gonadal dysgenesis (M/c cause of Primary Amenorrhea)*[Q] Turners syndrome: 45XO[Q] Pure gonadal dysgenesis: 46 XX[Q] Swyers syndrome: 46 XY[Q] Savage syndrome: Resistant ovary syndrome
Compartment III (Disorders of Anterior Pituitary)	Neoplasia Prolactinomas[Q]/Craniopharyngiomas[Q] Hypopituitary states – Simmond's disease[Q]/Chiari-Frommel syndrome[Q] Forbes Albright syndrome (Not very important)
Compartment IV (Disorders of CNS)	Kallmann syndrome[Q] (Amenorrhea + Anosmia)

Clinical Case 1

A 12 to 15 year female with normal secondary sexual characteristics complains of primary amenorrhea.

Solution: In all such cases 1st step is to see do USG or per Rectal examination to see uterus is present or not. This is because per vaginal examination is contraindicated in virgin females. Then proceed as shown in Flowchart 13.3.

Flowchart 13.3: When a female c/o primary amenorrhea with normal secondary sexual characteristic

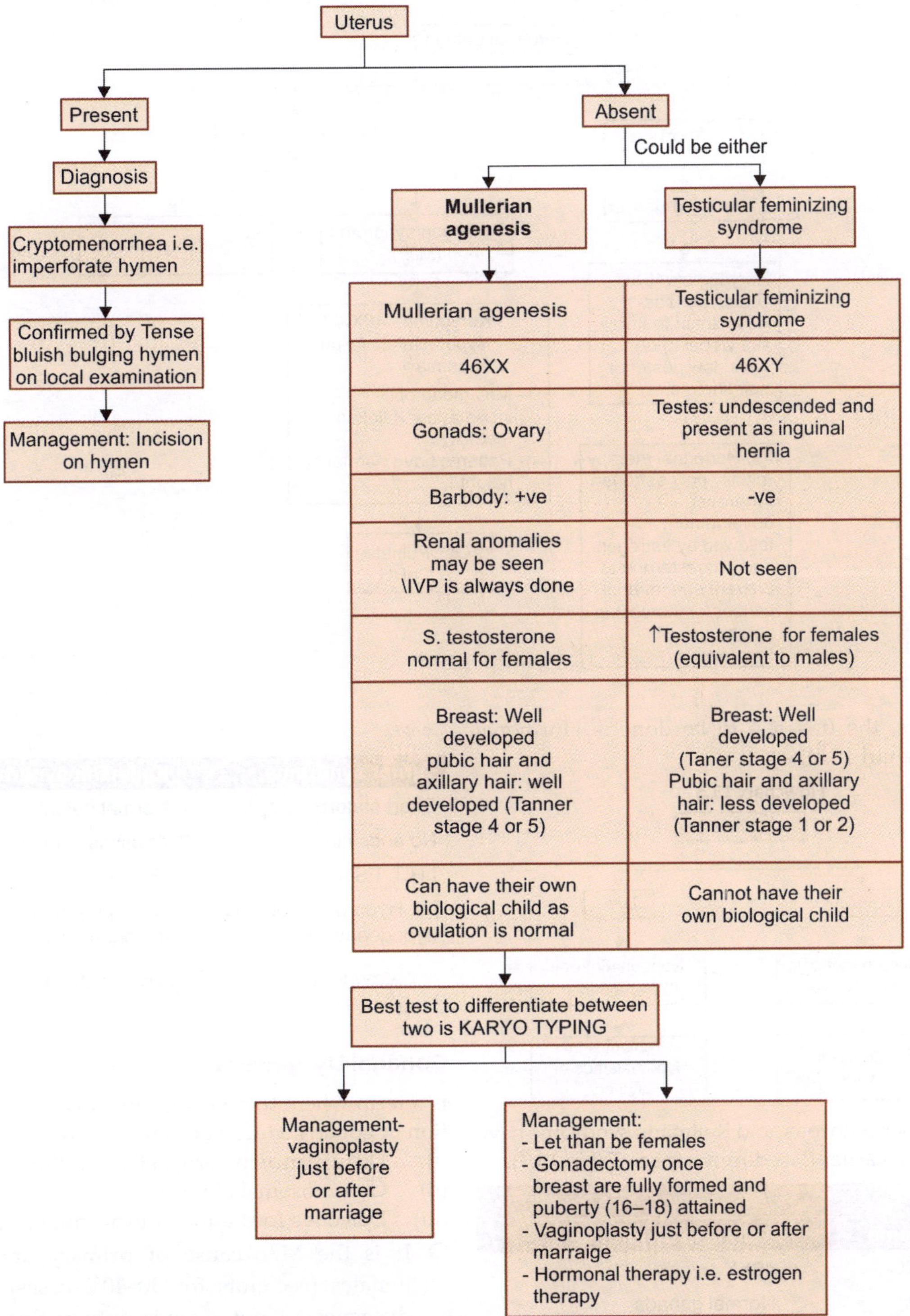

Note: Details of Mullerian agenesis & Testicular feminizing syndrome have been discussed earlier in book.

Clinical Case 2

A 12–15 years female with absent secondary sexual characteristics (i.e breast) C/O Primary amenorrhea.

Solution: In all such cases first thing to note is the height of the patient. Then proceed as shown in Flowchart 13.4

Flowchart 13.4: When a female c/o primary amenorrhea with absent secondary sexual characteristic

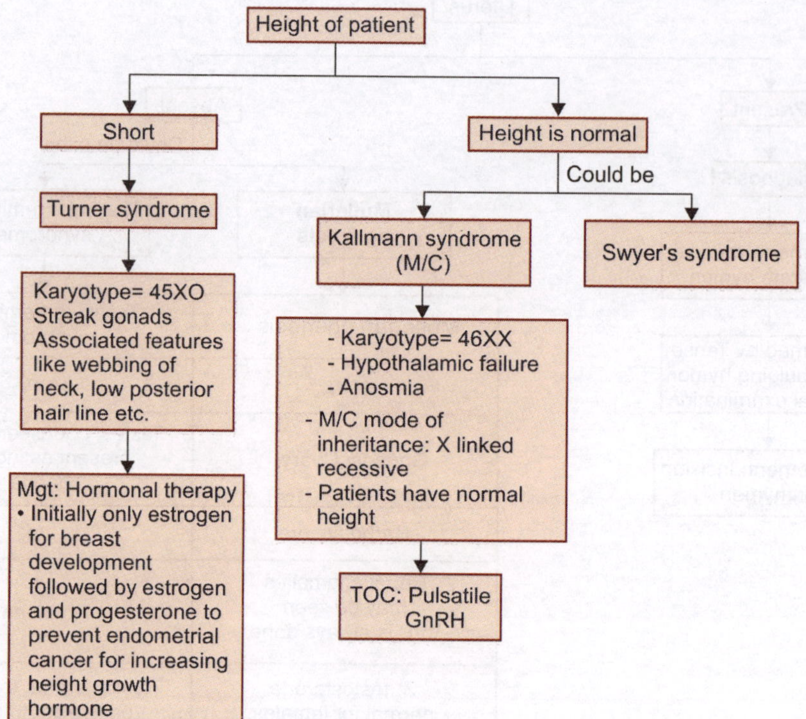

In these cases, the first test to be done is Hormonal profile (Flowchart 13.5).

Flowchart 13.5

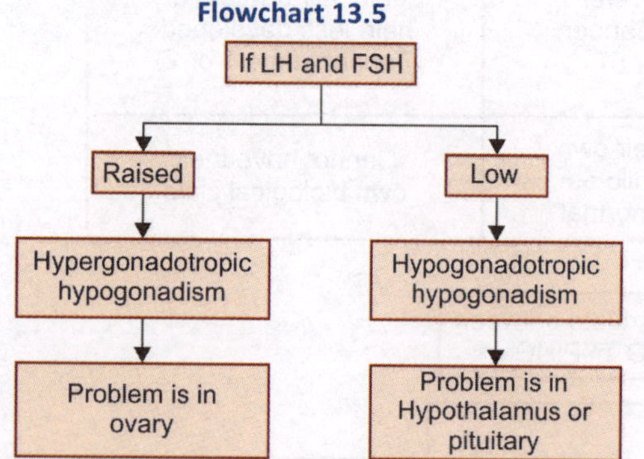

Details of Turner syndrome and Kallmann syndrome have been discussed earlier (For difference see Table 13.3).

Table 13.3

Turner syndrome	Kallmann syndrome
Genotype 45XO	46XX
Streak gonads	Normal gonads
Short stature	Normal height
No anosmia	Anosmia is present
LH ↑ FSH ↑	LH ↓ FSH ↓
i.e. Hypergonadotropic hypogonadism	i.e. hypogonadotropic hypogonadism

Now let us discuss Swyers syndrome/Pure Gonadal dysgenesis.

Gonadal Dysgenesis

Is a term where there is incomplete or defective formation of gonads which could be due to:

(i) Disturbance in germ cell migration
(ii) Chromosomal abnormality
(iii) Defective formation of urogenital ridge

- It is the M/c cause of primary amenorrhea in females (accounts for 30–40% cases). If Gonadal dysgenesis is not given in options then go for.
- Gonadal dysgenesis could be of several types:

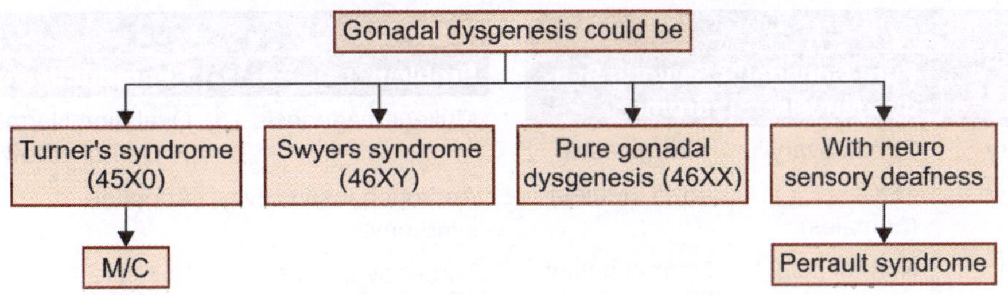

Turner Syndrome: Discussed in detail in chapter 6

Swyer Syndrome

It is an example of dysgenetic testis (Flowchart 13.6).

Flowchart 13.6: Swyer syndrome

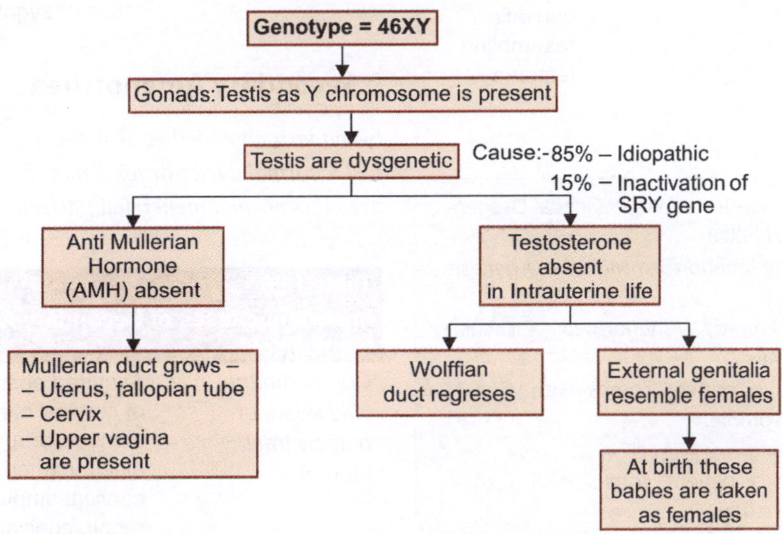

At puberty: Some testosterone is produced by adrenals but levels of testosterone are still low.

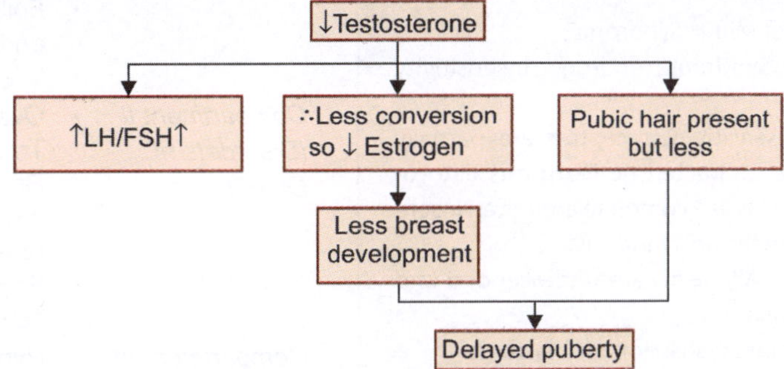

Since they have external genitalia resembling females so these babies are reared up as females and patients complain of primary amenorrhea at puberty obviously as ovaries are absent

Management: Dysgenetic gonads can develop germ cell tumor: **Gonadectomy has to be done as soon as diagnosis is made**

- Sexuality issue—let them be females
- For breast development—initially estrogen should be given alone and subsequently, estrogen and progestin therapy (cyclical) to maintain sexual maturation
- Pregnancy can be achieved by IVF using donor Oocytes. Pregnancy is not associated with any specific risk or complications.

Table 13.4

Turner's Syndrome	Pure Gonadal dysgenesis	Swyer's Syndrome
Gonads: Streak ovary	Streak ovary	Streak testis
Karyotype: 45XO (Females)	46XX (Females)	46XY (Males)
Height: Short stature	Normal height	Normal height
Associated abnormalities like webbing neck, CVS problems are present	Absent	Absent
Uterus present (hypoplastic)	Uterus present (hypoplastic)	Uterus present
External genitalia: Female (infantile)	Female	Ambiguous genitalia resembling females

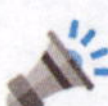

Important One Liners

- M/c cause of Primary Amenorrhea: Pure Gonadal Dysgenesis > Turner Syndrome (45XO)
- 2nd M/c cause of Primary Amenorrhea: Mullerian Agenesis (46XX)
- 3rd M/c cause of Primary Amenorrhea: Testicular Feminizing Syndrome (46XY)
- 1st Test to do when a patient comes with C/o 1° amenorrhea: Hormonal profile.
- Best Test is → Karyotyping
- 1st Test to do when a patient comes with C/o 2° amenorrhea: Hormonal study.
- Time for vaginoplasty: Just before or After marriage
- M/c method for doing vaginoplasty: McIndoe Vaginoplasty
- Indications of Vaginoplasty
  - Mullerian agenesis (or MRKH Syndrome)
  - Testicular Feminizing Syndrome (Androgen Insensitivity Syndrome)
- In partial androgen insensitivity, receptors are partially sensitive to androgens. Characteristic **feature is clitoromegaly**[Q]: Rest everything is like complete androgen insensitivity, i.e. Testicular feminizing syndrome.
- In complete and partial AIS: testis are undescended and present as Inguinal Hernia
- M/c tumor in undescended testis: Gonadoblastoma
- M/c malignant tumor in undescended tests: Seminoma
- Time for Gonadectomy (Removal of Testis):
  - In complete Androgen insensitivity syndrome—After Puberty (16 years)
  - In incomplete androgen insensitivity syndrome—As soon as diagnosis is made
  - In Swyers syndrome—As soon as diagnosis is made
- Worst Reproductive outcome: Androgen Insensitivity Syndrome. Their only way of having a child is by Adoption.

Table 13.5

Problem	Reproductive outcome
Mullerian agenesis	Ovulation Normal ∴ Do IVF followed by surrogacy
Androgen insensitivity syndrome	Adoption
Turner syndrome	Possible with IVF using donor oocytes but Pregnancy is contraindicated due to risk of aortic dissection or rupture
Kallmann syndrome	Hormonal Therapy
Swyers syndrome	They have uterus so do IVF with donor oocytes followed by implantation of zygotes in their own uterus

Secondary Amenorrhea

Secondary amenorrhea is defined as absence of menstruation for 3 normal cycles or for 6 months or more in a woman with previous normal menstrual pattern in absence of pregnancy...

– Leon Speroff 8th/ed, p436

Table 13.6
Important causes of Secondary Amenorrhea (Compartment wise)

Compartment I (Disorders of outflow tract/ uterus)	• Acquired obstruction (gynatresia) of cervical canal causing severe stenosis or atresia following electrocauterization, chemical burns, cervical amputation in Fothergill's repair, conization, CIN, or genital tuberculosis. • ***Asherman's syndrome***[Q] • Following excessive curettage or endometrial tuberculosis • V V F (cause unknown)
Compartment II (Disorders of Ovary)	• Ovary Tumor – ***PCOD***[Q] • Trauma – Surgical extirpation/ Radiotherapy • Infections – Mumps, Tuberculosis rarely pyogenic infections • **Premature ovarian failure** (i.e. before 40 years)
Compartment III (Pituitary)	• Hyperprolactinemia/**prolactin tumor/ prolactinoma** • Insufficiency as in Simmond's disease, Sheehan's syndrome • Empty sella syndrome
Compartment IV (Hypothalamus)	• GnRH deficiency • Vigorous exercise/excessive stress • Weight loss • Eating disorders – anorexia and Bulimia

Contd...

Contd...

Important causes of Secondary Amenorrhea (Compartment wise)	
	• Radiation • Pseudocyesis • Infection (TB) • Infiltrative disease (sarcoidosis)

Besides these some other causes of secondary amenorrhea are

- Pregnancy-M/c cause of secondary amenorrhea
- *Hypothyroidism*[Q] *(V. Imp. cause, should be ruled out in every case)*
- Hyperprolactinemia

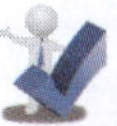

KEY POINTS

Levels of Prolactin and associated Menstrual disorders

Increased levels of prolactin adversely affect GnRH secretion which leads to amenorrhea. This is the reason for amenorrhea in prolactinomas and during lactational period.

- Diabetes
- Tuberculosis
- Renal disease/liver disease
- Addison disease/Cushing's syndrome/acromegaly
- Drugs (phenothiazines, reserpine, antidepressants, OCPs).
- Malabsorption syndrome
- AIDS

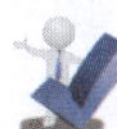

KEY POINTS

Pregnancy is a cause of secondary amenorrhea as well as physiological amenorrhea.

- **Causes of physiological amenorrhea**
  - Before puberty.
  - After menopause
  - During pregnancy
  - During lactation.
- Lactation leads to amenorrhea as hypothalamic GnRH secretion is suppressed by negative feedback of excess prolactin, thereby lowering FSH and LH levels.

Asherman's Syndrome

- First described by Joseph Ashermann and was called as amenorrhea traumatica.
- It is amenorrhea due to intrauterine synechiae formation and the endometrium is defective.
- **M/c cause** of Asherman's syndrome is vigorous uterine curettage in postpartum period but the syndrome can also occur after myomectomy, cesarean section, and tubercular endometritis.
- Patient complains of less menstrual blood loss called as Hypomenorrhea (characteristic feature) or secondary amenorrhea.
- **IOC** = Hysteroscopy
- **Other Ix** = HSG which shows honeycomb appearance.
- **Management**
  Hysteroscopic adhesiolysis followed by insertion of intra uterine balloon catheter to prevent reformation of synechiae for (7–10 days) and cyclical estrogen and progesterone (to rebuild the endometrium).

Sheehan's Syndrome

- *It is the syndrome which results from acute ischaemic necrosis of most of the anterior pituitary*[Q] *due to spasm in its arterioles occurring at the time of severe hemorrhage or shock complicating childbirth.*
- Only the anterior pituitary is affected because in parturient woman, blood supply to the pituitary gland is modified to the advantage of the posterior lobe and disadvantage of the anterior lobe so, when spasm occurs, posterior lobe is protected.
- When 75% of anterior pituitary is destroyed, manifestations of Sheehan's syndrome appear and when 95% is destroyed - fully developed Simmond's syndrome is seen.
- Deficiencies in GH, LH, FSH and prolactin are more common. Later on ACTH and TSH deficiencies occur.

Clinical Features

Symptoms[Q]

- Failure of lactation after delivery[Q] (due to ↓ Prolactin) - M/c presentation
- Secondary amenorrhoea[Q] (↓ LH/↓ FSH)
- Loss of libido[Q]
- Increased sensitivity to cold (hypothyroidism)[Q] (↓ TSH)

Signs

- Absence of axillary sweating[Q]
- Loss of axillary and pubic hair[Q] (Signs of adrenal cortical failure)
- Decrease in skin pigmentation[Q]
- Anemia due to lack of pituitary erythropoietic factor
- Weakness, lethargy[Q]
- Hypothyroidism[Q] and hypothermia[Q]
- Hyponatremia
- Hypoglycemia[Q] (due to decreased insulin tolerance)[Q]
- All genital organs show atrophy, uterus is smaller than in postmenopausal women[Q] as there is decrease in FSH, LH and estrogen although dormant ovaries retain their ova till menopause[Q]

Diabetes insipidus is never seen

Lab Investigation

Most common is prolactin deficiency along with decreased levels of FSH[Q], LH[Q], TSH[Q], ACTH[Q], oestrogens[Q], and urinary 17-keto steroids[Q]

Management

The treatment of Sheehan's syndrome includes: *Life-long hormone substitute of estrogen, progesterone, thyroid, and adrenal hormone.*

Premature Menopause

Is defined as secondary amenorrhoea before 40 years of age, due to ovarian failure. It is clinically defined as secondary amenorrhea for at least 3 months with raised FSH, raised FSH/LH ratio and low E_2 levels in a women under 40 years of age.

Prolactinoma

- M/C pituitary adenomas
- Types:
  - Microadenoma (<1 cm) (M/c)
  - Macroadenoma (>1 cm)
- Patients have increased prolactin which decreases GnRH, leading to 2° amenorrhea
- Due to increased prolactin, galactorrhea is seen
- Due to mass effects of the tumor–(as the tumor lies near optic chiasma)–visual disturbances (M/c = bitemporal hemianopsia, i.e. tunnel vision) and headaches are complained of
- M/c presentation of Hyperprolactinemia is infertility

Management: Cabergoline 0.25 mg twice week for microadenoma.

Macroadenoma—Initial treatment is cabergoline. If there is no response or if tumor is >3 cms and patient desires pregnancy then surgery is done.

Remember

- DOC for increased prolactin is cabergoline
- DOC for increased prolactin in infertile females is Bromocriptine (as it induces ovulation also)

Work up for a case of Secondary Amenorrhea (see Flowchart 13.7)

Flowchart 13.7: Workup of case of secondary amenorrhea

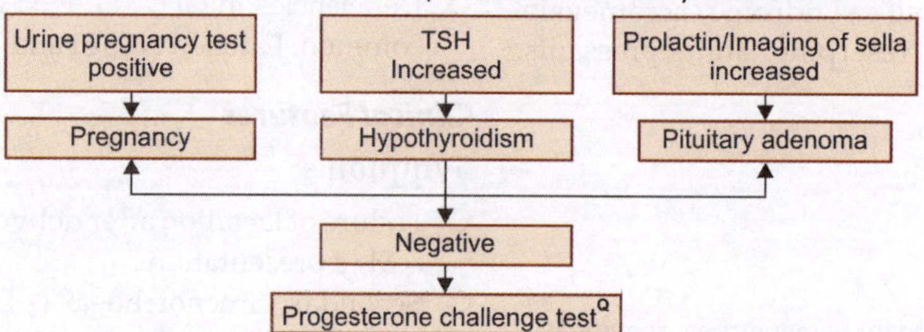

Purpose: To assess the level of endogenous estrogen and competence of outflow tract.
Method: Progesterone totally devoid of estrogenic activity (like MDPA, micronized progesterone) is given for 5 days and then withdrawn.

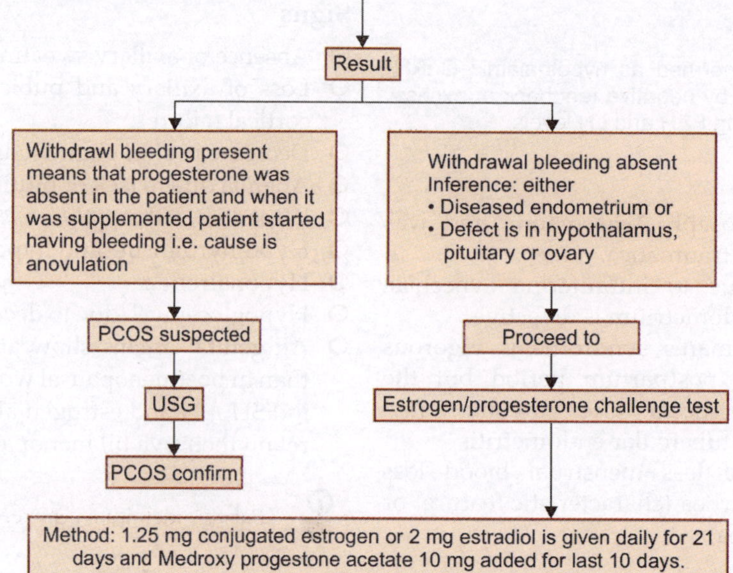

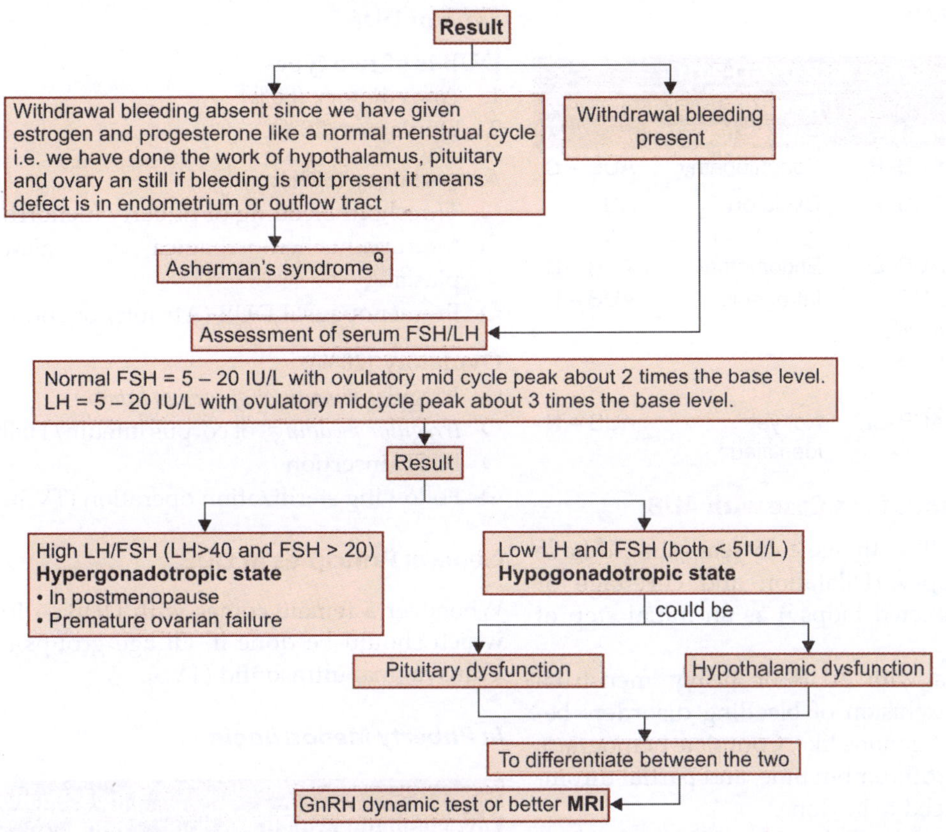

Note: Friends it is quite difficult to understand the above chart in one go, you will have to go through it 3–4 times to understand it well.

Characteristics of Normal Menstrual Cycle

Table 13.7: Normal Characteristics of Menstrual Cycle

Normal length of cycle	24 days–38 days (study based) or 21–35 days (population based) ($\pm$5 variation)
Average length	28 days (This is seen only in 15% of females)
Number of days of bleeding Average days	2–7 days 4–6 days
Normal blood loss Average blood loss	5-80 mL 30 mL (pg 594 Leon Speroff 8/e) (If this is not given in options: 2nd best = 35 mL 3rd best = 50 mL

Atypical Uterine Bleeding *(Ref: Leon Speroff 8th/ed, p592)*

Any deviation from above is called as **atypical uterine bleeding (AUB)**

AUB can be:

- **Menorrhagia:** Abnormally long or heavy menses. But cycles are regular
  - Blood loss ≥85 mL
  - Number of days of bleeding > 7 days
- **Hypomenorrhea:** Less bleeding with regular cycles
  - Blood loss < 5 mL
  - Number of days of bleeding < 2 days
- **Polymenorrhea:** Frequent cycles, occurring at short intervals.
- **Oligomenorrhea:** Infrequent cycles, occurring at long intervals.
- **Amenorrhea:** Absent menses
- **Metrorrhagia:** Bleeding occurring at irregular intervals

In order to create universally accepted nomenclature to describe abnormal uterine bleeding, International Federation of Gynecology and Obstetrics (FIGO) and American College of Obstetricians and Gynecologists (ACOG) introduced newer system of terminology to describe AUB.

The newer classification system is known by the acronym PALM-COEIN (FIGO-2011). It is used to classify the abnormal uterine bleeding on the basis of etiology.

Etiopathology of AUB

Classification of AUB (FIGO-2011)			
Structural causes (PALM)		**Nonstructural systemic causes (COEIN)**	
• **P**olyp	AUB–**P**	Coagulopathy	AUB – **C**
• **A**denomyosis	AUB–**A**	Ovulatory dysfunction	AUB – **O**
• **L**eiomyoma	AUB–**L**	Endometrial	AUB – **E**
– Submucosal myoma	AUB–L SM	Iatrogenic	AUB – **I**
– Other myoma	AUB–**LO**		
• **M**alignancy and hyperplasia	AUB–**M**	Not yet identified	AUB – **N**

Management Options for a Case with AUB

- Women with AUB with age ≥ 45 years should have endometrial biopsy (Dilatation and curettage or hysteroscopy directed biopsy) as an initial step of management.
- Adolescent girls with AUB or heavy menstrual bleeding need exclusion of bleeding disorders besides other investigations like, Complete hemogram, platelet count, prothrombin time, and partial thromboplastin time need to be done.
- In adolescent females Dilatation and curettage is never done.

DUB – Dysfunctional Uterine Bleeding

Definition

DUB is defined as a state of abnormal uterine bleeding without any clinically detectable organic pelvic pathology.

Causes of DUB

See Flowchart 13.8

Type of DUB

DUB is of two types:

1. Anovulatory (80%)
2. Ovulatory (20%)

Anovulatory (80%):

- Threshold bleeding of puberty menorrhagia
- Metropathia hemorrhagica[Q]/cystic glandular hyperplasia[Q]
- Premenopausal DUB (Atrophy of endometrium).

Ovulatory (20%):

- *Irregular ripening*[Q] *of corpus luteum*
- *Irregular shedding*[Q] of corpus luteum/Halban's disease
- IUCD insertion
- Following sterilization operation (TVS).

General Principles in DUB

Whenever a female comes with DUB → Investigations which should be done in all age groups are TSH and Transvaginal ultrasound (TVS).

In Puberty Menorrhagia

Investigations which are done	Investigations never done
• TVS • TSH • Bleeding profile • S. progesterone level between 22–24 days of cycle (≥3 ng/dL, indicates ovulation has occurred). • Pregnancy test-If patient is sexually active • Culture for gonorrhoea and chlamydia	• Pervaginal examination • Dilatation and curettage

Flowchart 13.8: Causes of AVB

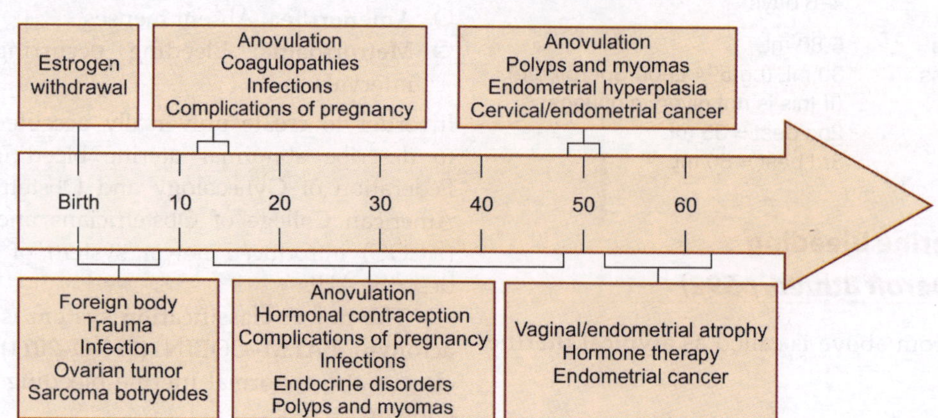

In Reproductive Age

Investigations done

- TSH
- TVS
- Pregnancy test
- S. progesterone level on day 22–24 of cycle (≥ 3 ng/dL, means ovulation has occurred)
- Endometrial biopsy
- Hysteroscopy
- MRI

M/c cause of DUB is anovulatory bleeding

Management

Management of Anovulatory Bleeding

Mainstay of therapy is-Progestin Therapy

- In anovulatory DUB, since there is no ovulation—progesterone is low but estrogen is normal which proliferates the endometrium(hyperplasia) which eventually sheds bringing about DUB. Progestin is a powerful anti-estrogen. It stimulates 17B-hydroxysteroid dehydrogenase and sulfonyl transferase activity, the enzymes that convert estradiol to estrone which is rapidly cleared from the body.
- Progesterone further downregulates estrogen receptors.

  Thus progesterone can control anovulatory DUB effectively. The only point to remember is that progesterone can only act, on uterus which has been primed by estrogen.

  ∴ **Progesterone treatment is unlikely to be effective in patients with thin, attenuated or denuded endometrium.**

  Progesterone therapy should be given in the last 12–14 days of cycles for anovulatory DUB and for bringing about regression of endometrial proliferation caused by estrogen. Drug = Cyclical Medroxy progesterone acetate 5–10 mg × Last 12–14 days of cycle.

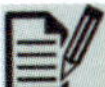

Important Concept

There for DOC for Anovulatory DUB in young girls females who are not sexually active = cyclical progesterone.

For those who are sexually active and are having anovulatary DUB want contraception also:

2 choices—Estrogen + Progestin i.e. OCP

—DMPA-injection (150 mg every 3 months)

For severe acute bleeding with thick endometrium treatment options include:

1. High dose progesterone alone, continuously from Day 1 of cycle

   E.g. Megesterol 20–40 mg oral

   Medroxy progesterone acetate 10–20 mg twice daily

Contd...

Contd...

2. OCP's—2 to 3 tablets daily

   This should be continued for 2 weeks even though bleeding stops in 48 hours

For severe acute bleeding with thin, denuded endometrium, in hemodynamically unstable patients

1. High dose estrogen alone: Conjugated estrogen 25 mg every 4 hrs till bleeding subsides for up to 24 hours. Drawback is it may increase the risk of thromboembolism.

Management of Ovulatory Bleeding

- NSAID's
- Estrogen and progesterone pills
- LNG-IUCD-Mirena
- Tranexamic acid
- GnRH agonist

Uterus Conserving Surgeries for DUB -Endometrial Ablation/Resection

The various surgeries included in Endometrial Ablation are:

- Laser (Nd:YAG) endometrial ablation
- Transcervical resection of endometrium (TCRE)
- Cryo ablation
- Microwave ablation
- Thermal balloon.

Indications

- Failed medical treatment
- Women who do not wish to preserve menstrual or reproductive function
- Uterus—normal size or not bigger than 10 weeks pregnancy size
- Small uterine fibroids (< 3 cm) - use microwave ablation
- Women who want to avoid longer surgery
- Woman who prefers to preserve her uterus.

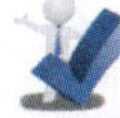

KEY POINTS

In endometrial ablation surgeries, whole of endometrium is destroyed, thus, it should not be done in females who desire future pregnancy.

Prerequisites

- Patient's family should be complete
- There should be no evidence of malignancy

Technique

- **Laser ablation** of the endometrium using the Nd:YAG laser through hysteroscope is an alternative to hysterectomy. It is employed as an elective alternative to hysterectomy or when hysterectomy has been medically contraindicated. Tissue destruction to a depth of 4–5 mm produces a therapeutic Asherman's syndrome and amenorrhea.

- **In Uterine thermal balloon**: Endometrium is destroyed using a thermal balloon with hot normal saline (87°C) for 8–10 minutes. No dilatation of the cervical canal is needed. This procedure is suitable for women who are not suitable for general anesthetic or long duration surgery. The success rate is similar to TCRE. No pretreatment endometrial thinning is required. This is considered as a first line therapy and is done as a day care basis.
- **Microwave endometrial ablation**: Endometrial tissue up to a depth of 6 mm is ablated. Temperature in the region is 75–80°C.

  Novasure: Endometrial ablation is done using a bipolar radio frequency mounted on an expandable frame.

  Radio frequency energy vaporizes or coagulates the endometrium up to the myometrium. The procedure is quick, simple, and safe. Women with uterine cavity < 4 cm, PID, cesarean delivery are contraindicated.
- **Transcervical resection of the endometrium (TCRE)** through continuous flow resectoscope is quicker and less costlier than laser ablation. It can be carried out even under paracervical block. Resectoscope loop must remove the basal layer of endometrium along with superficial layer of myometrium, otherwise regeneration of endometrium causes failure of operation.

  Result: Ablation of endometrium up to a depth of 4–5 mm using laser, roller ball, thermal balloon, microwave, is an effective method. Resection of endometrium up to the basal layer is also a quicker and less costlier method. Overall, amenorrhea occurs in 30–40% of women, about 50% have decreased bleeding and 10% may need repeat procedure or hysterectomy.

Complication

Most important is uterine perforation and fluid absorption leading to fluid overload.

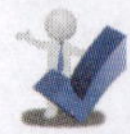

KEY POINTS

Contraindications of endometrial ablation
- Pregnancy
- Acute pelvic infection
- Endometrial hyperplasia
- Genital cancer
- Women wishing to preserve fertility
- Expectation of amenorrhea
- IUCD in place

Hysterectomy

Hysterectomy is not recommended as a first line therapy for heavy menstrual bleeding (HMB) or DUB. However, hysterectomy is justified when the conservative treatment fails or contraindicated and the blood loss impairs the health and quality of life. Presence of endometrial hyperplasia and atypia on endometrial histology is an indication for hysterectomy.

Metropathia Hemorrhagica

- *It is a specialized form of DUB.*
- Mostly seen in premenopausal women.
- ***Maximum age incidence:*** Between ages 40–45 years.

Pathophysiology (See Flowchart 13.9)

Flowchart 13.9: Pathophysiology of metropathia hemorrhagica

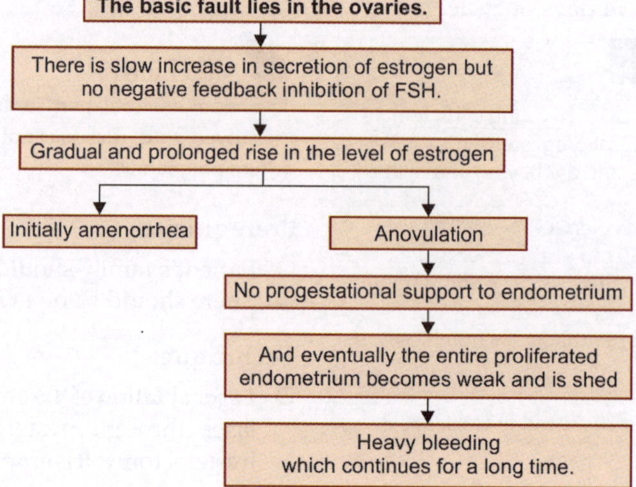

Changes in the Uterus: Symmetrical enlargement of the uterus to a size of 8–10 weeks due to hypertrophy of muscles.

Microscopic appearance:

- Hyperplasia of all endometrial components.
- Intense **cystic glandular hypertrophy.**[Q]
- Some glands are small and some large giving appearance of *"swiss cheese"*.[Q]
- Glands are empty and lined by columnar epithelium.
- Secretory changes are absent.[Q] (no cork screw glands seen)
- Follicular cysts containing estrogen present on ovaries.

Signs and Symptom: Patient complains of prolonged amenorrhea (of 6–8 weeks) followed by excessive painless bleeding (anovulatory bleeding).

Treatment: It is best treated by progestogen.

Postmenopausal Bleeding

- It is **defined** as any bleeding which occur in a middle-aged female after 12 months of amenorrhea.
  - M/C cause: Endometrial atrophy
  - Other causes: HRT, endometrial polyps, endometrial hyperplasia, endometrial cancer, cervical cancer

Table 13.8

Cause of Postmenopausal Bleeding	Percentage
Endometrial atrophy (MC)	60–80%
Estrogen Replacement therapy	15–25%
Endometrial Polyps	2–12%
Endometrial hyperplasia	5–10%
Endometrial cancer	10%

  - **M/C cancer, causing post-menopausal bleeding:** In developed countries Ca endometrium
  - **M/C cancer, causing post-menopausal bleeding in India:** Ca cervix
  - M/C cancer causing postmenopausal bleeding worldwide: Cancer cervix
  - **% of post-menopausal bleeding patients who have endometrial cancer:** 10%
- **First investigation to be done,** when a patient comes with post-menopausal bleeding: TVS.

Flowchart 13.10: Investigation in a patient c/o Primary amenorrhea

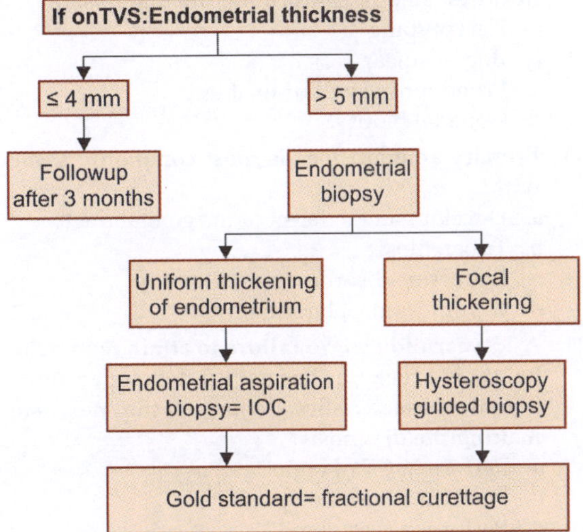

Investigation of choice in post-menopausal bleeding: Endometrial biopsy.

Gold standard investigation: Fractional curettage.

NEW PATTERN QUESTIONS

N1. A 5-year-old girl complains of failure to attain menarche. Her height is 4 feet inches, secondary sexual characteristics are absent. What is the next best step in making a diagnosis?
a. Perform a CT of brain
b. Perform a hormone profile
c. Do a karyotype
d. Do a TVS

N2. In the same question, if on USG uterus and vagina are seen LH and FSH levels are high. What is the next best step in conforming the diagnosis?
a. Karyotyping
b. Buccal smear
c. Progesterone withdrawal test
d. Gonadal biopsy

N3. Primary amenorrhoea is most commonly associated with:
a. Developmental defect of the genital tract
b. Tuberculosis
c. Endocrine disorders
d. Chromosomal abnormality

N4. A 15-year-old girl c/o failure to attain menarche. Her height is 4 feet. She has not yet developed secondary sexual characteristics. What is the next step in making the diagnosis?
a. Perform a CT of brain
b. Perform a hormone profile
c. Perform a Karyotype
d. Perform an USG scan

N5. In the same question if USG shows uterus and vagina. FSH and LH levels are high. What is the best step in confirming the diagnosis?
a. Perform a CT
b. Perform a Karyotype
c. Perform a buccal smear
d. Perform progesterone withdrawal test

N6. In the same question—what is the best treatment option of karyotype XO is confirmed?
a. Long term treatment with estrogen
b. Removal of streak gonads
c. Treatment with growth hormone for 6 months
d. Treatment with estrogen x 1 year and maintenance with estrogen and progesterone

N7. A 14-year-old girl presents with primary amenorrhea and monthly lower abdomen pain. She has good secondary sexual characteristics with axillary and pubic hair. Examination of the external genitalia reveals a bulging bluish membrane. Most appropriate next step in diagnosis:
a. Perform a hormonal profile
b. Perform a karyotype
c. Perform a laparoscopy
d. Perform an USG

N8. A 30-year-old athlete complains of amenorrhea for 1 year. Her BMI is 20 kg/m^2. LH and FSH are in low normal range. Clinical and USG findings are normal. Most likely cause is:
a. Depression
b. Excessive exercise
c. Premature menopause
d. Anorexia nervosa

N9. A 30-year-old athlete complains of amenorrhea for 1 year. Her BMI is 20 kg/m^2 Her:
FSH = 60 IU
LH = 55 IU
USG = Normal
Clinical examination—Normal
Most likely cause is:
a. Depression
b. Excessive exercise
c. Premature menopause
d. Anorexia nervosa

N10. In an infant who has clitoral enlargement and some degree of labial fusion. What is the first step in arriving at the diagnosis?
a. Perform a karyotype
b. Perform an USG scan
c. Perform blood 17 (OH) progesterone levels
d. Perform serum testosterone levels

N11. In the same question if karyotype is 46XX, then what is the next step in diagnosis?
a. USG scan
b. Laparoscopy
c. Blood 17 (OH) progesterone levels
d. Serum testosterone levels

N12. Withdrawal bleeding following administration of progestogen in a case of secondary amenorrhea indicates all *except*:
a. Absence of pregnancy
b. Production of endogenous estrogen
c. Endometrium is responsive to estrogen
d. Defect in pituitary gonadal axis

N13. Abnormal uterine bleeding is/are:
a. Blood loss of more than 80 mL
b. Cycle duration is more than 35 days or less than 21 days
c. Bleeding period lasting 7 days or more
d. Irregular bleeding during a regular cycle

N14. Metrorrhagia is produced by the following except:
a. Fibroid polyp
b. CA endometrium
c. IUD
d. Intramural fibroid

N15. In DUB, there is:
a. Increased estrogen
b. Decreased receptors of progesterone
c. Decreased receptors of estrogen
d. Pituitary imbalance of hormones

N16. Halban's disease is due to:
a. Persistent corpus luteum
b. Deficient corpus luteum
c. Persistent trophoblast
d. Deficient trophoblast

N17. Anita 15-year-old, complains of heavy periods since 2 months. O/E: wt 40 kg and BP 120/80 mm Hg. All of the following investigations are indicated, *except*:
a. S. TSH
b. Platelet count
c. Bleeding and clotting time
d. Estradiol levels

N18. The following are the features of anovular menstruation *except*:
a. The only symptom may be failure of conception
b. It is usually associated with painless periods
c. May be associated with premenstrual syndrome
d. May be associated with DUB

N19. Most common endometrial pattern in dysfunctional uterine bleeding:
a. Normal
b. Hyperplastic with Swiss-Cheese pattern
c. Nonsecretory
d. Atrophic

N20. Most common cause of menorrhagia in childbearing period:
a. Fibroid
b. Dysfunctional uterine bleeding
c. Pelvic endometriosis
d. Adenomyosis

N21. Metropathica hemorrhagica is best treated by:
a. Curettage of uterus b. Progestogen
c. Estrogen d. Clomiphene

N22. Swiss-Cheese pattern of endometrium is seen in:
a. Endometrial hyperplasia
b. Endometrial cancer
c. Metropathia haemorrhagica
d. H. mole

N23. The investigation of choice in a 55-year-old post-menopausal women who has presented with post-menopausal bleeding is:
a. Pap smear
b. Fractional curettage
c. Transvaginal ultrasound
d. CA-125

N24. The most common source of vicarious menstruation is:
a. Heart b. Lungs
c. Nose d. Kidney

N25. Routine endocrine evaluation of a woman with secondary amenorrhea consists of all except:
a. FSH b. TSH
c. ACTH d. Prolactin

PREVIOUS YEAR QUESTIONS

1. **A 13-year-old young girl presents in the casualty with acute pain in the lower abdomen. She has history of cyclical pain for last 6 months and she has not attained her menarche yet. On local genital examination, a tense bulge in the region of hymen was seen. The most probable diagnosis is:** *(AIIMS May 06)*
   a. Mayer-Rokitansky-Küster-Hauser syndrome
   b. Testicular feminization syndrome
   c. Imperforate hymen
   d. Asherman's syndrome
2. **The commonest cause of primary amenorrhoea is:** *(AIIMS Nov 03)*
   a. Genital tuberculosis
   b. Ovarian dysgenesis
   c. Mullerian duct anomalies
   d. Hypothyroidism
3. **Which is not primary amenorrhea?** *(AI 09/AI 2011/AIIMS May 2010)*
   a. Sheehan's syndrome
   b. Kallmann's syndrome
   c. Mayer Rokitansky Koster Hauser syndrome
   d. Turner syndrome
4. **A woman has 2 kids. She presents with galactorrhea and amenorrhea for 1 year. The most probable diagnosis is:** *(AIIMS May 02)*
   a. Pregnancy
   b. Pituitary tumor
   c. Sheehan's syndrome
   d. Metastasis to pituitary from other carcinoma
5. **Mrs. Sinha having her youngest child of 6 years age presents to her family physician with complaints of pruritis vulvae and amenorrhea. On examination she is found to have loss of pubic and axillary hairs, patch of vitiligo and hypotension. She is lethargic and has cold intolerance. She has got multiple skin infections and anemia. All of the following should be used to treat her, *except*:** *(AIIMS Nov 01)*
   a. Cortisol   b. Insulin
   c. Ethinyl estradiol   d. Thyroid extract
6. **Hypothalamic amenorrhea is seen in:** *(AIIMS Nov 01)*
   a. Asherman syndrome
   b. Stein-leventhal syndrome
   c. Kallmann syndrome
   d. Sheehan's syndrome
7. **Primary amenorrhoea with anosmia is seen in:** *(AIIMS June 00)*
   a. Kallmann syndrome
   b. Laurence Moon Biedl syndrome
   c. Foster-Kennedy syndrome
   d. Sheehan's syndrome
8. **A 19-year-old patient complains of primary amenorrhea. She had well developed breast and public hair but on examination there was absence of uterus and vagina. Likely diagnosis is:** *(AIIMS Nov 2010)*
   a. XYY   b. Mullerian agenesis
   c. Gonadal dysgenesis   d. Klinefelter syndrome
9. **A 35-year-old lady is not having her menses for last 4 months. She has high serum FSH and LH level with low estradiol. The likely cause is:** *(AIIMS Nov 99)*
   a. Panhypopituitarism
   b. Polycystic ovarian disease
   c. Exogenous estrogen administration
   d. Premature menopause
10. **A 30-year-old woman para 2 + 0, hypertension have menorrhagia. Which is best treatment for her?** *(AIIMS May 2011)*
    a. Combined pills
    b. Mirena
    c. Hysterectomy
    d. Transcervical resection of endometrium
11. **A 45 years old lady presented with dysfunctional uterine bleeding. On transvaginal USG thickness of endometrium was found to be 8 mm. What should be the nest step in the management of this patient?** *(AIIMS Nov 08/AIIMS Nov 2011)*
    a. Histopathology   b. Hysterectomy
    c. Progesterone   d. OCP
12. **Raja Devi 45 years old women present with history of poly-menorrhea for last six months. The first line of management is:** *(AI 02)*
    a. Hysterectomy
    b. Progesterone for 3 cycles
    c. Dilatation and curettage
    d. Oral contraceptive for 3 cycles
13. **In a 45 years old lady with DUB for 6 months duration best line of management is:** *(AIIMS June 00)*
    a. Progesterone for 6 months
    b. OCP for 6 months
    c. Dilation and curettage
    d. Hysterectomy
14. **Commonest cause of post menopausal bleeding in India is:** *(AI 07, AIIMS May 07)*
    a. Ca endometrium   b. Ca cervix
    c. Ca vulva   d. Ovarian tumour
15. **A teenage girl presented in OPD with moderate acne and history of irregular menses. What treatment will you give?** *(AIIMS Nov 2010)*
    a. Oral isotretinoin
    b. Oral acitretin
    c. Oral minocycline
    d. Cyproterone acetate

16. Primary Amenorrhea: *(PGI Dec 08)*
a. Absence of Menarche by 14 years without secondary sexual characters
b. Absence of Menarche by 16 years with secondary sexual characters
c. Absence of secondary sexual characters by years

17. Causes of secondary amenorrhea are: *(PGI June 01)*
a. Turner's syndrome
b. Endometriosis
c. Asherman's syndrome
d. Thyroiditis
e. PCOD

18. Lady recovered from severe PPH, complains of failure of lactation and menstruation, which of the following can be seen? *(PGI Dec 08)*
a. Increased excretion of Na^+
b. Retention of Water
c. Increased Prolactin
d. Increased GnRH
e. Increased TSH

19. A patient with amenorrhea had bleeding after giving a trial of progesterone. This implies: *(PGI Dec 01)*
a. Sufficient estrogen
b. Sufficient progesterone
c. Normal ovarian function
d. Intact endometrium
e. Intact pituitary axis

20. Positive progesterone challenge test in a patient of secondary amenorrhea, seen in: *(PGI June 04)*
a. Asherman Syndrome
b. Endometrial TB
c. Hypopituitarism
d. Premature ovarian failure
e. PCOD

21. Withdrawal bleeding with progesterone seen in otherwise amenorrheic woman due to: *(PGI Dec 97)*
a. Hypogonadotrophic hypogonadism
b. Anovulation
c. Ovarian failure
d. TB endometritis

22. In a case of secondary amenorrhea who fails to get withdrawl bleeding after taking E and P, the fault lies at the level of: *(PGI June 05)*
a. Pituitary b. Hypothalamus
c. Ovary d. Endometrium

23. Child with primary amenorrhea with negative progesterone challenge test but positive combined progesterone and estrogen test. Diagnosis may be: *(PGI June 07)*
a. Mullerian agenesis b. PCOD
c. Asherman syndrome d. Prolactinoma

24. Average blood loss in normal menstruation: *(PGI June 05)*
a. 50 mL b. 80 mL
c. 100 mL d. 120 mL
e. 10 mL

25. Menorrhagia is defined as blood loss per vagina more than: *(AIIMS Nov 99)*
a. 80 mL b. 110 mL
c. 150 mL d. 50 mL

26. Polymenorrhoea Means: *(PGI Dec 08)*
a. Menses < 21 days b. Menses >35 days
c. Painful menses d. DUB

27. Initial evaluation in adolescent with abnormal uterine bleeding: *(PGI June 05)*
a. Haemogram b. Platelet count
c. USG d. D & C
e. Examination under anesthesia

28. Most common cause of puberty menorrhagia: *(PGI June 07)*
a. Anovulation b. Malignancy
c. Endometriosis d. Bleeding disorder

29. Puberty menorrhagia is treated by: *(PGI June 02)*
a. Progesterone
b. Progesterone and estrogen
c. GnRH analogues
d. Danazol
e. Surgery

30. Causes of dysfunctional uterine bleeding can be: *(PGI Dec 01)*
a. Uterine polyp
b. Fibroid
c. Granulosa cell tumour
d. Irregular ripening of endometrium
e. Irregular shedding of endometrium

31. The most common histological finding of endometrium in DUB is: *(PGI June 99)*
a. Hypertrophic
b. Hyperplastic
c. Cystic glandular hyperplasia
d. Dysplastic

32. Treatment of DUB in young female is: *(PGI 95)*
a. Hormones b. Radiotherapy
c. D & C d. Hysterectomy

33. Treatment for 32 years old multipara with dysfunctional uterine bleeding (DUB) is: *(PGI Dec 00)*
a. Progesterone b. Danazol
c. Prostaglandins d. Endometrial ablation
e. Hysterectomy

34. A 45-year-old female presenting with dysmenorrhoea and menorrhagia most probably has: *(PGI Dec 97)*
a. DUB b. Endometriosis
c. Fibroid d. Endometrial Ca

35. All are causes of postmenopausal bleeding *except*: *(PGI Dec 00)*
a. Carcinoma *in situ* of cervix
b. Ca. endometrium
c. Ca. ovary
d. Ca. fallopian tube

36. Post-menopausal bleeding is associated with all *except*: *(PGI Dec 04)*
a. Ca cervix b. CIN
c. Ca ovary d. Endometrial Ca
e. Ca fallopian tube

37. A woman of 50 years who attained menopause, coming with one episode of bleeding P/V. Which of the following to be done? *(PGI June 09)*
a. Assess for H/o HRT b. Hysterectomy
c. PAPs smear d. Endometrial biopsy
e. TVS

38. Evaluation of a patient with post-menopausal bleeding is done by: *(PGI June 05)*
a. Pap smear b. USG
c. Endometrial biopsy d. Dilatation & curettage

39. Cryptomenorrhea occurs due to: *(AI 95)*
a. Imperforate hymen b. Asherman's syndrome
c. Mullerian agenesis d. All

40. A 35-year-old mother of two children is suffering from amenorrhea from last 12 month. She has a history of failure of lactation following second delivery but remained asymptomatic thereafter. Skull X-ray shows empty sella diagnosis is: *(AI 02)*
a. Menopause
b. Pituitary tumor
c. Sheehan's syndrome
d. Intraductal papilloma of breast

41. A 35-year-old female patient Radha having children aged 5 and 6 years has history of amenorrhea and galactorrhea. Blood examination reveals increased prolactin. CT of head is likely to reveal: *(AI 02)*
a. Pituitary adenoma
b. Craniopharyngioma
c. Sheehan's syndrome
d. Pinealoma

42. In a woman presenting with amenorrhea headache, blurred vision and galactorrhea appropriate investigation: *(AI 97)*
a. Prolactin levels b. LH
c. FSH d. HCG

43. Primary amenorrhea with absent uterus, normal breasts and scanty pubic hair is seen in: *(AI 2010)*
a. Mayer Rokitansky Kuster Hauser Syndrome
b. Turner Syndrome
c. Noonan Syndrome
d. Testicular feminizing syndrome

44. A patient had a spontaneous abortion, then she came with amenorrhea and FSH 6 IU/mL. What the most probably diagnosis? *(AI 10)*
a. Ovarian failure b. Uterine Synechiae
c. Pregnancy d. Pituitary failure

45. Lactational amenorrhea is due to:
a. Prolactin induced inhibition of GnRH
b. Prolactin induced inhibition of FSH
c. Oxytocin induced inhibition of GnRH

46. All of the following conditions are associated with primary amenorrhea *except*: *(AI 97)*
a. Testicular feminization syndrome
b. Stein-Leventhal syndrome
c. Turner's syndrome
d Mayer Rockitansky Kuster Hauser Syndrome

47. The most common cause of secondary amenorrhea in India is: *(AI 05)*
a. Endometrial tuberculosis
b. Premature ovarian failure
c. Polycystic ovarian syndrome
d. Sheehan's syndrome

48. Evidence based treatment for menorrhagia is all *except*: *(AI 09/AIIMS May 2010)*
a. OCPS
b. Progesterone for three months cyclically
c. Tranexamic acid
d. Ethamsylate

49. Which of the following is not indicated in menorrhagia: *(AI 02)*
a. NSAID's b. Clomiphene
c. Norethisterone d. Tranexamic acid

50. Which of the following statements is true about Swyer syndrome? *(AIIMS Nov 2015)*
a. Can be fertile with surrogacy
b. Can be fertile with ovum donation
c. Presents with primary fertility
d. Gonadectomy is indicated for all patients

51. Which of these is seen in Asherman syndrome:
a. Oligomenorrhea *(AIIMS Nov 2015)*
b. Hypomenorrhea
c. Metromenorrhagia
d. Polymenorrhea

52. A 18-year-old girl presented to the gynecology OPD with amenorrhea. On examination she was found to have Tanner's Stage V breasts and no pubic and axillary hairs. Ultrasound revealed absent uterus and nondeveloped gonads. What is the likely diagnosis?
a. Androgen insensitivity Syndrome *(AIIMS May 2015)*
b. Turner's syndrome
c. Cryptomenorrhea
d. Mayer-Rokitansky-Küster-Hauser syndrome

53. A mother brings her 19 years old daughter to your clinic with complaint that she has not started having menses. General examination reveals normally developed breasts and pubic hair. On pelvic examination, vaginal ending is blind and uterus is not palpable. Which of the following do you suspect?
a. Mullerian agenesis b. Asherman syndrome
c. Gonadal dysgenesis d. Turner's syndrome

54. A young female presented to you with primary amenorrhea. Examination reveals normal breast development and absent axillary hairs. Pelvic examination shows a normally developed vagina with clitoromegaly. On ultrasound, gonads are visible in the inguinal region. What is the most likely diagnosis?
a. Complete androgen insensitivity syndrome
b. Partial androgen insensitivity syndrome
c. Mayer Rokitansky Kuster Hauser syndrome
d. Gonadal dysgenesis

55. True about primary amenorrhoea: *PGI May 2016*
a. In Rokitansky-Kuster-Hauser syndrome, FSH is normal
b. In Turner syndrome, FSH is decreased
c. In Kallman syndrome, FSH is increased
d. In Kallman syndrome, LH is reduced

56. A patient presents with galactosemia and amenorrhea and high prolactin levels. MRI shows microadenoma of pituitary. All of the following will be seen in this patient *except*: *JIPMER December 2016*
a. High esterol b. Low costirol
c. Low FSH d. Low GnRH

57. Causes of abnormal bleeding is/are:
a. Hypothyroidism *PGI November 2011*
b. Asherman syndrome
c. Senile endometritis
d. Turner syndrome
e. Cervical polyp

58. A 15-year-old adolescent girl with primary amenorrhea and cyclical lower abdomen pain lasting for 2 days every 28 days. Normal secondary sexual characteristics. P/R reveals anterior swelling. Most probable diagnosis is: *JIPMER May 2016*
a. Cervical incompetence
b. Imperforate hymen
c. Mullerian agenesis
d. Pregnant with placenta previa

59. False statement regarding Sheehan syndrome: *JIPMER May 2016*
a. Regression of secondary sexual characteristics
b. Pituitary enlargement occurs
c. Hyponatremia
d. Somatotropin replacement done

60. A 18-years-old girl presents with history of primary amenorrhea. On examination, she has normal breast but vagina ends in a little pouch. Most probable diagnosis is: *JIPMER November 2015*
a. Complete androgen insensitivity syndrome
b. Testicular feminizing syndrome
c. MRKH syndrome
d. Turner syndrome

61. A 20-year-old short statured female comes to OPD with H/O primary amenorrhea. On examination she has webbing of neck, normal female external and internal genitalia. Breast development and public hair are absent. A diagnosis of Turner syndrome is made. However, the consultant still asks for her genetic phenotyping to rule out Y chromosome because: *JIPMER November 2015*
a. It's a routine procedure
b. Individuals harbouring Y chromosomes are at risk for germ cell malignancies
c. Diagnosis of Turner syndrome can be confirmed only if there is no Y chromosome
d. Individuals with Y chromosome should be reared as males

62. The presentation of Ashermann syndrome typically involves: *JIPMER November 2015*
a. Hypomenorrhea
b. Oligomenorrhea
c. Menorrhagia
d. Metrorrhagia

63. DUB treatment includes: *PGI May 2011*
a. NSAID
b. Progesterone
c. Tranexamic acid
d. Low dose OCP
e. Conjugated estrogen

64. Correct statement about menstruation: *PGI November 2011*
a. Polymenorrhoea means episodes of menstruation at intervals less than 21 days
b. Oligomenorrhea is scanty, regularly speed bleeding cyclic menstruation
c. Menorrhagia: very large amount of regularly spaced bleeding
d. Secondary amenorrhea - no bleeding for >12 weeks who have previously menstruated
e. Post-menopausal bleeding occurs after 1 year of stoppage of menses.

65. Which of the following statements is/are true:
a. Primary amenorrhea is failure of onset of menstruation beyond age of 14 years
b. Secondary amenorrhea is failure of occurrence of menstruation for 12 months who have previously menstruated
c. Polymenorrhoea is menstruation at less than 28 days
d. Oligomenorrhea is menstruation at intervals of more than 35 days
e. Primary amenorrhea is failure of onset of menstruation beyond age of 15 years in presence of secondary sexual characteristics

66. Abnormal uterine bleeding is/are: *PGI May 2013*
a. Blood loss more than 80 mL
b. Cycle duration more than 35 days or less than 21 days
c. Bleeding for more than 7 days
d. Irregular bleeding during regular cycle

67. What is the best treatment option for Metropathia haemorrhagica? *(AIIMS May 2019)*
a. Cyclical progesterone
b. Hysterectomy
c. Uterine artery embolization
d. Dilatation and curettage

68. Cork screw glands is/are absent in: *(PGI May 2019)*
a. Halban's disease
b. Metropathia haemorrhagica
c. Irregular ripening
d. PCOS
e. Ovarian neoplasms

ANSWERS TO NEW PATTERN QUESTIONS

N1. Ans. is b, i.e. Perform a hormone profile

N2. Ans. is a, i.e. Karyotyping

The patient has short stature and secondary sexual characteristics are absent:

If secondary sexual characteristics are absent, it means there is less of estrogen. This could be due to a problem in ovary or hypothalamus and pituitary.

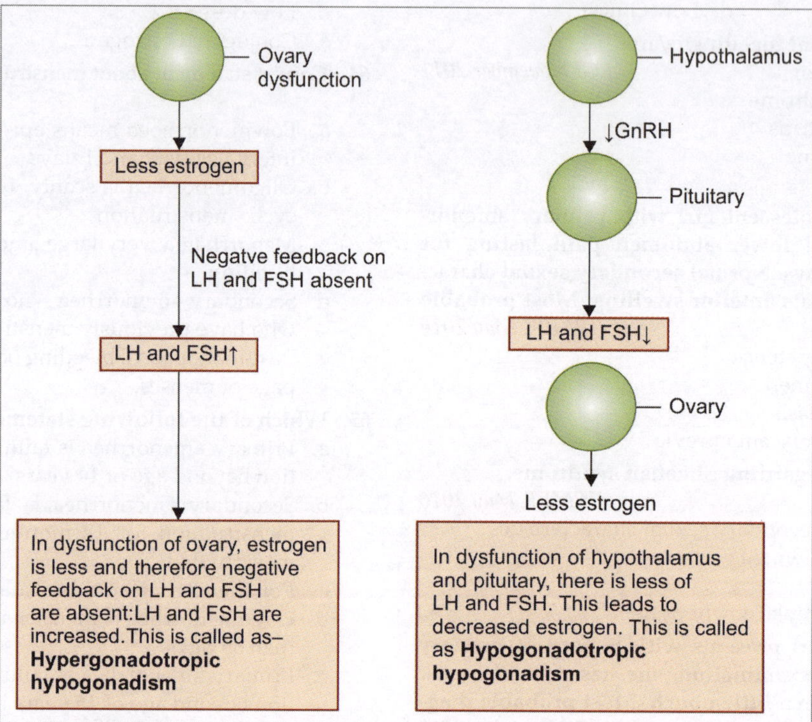

So the first step would be to identify the type of hypogonadism ∴ Ans for N1 is perform a hormonal profile then the next step would be karyotyping (Ans N2).

Best test for 1° amenorrhea: Karyotyping
This is because:
M/c cause of 1° amenorrhea Gonadal dysgenesis: Turner syndrome (45XO)
2nd cause of 1° amenorrhea: Mullerian agenesis (46XX)
3rd cause of 1° amenorrhea: Testicular feminizing syndrome (46XY)
All 3 can be differentiated by karyotyping

In this question:

1. Pt has decreased estrogen→Absent secondary sexual characteristics
2. Short stature
3. ↑LH and ↑ FSH

Most probably it is a case of Turner syndrome (45XO)

N3. Ans. is d, i.e. Chromosomal abnormality

See previous question for explanation

N4. Ans. is b, i.e. Perform a hormonal profile

N5. Ans. is b, i.e. Perform a karyotype

As discussed earlier: 1st step in primary amenorrhea is to identify the site of lesion by doing Hormonal profile (Ans N4)

In question N5: LH and FSH are high

USG: shows uterus and vagina are present

Pt has short height (4 feet)
No secondary sexual characteristics
Now since LH and FSH are high and estrogen is low (as secondary sexual characteristics are absent)
∴ It is a case of hypergonadotropic hypogonadism—so most probably it is Turners syndrome. This can be confirmed by doing karyotyping.
So as I have told earlier—Always remember in Primary amenorrhea

1st Test: Hormonal Profile
Best Test: Karyotyping

N6. Ans. is d, i.e. Treatment with estrogen x1 year and maintenance with estrogen and progesterone

1st step in management of all cases of primary amenorrhea is reassurance and explanation of the condition. The patient and the parents should understand future prospects.
Best treatment in Turners Syndrome is to give **estrogen for 1 year (to promote breast development)**, followed by long term treatment with estrogen and progesterone.
This will result in monthly withdrawal bleeding. Sexual activity is normal: as vagina is present
Therapy with Growth hormone can increase height if it is given before estrogen therapy.
There is no need to remove streak gonads.
Pregnancy is possible with IVF using Donor Oocytes but is contraindicated due to risk of aortic rupture and dissection.

N7. Ans. is d, i.e. Perform an USG

This patient has imperforate hymen as she has monthly abdominal pain, good secondary sexual characteristics and a bulging bluish membrane (due to collection of blood in vagina) is seen.
Most appropriate next step is to do an USG to confirm the presence of uterus, cervix and vagina.

N8. Ans. is b, i.e. Excessive exercise

This athlete has BMI = 20 kg/m^2, i.e. she is underweight
Her FSH and LH are in low normal range
All these findings point towards that either there is a problem in hypothalamus or pituitary.
One of the causes of hypothalamic amenorrhea is excessive exercise which is the most probable cause in this case.

N9. Ans. is c, i.e. Premature menopause

In the athlete =Aged 30 years
BMI = 20 kg/m^2 (decreased)
FSH = 60 IU (increased)
LH = 55 IU(increased)

Clinical state	Serum FSH	Serum LH
Normal adult female	5–20 IU/L	5–20 IU/L
Hypogonadotropic State: Prepubertal, hypothalamic or pituitary dysfunction	< 5 IU/L	<5 IU/L
Hypergonadotropic State: Postmenopausal or ovarian failure	> 20 IU/L	> 40 IU/L

This indicates hypergonadotropic problem which means site of lesion is ovary. The only ovarian cause given in the question is premature menopause (i.e. menopause in a female < 40 years).

N10. Ans. is a, i.e. Perform a karyotype

A child born with ambiguous genitalia could be a female who has been exposed to androgens like in case of congenital adrenal hyperplasia or a male who is undermasculinized or a true hermaphrodite.
Therefore first step in diagnosis is to perform a karyotype.

N11. Ans. is c, i.e. Blood 17(OH) progesterone levels since the karyotype is 46XX and patient has ambiguous genitalia. Most probable cause is congenital adrenal hyperplasia.

Screening test for congenital adrenal hyperplasia-17(OH) progesterone levels.
Confirmatory test = ACTH stimulation test

N12. Ans. is d, i.e. Defect in pituitary gonadal axis *Ref: Dutta Gynae 6th/ed, p467; Leon Speroff 7th/ed, p404-409*

As discussed earlier withdrawl bleeding following administration of progesterone suggests:

- The uterus is sufficiently primed with estrogen, i.e. production of endogenous estrogen is normal which means. Ovaries and hypothalamic pituitary axis are functioning normally.
- The outflow tract (uterus) is normal and endometrium is responsive to estrogen.
- There is a defect in production of progesterone (so pregnancy ruled out).

N13. Ans. is all.

Any uterine bleeding outside the normal volume, duration, regularity or frequency is considered **abnormal uterine bleeding (AUB).** Nearly 30% of all gynecological outpatient.

Abnormal menstrual bleeding pattern have been traditionally expressed by terms like menorrhagia, metrorrhagia, polymenorrhea, and oligomenorrhea. In order to create an universally accepted nomenclature to describe abnormal uterine bleeding, International Federation of Gynecology and Obstetrics (FIGO) and American College of Obstetricians and Gynaecologists (ACOG) introduced newer system of terminology to describe AUB. The newer classification system is known by the acronym PALM-COEIN (FIGO-2011). It is used to classify the abnormal uterine bleeding on the basis of etiology. Polyp, adenomyosis, leiomyoma, malignancy and coagulopathy, hyperplasia, ovulatory dysfunction, endometrial, iatrogenic, and not yet classified are the different etiological factors expressed by one (or more) letters.

The term dysfunctional uterine bleeding (DUB), discussed above is a type of AUB, whereas no systemic or locally identifiable structural cause is found.

Etiopathology of AUB

The common causes of abnormal uterine bleeding with the PALM-COEIN classification are shown below. The letter within the parenthesis indicate the pathology.

Classification of AUB (FIGO-2011)

Structural causes (PALM)		Nonstructural systemic causes (COEIN)	
• Polyp	AUB–**P**	Coagulopathy	AUB – **C**
• Adenomyosis	AUB–**A**	Ovulatory dysfunction	AUB – **O**
• Leiomyoma	AUB–**L**	Endometrial	AUB – **E**
– Submucosal myoma	AUB– **L SM**	Iatrogenic	AUB – **I**
– Other myoma	AUB–**LO**		
• Malignancy and hyperplasia	AUB–**M**	Not yet identified	AUB – **N**

N14. Ans. is d, i.e. Intramural fibroid *Ref: Dutta Gynae 6th/ed, p186*

Metrorrhagia: It is defined as irregular, acyclical bleeding from uterus, amount of bleeding is variable. Metrorrhagia also includes irregular bleeding in the form of contact bleeding or intermenstrual bleeding.

Menometrorrhagia: When the bleeding is so irregular and excessive that the menstruation cannot be identified.

Common causes of metrorrhagia are:

- Fibroid polyp
- Ca cervix and Ca endometrium
- Urethral caruncle
- Breakthrough bleeding in pill users
- IUCD in utero
- Decubitus ulcer

> ***Note:*** Fibroids lead to menorrhagia
> Fibroid polyp lead to metrorrhagia

N15. Ans. is a, i.e. Increased estrogen *Ref: Shaw 15th/ed, p301*

DUB is mainly anovulatory:

Bleeding occurs due to the hypertrophy and hyperplasia of the endometrium induced by a high titer of estrogen in the circulating blood is absence of progesterone.

This is the reason why initially due to lack of progesterone patients complain of amenorrhea and later on, due to excessive estrogen they complain of excessive bleeding.

N16. Ans. is a, i.e. Persistent corpus luteum *Ref: Shaw 15th/ed, p307; Jeffocate 7th/ed, p604; Dutta Gynae 6th/ed, p178, 5th/ed, p184*

Halban's disease:

- Rare, self-limiting process.
- Also called irregular shedding.
- It is due to persistent corpus luteum[Q] due to incomplete withdrawl of LH even on 26 in day of cycle. The CL continues to secret progesterone
- Menstruation comes on time, is prolonged but not heavy. Slight bleeding continues intermittently for several days after proper flow.
- ***On D & C done on 5–6th of cycle*** – endometrial tissue shows presence of progestational changes (proliferative endometrium) along with secretory endometrium.

Pregnanediol is found in urine during menstruation.

- *Treatment* – spontaneous cure or NSAIDs for 6 months.

Also know-Irregular ripening of corpus luteum-

- It is due to poor formation and function of corpus luteum.[Q]
- The endometrium is without adequate hormonal support, so slight losses or spotting occur for many days before the proper flow starts.

Diagnosis:

- Serum progesterone <5 ng/mL (or urinary pregnanediol <3 mg) in luteal phase.
- Endometrial study prior to or soon after spotting reveals patchy areas of secretory changes amidst proliferative endometrium.

Management: Administration of progestogens in premenstrual phase.

N17. Ans. is d, i.e. Estradiol levels *Ref: Dutta Gynae 6th/ed, p55*

Important causes of puberty menorrhagia are:

- HPO axis immaturity (anovulation)
- Bleeding disorders
- Endocrinological causes

Hence TSH, platelet count and BT/CT are done S. estradiol levels are of no utility in the workup of this patient.

Note: Always rule out bleeding disorder in patients of puberty menorrhagia.

N18. Ans. is c, i.e. May be associated with premenstrual syndrome *Ref: Dutta Gynae 6th/ed, p182*

Premenstrual syndrome is associated with ovulatory menstrual cycle. Rest all features are of anovulatory cycle.

N19. Ans. is a, i.e. Normal *Ref: Dutta Gynae 6th/ed, p189*

N20. Ans. is b, i.e. Dysfunctional uterine bleeding *Ref: Dutta Gynae 6th/ed, p185*

Common causes of menorrhagia:

- Dysfunctional uterine bleeding
- Fibroid uterus
- Adenomyosis
- Chronic tubo-ovarian mass

N21. Ans. is b, i.e. Progestogen *Ref: Dutta Gynae 5th/ed, p184,187, 6th/ed, p*

As discussed in the preceding text ***metropathica hemorrhagica*** *is a type of anovulatory DUB, hence logically speaking it should be best treated by progesterone therapy.*

It is mostly seen in premenopausal women.

Patients complain of a variable period of amenorrhea followed by excessive painless bleeding.

On HPE-cystic glandular hyperplasia, Swiss cheese pattern is seen, and secretory changes are absent

Treatment:

- In DUB due to anovular causes: Progesterones are the mainstay of therapy.
- They diminish the effects of estrogen on target cells by inhibiting oestrogen receptors.

N22. Ans is c, i.e. Metropathia haemorrhagica

See the text for explanation

N23. Ans. is b, i.e. Fractional curettage *Ref: Dutta Gynae 6th/ed, p 560*

In postmenopausal bleeding:

1st Investigation: TVS
IOC: Endometrial biopsy
Gold standard: Fractional curettage

Since endometrial biopsy is not given in options:-
Best answer is Fractional curettage

N24. Ans. is c, i.e. Nose *Ref: Jeffcoate 7th/ed, p 634*

Vicarious menstruation is a rare condition in which extragenital bleeding occurs at regular intervals corresponding to menstrual period. The commonest form of vicarious bleeding is epistaxis and this is a feature in 30% cases. Other sites affected are alimentary tract, lungs, breast, gums, lips, kidney, rectum, retina and conjunctiva.

It occurs most often at the extremes of menstrual life and in individuals with nervous and vascular instability. It ceases with menopause.

The epithelium over the inferior turbinate bones is already influenced by estrogen and so epistaxis is most common form of vicarious menstruation.

N25. Ans is c, i.e. ACTH *Ref: Leon Sproff 8th/ed, p475*

The routine endocrine evaluation of women with amenorrhea includes measurement of serum TSH, prolactin and FSH. Women with pituitary macroadenoma require additional evaluation, including a serum free T4, IGF-1 and morning cortisol level.

ANSWERS TO PREVIOUS YEAR QUESTIONS

1. **Ans. is c, i.e. Imperforate hymen** *Ref: Shaw 15th/ed, p96-97*
   A young girl who has not attained menarche but has history of cyclical pain for last 6 months, presenting to casualty with acute abdomen and on examination a tense bulge in the region of hymen – clearly point towards "Imperforate hymen" as the diagnosis. For details see the preceding text.
2. **Ans. is b, i.e. Ovarian dysgenesis** *Ref: Leon Speroff 7th/ed, p420; Shaw 15th/ed, p284*
   - Most common cause of Primary Amenorrhea = *Gonadal dysgenesis[Q]/ovarian dysgenesis/Turners syndrome*
   - 2nd most common cause of Primary Amenorrhea = *Mullerian agenesis (Mayer Rokitansky Kuster Hauser Syndrome).[Q]*

   "Mullerian agenesis is a relatively common cause of primary amenorrhea, more frequent than congenital androgen insensitivity and second only to gonadal dysgenesis." *Ref: Leon Speroff 7th/ed, p420*
   - 3rd most common cause is testicular feminizing syndrome.
3. **Ans. is a, i.e. Sheehan's syndrome** *Ref: Shaw 14th/ed, p256-257*
   - Kallmann's syndrome is due to hypothalamic dysfunction characterized by a deficiency of gonadotropin releasing hormone (GnRH) causing a hypogonadotrophic hypogonadism. This is associated with anosmia. It can occasionally be associated with optic problems, such as color blindness or optic atrophy, nerve deafness, cleft palate, cryptorchidism, renal agenesis, and mirror movement disorder.
   - MRKH syndrome, also known as Mullerian agenesis is due to anatomical absence of uterus. *This is the second most common cause of primary amenorrhea.*
   - Turner's syndrome is a type of gonadal dysgenesis *and is overall the most common cause of primary amenorrhea*
   - Sheehan's syndrome is postpartum pituitary necrosis. It leads to secondary amenorrhea and not primary amenorrhea.
4. **Ans. is b, i.e. Pituitary tumor**
   Ref: Novak 14th/ed, p1104, 1109; Harrison 17th/ed, p2205-2206; Williams Gynae 1st/ed, p338 Onwards

   The female in the question is presenting with galactorrhea and amenorrhea for 1 year which raises the suspicion for pituitary tumor i.e. prolactinoma/pituitary adenoma.

Pituitary Adenomas:
- Most common Pituitary adenoma is Prolactinomas.

Microadenomas	Macroadenomas
< 1 cm in diameter[Q] Female–male ratio = 20:1[Q] 5% of microadenomas progress to macroadenomas. 30% resolve spontaneously	> 1 cm in diameter[Q] Female–male ratio = 1:1[Q] Prolactin levels > 100 μg/L

Presentation:

Women present with:
- Galactorrhea[Q]
- Features of hypogonadism: *(as prolactin inhibits GnRH)*
  - *Amenorrhea[Q] / Oligomenorrhea*
  - Delayed puberty, Anovulation
  - *Infertility[Q]*

Men present with:
- Impotence
- Loss of libido
- Infertility.

In both sexes, they can cause symptoms due to mass effects of the tumor:
- Cavernous sinus syndrome consisting of:
  - Headaches
  - Visual defects *(Most common Bitemporal hemianopsia)*
  - Cranial nerve palsies especially III, IV, and VI
- Raised serum prolactin levels
- X-Ray sella shows space occupying lesion.

Investigations: In all cases of hyperprolactinemia:
- MRI should be performed
- TSH levels should be measured.

Management:

Microadenoma with no desire of fertility:
- Asymptomatic patients with microadenomas rarely progress to macroadenomas and are managed conservatively.
- If patient has osteopenia, (due to hypoestrogenemia caused by ↑ Prolactin levels) = estrogen replacement or OCP's.
- Monitor patients with regular serial prolactin levels and MRI (every 12 months).

For symptomatic microadenomas:

- Medical management by dopamine agonist viz cabergoline (which increase dopamine levels, thus decreasing prolactin levels) is the mainstay of therapy.
- Other dopamine agents like Bromocriptine, pergolide, lisuride (both ergot derivatives) and quinagolide (non ergot derivative) can also be used.

Macroadenomas: Long-term cabergoline therapy with periodic serum prolactin measurements (6 monthly) and MRI (6 monthly).

Surgery indications:

Tumors unresponsive to Bromocriptine

Tumor > 3 cms and female wants to conceive.

5. **Ans. is b, i.e. Insulin** *Ref: Jeffcoate 7th/ed, p582-583*

Well friends let's first diagnose the disorder with which Mrs. Sinha is suffering, then only we can debate about its management.

- The anterior pituitary hormones are affected in order = GH, FSH and LH, TSH, and ACTH
- In the question: **Mrs. Sinha has:**
  - Amenorrhea: due to ↓ FSH/LH
  - Cold intolerance
  - Hypotension *due to ↓ TSH*
  - Loss of axillary hair
  - Loss of pubic hair *due to ↓ ACTH (Adrenal cortical failure)*
  - Decreased skin pigmentation (vitiligo)

All these can be explained by: Sheehan's syndrome (and the question also says her youngest son is 6 years old which should hint at something: ***Remember -*** in **AIIMS** they have a meaning for each and every word).

Sheehan's syndrome is characteristically caused by ischemic necrosis of most of the anterior pituitary which results from spasm in its arterioles occurring at the time of severe haemorrhage or shock (usually postpartum) complicating child birth.

"The syndrome may develop slowly over 8–10 years time." *Ref: Dutta Gynae 6th/ed, p465*

The treatment of Sheehan's syndrome includes: Lifelong hormone substitute including estrogen, progesterone, thyroid, and adrenal hormone. *– Internet link www.nlm.nih.gov/medlineplus/ency/article/001175.htm.*

Replacement therapy with appropriate hormones including corticosteroid and thyroid are needed

Dutta Gynae 6th/ed, p465

6. **Ans. is c, i.e. Kallmann syndrome** *Ref: Shaw 15th/ed, p284; Harrison 17th/ed, p2198*

Kallmann syndrome is congenital GnRH deficiency along with anosmia or hyposmia. This is an hypothalamic cause of primary amenorrhea.

7. **Ans. is a, i.e. Kallmann syndrome** *Ref: Shaw 15th/ed, p70; Harrison 17th/ed, p2198*

Friends, you know the answer to this question quite well. Here I would like to point out that in solving PGMEE Questions of previous years, it is not only important to know the correct answer with its details, it is equally important to know the details of incorrect options (as Questions might be asked on these incorrect options in future).

So, let's know:

Laurence Moon Biedl Syndrome

It is an autosomal recessive disorder characterized by GnRH deficiency (hypogonadism) (FSH < 40 mIU/mL) and associated with:

- Obesity
- Mental retardation
- Polydactyly
- Retinitis Pigmentosa

Sheehan's syndrome: described in detail earlier

Foster Kennedy Syndrome: ***Do not get confused with this option:*** It is the same Foster Kennedy Syndrome as you have read in Ophthalmology, characterized by papilloedema in one eye and optic atrophy in the other. It results from raised intracranial pressure and simultaneous optic nerve compression secondary to tumor - classically, a meningioma of the olfactory groove, or more commonly, due to meningioma of the sphenoid wing.

8. **Ans. is b, i.e. Mullerian agenesis** *Ref: Jeffcoates 7th/ed, p197-198; Leon Speroff 7th/ed, p455-457,460-461,1261-1262*

In the question a 19-year-old girl is presenting with primary amenorrhea, she has well developed breast and public hair but on examination uterus and vagina are absent. Since her breast and public hair both are well developed- this means her secondary sexual characteristics are well developed.

This means in this female amount of estrogen is adequate, which means she has normally functioning ovaries.

Thus, options **XYY** (presence of Y Chromosome means- gonads are testis), **Klienfelter's syndrome** (genotype = 47XXY- again since Y chromosome is present, gonads are testes i.e. they are males) are ruled out and in gonadal dysgenesis–

gonads are incompletely formed and are streak gonads, M/c example is Turner's syndrome - genotype 45XO. Since gonads are streak, therefore estrogen is insufficient so secondary sexual characteristics are not well developed. In Turners thus by exclusion, our answer is **option b-** i.e. **Mayer-Rokitansky-Küster-Hauser syndrome.**

"Patients with mullerian agenesis, typically present in late adolescence or as young adults, well after menarche was expected, with primary amenorrhea as their only complaint. They exhibit normal, symmetrical breast and public hair development, no usable vagina and have no symptoms or signs of cryptomenorrhea because the rudimentary uteri contain no functional endometrium."

Ref: Leon speroff 8th/ed, p455

9. **Ans. is d, i.e. Premature menopause** *Ref: Shaw 14th/ed, p60*

- *Premature menopause is defined as secondary amenorrhea before 40 years of age, due to ovarian failure. It is clinically defined as secondary amenorrhea for atleast 3 months with raised FSH, raised FSH/LH ratio and low estrogen levels in a women under 40 years of age.*
- *In case of PCOD or Stein-Leventhal syndrome,* estrogen level is normal, LH is raised, LH/FSH ratio is raised.
- Panhypopituitarism leads to decreased LH and FSH levels which in turn leads to decreased estrogen.
- Exogenous oestrogen reduces FSH and LH by its feedback mechanism.

Conditions	Gonadotropins (LH, FSH)	Estrogen
Premature menopause	Both increased	Decreased
Pan hypopituitarism	Both decreased	Decreased
Exogenous estrogen	Both decreased	Increased
PCOD	LH increased, FSH normal	Increased

Remember: For diagnosis of premature ovarian failure serum FSH levels should be > 40 mIU/mL on 2 occasions, atleast 1 month apart.

10. **Ans. is b, i.e. Mirena** *Ref: Novak 15th/ed, p788; Williams Gynae 1st/ed, p187-188*

We have discussed in the preceding text, management options for females of reproductive age group -

In this particular question, female is 30 years old i.e. very young so we should not choose hysterectomy or endometrial ablation as the management of choice because in future she might desire pregnancy.

Patient is hypertensive, hence OCPs are contraindicated, so our answer by exclusion is Mirena which is logically also correct , as this patient has 2 children so she may not desire pregnancy presently.

Thus, Mirena serves 2 purposes in this female-

I. Controls bleeding
II. Contraceptive benefit.

In future, if she desires pregnancy, she may get mirena removed.

Our answer is further supported by the following lines -

"The LNG IUS can be used in all women as a first line of treatment of menorrhagia inplace of oral medications. It is particularly useful in reproductive aged women who desire contraception." *Ref: Williams Gynae 1st/ed, p188*

"Heavy menstrual bleeding that doesnot respond to oral medication may be managed by endometrial ablation using coagulation, resection or vaporisation provided that patient is willing to forgo future fertility. ***Alternatively if future fertility is desired, a levonorgestrel releasing intrauterine device can provide virtually equal clinical outcome."*** *Ref: Novak 15th/ed, p788*

11. **Ans. is a, i.e. Histopathology** *Ref: Williams Gynae 1st/ed, p 180*

A 45 years old lady is presented with DUB:

- Chances of endometrial hyperplasia/neoplasia are high.
- TVS findings show thickness of endometrium as 8 mm, so obviously next step would be to an endometrial biopsy, i.e. histopathological examination.

12. **Ans. is c, i.e. Dilatation and curettage** *Ref: CGDT 9th/ed, p629; Jeffcoate 7th/ed, p610*

13. **Ans. is b, i.e. OCP for 6 months**

Friends, I have given these *questions (12 and 13)* together, so that you understand the difference between the two.

Question 12 asks: Polymenorrhea in a 45 years old woman for 6 months – first line of management.

Whereas question 13 asks -DUB in a 45 years old woman for 6 months – best line of management.

As far as first line of management is concerned if such a patient comes to me, definitely I would investigate the patient to rule out endometrial cancer. I would perform biopsy but since it is not given, I will do for D&C.

"In the later reproductive years, even more care must be given to exclude pathological cause because of the possibility of endometrial cancer. Aspiration, curettage, or both should clearly establish anovulatory or dyssynchronous cycles as the cause before hormone therapy is started." *Ref: Jeffcoate 7th/ed, p609*

"Above 40, anovulatory DUB is again the commonest cause, but endometrial malignancy must be excluded and so endometrial sampling is performed as a first line investigation." *Ref: Text book of Gynae Shiela Balakrishnan 1st/ed, p58*

As far as the therapy is concerned, in perimenopausal age group–

"In this age group, anovulatory DUB is definitely more common, but endometrial pathology, especially endometrial malignancy must be ruled out" *Ref: Text book of Gynae Sheila Balakrishnan 1st/ed, p56*

And as we know in anovulatory DUB – medical therapy of choice is - Progesterone

As far as D & C is concerned: dilatation and curettage is basically for diagnostic purpose, its therapeutic benefit is very short lived

"Therapeutic curettage is of no value in the treatment of polymenorrhea."

Ref: Jeffcoate 7th/ed, p610

For hysterectomy-

The place of surgery in the treatment of excessive bleeding without an organic basis varies with the age of the patient; it should be a last resort in young girls but may be considered earlier in women above the age of 40 years. Nevertheless, in the latter group it is good practice to exclude organic disease by ultrasound and endometrial aspiration, to try medical therapy, and proceed to hysterectomy if the response is inadequate or not sustained.

Ref: Jeffcoate 6th/ed, p575

When the patient is above 40 years of age, and when the hemorrhage fails to respond to simpler measure, hysterectomy is indicated. It is the treatment of choice in all cases of persistent or recurrent postmenopausal bleeding for which there is no obvious cause.

Ref: Jeffcoate 7th/ed, p611

From above lines it is clear that hysterectomy is the last resort, first medical management is tried in perimenopausal females.

Hysterectomy personally I feel is not the best treatment as it is a major surgery, has its own complications and high rate of morbidity. I will not advise hysterectomy to all patients who come to me with the complain of DUB I will advise medical therapy and then proceed to hysterectomy if it fails. This is what we do in general practice.

Management protocol of DUB in perimenopause females

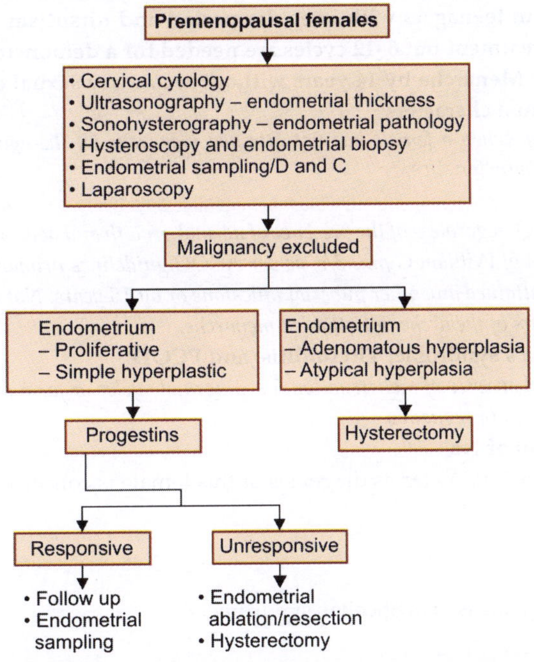

14. Ans. is b, i.e. Ca cervix *Ref: Gynae. for PG's by Bijoy Sree Sen Gupta 2nd/ed, p156-157; Shaw 15th/ed, p392; Jeffcoate 7th/ed, p471*

Friends, all the options given in the question can cause postmenopausal bleeding. The main question is most common cause in India –

"In the developed world Post Menopausal Bleeding (PMB) is a frequent presentation of endometrial carcinoma. The scenario is different in the developing world where carcinoma cervix is still the leading malignancy of the genital tract and the leading cause of PMB." *Ref: Bijoy Sree 2nd/ed, p156*

Remember:
- M/c cancer causing postmenopausal bleeding in India: Ca Cervix
- M/c cancer causing postmenopausal bleeding world wide: Ca cervix
- M/c cancer causing postmenopausal bleeding in developed countries: Ca endometrium.
- M/c cause of postmenopausal bleeding: Endometrial atrophy

Causes of Post Menopausal Uterine Bleeding with their frequency of occurrence. *Ref: Novak 15th/ed, p1256,427*

Table 35.3, p 1256 Cause	Percentage
Endometrial atrophy (MC)	60–80%
Estrogen Replacement therapy	15–25%
Endometrial Polyps	2–12%
Endometrial hyperplasia	5–10%
Endometrial cancer	10%

15. **Ans. is d, i.e. Cyproterone acetate** *Ref: Read Below*

A teenage girl is presenting with H/O irregular menses and acne both of which could mean excessive androgen production in females, so the best treatment would be to give her OCP's with progesterone belonging to 3rd or 4th generation
3rd generation progesterone: Desogestrel, Gestodene, Norgestimate.
4th generation: Cyproterone acetate

Anti-androgens Cyproterone acetate: It is an antiandrogen which inhibits gonadotropin secretion and interferes with androgen action on the target organs by competing for the androgen receptors.
It should be administered along with ethinyl-estradiol to prevent menstrual irregularities and ovulation. It is available as combined estrogen – progestin oral contraceptive (2 mg cyproterone acetate and 35 μg ethinyl estradiol as (Ginette or Diane 35)

"A combined pill containing 35 mcg ethinyl estradiol and 2 mg of an anti-androgen cyproterone acetate (Diane 35 or Ginette) is the drug of choice in teenagers with irregular period and hirsutism. The effect on acne and seborrhea is evident shortly after starting treatment but 6–12 cycles are needed for a demonstrable effect on hirsutism.

16. **Ans. is a and b, i.e. Absence of Menarche by 14 years without secondary sexual characters; and Absence of Menarche by 16 years with secondary sexual characters** *Ref: Shaw 15th/ed, p284*

Primary amenorrhea is a condition when a female has not attained menarche by the age of 14 years in the absence of growth or development of secondary sexual characteristics.

OR

No menarche by the age of 16 yearsQ regardless of the presence of normal growth and development of secondary sexual characteristics. But remember as per recent edition of William Gynae 3/e, as per ACOG guidelines primary amenorrhea is when a female by age 13 has neither had menarche nor has attained any other pubertal milestone or by 15 years. Not attained menarche. But has attained other pubertal milestone. or within 3 years of thelarche not attained menarche.

17. **Ans. is c, d and e, i.e. Asherman's syndrome; Thyroiditis; and PCOD** *Ref: Shaw 14th/ed, p259-260*

Secondary amenorrhea is defined as absence of menstruation for 3 normal cycles or for 6 months or more in a woman with previous normal menstrual pattern in absence of pregnancy *Ref: Williams Gynae p365*

18. **Ans. is a, i.e. Increased excretion of Na$^+$** *Ref: Read below*

Now, friends this is a tricky question. As far as diagnosis of this female is concerned there is no doubt that she is having Sheehan's syndrome.

As discussed earlier in next–

Levels of prolactin
Levels of GnRH
Levels of TSH } are all decreased in Sheehan syndrome

Along with this, level of ACTH is also decreased.

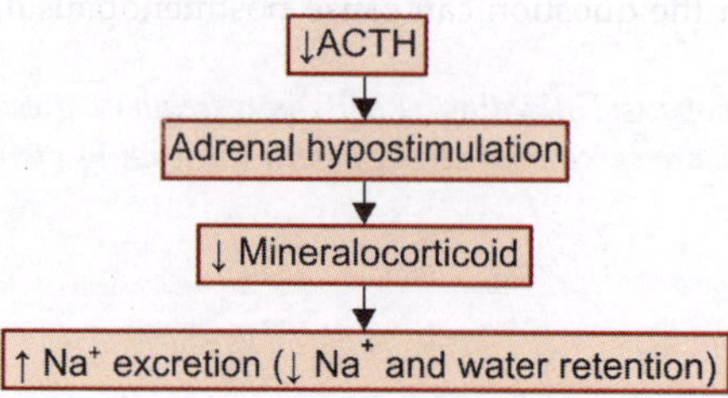

19. Ans. is a, d and e, i.e. Sufficient estrogen; Intact endometrium; and Intact pituitary axis

Ref: Dutta Gynae 5th/ed, p447, 6th/ed, p469; Leon Speroff 7th/ed, p404-409

20. Ans. is e, i.e. PCOD

21. Ans. is b, i.e. Anovulation *Ref: Dutta Gynae. 5th/ed, p447; Williams Gynae 1st/ed, p377*

If a patient is having positive progesterone challenge i.e. bleeding occurs after giving progesterone it means:

If withdrawal bleeding occurs, it proves— (i) The intact hypothalamopituitary ovarian axis and (ii) There is adequate endogenous estrogens (serum E2 level more than 40 pg/mL) to promote progesterone receptors in the endometrium, (iii) Anatomically patent outflow tract and (iv) Endometrium is responsive.

The defect lies in production of progesterone (as when progesterone is supplemented from outside, it results in withdrawal bleeding) and since progesterone is produced mainly by corpus luteum, so, the defect is anovulation.

The main cause of Anovulation in a case of 2° amenorrhea is polycystic ovarian disease.

22. Ans. is d, i.e. Endometrium *Ref: Dutta Gynae 5th/ed, p447*

Read the question carefully, it says absence of withdrawl bleeding after estrogen-progesterone challenge test.

Estrogen-progesterone challenge test

Procedure: Ethinyl estradiol (.02 mg) or conjugated equine estrogen (1.25 mg) is given daily for 25 days. MDPA 10 mg daily is added from day 15 to 25 (Alternatively estrogen is given for 21 days and progesterone is added in last 5 days).

↓ The test creates a condition similar to normal menstrual cycle

Withdrawl bleeding occurs	No withdrawl bleeding
Means endometrium and outflow tract are normal and if provided by normal hormonal levels, results in menstruation. Defect lies in production of estrogen i.e. either in ovary[Q]/ Pituitary[Q]/Hypothalamus	***Means their is a defect in endometrium***[Q] or outflow tract[Q] (As despite normal hormonal sequence no bleeding occurs).

23. Ans. is d, i.e. Prolactinoma *Ref: Dutta Gynae 6th/ed, p467*

This child is presenting with primary amenorrhea with:

- Negative progesterone challenge test - which rules out PCOD (which may sometimes manifest as primary amenorrhea)
- When next step was done i.e., estrogen, progesterone combined test – It comes out to be positive i.e., compartment I system (uterus, endometrium and outflow tract) is normal if properly stimulated by estrogen which rules out mullerian agenesis and Ashermann's syndrome.
- Positive estrogen progesterone combined test means the defect is in the production of estrogen i.e., either ovaries, pituitary, or hypothalamus.

So from the given options we have to look for a cause which involves either of the above sites, which in this case is prolactinoma.

24. Ans. is a, i.e. 50 mL *Ref: Novak 14th/ed, p461; Shaw 15th/ed, p283*

25. Ans. is a, i.e. 80 mL *Ref: Shaw 15th/ed, p283*

26. Ans. is a and d, i.e. Menses <21 days; and DUB *Shaw 15th/ed, p283*

Characteristics of menstrual cycle and all terms have been discussed in text.

27. Ans. is a, b and c, i.e. Haemogram; Platelet count; and USG *Ref: Novak 14th/ed, p450-454,15th/ed, p390-397; Dutta Gynae 6th/ed, p55*

28. Ans. is a, i.e. Anovulation

29. Ans. is a, b and c, i.e. Progesterone; Progesterone and estrogen; and GnRH analogues

Ref: Shaw 15th/ed, p302; Novak 15th/ed, p394-397; Dutta Gynae 6th/ed, p

Puberty menorrhagia is excessive cyclical regular bleeding occurring in adolescents.

Most of the adolescent females have irregular periods for a variable period following menarche due to anovulatory cycles. Anovulatory bleeding can be too frequent, prolonged or heavy particularly after a long interval of amenorrhea.

Physiology:

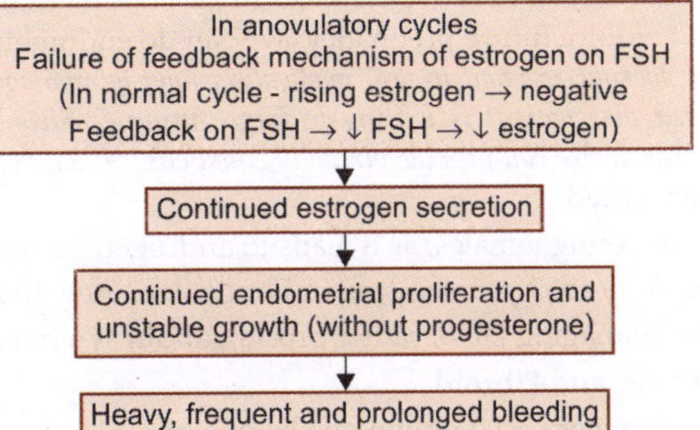

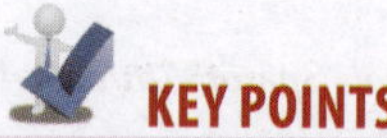

KEY POINTS

Causes of puberty menorrhagia-
Most common cause - anovulation
IInd most common cause is – Bleeding disorders - blood dyscrasias and coagulation disorders.

Management: It is like anovulatory DUB
i. With progesterone alone
ii. With estrogen and progesterone
iii. Only estrogen in case of uncontrollable bleeding.

Role of dilatation and curettage in puberty menorrhagia: *"D & C is done only in rare cases of puberty menorrhagia - when intrauterine clots are seen on USG (as the cause of bleeding) to rule out endometrial tuberculosis."* *Ref: Novak 15th/ed, p396*

"If a girl fails to respond to hormonal therapy curettage of endometrium is necessary to rule out genital tuberculosis which is seen in 4% of these young girls." *Ref: Shaw 14th/ed, p271*

D & C is not a part of initial evaluation in adolescents (so, **option "d"** ruled out).

Use of GnRH analogues:

"For adolescent patients with coagulopathies or malignancy requiring chemotherapy, long term therapeutic amenorrhea with menstrual suppression using GnRH analogues can be achieved." *Ref: Novak 14th/ed, p454,15th/ed, p397*

30. Ans. is d and e, i.e. Irregular ripening of endometrium; and Irregular shedding of endometrium *Ref: Shaw 15th/ed, p301-302 Table 22.2*

DUB is defined as a state of abnormal uterine bleeding without any clinically detectable organic pelvic pathology.

DUB is of 2 types:
1. Anovulatory (80%)
2. Ovulatory (20%)

Anovulatory (80%):
- Threshold bleeding of puberty menorrhagia
- Metropathia hemorrhagica[Q]/cystic glandular hyperplasia[Q]
- Premenopausal DUB (Atrophy of endometrium).

Ovulatory (20%):
- *Irregular ripening[Q] of corpus luteum*
- *Irregular shedding[Q] of corpus luteum*
- IUCD insertion
- Following sterilization operation.

31. Ans. is b, i.e. Hyperplastic *Ref: Dutta Gynae 6th/ed, p189*

Endometrial pattern in DUB
- Normal secretory endometrium = 60%
- Hyperplastic endometrium = 30%
- Irregular shedding, Irregular ripening, Atrophic pattern } = 10%

Since normal secretory endometrium is not given in options so, we will see 2nd most common which is hyperplastic endometrium.

32. Ans. is a, i.e. Hormones *Ref: Dutta Gynae 5th/ed, p187; Novak 14th/ed, p465*

Treatment of DUB in young females is always hormonal.

33. Ans. is a and d, i.e. Progesterones; and Endometrial ablation *Ref: Novak 15th/ed, p788; Williams Gynae 1st/ed, p187*

Now in this question, patient is 32 years old and is multiparous- so LNG- IUCD will be best option for her i.e option a-progesterones is correct.

Since, it is a multiple choice question so here we can also mark endometrial ablation as correct option, because she is multiparous and if she doesnot require future pregnancy -we can do endometrial ablation.

"Heavy menstrual bleeding that doesnot respond to oral medication may be managed by endometrial ablation using coagulation, resection or vaporization provided that patient is willing to forgo future fertility. Alternatively, if future fertility is desired, a levonorgestrel releasing intrauterine device can provide virtually equal clinical outcome." *Ref: Novak 15th/ed, p788*

As far as other options are concerned-

Danazol-it should not be used in young females, as it leads to androgenic side effects

Hysterectomy-it should not be done at 32 years unless and until absolutely indicated.

Prostaglandins-are not used for managing DUB, rather prostaglandin synthetase inhibitors are used.

34. Ans. is b and c, i.e. Endometriosis; and Fibroid *Ref: Read Below, Shaw 15th/ed, p302-303*

Well friends, here we will have to weigh each option one by one.

Option "a": DUB *Ref: Shaw 14th/ed, p271-272*

- Metropathia hemorrhagica is seen in age group of 40–45 years which coincides with the age of the patient given in the question.
- But in DUB (as 80% cases are due to anovulatory bleeding) pain is characteristically absent. Bleeding is always painless and acyclical and continues for 2–8 days. In about half the cases, it is preceded by a short period of amenorrhea (metropathia hemorrhagica).

  So, **option "a"** is ruled out.

Option "b": Endometriosis

- Dysmenorrhea (secondary and progressive in nature) and menstrual irregularities including menorrhagia are specifically seen in endometriosis. *Ref: Shaw 15th/ed, p468-469*
- As far as age is concerned.

  "Active endometriosis is seen most commonly between the ages of 30 and 40 years. It can however occur at any time between the menarche and the menopause, even before the age of 20 years." *Ref: Jeffcoate 7th/ed, p368*

  So, endometriosis is one of the possible differential diagnosis.

Option "c": Fibroid

- *Age group:* Seen in women of child bearing age group. Seen in 40% of women above the age of 40 years.
- Fibroids most commonly cause symptoms between the ages of 35 and 45 years. (So age is consistent with the patients age).
- *Fibroid uterus causes menorrhagia and dysmenorrhea. So, the possibility of fibroid is high.* *Ref: Shaw 15th/ed, p357*

Option "d": Endometrial carcinoma

- It is not a case of endometrial Ca because, endometrial Ca is common in 55–60 years. *Ref: Shaw 15th/ed, p416*
- Patient presents with irregular and heavy cycles.
- The lower abdominal pain in advanced stage is due to parametrial involvement. *(Not dysmenorrhea)*

Ref: Shaw 15th/ed, p418; Jeffcoate 7th/ed, p508

35. Ans. is a, i.e. Carcinoma *in situ* of cervix

36. Ans. is b, i.e. CIN *Ref: Novak 14th/ed, p490; CGDT 10th/ed, p577-578; Jeffcoate 7th/ed, p614*

Postmenopausal bleeding is defined as bleeding which occurs after 12 months amenorrhea in a middle aged women.

Causes of Post Menopausal Bleeding:

- Exogenous estrogen (HRT)
- Vaginitis - tubercular, candida, chlamydia, senile
- Endometrial hyperplasia
- Cervical cancer
- Uterine sarcoma
- DUB - ovulatroy/anovulatory ulcer/Foreign body
- Bleeding from urethera, bladder, rectum which is mistaken for vaginal bleeding.
- Endometritis - tubercular, senile pyometra & hematometra
- Endometrial/cervical polyp
- Endometrial cancer (correct option)
- Ovarian cancer (correct option)
- Fallopian tube carcinoma
- Injuries - direct trauma / Decubitus

As far as Fallopian tube carcinoma is concerned. Most common age group = 50–60 years.

Most common symptom: Watery discharge which tracks from the tube through the uterus and vagina (hydrops tubal profluens).It is typically colourless, profuse in amount and escapes continuously or in gushes. The discharge ultimately becomes blood stained from ulceration of growth and female presents as *post menopausal bleeding*. (correct option).

Cervical cancer is a cause of postmenopausal bleeding, but cervical carcinoma in situ which is seen at 25–35 years of age and CIN which is seen in women in their 20's is not a cause of post menopausal bleeding.

Remember:

"CIN is most commonly detected in women in their 20's, peak incidence of carcinoma in situ is in women aged 25 – 35, while incidence of cervical cancer rises after the age of 40." *Ref: CGDT 10th/ed, p833*

37. Ans. is a, c, d, and e, i.e. Assess for H/o HRT; Papsmear; Endometrial biopsy and TVS

38. Ans. is a, b, c and d, i.e. Pap smear; USG; Endometrial biopsy; and Dilatation & curettage

Ref: CGDT 10th/ed, p577-578; Novak 15th/ed, p427,1256

As discussed in the preceeding test whenever is postmenopausal female comes with bleeding

1st step: TVS/USG

2nd step: IOC : endometrial biopsy

(It has replaced D&C, but at places where endometrial biopsy is not available, still D&C is done)

Gold standard: Fractional curettage

Apart from this:

"A pap test is essential when post-menopausal bleeding is noted, although the pap test is an insensitive diagnostic test for detecting endometrial cancer." *Ref: Novak 15th/ed, p427*

39. Ans. is a, i.e. Imperforate hymen *Ref: Dutta Gynae 6th/ed, p450; Shaw 15th/ed, p96-97*

- Cryptomenorrhea is defined as occurrence of menstrual symptoms without external bleeding.
- Menstrual blood fails to come out from genital tract due to obstruction in the outflow passage.
- **Causes:**

Congenital	Acquired
Imperforate hymen (commonest) Transverse vaginal septum Atresia of upper third vagina & cervix	Cervical stenosis following: • Amputation • Cauterization • Conization • 'Radium' treatment for malignant conditions

40. Ans. is c, i.e. Sheehan's syndrome *Ref: Williams Gynae 1st/ed, p374; Leon Speroff 7th/ed, p438; Jeffcoate 7th/ed, p582-583*

Friends, here before arriving to any diagnosis lets first see the causes of:

Empty Sella:

- Congenital incompleteness of the sellar diaphragm.
- Secondary to surgery/radiotherapy or infarction of pituitary tumor.
- Secondary to infarction and necrosis of pituitary gland.

Now from the given causes: either pituitary tumor or Sheehan's syndrome can cause an empty sella on X-ray.

Pituitary tumours (micro/macroadenoma) are prolactin secreting tumors and hence, cause galactorrhea (not lactational failure) with amenorrhea and are so, ruled out.

So, the obvious answer by exclusion is Sheehan's Syndrome.

Remember

Amenorrhea

With failure to lactate → Think sheehan's syndrome

With galactorrhea, headache and blurring of vision → Think prolactinoma

Sheehan's syndrome:

- *It is the syndrome which results from ischemic necrosis of most of the anterior pituitary[Q] due to spasm in its arterioles occurring at the time of severe hemorrhage or shock, complicating childbirth.*

Clinical Features: Symptoms[Q]

- Failure of lactation after delivery[Q]
- Secondary amenorrhea[Q]
- Loss of libido[Q]
- Increased sensitivity to cold (hypothyroidism)[Q]

41. Ans. is a, i.e. Pituitary adenoma *Ref: Novak 14th/ed, p1104,1109; Harrison 17th/ed, p2205-2206; Williams Gynae 1st/ed, p 338 onwards*

See the explanation in previous question.

42. Ans. is a, i.e. Prolactin levels *Ref: Harrison 17th/ed, p2205; Williams Gynae 1st/ed, p338-340*

See the explanation of Q 40.

43. Ans. is d, i.e. Testicular feminizing syndrome *Ref: Novak 14th/ed, p1037-1038*

The patient is presenting with primary amenorrhea along with well developed breast and scanty pubic hair and axillary hair -leave no doubt regarding Testicular feminizing syndrome as the diagnosis. For details see chapter-sexuality ansd intersexuality of the guide.

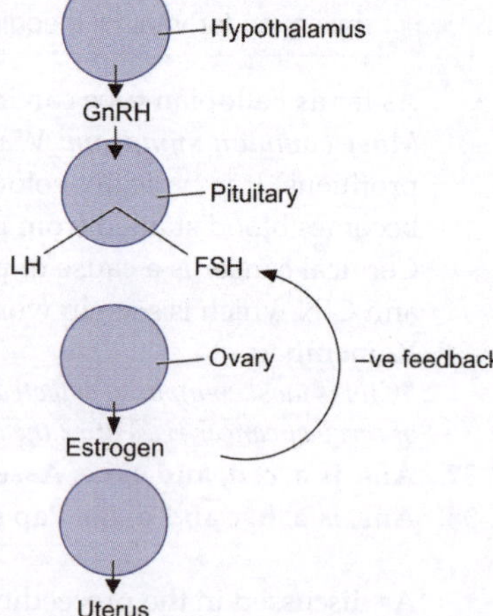

44. Ans. is b, i.e. Uterine Synechiae *Ref: Leon speroff 7th/ed, p415-425, 8th/ed, p443 for FSH significance and 459 for asherman syndrome*

Explanation:

Normal FSH values range from 5 to 20 mIU/mL. In the question, FSH levels are 6 mIU/mL, that means this is a case of secondary amenorrhea with normal FSH values.

- In case of pituitary failure – as is evident from the flow diagram → values of FSH should be lower than the normal values. So **Option 'd'** is ruled out
- Incase of ovarian failure → estrogen is deficient so negative feedback on FSH will be absent, thus values of FSH will be more than normal. In case of ovarian failure/menopause, FSH is above 40 m IU/mL so **option a** is also ruled out.
- Normal FSH and amenorrhea point towards uterine pathology. The patient had a spontaneous abortion following which a curettage is generally required which would be responsible for intrauterine synechiae (Asherman's Syndrome). Thus, the most probable diagnosis is uterine synechiae.

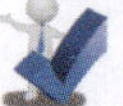

KEY POINTS

Remember

Hyperprolactinemia leads to decreased levels of FSH.

45. Ans. is a, i.e. Prolactin induced inhibition of GnRH

Ref: Leon Speroff 7th/ed, p582; John Hopkins Manual of Obs And Gynae 4th/ed, p472

- In breastfeeding females, prolactin levels are increased in response to suckling stimulus of breast feeding.
- Besides Prolactin, FSH concentrations are normal and LH concentrations are low.
- Despite the presence of gonadotropin the ovary during lactational hyperprolactinemia does not display follicular development and does not secrete estrogen.
- These observations suggest that high concentrations of prolactin can work at both central level (by inhibiting pulsatile secretion of GnRH) and peripheral level i.e. ovarian sites (by inhibiting synthesis of progesterone and by changing testosterone/dihydrotestosterone ratio i.e. increasing local antiestrogen concentrations) to produce lactational amenorrhea and anovulation.
- The principle of GnRH suppression by prolactin is reinforced by the demonstration that, treatment of amenorrheic, lactating women with pulsatile GnRH, fully restores pituitary secretion and normal ovarian cyclic activity.

46. Ans. is b, i.e. Stein-Leventhal syndrome *Ref: Shaw 15th/ed, p284-285*

The **Stein-Leventhal Syndrome** *also known as* **Polycystic Ovarian Disease (PCOD)** *is an important cause of Secondary Amenorrhea in young women.*

Testicular Feminizing syndrome, Turners syndrome and Mayer Rokitansky Kuster Hauser syndrome are causes of Primary amenorrhea.

47. Ans. is a, i.e. Endometrial tuberculosis *Ref: Read below*

In a country like India where most of the population belongs to middle, lower middle, and lower class: Endometrial tuberculosis seems to be the most common cause of secondary amenorrhea.

48. Ans. is d, i.e. Ethamsylate *Ref: Williams Gynae 1st/ed, p187*

49. Ans. is b, i.e. Clomiphene

Ref: Dewhurst's Textbook of Obs. & Gynae. 7th/ed, p401; Gyanaecology by Soutter – Stanton 2nd/ed, p435; Shaw 12th/ed, p242

Medical Management of Menorrhagia:

A. Prostaglandin synthetase inhibitor	B. Antifibrinolytic	C. Hormones
• Mefenamic Acid	• Tranexamic acid	• Progesterones • Estrogen • OCP's • Danazol/Gestrinone (androgen) • GNRH analogues

NSAID's

- ***Rationale:*** Its use stems from the suspected role of prostaglandins in the pathogenesis of DUB.
- ***Advantages:*** – It is required only during menstruation
  – It provides relief from dysmenorrhea
- ***Tranexamic acid:*** It is an antifibrinolytic drug which exerts its effects by reversibly blocking lysine binding sites on plasminogen. The resulting decreased plasmin levels diminish fibrinolytic activity within endometrial vessels to prevent bleeding.

"Clinically, the drug has been shown effective to reduce bleeding in upto half of the women with DUB related to menorrhagia."

Ref: Williams Gynae 1st/ed, p187

According to latest RCOG guidelines tranexamic acid is the first line DOC for menorrhagia

Progesterone's

"With the introduction of potent orally active progestins, they be came the mainstay in the management of DUB in all age groups and practically replaced the isolated use of oestrogens and androgens." *Ref: Dutta Gynae 5th/ed, p187*

Estrogen: High dose estrogen therapy may be useful in controlling acute bleeding episodes because it promotes rapid endometrial growth to cover denuded surface. Conjugated equine estrogens are administered orally at dosages up to 10mg daily given in four divided doses. Similarly the drug can be given intravenously in 25 mg doses every 4 hours for up to 3 doses. Once bleeding has slowed, patients can be transitioned to an oral taper using COCs.

Androgens – Danazol – It is suitable for recurrent symptoms and in patients waiting for hysterectomy. A smaller dose tends to minimize the blood loss and higher dose produces amenorrhea.

Gestrinone – can also be used like Danazol.

Mifepristone – It is an antiprogesterone. It inhibits ovulation and induces amenorrhea but is not commonly used for DUB (this drug is not mentioned in *Williams Gynae* for management of DUB)

Gonadotropin Releasing hormone agonists (GnRH agonist) – Its subtherapeutic doses decrease the blood loss whereas therapeutic doses produce amenorrhea.

It is valuable for short term use in severe DUB, particularly if the woman is infertile and wants pregnancy.

- As far as ethamsylate is concerned:
  - It is an hemostatic agent but its action and efficacy is inconsistent.
  - Though in some books it is given ethamsylate may be used but *Williams Gynae.* specifically says:
    "Because of its inconsistent efficacy, in United States ethamsylate does not have a clinical role the treatment of menorrhagia."

Ref: Williams Gynae 1st/ed, p187

50. Ans. is b, i.e. Can be fertile with ovum donation *Ref: Shaw's Textbook of Gynecology 15th/ed, p145*

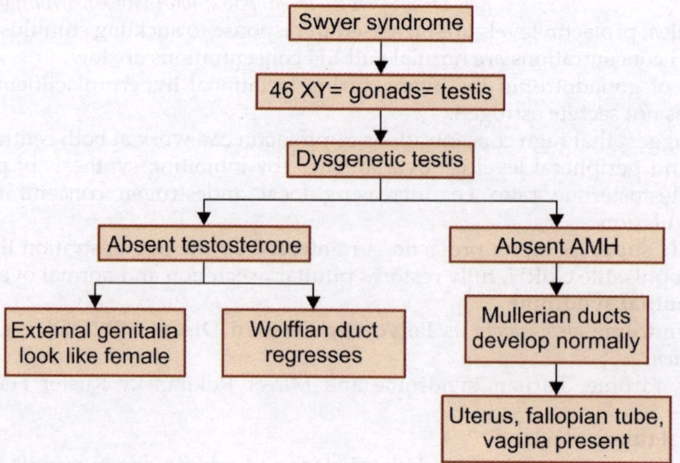

51. Ans. is b, i.e. Hypomenorrhea *Ref: Shaw's Textbook of Gynecology 15th/ed, p250*

52. Ans. is a, i.e. Androgen insensitivity syndrome *Ref: Williams Obstetrics 24th/ed, p149*

The patient at 18 years of age is presenting with:

- Amenorrhea
- Tanner stage V of breast
- No pubic and axillary hair
- USG shows absent uterus and non-developed gonads.

All these findings point towards Androgen insensitivity syndrome.

53. Ans. is a, i.e. Mullerian agenesis

In this case patient is C/O primary amenorrhea and

(i) Has normal breast and normal pubic hair (i.e. Turner syndrome and, Gonadal dysgenesis ruled out).
(ii) She has 1° primary amenorrhea (rules out Asherman Syndrome)

Thus by exclusion our answer is Mullerian agenesis.

54. Ans. is b, i.e. Partial androgen insensitivity syndrome

In the question patient has 1° amenorrhea:

- Breast development is normal and absent axillary hair. (This means it cannot be Mayer-Rokitansky-Küster-Hauser syndrome—where Breast and pubic as well as axillary hair are well developed and it cannot be Gonadal dysgenesis as none of the secondary sexual characteristics are developed in it).
  We are left with 2 options:
  Option a—Complete androgen insensitivity
  Option b—Partial androgen insensitivity
  In both these conditions—Breast development will be normal and pubic hair and axillary hair will be absent but clitoromegaly will be seen in partial androgen insensitivity only.

55. Ans. is a and d, i.e. In Rokitansky-Kuster-Hauser syndrome, FSH is normal and In Kallman syndrome LH is reduced.

In MRKH Syndrome-Ovaries are normal so estrogen is normal, so negative feedback of estrogen on FSH is normal, hence levels of FSH are normal

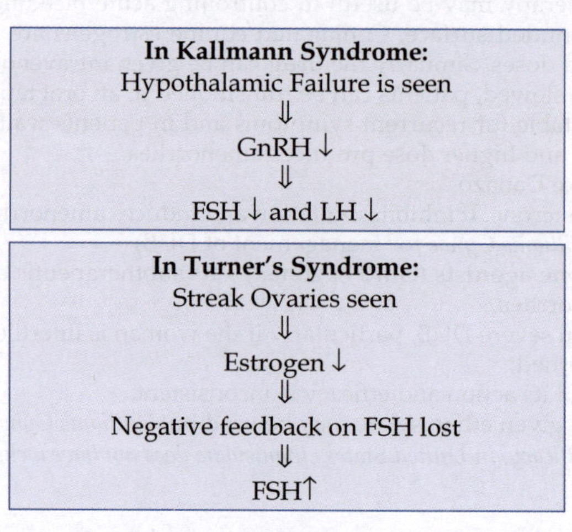

56. **Ans. is a, i.e. High esterol**

Now this patient is having a pituitary tumor secreting prolactin. Prolactin has a negative feedback on GnRH. Therefore, there will be

- Low GnRH
- Low LH
- Low FSH
- Low sex steroids

57. **Ans. is a, b, c and e, i.e. Hypothyroidism; Asherman syndrome; Senile endometritis; and Cervical polyp**

Causes of abnormal uterine bleeding are:

P = polyps (i.e. option e)
A = Adenomyosis
L = Leiomyoma
M = Malignancy
C = Coagulopathy
O = Ovulatory dysfunction
E = Endometrial (option b and c)
I = Iatrogenic
N = Not yet identified

Any thyroid problem should always be ruled in all cases of AUB.

58. **Ans. is b, i.e. Imperforate hymen**

1° amenorrhea with cyclical abdominal pain with normal secondary sexual characteristics and an anterior swelling (bulge) on P/R examination (in other words uterus is present) indicate imperforate hymen.

- Cervical incompetence and pregnancy with placenta previa are not causes of 1° amenorrhea.
- It cannot be Mullerian malformation as uterus is palpable on P/R examination

Note: This is a 15-year-old girl i.e. a virgin & so we do not do per vaginal examination in her.

59. **Ans. is b, i.e. Pituitary enlargement occurs**

- Sheehan syndrome is postpartum necrosis of anterior pituitary gland due to acute excessive blood loss (even after PPH). Hence obviously there will not be pituitary enlargement
- Now since anterior pituitary gland is increased so all hormones released by it will decrease i.e. LH/FSM (so there will be decreased estrogen & regression of secondary sexual characteristics.

  ACTH decreases hence there is hyponatremia and decreased cortisol production.

60. **Ans. is c, i.e. MRKH syndrome**

Primary amenorrhea with:

- Normal breast i.e. normal secondary sexual characteristic
- But a small vaginal pouch indicates MRKH

  Presence of normal breast rules out Turner's syndrome & presence of vaginal pouch rules out androgen insensitivity syndrome

61. **Ans. is b, i.e. Individuals harbouring Y chromosomes are at risk for germ cell malignancies**

Ref: Williams Gynae 3rd/ed, p383

Patients with gonadal dysgenesis such as Turner syndrome are considered for karyotyping. If It shows presence of Y chromosomes, then bilateral oophorectomy because of increased risk of ovarian germ cell tumors.

62. **Ans. is a, i.e. Hypomenorrhea** *Ref: Williams Gynae 3rd/ed, p372*

"Depending on the degree of scaring, patients may decrease amenorrhea, in less severe cases, hypomenorrhea or recurrent pregnancy loss due to inadequate placentation." *Ref: Williams Gynae 3rd/ed, p372*

63. **Ans. is a, b, c, d and e i.e. NSAID; Progesterone; Tranexamic acid; Low dose OCP; Conjugated estrogen (See the text for explanation)**

64. **Ans. is a, b, c, d and e, i.e. Polymenorrhoea means episodes of menstruation at intervals less than 21 days; Oligomenorrhea is scanty, regularly speed bleeding cyclic menstruation; Menorrhagia: very large amount of regularly spaced bleeding; Secondary amenorrhea – no bleeding for >12 weeks who have previously menstruated; Post-menopausal bleeding occurs after 1 year of stoppage of menses.**

65. **Ans. is d and e, i.e. Oligomenorrhea is menstruation at intervals of more than 35 days; Primary amenorrhea is failure of onset of menstruation beyond age of 15 years in presence of secondary sexual characteristics**

66. **Ans. is a, b, c and d i.e. Blood loss more than 80 mL; Cycle duration more than 35 days or less than 21 days; Bleeding for more than 7 days; Irregular bleeding during regular cycle (See the text for explanation)**

Ref: Williams Gynae 3rd/ed, p369

67. **Ans. is a, i.e. Cyclical progesterone**

Metropathia haemorrhagica

- It is a special form of dysfunctional uterine bleeding
- It is characterized by thickening of the endometrium and cystic follicles in one or both ovaries
- It is most commonly seen in women over 40 years of age, however it may also develop in young girls.

Clinical findings:

- Most common complaint is continuous vaginal bleeding which may last for weeks
- Bleeding is always painless since it is anovulatory.

It is subdivided into 4 types based upon the menstrual history:

- Type 1: Occurs in 50% cases; continuous vaginal bleeding is preceded by amenorrhea of about 8 to 10 weeks
- Type 2: Bleeding follows normal pattern and occurs at the normal expected time
- Type 3: Bleeding may be preceded by menorrhagia
- Type 4: There is a uptic glandular hyperplasia and there is absence of secretory endometrium with absence or cave screw glands

Differential diagnosis are—ectopic gestation and miscarriage:

Treatment: Cyclical progesterone therapy.

68. **Ans. is b, i.e. Metropathia haemorrhagica**

Metropathia haemorrhagica (Shroeder's Disease) *Shaw's Gynae 17th/ed, p133; Dutta Gynae 7th/ed, p155*

- The characteristic feature of endometrium in Metropathia haemorrhagica is **cystic glandular hyperplasia.**
- Another important feature is absence of secretory endometrium with **absence of corkscrew glands.**
- Endometrium is usually thick and polypoidal.
- Thin polyp projection into the uterine cavity.

"**Halban's disease** (Irregular shedding): It is rare and self-limited. Irregular shedding is due to persistent corpus luteum"

– Shaw's Gynae 17th/ed, p139

"**Irregular ripening**: It is an ovulatory bleeding due to deficient corpus luteum function" *–Shaw's Gynae 17th/ed, p139*

CHAPTER 14A

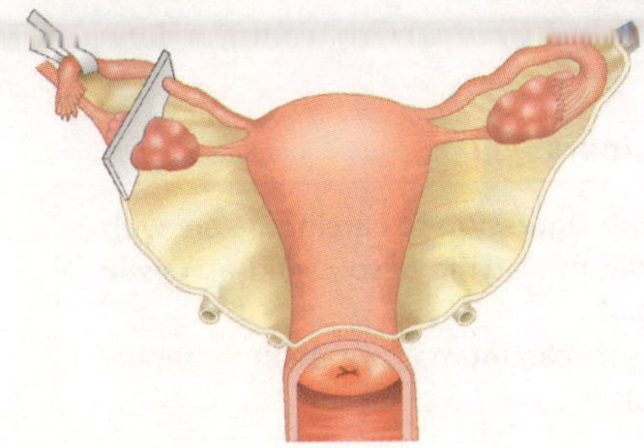

Gynecological Oncology: Uterine Cancer

Endometrial Hyperplasia

Endometrial Hyperplasia is defined as endometrial thickening with proliferation of regularly sized and shaped glands and an increased gland to stroma ratio.

Due to excessive estrogen, there is Hyperproliferation of endometrium and when this entire endometrium sheds, it leads to excessive bleeding.

They are clinically important because:

- They cause abnormal bleeding.[Q]
- Either precede or occur simultaneously with endometrial carcinoma.

Types of Endometrial Hyperplasia

Endometrial Hyperplasia can be

1. Simple
2. Complex (Table 14A.1)

Table 14A.1: Endometrial Hyperplasia

Simple	Complex
• It results from circumstance in which there is prolonged, increased estrogen production: i. Follicular cysts of ovary[Q] ii. PCOD[Q] iii. Granulosa and Theca cell tumors of ovary[Q] iv. HRT[Q] In perimenopausal age they are associated with glucose intolerance.[Q]	• Less obviously connected with increased estrogen • Mostly, cause is unknown • Can be associated with: – PCOD[Q] – Glucose intolerance[Q]
Pathology • Glands are large, cystic with increased glands/stromal ratio[Q] • Scanty mitosis[Q] • Glands lined by columnar[Q] epithelium • Stroma is sparsely cellular	**Pathology** Glands number is increased, size is increased and Glands are thrown into folds **(over crowding of glands)** • Numerous mitosis[Q] • Glands are lined by stratified squamous epithelium[Q] • Stroma is densely cellular[Q]

The simple and complex hyperplasia can be further divided into 2 categories:

- Without atypical cells
- With atypical cells

Hence there are 4 main types of endometrial hyperplasia as per WHO:

1. Simple hyperplasia without atypical cells.
2. Complex hyperplasia without atypical cells
3. Simple hyperplasia with atypical cells
4. Complex hyperplasia with atypical cells

KEY POINTS

Characteristics of Atypical cells

- Large in size[Q]
- Loss of polarity[Q]
- Irregular shape[Q]
- Hyperchromatic nucleus[Q] and prominent nucleoli[Q]
- Altered nucleus cytoplasmic ratio.[Q]

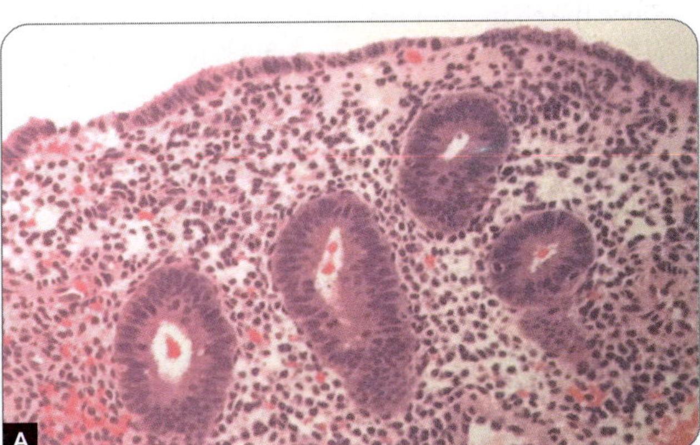

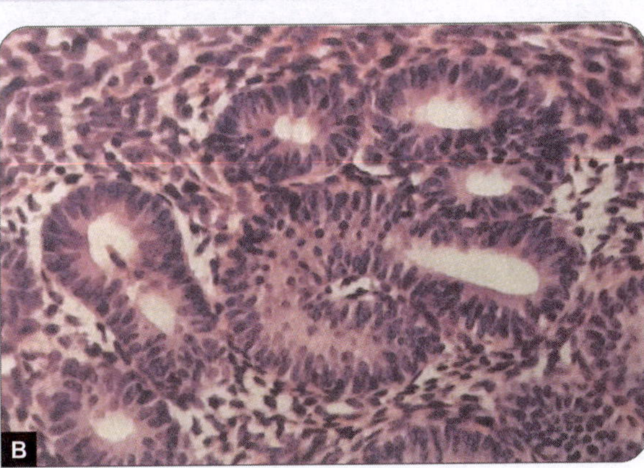

Figs. 14A.1A and B: (A) Normal proliferative endometrium; (B) Simple hyperplasia

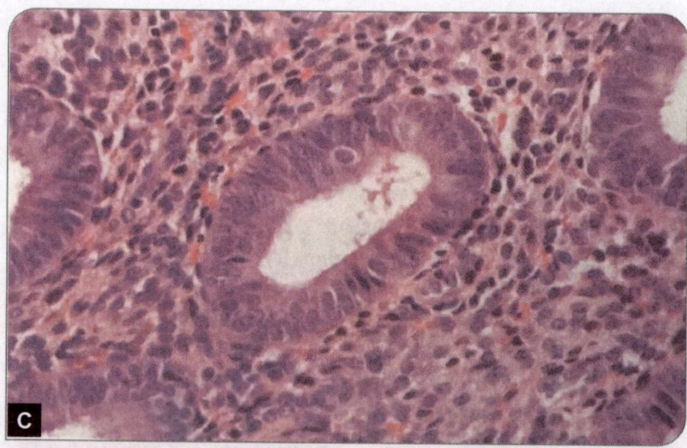

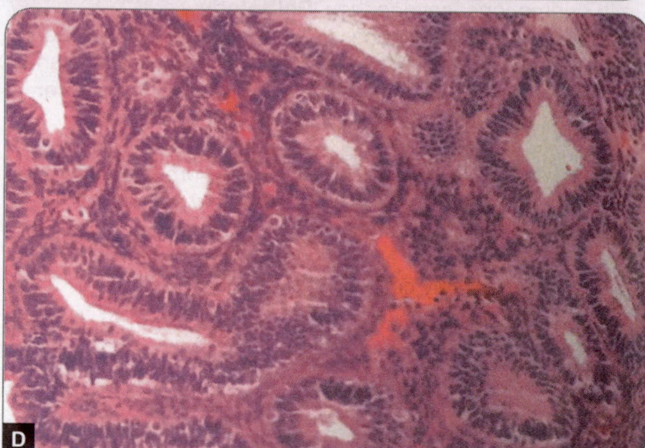

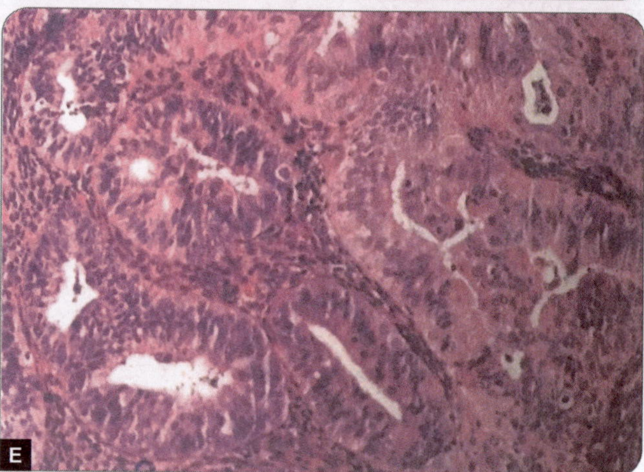

Figs. 14A.1C to E: (C) Simple hyperplasia with atypia; (D) Complex hyperplasia; (E) Complex hyperplasia with atypia

Chances of Progression to Carcinoma

Table 14A.2

Type of hyperplasia	Progression to cancer
• Simple without atypia	1%[Q]
• Complex without atypia	3%[Q]
• Simple with atypia	8%[Q]
• Complex with atypia	29–30%[Q]

Important One Liners

- **Minimum chances of progression to carcinoma** are with simple hyperplasia without atypia (also called as **Cystic Glandular Hyperplasia**).
- **Maximum chances of carcinoma are** with complex hyperplasia with atypia.[Q]

Diagnostic Protocol

Whenever a female comes with C/O excessive bleeding. The first investigation to do is Transvaginal, ultrasound.

On TVS: Measure endometrial thickness as increased estrogen leads to endometrial proliferation).

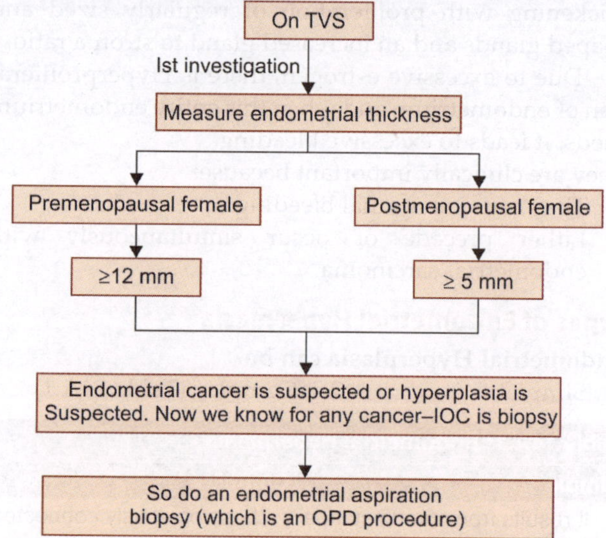

Management of Endometrial Hyperplasia

Depends on the patient's age and the presence or absence of cytological atypia.

Non-atypical Hyperplasia

Since the chances of malignancy in this category are less (1% for simple hyperplasia and 3% for complex), hence they are managed medically:

- **Premenopausal women**: Progesterone therapy:
  Options:
  - Medroxyprogesterone acetate for 21 days a month daily for 3 months.
  - Progesterone containing IUCD.
- **Perimenopausal women:**
  Periodic oral progesterone like medroxyprogesterone acetate 5–10 mg or 200 mg micronized progesterone (200 mg) daily **for 14 days of each month.** This treatment should be followed after 3–4 months with aspiration curettage.

Atypical Hyperplasia

In this category chances of malignancy are high (simple-8%, complex-30%, hence they are managed surgically).

- **Ideal treatment is**–Hysterectomy
- **Premenopausal women willing to preserve fertility**: High dose progesterone therapy **(megestrol)** after full information of risk of a undiagnosed cancer or progression to cancer. In these cases periodic TVS and endometrial biopsy is necessary.

Extra Edge

Apart from WHO classification of Endometrial Hyperplasia. There is another term which is different from endometrial Hyperplasia & that is **Endometrial Intraepithelial Neoplasia:**

Diagnosis of EIN requires following

- Glandular volume more than stroma
- Cytological demarcation from surrounding normal glands.
- Lesions with largest diameter ≥1 mm
- Exclusion of confounding processes like hormonal effect. EIN and Endometrial Hyperplasia are not same EIN has resemblance to atypical endometrial Hyperplasia

Endometrial Carcinoma

Epidemiology

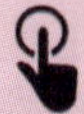

- M/c Cancer in females worldwide: Breast cancer
- M/c Cancer in females in developing countries: Breast cancer
- M/c female genital tract worldwide: Cancer cervix
- M/c female genital tract in developing countries: Cancer cervix.
- M/c female genital tract in developed countries: Cancer endometrium

- Mean age of presentation is 60 years: Peak incidence occurs from 55 to 70 years
- Majority are diagnosed early
- 5 years survival for stage I disease is more than 90%
- Overall 5 years survival for all stages is 60–70%

Risk Factor

Endometrial cancer occurs as a result of unopposed estrogen exposure in body. It is an Estrogen dependent tumor. Hence it is more common in obese, nulliparous females.

Mnemonic

Family Has OLD AUNTIS

Family	Family history (all 1st degree relative have increased chances)
Has	Hypertension
O	Obesity
L	Late menopause/Early menarche
D	Diabetes
A	Atypical endometrial hyperplasia
U	Unopposed estrogen or increased estrogen in body as in: HRT, fibroid, PCOD and feminizing ovarian tumors
N	Nulliparity
T	Therapy: Tamoxifen therapy and radiation therapy
I	H/O Infertility/menstrual irregularity
S	Senile endometritis/pyometra

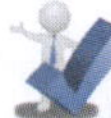

KEY POINTS

- Whenever there is an **obese** female with **diabetes** and **Hypertension**, there are increased chances of endometrial cancer. This is called as the **CORPUS CANCER Syndrome**.
- Estrogen replacement without concomitant progesterone carries a relative risk of 4.5 to 8 & persists for 10 years after treatment is stopped.
- BMI > 30 kg/m^2 will triple the risk of endometrial cancer
- A woman taking Tamoxifen has an annual risk of 2 in 1000 of developing endometrial cancer.
- Tamoxifen is an SERM. It has both estrogenic and antiestrogenic actions. It has antiestrogenic action on breast & is thus used in treatment of breast cancer. But it has estrogenic action on endometrium and this can lead to Endometrial cancer.
- Women with HNPCC syndrome have 40% risk of developing endometrial cancer by the age of 70 years.
- OCP's decrease endometrial cancer risk by 40%, even uptil 15 years after discontinuation and the protection increases with the length of use.

Approximately 5% of endometrial cancer is hereditary, with majority of these presenting as a part of the **Lynch II or Hereditary Non Polyposis Colorectal Cancer (HNPCC) syndrome.** Besides endometrial cancer, individuals in this family are at increased risk of **colorectal cancer**, **ovarian**, urinary, biliary, gastric and small intestinal cancer. Abnormal bleeding at any age should be evaluated by tissue biopsy in women of HNPCC families. Routine surveillance may consist of yearly USG and endometrial biopsy commencing at the age of 30–35.

Protective Factors

- Oral contraceptive pills (combined pills with addition of progesterone to HRT)
- Smoking (as it decreases levels of estrogen, decreases weight and is associated with earlier age of menopause)
- Multiparity
- Physical exercise.

Classification

- Adenocarcinoma/endometrioid (most common 80%). ***Note:*** Uterus is lined by columnar epithelium hence logically speaking also, the most common to occur in uterus is adenocarcinoma
- Adenosquamous carcinoma (15%) or adenocarcinoma with squamous differentiation
- Papillary serous adenocarcinoma
- Mucinous adenocarcinoma
- Clear cell carcinoma.

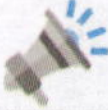

Important One Liners

- **M/C variety of endometrial cancer** is adenocarcinoma
- **Most malignant variety** is clear cell carcinoma and papillary serous tumor.
- Mucinous variety of endometrial CA needs to be differentiated from Adeno CA of endocervix. It is done by using **vimentin stain.**

Adenocarcinoma is further divided into 3 grades:

Grade	Called as	Definition
1.	Well differentiated	≤ 5% undifferentiated cells
2.	Moderately differentiated	6–50% undifferentiated cells
3.	Poorly differentiated	≥ 50% undifferentiated cells

Histology of Endometrial Cancer

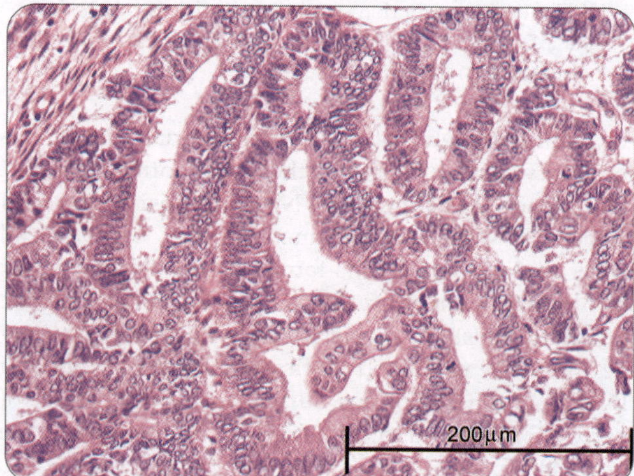

Fig. 14A.2: Histology of uterine cancer.

- Histological criteria for diagnosis of endometrial Ca (Fig. 14A.2)
- Back to back arrangement of glands[Q]
- **Desmoplastic stroma**
- Excessive papillary pattern
- Squamous cell differentiation

Histological Differences in Endometrial Cancer

On the basis of histology endometrial cancer can be classified into two main types:

Table 14A.3

Features	Type I (Endometrioid) (80%)	Type II (Nonendometrioid) (20%)
Specific subtypes	Endometrioid, Adenocarcinoma grade 1, 2	Papillary serous, clear cell, Adenocarcinoma grade 3
Prognosis	Good	Bad
	M/C	Less Common
Unopposed estrogen	Present	Absent
	Seen in obese females	Seen in thin females
Menopausal status	Pre and perimenopausal	Postmenopausal
Race	White	Black
Hyperplasia	Present	Absent
Grade	Low	High
Behavior	Stable	Aggressive
Associated gene alteration	pTEN/Kras	p53, HER2/neu

The MIC variety of Endometrial cancer is Aderocarcinoma. Aderocarcinoma is further divided into 3 grades.

Papillary Serous Cancer

- Seen in 5-10% of endometrial cancers
- Associated with BRCA 1 & BRCA 2 gene
- It metastasizes early by spreading through peritoneum therefore in its staging-omentectomy and peritoneal biopsy should also be done.

Clear Cell Carcinoma

- It accounts for < 5% of all endometrial carcinomas
- Most characteristic histological finding is presence of **"hobnail cells"**
- It characteristically occurs in older women and is a very aggressive type of endometrial cancer
- Prognosis is similar to or worse than papillary serous carcinoma
- In staging: Omentectomy and peritoneal biopsy should also be done.

Clinical Features

- Irregular vaginal bleeding: **M/c complaint or symptom.** If it is not given in options then go for postmenopausal bleeding
- Postmenopausal bleeding: **Most specific complaint**

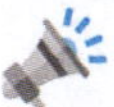

Important One Liners

Post menopausal bleeding is any bleeding which occurs in a postmenopausal female after ≥ 12 months of amenorrhea.

Novak Gynae 15/ed, p1250

Cause of bleeding	Patient age
Endometrial atrophy	60–80%
HRT	15–25%
Endometrial polyp	2–12%
Endometrial hyperplasia	5–10%
Endometrial cancer	10%

- M/C cause of postmenopausal bleeding—senile endometritis.
- M/C cancer causing post menopausal bleeding-In India-Cancer cervix
- M/C cancer causing postmenopausal bleeding in developed countries – Endometrial cancer
- Percentage of postmenopausal bleeding patients who have endometrial cancer is 10%.

Some Extra Symptoms

- Discharge per vagina (1%):
  - Brown, watery offensive discharge
  - Watery discharge free from blood (hydrorrhea[Q]).
- Pelvic pressure/discomfort
- Referred pain in hypogastrium or both iliac fossae **(Simpson's pain)**
  Pain is not severe and tends to occur at the same time each day, lasting only 1-2 hours
- In some older patients, bleeding may not occur due to cervical stenosis, causing hematometra/ pyometra.

Symptoms not Seen in Endometrial Cancer

Since in Endometrial cancer the M/C variety is Endometrioid variety or Type 1 tumors & that is M/C in obese females.

Hence the general symptoms which are oftenly associated with all cancers are not seen in Endometrial cancer like:

- Loss of appetite
- Loss of weight
- Cachexia

Investigations

- **Screening:** Routine screening for Ca endometrium is not done, as Pap smear is positive only in 50% of patients of Ca endometrium
- In patients of HNPCC—chances of malignancy are high: Hence screening is required[Q]. **Screening method** in these patients include:
  - **Pelvic examination, endometrial sampling and TVS done** every 6 or 12 monthly.
  - Screening begins at age of 35 years.
- Best screening method in these patients is fractional curettage
  - **Best method to prevent Cancer in these patient is**—Prophylactic Hysterectomy with Bilateral Salpingo-Oophorectomy after completing childbirth.

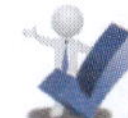

KEY POINTS

Remember:

- **Whenever a female C/O bleeding or if a female postmenopausal bleeding:** 1st investigation is TVS, so 1st investigation in endometrial cancer is also TVS
- IOC in endometrial cancer is endometrial aspiration biopsy.
- **Gold standard for diagnosing endometrial cancer-** Fractional curettage.

TVS

Whenever a patient comes with bleeding, 1st step is to do is TVS. If endometrial thickness is **less than or equal to 5 mm, further** testing may be deferred. But if their is recurrence of bleeding, a tissue diagnosis is essential.

If on TVS:

- Endometrial thickness is ≥5 mm
- Fluid is present in uterus
- Polypoidal mass seen

It indicates further testing is needed (*See* Flowchart 14A.1).

Flowchart 14A.1

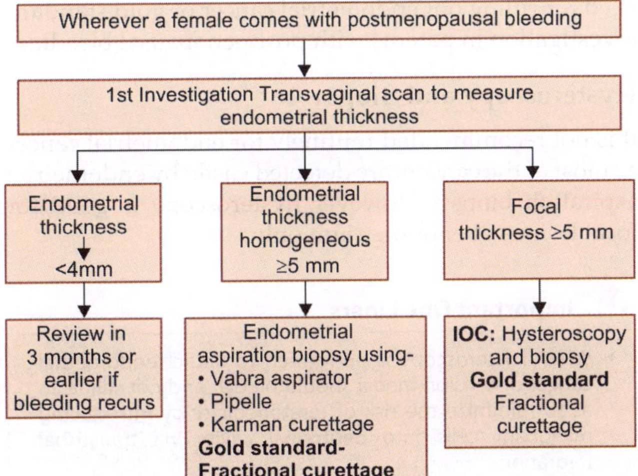

Endometrial Aspiration Biopsy

It is the **IOC for endometrial cancer**. Diagnostic accuracy: 92–98%

Endometrial aspiration biopsy can be performed in outpatient setting as it does not require any anesthesia and has the advantage of being simple, quick, safe, inexpensive, convenient. It is combined with endocervical curettage to rule out cancer cervix. It is done using a **Vabra aspirator (Fig. 14A.4), Karman curette, or Pipelle endometrial sampler (Fig. 14A.3).**

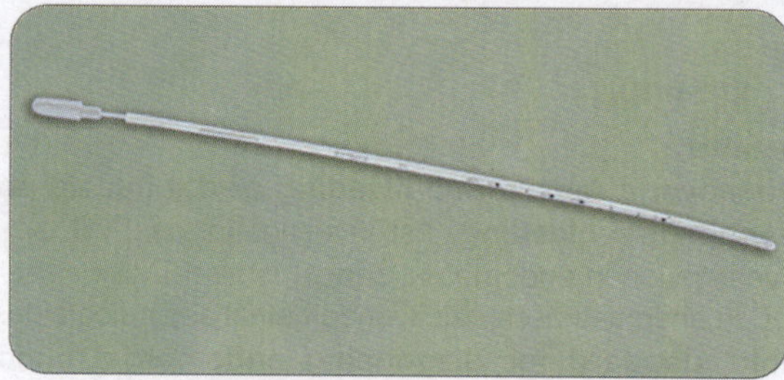

Fig. 14A.3: Pipelle endometrial sampler.

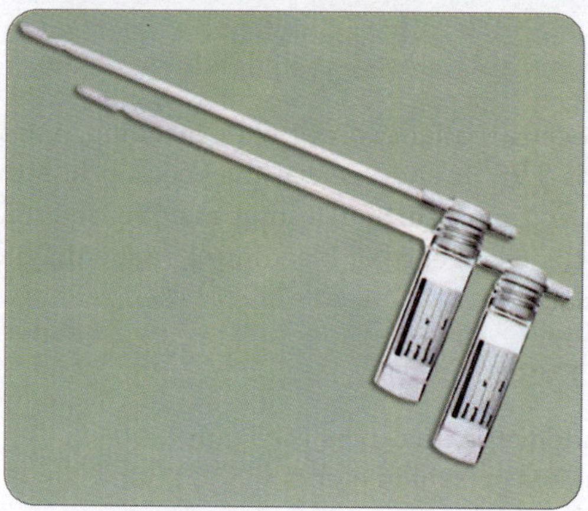

Fig. 14A.4: Vabra aspirator

Fractional Curettage

Fractional curettage is the **Gold standard investigation** used for ruling out endometrial cancer or gold standard investigation in patents with postmenopausal bleeding.

Hysteroscopy and Biopsy

It is not recommended routinely for endometrial cancer as most of the cancers are detected easily by endometrial aspiration biopsy. However hysteroscopy is good for focal lesions of endometrium only.

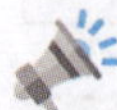

Important One Liners

- When hysteroscopy is performed to detect endometrial cancer distension media should be CO_2 and not saline so as to minimize the risk of teratogenicity by introducing malignant cells into peritoneal cavity via transtubal migration.

Role of other Investigations in Endometrial Cancer

Role of MRI in Endometrial Cancer: It helps in

- Determining the thickness of myometrial involved
- Gives information about Lower uterine segment involvement
- Gives information about cervical involvement

Role of CT

CT is generally not done in Endometrial cancer. It is done, it tells about

- Metastasis
- Pelvic involvement
- Lymph node involvements

Staging

- **Staging for endometrial cancer is done surgically,** and because many patients have early-stage diseases at the time of diagnosis, this is often the only intervention necessary.

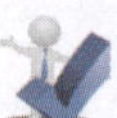

KEY POINTS

What do you understand by surgical staging:

- Surgical staging means once the diagnosis of Endometrial Cancer is made on Biopsy
- Do surgery send the sample for Histopathological examination histopathologist tells the stage, then post operative management is done.

Note: Surgical staging is done in Endometrial cancer and ovarian cancer.

Steps in Surgical Staging of Endometrial Cancer

- 1st step: Do MRI to know the depth of myometrial involvement
- 2nd step: Do surgery: The surgery done in Endometrial cancer is TAH + BSO i.e Total abdominal hysterectomy and Bilateral salpingo-oophorectomy.

Note: If while doing surgery- it is seen that cervix is also involved then instead of doing TAH + BSO, Wertheim's hysterectomy (Type II Hysterectomy) is done

- If while doing surgery, it is seen that cancer has spread beyond cervix and Wertheim's Hysterectomy is practically not feasible then a debulking surgery should be done.
- 3rd step: Lymph node dissection for LN dissection see Flowchart 14A.2.

Flowchart 14A.2: Lymph node dissection in endometrial cancer

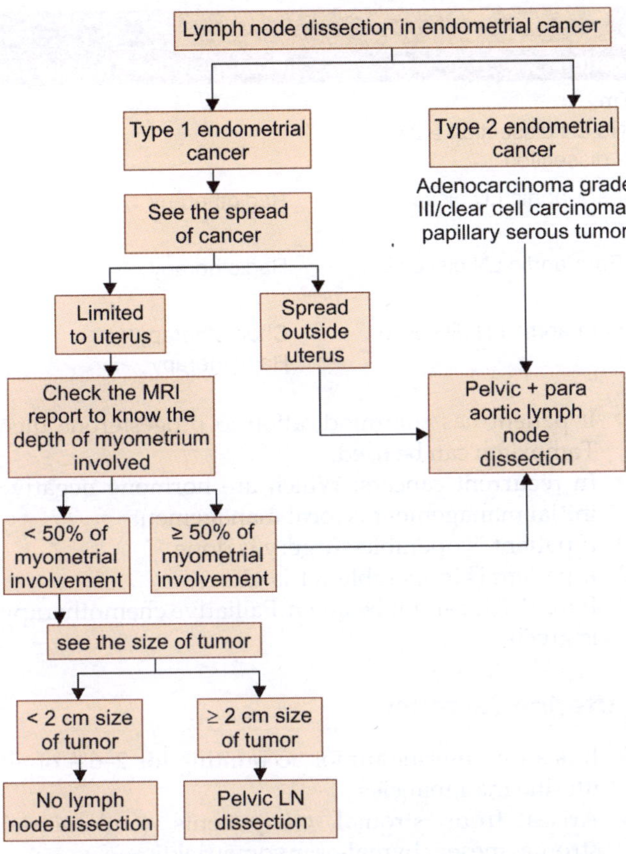

Spread

- **Most common** mode of spread is **direct extension.**[Q]
- Lymphatic spread occurs to pelvic and para-aortic nodes
- Hematogenous spread (usually to lungs) is rare.
- Remember: In all Gynae cancer Endometrial/ Ovarian cancer climax:- superficial inguinal
  M/C site of Recurrence of Endometrial cancer vagina
- With the above procedures; Omentectomy and peritoneal biopsy is done in case of **papillary serous** tumor and clear cell carcinoma.

FIGO Staging of Ca Endometrium (2009)

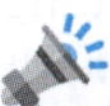

Important One Liners

- In all gynecological cancers FIGO staging system is being followed except in cancer vulva where both FIGO and TNM staging can be done.

Table 14A.4

Stage		
Stage I	=	Cancer confined to uterus
Stage IA	=	< 50% of myometrium involved.
Stage IB	=	50% or more of myometrium involved.
Stage II	=	Cancer spreads to cervix and endocervical stroma involved. (***Note***: Endocervical glandular involvement is now considered stage I).
Stage III	=	Cancer spreads beyond uterus and cervix
Stage IIIA	=	Tumor invades serosa or adnexa. Positive cytology has to be reported separately without changing the stage.
Stage IIIB	=	Vaginal and/or parametrial involvement
Stage IIIC1	=	Pelvic lymph nodes involved
Stage IIIC2	=	Para-aortic lymph nodes involved
Stage IV	=	Metastasis A: Regional metastasis to bladder or rectum B: Distant metastasis or superficial inguinal lymph node involved

Management

Principle of Management

- Remember–In cancer endometrium, staging is surgical.

In Surgery:

- TAH + BSO done till stage I
- Wertheim's hysterectomy is done when cervix is involved i.e in stage 2
- Debulking surgery is done in stage 3 & 4

For LN dissection

- In Type II varieties always pelvic & para-aortic lymph node dissection
- In Type 1, if cancer spreads outside uterus i.e from stage. II onwards always do Pelvic + para aortic LN dissection.
- If cancer is limited to uterus:- and:- ≥ 50% of myometrium is involved ie stage 1 B then pelvic & para aortic LN dissection is done.
- If < 50% of myometrium is, involved i.e. stage IA, In stage IA:- size of TM = ≥ 2 cm: do pelvic LN dissection.
- If < 2 cm size: No LN dissection.
- Thus treatment is mainly postoperative management

Postoperative Management

The postoperative management of choice in Endometrial cancer is Radiotherapy.

There are 2 exceptions to this:

1. In stage IA grade 1 and grade 2: No postoperative Therapy is given (Many times this question has been asked)
2. In stages III/IV: postoperative therapy of choice is: Chemotherapy + Radiotherapy (Doxorubicin or Adriamycin + Paclitaxel or Taxol + cisplatin or Platinol forming TAP chemotherapy.

Stagewise Management of Endometrial Cancer

Table 14A.5

Stage	Surgery	LN dissection	Postoperative Therapy
Stage 1 A Grade I & grade II	TAH + BSO	Size of Tm < 2 cm: No LN dissection ≥ 2 cm: pelvic LN dissection	—
Stage IA grade III Stage IB	TAH + BSO	Pelvic + para-aortic LN dissection	Radiotherapy
Stage II (cervix involved)	Wertheim's hysterectomy	Pelvic + Para aortic LN dissection	Radiotherapy
Stage III and stave IV	Debulking surgery	Pelvic + para aortic LN dissection	Chemotherapy +/– Radiotherapy

Prognostic Factors in Endometrial Cancer

- **Most important prognostic** factor is **lymph node metastasis.**[Q]
- **Age** at diagnosis (older the patient poorer the prognosis).
- **Stage of** the disease.[Q]
- **Histologic type** (endometrioid adenocarcinoma have good prognosis, clear cell carcinoma have poor prognosis).[Q]
- **Histologic grade.**[Q]
- **Myometrial penetration** (Increasing depth of invasion is associated with increasing likelihood of extrauterine spread and recurrence).
- **Extension to cervix**–Involvement of cervix, isthmus or both is associated with increased risk of extrauterine disease and lymph node metastasis.
- **Role of peritoneal cytology is controversial.**
- **Tumor size** (≥2 cm–means more lymph node metastasis).
- **Hormone receptor status (receptor positive–better prognosis).**
- Ploidy status: Aneuploid have got better prognosis compared to diploid tumors.
- Oncogene expression: HER: 2/neu, k-ras poor prognosis.

Recurrent Endometrial Cancer

- **M/c time of recurrence** is within first two years
- **M/c site of recurrence** = Vagina > pelvis
- **M/c symptom of local recurrence** vaginal bleeding
- **M/c symptom of pelvic recurrence** – pelvic pain
- **M/c site of extrapelvic recurrence** – Lung, lymph node (aortic), Liver, brain and bones

Management

- For patients with recurrent endometrioid tumors with hormone receptors positive, **initial treatment is progestin.**
- If patient has contraindication to progesterone then Tamoxifen can be used.
- In recurrent cancers: Which are hormone negative initial management is local management
- If patient is operable-surgery is done
- If patient is inoperable-RT is given
- If local T/t cannot be given-Palliative chemotherapy is given.

Uterine Sarcoma

- It is a rare uterine tumor accounting for 2–6% of all uterine malignancies
- Arises from stromal components (endometrial stroma, mesenchymal or myometrial tissues)
- Mostly seen in post menopausal age group
- There are three main varieties of uterine sarcoma (Table 14A.6)
- Vaginal bleeding is most common presenting symptom
- Behaves more aggressively and is associated with poorer prognosis
- 5-year survival rate – 35%.

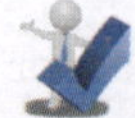

KEY POINTS

Uterine sarcomas may be pure (single cell type) or mixed (more than one cell type). The tumor is termed homologous when the tissue elements are native (e.g. smooth muscle or heterologous when tissue elements are not native (cartilage, striated muscle, bone). This is due to totipotent nature of endometrial stromal cells.

Treatment

First step is always exploration. TAH + BSO (done in all patients except premenopausal females with leiomyosarcoma where we do not do bilateral salpingo-oophorectomy) followed by chemotherapy. (Doxorubicin, Ifosfamide, Paclitaxel, carboplatin).

Novak 15th/ed, p1292

Staging of Sarcoma

Uterine sarcomas were staged previously as endometrial cancers, which did not reflect their clinical behavior. Now they are staged as follows:

Stage IA = Tumor limited to uterus < 5 cm
Stage IB = Tumor limited to uterus > 5 cm
Stage IIA = Adnexal involvement
Stage IIB = Tumor extends to extrauterine pelvic tissue
Stage IIIA = Tumor invades one site of abdominal tissue
Stage IIIB = Tumor invades more than one site of abdominal tissues
Stage IIIC = Metastasis to pelvic and/or para-aortic lymph nodes
Stage IVA = Tumor invades bladder and/or rectum
Stage IVB = Distant metastasis.

Table 14A.6: Varieties of Uterine Sarcoma

Endometrial Stromal Sarcoma (ESS)	Leiomyosarcoma	Carcinosarcoma (Mixed Mullerian Tumor)
• Arises from stromal cells • Least aggressive of the sarcomas • M/c age = Perimenopausal and postmenopausal females	• Occurs when fibroid becomes malignant • (0.1–0.5%) fibroids undergo malignancy • M/c age = 43–53 years • Differentiating feature of leiomyosarcomas is > 10 mitosis 10 high power field.	• M/c variety • M/c age = 62 years • M/c - postmenopausal bleeding • M/c mode of spread - Blood borne • Most aggressive sarcomas
	• No whorled appearance and no capsule	• M/c type of cells seen MMT are spindle cells.

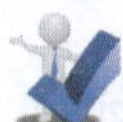

KEY POINTS

Mixed Mullerian tumors are diagnosed on the basis of **ten or more mitotic figures per ten high power fields (HPFs).** Those tumors with 5 to 10 mitotic figures per 10 HPF s are referred to as smooth muscle tumors of uncertain malignant potential. Tumors with < 5 mitotic figures per 10 HPFs and little cytological atypia are classified as cellular leiomyosarcomas.

Embryonal Rhabdomyosarcoma

- Most common malignant tumour of the genital tract in girls.
- Mostly arises from the submucosa of cervix or vagina.
- **Age:** 90% cases occur before the age of 5, peak incidence at 2 years of age.
- **Hallmark:** Pinkish, grape like polypoidal soft growth arising from the cervix.
- **Clinical features:** Blood stained watery vaginal discharge is the main symptom.
- **Treatment:** Initial staging with chest X-ray and CT scan.
- **Later:** Chemotherapy (VAC-Vincristine, Actinomycin D and Cyclophosphamide) followed by surgery is the treatment of choice.
- **Prognosis:** Poor.
- **Recurrence:** Common.

NEW PATTERN QUESTIONS

N1. Endometrial hyperplasia is often associated with:
a. Cystic teratoma b. Endodermal tumor
c. PCOS d. Sertoli Tumor cell

N2. TOC of endometrial hyperplasia without atypia in a 32-year-old female:
a. Hysterectomy b. OCP
c. Medroxyprogesterone d. GnRH analog

N3. The following are precursors of endometrial carcinoma except:
a. Atypical adenomatous hyperplasia
b. Atrophic endometrium
c. Adenocarcinoma in situ
d. Cystic hyperplasia

N4. Most malignant variety of endometrial carcinoma:
a. Endometrioid b. Papillary serous
c. Clear cell carcinoma
d. Adenosquamous carcinoma

N5. M/C cause of postmenopausal bleeding:
a. HRT b. Endometrial atrophy
c. Endometrial cancer d. Cervix cancer

N6. Percentage of postmenopausal bleeding patients who have endometrial cancer:
a. 5% b. 10%
c. 20% d. 25%

N7. A 52-year-old menopausal female (Menopause: 3 years back) presents with single episode of postmenopausal bleeding TVS shows endometrial thickness of 3 mm. What is the most appropriate step in management?
a. Perform fractional curettage
b. Perform Hysteroscopy and biopsy
c. Perform pipelle aspiration
d. Review in 3 months or earlier if bleeding occurs
e. Do TAH

N8. A 52-year-old menopausal female presents with single episode of postmenopausal bleeding. TVS shows endometrial of uniform thickness of 6 mm. What is the most appropriate step in management?
a. Perform fractional curettage
b. Perform hysteroscopy and biopsy
c. Perform pipelle aspiration
d. Do TAH

N9. A 54-year-old female who had attained menopause 2 years back, complains of single episode of bleeding. TVS shows endometrial thickness of 4 mm with an area of focal thickness of 6 mm. What is the most appropriate next step in management?
a. Perform fractional curettage
b. Perform hysteroscopy and biopsy
c. Perform pipelle aspiration
d. Renew in 3 months or earlier if bleeding recurs

N10. Screening is not done for following cancer:
a. Cancer cervix b. Cancer breast
c. Cancer ovaries d. Cancer endometrium

N11. A 65-year-old women presents with postmenopausal bleeding. Biopsy shows grade 2 endometrioid carcinoma at the fundus of uterus. She has uncontrolled diabetes and hypertension. What is the most appropriate next step in management?
a. Perform MRI scan
b. Perform TAH + BSO
c. Perform TAH + BSO + pelvic and paraaortic lymph node dissection
d. Surgery followed by RT

N12. A 54-year-old female presents with postmenopausal bleeding. Biopsy shows endometrioid variety of endometrial cancer of 1 cm in the uterine fundus histology shows grade 1 tumor. MRI shows <50% of myometrial involvement. Next step in management is:
a. TAH + BSO
b. TAH + BSO with pelvic lymphadenectomy
c. TAH + BSO with pelvic and paraarotic lymphadenectomy
d. TAH + BSO followed by RT

N13. A 52-year-old female has endometrial cancer of endometrioid variety stage Ia grade II limited to endometrium. The tumor has not spread outside the uterus. Size of tumor is 3–4 cm. What is the most appropriate management?
a. TAH + BSO
b. TAH + BSO with pelvic lymphadenectomy
c. TAH + BSO with pelvic and para aortic lymphadenectomy
d. TAH + BSO followed by RT.

N14. A 56-year-old female presents with postmenopausal bleeding. A diagnosis of grade II clear cell carcinoma is made. MRI reveals < 50% of myometrial invasion:
a. TAH + BSO
b. TAH + BSO with pelvic lymphadenectomy
c. TAH + BSO with pelvic and para-aortic lymphadenectomy
d. TAH + BSO followed by RT

N15. Drug useful in stage III & IV of endometrial cancer:
a. Danazol b. Cisplatin
c. Levonorgestrel d. Busulfan

N16. Primary carcinoma body of the uterus may be of following types except:
a. Adenocarcinoma
b. Adenosquamous carcinoma
c. Clear cell type
d. Large cell keratinizing type

N17. Increased risk of endometrial cancer in HNPCC syndrome on Lynch II is M/C associated with alteration in gene:
a. MSH 2 b. MSH 6
c. MLH 1 d. PMS 1

N18. In a 65-year-old female with adenocarcinoma of endometrium, the most important prognostic factor is:
a. Lymph node status
b. Ca 125 levels
c. Histologic variety of tumor
d. Stage of cancer

N19. Corpus Cancer syndrome constitutes:
a. Diabetes + MI + obesity + Endometrial Cancer
b. Diabetes + hypertension + obesity + Endometrial Cancer
c. Diabetes + obesity + MI + Ovarian Cancer
d. Diabetes + stroke + Hypertension + Endometrial Cancer

N20. Type 2 Endometrial Cancer is associated with all *except*:
a. Bad prognosis
b. M/c in black female
c. Associated with PTEN mutation
d. M/c in menopausal females

N21. The only clinically useful Tumor marker in management of Endometrial Cancer is:
a. CA125 b. CA19-9
c. Inhibin d. LDH

N22. M/c site of hematogenous spread of Endometrial Cancer:
a. Liver b. Lungs
c. Brain d. Lymph nodes

N23. Indications of Hormone Therapy in Endometrial Cancer are all *except*:
a. As a primary therapy in females with C/I to surgery
b. Young premenopausal female who desire fertility, it is used as primary treatment
c. As an adjuvant therapy in women with advanced and recurrent disease
d. In females with increased size of tumor

N24. Hormone therapy without surgery is indicated in:
a. Young females with stage 1 grade 1 tumors
b. Young females with stage 1 grade 2 tumors
c. Young females with stage 2 grade 1 tumors
d. Young females with stage 2 grade 2 tumors

N25. For staging of papillary serous carcinoma, procedure done in addition to normal staging procedure followed in Adenocarcinoma:
a. Infracolic omentectomy
b. Appendicectomy
c. Inspection and palpation of abdominal organs
d. Cholecystectomy

PREVIOUS YEAR QUESTIONS

1. **The risk of endometrial cancer is highest with the following histological pattern of endometrial hyperplasia:** *(AIMS May 06)*
   a. Simple hyperplasia without atypia
   b. Simple hyperplasia with atypia
   c. Complex hyperplasia without atypia
   d. Complex hyperplasia with atypia
2. **The risk of complex hyperplasia of endometrium with atypia progressing to malignancy in a postmenopausal woman is:** *(AIIMS 04, 05)*
   a. 3% b. 8%
   c. 15% d. 28%
3. **Percentage change of cystic glandular hyperplasia turning to malignancy:** *(PGI June 05)*
   a. 0.1% b. 2%
   c. 1% d. 10%
   e. 15%
4. **Endometrial hyperplasia is seen in:** *(AI 04)*
   a. Endodermal sinus tumor
   b. Dysgerminoma
   c. PCOD
   d. Ca cervix
5. **What is the ideal treatment for a 55-year-female with simple hyperplasia of endometrium with atypia?**
   a. Simple hysterectomy *(AI 08)*
   b. Medroxyprogesterone acetate (MPA)
   c. Levonorgestrel (LNG)
   d. IUCD
6. **All of the following are known risk factors for development of endometrial carcinoma except:**
   a. Obesity *(AI 03, 02)*
   b. Family history
   c. Use of hormone replacement therapy
   d. Early menopause
7. **Risk for endometrial cancer is/are:** *(PGI 04, 00)*
   a. Obesity
   b. Pregnancy before 20 years age
   c. PCOD
   d. Combined OC pills
   e. Premature menopause
8. **All are the risk factors for endometrial carcinoma *except*:** *(PGI June 09)*
   a. Multiparity
   b. Obesity
   c. Early menopause
   d. Unopposed estrogen therapy
   e. Hypertension
9. **Long-term tamoxifen therapy may cause:** *(AI 99, 98; PGI 99)*
   a. Endometrium Ca b. Ovary Ca
   c. Cervix Ca d. Vagina Ca
10. **Which of the following is not seen with corpus cancer syndrome in cancer endometrium?** *(AIIMS Nov 2010)*
    a. Multiparity b. Diabetes mellitus
    c. Hypertension d. Obesity
11. **A 50-year-old woman, nulliparous, diabetic and obese presenting with post-menopausal bleeding likely diagnosis is:** *(PGI 99)*
    a. Carcinoma in situ of cervix
    b. Carcinoma endometrium
    c. DUB
    d. None of the above
12. **True about endometrial carcinoma:** *(PGI 01)*
    a. Predisposed by diabetes mellitus, hypertension and obesity
    b. Adenosquamous type is most common
    c. Commonly associated with Ca cervix
    d. Common age group affected is between 20 and 40 years
13. **Which of the following is/are true about endometrial carcinoma:** *(PGI Nov 2014)*
    a. Less aggressive in postmenopausal women
    b. More common in diabetes
    c. Common after 40 years of age
    d. Associated with PCOD
    e. Associated with hereditary nonpolyposis colorectal cancer syndrome (HNPCC)
14. **The most malignant endometrial carcinoma is:**
    a. Adenocarcinoma *(JIPMER 03)*
    b. Adenoacanthoma
    c. Mixed adenosquamous carcinoma
    d. Clear cell carcinoma
15. **Investigation of choice in a 55-year-old postmenopausal woman who has presented with postmenopausal bleeding:** *(AI 06, 98)*
    a. Pap smear
    b. Fractional curettage
    c. Transvaginal ultrasound
    d. CA - 125 estimation
16. **Diagnosis of Endometrial carcinoma can be made from:** *(PGI May 2015)*
    a. Papanicolaou smear
    b. Fractional curettage
    c. Aspiration cytology from uterine
    d. Hysteroscopy and biopsy
    e. Colposcopy
17. **The stage of cancer endometrium with invasion of 10 mm of myometrium is:** *(AI 00)*
    a. Ia b. Ib
    c. IIb d. IIa
18. **Carcinoma endometrium with positive superficial inguinal lymph node status is classified as stage:** *(AI 99)*
    a. I b. II
    c. III d. IV

19. True about endometrial carcinoma in clinical stage III: *(PGI June 09)*
a. Vaginal metastasis
b. Para-aortic lymph node involvement
c. Pelvic lymph node involvement
d. Peritoneal involvement
e. Inguinal lymph node involvement

20. Lymph nodes not involved in Ca endometrium is: *(AIIMS 97)*
a. Para-aortic b. Presaral
c. Inferior mesenteric d. Inguinal

21. A perimenopausal lady with well differentiated adenocarcinoma of uterus has more than half myometrial invasion, vaginal metastasis and inguinal lymph node metastasis. She is staged as: *(AIIMS 96, 03)*
a. Stage IIIB b. Stage IIIC
c. Stage IVA d. Stage IVB

22. A lady presented with carcinoma endometrium involving >50% of myometrium extending to vagina and positive peritoneal cytology but no involvements of para aortic and preaortic nodes. What is the stage of disease? *(AIIMS Nov 2010)* *(May 2012)*
a. III A b. III B
c. III C1 d. III C2

23. Stage III B endometrial Ca-true is/are: *(PGI June 08, Dec 06)*
a. Vaginal metastasis
b. Lymph node metastasis
c. Bowel involvement
d. Lung metastasis
e. Serosa involved

24. Stage-IIIB endometrial carcinoma true is/are: *(PGI June 08; 09)*
a. Vaginal metastasis
b. Lymph node metastasis (paraaortic)
c. Pelvic lymph node involvement
d. Positive peritoneal cytology
e. Rectal invasion

25. Choice of adjuvant treatment for endometrial carcinoma stage I A grade I is: *(AI 04)*
a. Radiotherapy
b. Chemotherapy
c. Chemotherapy + Radiotherapy
d. No treatment

26. The following are indications for postoperative radiotherapy in a case of carcinoma endometrium except: *(AIIMS 04, 05)*
a. Myometrial invasion of more than half thickness
b. Positive lymph nodes
c. Endocervical involvement
d. Tumor positive for estrogen receptors

27. Indication for radiotherapy in carcinoma endometrium include all except: *(AIIMS Nov 07)*
a. Pelvic node involvement
b. Deep myometrial involvement
c. Enlarged uterine cavity
d. Poor differentiation

28. Indication of adjuvant radiotherapy in Ca endometrium is/are: *(PGI 05)*
a. Cervical involvement b. Lymph node involvement
c. Carcinoma in situ d. Papillary serous tumor
e. Estrogen receptor positive

29. Which of the following direct lymph node dissections in endometrial carcinoma? *(PGI May 2014)*
a. Penetration into half of myometrium
b. Clear cell carcinoma
c. Fundal involvement
d. Peritoneal metastasis
e. Papillary serous carcinoma

30. An 80-year-old female who has never taken estrogen, develops pink vaginal discharge. An endometrial biopsy shows an adenocarcinoma of the endometrium. Papanicolaou smear is negative. Of the following what is the most important indicator of prognosis? *(AI 04)*
a. Body habitus b. Level of CA–125
c. Nutritional status d. Histologic type of tumor

31. Following can cause endometrial cancer: *(AP 2008)*
a. Metropathia hemorrhagica
b. Gynandroblastoma
c. Dysgerminoma
d. All of the above

32. A female patient has adenocarcinoma uterus along with sarcoma of uterus. It is known as: *(AIIMS June 00)*
a. Homologous sarcoma
b. Sarcoma uterus
c. Mixed Müllerian carcinogenesis
d. Heterologous sarcoma

33. All are true regarding sarcoma botryoides except: *(PGI 01)*
a. Seen in vagina
b. Grape like clusters are seen
c. Seen in elderly women
d. It is an adenocarcinoma
e. Familial incidence is common

34. True statement regarding sarcoma botryoides: *(PGI May 2010)*
a. Involvement of vagina
b. Grape like growth seen
c. Common in old age
d. Malignant

35. True statement(s) regarding investigation in endometrial cancer: *(PGI Nov 2016)*
a. MRI is superior to CT in detecting myometrial involvement
b. CT is superior to MRI in detecting omental metastasis
c. USG is initial investigation to be performed
d. USG is the best investigation

36. An obese diabetic woman presents with menorrhagia. Curette from Endometrium shows Endometrial cancer. Which gene is associated with it? *(JIPMER Dec 2016/Nov 2017)*
a. p53 b. CDH-4
c. PTEN d. CYMC

37. An obese diabetic & hypertensive patient presents to Gynae OPD with postmenopausal bleeding and was diagnosed with Endometrial cancer with invasion of ≥50% of myometrium with extension to vagina, but no involvement of pelvic or para-aortic LN. What is the stage? *(JIPMER May 2017)*
a. Stage 2A b. Stage 3A
c. Stage 2B d. Stage 3B

ANSWERS TO NEW PATTERN QUESTIONS

N1. Ans. is c, i.e. PCOS

See the text for explanation

N2. Ans. is c, i.e. Medroxyprogesterone acetate

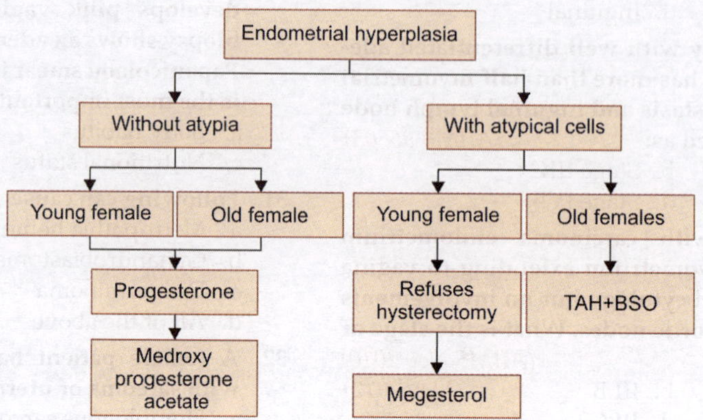

N3. Ans. is b, i.e. Atrophic endometrium

Premalignant Lesions of endometrial cancer

1. Simple hyperplasia (cystic glandular hyperplasia and complex hyperplasia with or without atypia)
2. Carcinoma in situ

N4. Ans. is c, i.e. Clear cell carcinoma

Most malignant variety of endometrial cancer: Clear cell carcinoma > papillary serous tumor

Most common variety is: Endometrioid (Adenocarcinoma)

N5. Ans. is b, i.e. Endometrial atrophy *Ref: Novak 15th/ed, p1256)*

N6. Ans. is b, i.e. 10%

Postmenopausal bleeding	
Cause	**Percentage**
Endometrial atrophy (M/C)	60–80
ERT	15–25%
Endometrial polyp	2–12
Endometrial hyperplasia	5–10%
Endometrial cancer	10%

N7. Ans. is d, i.e. Review in 3 months or earlier if bleeding occurs

N8. Ans. is c, i.e. Perform pipelle aspiration

N9. Ans. is b, i.e. Perform hysteroscopy and biopsy

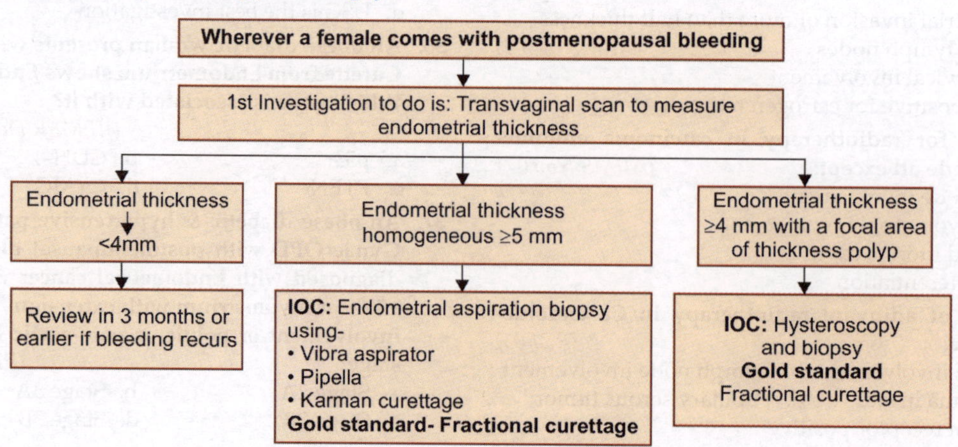

N10. Ans. is d, i.e. Cancer endometrium

Cancer endometrium

- No universal screening
- Screening done only in HNPCC syndrome
- Screening method in them – Pelvic examination
  – TVS
  – Endometrial sampling
- Best screening method of them – Fractional curettage
- Age of screening = ≥ 35 years
- Best method to prevent cancer = TAH + BSO once family is complete in these patients

N11. Ans. is a, i.e. Perform MRI scan:

Surprised by the answer 1 well, in the question it is given, Tumor is located in fundus, endometrioid variety, Grade 2 – but noting has been said about myometrial involvement. hence we cannot plan staging laparotomy. Because we do not know whether we have to perform lymph node dissection or not so we will first do MRI → to know extent of myometrial involvement & then decide next step ***"USG and MRI can be used to assess myometrial invasion pre-operatively with a fairly high degree of accuracy. This information may be of use in planning the surgical procedure with regard to whether lymph node sampling should be taken.*** *Ref: Novak 15th/ed, p1264.*

N12. Ans. is a, i.e. TAH + BSO

N13. Ans. is b, i.e. TAH + BSO with pelvic lymphadenectomy

N14. Ans. is c, i.e. TAH + BSO with pelvic and para-aortic lymphadenectomy

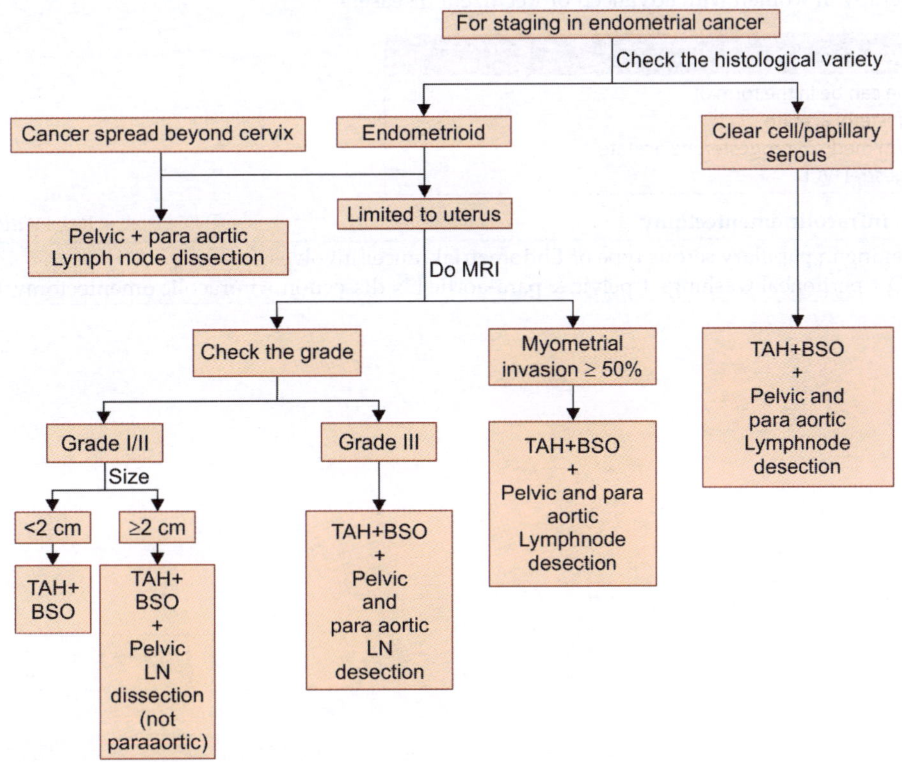

N15. Ans. is b, i.e. Cisplatin

Chemotherapy used in Endometrial cancer is cisplatin + Paclitaxel + Doxorubicin

N16. Ans. is d, i.e. Large cell keratinizing type

See the text for explanation

N17. Ans. is c, i.e. MLH 1 *Ref: Novak 15th/ed, p1252*

- Gene mutation M/C responsible for Endometrial cancer in HNPCC syndrome, i.e. lynch II syndrome is MLH 1
- Gene mutation M/C responsible for colon cancer in HNPCC syndrome – MSI.

N18. Ans. is d, i.e. Stage of cancer

Most important prognostic factor in endometrial cancer is is stage of disease.

N19. Ans. is b, i.e. Diabetes + Hypertension + Obesity + Endometrial Cancer
See the text for explanation.

N20. Ans. is c, i.e. Associated with PTEN mutation

Type 2 Endometrial cancer is associated with p53 gene mutation.

For more details see the text.

N21. Ans. is a, i.e. CA125 *Ref: Williams Gynae 3rd/ed, p708*

"The only clinically useful tumor marker in management of Endometrial Cancer is CA125 levels. Preoperatively an elevated level indicates the possibility of more advanced disease. In practice, it is most useful in patients with advanced disease or serous subtype to assist is monitoring response to therapy or during post treatment surveillance."

N22. Ans. is b, i.e. Lungs *Ref: Williams Gynae 3rd/ed, p713*

"Hematogenous dissemination most commonly results in metastases to lungs and less commonly to liver, brain, bone and other sites."

N23. Ans. is d, i.e. In females with large size of tumor *Ref: Williams Gynae 3rd/ed, p716*

N24. Ans. is a, i.e. Young females with stage 1 grade 1 tumors *Ref: William Gynae 3rd/ed, p717*

Hormonal Therapy in Endometrial cancer

- One of the unique characteristics of Endometrial Cancer is its Hormone Responsiveness.

Thus, Progesterone can be used as Primary treatment. 1. For women in whom surgery is C/I 2. Young premenopausal patients who desire fertility.

Note: Hormone therapy without Hysterectomy to given in stage 1 grade 1 females who desire fertility. In grade 2 tumors, further testing is necessary to asses the disease & then decision is made. Hormone Therapy/Progestone is used as an adjuvant therapy in women with advanced or Recurrent disease.

Also Know

Progesterone can be in the form of
1. Oral Megesterol acetate
2. Oral or 1/m medroxyprogesterone acetate
3. Levonorgestrel IVCD

N25. Ans. is a, i.e. infracolic omentectomy *Ref: Williams Gynae 3rd/ed, p716*

Surgical staging in papillary serous type of Endometrial cancer involves: TAH + BSO + peritoneal washings + pelvic & para-aortic LN dissection + infracolic omentectomy + peritoneal Biopsies.

ANSWERS TO PREVIOUS YEAR QUESTIONS

1. **Ans. is d, i.e. Complex hyperplasia with atypia**
2. **Ans. is d, i.e. 28%**
3. **Ans. is c, i.e. 1%** *Ref: Jeffcoate 7th/ed, p422-3; Novak 14th/ed, p1346; 15th/ed, p1252-3; Williams Gynae 1th/ed, p689*
   See the text for explanation
4. **Ans. is c, i.e. PCOD** *Ref: Jeffcoate 7th/ed, p422-3*
   Endometrial hyperplasia specially simple hyperplasia results from circumstances in which there is prolonged, increased estrogen production example:
   - Follicular cysts of ovary
   - PCOD
   - Granulosa and theca cells
   - HRT.
5. **Ans. is a, i.e. Simple hysterectomy** *Ref: Jeffcoate 7th/ed, p425; Williams Gynae 1st/ed, p691*
   Management of Atypical Endometrial Hyperplasia:
   "Hysterectomy is the best treatment for women at any age with atypical endometrial hyperplasia because the risk of concurrent subclinical invasive disease is high." ... Williams Gynae 1st/ed, p691
   "In presence of atypia, response to progesterone therapy is poor and relapse rate is high. Nearly one-third of them will progress to cancer and one-fourth may already have associated undiagnosed cancer. In women approaching or past menopause, hysterectomy is a safer choice in those with complex or atypical hyperplasia." ... Jeffcoate 7th/ed, p425
6. **Ans. is d, i.e. Early menopause**
7. **Ans. is a and c, i.e. Obesity; and PCOD**
8. **Ans. is a and c, i.e. Multiparity; and Early menopause**
   Ref: Shaw 15th/ed, p416-7; Williams Gynae 1st/ed, p688; Novak 14th/ed, p1345, 15th/ed, p1251-2
   See the text for explanation
9. **Ans. is a, i.e. Endometrium Ca** *Ref: Shaw 15th/ed, p417, Novak 14th/ed, p1345, 15th/ed, p1251-2*
   Long-term tamoxifen therapy is a predisposing factor for endometrial hyperplasia and cancers.

   Malignancies caused by long-term tamoxifen therapy:
   - Carcinoma endometrium—it is the most common carcinoma associated with it.
   - Uterine sarcoma.
   - Rarely liver cancer with long-term high dose.

   Nonmalignant effects of tamoxifen on uterus:
   - Endometrial hyperplasia
   - Endometriosis
   - Fibroid uterus
   - Ovarian cysts
   - Menstrual irregularities or amenorrhea.
10. **Ans. is a, i.e. Multiparity** *Ref: Jeffcoates 7th/ed, p504, Dutta Gynae 5th/ed p351*
    Combination of diabetes, obesity and hypertension in association with endometrial carcinoma is called as the **Corpus Cancer Syndrome**.
11. **Ans. is b, i.e. Carcinoma endometrium** *Ref: Jeffcoate 7th/ed, p503; Novak 14th/ed, p1349*
    A 50-year-old woman **nulliparous, diabetic** and **obese** (all predisposing factors for carcinoma endometrium) female is presenting with postmenopausal bleeding (most specific complaint in Ca endometrium). The most likely diagnosis is carcinoma endometrium.
12. **Ans. is a, i.e. Predisposed by diabetes mellitus, hypertension and obesity** *Ref: Jeffcoate 7th/ed, p503-5; Shaw 15th/ed, p417 for option a, 418 for option b, 416 for option c & option d; Novak 14th/ed, p1345, 15th/ed, p1256-7*
    Endometrial cancer:
    - Lets see each option regarding endometrial cancer one by one:
      - Predisposed by diabetes mellitus, hypertension and obesity-correct
      - Adenosquamous type is most common–incorrect as the most common variant is adenocarcinoma
      - Commonly associated with cancer cervix incorrect as cancer cervix and endometrial cancer are not related to each other.
      - Common age group affected is between 20 and 40 years incorrect as endometrial cancer occurs in postmenopausal females (6th–7th decade).
13. **Ans. is b, c, d, and e. i.e. More common in diabetes; Common after 40 years of age; Associated with PCOD; and Associated with HNPCC.**

In this question - no option needs explanation except option a which says, less aggressive in postmenopausal females. This is incorrect

"In general, younger women with endometrial cancer have a better prognosis than older women."
"Increasing age appears to be independently associated with disease recurrence in endometrial cancer." *Novac 15/ed, p 1266-1267*

14. Ans. is d, i.e. Clear cell carcinoma *Ref: Devita cancers 8th/ed, p1545, Table 42.3.2; Dutta Gynae 4th/ed, p334; Novak 14th/ed, p1354; Williams Gynae 1th/ed, p9691*

Clear cell carcinoma:
- It accounts for < 5% of all endometrial carcinoma.
- Most characteristic histological finding is presence of "hobnail cells".
- It characteristically occurs in older women and is very aggressive type of endometrial cancer.
- Prognosis is similar to or worse than papillary serous carcinoma.

Remember

Remember M/C variety of endometrial cancer = Adenocarcinoma
Most malignant is clear cell carcinoma followed by Papillary serous variety.

15. Ans. is b, i.e. Fractional curettage *Ref: Devita Cancers 8th/ed, p1546,344; Jeffcoate 7th/ed, p509; Novak 14th/ed, p1350; 15th/ed, p1257-8; Bijoy Sree Sen Gupta 2nd/ed, p616-7; Dutta Gynae 5th/ed, p344*

For postmenopausal bleeding
- 1st investigation: TVS
- IOC: Endometrial aspiration biopsy
- Gold standard: Fractional curettage

Now since endometrial aspiration biopsy is not given in the options, we will go for fractional curettage

16. Ans is b, c and d i.e. Fractional curettage; Aspiration cytology from uterus; and Hysteroscopy and biopsy.

Ref: Dutta Gyne, 5th/ed, p356-357

"Endometrial carcinoma: Pap smear is only 50% sensitive and not reliable" *- Shaw's Gynecology 16/e p510.*
"Colposcopy is used for cervical cancer. Aim- to study cervix when pap smear detects abnormal cells, to locate abnormal areas & take a biopsy, to study the extent of abnormal lesions, conservative surgery under colposcopic guidance & follow-up of conservative therapy cases."- Shaw's Gynecology 16/e p490.

17. Ans. is b, i.e. Ib *Ref: Novak 15th/ed, p1265; Shaw 15th/ed, p420*

In stage IA–Tumor is confined to uterus and either it is limited to endometrium or less than half of myometrium is involved.

Stage IB–Tumor confined to uterus with more than or equal to half of myometrial invasion

Thickness of 10 mm means more than half of myometrium, i.e. stage Ib.

18. Ans. is d, i.e. Stage IV *Ref: Novak 15th/ed, p1265; Shaw 15th/ed, p420*

In general inguinal lymph node metastasis are very frequently asked in exams:

Remember

- In Ca endometrium–Inguinal LN are involved in stage IV B
- In Ca ovary–Inguinal LN are involved in stage IV B.
- In Ca cervix–Lymph nodes rarely involved & if involved— it is stage IV B.
- In vulva cancer–Sentinel lymph nodes, i.e., first lymph nodes involved are–inguinal lymph node.

19. Ans. is a, b, c and d, i.e. Vaginal metastasis; Para-aortic lymph node involvement; Pelvic lymph node involvement; and Peritoneal involvement *Ref: Novak 15th/ed, p1265; Shaw 15th/ed, p420*

Kindly see FIGO staging given in preceding text.

20. Ans. is c, i.e. Inferior mesenteric *Ref: AJCC Cancer Staging Manual 6th/ed, p267*

Lymphatic drainage of uterus: ∴ Lymph nodes involved in ca endometrium. ... *BDC Vol II, 3th/ed, p319*

- Upper lymphatics (from fundus) – Para-aortic
- From cornua – Superficial inguinal nodes.
- Middle lymphatics (from body) – External iliac nodes.
- Lower lymphatics (from cervix) – External iliac node, Internal iliac nodes.

Besides these other regional lymph node involved in CA endometrium are:

- Parametrial LN
- Presacral LN
- Pelvic LN
- Obturator.

21. Ans. is d, i.e. Stage IV B *Ref: Novak 15th/ed, p1265; Shaw 15th/ed, p420*

The lady in above question has cancer spread to inguinal lymph nodes, i.e. stage IVB.

22. Ans. is b, i.e. III B *Ref: Williams Gynae 2th/ed, p830; shaw 15th/ed, p420; Novak 15th/ed, p1265*

As discussed earlier, 50% myometrial invasion means stage IC, positive peritoneal cytology puts it in stage III A Vaginal metastasis means stage III B cancer and since this is the highest stage.

Therefore, this patient has endometrial cancer belonging to stage III B.

23. Ans. is a and e, i.e. Vaginal metastasis; and Serosa involved

24. Ans. is a and d, i.e. Vaginal metastasis; and Positive peritoneal cytology *Ref: Novak 15th/ed, p1265; Shaw 15th/ed, p420*

Before answering these questions I want all of you to quickly revise staging of Ca Endometrium.

- Vaginal metastasis means stage IIIB[Q]
- Lymph node involvement is seen from stage IIIC onwards.
- Bowel involvement / rectal involvement means stage IVA.
- Lung metastasis means stage IV B.
- Serosa involvement/ positive peritoneal cytology means stage III A. The question is about stage IIIB, so everything involved before it is also included.

25. Ans. is d, i.e. No treatment *Ref Shaw 15th/ed, p420; Novak 15th/ed, p1275*

As discussed in preceding text – Stage Ia grade 1 and grade II require no postoperative treatment.

26. Ans. is d, i.e. Tumor positive for estrogen receptors

27. Ans. is c, i.e. Enlarged uterine cavity

28. Ans. is a, b and d, i.e. Cervical involvement; Lymph node involvement; and Papillary serous tumor

Ref: COGDT 9th/ed, p924; Shaw 15th/ed, p420; Novak 15th/ed, p1275; Onwards

Indications of adjuvant radiotherapy:

- Extrauterine extension.
- Lower uterine or cervical involvement.
- Papillary serous or clear cell histology.
- Poor histologic differentiation (Grade III).
- Myometrial penetration greater than 1/2 of thickening.
- Pelvic node involvement.

Tumor positive for estrogen receptors suggest well differentiated disease. So no adjuvant radiotherapy is recommended.

29. Ans. is a, b and e, i.e. Penetration into half of myometrium; Clear cell carcinoma; and Papillary serous carcinoma

Ref: Novak 15th/ed, p1271

Indications for lymph node (pelvic and Para-aortic) dissection in endometrial cancer

1. Tumor histology:
   - Clear cell carcinoma
   - Papillary serous carcinoma
   - Squamous carcinoma
2. Adenocarcinoma (endometrioid) III.
3. More than half of myometrial invasion
4. Isthmus-cervix extension
5. Extrauterine disease.
6. Tumor size > 2 cm

Note: In absence of these factor only bilateral pelvic lymphadenectomy is performed if the tumor size is greater than 2 cm.

Lymphadenectomy is altogether omitted for patient with above risk factors absent, absence of cervical involvement and tumor size less than 2 cm.

30. Ans. is d, i.e. Histologic type of tumor *Ref: John Hopkins Manual of Obs & Gynae 4th/ed, p564; Novak 15th/ed, p1266–8*

"The most significant prognostic factors for recurrence and survival are stage, grade and depth of myometrial invasion. Age, histologic type, LVSI and progesterone receptor activity also have prognostic significance."

... John Hopkins Manual of Obs & Gynae 4th/ed, p564

31. Ans. is a, i.e. Metropathia hemorrhagica *Ref: Shaw 14th/ed, p340,341,338; Dutta Gynae 5th/ed, p184 for option a*

Endometrial cancer is mainly caused by excessive estrogen

- Metropathia hemorrhagica is the same as cystic glandular hyperplasia and is a causative factor for endometrial cancer. *Ref: Dutta Gynae 5th/ed, p184*
- Gynandroblastoma is a virilizing tumor which secretes androgens (not estrogens) and so does not lead to endometrial cancer *Ref: Shaw 14th/ed, p34*
- Dysgerminoma is a neutral tumor which does not secrete either male or female sex hormones but secretes placental alkaline phosphatase, LDH and BHCG and therefore does not lead to endometrial cancer. *Ref: Shaw 14th/ed, p3386*

32. Ans. is c, i.e. Mixed Müllerian carcinogenesis *Ref: COGDT 10th/ed, p866*

Mixed Mullerian carcinoma is a mixture of both carcinomatous and sarcomatous element.

- Represent 50% of all uterine sarcoma.
- Most common combination is of serous carcinoma with endometrial sarcoma.
- Most commonly occur in postmenopausal women.

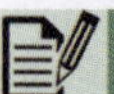

Remember

- Most common histologic type of uterine sarcoma is carcinosarcoma.[Q]
- Most common symptom of uterine sarcoma is bleeding.
- Surgery is main stay of treatment followed by chemotherapy.

Also Know

Heterologous tumors: If sarcoma component of mixed Müllerian tumors mimic extra uterine tissue (viz – striated muscle cell, cartilage, adipose tissue and bone) it is known as *Heterologous tumor*.

Homologous tumor: If mesenchymal/sarcomatous component of mixed Müllerian tumor consists of malignant endometrial or smooth muscle differentiation, the term homologous is used.

33. Ans. is c, d and e, i.e. Seen in elderly women; It is an adenocarcinoma; and Familial incidence is common *Ref: Robbin's Pathology 7th/ed, p1071–2*

34. Ans. is a, b and d, i.e. Involvement of vagina; Grape like growth seen; and Malignant *Ref: William Gynae 1st/ed, p683*

Embryonal Rhabdomyosarcoma is the most common malignancy of the vagina in infants and children.

Most common subtype of embryonal rhabdomyosarcoma is sarcoma botryoides

Seen in infants and children less than 5 years of age.

"This rare tumor develops almost exclusively in girls younger than 5 years, although vaginal and cervical sarcoma botryoides have been reported in females aged 15 to 20 years." *Ref: William Gynae 1st/ed, p683*

"Sarcoma botryoides are usually seen in patients who are younger than 5 years of age." *Ref: COGDT 10th/ed, p831*

In infants and children, sarcoma botryoides is usually found in vagina, in reproductive age females rhabdomyosarcoma is seen within the cervix and after menopause within the uterus.

35. Ans. is a, b and c, i.e MRI is superior to CT in detecting myometrial involvement, CT is superior to MRI in detecting metastasis and USG is initial investigation to be performed.

- **Role of Imaging is endometrial cancer**
  - **CT** is useful in assessing pelvic anatomy (which includes omental metastasis, visualizing enlarged lymph nodes in the pelvis and periaortic areas and diagnosing distant metastasis in liver and lymph nodes
  - **MRI** is particularly useful is identifying myometrial invasion, lower uterine segment or cervical involvement.
  - In endometrial cancer- M/C presentation is irregular vaginal bleeding

    Whenever a patient C/O bleeding- 1st investigation to be done is TVS

On TVS = If endometrial thickness

⇓

≥ 5 mm in post menopausal

⇓

IOC : Endometrial aspiration biopsy using Pipelle, Novak curette and Vabra aspirator

⇓

Gold standard = Fractional curettage

36. Ans. is a, i.e. p 53

37. Ans. is d, i.e. Stage 3B.

Since is this patient vagina is involved but pelvic and paraaortic lymph nodes are not involved, hence it is stage 3B.

REVIEW/PRACTICE QUESTIONS

1. **M/C Variety of Endometrial cancer**
   a. Squamous cell b. Adenocarcinoma
   c. Adeno-squamous d. Clear cell carcinoma
2. **Most malignant variety of endometrial cancer:**
   a. Clear cell carcinoma b. Adenocarcinoma
   c. Adeno squamous d. Squamous cell
3. **Chemotherapy used in Endometrial cancer:**
   a. Doxorubicin, Paclitaxel, Cisplatin
   b. Doxorubicin, 5F-U, Cyclophosphamide
   c. Cisplatin, Paclitaxel, 5-F-U
   d. Doxorubicin, etoposide, methotrexate
4. **M/c Route of spread of Endometrial cancer:**
   a. Direct spread
   b. Lymphatic
   c. Hematogenous
   d. Retrograde transtubal transport
5. **M/C site of recurrence of Endometrial cancer**
   a. Pelvis b. Vagina
   c. Ovary d. Lungs.
6. **M/c cause of postmenopausal bleeding:**
   a. Cancer endometrium b. Cancer cervix
   c. Endometrial atrophy d. HRT
7. **% of PMB patients with Endometrial cancer**
   a. 5% b. 10%
   c. 25% d. 60%
8. **M/C Cause of pyometra:**
   a. Endometrial cancer b. Cancer cervix
   c. Severe endometritis d. Cervical steronism
9. **Postoperative management for stage IA grade 1, Endometrial cancer:**
   a. Chemotherapy b. Radiotherapy
   c. Hormone therapy d. None of the above
10. **Screening for endometrial cancer is done in:**
    a. Obese females
    b. Females with
    c. Females >60 years
    d. Females with previous H/O breast cancer
11. **Gold standard for Endometrial cancer:**
    a. TVS
    b. Hysteroscopy
    c. Endometrial aspiration biopsy
    d. Fractional curettage
12. **Endometrial biopsy is indicated, if endometrial thickness is………… in a postmenopausal female:**
    a. $\geq$4 mm b. $\geq$5 mm
    c. $\geq$6 mm d. $\geq$7 mm
13. **TOC for simple Hyperplasia of endometrium without atypia:**
    a. TAH b. TAH + BSO
    c. Progesterone d. Estrogen
14. **Lymph nodes commonly involved in Endometrial cancer:**
    a. Femoral b. Para aortic
    c. Inguinal d. Both a and b
15. **Mainstay of treatment in stage 3 endometrial cancer:**
    a. Surgery b. RT
    c. CT d. Hormone therapy
16. **A 55-year-old postmenopausal lady with simple endometrial hyperplasia with atypia. What is the management?** *(AIIMS Nov 2018)*
    a. Hysterectomy
    b. Mirena
    c. Progestin
    d. Estrogens
17. **When would you do trans-vaginal sonography in post-menopausal bleeding if endometrial thickness is?** *(AIIMS May 2018)*
    a. 5 mm b. 7 mm
    c. 4 mm d. 9 mm
18. **Histopathology of endometroid carcinoma Type 2 includes:** *(PGI December 2018)*
    a. Endometroid b. Squamous
    c. Mucinous d. Papillary serous
    e. Clear cell
19. **Risk factors for endometrial carcinoma include:** *(PGI December 2018)*
    a. Familial non-polyposis cancer syndrome
    b. Early menopause
    c. OCPs
    d. Tamoxifen therapy
    e. Infertility

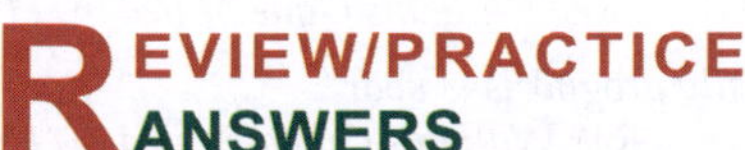

REVIEW/PRACTICE ANSWERS

1. **Ans. is b, i.e. Adenocarcinoma** *Ref: William Gynae 3rd/ed, p710*
2. **Ans. is a, i.e. Clear cell carcinoma** *Ref: William Gynae 3rd/ed, p710*
3. **Ans. is a, i.e. Doxorubicin, Paclitaxel, Cisplatin** *Ref: William Gynae 3rd/ed, p715*
4. **Ans. is a, i.e. Direct spread** *Ref: William Gynae 3rd/ed, p712*
5. **Ans. is b, i.e. Vagina** *Ref: M/c is vagina followed by pelvis*

6. **Ans. is c, i.e. Endometrial atrophy** *Ref: Novak 13rd/ed, p1256*
7. **Ans. is b, i.e. 10%** *Ref: Novak 15/e pg 1256*
8. **Ans. is c, i.e. Severe endometritis**
9. **Ans. is d, i.e. None of the above**
10. **Ans. is b, i.e. Females with** *Ref: William Gynae 3rd/ed, p707*
11. **Ans. is d, i.e. Fractional curettage**
12. **Ans. is b, i.e. ≥ 5 mm**
13. **Ans. is c, i.e. Progesterone**
14. **Ans. is b, i.e. Para aortic**
15. **Ans. is a, i.e. Surgery**

    Pelvic and para-aortic LN are mainly involved.
16. **Ans. is a i.e. Hysterectomy**
    - As discussed in chapter 14A, women with atypical hyperplasia should undergo a total hysterectomy because of the risk of underlying malignancy or progression to cancer.
    - A laparoscopic approach to total hysterectomy is preferable to an abdominal approach as it is associated with a shorter hospital stay, less postoperative pain and quicker recovery.
    - Postmenopausal women with atypical hyperplasia should be offered bilateral salpingo oophorectomy together with the total hysterectomy.
17. **Ans. is a i.e. 5 mm**

Flowchart: Investigation in a patient c/o Primary amenorrhea

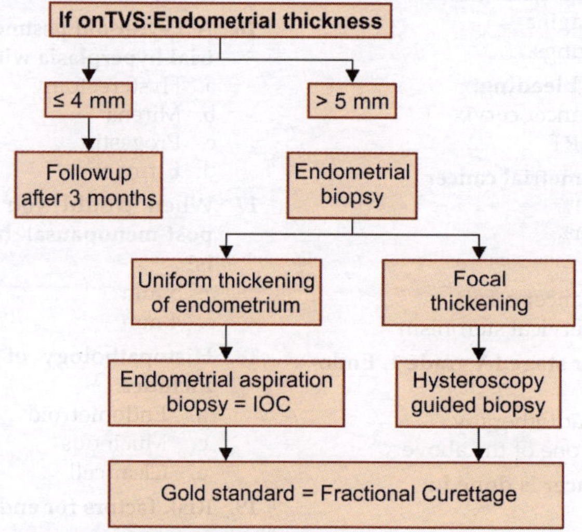

18. **Ans. is b, d and e, i.e. Squamous; Papillary serous; and Clear cell**

    As discussed in chapter on Endometrial Cancer: Endometrial cancer can be categorized as Type 1 and Type 2 cancers.

    Type 2 cancers include (have bad prognosis)
    - Serous type
    - Clear cell carcinoma
    - Endometroid grade 3 only. But in general endometroid is taken as Type 1 cancer

    Type 1 cancers include
    - Mucinous variety: *"Almost all are stage 1 grade 1 lesion and carry a good prognosis"* *Ref: Williams Gynae 3rd/ed, p710*
    - Endometrioid variety: *"This is the M/C histologic type of endometrial cancer and accounts for more than 75% of cases."* *Ref: Williams Gyne 3rd/ed, p711*

    This is type 1 tumor: *"Squamous cell carcinoma of endometrium have been reported. Typically prognosis is poor"* *Ref: Williams Gynae 3rd/ed, p712*

    These lines indicate that squamous cell carcinoma belongs to Type 2 variety as they are associated with bad prognosis.
19. **Ans. is a, d and e, i.e. Familial non-polyposis cancer syndrome; Tamoxifen therapy; and Infertility**

    Ref: Shaw's gyne 15th/ed, p416-20; Dutta's gyne 5th/ed, p341-47; Novak gyne 14th/ed, p1344-45

    Early menopause and OCPs are protective factors. Other 3 are risk factors.

    See chapter on Endometrial Cancer for more details.

CHAPTER 14B

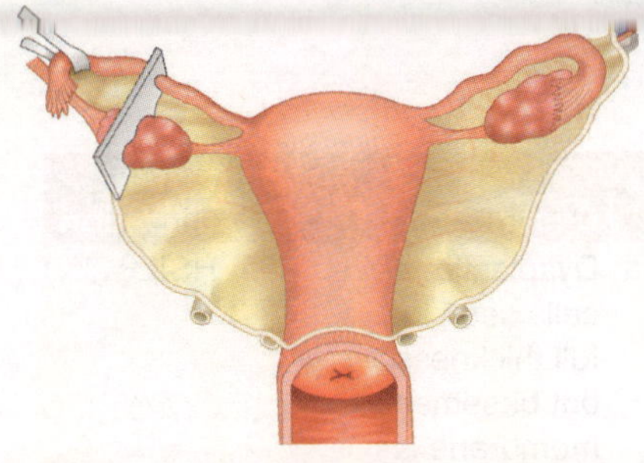

Gynecological Oncology: CIN, Cancer Cervix

General Considerations

Anatomy of Cervix

- The Endocervix is lined by single layer of columnar epithelium (called as glandular epithelium as it produces mucus & its deep infolding appear histologically similar to glandular tissue) and exocervix is covered by squamous epithelium. The place at which columnar epithelium of endocervix changes to squamous epithelium of exocervix is the **Squama-Columnar Junction or Transformation Zone.**
- The original **SC junction** is generally located at external os but it rarely remains restricted to it. Instead it is a dynamic point which changes in response to puberty, pregnancy, menopause and hormonal stimulation.

Transformation zone moves:

Inside, into endocervix	Moves out in:
With age Progesterone only pills	• Pregnancy • Puberty • OCP users

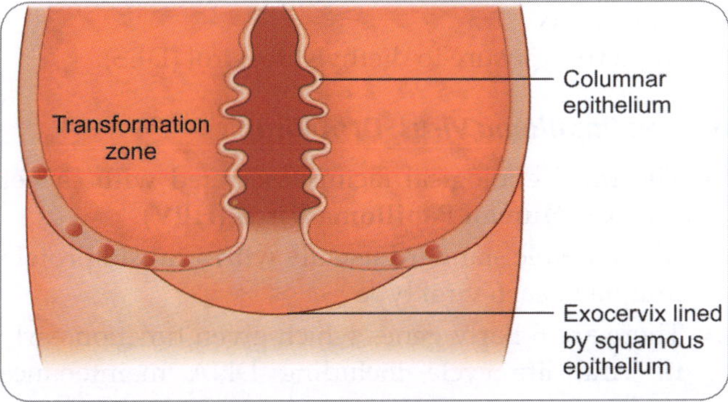

Fig. 14B.1: Parts of cervix

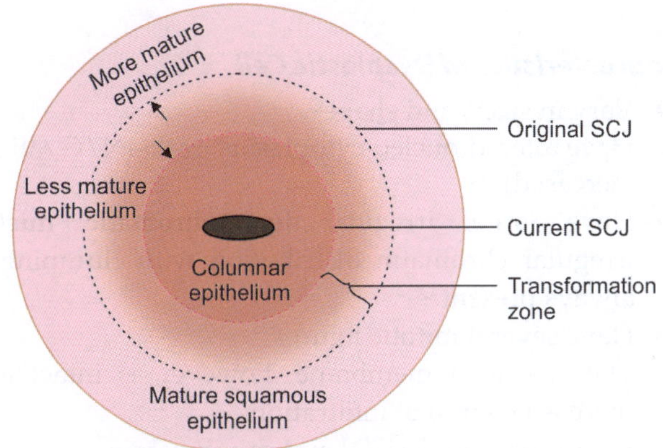

Fig. 14B.2: Diagram of PS view of cervix

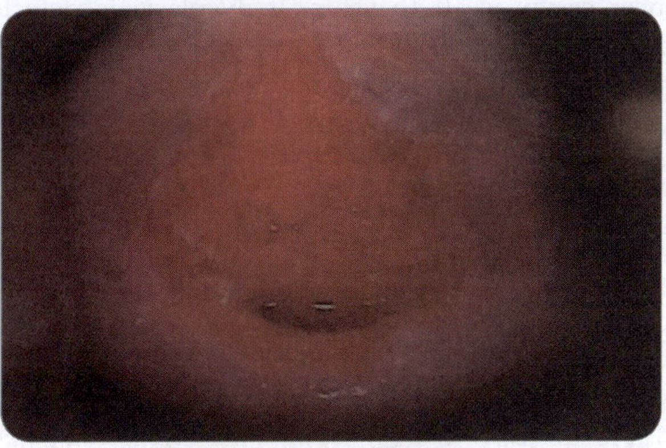

Fig. 14B.3: Photograph of PS view of cervix

Metaplasia and Dysplasia

In all females: the columnar epithelium of endocervix changes into squamous exocervix. This change is called as **Metaplasia**.

Metaplasia is:	– Physiological – Not premalignant – Occurs in all young females
Metaplastic cells are	– Normal cells – No nuclear atypia

In presence of infection/any other oncogenic stimuli, instead of metaplasia, dysplasia occurs (see flowchart 14B.1).

Dysplasia	- Is Pathological - Premalignant

Flowchart 14B.1

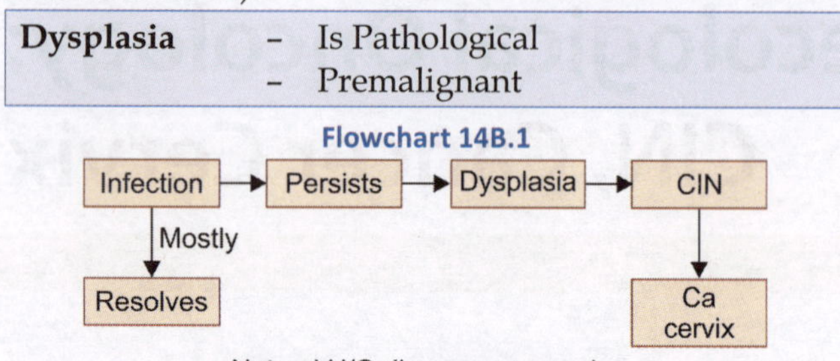

Natural H/O disease progression in Ca cervix

Characteristics of Dysplastic Cell

- Vary in size[Q], and shape[Q].
- Have altered nucleo-cytoplasmic ratio (N/C ratio is increased).[Q]
- Have large, irregular **hyperchromatic nuclei,** irregular chromatin distribution with clumping is always present.[Q]
- Have several mitotic figures.
- The basement membrane, however, is intact and there is no stromal infiltration.
- Dysplasia leads to CIN and cancer cervix.

Note: Time interval for dysplasia to change into invasive cancer cervix is 10–15 years. If dysplasia is detected during this time and treated, Ca cervix can be prevented. That is why universal screening of cancer cervix by pap smear is recommended.

CIN

Depending on the thickness of cervical epithelium, which has become dysplastic CIN can be classified as:

Tale 14B.1: Classification of cervical intraepithelial lesions

WHO	CIN	Description	Bethesda classification
Mild dysplasia	CIN I	Dysplastic cells seen in lower 1/3 of epithelial lining of cervix	LSIL[Q]
Moderate dysplasia	CIN II	Dysplastic cells seen in 2/3 of epithelial lining of cervix	HSIL[Q]
Severe dysplasia	CIN III	Dysplastic cells seen in more than 2/3 of epithelial lining of cervix	HSIL[Q]
Carcinoma in situ	Carcinoma in situ	Dysplastic cells seen in full thickness but basement membrane is intact	HSIL[Q]
In Invasive carcinoma	Ca cervix	Breach of Basement membrane seen	

Note: LSIL = Low squamous intraepithelial lesion.
HSIL = High squamous intraepithelial lesion.

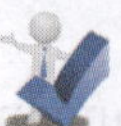

KEY POINTS

- M/C site for CIN is: Transformation zone
- Anterior lip of cervix is twice as likely to develop CIN as the posterior lip and CIN rarely originates in the lateral angles.
- CIN can be identified by microscopic examination of cervical cells in a cytology smear stained by papinacalou.

Factors Predisposing to CIN/Ca Cervix

- **Human Pappiloma virus infection** (*most important*)
- **Factors increasing the risk of sexually transmitted infections-**
  - Coitus before 18 years of age[Q]
  - Increasing age
  - Multiple sex partners[Q]
  - Multiparity[Q]
  - Poor personal hygiene[Q]
  - Poor socioeconomic status[Q]
- Smoking[Q] (predisposes to squamous cell CA).
- Immunosuppressed individuals[Q]
- Women on OCP[Q] or progesterone therapy for long time, are predisposed to *adenocarcinoma* of endocervix
- In utero exposure to diethylstilbestrol (DES).

Human Papilloma Virus: DNA Virus

- The M/C etiological factor associated with cancer cervix is **Human Papilloma Virus (HPV)**.
- It is a double standard usually with a capsid protein unique to each viral type
- There are 6 Early genes which given function early in viral life cycle including DNA maintenance replication & transcription
- Early genes are expressed in lower epithelial layers.

- The two late genes envolve major (L1) & minor (L2) capsid protein. These genes are expressed in superficial layers. Sequential HPV gene expression is synchronous with and dependent on squamous epithelial differentiation. Thus completion of viral cycle takes place only within an intact, fully differentiating squamous epithelium. Thus, makes HPV culture difficult.
- **High risk HPV** include 16, 18, 31, 33, 35, 39, 45, 52, 56, 58, 59, 68.
- **Low risk HPV** associated with **genital warts** and laryngeal papillomas are **subtypes 6 and 11.**
- Almost 80% women are infected by HPV at some point in their lives.
- Epidemiological studies have shown that HPV infection is the M/C STD.
- HPV is epitheliotropic. A new infection occurs when L1 & L2 capsid protein bind to epithelial basement membrane permitting entry of HPV viral particle into epithelial cell. It infects basal epithelial cells. The cytological changes were first recognised by **Koss** and **Durfee in 1956** and are called as **koilocytosis.**
- Viral proteins required for malignant **transformation are E6** and **E7 oncoproteins.**
- E6 gene acts on tumor suppression protein p53, E7 acts through Retino blastoma tumor suppression protein.
- Viral proteins required for replication are **E1** and **E2.**
- **HPV DNA detection is used along with pap smear as a screening procedure** in females more than 30 years of age.
- **Polymerase chain reaction (PCR) or southern blot or hybrid capture technique** is used for HPV DNA detection.

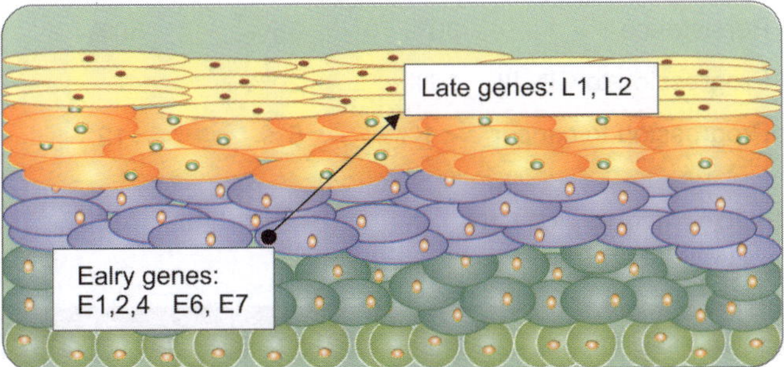

Fig. 14B.4: Early and late genes of HPV

Koilocytosis

- A common feature to both high and low risk HPV infection is the appearance of koilocytes in the differentiated layers of squamous epithelium.
- **Koilocytes are epithelial cells** that contain accentric, hyperchromatic, moderately **enlarged nucleus that is displaced by large perinuclear vaucole.**

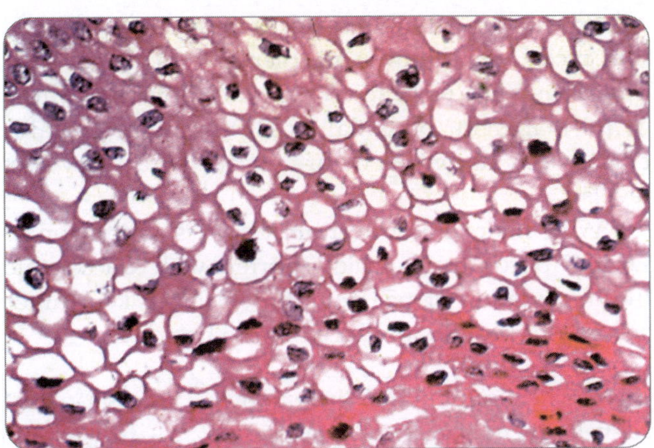

Fig. 14B.5: Koilocytosis—see the large perinuclear vaucole

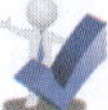

KEY POINTS

- M/C HPV subtype associated with Ca cervix is HPV-16.
- M/C is HPV 18 (13.1)
- M/C is HPV 45
- HPV subtype most specific for Ca cervix is HPV-18.
- M/C HPV found is low grade lesions & in women without neoplasia HPV-16
- M/C HPV subtype associated with squamous cell carcinoma is HPV-16.
- M/C HPV subtype associated with adenocarcinoma is HPV-18.
- M/C age for HPV non-infection is 20-24 years
- HPV injfection this is Mic STD in US
- On most females thus infection cells. For development of cervical cancer– it is presented HPV infection that is required.

Flowchart 14B.2

The natural history of genital HPV infection

Genital HPV infection causes various outcomes (Flowchart 14B.2).

Latent infection refers to that in which cells are infected but HPV remains quiescent. The virus remains below detectable levels.

Productive infection are characterized by viral life cycle completion and plentiful production of infectious viral particles. These infections have little or no malignant potential as HPV genome remains episomal & its oncogene are expressed at very low levels.

With neoplastic infection:_There is expression of E6 & E7 oncoproteins which interfere with & accelerate the degradation of p53 & pRb, which are key tumor suppressor proteins produced by the host.

Note: Persistent HPV infection is necessary for development of cervical neoplasia.
- A minority of HPV infections become persistent but most young women (65%) with HPV 16/18 infections lasting for ≥6 months will develop SIL.
- The risk of progression to high grade neoplasia increases with age.
- Cell mediated immunity plays the largest role in HPV persistence.

Diagnosis of HPV Infection

- HPV infection is suspected based on clinical lesions or results of cytology, histology, and colposcopy, all of which are subjective and often inaccurate. Moreover, serology is unreliable and cannot distinguish past from current infection (Dillner, 1999).
- As noted HPV culture is not feasible. Thus, diagnosis is confirmed only by the direction detection of HPV nucleic acids by methods that include in situ hybridization, nucleic acid amplification testing (NAAT), polymerase chain reaction (PCR), or others (Molijin, 2005).
- Currently, four HR HPV tests are approved by the Food and Drug Administration (FDA) for clinical use, and all use NAAT to detect any of the 13 or 14 HR HPV types.
- Two of these tests report specifically the presence of HPV 16 or HPV 18 to aid risk stratification and customized management.
- Due to clinical test limitations, a negative test result does not exclude HPV infection. Therefore, these tests are not indicated or useful for routine STD screening.
- LR HPV testing has no indication and can lead to inappropriate expense, further evaluation, and unnecessary treatment.

Namely, appropriate **clinical uses for HR HPV testing include**: contesting with cervical cytology screening in women aged 30 years or older, triage or surveillance of certain abnormal cytology results and untreated CIN, and posttreatment surveillance (Davey, 2014). One HR HPV test (Cobas HPV test) was recently FDA approved as a stand-alone screening test for cervical cancer for women 25 years of age and older.

If typical genital warts are found in a young woman or if high-grade cervical neoplasia or invasive cancer is identified by cytology or histology, then HPV infection is assumed, and HPV testing is unnecessary. Because of high HPV prevalence improving women (less than age 25), HR HPV testing for cervical cancer screening is not recommended. HPV testing is not FDA approved for use in women after TAH.

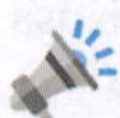
Important One Liners

Cancers caused by HPV	
Females	**Males**
Ca cervix	Penile Ca
Ca vagina	Anal Ca
Ca vulva	Oral Ca

Rate of Progression of CIN (Table 14B.2)

William Gynae pg 631

	CIN I	CIN II	CIN III
Regression to normal	60%	40%	30%
Persistence	30%	35%	50%
Progression to CIN III	10%	20%	—
Progression to cancer	< 1%	5%	>12

Epidemiology of CIN

Age

Table 14B.2	
CIN	M/c in 20–30 years
Ca in situ	30–35 years.
Ca cervix	Bimodal peak
	1st peak seen at 35–39 years.
	2nd peak seen at 55–60 years.

Diagnosis

See Flowchart 14B.3

Flowchart 14B.3

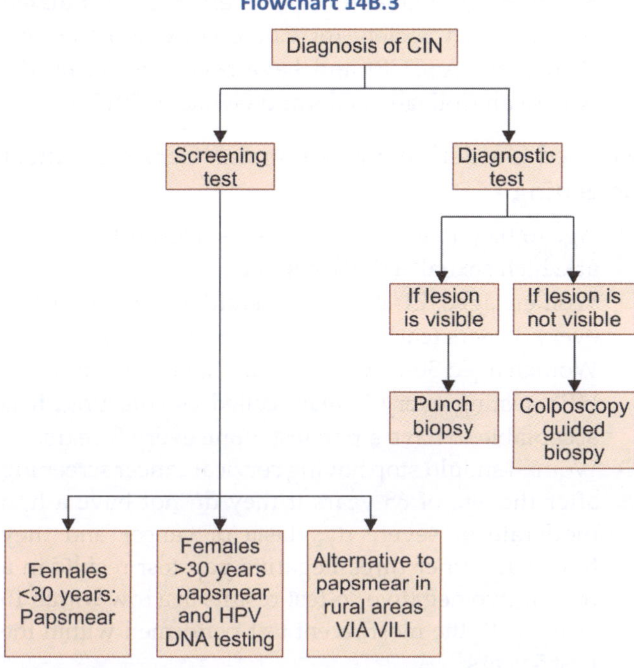

HPV DNA testing

- In 2003, the FDA first approved an HPV test for use with cytology for cervical cancer screening in women 30 years and older. The combination of HR HPV testing with cytology is referred to as contesting. This strategy is not currently endorsed for women younger than 30 due to the high prevalence of HRHPV infection in this age group and the resultant lack of test specificity.
- HPV testing is usually performed from the residual LBC specimen after the cytology slide is prepared.
- Testing is performed only for HR HPV types. As noted earlier, there is no clinical role for LR HPV testing.
- The combination of HPV testing with cytology increases the sensitivity of a single screening test for high-grade neoplasia to nearly 100 percent and leads to earlier detection and management of HSIL.
- The lack of sensitivity for cervical adenocarcinoma seen with traditional cytology testing also supports HPV testing use of primary screening.
- Due to high negative predictive value for high-grade neoplasia, slow progression of new HPV infection to neoplasia, and increased cost, contesting is repeated at 5-year intervals if both cytology and HPV test are negative.

Cytology

- Papsmear
- Liquid based cylotogy

Pap Smear (Exfoliative Cytology)

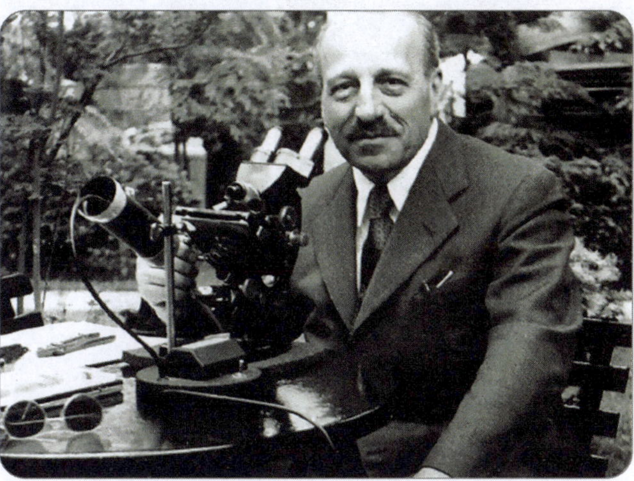

Fig. 14B.6: Georgis Papanicolou

- Pap smear is named after Georgis Papanicolaou (Fig. 14.B6)
- **Time for initiating pap smear:** 21 years of age **regardless of the age of first sexual intercourse.** (Even if a female had her first intercourse at 17 years)
- **Instrument used:** Ayers spatula and endocervical brush (Figs. 14B.7A and B)
  - **Method:** The concave end of ayers spatula is rotated through 360° over portio vaginalis of cervix and 1st slide is prepared by rotating it attendance. The ayers spatula can be wooden or plastic. These days only plastic spatula based.
  - With cytobrush, 2nd slide is prepared from endocervix. It is rotated by one quater or one half of them
  - For liquid based cytology cervical bloom is used. It has long bustless & short bustless five rotations in same due clear are recommended to sampling Ecto & Endo cervix simultaneously.
  - Control slide prepared from posterior wall/ posterior fornix of vagina from the other end of Ayer spatula

Important One Liners

- For hormonal study, sample is taken from the lateral wall of vagina
- For cytological study, (Pap smear) sample is taken from the posterior wall of vagina.

- **Fixative used:** 95% ethyl alcohol.
- The slide should not be left for air drying

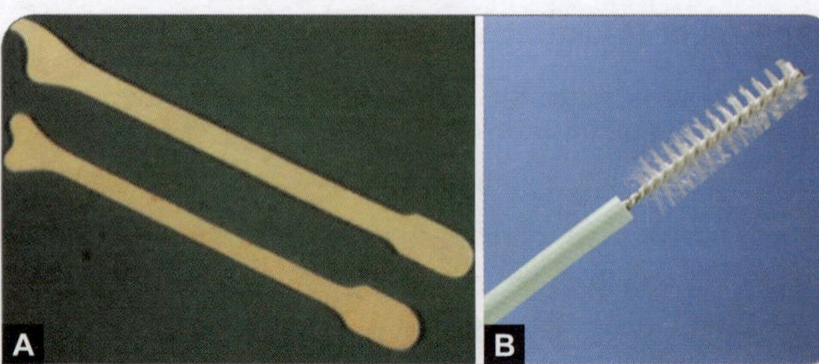

Figs. 14B.7A and B: Ayers spatula and endocervical brush

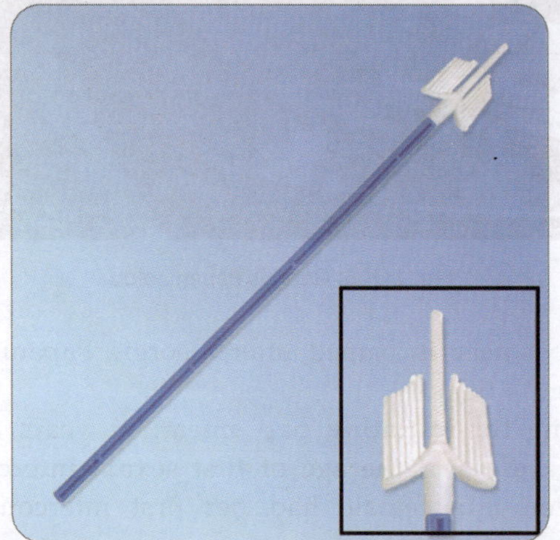

Fig. 14B.8: Cervical brush for liquid pap smear

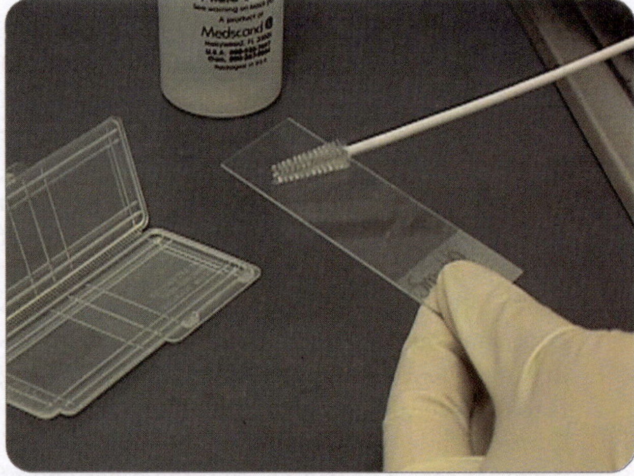

Fig. 14B.9: Method of taking sample in conventional pap smear

> *Note:* **Liquid base cytology is being used now a days.** Preservative used in liquid based cytology is Methanol. Instrument used is cervical brush (Fig. 14B.9).

Patient Preparation for Pap Smear

- Pap smear should be done approximately 2 weeks after (10–18 days) first day of last mensual period
- No douche, tamoon, jelly or, inter course for 48 hrs prior to test
- Screening guidelines for cancer cervix are formulated by American Society for Colposcopy and Cervical Pathology (ASCCP) and have been revised by the American College of Obs and Gynae in 2013.

Revised Guideline for Pap Smear: Cervical Cancer Screening

- Age to begin pap smear: 21 years irrespective of age at which sexual activity begins.
- Women aged 21-29 years should have a pap test every 3 years (earlier it was done annually)
- Women aged 30-65 years should have a pap test and HPV testing every 5 years called as cotesting. It is acceptable to have a pap test alone every 3 years.
- Women should stop having cervical cancer screening after the age of 65 years if they do not have a h/o moderate or severe dysplasia or cancer and they have had either three negative pap test results in a row or two negative co-test results in a row within 10 years, with the most recent test performed within the past 5 years.
- In patients who have detected HIV infection even before 21 years of age, in them pap testing is begun at earlier age and repeated in 6 months as per CDC 2015 guidelines but as per ACOG 2012, in illeal screening. In all females begins at 21 years. But both agree that in women with HIV infection (>21 years), annual screening is done. It is uncertain whether HIV positive females can discontinue screening after 65 years.
- Women with prior treatment for CIN2, CIN3, AIS or cervical cancer should continue routine screening for atleast 20 years.
- All guidelines recommend against pap screening in women who have undergone total hysterectomy for benign design if there is no past history of high grade CIN or cervical cancer.
- If hysterectomy was done in women with H/O high grade cervical intraepithelial neoplasia, ACOG recommends cytology of vaginal cuff every 3 years for 20 years after initial -3 pap test in first 2 years post hysterectomy.

Pap Smear Results

For understanding papsmear results—it is important to remember that squamous epithelium of vagina and exocervix has 3 main layers:

- Superficial cell layer (Figs. 14B.10A to D)
- Intermediate cell layer
- Basal and parabasal layer

The normal appearance of layers is shown in Figures 14B.10A to D

Initial Screening

Figs. 14B.10A to D: (A) Superficial cells; (B) Intermediate cells; (C) Parabasal cells; (D) Basal cells

Important Concept

Superficial cells:
- Largest epithelial cells
- Eosinophilic (pink in color)
- Nucleus is small, pyknotic
- These cells predominate when estrogen is the predominant hormone e.g. first half of menstrual cycle

Intermediate Cells:
- May be small/large
- Basophilic (blue in color)
- Round nuclei
- Cells size is twice the size of parabasal cells
- These cells predominate when progesterone is predominant hormone e.g. pregnancy or second half of menstrual cycle

Parabasal Cells:
- Small round cells with indistinct outline and large round nuclei and small amount of cytoplasm
- These cells predominate when their is no hormonal predominate e.g. Menopause

The pap smear report can have the following terminologies as per the Bethesda system (from 1 to 7):

1. **Within normal limits** (Fig. 14B.13)
2. Infection [organism should be specified – Trichomonas (14B.14), actinomyces and candida (14B.15), Herpes
3. Reactive and Reparative changes (Inflammatory, atrophic)
4. Atypical squamous cells of undetermined significance (ASC-US) (14B.16A)
5. Low grade squamous intraepithelial lesion (LSIL) (14.B.16B)
6. High grade squamous intraepithelial lesion (HSIL) (14B.17)
7. Squamous cell carcinoma (14B.18)

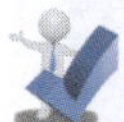

KEY POINTS

The Bethesda Classification System is based on cytological results of a pap test that permits the examination of cells but not tissue structure. The diagnosis of cervical intraepithelial neoplasia (CIN) or cervical carcinoma requires a tissue sample, obtained by biopsy of suspicious lesions (done during colposcopy), to make a histologic diagnosis .That is why pap smear should always be followed by colposcopy or punch biopsy to confirm the diagnosis.

Alternatives to cytology

VIA: **Vis**ual **insp**ection of cervix with 5% **acetic acid**. When acetic acid is applied, dysplastic cells start appearing white (stained). Hence VIA is considered positive if well defined, opaque acetowhite areas are visible near the border of squamo-columar junction, one minute after application of acetic acid (Fig. 14B.11).

VILI: (That is visual inspection with Lugol's Iodine.) Normal vaginal epithelial cells have glycogen

& when lugols iodine is applied, they appear brown or mahogany in colour (stained). But dysplastic cells don't take up iodine & remain unstained, i.e. yellow in colour (Fig. 14B.12).

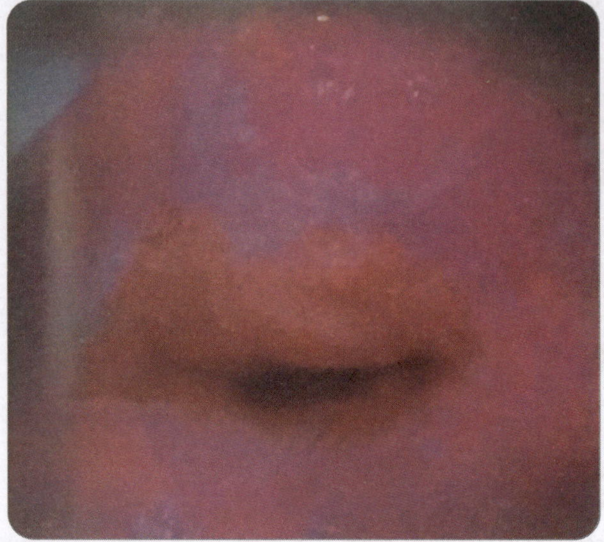

Fig. 14B.11: Cervix after application of acetic acid. Several areas of acetowhite change adjacent to the squamocolumnar junction are apparent

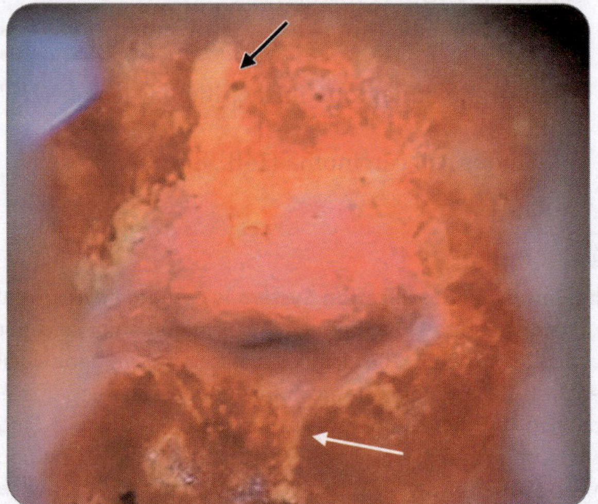

Fig. 14B.12: Same cervix after application of lugoi iodine solution. Nonstaining of the lesions at the 10 to 11 'O' clock positions is seen (Black arrow), while there is partial iodine uptake of acetowhite areas along the posterior SCJ (White arrow)

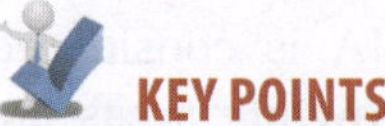

KEY POINTS

- Schilers iodine = 0.3%
- Lugols iodine = 5%
- VIA: Positive means areas white in colour
- VILI positive means areas which are unstained

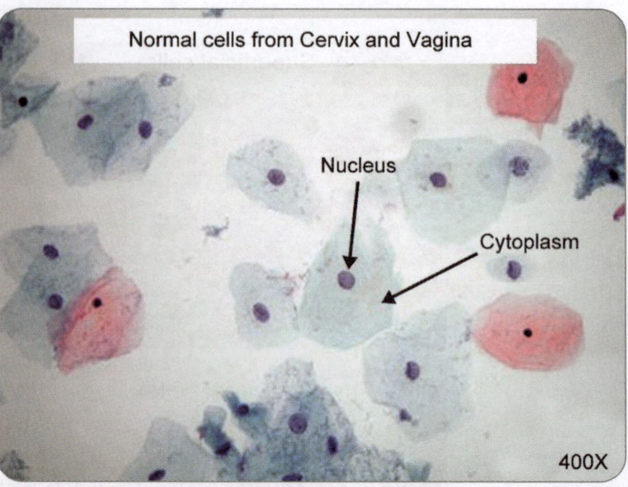

Fig. 14B.13: Normal pap smear all the types of cells. Depending on the cell which predominates we can know which hormone predominates for hormonal study

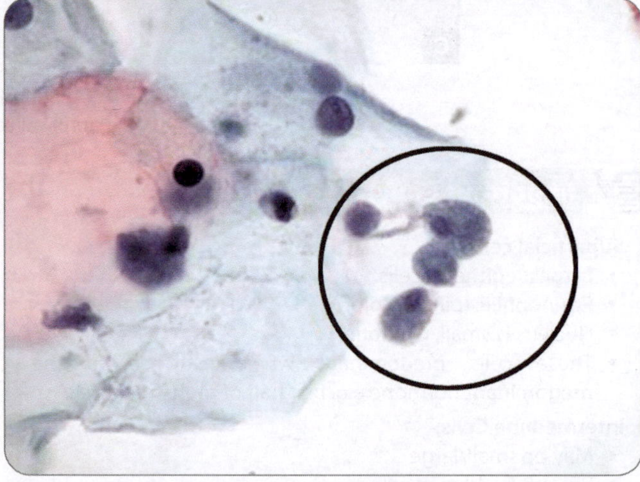

Fig. 14B.14: Papsmear showing Trichomonas infection

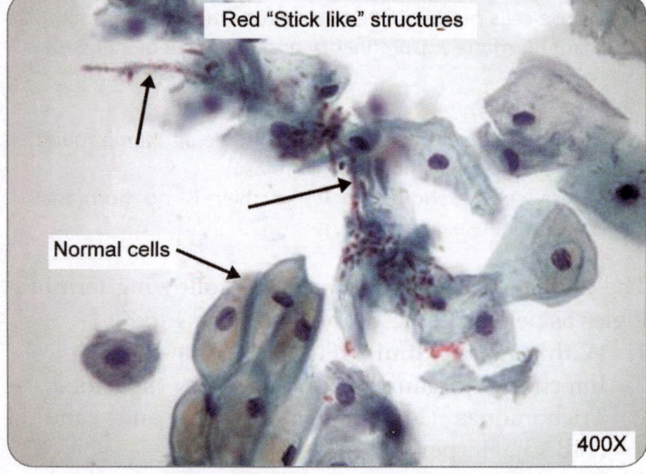

Fig. 14B.15: Papsmear showing Candida infection

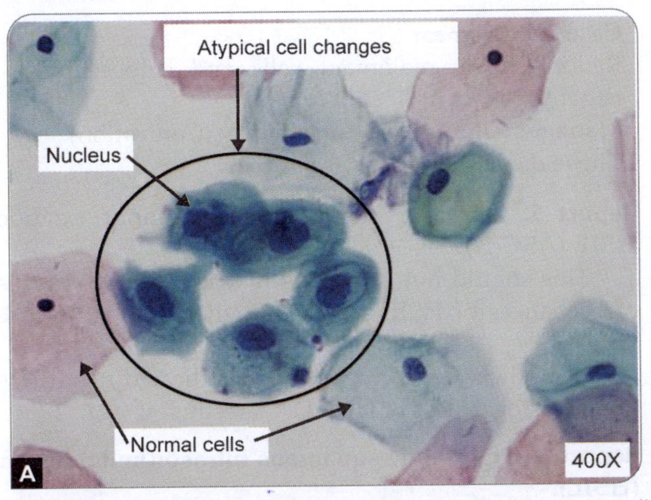

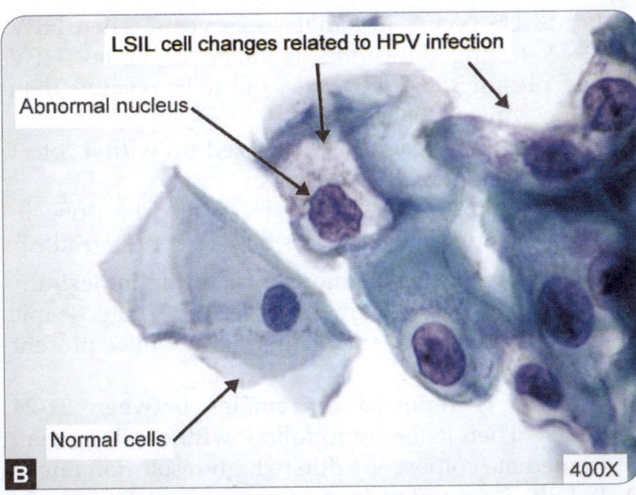

Figs. 14B.16A and B: (A) Papsmear showing Atypical Squamous Cells (ASC). The cells inside the circle contain slightly enlarged and darker nuclei compared to the normal cells from the cervix. (B) Papsmear showing LSIL. The LSIL cells seen here have a fair amount of cytoplasm but enlarged, dark nuclei compared to a normal cell

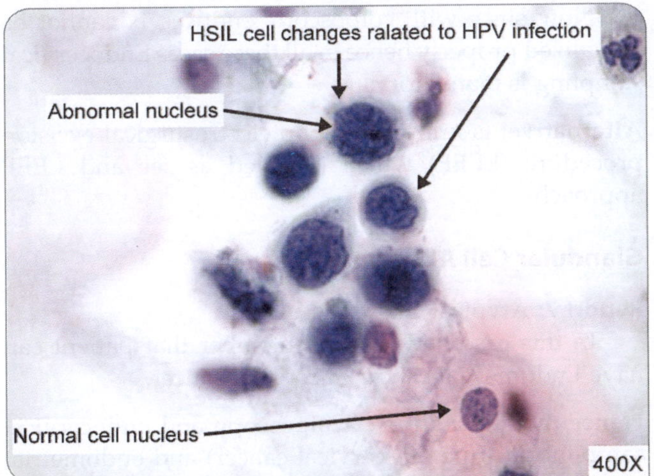

Fig. 14B.17: Papsmear showing HSIL. The HSIL cells seen here contain very little cytoplasm. The nuclei are wrinkled and dark compared to a normal cell

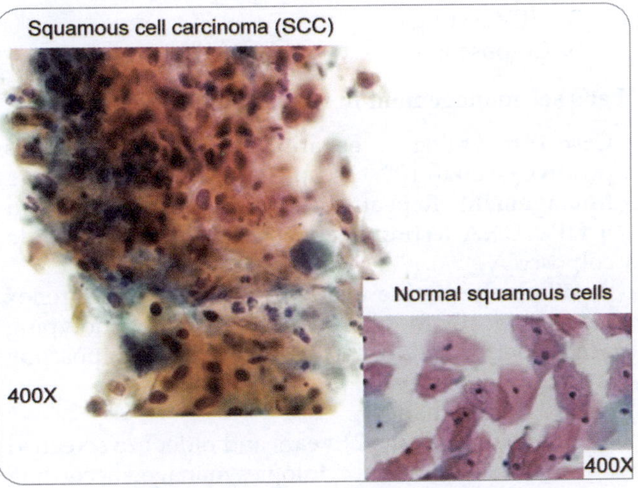

Fig. 14B.18: Papsmear showing Squamous cell carcinoma (SCC)

Management Strategies of Various Cytological Abnormalities

Now once Pap Test Result come: Management depends on Report.

Report 1: Unsatisfactory Pap Test

Repeat Pap test in 2 to 4 months.

Report 2: Infection:

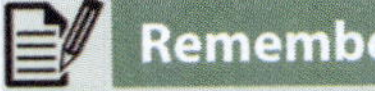

Infections which can be detected by Pap test are:

1. HPV
2. Bacterial vaginosis
3. HSV
4. Trichomonas vaginalis
5. Candida

Pap smear cannot detect

- Chlamydia

Management: Treatment with antibiotics.

Repeat Pap test in 2-4 months.

Epithelial cell Abnormality Management

Report 3: M/C cytological abnormality is ASC-US (i.e. atypical squamous cells of unknown significance).

- The term indicates cells that suggest SIL (squamous intraepithelial lesion but do not fulfil all criterias).
- An ASC-US often precedes the diagnosis of CIN2 & CIN3 but the risk is only 5-10%.

Cancer is found only in 1-2 per thousand.

- If ASCUS occurs in females between 21-24 years then repeat Pap Test and if it also comes abnormal then colposcopy is done.

- If ASCUS occurs in females ≥25 years: Then HPV DNA testing done (this is called as Reflex HPV DNA testing) and if it comes out to be positive then colposcopy is done.
  HPV negative results are followed up with a cotest in 3 years in females ≥25 years.
  Note: Reflex HPV DNA test can also be done in females between 21-24 years but is not preferred.

Report 4: Low grade squamous intraepithelial lesion: This should be followed by colposcopy (i.e. colposcopic biopsy) as most of times no visible lesion will be present to take punch biopsy.

- **If LSIL is reported in females between 21-24 years:** Then its better to follow with cytology than immediate colposcopy due to high resolution rate.
- If LSIL is reported in postmenopausal females in whom HPV test was not done:
  Options include:
  1. Repeat cytology at 6-12 months
  2. HPV testing
  3. Colposcopy

Let's see management in some special cases

Case 1: If cytology is negative and HPV DNA test is positive (seen in 10% cases).
Management: Repeat contesting in 12 months. But if HPV DNA testing is persistently positive then do colposcopy.
Another alternative available these days: A reflex test specifically for HPV-16 and 18 called genotyping can be performed. If positive, immediate colposcopy is recommended.
Case 2: In Pregnancy:

- Pregnant patients 21 years and older are screened and their abnormal cytologies managed according to guidelines for the general population. However, deferred evaluation of ASCUS and LSIL cytologies until at least 6 weeks postpartum is acceptable. If Pap test shows HSIL, adenocarcinoma in situ or suspected malignancy then colposcopy is done.
- When indicated, the goal of colposcopy is to exclude invasive cancer.
- Colposcopy and ectocervical biopsy are safe and accurate during pregnancy.
- Endocervical and endometrial sampling are not performed during pregnancy to avoid amnionic membrane rupture and infection. If colposcopy fails to confirm malignancy but pap test shows HSIL, then diagnostic conisation may be necessary. Many experts recommend delaying conisation uptil 2nd trimester.
- Preinvasive neoplasia is not treated but further is reevaluated postpartum. This is because lesion progression is typically slow and lesion grade may change during delivery and puerperal remodelling.

Case 3: Pap smear
Report shows malignant cells and colposcopy is negative.
Management: Earlier: Cone biopsy (Conization)
These days: Endocervical sampling

Report 5: Atypical squamous cells cannot exclude HSIL (ASC-H).

This should not be confused with ASC-US. In this case chances of HSIL are 25% (higher than ASC-H & LSIL).

In all these cases colposcopy is indicated regardless of age or regardless of HPV DNA testing.

Report 6: High grade squamous intraepithelial lesion (HSIL).

In all these cases: Biopsy is mandatory by colposcopy (if lesion is not visible) or by punch biopsy (if lesion is visible).

Now since with colposcopy endocervix cannot be visualized properly hence in all these cases Endocervical sampling is mandatory.

Alternative: Is immediate loop electrosurgical excision procedure (LEEP) which is called as see and LEEP approach.

Glandular Cell Abnormalities

Report 7: Atypical Glandular cells

In this case one has to remember that patient can have Endometrial cancer or cervical cancer.

Hence management is: Colposcopy and endocervical sampling (to rule out cervical cancer) and endometrial sampling (to rule out endometrial cancer)

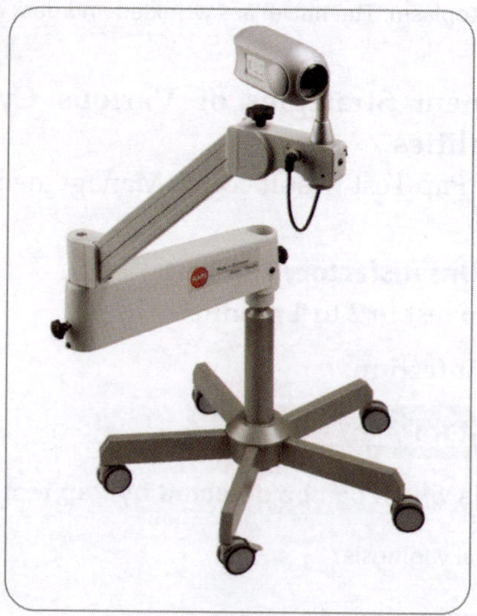

Fig. 14B.19: Colposcope

Colposcopic Directed Biopsy

- **Colposcopy is the Gold standard technique for evaluation of an abnormal cervical cytology smear/ pap smear.**
- It is an outpatient procedure that is simple, quick well tolerated and does not require any anesthesia.
- It allows examination of the lower genital tract and anus with a microscope
- Minimum (magnification with colposcope = 5 times).
- Maximum magnification = 30 times
- Focal length = 30. (Fig. 14B.19)
- Sensitivity = 50–80%

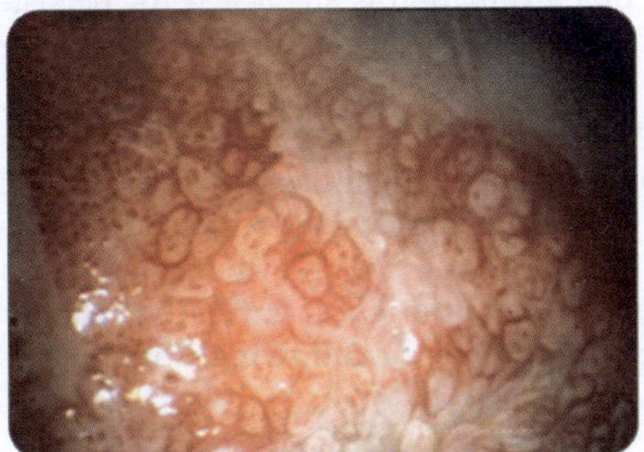

Fig. 14B.20: Mosaic blood vessels on colposcopy

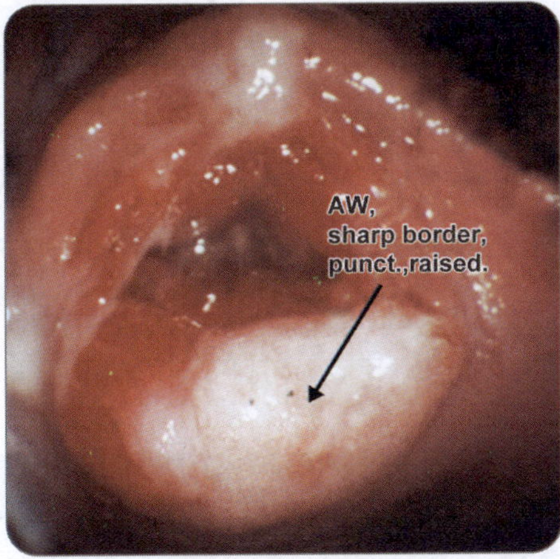

Fig. 14B.21: Acetowhite area on colposcopy

Method

- The first step is to visualize cervix under magnification without applying anything.
- Any white area visible before applying acetic, acid is **leukoplakia**. Biopsy sample should be taken from it.
- Biopsy sample should also be taken from any rough area or raised area of cervix.
- Any abnormal blood vessel pattern viz **mosaic, reticular** blood vessels, **comma-shaped** blood vessels or **punctate blood vessels** should be biopsied (Fig. 14B.20).
- Then 3-5% acetic acid should be applied on cervix gently but liberally.

General colposcopic examination has 3 components:

(1) Cervical visualization.
(2) SCJ visibility
(3) TZ Classification

As per IFCPC classification TZ is of 3 types:

Type 1: TZ that is entirely ectocervical

Type 2: TZ that has endocervical component but is visible on colposcopy.

Type 3: TZ that has endocervical component but is not completely visualized.

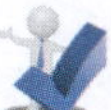

KEY POINTS

Limitation of colposcopy Upper 2/3rd of endocervix is not visualized by colposcopy hence for detecting adenocarcinoma, endocervical curettage is done

Principle

- *Application of acetic acid to normal epithelium:* Glycogen producing epithelium of cervix does not produce any effect and it appears pink during colposcopy.
- *Application of acetic acid to dysplastic epithelium:* When acetic acid is applied to dysplastic epithelium which have large nuclei with abnormally large amounts of chromatin (i.e. protein), acetic acid coagulates the proteins of the nucleus and cytoplasm, making the proteins opaque and white, therefore, dysplastic cells and cancerous cells appear white [called as **Aceto white areas**. (Fig. 14B.21)]
- *Application of acetic acid to metaplastic epithelium:* The immature metaplastic cells have large nuclei and also show some effects of the acetic acid. Since metaplastic epithelium is very thin, it does not appear white but instead appear grey and filmy.

Indications of Colposcopy ... *Shaw 14th/ed, p362*

- Abnormal pap smear cytology
- To locate abnormal areas[Q]
- To obtain directed biopsies[Q]
- Conservative therapy under colposcopy guidance[Q]
- For follow up of cases treated conservatively[Q]

Absolute Contraindications	Relative contraindications
None	Anticoagulant therapy if patient requires biopsy
	Upper or lower reproductive tract infection
	Uncontrolled severe hypertension
	Uncooperative or overly anxious patient

Cone Biopsy/Conization (Fig. 14B.22)

- It involves removal of a cone of the cervix which includes exocervix, entire squamocolumnar junction, and considerable part of endocervix.
- It is done in OT
- Procedure is done under general anaesthesia.
- The tissue so obtained is divided into 12 to 16 segments and each one blocked and sectioned separately.
- **Cone biopsy or conization is both a diagnostic as well as therapeutic procedure.**

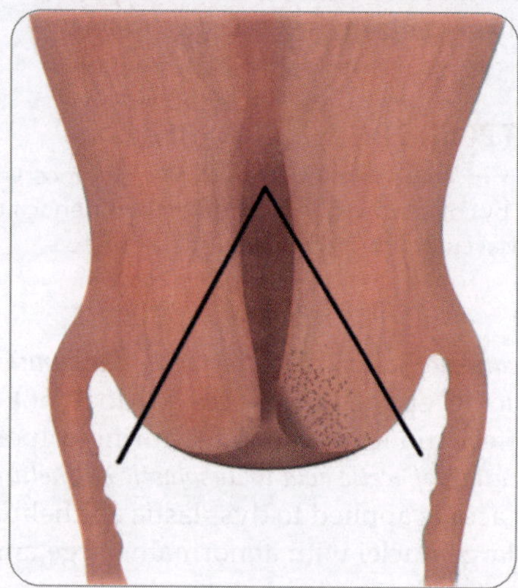

Fig. 14B.22: Cone biopsy

Table 14B.4: Indications of Cone biopsy

Diagnostic	Therapeutic
Limits of the lesion can not be visualised with coloposcopy.Q	Cancer in situ in young females
The squamocolumnar junction is not seen at colposcopyQ	Cancer cervix Stage 1A1 in young females
Endocervical curettage is positive in HSIL	
Microinvasive carcinoma or adenocarcinoma in situ is suspected based on biopsy, colposcopy or cytology results	
Lack of correlation between papsmear and colposcopy results.	

Complications of Cone Biopsy

- BleedingQ (M/C complication)
- InfectionQ
- Cervical stenosisQ
- Incompetent osQ

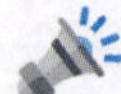

Important One Liners

Cone biopsy can lead to incompetent os and subsequent recurrent second trimester abortions.

Ectocervical Biopsy

Under direct colposcopic visualization, suspicious lesions are biopsied using, cervical biopsy forceps. Generally, cervical biopsy does not require an Anesthetic agent. Thickened Monsel solution (ferric subsulfate) or a silver nitrate applicator are applied with pressure to the biopsy site, providing hemostasis if need. Heavier bleeding is rare and can be controlled with direct pressure or brief vaginal packing.

The American College of Obstetricians and Gynecologists (2013) recommends biopsy of Acetowhite lesions regardless of colposcopic impression, and repeat colposcopic evaluation is suggested for persistent low grade cytologic abnormalities or HPV positive results.

Endocervical Sampling

For non-pregnant patients, endocervical sampling by curettage or brushing evaluates the endocervical canal epithelium that lies beyond the coloscopie's view. **Endocervical sampling is currently recommended during coloscopy in the following situations.**

Result

Colposcopy report is a histopathology report

Flowchart 14B.4

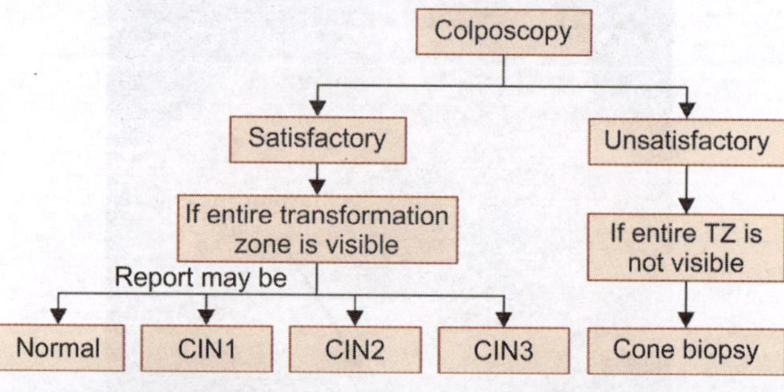

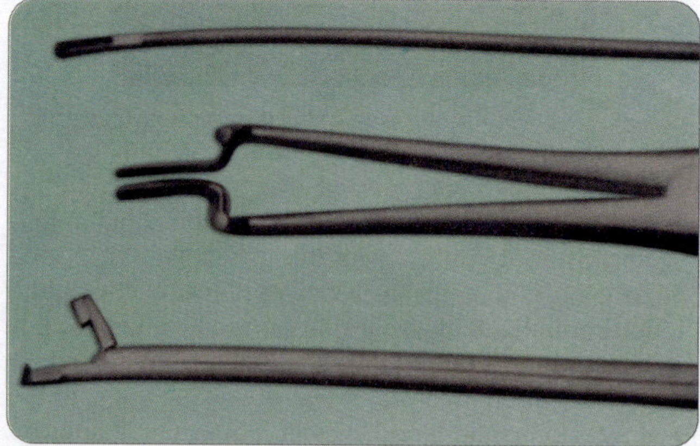

Fig. 14B.23: Tools used for cervical evaluation and biopsy. From top to bottom: Endocervical curette, endocervical speculum and cervical biopsy forceps

- Colposcopy is inadequate, or colposcopy is adequate but no lesion is identified. Endocervical sampling is acceptable in other cases at provider discretion.
- Initial evaluation of ASC-H, HSIL, AGC, or AIS cytology test results.
- Surveillance 4 to 6 months after excisional therapy if specimen margins are positive for HSIL.
- Surveillance after conization for AIS has been performed in women wishing fertility preservation. Negative endocervical curettage results and reassurance to this management (Schorge, 2003).

Endocervical sampling can be performed by either curettage or brushing. Endocervical curettage is performed by introducing an endocervical curette 1 to 2 cm into the cervical canal. The length and circumference of the canal is firmly curetted, carefully avoiding sampling of the ectocervix or the lower uterine segment.

Management of CIN

Preventive Measures

HPV vaccines

- HPV vaccines have been developed from the **inactivated capsid coat of the virus.**
- **HPV vaccines were earlier of two types. During its Feb 2015, meeting Advisory Committee on Immunization Practises (ACIP) recommended 9-valent HPV vaccine (9V HVP) as one of the three vaccines for preventive HPV (Table 14B.3).**

Table 14B.3: HPV vaccines

Characteristic	Bivalent (2V HPV)	Quadrivalent (4V HPV)	9 Valent (9V HPV)
Brand name	Cervirax	Gardasil	Gardasil-9
HPV subtypes	16, 18	6, 11, 16, 18	6, 11, 16, 18, 31, 33, 45, 52, 58
Protects against	CIN, Ca cervix	Anogenital warts, CIN, Ca cervix	Anogenital warts CIN, Ca cervix, vulva intraepithelial neoplasia, vaginal intraepithelial neoplasia
Manufacturer	GlaxoSmithiKline	Merck & Co	Merck & Co
Manufacturing	Trichoplusia insect line infected with L1 encoding baculovirus	Saccharomyces cerevisiae expressing L1	Saccharomyces cerevisiae expressing L1
Adjuvant	500 mcg aluminium hydroxide with monophosphoryl lipid A	225 mcg $Al(OH) PO_4SO_4$	500 mcg $Al(OH) PO_4SO_4$
Dose	0.5 mL	0.5 mL	0.5 mL
Administration	1/m	1/m	1/m
Administered to males or females	Only females	Both males and females	Both males and females
Age in females Ideal age range	11-12 years 9-26 years	11-12 years 9-26 years	11-12 years 9-26 years
Age in males Ideal age range	×	11-12 years 9-26 years	11-12 years 9-15 years—FDA approved 9-26 years—ACIP recommendation

Common points related to all vaccines:

- All the vaccines are recombinant vaccines composed of virus-like particles (VLPs) and are not infectious since they do not contain viral DNA.
- For girls and boys aged 9–14 years, a two-dose schedule (0.5 mL at 0 and 5–13 month) is recommended. If the second vaccine dose is administered earlier than 5 months after the first dose, a third dose is recommended.
- For those aged 15 years and above, and for immunocompromised patients irrespective of age, the recommendation is for three dose (0.5 mL at 0, 1, 6 months).
- WHO has reviewed the latest data and concluded that there is no safety concern regarding HPV vaccines.

Contraindications

- Pregnancy
- Hypersensitivity

Important points:

- For population who are seronegative and HPV-DNA negative for HPV 16 and HPV 18 at vaccination and have received all three dosages of vaccine, the efficacy is 100%.

- This protection is documented to last for 6.4 years to 7.5 years after vaccination
- To increase the period of efficacy they are combined with an adjuvant.

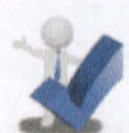

KEY POINTS

Screening practises should remain same in both vaccinated and unvaccinated persons.

Definitive Treatment of CIN

Options

Table 14B.4: Management options in CIN

Ablative methods	Surgical Excisional methods
• Cryosurgery • Laser ablation or vaporization	• Large loop excision of transformation zone (LLETZ) or loop electroexcisional procedure.(LEEP) • Conization • Hysterectomy
Aim: To destroy the entire transformation zone of the cervix (upto to a depth of 6–8 mm from the surface).	
Major disadvantage is that follow up with histopathological examination, is not possible after the procedure as squamocolumnar junction recedes into the endocervix.	

Comparison of Ablative Techniques for Managing CIN (Table 14B.5)

Ablative techniques for CIN management. *See* **Table 14B.5.**

Cryotherapy (Fig. 10B.16)	CO_2 Laser
• Destroys the surface epithelium of cervix by crystallising intracellular water. • Aim should be to produce an ice ball that extends 5-10 mm beyond the margin of lesion.	• Best method to treat CIN I/II if it extends to vaginal fornices.
• Temp = –20 to –30 – Agent used = N_2O (–89) or CO_2 (–65)	
• Depth of destruction = 5 mm. • (Method = freeze – thaw – freeze = 3 min- 5 min- 3 min).	• Depth of destruction = 7 mm.
• Can be used only if, lesion is on ectocervix. (Not on endocervix.)	• Major advantage: It can be used if vaginal extension of CIN is present.
• No evidence of microinvasive/ invasive cancer. • Vagina is not involved.	• No evidence of microinvasive invasive cancer.
• Postoperative complication **M/C:** vaginal discharge **others:** cervical stenosis or cervical dystocia (uncommon)	• No vaginal discharge

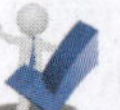

KEY POINTS

Criteria for employing ablative methods for treating CIN:
- Entire lesion should be visualised within the transformation zone (TZ)
- No evidence of microinvasion or macroinvasion.
- No endocervical glandular involvement
- No discrepancy in cytology, colposcopy and biopsy report.

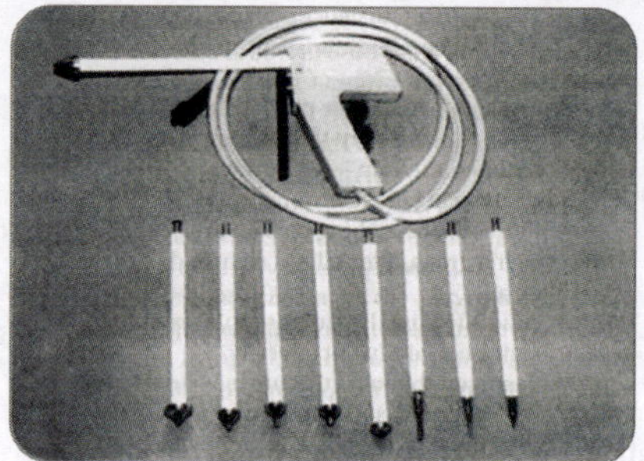

Fig. 14B.24: Cryosurgery probe

LEEP (Loop electro excisional procedure)/LLETZ [Large loop excision of transformation zone (Fig. 14B.17)]

- A loop of very thin stainless steel wire is used for excision of the transformation zone. The tissue effect of electricity depends on size of loop and wattage. If a low power or large diameter wire is used, effect is electrocautery and tissue damage is more. If high watt (35-55 W) & small loop (0.5 mm) is used effect is electrosurgical.
- Done under local anaesthesia
- It is an OPD procedure. No training is needed to perform it.
- Tissue upto a depth of 10 mm or more can be removed and sent for histopathological examination.
- Complications are minimal.

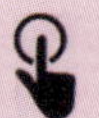

Currently, it is the method of choice for treating CIN II and CIN III at any age and irrespective of the number of children the female has.

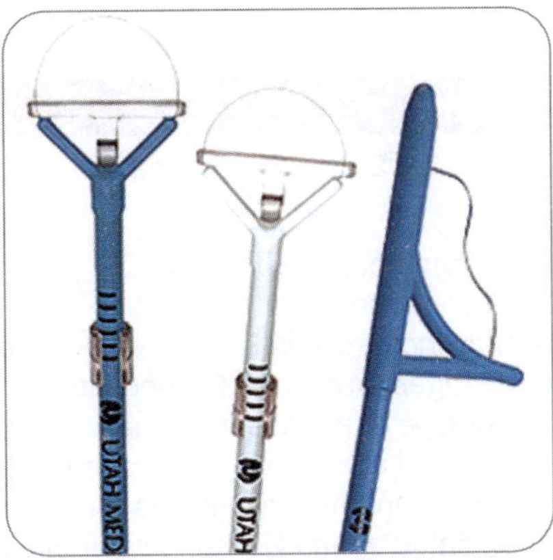

Fig. 14B.25: LEEP wires

Management of CIN at a Glance

- **CIN I** – observation. Do cotesting after 12 months
- If negative do routine screening
- In patients <25 years pap smear as done alone at 12 months & 24 months
  Note: If CIN I occurs in adolescent age group - follow up with annual cytology. In these patients follow up with HPV - DNA is not useful.
  CIN I Normally regresses within 2 years, if it persists for ≥ 2 years then treatment needed
- **CIN I persists for 2 years** – Cryotherapy.
- If patient, if <25 years, treatment is not, recommended ever if CIN I is present
- In patients <25 years pap smear is done alone at 12 months & 24 months
- **CIN II** – LEEP (in young females: repeat pap + coloscopy at 6 months man treatment is preferred)
- **CIN III** – LEEP (any age group)
- **Recurrent CIN III** – Hysterectomy
- **CIN extending to vaginal fornices** – Laser ablation.

Indications of Doing Hysterectomy Incase of CIN: Earlier, it was TOC for treating CIN in females ≥ 40 years but now it is done only if:

- Female has other associated gynecological problems (fibroid, prolapse) which need hysterectomy
- **Adenocarcinoma in situ in females**
- Recurrent/repetitive CIN 2/3 despite less invasive treatment in females who have completed their family.
- Patients not willing for follow-up.

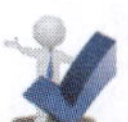

KEY POINTS

LEEP/LLETZ is the best management of CIN III in all age groups. Earlier in females < 40 yrs: LEEP was the procedure of choice and in females > 40 yrs hysterectomy was the choice but now for all age groups TOC is LEEP/LLETZ.

Cancer Cervix

Epidemiology

- Cervical cancer is overall the most common gynaecological malignancy in the world, and the second most frequently diagnosed cancer in women worldwide after breast cancer *(John Hopkins Manual of Obs and Gynae. p 541)*
- M/c age group-Bimodal peak = 1st peak seen at 35–39 years; 2nd peak seen at 60 to 65 years.
- M/c in low socioeconomic status.

Risk Factors for Ca CX

Same as CIN

Note

- Familial inheritance is not seen in cancer cervix.
- Early menarche and late menopause are not risk factors for cancer cervix

Early age of intercourse is a risk factor for Ca cervix

Screening

i. By paps test (as discussed)
ii. Downstaging for cervical cancer is defined as "the detection of the disease at an earlier stage when it is still curable. Detection is done by nurses and other paramedical health workers using a simple speculum for visual inspection of the cervix". Compared to cytological screening it is suboptimal. But in places where prevalence of cancer is high and cytological screening is not available, "downstaging screening" is useful. The strategy is, however, not expected to lower the incidence of cancer cervix, but it can certainly minimize the cancer death through early detection.

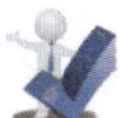

KEY POINTS

Down staging of ca cervix is done by per speculum examinations

- **Site:** M/C site for cancer cervix will be where cells are changing from one type to other, i.e. **transformation zone**.
- **M/C histological variety** of cancer cervix is squamous cell carcinoma.
- Since endocervix is lined by columnar epithelium, hence adenocarcinoma can also be seen.
- **M/C site for adenocarcinoma is endocervix.**

Histology

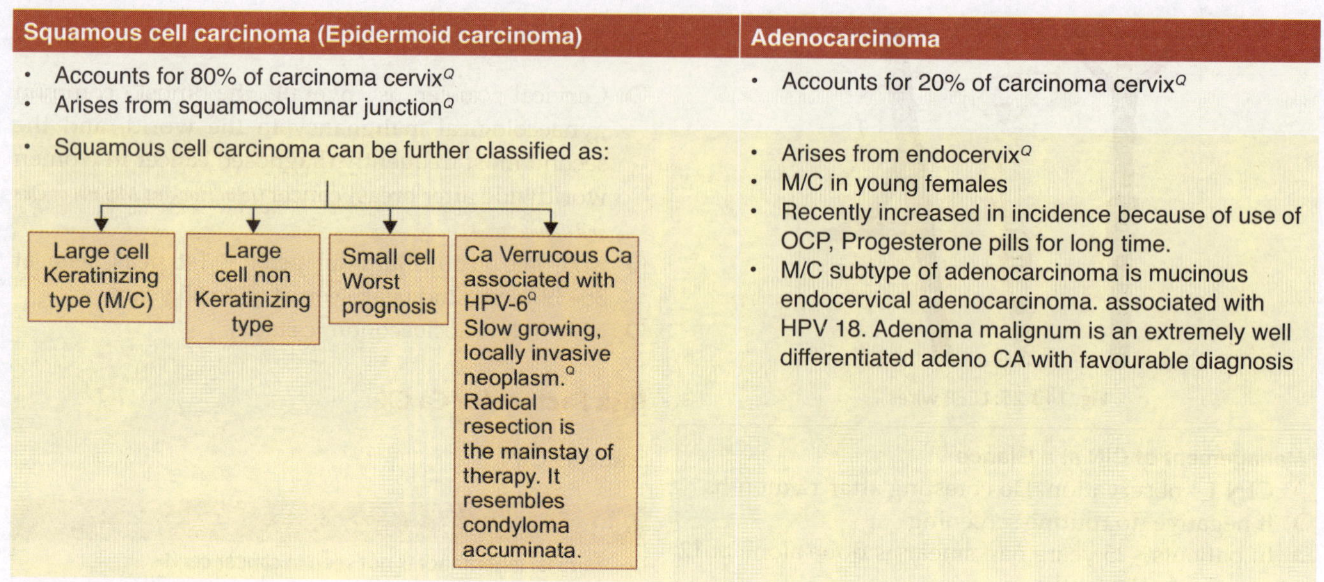

Squamous cell carcinoma (Epidermoid carcinoma)	Adenocarcinoma
• Accounts for 80% of carcinoma cervix[Q] • Arises from squamocolumnar junction[Q] • Squamous cell carcinoma can be further classified as: – Large cell Keratinizing type (M/C) – Large cell non Keratinizing type – Small cell Worst prognosis – Ca Verrucous Ca associated with HPV-6[Q] Slow growing, locally invasive neoplasm.[Q] Radical resection is the mainstay of therapy. It resembles condyloma accuminata.	• Accounts for 20% of carcinoma cervix[Q] • Arises from endocervix[Q] • M/C in young females • Recently increased in incidence because of use of OCP, Progesterone pills for long time. • M/C subtype of adenocarcinoma is mucinous endocervical adenocarcinoma. associated with HPV 18. Adenoma malignum is an extremely well differentiated adeno CA with favourable diagnosis

Clinical Features

Symptoms

- **Bleeding per vagina: Most common symptom is** irregular vaginal bleeding. **Most specific symptom-** postcoital bleeding.
- **Discharge:** It is at first creamy and later becomes dirty brown in colour and is very offensive.[Q] The odour is caused by infection of necrotic tissue with saprophytes.

Symptoms of Advanced Stage

- Deep pelvic pain[Q] often unilateral and radiating to hip or thigh.
- Urinary incontinence, dysuria, increased urinary frequency, ureteric colic.
- Rectal pain
- Low backache/Flank pain due to hydronephrosis.
- Triad of sciatic pain, leg edema and hydronephrosis is associated with extensive pelvic involvement by tumor.
- **Weight loss, anorexia, malaise, etc.**

Signs

- Four cardinal signs:
  - Hardness[Q]
  - Friability[Q]
  - Fixation[Q]
  - Bleeds on touch[Q]

Complications

Mnemonic: Private FUND *Ref: Jeffcoates 7th/ed, p472*

Private	Pyometra
F	Fistula: – Vesico vaginal – Vesico cervical – Recto vaginal
U	Uraemia
N	Nephrosis: – Hydronephrosis – Pyonephrosis
D	Death *(most common cause of death is uraemia).*

Important One Liners

- M/C cause of death in patients of Ca cervix is renal failure.
- IInd M/C common cause of death is haemorrhage.

Mode of Spread

- **M/C is lymphatic spread:** M/c site of Spread is Lymph nodes. The lymph nodes involved in cancer cervix are:

Primary group	Secondary group
	Common iliac
H = Hypogastric/Internal	Para aortic
O = Obturator	Inguinal
P = Paracervical/ureteric lymph node	
E = External iliac	

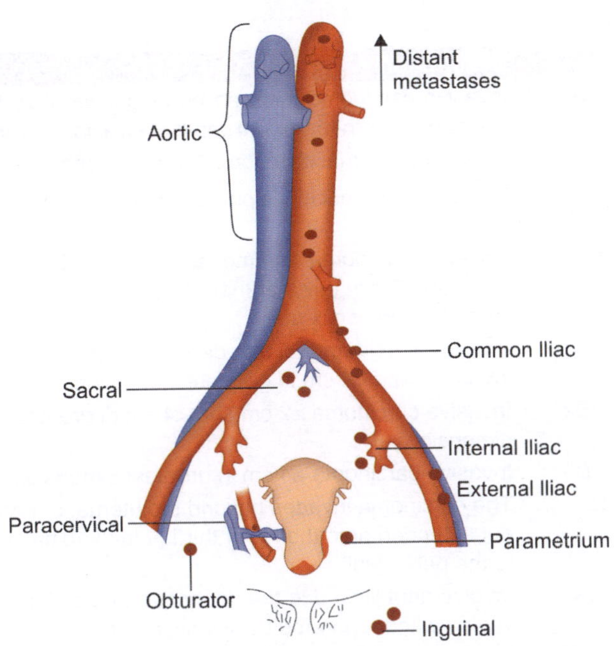

Fig. 14B.26: Lymphatic drainage of cervix

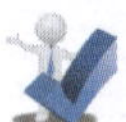

KEY POINTS

- **M/C lymph node involved in Ca cervix is** obturator LN
- **Sentinel lymph node is-Para** cervical or ureteric LN

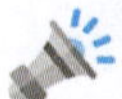

Important One Liners

Sentinel lymph node biopsy is most useful in which gynaecological cancer-Vulval cancer > cervical cancer.

- **Other Routes: Direct and hematogenous spread**

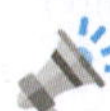

Important One Liners

- **M/C route of spread—Lymphatic**
- **M/C site involved is: Lymphnodes**
- **M/C site involved in hematogenous spread—lungs**

Papnicolaou Test and Cervical Biopsy

Histologic reevaluation of cervical biopsy is the primary tool to diagnose cervical cancer. Although Papanicolaou (Pap) tests are performed extensively to screen for this cancer, this test does not always detect cervical cancer. Specifically, Pap testing has only 50 to 80 percent sensitivity for detecting high-grade lesions.

Thus the preventive power of Pap testing lies in regular serial screening. Moreover in women who have stage 1 cervical cancer 30 to 50 percent of single cytologic obtained are as positive for cancer.

Hence Pap are read as positive for evaluation of a suspicious lesion is discouraged. Instead these lesions are directly biopsied with Tischler biopsy forceps or kevorkian curette.

When possible biopsy are taken from the tumor periphery, as central portions often contain only necrotic tissue, which will fail to yield a diagnosis. Moreover, biopsies ideally include underlying stroma, so that invasion, if present, can be assessed.

If abnormal Pap test finding are noted, colposcopy is often performed, and adequate cervical and endocervical biopsies are obtained. In some cases, cold knife conization is needed for this.

Diagnosis and Evaluation

Until now, the FIGO staging was based mainly on clinical examination with the addition of certain procedures that were allowed by FIGO to change the staging.

Physical examination	Radiological studies	Procedure
• Palpate lymph node	• Chest X-ray	• Biopsy
• Examine vagina	• Skeletal X Ray	• Conisation
• Bimanual rectovaginal examination	• IVP	• Endocervical Curettage
	• Barium enema	• Colposcopy
		• Hysteroscopy
		• Cystoscopy
		• Proctoscopy

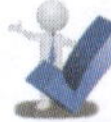

KEY POINTS

Remember

USG/CT scan /MRI/PET scan and lymphangiography were not included in the investigations earlier approved by FIGO.

In 2018, this has been revised by the FIGO Gynecologic Oncology Committee to allow imaging and pathological findings, where available, to assign the stage.

FIGO has recommended all investigation including:

- USG
- **MRI**: Best method of neurological assessment of primary tumors greater than 10 mm
- **CT scan**
- **PET scan**: Best for detecting Nodal metastases

Contd...

Contd...

- FIGO no longer mandates any biochemical investigations or investigative procedures; however, in patients with frank invasive carcinoma, a chest X-ray, and assessment of hydronephrosis (with renal ultrasound, intravenous pyelography, CT or MRI) should be done.
- The bladder and rectum are evaluated by cystoscopy and sigmoidoscopy only if the patient is clinically symptomatic. Cystoscopy is also recommended in cases of a barrel-shaped endocervical growth and in cases where the growth has extended to the anterior vaginal wall.
- Suspected bladder or rectal involvement should be confirmed by biopsy and histologic evidence. Bullous edema alone does not warrant a case to be allocated to stage IV

FIGO Staging of Cancer Cervix (Earlier)

Stage I: Carcinoma confined to cervix (extension to corpus is disregarded)

A = Microscopic cancer (<5 mm depth and <7 mm wide)

A1 = ≤ 3 mm deep.

A2 = >3 to <5 mm deep.

B = **Clinically visible lesion**

B1 = ≤ 4 cms in size

B2 = ≥ 4 cms in size

Stage II: Carcinoma involves upper 2/3rd of Vagina

A = Parametrium not involved

A1 = Clinically visible lesion ≤ 4 cm

A2 = Clinically visible lesion > 4 cm

B = Parametrium involved

Stage III: Carcinoma involves lower 1/3rd of Vagina

A = Pelvic side wall not involved

B = Pelvic sidewall involved/non functioning kidney, hydronephrosis, hydroureter

Stage IV: Metastasis of the carcinoma

A = Regional Metastasis (bladder and/or rectum involved)

B = Distant metastasis or superficial inguinal lymph nodes involved

FIGO Staging 2018 of Cancer Cervix

Table 14B.6: FIGO staging of cancer of the cervix uteri (2018).

Stage	Description
I	The carcinoma is strictly confined to the cervix (extension to the uterine corpus should be disregarded)
IA	Invasive carcinoma that can be diagnosed only by microscopy, with maximum depth of invasion <5 mm[a]
IA1	Measured stromal invasion ≥3 mm in depth
IA2	Measured stromal invasion ≥3 mm and <5 mm in depth
IB	Invasive carcinoma with measured deepest invasion ≥5 mm (greater than Stage IA), lesion limited to the cervix uteri[b]
IB1	Invasive carcinoma ≥5 mm depth of stromal invasion, and <2 cm in greatest dimension
IB2	Invasive carcinoma ≥2 cm and <4 cm in greatest dimension
IB3	Invasive carcinoma ≥4 cm in greatest dimension
II	The carcinoma invades beyond the uterus, but has not extended onto the lower third of the vagina or to the pelvic wall
IIA	Involvement limited to the upper two-thirds of the vagina without parametrial involvement
IIA1	Invasive carcinoma <4 cm in greatest dimension
IIA2	Invasive carcinoma ≥4 cm in greatest dimension
IIB	With parametrial involvement but not up to the pelvic wall
III	The carcinoma involves the lower third of the vagina and/or extends to the pelvic wall and/or causes hydronephrosis or nonfunctioning kidney and/or involves pelvic and/or para-aortic lymph nodes[c]
IIIA	The carcinoma involves the lower third of the vagina with no extension to the pelvic wall
IIIB	Extension to the pelvic wall and/or hydronephrosis or nonfunctioning kidney (unless known to be due to another cause)
IIIC	Involvement of pelvic and/or para-aortic lymph nodes, irrespective of tumor size and extent (with r and p notations)[c]
IIIC1	Pelvic lymph node metastasis only
IIIC2	Para-aortic lymph node metastasis
IV	The carcinoma has extended beyond the true pelvis or has involved (biopsy proven) the nucosa of the bladder or rectum. (A bulluos edema, as such does not permit a case to the allotted to Stage IV)
IVA	Spread to adjacent pelvic organs
IVB	Spread to distant organs

When in doubt, the lower staging should be assigned.

[a]Imaging and pathology can be used, where available, to supplement clinical findings with respect to tumor size and extent, in all stages.

[b]The involvement of vascular/lymphatic spaces does not change the staging. The lateral extent of the lesion is no longer considered.

[c]Adding notation of r (imaging) and p (pathology) to indicate the findings that are used to allocate the case to stage IIIC. Example: If imaging indicates pelvic lymph node metastasis, the stage allocation would be stage IIIC1r, and if confirmed by pathologic findings, it would be stage iiIC1p. The type of imaging modality or pathology technique used should always be documented.

Microinvasive Disease

Diagnosis of Stage IA1 and IA2 is made on microscopic examination of a LEEP (loop electrosurgical excision procedure) or cone biopsy specimen, which includes the entire lesion. It can also be made on a trachelectomy or hysterectomy specimen. The depth of invasion should not be greater than 3 mm or 5 mm, respectively, from the base of the epithelium, either squamous or glandular, from which it originates.

- The horizontal dimension is no longer considered in the 2018 revision as it is subject to many artefactual errors. Note must be made or lymphovascular space involvement, which does not alter the stage, but may affect the treatment plan.
- Extension to the uterine corpus is also disregarded for staging purposes as it does not in itself after either the prognosis or management. The margins should be reported to be negative for disease. If the margined of the cone biopsy are positive for invasive cancer, the patient is allocated to stage IB1.

Clinically visible lesions and those with lager dimensions are allocated to stage IB, subdivided in the latest staging as IB1. 1B2 and IB3 based on the maximum diameter of the lesion

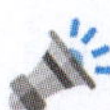

Important One Liners

Involvement of ureter & kidney: Stage IIIB
- Involvement of bladder: IVA
- Bullous edema of bladder does not mean cancer has metastasized to bladder. It occurs due to obstruction of ureter & indicates Stage IIIB not IVA

Management of Cancer Cervix

Principle

- All stages of cancer cervix (I-IV) are radiosensitive
- Stages of Ca cervix that are operable (Radical/ Wertheim's hysterectomy) are IA1, IA2, IB2, and IIA1
- Stages IA1, IA2, IB1, IB2 and IIA1 are radiosensitive and surgically operable, but surgery is preferred over radiotherapy for these stages because of the following reasons:
  - Preservation of ovarian function
  - Preservation of vagina for coital function
  - Psychological benefit to the patient
- Stages IB3 and IIA2 are treated by radiation
- Stages **IIB-IV** are not operable and have to be treated with radiotherapy only
- In squamous cell cancers, before giving radiotherapy, a chemotherapeutic agent is given to increase the sensitivity of the cells to radiation called as **radiosensitiser**. In cancer cervix **cisplatin is used as a radiosensitiser**, so **from stages IIB to IVA-management of choice is chemoradiation.**

  Use of cisplatin has resulted in reduction in local recurrence and distant metastasis.

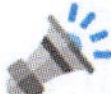

Important One Liners

Radiation therapy should not be used in patients with diverticulosis, pelvic or tubo ovarian abscess.

Also Know

Radical Trachelectomy
- **Radical trachelectomy-involves removal of 80% cervix, parametria** (Mackenrodts **ligaments) and vaginal cuff** along **with pelvic lymphadenectomy**
- Radical trachelectomy is an option for women with stage IA2 and IB1 disease who desire uterine preservation and fertility.
- **Indication** of doing trachelectomy-Low risk disease
- Negative nodes
- Size of tumor <2 cm
- A cerclage is done between uterus and vagina after the procedure
- If patient conceives after trachelectomy-do cesarean section.

Management of Cervical Cancer

Management of cervical cancer is primarily by surgery or radiation therapy, with chemotherapy a valuable adjunct.

Surgical Management

Surgery is suitable for early stages, where cervical conization, total simple hysterectomy, or radical hysterectomy may be selected according to the stage of disease and extent of spread of cervical cancer. Annexure–12 shows the types of radical hysterectomy. In stage IVA, there is a place for pelvic exenteration in selected cases.

Microinvasive Cervical Carcinoma: FIGO Stage IA

Stage IA1

Young females: The treatment is completed with cervical conisation unless there is lymphovascular space invasion (LVSI) or tumor cells are present at the surgical margin.

Older females: In women who have completed childbearing or elderly women, total extrafascial hysterectomy. Type 1 hysterectomy is recommended. Any route can be chosen, i.e. abdominal, vaginal, or laparoscopic.

Stage IA2/or IA1, with LVSI

Older females: Since there is a small risk of lymph node metastases in these cases, pelvic lymphadenectomy is performed in addition in type radical hysterectomy.

Young females: When the patient desires fertility, she may be offered a choice of the following: (1) cervical conisation with laparoscopic (or extra-peritoneal) pelvic lymphadenectomy, or (2) radical abdominal, vaginal, or laparoscopic trachelectomy with pelvic lymphadenectomy.

Post-treatment Follow-up

Follow-up with 3 monthly Pap smears for 2 years, then 6 monthly for the next 3 years is recommended after treatment after treatment of microinvasive carcinoma. With normal follow up at years, the patient can return to the routine screening schedule according to the national guideline.

FIGO Stage IB1

FIGO stage IB1 is considered as low risk with the following criteria: largest tumor diameter less than 2 cm, cervical stormed invasion less than 50%, and no suspicious lymph nodes on imaging.

- **In older females.** The standard management is a type 3 radical hysterectomy. Pelvic lymphadenectomy should always be included.

In younger females desiring fertility, a radical trachelectomy can be done for stage IA2-IB1 tumor measuring less than or equal to 2 cm.

FIGO Stage IB2 and IIA1

- IN FIGO stage IB2 and IIAI cervical cancer, surgery or radiotherapy can be chosen as the primary treatment depending on the other patient factors and local resources as both have similar outcomes.
- But as discussed surgery is preferred. The preservation of ovarian and sexual function makes surgery the preferred mode in younger women.
- In this case whether female is young or old. Type C radical hysterectomy represents a basic procedure for the treatment of cervical cancer, along with pelvic lymphadenectomy.
- Lymphadenectomy constitutes one of the bases of this surgical procedure, and the extent of regional lymph node excision induces the parametrial nodes, obturator nodes, external, internal, and common ilia nodes.
- The route of surgery may be laparotomy or minimally invasive surgery, either laparoscopic or robotic. The IACC trial compared the overall survival with open, surgery versus laparoscopy or robotic surgery in early stage cervical cancer. They concluded that hysterectomy by minimally invasive route was associated with higher rates of recurrence than the open approach in early-stage cervical cancer patients. Further studies may be required to further confirm these findings.

FIGO Stage IB3 and IIA2

In stage IB2 and IIA2, the tumors are larger and the likelihood of high risk factors such as positive lymph nodes, positive parametria, or positive surgical margins that increase the risk of recurrence and require adjuvant radiation after surgery are high.

In all these cases, concurrent platinum-based chemoradiation (CCRT) is the preferred treatment option. It has been demonstrated that the prognosis is more favorable with CCRT, rather than radiotherapy alone.

In areas where radiotherapy facilities are scarce, neoadjuvant chemotherapy (NACT) has been used with the poal of:

- Down-staging of the tumor to improve the radical curability and safety of surgery
- Inhibition of micrometastasis and distant metastasis. There is no unanimity of view.

The extent of surgery after NACT remains the same, i.e. radical hysterectomy and pelvic lymphadenectomy.

Stage II B-IV: Always CCRT concurrent platinum based chemoradiation

FIGO Stage IVA or Recurrence

Rarely, patients with IVA disease may have only central disease without involvement to the pelvic sidewall or distant spread. Such cases, or in case of such a recurrence, pelvic exenteration can be considered but usually has poor prognosis

Postoperative Management of Cancer Cervix

Once surgery is performed in cancer cervix, patient is reassessed for the presence or absence of risk factors see Table 14B.7:

Table 14B.7

Intermediate Risk Factors	High Risk Factors
• Large tumor size	• Positive or close margins
• Cervical stromal invasion to middle or deep one third (> 1 cms)	• Positive lymph nodes
• Lymph vascular space invasion **(3S)**	• Microscopic parametrial involvement **(3P)**

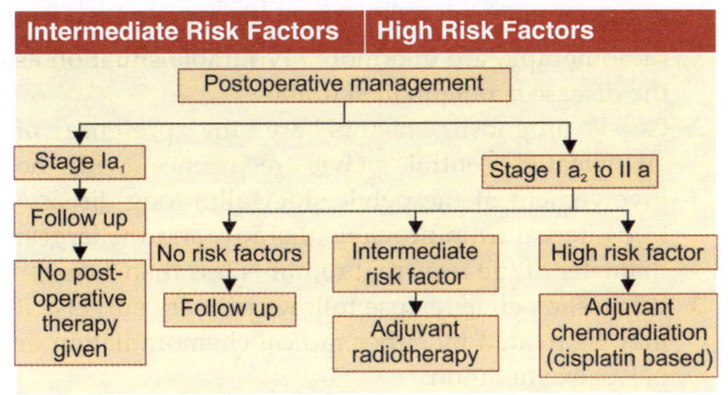

Radiation in Cancer Cervix

Radiation treatment plan in cancer cervix consists of a combination of:

i. **External beam radiotherapy (EBRT)**
   - Isotope used Cesium
   - ERBT is done to treat the regional lymphnodes and to decrease the tumour volume.

ii. **Brachytherapy:**

- EBRT is followed by brachytherapy delivered by intracavitary application to provide a treatment boost to the central tumour.
   - Intracavitary therapy alone may be used in patients with early disease with negligible incidence of lymph node metastasis
   - Isotopes used:
     - Low-dose rate technique Cs-137
     - High-dose rate techniques Ir-192.
   - **Intensity modulated radiation therapy (IMRT)** computer-generated algorithms that accurately distinguish between target treatment volumes and normal tissue.
   - Two important reference points in the brachytherapy of cancer cervix are:

	Point A	Point B
Location	2 cm above and 2 cm lateral to external os	2 cm above and 5 cm lateral to external os
Structure present	Paracervical/parametrial lymph node	Obturator lymph node
Dose of radiation	8000 cGy or 80 Gy	6000 cGy or 60 Gy

ABS criteria (American Brachytherapy Society):

- **Point A:** Early stae—Dose 80–85 Gy
  Locally advanced - stage (≥ IB2) = 85–90 Gy
- **Point B:** Early stage—50–55 Gy
  Late stage—55–60 Gy

Note: In routine pelvic radiation - inguinal lymphnodes are not included.

Comparison Between Surgery and Radiotherapy for Management of Cancer Cervix

	Surgery	Radiation
Survival	85%	85%
Serious complications	Urological fistulas1-2%	Intestinal and urinary strictures and fistulas 1.4–5.3%
Vagina	Initially shortened but may lengthen with regular intercourse	Fibrosis and possible stenosis, particularly in postmenopausal patients
Ovaries	Can be conserved	Destroyed
Chronic effects	Bladder atony in 3%	Radiation fibrosis of bowel and bladder in 6–8%
Surgical mortality	1%	1% (from pulmonary embolism during intracavitary therapy)

Carcinoma Cervix in Pregnancy

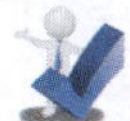

KEY POINTS

- Cervical cancer is the M/C malignancy in pregnancy.
- Symptoms of cervical cancer in pregnant and non pregnant women remain same

- PAP smear should be performed ideally on all pregnant women at the first antenatal visit and if required colposcopy and biopsy should be done. Punch biopsy can also be performed any time during pregnancy
- If there is a need to perform a diagnostic cone biopsy, it should be done in second trimester - (12-20 weeks)
- **CIN 1, 2 & 3** can be managed after pregnancy, vaginal delivery is possible
- Treatment modalities for Ca cervix are same as in nonpregnant women
- Cervical stage is the most important prognostic factor for cervical cancer during pregnancy
- **Stage 1A1:** vaginal delivery and then simple extrafascial hysterectomy or therapeutic conization after 6 weeks postpartum.If cesarean is being done it can be followed by hysterectomy directly.
- **Stage 1A2:** vaginal delivery and then wertheims hysterectomy and pelvic lymph node dissection after 6 weeks or immediately after cesarean section.
- **Stage, 1B, IIA:** If detected in first trimester = immediate Wertheim's hysterectomy on pregnant uterus.
- If detected in late second or third trimester: wait (treatment can be delayed up to 4-6 weeks) for fetal lung maturity and then classical caesarean section followed immediately by Wertheim's hysterectomy

- **Stage IIB-IV** : If detected in first trimester: Immediate radiotherapy (patient will spontaneously abort before 4000 cGY are delivered.
  If detected in late second or third trimester wait for fetal maturity, classical caesarean section and then radiotherapy begun postoperatively.

Stump Carcinoma
- Rare these days
- Earlier it was common when subtotal hysterectomy was done.
- It developed 2 years after hysterectomy.
- Incidence = 1%.

Treatment
- Early stages – surgery – Radical parametrectomy with upper vaginectomy and pelvic lymphadenectomy, i.e. cervix + upper vagina + parametrium + LN removed.
- Advanced stages – Radiotherapy.

Recurrent Disease

Recurrence may occur locally in the pelvic or para aortic, the patient may develop distant metastases, or there may be a combination

Local Recurrence

- The pelvic is the most common site of recurrence and patients who have only locally recurrent disease after definitive therapy, whether surgery or radiotherapy, are in a more favourable situation as the disease is potentially curable.
- Good prognostic factors are the presence of an isolated central pelvic recurrence with no involvement of the pelvic sidewall a long disease-free interval from previous therapy, and the largest diameter of the recurrent tumor is less than 3 cm.
- When the pelvic relapse follows primary surgery, it may be treated by either radical chemoradiation or pelvic exenteration.
- Confirmation of recurrence with a pathologic specimen obtained by biopsy is essential prior to proceeding with either therapy.
- The extent of recurrent disease and involvement of pelvic lymph nodes are prognostic factors for survival.
- Concurrent chemotherapy with either cisplatin and/or 5-fluorouracil may improve outcome.
- Pelvic exenteration may be feasible in some patients in whom there is no evidence of intraperitoneal or extrapelvic spread, and there is a clear tumor-free space between the recurrent disease and the pelvic sidewall.

A PET/CT scan is the most sensitive noninvasive test to determine any sites or distant disease, and should be performed prior to exenteration, if possible.

NEW PATTERN QUESTIONS

N1. All are true about TZ *except*:
a. It is a dynamic point
b. CIN originate from TZ
c. Gland openings & Nabothian cyst mark the original SCJ
d. SCJ is limited to external os

N2. Transformation zone moves out under the influence of all *except*:
a. Age
b. Pregnancy
c. OCP's
d. Puberty

N3. Feature of dysplastic cell are all *except*:
a. Decreased nucleocytoplasmic ratio
b. Several mitotic figures seen
c. Vary in shape and size
d. Irregular chromatin distribution with clumping

N4. All of the following are risk factors for cancer cervix *except*:
a. Early age of intercourse
b. Early menarche
c. Smoking
d. Multi parity

N5. All are true with regards to Adeno carcinoma of cervix *except*:
a. M/C site Transformation zone
b. M/C in young females
c. M/C in OCP users
d. Associated with HPV-18

N6. All are true with regards to HPV *except*:
a. It is epitheliotropic
b. Viral proteins needed for malignant transformation are E6, E7
c. Viral protein needed for replication E_1, E_2
d. E6 acts via Retinoblastoma gene

N7. Pap smear is useful in the diagnosis of all *except*:
a. Gonorrhea
b. Trichomonas vaginalis
c. Human papilloma virus
d. Inflammatory changes

N8. All of the following are screening methods for CIN *except*:
a. Colposcopic guided biopsy
b. Pap smear
c. HPV DNA testing
d. Visual inspection with acetic acid

N9. Colposcopic features suggestive of malignancy are all *except*:
a. Condyloma
b. Vascular atypyia
c. Punctation
d. White epithelium

N10. A patient complaints of post coital bleed; no growth is seen, on per speculum examination; next step should be:
a. Colposcopy biopsy
b. Conisation
c. Repeat pap smear
d. Culdoscopy

N11. A 50-year-old women present's with post coital bleeding. A visible growth on cervix is detected on per speculum examination. Next investigation is:
a. Punch biopsy *(AI 01)*
b. Colposcopic biopsy
c. Pap smear
d. Cone Biopsy

N12. A 45-years-old lady complains of contact bleeding. She has positive pap smear. The next line of management is: *(AIIMS 99)*
a. Colposcopy directed biopsy
b. Cone biopsy
c. Repeat pap smear
d. Hysterectomy

N13. A 30-year-old female undergoes pap smear. Her report shows presence of atypical squamous cells of unknown significance. What is the next best step in management?
a. Repeat pap smear in 6 months
b. Repeat pap smear in 2 years
c. Perform colposcopy
d. Do HPV-DNA testing

N14. In continuation to QN13, HPV DNA testing shows infection with high risk HPV types. What is the next step in management?
a. Perform colposcopy
b. Perform cryotherapy
c. Perform LEEP
d. Repeat smear and HPV test in 1 year

N15. Rekha a 45-year-old woman has negative pap smear with +ve endocervical curettage. Next step in management will be:
a. Colposcopy
b. Vaginal hysterectomy
c. Conization
d. Wertheim's hysterectomy

N16. A 35-year-old P_2C_2 female has CIN grade III confirmed on papsmear and Colposcopy. Next step in management is:
a. Conization
b. LEEP
c. Cryosurgery
d. Hysterectomy

N17. A 45-year-old P_2L_2 female has CIN grade III confirmed on papsmear and colposcopy. Best management:
a. Conization
b. LEEP
c. Cryosurgery
d. Hysterectomy

N18. A 35-year-old P_2L_2 female has CIN extending to vaginal fornix, confirmed on colposcopy Best management:
a. Conization
b. LEEP
c. Cryosurgery
d. Laser

N19. M/C Variety of cancer cervix:
a. Large cell Keratinizing
b. Large cell non Keratinizing
c. Small cell
d. Verrucous cancer

N20. M/C site of metastasis of Ca cervix is:
a. Lymph node b. Lungs
c. Bone d. Abdominal cavity

N21. A patient of Ca cervix presents with:
a. Menorrhagia b. Metrorrhagia
c. Polymenorrhae d. Amenorrhea

N22. A 55-year-old woman is diagnosed with invasive cervical carcinoma by cone biopsy. Pelvic examination and rectal examination reveal the parametrium is free of disease but upper part of vagina is involved with tumor. IVP and sigmoidoscopy are negative but CT S can of abdomen and pelvis shows grossly enlarged pelvic and para aortic nodes. This patient is classified as stage:
a. IIa b. IIb
c. IIIa d. IIIb
e. IIIc

N23. An intravenous pyelogram (IVP) showing hydronephrosis in the work up of a patient with cervical cancer otherwise confined to a cervix of normal size would indicate stage:
a. I b. II
c. III d. IV

N24. All are signs of inoperability of carcinoma of cervix *except*:
a. Fixity of cervix and parametrium to lateral pelvic wall
b. Presence of extra pelvic metastasis
c. Involvement of bladder
d. Tumor size >4 cms

N25. If stage Ib cervical cancer is diagnosed in a young woman, while performing radical hysterectomy which structure would you not remove:
a. Uterosacral and uterovesical ligament
b. Pelvic LN
c. Both ovaries
d. Upper third of vagina

N26. Point B in the treatment of carcinoma cervix receives the dose of:
a. 7000 cGy b. 6000 cGy
c. 5000 cGy d. 10,000 cGy

N27. A 55-year-old lady diagnosed with cancer cervix and treated with radiotherapy, develops uremia. M/C cause of uremia in this patient is:
a. Radiation nephritis
b. B/L ureter invasion
c. Ureteric stenosis due to radiation
d. CRF

N28. The following statements are related to the treatment of carcinoma cervix stage 1B *except*:
a. Surgery and radiotherapy have got almost equal 5-year-survival rate
b. Surgery has got higher morbidity than radiotherapy
c. Radiotherapy has got few limitations
d. In younger age group, radiotherapy is preferred

N29. Poor prognostic factor in the management of cancer cervix are all *except*:
a. Young age
b. Well differentiated squamous cell carcinoma
c. Hydroureter
d. Aderocarcinoma

N30. A 47-year-old female is diagnosed with cervical cancer. Which lymph node would be first involved in metastatic spread of this disease beyond the cervix and uterus:
a. Internal iliac lymph node
b. Obturation node
c. External iliac node
d. Paracervical node

N31. Advantages of surgery over radiotherapy in CA cervix are all *except*:
a. Low mortality
b. Conservation of ovaries
c. Preservation of cortal function
d. None

N32. A 30-year-old woman with one child is found to have preclinical invasive disease of cervix penetrating to a depth of 4 mm and 7 mm wide She wishes to preserve fertility. What is the most appropriate right:
a. Chemoradiation
b. Cone biopsy
c. Radical trachelectomy with pelvic LN dissection
d. Radical trachelectomy

N33. A 35-year-old woman with one child is found to have a visible cervical lesion measuring 2 cms. Biopsy shows squamous cell carcinoma of cervix. The lesion is confined to cervix. She wants to preserve her fertility. What is the most appropriate treatment?
a. Chemoradiation
b. Cone biopsy
c. Radical tracheostomy with lymph node dissection
d. Radical tracheostomy

N34. Management of CIN1 first diagnosed in a female of 22 years on Pap smear and colposcopy:
a. Do at HPV DNA testing
b. Pap smear + HDN DNA testing
c. LEEP
d. Repeat Pap smear after 12 months

N35. Management of persistent CIN1 in a female ≥26 years follow-up:
a. LEEP
b. Cryosurgery
c. Do HPV+ Pap smear
d. Hysterectomy

PREVIOUS YEAR QUESTIONS

CIN

1. **True about CIN:** *(PGI Dec 04)*
   a. Premalignant lesion
   b. HPV predisposes
   c. Pap smear can detect it
   d. Chlamydia infection can predispose
   e. Occurs at squamocolumnar junction
2. **A patient is diagnosed to have CIN II. She approaches you for advice. You can definitely tell her the risk of malignancy as:** *(AI 98; AIIMS 01)*
   a. 15% b. 60%
   c. 30% d. 5%
3. **All of the following changes are seen in dysplasia of squamocolumnar junction, *except*:** *(AIIMS 97)*
   a. Breaking of basement membrane
   b. Change of epithelium
   c. Hyperchromatic nuclei
   d. Increased mitotic figure
4. **In a cervix low grade squamous intraepithelial lesion (LSIL) in Bethseda system includes:** *(PGI May 2010)*
   a. CIN 1 b. CIN 2
   c. CIN 3 d. Squamous metaplasia
5. **Acetic acid staining of cervix shows following *except*:** *AIIMS May 02)*
   a. Squamous dysplasia
   b. Cervical carcinoma in situ
   c. Cervical polyp
   d. Cervical dysplasia
6. **In colposcopy following are visualised *except*:**
   a. Upper 2/3rd endocervix
   b. Cervical carcinoma in situ
   c. Cervical polyp
   d. Cervical dysplasia
7. **All of the following are indications of colposcopy:** *(PGI Dec 05)*
   a. Suspicious pap smear
   b. Obvious mass seen
   c. Suspected invasive carcinoma
   d. Patient who refuse biopsy
8. **Pap smear of Lelawati 45-years female shows CIN grade III. Which of the following is the next step in management:** *(AIIMS)*
   a. Punch biopsy
   b. Large loop excision
   c. Colposcopy directed biopsy
   d. Cone biopsy
9. **A 40-year-old multiparous woman is detected to have CIN-2 by Pap smear. What is the next step in management** *(JIPMER Nov 2014)*
   a. Conization b. Hysterectomy
   c. Colposcopy d. Repeat Pap smear
10. **High-Grade Squamous Intraepithelial Lesions (HSIL) are found on pap smear. Next step(s) of management:** *(PGI May 2017)*
    a. Colposcopic study and biopsy of suspicious lesions
    b. Hysterectomy
    c. Radiotherapy
    d. Liquid based cytology
    e. HPV DNA testing
11. **Cone biopsy is indicated in all the following conditions *except*:** *(AIIMS)*
    a. Indefinite diagnosis on colposcopy
    b. CIN-III
    c. Cervical metaplasia
    d. Microinvasive carcinoma
12. **Cone biopsy of cervix is indicated in all cases showing:** *(PGI 04)*
    a. Parametrial invasion
    b. Abnormal pap smear
    c. Endometrial Ca
    d. Endocervical curettage positive
    e. Clear cell Ca
13. **True about low grade squamous intraepithelial lesions:** *(PGI May 2016)*
    a. Confined to the lower 1/3 of the epithelium of cervix
    b. All cases are treated by cryotherapy
    c. 30% progress to invasive cancer in 10 years
    d. It is kept under observation with PAP smear of HPV DNA tests
14. **A woman undergoes Pap smear. Cytology shows atypical squamous cells of unknown significance. Next line of management will be** *(PGI Nov 2011)*
    a. Repeat Pap
    b. Cervical biopsy
    c. HPV DNA testing
    d. LEEP
    e. Colposcopy
15. **Therapeutic conisation is indicated in:** *(AIIMS)*
    a. Microinvasive carcinoma
    b. CIN (III)
    c. Unsatisfactory colposcopy with cervical dysplasia
    d. Cervical metaplasia
16. **Young lady comes with mild erosion of cervix and pap smear shows dysplasia, next step is:** *(PGI Dec 98)*
    a. Antibiotics b. Colposcopy
    c. Cryosurgery d. Conization
17. **A 35-year-old lady with post coital bleeding management is:** *(AIIMS Nov 09; May 08)*
    a. Clinical examination and pap smear
    b. Visual examination with lugol iodine
    c. Visual examination with acetic acid
    d. Colposcopy

18. A 55-year-old lady presenting to out patient department (OPD) with postcoital bleeding for 3 months has a 1 × 1 cm nodule on the anterior lip of cervix. The most appropriate investigation to be done subsequently is: *(AI 03)*
a. Pap smear
b. Punch biopsy
c. Endocervical curettage
d. Colposcopy

19. Meena 45-years-old female presents with post coital bleeding. On per speculum examination a friable mass is found in cervix. Next step in management is: *(AIIMS Nov)*
a. Colposcopy directed biopsy
b. 6 monthly pap smear
c. Only observation
d. Punch biopsy

20. Investigation of choice in postcoital bleeding in a 60-year-old lady is: *(AIIMS 96, 97; AI 96)*
a. Pap smear b. Colposcopy and biopsy
c. Pelvic ultrasound d. Cone excision of cervix

21. A 40-year-old woman presents with abnormal cervical cytology on PAP smear suggestive of CIN (III). The next best step in management is: *(AI 2010)*
a. Hysterectomy
b. Colposcopy and LEEP
c. Colposcopy and cryotherapy
d. Conization

22. A female 35 years P3 L3 with CIN III on colposcopic biopsy what would you do? *(AI 09)*
a. LEEP b. Conization
c. Hysterectomy d. Cryotherapy

23. Which of the following statements is not true about cervical cancer screening guidelines according to WHO? *(AIIMS Nov 2016)*
a. Pap smear should be repeated yearly in women of reproductive age group
b. HPV test should be done five yearly in women between age of 30 and 49 years
c. Visual inspection with acetic acid is more reliable at older age as it becomes easier to identify the transformation zone with age
d. Pap smear can be repeated less frequently if it comes out negative for 3 consecutive years

Carcinoma Cervix

24. True about Ca cervix: *(PGI Dec 06)*
a. 90% associated with HPV
b. Nulliparity
c. OCP
d. Immunocompromised patients

25. Predisposing factors for Ca cervix: *(PGI Dec 08)*
a. Multiple sex partners b. Genital warts
c. HPV 16, 18 d. Virginity
e. Late menarche

26. Risk factors for Ca Cervix: *(PGI May 2011)*
a. HPV
b. Monogamy
c. Late age at 1st inter course
d. Smoking
e. Immunosuppression

27. Carcinoma cervix is more common in: *(PGI 01)*
a. HIV patient b. Multiparity
c. Smoking d. Nulliparity
e. Family history

28. Which of the following is not a risk factor for CA cervix? *(AIIMS Nov 2013)*
a. Low parity
b. Multiple sexual partner
c. Early sexual intercourse (< 16 years)
d. Smoking

29. M/C agent responsible for Ca cervix is: *(AI 07)*
a. HPV 16 b. HPV 18
c. HPV 31 d. HPV 36

30. HPV associated with adenocarcinoma of cervix: *(PGI 05)*
a. Type 6 b. Type 18
c. Type 11 d. Type 42

31. Adenocarcinoma of cervix is associated with: *(PGI Nov 2010)*
a. HPV 6
b. HPV 11
c. HPV 16
d. HPV 18
e. HPV 51

32. Most common type of human papilloma virus causing Ca cervix are: *(PGI 03)*
a. 16 and 18 b. 1 and 33
c. 6 and 11 d. 2 and 14
e. 2 and 5

33. High risk HPV includes: *(PGI 02)*
a. Type 16 b. Type 18
c. Type 11 d. Type 12

34. HPV type least commonly associated with carcinoma cervix: *(PGI Nov 2012)*
a. 6 b. 11
c. 16 d. 18
e. 33

35. Cervix carcinoma arises from: *(PGI Dec 08)*
a. Squamocolumnar junction
b. Isthmus
c. Cervical lip
d. Internal os

36. Earliest symptom of carcinoma cervix is: *(PGI 99)*
a. Irregular vaginal bleeding
b. Post coital bleed
c. Foul smelling discharge
d. Pain

37. A case of carcinoma cervix is found in altered sensorium and is having hiccups. Likely cause is: *(AI 01)*
a. Septicemia b. Uremia
c. Raised ICT d. None of the above

38. Which investigation is not done in FIGO staging of CA cervix? *(AIIMS 96)*
a. Cystoscopy
b. Chest X-ray
c. Pelvic ultrasound
d. IVP

39. All of the following investigations are used in FIGO staging of carcinoma cervix *except*: *(AIIMS Nov 08)*
a. CECT
b. Intravenous pyelography
c. Cystoscopy
d. Proctoscopy

40. Carcinoma cervix extends upto lateral pelvic wall. The stage would be: *(AI 97)*
a. Stage I
b. Stage II
c. Stage III
d. Stage IV

41. Which is/are feature(s) of stage Ib2 cancer cervix? *(PGI Nov 12)*
a. Microinvasive carcinoma with stromal invasion <3 mm
b. Microinvasive carcinoma with stromal invasion <5 mm
c. Microinvasive carcinoma with 6 mm carcinoma with stromal invasion >5 mm
d. Size of lesion ≤ 4 cm
e. Size of lesion > 4 cm

42. In Ca cervix lymphatic spread involve which of the following lymph node/nodes: *(PGI 02)*
a. Obturator LN
b. External iliac LN
c. Inguinal LN
d. Femoral LN
e. Hypogastric LN

43. A 42-year-old female P3 + 0 + 0 + 3 is found to have carcinoma in situ. Best treatment would be: *(AI 97)*
a. Hysterectomy
b. Wertheim's hysterectomy
c. Conisation
d. Wait and watch

44. False statement about treatment of Ca cervix: *(PGI June 05)*
a. Radiotherapy is helpful in all stages
b. Prognosis of surgery good if done in early stages
c. When radiotherapy is given, para-aortic LNs should be included
d. Chemotherapy is reserved for late stages
e. From stage Ib onwards same prognosis with surgery and RT

45. A lady undergoes radical hysterectomy for stage Ib cancer cervix. It was found that cancer extends to lower part of body of uterus and upper part of cervix next step of management will be: *(AIIMS May 2010)*
a. Chemotherapy
b. Radiotherapy
c. Chemoradiation
d. Follow-up

46. In cancer cervix management includes: *(PGI Nov 2013)*
a. Radiotherapy
b. Wertheim's hysterectomy
c. Pap smear
d. CT abdomen
e. Cervical biopsy

47. HPV commonly associated with cancer cervix is: *(PGI Nov 2012)*
a. 6
b. 11
c. 16
d. 18
e. 35

48. Treatment of Ca cervix stage IB includes: *(PGI Nov 10)*
a. Surgery
b. Chemotherapy
c. Radiotherapy
d. Cryotherapy
e. Leep

49. Treatment of stage IIa cervical cancer includes: *(PGI Nov 12)*
a. Radical hysterectomy
b. Radical hysterectomy with pelvic lymph node dissection
c. Total abdominal hysterectomy with B/L salphingo oophorectomy
d. Chemoradiation

50. Treatment of stage III B carcinoma cervix is: *(AIIMS Nov 2010/AIIMS May 2012 Nov 2012)*
a. Wertheim procedure
b. Schauta's procedure
c. Chemotherapy
d. Intracavitary brachytherapy followed by external beam RT

51. True statement regarding Ca cervix involving parametrium but not pelvic involvement: *(PGI May 2010)*
a. Stage II A
b. Stage II B
c. Radiotherapy should be given
d. Hysterectomy can be useful
e. Staging should be done after cystoscopy

52. Cervical cone biopsy in a case of carcinoma cervix causes all, *except*: *(AIIMS May 94)*
a. Bleeding
b. Cervical stenosis
c. Infection
d. Spread of malignancy

53. A 55-year-old woman was found to have Ca cervix, FIGO stage 2–3, locally advanced. What would be the management? *(AIIMS May 2012)*
a. Surgery plus chemotherapy
b. Radiotherapy plus chemotherapy
c. Chemotherapy
d. Radiotherapy plus HPV vaccine

54. HPV triage strategy includes all *except*:
a. Conventional pap smear
b. Liquid based cytology
c. Hybrid capture 2 for HPV DNA
d. Colposcopy

55. Nulliparous women have high risk of following cancer: *(PGI May 2015)*
a. Cervical cancer
b. Vaginal cancer
c. Breast cancer
d. Ovarian cancer
e. Endometrial Ca

56. In a woman diagnosed with cervical cancer, all of the following investigations are included in FIGO staging *except*: *(JIPMER May 2017)*
a. IVP
b. CT abdomen
c. Cystoscopy
d. Chest X-ray

57. Stage IIB cervical cancer. Best line of management is: *(JIPMER 2017)*
a. Type 3 Hysterectomy
b. Chemotherapy
c. Radiation therapy
d. Chemoradiation

58. Lymph nodes excluded in external radiation therapy of cancer cervix *(PGI May 2012, PGI Nov 2016)*
a. External iliac LN
b. Internal Iliac LN
c. Sacral LN
d. Obturator LN
e. Common iliac LN

59. Tue regarding vaccination for HPV: *(PGI Nov 2012)*
a. Both bivalent and quadrivalent are available
b. Two doses are given
c. Target group is age 20-45 years
d. Most common HPV causing cancer cervix is 16 & 18

60. True about staging of cervical cancer: *(PGI June 2009)*
a. Staged clinically
b. When there is a doubt regarding staging, earlier staging is selected
c. Carcinoma extending beyond cervix to pelvic side wall is stage II
d. Stage II includes cancer extending uterus
e. Identification of para aortic LN in clinical stage I makes it stage IV

61. Risk factors for cancer cervix: *(PGI Dec 2008)*
a. Virginity
b. Multiple sex partners
c. Genital warts
d. Circumscribed partners
e. Late menarche

62. True about stage IB cervix carcinoma management: *(PGI Nov 2015)*
a. Radiotherapy alone
b. Simple hysterectomy done
c. Primary chemoradiation
d. Wertheim's hysterectomy + pelvic lymphadenectomy
e. Simple hysterectomy + equivalent chemotherapy

63. Screening test for cervical cancer includes: *(PGI Nov 2015)*
a. HPV serology b. Cervical biopsy
c. Colonoscopy d. Cytology
e. Conisation

64. A 40-year-old female was diagnosed with CIN-3. What will be the management? *(AIIMS Nov 2018)*
a. Trachelectomy
b. Hysterectomy
c. Conization
d. Colposcopy + LEEP

65. The given below instrument used in which procedure? *(AIIMS Nov 2019)*

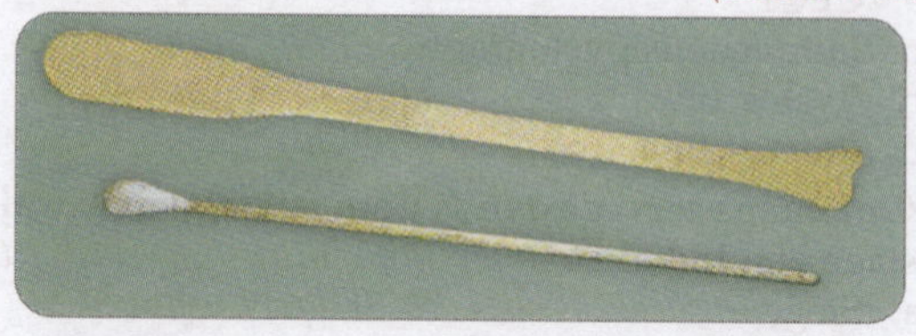

a. PAP b. VIA
c. VILI d. Colposcopy

66. A 16-year-unmarried girl came for vaccination against cervical cancer. Which vaccine to be given? *(AIIMS Nov 2019)*
a. Gardasil b. Rabivac
c. Biovac d. Tvac

67. A 35 years old lady presents with post-coital bleed. On examination, there is presence of cervical hypertrophy and anterior erosion with a healthy vagina. What will be next step in management? *(AIIMS May 2019)*
a. PAP smear
b. Conization
c. Four quadrant biopsy
d. Hysterectomy

68. Stage 3 cervical carcinoma (FIGO staging) is: *(PGI December 2018)*
a. Involving lower 1/3rd of vagina
b. Involving upper 2/3rd of vagina
c. Involving medial 1/3rd of parametrium/complete parametrium
d. Involving medial half of parametrium
e. Involving pelvic wall

69. Management options of HSIL on pap smear includes: *(PGI December 2018)*
a. Colposcopic biopsy and curettage
b. HPV DNA
c. HPV vaccination
d. Liquid based cytology
e. Hysterectomy

ANSWERS TO NEW PATTERN QUESTIONS

N1. Ans. is d, i.e. SCJ is restricted to external os.

As discussed Squamo Columnar Junction (SCJ) is a dynamic point & is not restricted to External os

N2. Ans. is a, i.e. Age. *Ref: Novaks 15th/ed, p576-578*

Squamocolumnar insction/Transportation zone
- SCJ is found in external os in neonates
- **But it is a dynamic part & does not remain restricted to it. It moves with age and hormonal influence.**
- **The original SC Junction is marked by the presence of nobothian cysts and glandular openings.**

The TZ moves inside (not out) with age.
It moves out
In pregnancy
At puberty
With OCp use
- M/c site of origin of CIN or cancer cervix is **Transformation Zone.**

N3. Ans. is a, i.e. Decreased nucleocytoplasmic ratio.

In dysplastic cells nucleo cytoplasmic ratio is increased.

N4. Ans. is b, i.e. Early menarche *Ref: Novak 15th/ed, p1305*

Early Menarche and Late menopause are risk factors for endometrial cancer and ovarian cancer, not cervical cancer. Likewise familial inheritance plays a role in ovarian cancer and endometrial cancer, not cervical cancer.

N5. Ans. is a, i.e. M/C site is transformation zone.

M/c cancer cervix = squamous cell cancer
M/c site of cancer cervix = Transformation zone

Adenocarcinoma of cervix
- M/c in young females
- M/c in OCP users
- Associated with HPV-18
- M/c site : Endocervix

N6. Ans. is d, i.e. E6 acts via Retinoblastoma gene *Ref: Novak 15th/ed*

E6 acts via tumor suppression gene–p53
E7 acts through Retinoblastoma gene.

N7. Ans. is a, i.e. Gonorrhea *Ref: Novak 15th/ed, p585*

- The pap test was first performed by Georgs Papinkalou
- It is used as a screening test for CIN and cancer cervix.

It can also detect a number of infection like:
- Trichomonas
- Candida
- Actinomyces
- Herpes simplex virus
- Koilocytosis of human papillonea viruses

***Note*: Pap test cannot detect gonorrhea and chlamydia.**[Q]

N8. Ans. is a, i.e. Colposcopic guided biopsy.

Screening methods	Diagnostic method
Papsmear (conventional/liquid based)	Lesion visible = Punch biopsy
VIA (visual inspection with acetic acid)	Lesion not visible = Colposcopy/colposcopic biopsy
VILI (visual inspection with lugols iodine)	Cone biopsy
Automated image guided slide screening system (EDA approved)	
HPV DNA Testing	

N9. Ans. is 'a' i.e. Condyloma.

Abnormal features on colposcopy which need to be biopsied.

Before applying acetic acid	• Leukoplakia • Rough area
After applying acetic acid	• Aceto white area • Abnormal (atypical) vascular pattern – Reticular pattern – Mosaic pattern – Punctate pattern

N10. Ans. is c, i.e. Repeat Pap smear

See explanation of N12.

N11. Ans. is a, i.e. Punch biopsy

See explanation of N12.

N12. Ans. is a, i.e. Colposcopy directed biopsy

Friends there are 2 situations in questions N10, N11, N12.

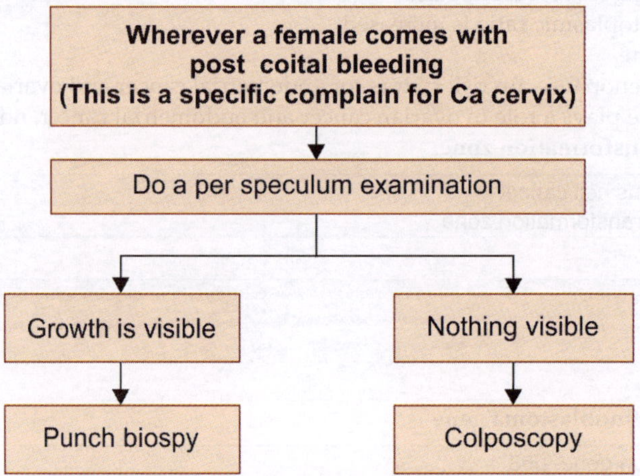

(ii) When a female comes to you with abnormal papsmear.

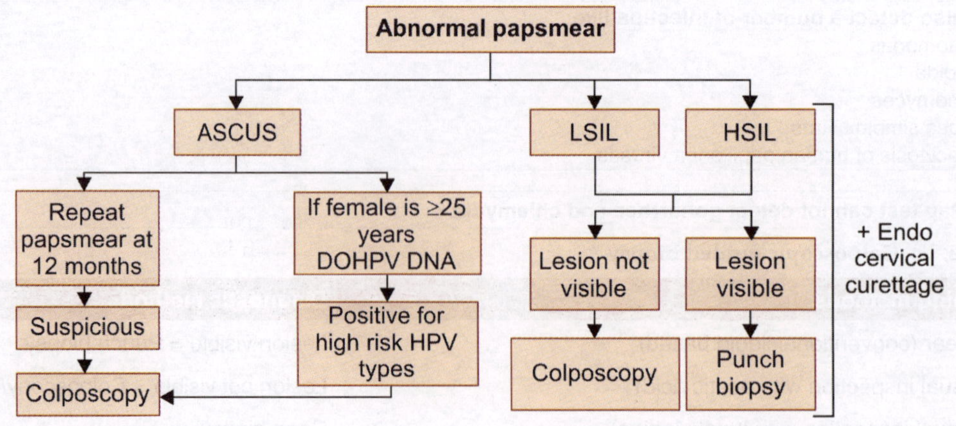

In LSIL: Endocervical curettage is optional

In HSIL = Endocervical curettage is mandatory.

N13. Ans. is d, i.e. Do HPV DNA testing. *Ref: Williams Gynae 3rd/ed, p636*

N14. Ans. is a, i.e. Perform colposcopy.

Management of ASCUS

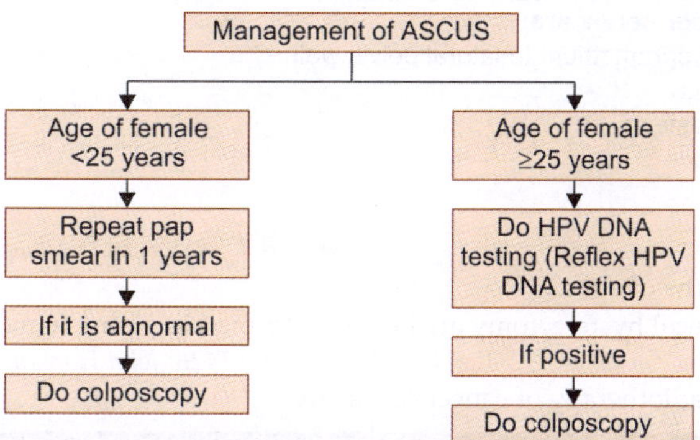

N15. Ans. is c, i.e. Conization.

Whenever endocervical curettage is positive, it could mean adeno carcinoma of endocervix. ∴ it should be followed by cone biopsy/conization as by colposcope upper part of endocervix cannot be visualized.

N16. Ans. is b, i.e. LEEP.

See explanation of N18.

N17. Ans. is b, i.e. LEEP.

See explanation of N18.

N18. Ans. is d, i.e. Laser.

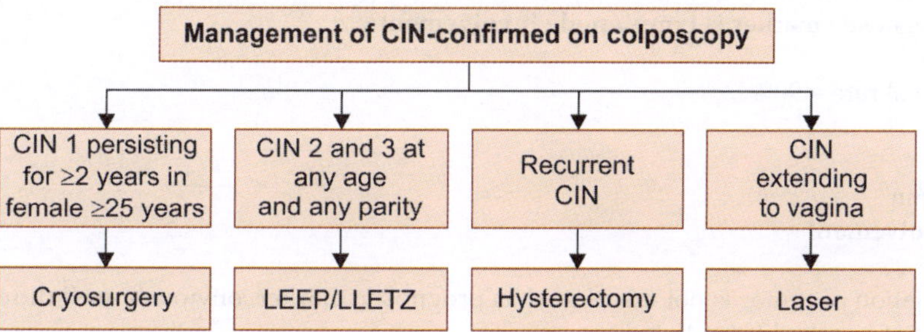

N19. Ans. is a, i.e. Large cell keratanizing. *Ref: Novak 15th/ed, p1210*

See the text for explanation.

N20. Ans. is a, i.e. Lymph nodes.

M/C route of spread of Ca Cervix: Lymphatics
M/C site of metastasis: Lymph nodes
M/C site of metastasis by hematogenous route: Lungs.

N21. Ans. is b, i.e. Metrorrhagia.

Cancer cervix presents most commonly as irregular vaginal bleeding i.e. Metrorrhagia.

N22. Ans. is e, i.e. Stage IIIC

Now here – in this patient

On examination – Parametrium is not involved and upper part of vagina is involved so stage will be IIa – clinically.

Remember cervical cancer is still staged clinically by using investigations recommended by FIGO.

CT scan results, earlier were not reommended by FIGO but now it is taken into consideration, it shows pelvic & para-aortic nodes involved i.e. Stage IIIC2.

N23. Ans. is c, i.e. Stage III

Now here - the investigation done is IVP which is one of the recommended investigations by FIGO therefore results of IVP are important for staging. By definition, a positive IVP would mean ureter is involved i.e. extension to pelvic side wall and i.e. Stage IIIB.

Such staging applies even if there is no palpable tumor beyond the cervix.

N24. Ans. is None *Ref: (Read below)*

> **Signs of inoperability of cancer cervix are:**
> a. Complete fixity of cervix and parametrium to lateral pelvic wall
> b. Extensive infiltration of vagina
> c. Presence of extrapelvic metastasis
> d. Extensive infiltration of bladder
> e. Presence of VVF.

N25. Ans. is c, i.e. Both ovaries *Ref: Textbook of Gynacecology sheila Balakrishnan 1st/ed, p255*

Cancer cervix rarely involves the ovaries.

∴ When radical/modified radical hysterectomy are being performed in young females, ovaries should not be removed.

N26. Ans. is b, i.e. 6000 cGy *Ref: Novak, 14th/ed, p1428; John Hopkins manual of Obs and Gynae 4th/ed, p554*

Two important points in the radiotherapy of cancer cervix are

	Point A	Point B
Location	2 cm above and 2 cm lateral to external os	2 cm above and 5 cm lateral to external os
Structure present	**Paracervical/parametrial lymph node**	Obturator lymph node
Dose of radiation	7000 – 8000 cGy	4000-6000 cGy

N27. Ans. is b, i.e. B/L ureter invasion.

M/C cause of uremia in cancer cervix is B/L ureteric invasion.

N28. Ans. is d, i.e. In younger age group, radiotherapy is preferred *Ref: Dutta Gynae 6th/ed, p195*

As explained in the text, in younger age group we prefer surgery with preservation of ovaries and not radiotherapy

N29. Ans. is b, i.e. Well differentiated squamous cell carcinoma prognostic factors for Ca cervix

Most important prognostic **marker is lymph node involvement**

Others: Size of Tm

Size < 2 cm = Survival rate = 90%

> 2 cm = 60%

> 4 cm = 40%

- **Depth of invasion**
- **Parametrial involvement**
- **Age of patient**

Although differentiation of tumor is not mentioned as prognostic marker, obviously well differentiated tumor is a good prognostic marker not poorly differentiated tumor.

N30. Ans. is d, i.e. Paracervical node

Sentinel LN in cancer cervix: paracervical/ureteric lymph node

M/C LN involved in cancer cervix: obturator.

N31. Ans. is a i.e. Low mortality *Ref: Novars 15th/ed, p1326*

Mortality is same for both surgery and radiation.

Comparison of surgery and radiation in cancer cervix		
Parameter	Surgery	Radiation
Survival	85%	85%
Mortality	1%	1% (due to pulmonary embolism)
Serous complication	Urological fistula (1–2%)	Intestinal and urinary stricture and fistula (1–5%)
Vagina/coital function	Normal	Fibrosed ∴ Coital function hampered
Ovaries	Can be conserved	Destroyed
Chronic complication	Bladder atony 3%	Radiation fibrosis of bladder and bowel 6–8%

N32. Ans. is c, i.e. Radical trachelectomy with pelvic lymph mode dissection:

This female is having cancer, 4 mm deep and 7 mm wide, i.e. stage Ia_2 of the cancer.

In stage Ia_2 if a female wishes to preserve fertility, radical trachelectomy along with lymph mode dissection or conization with pelvic lymph node dissection is best management.

N33. Ans. is c, i.e. Radical tracheostomy with lymph node dissection.

In this case the female has cancer confined to cervix i.e. it is Stage I

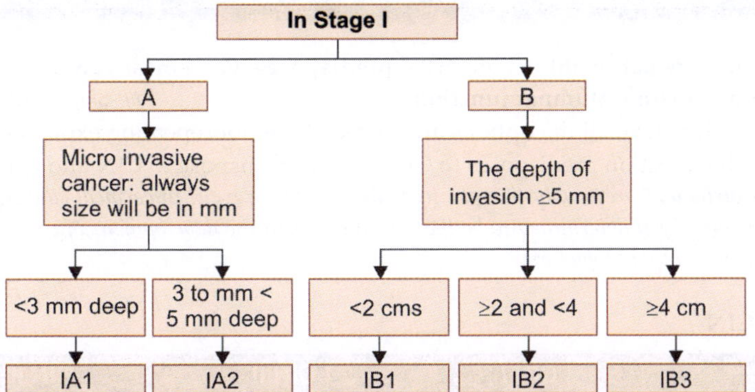

So this patient has cancer 2 cm is size which means IB2.

In young females with cancers ≤ 2 cms:- Management is Radical Trachelectomy with lymph node dissection.
If her cancer would be >2 cms then do Type 3 hysterectomy.

Stage	Management in young female	Management in old females/no fertility needed
IA1 (without LVSI)	Cervical conization	Type 1 Hysterectomy
IA2 or IA1 with LVSI	Conization or Tracheostomy with pelvic lymph node dissection	Type 2 Hysterectomy with pelvic LN dissection
IB1	Radical tracheostomy (if size of tones ≤ 2 cms + Pelvic lymph node dissection	Type 3 Hysterectomy with pelvic LN dissection
IB2 & IIA1	Type 3 hysterectomy + LN dissection	Type 3 Hysterectomy + LN dissection (of parametrial nodes, Obturator node, external, internal and common iliac nodes)
IB3 & IIA2	Chemoradiation	

34. Ans. is d, i.e. Repeat Pap smear after 12 months

CIN1:

- Treatment is acceptable only if CIN1 persists for more than 2 years.
- In females under 25 years, treatment is not recommended even if it is persistent.

CIN1 Age	Condition	Management
Age ≥ 25 years	First diagnosed	Observation Cotest (Pap + HPV) after 12 months If it is negative, continue routine screening 3 years later..
Age 21-25 years	First diagnosed	Pap smear at 12 months & 24 months instead of cotesting
Age ≥ 25 years	CIN persists	Ablation (if Pap smear lacked HSIL or ASC-H) Colposcopic examination is adequate otherwise Excision
Age 21-25 years	CIN persists & Pap abnormality Sterus + HSIL	Monitoring at 6 monthly interval

35. Ans. is b, i.e. Cryosurgery

ANSWERS TO PREVIOUS YEAR QUESTIONS

1. **Ans. is a, b, c, d and e, i.e. Premalignant lesion; HPV predisposes; Pap smear can detect it; Chlamydia infection can predispose; and Occurs at squamocolumnar junction** *Ref: Shaw 15th/ed, p400; Novak 14th/ed, p1404*
   As discussed in the preceeding text, all the options are correct. I am not repeating explanation for all the options but just for option d, i.e. Chlamydia infection predisposes to CIN. STD's predispose to CIN and Chalmydia is an STD.
   "Infection with the herpes virus was previously thought to be the initiating event in cervical cancer; however, infection with human papilloma virus (HPV) has now been determined to be the causal agent in the development of cervical cancer, with herpes virus and Chlamydia trachomatis likely acting as cofactors." *Ref: Novak 14th/ed, p1404*
2. **Ans. is d, i.e. 5%** *Ref: William Gynae 3rd/ed, p????*
   Rate of progression of CIN

	CIN I	CIN II	CIN III
Regression to Normal	57	43	32
Persistence	32	35	56
Progression to CIS/CIN III	11	22	
Progression to cancer	< 1%	5%	>12%

3. **Ans. is a, i.e. Breaking of basement membrane** *Ref: Robbin's 7th/ed, p1076, Shaw 15th/ed, p400*
   Dysplasia: Represents a change in which there *is alteration in cell morphology and disorderly arrangement of the cells of the stratified squamous epithelium*. It is a premalignant lesion.
   Characteristics of Dysplastic cell:
   - Vary in size[Q], shape[Q] and polarity[Q].
   - Have altered nucleo-cytoplasmic ratio (N/C ratio is increased).[Q]
   - Have large, irregular **hyperchromatic nuclei** with marginal condensation of chromatin material.[Q]
   - **Have several mitotic figures.**
   - **The basement membrane, however, is intact and there is no stromal infiltration.**
4. **Ans. is a, i.e. CIN 1** *Ref: Shaw 15th/ed, p400*

   In Bethesda system:
   LSIL = CIN 1
   HSIL = CIN 2, CIN 3/Ca in situ
5. **Ans. is c, i.e. Cervical polyp.**
   As discussed in text, colposcopy or acetic acid can detect dysplasia and cancer in situ. With a colposcope you can see a polyp but it does not need acetic acid staining, hence it is ruled out
6. **Ans. is a, i.e. Upper 2/3 of endocervix.**
   Now do not get confused, in the previous question they were asking about acetic acid staining, but now they are saying simply colposcope.
   Colposcope is a magnifying instrument, so obviously you can see a polyp by it. See figure 38.10 of shaw Gynae pg 490, 16 edition in case of doubt.
   As discussed in the text a colposcope cannot visualize upper 2/3rd endocervix.
7. **Ans. is a and c, i.e. Suspicious pap smear and Suspected invasive carcinoma.**
8. **Ans. is c, i.e. Colposcopy directed biopsy**
   Ref: CGDT10th/ed, p837, 841; Harrison 17th/ed, p608; Williams Gynecology 1st/ed, p628, Table 29-6; William Gynae 3rd/ed, p629
9. **Ans. is c, i.e. Colposcopy**
10. **Ans. is a, i.e Colposcopic study and biopsy of suspicious lesions**
    As discussed in chapter 14 B, pap smear is a screening test, so whenever you get LSIL or HSIL on report you have to confirm it by doing a colposcopy and biopsy. If some growth is visible then instead of colposcopy, punch biopsy should be done.
    - Pap smear is only a screening test. To confirm we need to do a biopsy.
    - In all visible lesions punch biopsy should be done
    - In case of invisible lesion colposcopic directed biopsy is the gold standard. Thus in this case since it is not mentioned growth is visible so we do colposcopy guided biopsy.

HPV DNA testing is not recommended for HSL as in most of the cases it will be positive and that does not alter the management.

"If typical genital warts are found in young women or if HSIL or invasive cancer is identified on cytology or histology, then HPV infection is assumed, and HPV testing is unnecessary."

11. **Ans. is c, i.e. Cervical metaplasia**

As discussed metaplasia is a normal phenomenon occurring in all females so obviously cone biopsy is not done for it.

12. **Ans. is b, and d, i.e. Abnormal pap smear; Endocervical curettage positive**

13. **Ans. is a, & d, i.e. Confined to lower 1/3 of epithelium of cervix and It is kept under observation until Pap smear or HPV DNA test.**

Let's see each option here with respect to LSIL i.e. CIN1

(a) Confined to lower 1/3 of epithelium of cervix - correct

(b) All cases treated by cryotherapy - incorrect

As discussed in text, cryotherapy is done in persistent cases if female ≥ 25 years.

(c) 30% progress to invasive cancer - incorrect - as shown in table Ans 1:

- CIN1 = <1%
- CIN2 = 5%
- CIN3 = >12%

} Progress to cancer

(d) It is kept under observation with Pap smear or HPV DNA - Correct

14. **Ans. is a, i.e Repeat Pap, c i.e. HPV DNA testing, e i.e. Colposcopy** *Ref: William Gynae 3rd/ed, p636*

See explanation of Q13 for explanation

15. **Ans. is a, i.e. Microinvasive carcinoma** *Ref: Shaw 15th/ed, p405; Novak 14th/ed, p584-5; 15/ed, p604*

Cone biopsy or conization is both diagnostic as well as therapeutic procedure

Indications of Cone biopsy	
Diagnostic	**Therapeutic**
• Limits of the lesion cannot be visualised with coloposcopy.[Q]	• Ca in situ in young females
• The squamocolumnar junction is not seen at colposcopy[Q]	• Cancer cervix stage 1A1 in young females (microinvasive cancer)
• In endocervical curettage histological findings are positive for CIN - II or CIN - III[Q], CA in situ	
• Micro Invasive carcinoma or adenocarcinoma in situ is suspected based on biopsy, colposcopy or cytology results	
• *Lack of correlation between cytology, biopsy & colposcopy results.*	

Complications of cone biopsy

- Bleeding[Q] (M/C complication)
- Infection[Q]
- Cervical stenosis[Q]
- Incompetent os[Q]

16. **Ans. is a, i.e. Antibiotics** *Ref: Jeffcoate 7th/ed, p410-1; Dutta Gynae. 4th/ed, p250*

The erosion should first be treated with antibiotics and then pap smear repeated.

17. **Ans. is a, i.e. Clinical examination and pap smear.**

As discussed earlier, patient complaining of post cotal bleeding, should be investigated by colposcopy is as it is a specific symptom of cancer cervix. *Ref: Novak 15th/e p1305*

18. **Ans. is b, i.e. Punch biopsy**

Now since here lesion is visible and post coital bleeding is a specific complain of cancer cervix we do punch biopsy.

19. **Ans. is d, i.e. Punch biopsy**

20. **Ans. is b, i.e. Colposcopy and biopsy**

Now I know many of you might think answer as Pap smear, but the answer is Colposcopy or Biopsy.

Read what Williams has to say - in case cancer cervix is suspected (post vital bleeding means cancer cervix is suspected)

"Histology is the primary tool to diagnose cervical cancer. Although Pap test are performed extensively to screen for this cancer, this test does not always detect cervical cancer. Specifically, pap testing has only a 53 to 80% security for detecting high grade lesions on any single given test. Thus, preventive power of this lies in regular serial screening. Moreover, women who have stage 1 cervical cancer, only 30-50% of single cytological smears are positive for cancer. Hence, pap testing alone for evaluation of a suspicious lesion is discouraged. Instead these lesions are directly prepared. *Williams Gynae 3/e page 663*

21. **Ans. is b, i.e. Colposcopy and LEEP.**

The patient in the question has CIN (III) on pap smear. PAP smear is only a screening procedure and not diagnostic. Hence for confirming the diagnosis, we will have to do colposcopy followed by LEEP to treat it, if it is confirmed. This can be done in 2 steps or single step.

22. Ans. is a, i.e. LEEP *Ref: CGDT 10th/ed, p840; Jeffocate 7th/ed, p421*

As discussed in the previous question – Loop Electrosurgical Excision Procedure (LEEP) has now become the procedure of choice for treating CIN II and CIN III in all age groups. Therefore in this patient we will go for LEEP.

23. Ans. is a, i.e. Pap smear should be repeated yearly in women of reproductive age group.

See the text for explanation.

24. Ans. is a, c and d, i.e. 90% associated with HPV; OCP; and Immunocompromised patients

25. Ans. is a, b and c, i.e. Multiple sex partners; Genital warts and HPV 16, 18

26. Ans. is a, d and e, i.e. HPV; Smoking; and Immunosuppression

27. Ans. is a, b and c, i.e. HIV patient, Multiparity and Smoking. *Ref: CGDT 10th/ed, p834; Shaw 14th/ed, p359*

28. Ans. is a, i.e. Low parity

Factors Predisposing to CIN/Ca cervix:

- **Human Papilloma virus infection**
- **Sexually transmitted infections:**
  - Coitus before 18 years of age[Q]
  - Multiple sex partners[Q]
  - Multiparity[Q]
  - Poor personal hygiene[Q]
  - Poor socioeconomic status[Q]
- **Smoking[Q],**
- **Immunosuppressed individuals[Q]**
- **Women on OCP[Q], Progesterone therapy for long time are predisposed to *adenocarcinoma* of endocervix.**
- **In utero exposure to DES**

"HPV is central to the development of cervical neoplasia. HPV – DNA is found in 95% of all squamous cell carcinoma & 90% of all adenocarcinomas."

29. Ans. is a, i.e. HPV 16

30. Ans. is b, i.e. Type 18

31. Ans. is c, d, e, i.e. HPV 16, HPV 18, HPV 51

32. Ans. is a, i.e. 16 and 18 *Ref: Novak 14th/ed, p 568; 15th/ed, p 581; COGDT 10th/ed, p 843*

33. Ans. is a and b, i.e. Type 16; and Type 18 *Ref: Williams Gynae 1st/ed, p 619; Dutta Gynae 6th/ed, p 323*

34. Ans. is a and b i.e. 6 and 11.

MIC HPV always cancer cervix = HPV16

MIC HPV always cancer cervix = HPV18

High risk HPV include = HPV, 16, 18, 31, 33, 35, 39, 45, 51, 52, 56, 58, 59, 68 *Ref: Novak 15th/ed, p580;*

35. Ans. is a and c, i.e. Squamocolumnar junction and Cervical lip

Ref: Shaw 15th/ed, p 400; Novak 14th/ed, p564; Williams Gynae 1th/ed, p619

- M/C site for carcinoma cervix : Squamo columnar junction

"The anterior lip of cervix is twice as likely to develop CIN as the posterior lip and CIN rarely originates at lateral angles" *Ref: Novak 14/ed, p564*

- M/C site for adenocarcinoma of cervix is Endocervix.

36. Ans. is a, i.e. Irregular vaginal bleeding *Ref: Jeffcoate 7th/ed, p471; Williams Gynae. 1st/ed, p652*

"In its very early stage, invasive carcinoma of cervix causes no symptoms and is discovered accidently or as a result of routine search. Symptoms come with surface ulceration and consist only of irregular uterine bleeding or discharge or both. These being peri-or postmenopausal in half the cases. The first episode of bleeding commonly follows coitus, straining at stool or trauma." *Ref: Jeffcoates 7th/ed, p 471*

"For those with symptoms, however, early stage cervical cancer may create a watery, blood tinged vaginal discharge. Intermittent vaginal bleeding that follows coitus or douching may also be noted." *Ref: Williams Gynae. 1st/ed, p652*

The earliest symptom of invasive cervical cancer is usually abnormal vaginal bleeding, often following coitus or vaginal douching. This may be associated with clear or foul smelling vaginal discharge. *Ref: Devita 8th/ed, p1502*

Thus earliest symptom is irregular vaginal bleeding which usually follows coitus. So I am taking option 'a', i.e. irregular vaginal bleeding as the correct answer.

37. Ans. is b, i.e. Uremia *Ref: Jeffcoate 7th/ed, p472*

"The ultimate cause of death in their order of frequency and importance - uraemia cachexia associated with recurrent haemorrhage, infection and interference with nutrition, complication of treatment and remote metastasis to vital organs (rare)."

Hiccups and altered sensorium are nonspecific signs of uraemia and so the likely cause in this case is uraemia.

Also Know

Uraemia in carcinoma cervix occurs when tumor involves ureter and results in blockage.

- M/C cause of death in cancer cervix =Renal failure/uremia
- Second M/C cause of death in cancer cervix=Hemorrhage.

38. Ans. is c, i.e. Pelvic ultrasound

39. Ans. is a, i.e. CECT *Ref: Dutta Gynae. 5th/ed, p328, 6th/ed, p341; Novak 14th/ed, p1410*

Staging Procedures in Ca cervix (As recommended by FIGO)

Physical examination	Radiological studies	Procedure
• Palpate lymph node	• Chest X-ray	• Biopsy
• Examine vagina	• Skeletal X Ray	• Conisation
• Bimanual recto vaginal examination	• IVP	• Endocervical Curettage
• Barium enema		• Colposcopy • Hysteroscopy • Cystoscopy • Proctoscopy

Mnemonic: **BS$_4$C Exam**
B = **B**iopsy
C = **C**onization
S$_4$ = 4 types of scopy's
Exam = **E**ndocervical curettage

Note: USG, CECT, MRI, PET, Laparoscopy, Laparotomy and Lymphangiography are optional and were not included Earlier by FIGO these investigation were not recommended but now all are recommended.

40. Ans. is c, i.e. Stage III *Ref: Novak 15th/ed, p1317, Devita 8th/ed, p1501 Table 42-2-2 and p1503*

As discussed in the staging given in preceeding text carcinoma extending to pelvic wall means stage III.

41. Ans. is d, i.e. Size of lesion ≤ 4 cm

As per new staging IB2 is if size of lesion is <4 cm.

42. Ans. is a, b and e, i.e. Obturator LN; External iliac LN; and Hypogastric LN

Ref: Williams Gynae 1st/ed, p649; Devita 7th/ed, p1297

Primary group	Secondary group
H = Hypogastric/iliac nodes	Common iliac
O = Obturator	Para aortic
P = Presacral and parametrial	Inguinal
E = External iliac	

43. Ans. is a, i.e. Hysterectomy *Ref: Novak 15th/ed, p602*

Hysterectomy remains the preferred management for women with histological diagnosis of AIS on a specimen from a diagnostic excisional procedure.

A diagnosis of AIS from a punch biopsy or a cytological diagnosis of AIS is not sufficient to justify hysterectomy without a diagnostic excisional procedure.

Negative margins in an excisional specimen do not mean to lesion is completely excised.

If future fertility is desired, conservative excisional management is acceptable.

If conservative excisional procedure is performed and margins are involved or if endocervical sample at the time of excision shows AIS or CIN, reexcision is recommended.

Assessment at 6 months using a combination of cytology, colposcopy , HPV DNA testing and endocervical sampling is acceptable.

44. Ans. is c and e, i.e. When radiotherapy is given paraaortic LN should be included and From stage Ib onwards same prognosis with Surgery and Radiotherapy

Ref: Novak 14th/ed, p1417-8, 1436; 15th/ed, p1326, 1333; William Gynae 1st/ed, p658-9

I have discussed management of cancer cervix in detail in preceeding text.

Option "a": Radiotherapy is helpful in all stages. ... *Correct*

Option "b": Prognosis of surgery is good if done in early stages. ... *Correct*

Option "c": When radiotherapy is given para aortic LN should be included. It is incorrect as routine radiotherapy for cancer cervix does not include para aortic lymphnodes. If para aortic lymph nodes are involved then only extended field radiotherapy should be given.

"The routine use of extended field radiation for prophylactic para aortic radiation without documentation of distant metastasis to para aortic nodes was evaluated and is not practiced because of increased enteric morbidity associated with this treatment modality."

Ref: Novaks 15th/ed, p1326

Note:

- IOC to know whether para-aortic lymph nodes are evolved is PET/CT imaging studies.

- Radiotherapy for para aortic lymph nodes leads to bowel complications and to avoid these complications, extra peritoneal dissection of para aortic nodes is recommended and the dose of radiation should be reduced to 5000 cGy or less. When this approach is used, post radiotherapy bowel complications occur in <5% patients and 5 year survival rate is 15 – 26% in patients with positive para aortic nodes.

Option "d": Chemotherapy is reserved for last stages. ... *Correct*

Option "e": From stage 1B onwards same prognosis with surgery and RT.

The only data which I could get on this is:

"Stages 1B1,1B2 and 2A (size of lesion <4 cms)-these patients can be managed by surgery or primary chemoradiation. Several studies showed similar survival rates and outcomes. In bulky stages 1B2 and 2A2 -chemoradiation should be preferred but if patient wishes to conserve ovary then surgery should be done but it has increased morbidity because most of these patients have intermediate or high risk factors present for which post operative radiotherapy or chemoradiation has to be given." *Ref: Novak Gynae 15th/ed, p1333*

45. Ans. is d, i.e. Follow-up *Ref: Novak Gynae 14th/ed, p1436, 1426, 1418-1, 1408*

Postoperatively it was found that carcinoma extends to the lower part of uterus. Now this is a trap because uterine extension has no significance in cancer cervix and does not change the staging.

46. Ans. is a, b, d and e, i.e. Radiotherapy, Wertheim's hysterectomy, CT abdomen and Cervical biopsy

See the text for explanation

47. Ans. is c & d, i.e. HPV 16 and HPV 18

"Together HPVs 16 & 18 account for approximately 70% of cervical cancers worldwide, 68% of squamous cell carcinomas and 85% of adenocarcinomas." *Ref: Williams Gynae 3rd/ed, p628*

48. Ans. is a and c, i.e. Surgery and Radiotherapy *Ref: Novak Gynae 15th/ed, p1332; Devita 8th/ed, p1508-9*

Stage IB1 and IB2 is managed by surgery and IB3 by chemoradiation.

49. Ans. is b and d, i.e. Radical hysterectomy with pelvic lymph node dissection, Chemoradiation.

From stage IB3 and IIa2 onwards → management becomes chemoradiation. Stage IIa, is managed by radical hysterectomy with pelvic lymph node dissection.

50. Ans. is d, i.e. Intracavitary brachytherapy followed by external beam RT.

Ref: Novak 14th/ed, p1436, 1427; Shaw 15th/ed, p414

As discussed in the preceeding text, best treatment for stage III B of invasive cancer is chemoradiation. Since this option is not given - we will go for next best option, i.e. Radiotherapy

Generally from stage II a-IV A when radiotherapy is given - external beam pelvic radiation precedes brachytherapy. But again since we don't have this option, we are going for vice versa (which is not incorrect).

51. Ans. is b, c and e, i.e. Stage IIB: Radiotherapy should be given; Staging should be done after cystoscopy.

Ref: COGDT 10th/ed, p848-9; Novak 14th/ed, p1407-9; Shaw 15th/ed, p412-5

Cancer cervix involving the parametrium but not the pelvis refers to stage IIB (i.e. **option 'a'** is incorrect and **option 'b'** is correct).

Management of choice for stage II b is – chemoradiation (i.e. 5 days Radiotherapy along with cisplatin added on any one day). i.e. **option 'c'** is correct.

Surgery–(Radical/wertheims hysterectomy) is not done for stage IIb. (i.e. **option 'd'** is incorrect).

Procedures done for Surgical staging of Ca cervix as advised by FIGO includes cystoscopy and thus cystoscopy should be done before staging (i.e. **option 'e'** is correct).

52. Ans. is d, i.e. Spread of malignancy *Ref: Shaw 15th/ed, p406; Jeffcoate 7th/ed, p421; Williams Gynae 1st/ed, p635*

Complications of Cone biopsy are:

- Hemorrhage[Q]
- Sepsis (infection)[Q]
- Cervical stenosis[Q]
- Pregnancy complications which include:
  - *Mid trimester abortions[Q]*
  - *Preterm labour[Q]*
  - *Cervical dystocia[Q]*

Also Know

- Cone biopsy should be done under general anaesthesia.
- The cone should include the entire outer margin and the endocervical lining but internal OS is spared.
- A small cone is preferred in younger women to avoid pregnancy complications.

53. Ans is b, i.e. Radiotherapy plus chemotherapy *Ref: Williams Gynae 2nd/ed, p787; Novak 14th/ed, p1436*

As discussed in detail in preceeding text best for cervical cancer of (stages II B to IV A) is chemoradiation (i.e. chemotherapy and radiotherapy), where by cisplatin is used as a radiosensitiser to increase the sensitivity of the cells to radiotherapy before giving radiotherapy.

Since in this question –chemotherapy + radiotherapy is given as one of the options, hence, we will mark it as the correct option.

54. Ans. is a, i.e. Conventional pap smear *Ref: Dutta Gynae 6th/ed, p323-4*

HPV triage strategy includes:

i. Pap smear test–by liquid based thin layer cytology

ii. Hybrid capture 2 for detecting HPV DNA

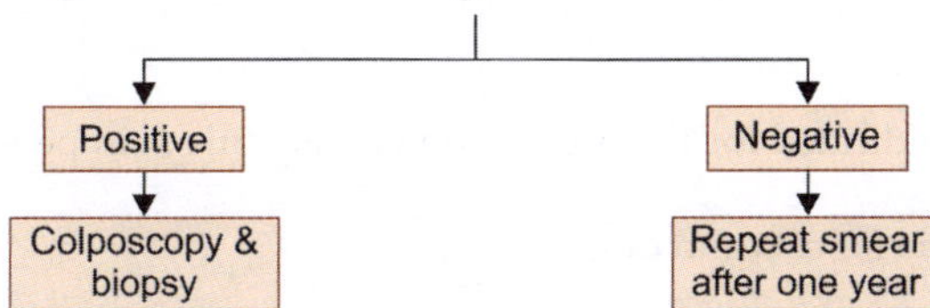

This triage strategy can detect CIN II and III lesions effectively and reduces the load of coloscopy clinic.

55. Ans. is c, d and e, i.e. Breast cancer, Ovarian cancer and Endometrial cancer.

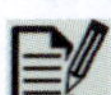

Remember

A simple funda- All hyperestrogenic conditions are M/C in nulliparous females.

Conditions M/C in Nulliparous Females
- PCOD
- Fibroid
- Endometriosis
- Endometrial hyperplasia
- Cancer endometrium
- Cancer ovary
- Cancer breast

56. Ans. is b, i.e CT scan of abdomen as per old guidelines

Ans is None as per new guidelines.

57. Ans. is d, i.e. Chemoradiation. See the text for explanation.

58. Ans. is e, i.e. Common iliac lymph nodes.

In external beam radiotherapy commonly involved lymph nodes are included:

1. Internal iliac LN
2. External iliac LN
3. Hypogastric LN
4. Obturator LN
5. Presacral LN

59. Ans. is a, b, & d i.e. Both bivalent and quadrivalent are available, Two doses are given & Most common HPV causing cancer cervix is 16 & 18.

See the text for explanation

60. Ans is a, and b, i.e. Staged clinically and When there is doubt regarding staging, earlier staging is selected.

Option a: Staged clinically—Correct

Option b: When there is doubt regarding staging, earlier staging is selected—Correct

Option c: Carcinoma extending beyond cervix to pelvic side wall is stage II—Incorrect (it is stage III)

Option d: Stage II includes cancer extending uterus—incorrect—Extension of cancer cervix to uterus is disregarded

Option e: Identification of para aortic LN in clinical stage I makes it stage IV—incorrect—It makes it stage IIIC.

61. Ans. is b, & c, i.e. Multiple sex partners and Genital warts.

See the text for explanation

62. Ans. is c, & d, i.e. Primary chemoradiation and Wertheim's hysterectomy + pelvic lymphadenectomy

See the text for explanation

63. Ans. is a, & d, i.e. HPV serology & Cytology.

Colposcopy, cervical biopsy & conization are diagnostic tests not screening test

64. Ans. is d i.e. Colposcopy + LEEP

As discussed in chapter 14B, any age of female, any party diagnosed with CIN3 should undergo LEEP.

65. Ans. is a, i.e. Pap smear *Ref: Shaw's Textbook of Gyne 16th/ed, p87*

- The image shown is that Ayer's spatula, which is used for preparing Pap smear.
- Ayres spatula and endocervical brush are used for Pap smear.

- **Method**: The concave end of Ayres spatula is rotated through 360° over transformation zone and 1st slide is prepared. With cytobrush 2nd slide is prepared from endocervix.
- The smear is then fixed using Ethyl alcohol (95%).

66. Ans. is a, i.e. Gardasil *Ref: Shaw's Textbook of Gyne 16th/ed, p495*

Gardasil is the vaccine of choice in this situation.

Other options:

- **Biovac**: It is freeze-dried live attenuated vaccine indicated for the prevention of Hepatitis A in persons of age 1 year or older
- **Rabivac**: It is monovalent inactivated rabies vaccine for cats and dogs.
- **Tvac**: It is tetanus vaccine

HPV vaccines

- HPV vaccines have been developed from the inactivated capsid coat of the virus.
- HPV vaccines were earlier of two types. During its Feb 2015, meeting Advisory Committee on Immunization Practices (ACIP) recommended 9-valent HPV vaccine (9V HVP) as one of the three vaccines for preventive HPV.

Characteristic	Bivalent (2V HPV)	Quadrivalent (4V HPV)	9 Valent (9V HPV)
Brand name	Cervarix	Gardasil	Gardasil-9
HPV subtypes	16, 18	6, 11, 16, 18	6, 11, 16, 18, 31, 33, 45, 52, 58
Protects against	CIN, Ca cervix	Anogenital warts, CIN, Ca cervix	Anogenital warts CIN, Ca cervix, vulva intraepithelial neoplasia, vaginal intraepithelial neoplasia
Manufacturing	Trichoplusia insect line infected with L1 encoding baculovirus	Saccharomyces cerevisiae expressing L1	Saccharomyces cerevisiae expressing L1
Adjuvant	500 mcg aluminium hydroxide with monophosphoryl lipid A	225 mcg $Al(OH) PO_4SO_4$	500 mcg $Al(OH) PO_4SO_4$
Dose	0.5 mL	0.5 mL	0.5 mL
Administration	1/m	1/m	1/m
Administered to males or females	Both males and females	Both males and females	Both males and females
Age in females ideal age range	11–12 years 9–26 years	11–12 years 9–26 years	11–12 years 9–26 years
Age in males ideal age range	11–12 years 9–26 years	11–12 years 9–26 years	11–12 years 9–15 years—FDA approved 9–26 years—ACIP recommendation

67. Ans. is a, i.e. PAP smear

Now in this question, Patient is coming with complaint of post coital bleeding. On local examination cervical hypertrophy and anterior erosion is seen.

Remember: In Cancer cervix: The most specific symptom is post coital bleeding.

Case: Whenever a female comes with post coital bleeding:

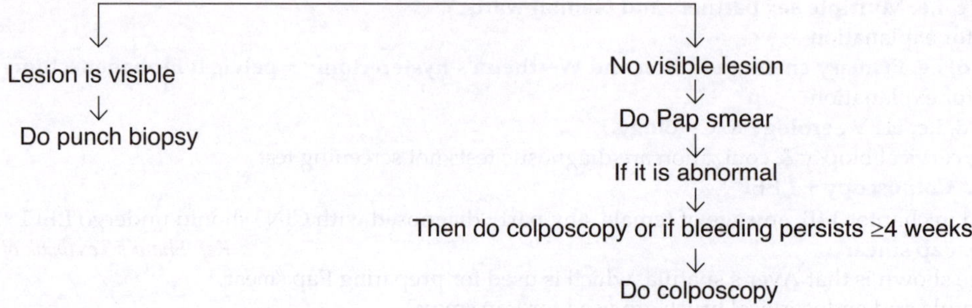

68. Ans. is a and e, i.e. Involving lower 1/3rd of vagina, and Involving pelvic wall

- Involving lower 1/3rd of vagina – stage IIIA
- Involving pelvic wall – stage IIIB

Other options

- Involving upper 2/3rd of vagina – stage IIA
- Involving medial 1/3rd of parametrium/complete parametrium – stage IIB
- Involving medial half of parametrium – stage IIB

69. Ans. is a, i.e. Colposcopic biopsy and curettage

In patients detected with HSIL:

Management is:

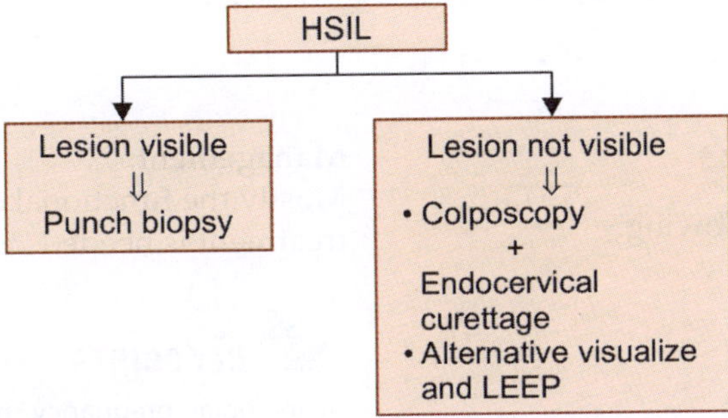

- Now HPV-DNA testing plays a role in those cases where there are atypical squamous cells not in case of HSIL.
- HPV vaccination is useful before exposure to human papilloma virus. It has no role in management of HSIL.
- Hysterectomy is not done in management of CIN these days. Even if we are thinking about hysterectomy, then the diagnosis needs to be confirmed by biopsy first. Just getting HSIL on pap smear, does not indicate hysterectomy.

CHAPTER 14C

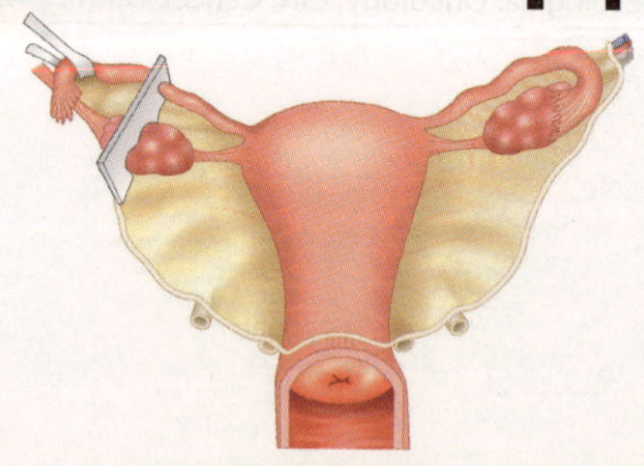

Gynecological Oncology: Ovarian Tumors

Ovarian Mass/Adnexal Mass

This term implus to any of the following:
(i) Functional ovarian cyst
(ii) Being tumor
(iii) Border line tumor
(iv) Malignant tumor

Lets deal with cell of the following categories separately:

1. Functional Cysts of Ovary

- They are these cysts which arise due to temporary hormonal disturbances
- These regress spontaneously
- M/C functional ovarian cyst: **Follicular cyst.**
- The follicular cysts are actually the stimulated follicles which did not undergo apeptosis during the cycle & continued to grow.
- A follicle is called as the cyst if it is ≥ 3 cm (30 mm).
- In the second half of menstrual cycle corpus luteum is formed which regresses in 12-14 days but if it fails to regress & becomes cystic or haemorrhagic, it is called as **corpus luteal cyst.**
- M/c cyst to Rupture:
  - Corpus luteal cyst

Also Know

Earlier it was recommended that females with functional cyst should be given combined oral pills for 3 months to hasten resolution. But evidence doesnot support its use now.

Ovarian Cysts in Pregnancy

"Theca luteal cyst is formed due to excessive HCG".

William gynae 3rd/ed, p219

Conditions where theca lutein cyst are formed:
- Molar pregnancy/gestational trophoblastic disease
- Twin pregnancy
- Ovulation induction with hCG or hMG
- Multifetal gestation
- Placentomegaly

Management:
Mostly the functional cyst resolve on their own. No treatment is needed

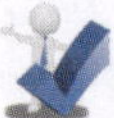

KEY POINTS

If in molar pregnancy, management of theca luteal cyst is asked– say nothing needs to be done
- Just manage molar pregnancy by suction evacuation.
- No special treatment of cyst is needed.

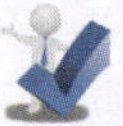

KEY POINTS

Complications of Ovarian Cyst
- Torsion (M/c tumor to undergo torsion – Dermoid cyst Management = immediate surgery → Detorsion and cystectomy, preserving the ovary)
- Rupture of cyst (M/c with corpus luteum cyst)
- Haemorrhage in cyst (M/c with serous cystadenoma)
- Infection: pseudomyxoma peritonei (M/c in mucinous cystadenoma)
- Malignancy (risk of malignancy is maximum in – Serous cystadenoma (40%)
  Least (1–2%) in dermoid cyst

(2) Benign Ovarian Tumors

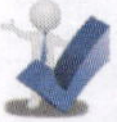

KEY POINTS

90% of all ovarian tumors in the reproductive age group are Benign. Physiological cysts are very common in this age group and must be considered as a possibility.

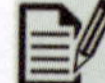

Points to Remember

High Risk Features of malignancy on USG:
(i) Bilateral
(ii) Solid mass/Multiocular cyst
(iii) Presence of thick septa (≥3 mm)
(iv) On surface: If papillary irregularties are present
(v) Presence of ascites
(vi) Presence of enlarged lymph nodes or matted bowel loops

Also Know

Risk of malignancy index (RMI)

RMI = U × M × value of CA125

U = Ultrasound score

M = Menopausal score

ULTRASOUND FINDINGS (1 point for each)

B = Bilateral

A =Ascites

M = Evidence of malignancy/metastases

S = Solid areas

U = 1 (for ultrasound scores of 0 or 1)

U = 3 (for ultrasound scores of 2-5)

MENOPAUSAL STATUS

- Postmenopausal: M = 3
- Premenopausal: M = 1

If **RMI>200:** Gynecologic Oncology referral is recommended as it is highly suggestive of malignancy.

V Imp

Indications for surgery on Adnexal mass

1. Any ovarian mass showing high risk features on USG
2. Size of ovarian mass ≥7 cm.
   Size of Adnexal mass ≥10 cm
3. Raised CA125 levels in Postmanopausal females (≥35 IU)

Note: In a Reproductive age female CA125 levels are not measured in a case of ovarian mass as CA125 levels can be raised due to many benign conditions like Endometriosis genital TB, PID. If the levels are ≥2000 IU: then it is significant.

4. In case of acute complications of cyst tumor like Torsion (M/c ovarian cyst/to undergo Torsion: Dermoid cyst)
5. For any diagnostic purpose

Case 1: Benign Mass in Reproductive age female.

No need for measuring CA125 levels

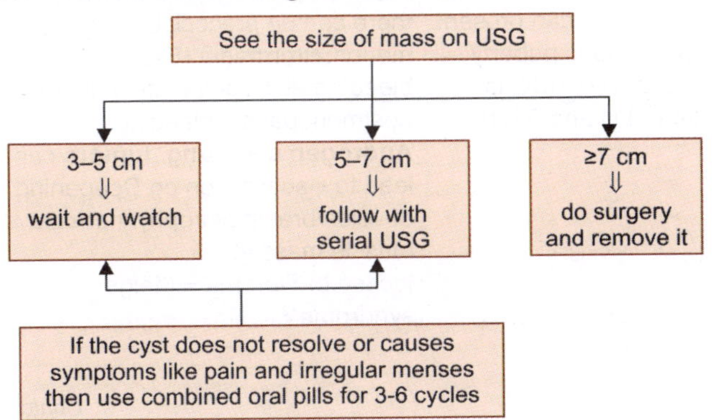

Case 2: Benign Mass in Extremes of age

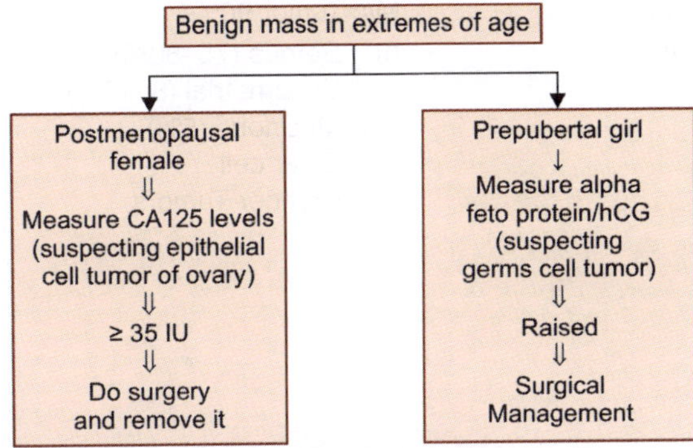

Case 3: Adnexal Mass in Pregnancy

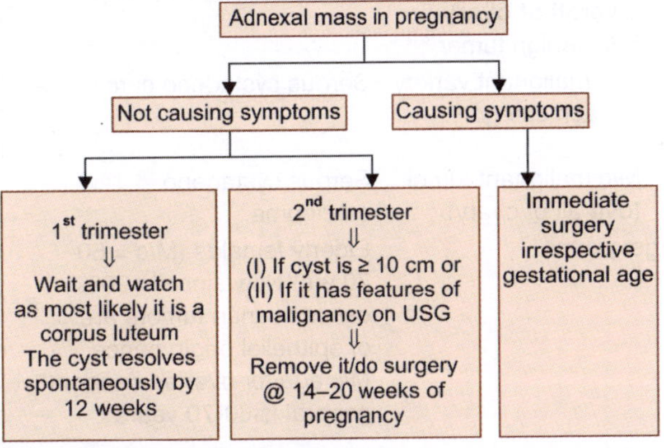

Important One Liners

- M/C ovarian cyst diagnosed in pregnancy- Dermoid cyst
- M/C ovarian tumor to undergo torsion in pregnancy- Dermoid cyst
- M/C time for ovarian cyst to undergo torsion in pregnancy- end of first trimester and/or puerperium

Important Concept

If an ovarian cyst is detected during puerperium: Management should be surgical removal as it will have high chances of undergoing torsion.

Also Know

Percentage of ovarian masses which become malignant:
In postmenopausal female = 30%
In premenopausal female = 7%

WHO Classification of Ovarian Tumors

Broad Categories:

(i) Epithelial cell tumors = 90%
(ii) Germ cell tumors = 5-8%
(iii) Sex cord tumors = 3%
(iv) Metastatic tumors = (Least common)

	Epithelial Cell Tumor	Germ Cell Tumor	Sex Cord Tumor
M/c Tumor	M/c Tumor 90%	5-8%	3%
Varieties	(i) Serous (75–80%) (ii) Endometrial (8–10%) (iii) Mucinous (5%) (iv) Clear cell (v) Brenner Tumors	Thank: Teratoma {Mature Immature = Dermoid cyst You=Yolk sac Tumor/ Endodermal sinus tumor C = Choriocarcinoma D = Dysgerminoma E = Embryonal tumor	A. Estrogen secreting tumors (i) Granulosa cell tumor (ii) Fibroma (iii) Thecoma B. Androgen secreting tumor (i) SERTO LI cell tumor (ii) LEYDIG cell tumor (iii) HILUS cell tumor C. Gynandroblastoma (both estrogen and androgen secreting
• M/c benign variety in the category	Serous cystadenoma	Dermoid cyst or mature cystic teratoma	
• **Overall of ovary**: M/c benign tumor		Dermoid cyst	
• M/c malignant variety in each category.	Serous cystadeno carcinoma	Recently it is Mature Teratoma (Earlier it was: Dysgerminoma)	
• M/c malignant tumor (overall of ovary)	Serous cystadeno carcinoma		
Age groups	Elderly females (M/c = 60-70 yrs) Now since in 90% cases ovarian tumors are of epithelial origin hence M/c age for ovarian caner in general is 60-70 years	Young females (10-20 years) Note: In age group 10-20 years, in 70% cases ovarian tumors are Germ cell Tumors). Hence if Question says:- M/c ovarian tumor in 10 – 20 years age group-GCT	Premenopausal female but it can be seen at any age group
U/L or Bilateral	Mostly B/L • Serous cystadenoma: 15-20% • Mucinous cystadenoma: 10% • Brener tumor: Mostly unilateral	Mostly U/L Incidence of bilaterality • Dysgermioma: 15-20% • Dermoid cyst: 10% • Yolk sac/Endodermal sinus tumor is 100% unilateral. Hence biopsy of opposite ovary is contraindicated	Mostly U/L Incidence of bilaterality in Granulosa cell tumor: ≤ 2%
Growth of tumor	Slow growing tumors	Rapidly growing tumors (Most Rapid is yolk sac tumor)	
Symptoms	Non specific symptoms: Nausea vomiting irritable Bowel syndrome Because of non specific symptoms, they are detected late In case of Mucinous tumors pseudomyoxma peretonei*1 In case of Brenner tumors*2 pseudo Meig syndrome.	• As they are rapid growing they present with subacute pain in abdomen • These tumors secrete hCG and so patient can present with precocious puberty (as α submit of hCG is similar to LH and FSH)	These are hormone secreting tumors **granulosa cells tumors secrete estrogen** so depending on age of patients there can be precocious puberty, menometrorrhagia (Excessive bleeding at irregular intervals) or postmenopausal bleeding. **Androgen secreting tumors** can lead to visualization eg Deepening of voice/breast astrophy/increase muscle mass etc Incase of Fibroma = Meigs syndrome*3

(*Note*: *1, *2, *3, all are discussed in detail, Later in the chapter).

Contd...

Contd…

	Epithelial Cell Tumor	Germ Cell Tumor	Sex Cord Tumor
Prognosis	Due to vague symptoms they will be detected at a late stage and so will have **bad prognosis**	**Better prognosis** • GCT with best prognosis is Dysgerminoma (very highly Radiosensitive and chemosensitive tumor • GCT with worst prognosis: Yolk sac Tumor	Best prognosis as it has very specific symptoms so detected at very early stage
Malignant potential	• Serous variety – Benign = 65% – Malignant 35-40% (serous cyst adenocar-cinoma) – Mucinous 25% = (mucinous adenocarcinoma) – Brenner = Mostly benign (<2% malignant) • Clear cell Tumor: Highly malignant • Endometrial tumor: – Low malignant potential – Lining epithelium has resemblance to Endometrium of uterus – When it becomes malignant it changes to Endometrial cancer – It is Associated with Endometriosis	• M/c malignant GCT: – Immature teratoma > Dysgerminoma • Most malignant GCT = Yolk sac tumor • Dermoid cyst becomes malignant < 2% cases & when it becomes malignant the M/c malignancy which occurs in squamous cell carcinoma (Not immature Teratoma)	Granulosa cell tumor: secretes estrogen which can lead to Endometrial hyperplasia (in 25–50% cases) or Endometrial cancer (in 5% cases)
Route of spread	M/c = Transcoelomic/ Transpertioneal spread 2nd M/c = Lymphatic 3rd = Hematogenous	M/c = Transcoelomic/ Transpertioneal spread 2nd M/c = Lymphatic 3rd = Hematogenous **Remember**: Dysgerminoma can metastaze to opposite ovary and lower vertebra	Lymph node metastasis is rare. Granulosa cell tumor is a slow growing tumor which remains confined to ovary for a long time but if it spreads then M/c site is opposite ovary
Staging method	Surgical staging (Details discussed late)	Surgical staging	Surgical staging
Management	Surgical staging (TAH + BSO or Debulking surgery) Followed by chemotherapy in all stages: except stage IA & IB grade I & grade II. Chemotherapy cisplatin or carboplatin + paclitaxel	Conservative surgery (unilateral salpingo oophorectomy) + Chemotherapy in all stages (No exception) chemotherapy of choice is B = Bleomycin E= Etoposide P = Cisplatin/Carboplatin	Depending on age → Young Female → Unilateral Salpingoophorectomy; Older Female → TAH + BSO • Surgery is followed by chemotherapy in stages III and IV only Chemotherapy of choice BEP.

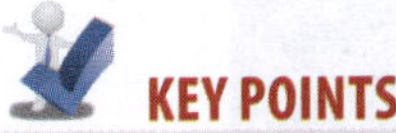

KEY POINTS

Ovary is most Radiosensitive pelvic organ but ovarian cancers are Radioresistant tumors hence there is no role of radiotherapy. Most radiosensitive ovarian tumor = Dysgerminoma

Detailed Discussion about Some Important Ovarian Tumors

Dermoid Cyst

- M/c benign tumor of ovary: Dermoid cyst
- M/c benign epithelial tumor of ovary: serous cyst adenoma
- M/c solid benign tumor of ovary: fibroma
- M/c benign tumor of ovary in pregnancy = dermoid cyst
- M/c malignant tumor of ovary in pregnancy = Dysgerminoma

2 Important Percentages to Remember in Dermoid Cyst

% of Bilaterality in Dermoid = 10%
% Chances of malignancy in Dermoid = <2%

- Age group = M/C = Reproductive age group. But it can be seen in postmenopausal females as well as new born girls.
- Dermoid cyst usually contains derivatives of ectoderm, endoderm and mesoderm. Most common element is ectodermal (present in 100% cases)
- Characteristically they are unilocular cyst containing hair and cheesy sebaceous material, teeth, bones, thyroid tissue and cartilage.
- It is lined by keratinized squamous epithelium
- On cross-section—they typically show an area of localised growth from which hair projects, teeth and bone are seen. It is called as Rokintansky protuberance or dermoid process (see Fig. 14C.4).
- Malignant change in a dermoid cyst occurs in 0.5-2% cases in patients more than 40 years. Most common malignancy which develops is, squamous cell carcinoma

Radiographic Features

Plain radiograph may show calcific and tooth components with in the pelvis (Fig. 14C.1) on raised area called as **Rokinstansky Protuberance**

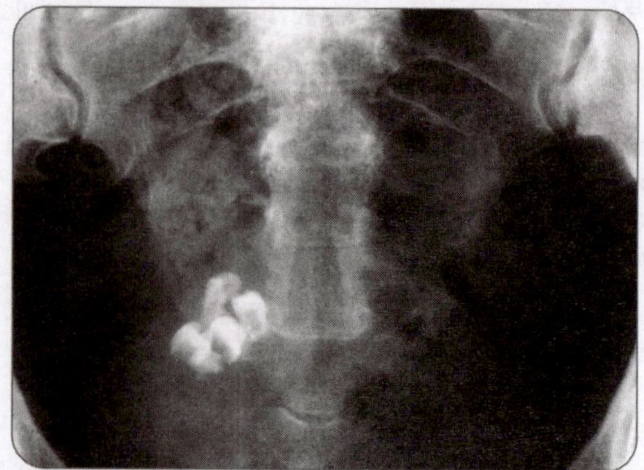

Fig. 14C.1: Radiograph of dermoid cyst showing calcific and tooth components within the pelvis

Pelvic Ultrasound

- Ultrasound is the preferred imaging modality. Most lesions are unilocular.
  The spectrum of sonographic features includes:
  - Most characteristics appearance: White ball appearance due to hair and sebum (Fig. 14C.2).
  - Multiple thin, echogenic bands caused by hair in the cyst cavity: **The dot-dash pattern** (Fig. 14C.3).
  - Hyperechoic Rokitansky nodule: Dermoid plug with shadowing (Fig. 14C.4).
- On Colour Doppler: No internal vascularity seen.

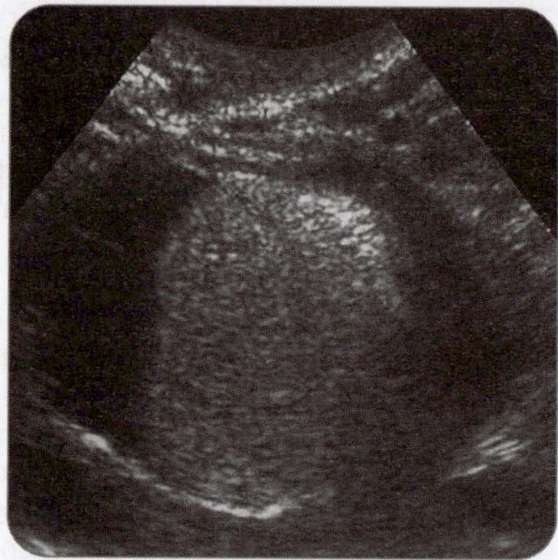

Fig. 14C.2: White ball appearance of dermoid cyst on USG

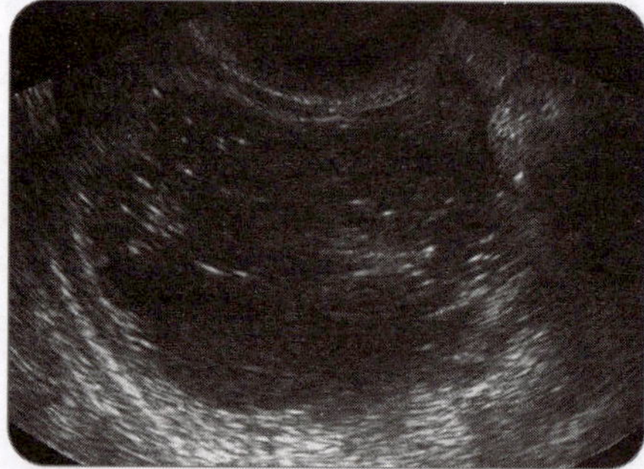

Fig. 14C.3: Dash and dot appearance of dermoid cyst on USG

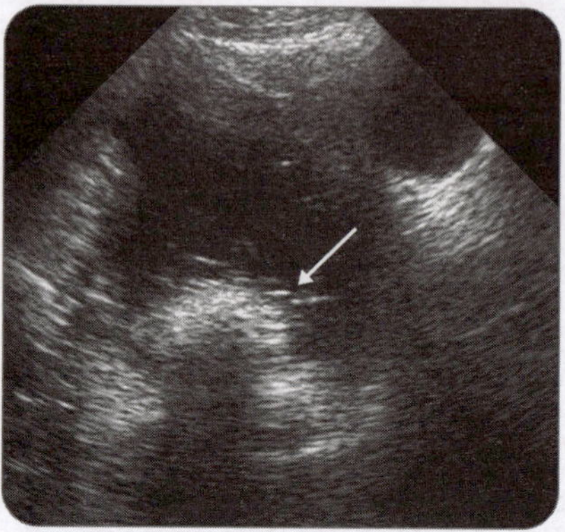

Fig. 14C.4: Rokintansky protuberance in dermoid cyst on USG

Benign Epithelial Tumors of Ovary

Serous cystadenoma	Mucinous cystadenoma	Brenners tumor
Resembles the epithelium of ovary or fallopian tube (Recent studies show that it resembles more like ciliated epithelium of fallopian tube)	Resembles glandular epithelium of cervix	Resembles the transitional epithelium
Percentage of bilaterality 20%	10%	Mostly unilateral
Malignant potential 40%	≤ 20%	Mostly benign (malignant less 2%)
Unilocular cyst (Thin walled) filled with clear fluid	Mostly multilocular cyst filled with mucinous fluid	Solid benign tumor with rubbery consistency
Histological pathological characteristic PSAMMOMA body	On cut section it gives a honey coob appearance. No other HP characteristic	Walthard cell rest and coffee bean nuclei
PSAMMOMA body has concentric fine granules seen on X-Ray		—
—	It is associated with pseudo myxoma peretonei	It is associated with pseudo Meig syndrome

Histopathological Examination

- **Histopathologically:** Serous tumors show presence of **psammoma bodies**. In histopathology of serous cystadenocarcinoma you will see papillary (finger like) structures and cystic spaces lined by ciliated epithelium. Their will be malignant cells (atypical cells showing mitosis) which will indicate it is cystadenocarcinoma. Now if the histopathological slide is predominantly blue it means it is serous cyst adenocarcinoma (Fig. 14C.5A) because in mucinous cystadenocarcinoma, there will be abundant mucinous cystoplasm, making it more white (Fig. 14C.5B).

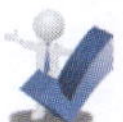

KEY CONCEPT

Benign Tumors of ovary are mostly cystic in consistency and malignant tumors are solid

2 exceptions are:

Solid Benign Tumors of ovary:

M/c Fibroma

2nd M/c = Brenner tumor

Other solid ovarian tumors are: Krukenberg tumors

Pseudomyxoma Peritonei

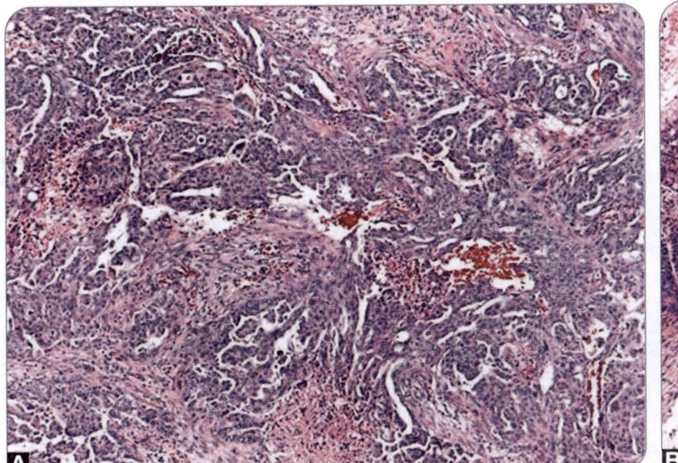

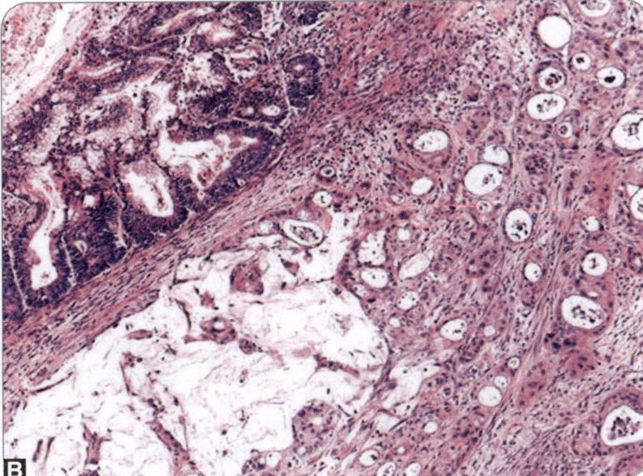

Figs. 14C.5A and B: (A) Serous cystadenoma; (B): Mucinous cystadenoma

Pseudomyxoma peritonei is a condition in which the neoplastic epithelium secretes large amounts of gelatinous mucinous material. So the peritoneal cavity is filled with mucinous material. It is most commonly seen secondary to:

- M/c appendicular carcinoma *(well differentiate carcinoma)*.
- Ovarian mucinous carcinoma; mucinous cystadenoma.
- Mucocoele of appendix (less commonly seen).

Even after removal of the ovarian tumors, these cells continue to secrete mucin.

Tendency of *recurrence* is present.

Prognosis is Poor:

Management: Hysterectomy with Bilateral salpingo-oophorectomy with removal of mucinous peritoneal implants along with appendix.

Meigs syndrome Combination of fibroma with ascites and hydrothorax, usually right sided is called as Meigs syndrome. Seen in 1-5% patients.

Criteria for diagnosis of Meig's syndrome

- Tumor must be ovarian, solid and benign–Fibroma
- Both hydrothorax and ascites must be present.
- Removal of the tumor must result in their spontaneous and permanent cure.

Pseudomeig syndrome: When ascites and hydrothorax occur with Brenner tumor, Thecoma and Granulosa Cell Tumor it is called as Pseudomeig syndrome.

Endometroid Tumor

- It is the ovarian epithelial cancer which has highest association with endometrial cancer (15 to 20%)
- It is also associated with endometriosis
- Have low malignant potential
- 40% are Bilateral

Important One Liners

- Ovarian cancer which has highest risk of endometrial cancer is **endometrioid epithelial ovarian cancer** (15–20% risk)

Clear Cell Carcinoma

- It an also be associated with **endometriosis**
- Always **high grade tumors** (grade 3 tumors)
- It is **chemoresistant**
- Histological characteristic is large epithelial cells with clear cytoplasm due to **glycogen**
- The clear cell carcinoma is histologically identical to that seen in uterus & vagina in females exposed to DES in utero.

Borderline Tumors

Also called as low malignant potential tumors

- Seen at younger age group 30–50 yrs (whereas malignant epithelial tumors are seen in ages 50–70 years)
- These tumors display malignant characteristic like:
  - Nuclear atypia present
  - Mitosis seen (<4/10 per high power filed)
  - Epithelial hyperplasia present

  But the characteristic which distinguishes term from malignant variety is:

  Absence of stromal invasion
- Approximately 10% of all epithelial tumors are borderline out of which 30% are mucinous variety.
- The tumors remain confined to single ovary for a very long time and are slow growing and thus have a good prognosis (5 year survival rate >99%)

Note: Up to 40% of serious borderline tumors may spread beyond ovary. But that does not necessarily near it has become malignant.

Management: Conservative surgery i.e unilateral salpingoophorectomy.

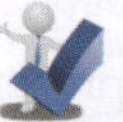

KEY CONCEPT

Conservative surgery in ovarian cancer is unilateral salpingo-oophorectomy which has only few indications. Rest in all cases radical surgery in the form of bilateral salpingo-oophorectomy with. Total Abdominal Hysterectomy is done.

Indications of conservative surgery in ovarian cancer:

1. Borderline tumors
2. Germ cell tumor
3. Sex cord tumor in young female
4. Epithelial cell tumors in early stages in young females.

MALIGNANT OVARIAN TUMORS

Etiology of Ovarian Cancers

There are 2 theories related to development of ovarian cancer:

i. **Excessive estrogen:** Ovarian cancer like endometrial cancer is an hyperestrogenic condition.

ii. **The theory of incessant ovulation:** Which means as the frequency of ovulation increases, risk of ovarian cancer also increases so based on these two theories the risk factors and protective factors for ovarian cancers are:

Risk factors	Protective factors
• Nulliparity • Obesity • Early menarche and late menopause • Clomiphene citrate or ovulation inducing drugs • Infertility/PCOD • Workers in asbestos factory • Dysgenetic gonads • HRT +/-	• Multiparity • Pregnancy • Exercise • Smoking as it inhibits enzyme aromatase • Anovulation • OCP's (as they bring about anovulation) • Breast feeding • Tubal ligation and Hysterectomy (as they do not allow ovary to get exposed to carcinogens)

Epidemiology

- Life time risk of developing ovarian cancer is 1 in 70 (1.4%)
- Ovarian cancer is fifth leading cause of cancer related death worldwide in females, after – lung > breast > colorectal > pancreatic > ovarian cancer
  - Peak incidence of invasive epithelial ovarian cancer is 56 to 60 years of age.[Q]
  - Average age for borderline tumors is 46 years.[Q]
- 5–10% of epithelial ovarian cancers have hereditary predisposition.[Q]
- **About 30% of ovarian neoplasia in postmenopausal women are malignant whereas only about 7% of ovarian epithelial tumors in premenopausal females are malignant.**[Q]

Hereditary Breast and Ovarian Cancer

- Most hereditary ovarian cancers are associated with mutations in **BRCA 1** located on chromosome 17. Small proportions have mutations in BRCA 2 gene located on chromosome 13.
- 5–10% ovarian tumors are hereditary
- The mutations are inherited in an autosomal dominant patterns

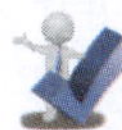

KEY POINTS

Women with BRCA gene mutations have a life time risk of breast cancer of 82%,

BRCA1 → Ovarian cancer (54%)

BRCA2 → Ovarian cancer (23%)

HNPCC → Ovarian cancer (15%)

Note: **Hereditary ovarian cancers occur in women approximately 10 years younger than those with nonhereditary tumors.**

- BRCA-1 is more carcinogenic than BRCA-2.
- **Lynch II Syndrome/HNPCC–hereditary non polyposis colorectal cancer (HNPCC)**
  It includes multiple adenocarcinomas and involves a combination of familial colon cancer (Lynch I); a high-rate of ovarian, endometrial, breast cancers; genitourinary cancer and hereditary nonpolyposis coli.
  Mutations associated with it are MSH2, MLH1, PMS1 & PMS2

Recommendations for Hereditary Cancer

Current recommendations for management of women at high risk for ovarian cancer are summarized as follows:

- Women who appear to be at high risk for ovarian or breast cancer should undergo genetic counseling and, if the risk appears to be substantial (i.e. a calculated risk of at least 10% in having a mutation in BRCA1 or BRCA2), may be offered genetic testing for BRCA1 and BRCA 2.
- Women who wish to preserve their reproductive capacity can undergo screening by transvaginal ultrasonography every 6 months, although the efficacy of this approach is not established.
- Oral contraceptives should be recommended to young women before they embark on an attempt to have a family but the risk of breast cancer and cervical cancer should be kept in mind.
- **Women who do not wish to maintain their fertility or who** have completed their **families should be recommended to undergo prophylactic bilateral salpingo-oophorectomy after the age of 35, but definitely by age 40 years**. These women should be counseled that this operation does not offer absolute protection, because peritoneal carcinomas can occur after bilateral salpingo-oophorectomy.

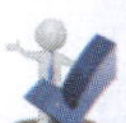

KEY POINTS

After bilateral salpingo-oophorectomy risk of:
- Ovarian cancer is decreased by 96%
- Breast cancer is decreased by 50% to 80%

- In women who have a strong family history of breast or ovarian cancer, annual breast screening should be performed beginning at age 30 years using a combination of magnetic resonance imaging (MRI), mammograms, and ultrasound. Ideally, these women should be followed in clinics that manage women at high risk for cancer.
- In women with HNPCC, hysterectomy is mandatory when performing prophylactic BSO because of coexisting endometrial cancer risk. In BRCA mutations it is not routinely recommended.

Malignant Epithelial Tumors:
- Associated with p 53 & Kras gene mutation
- The M/c gene mutation seen is p 53 gene mutation

Rest all details of epithelial tumors we have discussed in detail in the table.

Germ Cell Tumors

Dysgerminoma (Fig. 14C.7)

Points already discussed	New points to Remember
• 2nd M/c malignant GCT • It is the GCT with best prognosis • Most Radio sensitive ovarian tumor • M/c ovarian cancer in pregnancy	It is associated with dysgenetic gonads (i.e. gonads with Y chromosome present) e.g. Turners syndrome (45 × 0/46 XY) Swyers syndrome (46 XY) Testicular ferminizing syndrome (46 XY)

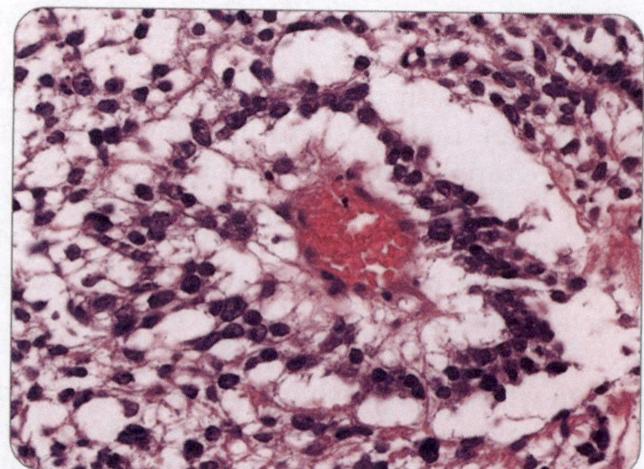

Fig. 14C.6: Schiller-Duval bodies. It consists of a central vessel surrounded by tumor cells—the whole structure being contained in a cystic space lined by tumor cells

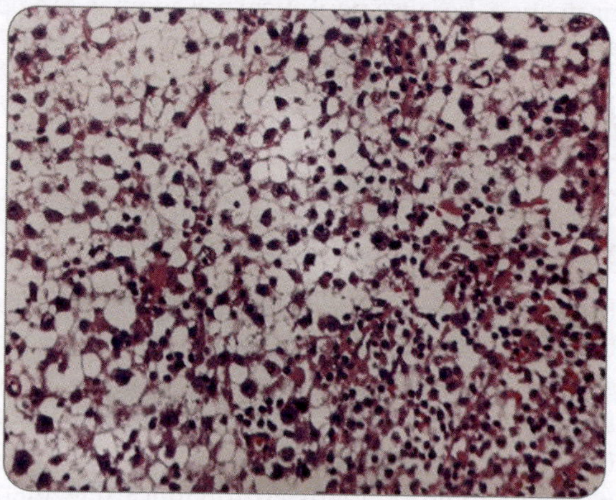

Fig. 14C.7: Histological characteristic of dysgerminoma. The ovary showing large round, ovoid or polygonal cells with abundant clear, very pale staining cytoplasm large and irregular nuclei and prominent nucleoli

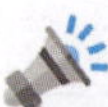

Important One Liners

- M/c ovarian tumor associated with dysgenetic gonads:- Gonadoblastoma
- M/c benign tumor associated with dysgenetic gonads = Gonadoblastoma
- M/c ovarian cancer (malignant) associated with dysgenetic gonads = Dysgerminoma

Tumor Marker: Placental alkaline phosphate + LDH

Appearance: (Fig. 14C.7)

Grossly: The dysgerminoma is solid, has a lobulated appearance & is pink/tan in colour.

On HPE = Large polyhedral cells rich in glycogen, with clear/white cytoplasm

- Large prominent nuclei
- Eosinophilic fibrous septa present

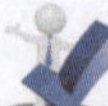

KEY POINTS

Dysgerminomas are also seen in phenotypic females with abnormal gonads like:

- Pure gonadal dysgenesis (46XY with bilateral streak gonads, Swyer syndrome)
- Mixed gonadal dysgenesis
- Testicular feminization syndrome (46XY)
- Klinefelter syndrome
- For patients in whom karyotype reveals Y chromosome, both ovaries should be removed although uterus may be left in situ for possible future embryo transfer.

Dysgerminoma in pregnancy

- M/c ovarian tumor detected during pregnancy - Dermoid
- M/c malignant tumor detected in pregnancy - Dysgerminoma.

Early stage dysgerminoma (Stage Ia)

- Tumor can be removed intact and pregnancy continued.

Advanced disease

- Continuation of pregnancy depends on the gestational age of fetus.
- Chemotherapy can be given in the second and third trimester in the same dosages as given for the nonpregnant patient without apparent detriment to the fetus.

Yolk Sac Tumor (Endodermal Sinus Tumor

Points already learnt	New points to learn
• It is the most malignant GCT • It is the GCT with the worst prognosis • It is unilateral in 100% cases	On Histopathological examination: Schiller–Duval bodies are present

Histopathology: Schiller–Duval body: (Fig. 14C.6)

- It is a central (Red) capillary surrounded by tumor cells. These cells are present in a cystic space

Tumor Marker: Alpha feto protein and antitrypsin.

Sex Cord Tumor: Granulosa Cell Tumor (Fig. 14C.8)

Points already learnt	New points to lean
• It is an estrogen secreting tumor • **At various age groups it has different presentations:** – Puberty–precocious puberty – Reproductive age – Menometrorrhagia – Menopausal age– Post menopausal bleeding • Best prognosis in all ovarian tumors.	On HPE: Call-Exner bodies seen. • The entire slide of HPE of granulosa cell tumor will be overcrowded with cells • Cells have scanty pale cystoplasma • Large nuclei with longitudinal slit i.e. coffee bean *nuclei* • *Cell–Exner body:* Small eosinophilic fluid spaces with rosette arrangement of cells around it.

Tumor Marker: Inhibin

Note: The etiology of SCST's is unknown but a single recurrent FOXL2 gene mutation is present in virtually all cases.

Masculanising Tumors

Arrhenoblastoma/ Androblastoma Hilus cell Tm	Adrenal cortical Tm/ Lipoid cell Tm of ovary	Gynandroblastoma
• Affect child bearing age group (10–35 years) **It includes :** • Sertoli Cell Tumor (SCT) • Leydig cell Tumor • Sertoli – Leydig cell Tumor	• Seen in postmenopausal females • Characterised by presence of Reinke's crystals	• Combination of granulosa cell tumor & arrheno blastoma

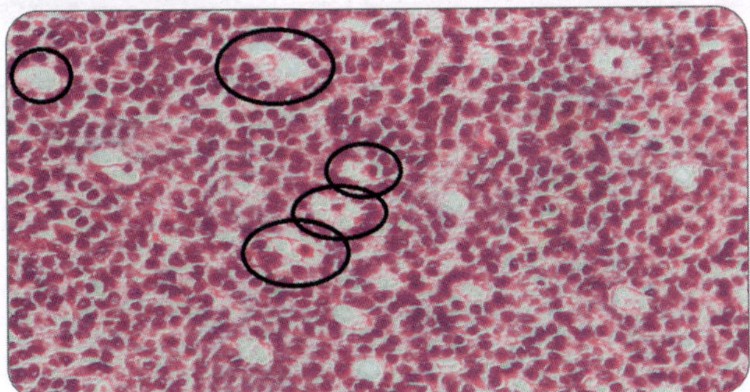

Fig. 14C.8: Call-Exner bodies are small eosinophilic fluid filled spaces between granulosa cells

Presentation : They are low grade malignancies.

All masculinizing tumors cause defeminization, followed by masculinization.

Patient complain of :
- Altered body contour
- Scanty and irregular menstruation followed by amenorrhoea
- Flattening of breast
- Increased hair growth – hirsutism
- Clitoromegaly
- Receding hair line
- Hoarseness of voice

Diagnosis: Serum Testosterone levels raised >200 ng/dL and increased androstenedione.

(DHEAS may be normal which helps to differentiate it from a masculinizing adrenal tumor)

Also know: Tumor Markers of Various Ovarian Cancer

Tumor	Tumor Marker
Epithelial nonmucinous tumor	CA125 Mainly alters Human epididymal pattern 4, OVA 1
Mucinous tumor	CA19-9, CEA
Yolk sac tumor	Alfa feto protein (Anti Trypsin alpha1
Choriocarcinoma	hCG
Dysgerminoma	LDH, alkaline phosphate
Embryonal carcinoma	hCG alpha feto protein
Granulosa cell tumor	Inhibin

Surgical Staging of Ovarian Cancer

Steps of Staging Surgical Laparotomy in Ovarian Cancer:
- Open the abdomen by a midline vertical incision (Remember: it is not a transverse incision)
- Look at all the organs
- Palpate all the organs and surfaces
- Take samples
  - Ascitic fluid is present
  - If no ascitic fluid is present then do saline wash & take the wash fluid
  - Pelvic lymphnodes
  - Scrapings of diaphragm
- Do biopsy (Multiple peritoneal biopsies)
- **Do surgery:**

TAH + BSO + Infracolic metectomy (*Note:* Not omental biopsy).

> **Also Know**
>
> In case of mucinous tumors one additional step, appendicectomy is done.
>
> **In case of advanced cancer:** TAH + BSO is replaced by Debulking surgery

FIGO Staging of Ovarian Cancer (2014)

Table 14C.1:

Stage I: Tumor confined to ovaries	
IA	Tumor limited to 1 ovary, capsule intact, no tumor on surface, negative washings.
IB	Tumor involves both ovaries rest like IA.
IC Tumor limited to 1 or both ovaries	
IC1	Surgical spill (Intra operative capsule rupture)
IC2	Capsule rupture before surgery or tumor on ovarian surface.
IC3	Malignant ascites or peritoneal washings.

Stage II: Tumor involves 1 or both ovaries with pelvic extension (below the pelvic brim) or primary peritoneal cancer	
IIA	Tumor spreads to uterus or Fallopian tubes
IIB	Spreads to other pelvic organs and pelvic nodes.

Stage III: Tumor involves 1 or both ovaries with cytologically or histologically confirmed spread to the peritoneum outside the pelvis and/or metastasis to the retroperitoneal lymph nodes		
IIIA (Positive retroperitoneal lymph nodes and/or microscopic metastasis beyond the pelvis.		
IIIA1	Positive retroperitoneal lymph nodes only Para-aortic	
	IIIA 1(i)	Metastasis ≤ 10 mm
	IIIA 1(ii)	Metastasis > 10 mm
IIIA2	Microscopic extrapelvic (above the brim) peritoneal involvement ± positive retroperitoneal lymph nodes	
IIIB	Macroscopic extrapelvic peritoneal deposit ≤ 2 cm with or without involvement of retroperitoneal lymph nodes includes extension to capsule of liver/spleen.	
IIIC	Macroscopic extrapelvic, peritoneal metastasis > 2 cm with or without involvement of retroperitoneal lymph nodes includes extension to capsule of liver/ spleen.	

Stage IV: Tumor involves 1 or both ovaries with cytologically or histologically confirmed spread to the peritoneum outside the pelvis and/or metastasis to the retroperitoneal lymph nodes	
IVA	Pleural effusion with positive cytology
IVB	• Hepatic and/or splenic parenchymal metastasis • Metastasis to extra-abdominal organs • Inguinal lymph nodes

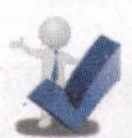

KEY POINTS

Inguinal lymph nodes are involved in—

Ca ovary – stage IVB

Ca Endometrium – stage IVB

Ca Cervix – stage IVB

Note:

In ovarian cancer

- Pelvic LN involved in stage – IIB
- Para-aortic LN involved in stage IIIA
- Inguinal LN involved in stage IVB

Management of Epithelial Ovarian Tumors

In ovarian cancers similar to endometrial cancer – staging is surgical i.e. Hysterectomy with Bilateral Salpingo Oophorectomy has already been performed. Therefore treatment basically consists of postoperative management. The preferred post operative treatment in ovarian tumors is chemotherapy. 6 cycles of carboplatin and paclitaxel and in advanced cases cisplatin and paclitaxel.

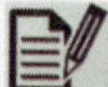

Definition

Debulking, also called **cytoreduction,** is defined as removal of as much tumor as possible during surgical exploration. Optimal cytoreduction implies that tumor nodules no larger than 1.5 cm in diameter are left behind and survival improves as the amount of residual diseases decreases.

Stagewise Management of Ovarian Tumors

Table 14C.2

Stage	Management
Low malignant potential tumors, i.e. stage I (A or B) Grade I and II	Surgical staging. No postoperative treatment required ***Note:*** In a young woman who wish to preserve fertility if intraoperative findings are consistent with stage I, unilateral salpingo oophorectomy may be performed. The uterus and the contralateral ovary can be removed later when the patient has completed child bearing.
Stage	**Management**
Stage I (A or B) Grade III and all grades of Stages IC and II	Surgical staging followed by three to six cycles of chemotherapy postoperatively (carboplatin and paclitaxel).
Advanced ovarian cancer – Stage III/IV	Cytoreduction or debulking surgery followed by six cycle of platinum based chemotherapy (cisplatin + paclitaxel preferred) each cycle given after 3 weeks.

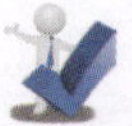

KEY POINTS

- Primary cytoreductive surgery, or debulking is central in the treatment of advanced disease because maximal cytoreduction is one of the most powerful predictor of survival in patients with advanced cancer. The determination of residual disease does not include the total volume of tumor cells left behind but rather the diameter of the largest single residual nodule.
- The 'gold standard' for identifying residual disease is second look laparotomy.

Neoadjuvant therapy i.e. initial treatment with chemotherapy followed by interval debulking surgery is also suggested.

Indications

- Patients with medical conditions which prohibit initial surgery.
- In patients in whom suboptimal debulking is likely.

Posttreatment Surveillance plan consists of physical examination with rectovaginal examination, CA-125 testing, and CT scan every 3 months for the first 2 years.

Metastatic Ovarian Carcinoma

First Type	Second Type *(Krukenberg Tumor)*
• They are metastatic tumors from Intestine, Gall bladder, pancreas, corpus, and cervix • They are most commonly bilateral • They have irregular surface • The method of ovarian infiltration is by surface implantation or retrograde implantation	• They are metastatic tumors from stomach (70%), large bowel (15%) and breast (6%) • They are always bilateral.[Q] • They have a smooth surface which may be slightly bossed. • Always arise by retrograde lymphatic spread.

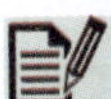

Most common

M/C cancer metastasizing to ovary in decreasing order

- Colon
- Breast
- GIT/stomach
- Appendiceal

Krukenberg Tumor

- Krukenberg tumor by definition ***represent carcinoma of stomach metastasised to ovary***. But the eponym is commonly used to denote any gastric cancer metastatic to ovary
- Tumor arise by *retrograde lymphatic spread*[Q] i.e. carcinoma cells pass from the stomach to the superior gastric lymphnode which also receive lymphatics from ovary.

Characteristics of Krukenberg Tumor

- Always bilateral[Q]
- Have smooth surface[Q]
- No tendency to form adhesions
- Freely mobile
- No infiltration through the capsule.
- Histologically tumor has signet ring cells in the background of myxomatous stroma.
- They retain the shape of normal ovary.[Q]
- Have waxy consistency.[Q]

Histological Characteristics of Ovarian Tumors

Table 14C.3

Feature	Associated tumor
Call-Exner bodies & coffee bean nuclei	Granulosa cell tumor
Schiller duval bodies	Endodermal sinus tumor
Reinke's crystal	Hilus cell tumor
Psammoma bodies	Serous epithelial tumors
Walthard cell nest	Brenner tumor
Signet ring cell	Krukenberg tumor
Hobnail cell	Clear cell tumor
Large polygonal cell with lymphocytic infiltration and fibrous septa	Dysgerminoma
Skin, teeth, cartilage	Teratoma

Tumor Markers of Ovarian Neoplasm

Table 14C.4

Ovarian tumor	Tumor marker
Epithelial cell Tumor-Serous variety	• CA 125 • Mucinous variety-Ca 19-9,CEA • Both serous and mucinous variety-OCCA, OCA
Germ cell tumors Choriocarcinoma = hCG Yuck sac Tm = AFP 1 and alpha 1 anti trypsin Dysgerminoma = LDH PL alkaline phosphatase Embryonal = AFP hCG	
Granulosa cell tumor	Inhibin

Important Points

Physical Characteristics Differentiating Benign and Malignant Ovarian Tumors

Table 14C.5

Benign	Malignant
M/C in reproductive age	M/C in extremes of age
History of pain present	Usually painless Pain is seen in last stages
Mostly unilateral	Mostly bilateral
Have cystic consistency	Variable consistency
Tender	Non tender (Old age adolescent age)

IOC to distinguish between Benign and Malignant tumor is ultrasound (TUS > ATAS)

Ultrasound Characteristics of Benign vs Malignant Ovarian Tumors

Table 14C.6

Physical examination	Benign tumor	Malignant tumor
Mobility	Mobile & smooth	Fixed, and have surface irregularities
Consistency	Cystic	Solid or firm
Laterality	Unilateral	Bilateral
Cul-de-sac	Smooth on P/V examination	Nodular on P/V examination
Radiography		
Size	Usually < 10 cm size	Any size
Septations	< 2 mm thickness	Multiple septations ≥ 3 mm in size
Calcification	Seen in teratoma	Usually absent
Omental caking	Absent	Seen
Ascites	Absent	Present
Intraoperative	Unilateral cyst with no adhesion Capsule intact	Solid areas with adhesion. Rupture may occur. Capsule is breached

NEW PATTERN QUESTIONS

N1. All of the following are germ cell tumors of the ovary *except*:
a. Teratoma b. Fibroma
c. Dysgerminoma d. Endodermal sinus tumor

N2. Sex cord stromal tumors of the ovary include all except:
a. Luteomas
b. Gynandroblastomas
c. Sertoli-Leydig cell tumors of the ovary
d. Theca-fibroma

N3. M/C functional cyst of ovary is:
a. Chocolate cyst b. Follicular cyst
c. Dermoid cyst d. Corpus luteal cyst

N4. Lutein cysts are associated with all *except*:
a. Gestational trophoblastic tumors
b. Clomiphene administration
c. Bilaterality
d. Use of OCP's

N5. Management of a 5 cm dermoid cyst which has undergone torsion at 10 weeks of pregnancy is:
a. Wait and watch b. Removal in 2nd trimester
c. Immediate removal d. Serial USG monitoring

N6. A 52-years-old postmenopausal female presents unilocular with a ovarian cyst of 6 cm with normal Ca125 levels management is:
a. USG guided ovarian tapping
b. Wait and watch
c. Surgery d. OCP

N7. M/C benign ovarian tumor is:
a. Serous cystadenoma b. Mucinous cystadenoma
c. Mature cystic teratoma d. Immature cystic teratoma

N8. Psammoma bodies are see in:
a. Serous tumors b. Brenner tumor
c. Fibroma d. Endodermal sinus tumor

N9. M/C cause of pseudomyxoma peritonei:
a. Mucocele of appendix
b. Mucinous cystadenoma
c. Mucinous cystadenocarcinoma
d. Appendix carcinoma

N10. Dash and dot appearance on USG is seen in:
a. Adenomyosis b. Dermoid cyst of ovary
c. Molar pregnancy d. Serous tumors of ovary

N11. Percentage chances of ovarian cancer, in first degree relatives, if a 65 years old female dies to ovarian cancer within first year of its detection:
a. 3% b. 10%
c. 15% d. No risk

N12. M/C gene mutation in epithelial cell ovarian tumors:
a. p 53 gene b. KRAS
c. BRCA d. PTEN

N13. M/C ovarian cancer associated with endometriosis:
a. Endometroid tumor b. Clear cell tumor
c. Germ cell tumor d. Brenner tumor

N14. Para-aortic lymph node involvement is seen in which stage of ovarian cancer?
a. Stage II A b. Stage II B
c. Stage III A d. Stage III B

N15. Germ cell tumor with the best prognosis:
a. Dysgerminoma
b. Teratoma
c. Endodermal sinus tumor
d. Embryonal carcinoma

N16. Malignant ovarian tumor seen in dysgenetic gonads:
a. Serous cystadenocarcinoma
b. Endodermal sinus tumor
c. Granulosa cell tumor
d. Dysgerminoma

N17. The following statements are related to Krukenberg tumor *except*:
a. It is always secondary
b. The most common primary site is pylorus of the stomach
c. The tumor is bilateral
d. 'Signet ring' looking cells are characteristic

N 18. Protective factor for ovarian cancer:
a. Nulliparity
b. Bilateral Tubectomy
c. Dysgenetic gonads
d. Woker of asbestos industry

N19. All of the following are features of Borderline tumors *except*:
a. Occurs in younger age
b. Mitotic figures < 9/10 per high power filed
c. Very good prognosis
d. Stromal invasion seen

N20. Bilateral ovarian tumor with pleural effusion is staged as:
a. Stage II A b. Stage III A
c. Stage IV A d. Stage IV B

N21. Largest benign ovarian tumor:
a. Serous cystadenoma b. Brenner tumor
c. Fibroma d. Mucinous cystadenoma

N22. All are correctly matched *except*:
a. Dermoid cyst: bone
b. Mucinous tumor: Psammoma bodies
c. Krukenberg tumor: Signet ring cells
d. Brenner tumor: Walthard and cell risk

N23. RMI value of ------- denotes possible malignancy:
a. > 200 b. > 250
c. > 300 d. > 350

N24. Favourable prognostic factors for ovarian cancer: are cell *except*:
a. Young age
b. Mucinous tumor
c. Well differentiated tumor
d. No ascites

N25. M/C ovarian tumor in a 15-year-old female:
a. Sex cord tumor b. Matastatic tumor
c. Germ cell tumor d. Epithelial tumor

PREVIOUS YEAR QUESTIONS

General

1. **Which of the following statement(s) is/are true about cysts in ovary except?** *(PGI May 2017)*
   a. Follicular cyst is least common among functional cyst
   b. Corpus luteal cysts are often associated with pregnancy
   c. Dermoid cysts are germ cell tumor
   d. Fibroma of ovary is associated with Meig's syndrome
   e. Theca Leutin cyst is seen in association with hydatiform mole and GnRH analogue use
2. **All of the following are known risk factors for the development of ovarian carcinoma except:** *(AIIMS 03)*
   a. Family history of ovarian carcinoma
   b. Use of oral pills
   c. Use of Clomiphene
   d. BRCA - 1 positive individual
3. **Which of the following strategy has been recommended to reduce the heredity risk for ovarian cancer in women with BRCA - 1 and BRCA - 2 mutations?** *(AIIMS 05)*
   a. Use of oral contraceptive pills
   b. Screening with transvaginal ultrasound
   c. Screening with CA - 125
   d. Prophylactic oophorectomy
4. **Most common ovarian tumor in less than 20 years is:** *(AIIMS 97)*
   a. Epithelial tumor
   b. Germ cell tumor
   c. Metastatic tumor
   d. Sexcord stromal tumor
5. **Which of the following is the most radiosensitive ovarian tumors?** *(AIIMS 97)*
   a. Dysgerminoma
   b. Dermoid cyst
   c. Serous cystadenoma
   d. Endodermal sinus tumor
6. **MC ovarian tumor in younger age group or M/C malignant Tm in young age group:** *(PGI June 05/04)*
   a. Dysgerminoma
   b. Dermoid
   c. Mucinous cystadenoma
   d. Fibroma
   e. Granulosa cell tumor
7. **All of the following are true about Borderline tumors except:**
   a. 10% of all epithelial tumors are borderline
   b. They have a good prognosis
   c. Metastases are common
   d. Absence of stromal invasion
8. **According to WHO classification of ovarian tumors, Brenner tumor of ovary belongs to:**
   a. Epithelial tumors
   b. Sex cord stromal tumors
   c. Germ cell tumors
   d. Metastatic tumors

Epithelial Cell Tumors

9. **Ovarian tumors are commonly arise from:** *(UP 05)*
   a. Stroma
   b. Surface epithelium
   c. Germinal epithelium
   d. Endoderm
10. **True about Brenner tumor:** *(PGI 03)*
    a. Usually bilateral
    b. Resembles fibroma
    c. Accounts for 20% of all ovarian tumors
    d. Common in postmenopausal age group
11. **A 25-year-old married nullipara undergoes laparoscopic cystectomy for ovarian cyst which on histopath reveals ovarian serous cystadenocarcinoma. What should be the next management?** *(AIIMS Nov 08)*
    a. Serial Ca-125 measurement and follow-up
    b. Hysterectomy and bilateral pingo oophorectomy
    c. Hysterectomy + Radiotherapy
    d. Radiotherapy
12. **Chemotherapeutic drug effective in the treatment of epithelial ovarian cancer is:** *(Karn 02)*
    a. Carboplatin
    b. Paclitaxel
    c. Cyclophosphamide
    d. Methotrexate Karnataka

Sex Cord Tumors

13. **Which of the following are masculinizing tumors of the ovary?** *(AI 97)*
    a. Granulosa cell tumor
    b. Dysgerminoma
    c. Dermoid Cyst
    d. Arrhenoblastoma
14. **Which of the following is correct regarding granulosa cell tumor of ovary?** *(AIIMS 96)*
    a. Common in puberty
    b. Associated with Ca endometrium
    c. Malignant change occur rarely
    d. It is bilateral
15. **True about granulosa cell tumors:** *(PGI Dec 05)*
    a. MC malignant tumor of ovary
    b. It secretes hormones
    c. Associated with endometrial hyperplasia
    d. Chemotherapy sensitive

Germ Cell Tumor

16. The most common pure germ cell tumor of the ovary: *(AI 05)*
a. Choriocarcinoma
b. Dysgerminoma
c. Embryonal cell tumor
d. Malignant Teratoma

17. Which of the following is the most common pure malignant germ cell tumor of the ovary? *(AIIMS 04, 05)*
a. Choriocarcinoma b. Gonadoblastoma
c. Dysgerminoma d. Malignant teratoma

18. Malignant germ cell tumors of ovary includes all of the following *except*: *(PGI 04)*
a. Choriocarcinoma b. Arrhenoblastoma
c. Brenner's tumor d. Serous cystadenoma
e. Teratoma

19. True about mature ovarian teratoma: *(PGI May 2016)*
a. Recurrence is common after excision
b. Contain hair, Teeth, bone & cartilage
c. Mostly benign
d. Torsion is common complication

20. Features of dysgerminoma are: *(PGI June 06)*
a. Unilateral
b. Post-menopausal
c. Virilising
d. Cut section gritty
e. ↑ AFP

21. True about dysgerminoma: *(PGI June 09)*
a. Radiosensitive
b. Most common malignant germ cell tumor
c. Bilateral
d. ↑ AFP
e. Common in postmenopause

22. True about dysgerminoma of ovary: *(PGI Dec 04)*
a. Blood spread seen
b. Schiller-Duval bodies seen
c. Increase alfa fetoprotein
d. Bleomycin, etoposide and cisplatin given
e. Radiosensitive

23. Chemotherapy for dysgerminoma is: *(AP 05)*
a. Cisplatin, etoposide, bleomycin
b. Cyclophosphamide, vincristine, prednisolone
c. Adriamycin, cyclophosphamide, cisplatin
d. Methotrexate, oncovin, cyclophosphamide

24. A 12-years-old female is admitted as a patient of dysgerminoma of right ovary 4 × 5 cm in size with intact capsule. Best treatment will be: *(AIIMS 01)*
a. Ovarian cystectomy
b. Oophorectomy on the involved side
c. Bilateral oophorectomy
d. Hysterectomy with bilateral salpingo oophorectomy

25. True about dermoid cyst of ovary: *(PGI 03)*
a. It is teratoma
b. Frequently undergo torsion
c. X-ray is diagnostic
d. Invariably turns to malignancy
e. Contains sebaceous material and hairs

26. True about Yolk sac tumor: *(PGI 02)*
a. Also called endodermal sinus tumor
b. Always have elevated AFP level
c. Schiller Duval bodies seen
d. Highly malignant
e. Arise from epithelial cells of ovary

27. True about endodermal sinus tumors: *(PGI Dec 05)*
a. Schiller Duval bodies seen
b. It is a benign tumor
c. ↑ hCG
d. It is seen in young individuals
e. It is a malignant tumor

Krukenberg Tumor

28. All of the following are true about Krukenberg's tumor *except*: *(AI 96)*
a. Has a rough surface
b. Shape of ovary is maintained
c. Usually bilateral
d. Arises usually form stomach carcinoma

29. Smt. Pushpa is a suspected case of ovarian tumors. On laparotomy bilaterally enlarged ovaries with smooth surface was seen: *(AIIMS 00)*
a. Granulosa cell tumor
b. Krukenberg tumor
c. Dysgerminoma
d. Primary adenocarcinoma

30. The following tumors commonly metastasise to the ovary, *except*: *(J & K 05)*
a. Malignant melanoma b. Stomach
c. Oesophagus d. Lymphoma

Presentation/Complication

31. A 55-year-old female presents with abdominal pain, distension, ascites and dyspnea. Her CA 125 levels are elevated. The most likely diagnosis is: *(AI 2012)*
a. Ca ovary b. Ca cervix
c. Ca lung d. Symphoma

32. Pain of ovarian carcinoma is referred to: *(AIIMS May 2010)*
a. Back of thigh
b. Cervical region
c. Anterior surface of thigh
d. Medial surface of thigh

33. True about Meig's syndrome: *(PGI Dec 06)*
a. Lymphatic dysplasia
b. 2–30 years age
c. Associated with ascites and pleural effusion
d. No treatment required

34. All are components of Meig's syndrome, *except*: *(AIIMS 97; AI 95)*
a. Pleural effusion
b. Ovarian tumor
c. Ascites
d. Pericardial effusion

35. Meig's syndrome is associated with: *(PGI 95, 99)*
a. Teratoma
b. Brenner tumor
c. Theca cell tumor
d. Fibroma

36. The most common complication of an ovarian tumor is: *(AI 95)*
a. Torsion b. Hemorrhage
c. Infection d. Hyaline change

37. Most common ovarian cyst to undergo torsion: *(AI 07)*
a. Benign cystic teratoma b. Dysgerminoma
c. Ovarian fibroma d. Brenner's tumor

38. Pseudomyxoma peritonei is seen in: *(PGI 98)*
a. Serous cystadenoma
b. Pseudomucinous cyst
c. Mucinous cystadenoma
d. Teratoma

39. The pseudomyxoma peritonei occurs as a complication of the following ovarian tumors: *(AIIMS May 06)*
a. Serous cystadenoma b. Mucinous cystadenoma
c. Dysgerminoma d. Gonadoblastoma

40. Attacks of flushing and cyanosis occur in which type of ovarian tumors? *(AIIMS 79; AMU 82)*
a. Struma ovarii
b. Krukenberg's tumor
c. Arrhenoblastoma
d. Carcinoid tumors of ovary
e. Granulosa cell tumor

Diagnosis

41. In a suspected case of ovarian cancer, imaging work up is required for all of the following *except*: *(AI 06)*
a. Detection of adnexal lesion
b. Characterization of lesion
c. Staging
d. Asses resectability

42. A 45-year-old female is having bilateral ovarian mass, ascites and omental caking on CT scan. There is high possibility that patient is having: *(AI 03)*
a. Benign ovarian tumor
b. Malignant epithelial ovarian tumor
c. Dysgerminoma of ovary
d. Lymphoma of ovary

43. Feature in USG suggestive of ovarian malignancy is: *(PGI 99)*
a. Papillary pattern b. Septations
c. Bilaterality d. Clear fluid

44. A 24-old-old woman presents with new onset right lower quadrant pain, and you palpate an enlarged, tender right adnexa. Which of the following sonographic characteristics of the cyst in this patient suggests the need for surgical exploration now instead to observation for one menstrual cycle?
a. Lack of ascites b. Unilocularity
c. Papillary vegetation d. Diameter of 3 cm

45. A 20-year-old young girl, presents with history of rapidly developing hirsutism and amenorrhea with change in voice. To establish a diagnosis you would like to proceed with which of the following tests in blood? *(AI 02)*
a. 17 OH progesterone
b. DHEA
c. Testosterone
d. LH + FSH estimation

46. A lady has ovarian mass, X-ray pelvis shows a radio-opaque shadow. The probable diagnosis is: *(AIIMS 98)*
a. Mucinous cyst adenoma
b. Serous cyst adenoma
c. Dysgerminoma
d. Dermoid cyst

47. A 20-year female presents with a ovarian mass 6 × 6 × 6 cm in size. Ultrasonography reveals solid structures in the mass. Her serum biomarkers such as AFP. Free beta-hCG and CA 125 are normal, however, her serum alkaline phosphatase was found to be elevated. The most likely diagnosis is: *(AIIMS Nov 2011)*
a. Dysgerminoma
b. Endodermal sinus tumor
c. Malignant teratoma
d. Mucinous cystadenocarcinoma

48. Smt. Pushpa is a suspected case of ovarian tumors. On laparotomy bilaterally enlarged ovaries with smooth surface was seen: *(AIIMS 00)*
a. Granulosa cell tumor
b. Krukenberg tumor
c. Dysgerminoma
d. Primary adenocarcinoma

49. Reinke's crystals are found in: *(AIIMS 95)*
a. Arrhenoblastoma b. Granulosa cell tumor
c. Dysgerminoma d. Hilus cell tumor

50. Which are seen in endodermal sinus tumor?
a. Schiller-duval bodies b. Reed-Sternberg cells
c. Reinke's crystals d. Russell bodies

Tumor Markers

51. In a case of Dysgerminoma of ovary one of the following tumor markers is likely to be raised: *(AI 05)*
a. Serum HCG
b. Serum alpha fetoprotein
c. Serum lactic dehydrogenase
d. Serum inhibin

52. Which is raised in dysgerminoma? *(AI 09)*
a. AFP b. LDH
c. hCG d. CA-A 19-9

53. All of the following are the markers for malignant germ cell tumors of ovary except: *(AIIMS 05)*
a. CA - 125 b. Alpha fetoprotein
c. β-hCG d. LDH

54. CA - 125 is a tumor marker for: *(AIIMS 97, 98)*
a. Carcinoma ovary b. Carcinoma endometrium
c. Carcinoma vagina d. Carcinoma cervix

55. CA - 125 is specifically associated with: *(PGI 02)*
a. Colon Ca b. Breast Ca
c. Ovarian Ca d. Bronchogenic Ca
e. Pancreatic Ca

56. CA - 125 is specific marker of: *(PGI 99)*
a. Choriocarcinoma
b. Teratoma
c. Epithelial cell carcinoma of ovary
d. Seminoma

57. **A lady with CA ovary in follow-up with raised CA 125 level, next step:** *(AIIMS May 08)*
    a. CT
    b. PET
    c. MRI
    d. Clinical exam and serial follow up of CA 125
58. **Placental alkaline phosphatase is marker of:** *(PGI 96)*
    a. Theca cell tumor
    b. Teratoma
    c. Choriocarcinoma
    d. Dysgerminoma
59. **Marker for granulosa cell tumor:** *(AIIMS May 08)*
    a. CA 19-9 b. Ca 50
    c. Inhibin d. Teratoma
60. **Markers of malignant ovarian tumour is/are:** *(PGI May 2016)*
    a. Inhibin
    b. Beta human chorionic gonadotropin
    c. Alpha fetoprotein (AFP)
    d. Pax 7
    e. NB/70K

Unilateral/Bilateral

61. **All of the following ovarian tumors usually occur bilaterally, *except*:** *(AIIMS 95)*
    a. Metastatic mass
    b. Dysgerminoma
    c. Cyst adenoma of ovary
    d. Dermoid cyst
62. **Bilateral germ cell tumor is:** *(AIIMS May 07)*
    a. Dysgerminoma
    b. Immature teratoma
    c. Embryonal cell carcinoma
    d. Endodermal sinus tumor
63. **Which ovarian tumor is likely to involve the opposite ovary by metastasis?** *(AI 96)*
    a. Granulosa cell tumor b. Dysgerminoma
    c. Gynandroblastoma d. Endodermal sinus tumor

Staging

64. **Surgical staging of ovarian Ca all done except:** *(AI 09)*
    a. Peritoneal washing b. Peritoneal biopsy
    c. Omental biopsy d. Palpation of organs
65. **Laparotomy performed in a case of ovarian tumor revealed unilateral ovarian tumor with ascites positive for malignant cells and positive pelvic lymph nodes. All other structures were free of disease. What is stage of the disease?** *(AI 03)*
    a. Stage II b b. Stage III a
    c. Stage III b d. Stage III c
66. **Bilateral ovarian cancer with; capsule breached; ascites positive for malignant cells. Stage is:** *(AI 01; AIIMS 07)*
    a. I b. II
    c. III d. IV
67. **A 55-year-old female patient has carcinoma ovary with bilateral involvement with ascitic fluid in the abdomen. The stage is:** *(AIIMS 99)*
    a. II b. III
    c. IV d. IC
    e. Dysgerminoma
68. **What is the stage of ovarian Ca with superficial liver metastasis with B/L ovarian mass?** *(PGI Dec 06)*
    a. Stage I b. Stage II
    c. Stage III d. Stage IV
    e. Ca in situ

Ovarian Cysts and Their Management

69. **All are true about serous cystadenoma of the ovary *except*:** *(UP 04)*
    a. Bilateral
    b. Unilateral
    c. Concentric calcification
    d. Multiloculated, sticky, gelatinous fluid
70. **A 35-year-old patient on USG shows 3 × 4 cm clear ovarian cyst on right side. Next line of management is:** *(PGI Dec 08)*
    a. Laparoscopy
    b. OC pills
    c. Wait and watch
    d. Ca-125 estimation
71. **Kruti, 56 years old, complained of pain in abdomen, with USG showing 4 cm bilateral ovarian mass with increased vascularity. Next line of managements:** *(AI 2007)*
    a. USG guided ovarian tapping
    b. Wait and watch
    c. Surgery
    d. OC pills x three cycles.

Pregnancy and Cysts

72. **Most common ovarian tumor in pregnancy is:** *(AIIMS 96)*
    a. Mucinous cyst adenoma
    b. Dermoid cyst
    c. Metastasis
    d. Dysgerminoma
73. **Which of the following ovarian tumor is most prone to undergo torsion during pregnancy?** *(AI 06)*
    a. Serous cystadenoma
    b. Mucinous cystadenoma
    c. Dermoid cyst
    d. Theca lutein cyst
74. **A 15 cms X 15 cms ovarian cyst has been diagnosed in an 8 weeks pregnant lady. Further Management includes:** *(PGI Nov 10)*
    a. Only follow up without surgical intervention
    b. Laparotomy at 14–16 weeks
    c. Cesarean delivery and ovariotomy at term
    d. Surgery after delivery
    e. Immediate operation
75. **Which is/are used in management of stage III ovarian cancer:** *(PGI Nov 12)*
    a. Debulking
    b. Mantle field irradiation
    c. Abdomino-pelvic radiotherapy is very effective
    d. Chemotherapy
    e. Cytoreduction

76. A 10-year-old girl presents with a mass in lower abdomen involving umbilical and the hypogastrium. On examination it is cystic and mobile and the examiner is unable to insinuate fingers between the mass and the pelvic bone. What is the likely diagnosis? *(AIIMS May 2015)*

a. Duplication of small intestine
b. Mesenteric cyst
c. Omental cyst
d. Ovarian cyst

77. True about Dysgerminoma: *(PGI May 2015)*

a. Rare tumor in pregnancy
b. Always b/l
c. Total abdominal hysterectomy is usually done
d. Unilateral salpingo-oophorectomy is generally done
e. Constitute 30% of all malignant germ cell tumor

78. A lady with abdominal mass was investigated. On surgery, she was found to have bilateral ovarian masses with smooth surface. On microscopy they revealed mucin secreting cells with signet ring shapes. Diagnosis? *(AIIMS May 2015)*

a. Dysgerminoma
b. Krukenberg tumor
c. Mucinous adenocarcinoma of the varies
d. Dermoid cyst

79. A 35-years-old female presented with an adnexal mass. CA125 was slightly raised, CA199 was normal and LDH was elevated. Tumor was resected and the gross and microscopic image were as given below. What is the most likely diagnosis? *(AIIMS Nov 2016)*

a. Papillary serous cystadenocarcinoma
b. Dysgerminoma
c. Teratoma
d. Choriocarcinoma

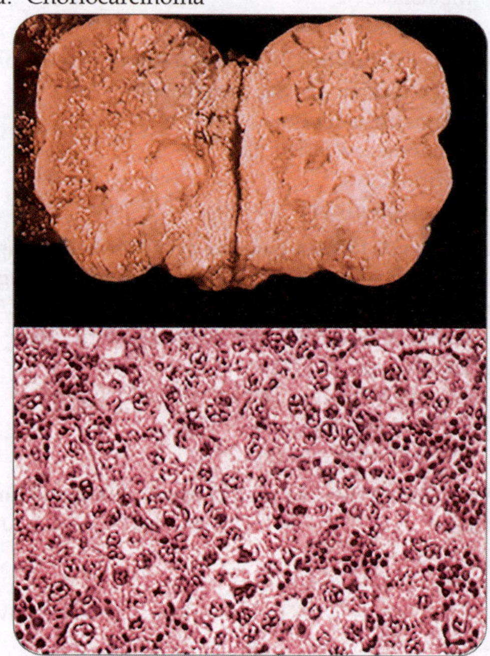

80. A patient presenting with an adnexal mass was operated and the following tumor was removed. What is the likely diagnosis? *(AIIMS Nov 2016)*

a. Mature teratoma
b. Dysgerminoma
c. Granulosa cell tumor
d. Mucinous adenocarcinoma

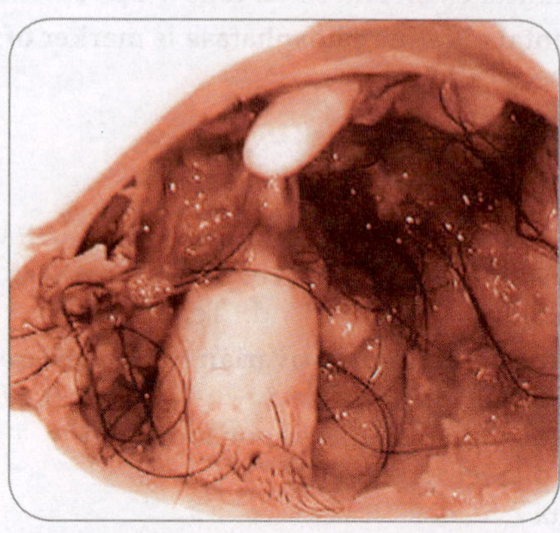

81. The following is the picture of the Pap smear of a 45- years-old female with left ovarian tumor in her late menstrual phase showing squamous cells. What is the likely histology of the tumor? *(AIIMS May 2016)*

a. Serous papillary carcinoma
b. Granulosa cell tumor
c. Mucinous adenocarcinoma
d. Dysgerminoma

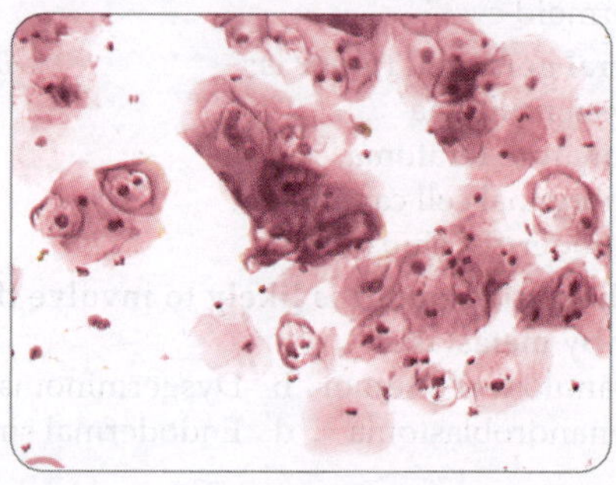

82. A 26-years-old female presented with mild pain in lower abdomen. She has had 2 full-term normal delivery earlier. Her last menstrual period was 3 weeks back. On pelvic examination, you find a palpable mass in the adnexa. On USG pelvis, you find a 5 cm ovarian cyst. What should be your next step? *(AIIMS May 2016)*

a. Observation and follow-up for cyst after 2–3 months
b. CA-125 levels
c. Diagnostic exploratory laparotomy
d. CECT of pelvis

83. Microscopic features of endodermal sinus Tumor is/are: *(PGI Nov 2011)*

a. Schiller Duval body
b. Intracellular and extracellular hyaline deposits
c. Granulosa granuloma cells with prominent nuclei
d. Spindle shaped cells or myxoid
e. Fibrous sheath

ANSWERS TO NEW PATTERN QUESTIONS

N1. Ans. is b, i.e. Fibroma
See the text for explanation.

N2. Ans. is a, i.e. Luteomas *Ref: Dutta Gynae 6th/ed, p 384*

SEX CORD Stromal Tumors
- Granulosa cell tumors
- Thecomas, fibromas
- Sertoli-Leydig cell tumors (androblastoma)
- Gynandroblastoma (mixed)

Sex cord stromal tumors constitute 6–10 percent of all ovarian neoplasms. Peak incidence is over the age of 50. As 15–30 percent of these tumors produce hormones, they are also known as *'functioning tumors'*.

N3. Ans. is b, i.e. Follicular cyst *Ref: COGDT 11th/ed, p26*
See the text for explanation.

N4. Ans. is d, i.e. Use of OCP's *Ref: Dutta Gynae 6th/ed, p 290*
Lutein cysts are usually bilateral and caused by excessive chorionic gonadotropin secreted in cases of gestational trophoblastic tumors. These may also be formed with administration of gonadotropins or even clomiphene to induce ovulation. These are usually lined either by theca lutein cells called theca lutein cyst or by granulosa lutein cells, called granulosa lutein cyst.
Spontaneous regression is expected within few weeks following effective therapy of the tumors with the gonadotropin level returning back to normal.

N5. Ans. is c, i.e. Immediate removal *Ref: COGDT 11/ed, page 24*
Thus female is presenting with ovarian cyst at 10 weeks and the cyst has undergone torsion.
Whenever a cyst undergoes torsion or any other complication, it should be removed immediately.

N6. Ans. is b, i.e. Wait and watch *Ref: Novaks 141th/ed, p1366*
In postmenopausal women with unilocular cyst measuring 7 or less with normal serum CA125 levels, expectant management is acceptable.

N7. Ans. is c, i.e. Mature cystic teratoma
M/C benign tumor of ovary is dermoid cyst, i.e mature cystic teratoma.
M/C benign epithelial tumor of ovary—serous cyst adenoma.

N8. Ans. is a, i.e. Serous tumor
See the text for explanation.

N9. Ans. is d, i.e. Appendix carcinoma
M/C cause of pseudomyxoma peritonei is appendix carcinoma.

N10. Ans. is b, i.e. Dermoid cyst of ovary
See the text for explanation.

N11. Ans. is d, i.e. No risk
If a postmenopausal female develops ovarian cancer, it is sporadic and hence there is no risk in 1st degree relative.
If one 1st degree relative of premenopausal female has ovarian cancer—risk is increased by 10%.
If two 1st degree relatives of premenopausal females have ovarian cancer—risk is increased by 35–40%.

N12. Ans. is a, i.e. p53 gene mutation
See the text for explanation.

N13. Ans. is b, i.e. Clear cell tumor
M/C ovarian cancer associated with endometrial cancer: Endometrioid tumor
M/C ovarian cancer associated with endometriosis: Clear cell carcinoma

N14. Ans. is c, i.e. Stage III A
In ovarian cancer
Pelvic lymph nodes are involved in stage II B
Para aortic lymph nodes are involved in stage III A
Inguinal lymph nodes are involved in stage IV B.

N15. Ans. is a, i.e. Dysgerminoma
GCT with best prognosis - dysgerminoma
GCT with worst prognosis - Endodermal sinus tumor

N16. Ans. is d, i.e. Dysgerminoma

M/C benign ovarian tumor seen in dysgenetic gonads is gonadoblastoma

M/C malignant ovarian tumour in dysgenetic gonads is dysgerminoma.

N17. Ans. is a, i.e. It is always secondary *Ref: Dutta Gynae 6th/ed, p387*

- Krukenberg tumor is generally a metastatic tumor to the ovary. But "Krukenberg tumor may be a primary tumor" *Ref: Dutta Gynae 6th/ed, p387*
- The most common primary sites from where metastases to the ovaries occur are gastrointestinal tract (pylorus, colon and rarely small intestine), gallbladder, pancreas, breast and endometrial carcinoma.
- These are usually bilateral tumors which maintain shape of the ovary. Histologically 'signet ring' looking cells are characteristic of Krukenberg tumor.
- In most patients with Krukenberg's tumors, the prognosis is poor. Median survival being less than a year. Rarely, no primary site can be identified and the Krukenberg's tumor may be a primary tumor.

Also know: Metastatic tumors from the GI tract can be associated with sex hormone (estrogen and androgen) production. Patient may present with postmenopausal bleeding.

N18. Ans is b, i.e. Bilateral tubectomy *Ref: William gynae 3/ed, p736*

"Tubal ligation and Hysterectomy are each associated with a substantial reduction in risk. Theoretically, any gynaecological procedure that precludes intants from reaching the ovaries via as caesarian from the lower genital tract might plausibly exert a similar protective effect." *Ref: Williams Gynae 3rd/ed, p736*

N19. Ans. is d, i.e. Stromal invasion *Ref: Shaw gynae 15th/ed, p373-374*

Malignant tumor has 2 characteristics different from borderline tumors:

(i) Stromal invasion present (it is absent in borderline tumor).

(ii) Mitosis ≥ 4/10 per high power field. (in borderline < 4/10 per high power)

N20. Ans. is c, i.e. Stage IV A: *Ref: Williams Gynae 3rd/ed, p750, Table 35.5*

See the text for explanation

N21. Ans. is d, i.e. Mucinous cystadenoma *Shaw 15th/ed, p375*

Mucinous Tumors:

"The tumors are not infrequent, can grow to a large size and after weigh as much as 5-10 kg and are often pedunculated" *Shaw Gynae 15th/ed, p375*

N22. Ans. is b, i.e. Mucinous tumor: psammoma body

Psammoma body is a histological characteristic of non mucinous epithelial tumors of ovary

N23. Ans. is a, i.e. > 200

See the text for expl.

N24. Ans. is b, i.e. Mucinous tumor *Ref: William gynae 3rd/ed, p753, Table 35-9*

Most Important favourable prognostic factors for ovarian cancer

1. Younger age
2. Cell type other than mucinous & clear cells
3. Well differentiated tumor
4. Small disease volume
5. No ascites

N25. Ans. is c, i.e. Germ cell Tumor. *Ref: Williams Gynae 3rd/ed, p761*

"GCT- These tumors are the most common ovarian malignancy diagnosed during childhood and adolescence, although only 1% of all ovarian cancers develop in these age groups. At age 20, however, the incidence of epithelial ovarian cancer begins to rise & exceeds that of germ cell tumors." *Ref: Williams Gynae 3rd/ed, p761*

ANSWERS TO PREVIOUS YEAR QUESTIONS

1. **Ans. is a. Follicular cyst is least common among functional cyst**

Ref: Shaw's 16th/444; Dutta Gynae 6th/289-90 Robert Shaw Gynae 4th/673

"Theca Lutein cysts are often found in association with hydatiform moles, choriocarcinoma, gonadotropin (hCG) or clomiphene therapy" *Ref: Shaw's Gynae 16th/ed, p430*

"The combination of an ovarian fibroma with ascites and hydrothorax, usually right side is known as Meig's syndrome".

Ref: Shaw's 16th/ed, p444

"Corpus luteal cyst: It may be often associated with pregnancy and persists for about 12 week's *Ref: Dutta Gynae 6th/ed, p290*

"Dermoid cyst arises from the germ cells arrested after the first meiotic division. *Ref: Dutta Gynae 6th/ed, p290*

Non-neoplastic Ovarian Masses

Functional ovarian cysts include follicular cysts, corpus luteum cysts, and theca lutein cysts.

- M/C functional cysts are follicular cysts
- All are benign and usually do not cause symptoms or require surgical management.
- Cigarette and marijuana smoking are associated with an increased risk of functional cysts, although the increased risk may be attenuated in overweight or obese women.
- Oral contraceptive use is associated with a decreased risk of developing ovarian cysts, although low-dose pills may have a smaller benefit, and oral contraceptives do not hasten the resolution of ovarian cysts.
- **Corpus luteum cysts** are less common than follicular cysts. Corpus luteum cysts may rupture, leading to a hemoperitoneum and requiring surgical management
- **Theca lutein cysts** are the least common of functional ovarian cysts. They are usually bilateral and occur with pregnancy, including molar pregnancies. They may be associated with multiple gestations, molar pregnancies, choriocarcinoma, diabetes, Rh sensitization, clomiphene citrate use, human menopausal gonadotropin–human chorionic gonadotropin ovulation induction, and the use of GnRH analogues.
- Most benign cystic teratomas (dermoid cysts) occur during the reproductive years, although dermoid cysts have a wider age distribution than other ovarian germ cell tumors; in some case series, up to 25% of dermoids occur in postmenopausal women, and they can occur in newborns" *Ref: Novak's Gynae 15thed pg 413*

2. **Ans. is b, i.e. Use of oral pills** *Ref: Shaw 15/e p 368, Wililams Gynae 3/e p218, CGDT 10th/ed, p871 - 872*

"Oral combined pills administered for 3 months resolves the cyst in most cases." *Ref: Shaw 15 e/ Pg 368*

"Potential factors, high dose COC's supplies ovarian activity and protect against cyst development. However in subsequent studies low dose pills COC's provided only modest protective effect." *Wililams Gynae 3rd/ed, p218*

3. **Ans. is d, i.e. Prophylactic oophorectomy**

Ref: Novak 14th/ed, p1471; Devita 7th/ed, p1369; Wililams Gynae 1st/ed, p718-719; Recent Advances in Gynae - Studs

Strategies for prevention of hereditary ovarian cancer

- Genetic testing for susceptibility to ovarian cancer is rapidly becoming integrated into the clinical practice of oncology. Strategies have been adopted to reduce the incidence of ovarian cancer in patient with BRCA-1 and BRCA-2 mutations.

a. **Prophylactic oophorectomy:**

"The only proven way to prevent ovarian cancer is surgical oophorectomy. As another possible site of disease among these high risk patients is fallopian tube therefore should be removed. IN BRCA 1 or BRCA-2 mutation carriers, prophylactic bilateral salpingo-oophorectomy (BSO) may be performed on either completion of childbearing or at age 40. In these patients, the procedure is approximately 90% effective in preventing epithelial ovarian cancer. In women with HNPCC, the risk reduction approaches 100%."

Ref: William Gynae 3/e p738

- Additional benefit of prophylactic oophorectomy is that the risk of breast cancer is reduced by 50-80%.

b. **Oral contraceptive pills:**

- Data received from a multicenter control of genetic screening centers indicates that the use of oral contraceptive pill is associated with 50% decreased risk for developing ovarian cancer in women who have mutation in either in BRCA - 1 or BRCA - 2. However there is short term increased risk of developing breast cancer.

c. **Role of screening with CA 125 and transvaginal ultrasound:**

"In BRCA1- BRCA2 mutation carriers who donot wish to undergo prophylactic surgery a combination of through pelvic examination, transvaginal sonographic examination and CA125 blood testing should be done". *Ref: Williams Gynae 1st/ed, p719*

- Best method of prevention: Prophylactic BSO at 35 years or as soon as family is complete, not later than 40 years.
- 2nd line: OCP's + screening
- Screening: TVS + Ca 125 started at 35 years and done every 6 or 12 months, breast screening by MRI and mammography at 30 years done annually.

4. Ans. is b, i.e. Germ cell tumor *Ref: Shaw 15th/ed, p376*

5. Ans. is a, i.e. Dysgerminoma *Ref: Bailey & Love 24th/ed, p221*

"Below the age of 20 years 60% of the tumors are of germ cell origin and in girls under the age of 10 years almost 85% are of germ cell origin and are invariably malignant."

In females with HNPCC gene mutation along with BSO, hysterectomy should also be done as there is an associated risk of endometrial cancer. In BRCA gene mutation Hysterectomy is not routinely recommended.

Remember

The most common malignant GCT Earlier was dysgerminoma but now its incidence has declined & it is the second most common malignant GCT.

"Because their incidence has declined by approximately 30 percent over the past few decades, dysgenia accurately accounts for only approximately one third of all malignant ovarian germ cell tumors." *Ref: Williams Gynae 3/ed, p762*

"Due to a 60 percent increased incidence during the past few decades, immature teratomas are now the M/C variant & account for 40 – 50% of all malignant ovarian germ cell tumors." *Ref: William gynae 3rd/ed, p765*

Most common germ cell tumor of ovary is dermoid cyst (mature teratoma). It is benign in nature.

Remember:

- Most common ovarian tumor (overall) – *Epithelial cell tumor.*
- Most common tumor in young woman is – *Germ cell tumor.* *Ref: Shaw 14th/ed, p555*
- Most common malignant tumor of ovary – *Serous cystadenocarcinoma.*
- Most common benign tumor of ovary (overall) – Dermoid cyst. *Ref: Williams Gynae 1st/ed, p219*
- Most common benign epithelial tumor of ovary – Serous cystadenoma. *Ref: Jeffcoate 7th/ed, p531*
- Most common germ cell tumor – Mature teratoma (Dermoid cyst).
- Most common malignant GCT – Immature teratoma > Dysgerminoma. *Ref: Williams Gynae 3/e p765*
- Most common ovarian tumor in pregnancy (but in remains undiagnosed) – Serous cystadenoma.
- Most Common benign tumor diagnosed in pregnancy – Dermoid cyst.
- Overall most common ovarian tumor diagnosed in pregnancy – Dermoid cyst.
- Most common malignant ovarian tumor detected during pregnancy – Dysgerminoma.
- Germ cell Tumor with best prognosis - Dysgerminoma
- Germ cell tumor with worst prognosis – endodermal sinus tumor
- Germ cell tumor which has maximum bilaterality – Dysgerminoma
- Germ cell tumor which presents as acute abdomen – Endodermal Sinus Tumor
- Most common ovarian tumor to undergo torsion during pregnancy – Dermoid cyst.
- Most common ovarian tumor to involve opposite ovary by metastasis – Granulosa cell tumor.
- Most radiosensitive ovarian tumor – Dysgerminoma.. *Ref: Bailey & Love 24th/ed, p221*
- Most rapidly growing ovarian tumor – Yolk sac Tm- (Endodermal Sinus Tumor)

Ovarian Tumor: Causing:

- *Pseudomyxoma peritonei* – Mucinous cystadenoma/Micinous cystadenocarcinoma
- *Meig's syndrome* – Ovarian fibroma
- *Pseudomeig's syndrome:* – Brenner's tumor
  – Granulosa cell tumor
  – Thecoma
- Ovarian tumor associated with hyperpyrexia and hypercalcemia
  – Mesonephroid tumor.
- Ovarian tumor arising from epithelium of urinary tract – Brenner Tm
- Feminizing tumors: – Granulosa cell tumor
  – Theca cell tumor
  – Fibromas
- Virilising tumor: – Androblastoma
  – Hilus cell Tm
  – Gynadroblastoma
  – Adrenal cortical tumor
- Largest benign ovarian tumor – Mucinous cyst adenoma
- Tumor with lymphocytic infilteration: – Dysgerminoma.

6. Ans. is a, i.e. Dysgerminoma *Ref: Shaw 15th/ed, p378, 377, 375, 379, 381*

Most common tumor at young age is Germ cell tumor. Amongst the options given, malignant germ cell tumor is Dysgerminoma so it will be our answer of choice.

The age incidence of tumors given in the options:

Dysgerminoma	– 10–20 years
Dermoid cysts	– Can occur at any age. Maximum age incidence in between 40–50 years.
Mucinus cystadenoma	– Between 30–60 years.
Granulosa cell tumor	– Mostly in postmenopausal or > 40 years.
Ovarian fibroma	– No particular age incidence.

7. **Ans. is c, i.e. Metastases are common** *Ref: Textbook of Gynacecology Sheila Balakrishnan 1st/ed, p255*
   See the text for exploration.
8. **Ans. is a, i.e. Epithelial tumors** *Ref: Textbook of Gynacecology Sheila Balakrishnan 1st/ed, p252*
   See the text for explanations.
9. **Ans. is b, i.e. Surface epithelium** *Ref: Shaw 14th/ed, p334*
   Epithelial tumors are derived from the ovarian surface epithelium. In general, epithelial tumors comprise 50-60% of all ovarian tumors but malignant epithelial tumors comprise 90% of all ovarian cancers.
10. **Ans. is b, and d, i.e. Resembles fibroma; and Common in postmenopausal age group** *Ref: Shaw 15th/ed, p376*
    Brenner tumor is also called as Transitional cell tumor:
    - It is a rare epithelial neoplasm of ovary resembling fibroma.[Q]
    - It is an essentially benign tumor.[Q]
    - Tumor is generally seen in women around menopause and is generally unilateral.[Q]
    - Cause menopausal bleeding and Pseudomeig syndrome (ascites and hydrothorax).[Q]
    - Malignant change is very rare.
    - Histologically it shows walthard cell rests of transitional cells[Q], cells have coffee bean nuclei, cut section is gritty.
11. **Ans. is a, i.e. Serial Ca-125 measurement and follow-up** *Ref: Novak 14th/ed, p1479-1480; 15th/ed, p1371*
    Here the patient is 25 years old nullipara and cystectomy sample shows serous cysadenocarcinoma - Probably the disease is limited to the ovary removed, hence to be called stage Ia.
    Doing an oophorectomy here will suffice as the patient is young and nullipara. Next step is to follow the patient with regular CA 125 estimations. Though the levels of CA 125 are not specific but in this condition where the follow up is after a known cause there is ample sensitivity.
    "Fertility preservation in early stage ovarian cancer - *The uterus and the contralateral ovary can be preserved in women with stage Ia, grade 1 to 2 disease who desire to preserve fertility. The conditions of the women should be monitored carefully with routine periodic pelvic examination and determinations of serum CA 125 levels. Generally, the other ovary and the uterus are removed at the completion of childbearing."* *Ref: Novak 14th/ed, p1479-1480; 15th/ed, p1371*
12. **Ans. is a and b, i.e. Carboplatin; and Paclitaxel** *Ref: Novak 14th/ed, p1493*
    As discussed in the text, combination chemotherapy of carboplatin and paclitaxel is best but if a patient cannot tolerate combination chemotherapy then only paclitaxel is given.
13. **Ans. is d, i.e. Arrhenoblastoma** *Ref: Shaw 15th/ed, p380-381*
    Masculinizing Tumors develop from Sex cord of Embryonic gonad and include
    - Arrhenoblastoma/Androblastoma/Hilus cell Tm
    - Adrenal cortical Tm/Lipoid cell Tm of ovary
    - Gynandroblastoma
14. **Ans. is b, i.e. Associated with Ca endometrium** *Ref: Shaw 15th/ed, p379; Novak 14th/ed, p1520-1521*
    Granulosa cell tumor is a sex cord tumor.
    - **Age:** It can be seen at any age. Most common before puberty and *after 40 years.* (Maximum incidence at 52 years). Hence option a i.e. it is common is puberty is incorrect *Ref: Williams Gynae 1st/ed, p747*
    - Tumor secretes estrogen which is responsible for clinical features like precocious puberty, menometrorrhagia and post menopausal bleeding.
    - They are low grade malignancies.
    - Almost always unilateral[Q] (B/L in < 2%) i.e. **option d incorrect**

    Malignant transformation:
    - Since they secrete estrogen, 25–50% are associated with *Endometrial hyperplasia.*
    - 5 per cent of tumors are associated with endometrial cancer.

    "There is a strong evidence that carcinoma of the endometrium may be associated with ferminizing tumors of the ovary in postmenopausal women." *Ref: Shaw 15th/ed, p380*
    Marker: Granulosa cell tumor secrete inhibin which is a useful marker for it.
    Prognosis: Is good with 5 year survival rate being 90%.
    Metastasis: It is peculiar in case of granulosa cell tumor, it first involves opposite ovary followed by metastasis in lumbar region.
15. **Ans. is b and c, i.e. It secretes hormones; and Associated with endometrial hyperplasia**
    Ref: Novak 14th/ed, p1520 - 1521, 15th/ed, p1408

- Most common malignant tumor of ovary is *Serous cystadenocarcinoma* **(Option "a"** is incorrect).
- Granulosa cell tumor secretes estrogen and so, in 25 - 50% cases is associated with endometrial hyperplasia. ***(Option "b"*** and *"c"* are correct).
- Surgery is the TOC.

Management: Surgery is the TOC. Type of surgery depends on age of occurrence.

Children and women of reproductive age → Unilateral salpingo-oophorectomy

Postmenopausal → TAH + BSO.

"There is no evidence that adjuvant chemotherapy will prevent recurrence of disease."

Ref: Novak 14th/ed, p1523, 15th/ed, p1408

"The mainstay of treatment for patients with an ovarian SCST (Sex Cord Stromal Tumors) is complete surgical resection due to their relative insensitivity to adjuvant chemotherapy or radiation." *Ref: Williams Gynae 2nd/ed, p892*

(So, **Option "d"** is incorrect)

16. Ans. is d, i.e. Malignant Teratoma

17. Ans. is d, i.e. Malignant Teratoma *Ref: Williams Gynae 3/ed, p765*

18. Ans. is b, c and d, i.e. Arrhenoblastoma; Brenner's tumor; and Serous cystadenoma

- *Most common germ cell Tumor – Mature teratoma or Dermoid cyst*Q (Benign in nature).
- *Most common malignant GCT – Immature teratoma > Dysgerminoma.*Q

"Due to 60% increased incidence during the past few decades, immature teratomas are now the M/c variant and account for 40 – 50% of all malignant GCT". *Ref: Williams Gynae 3rd/ed, p765.*

- *Most common benign Tumor of ovary – Dermoid cyst*Q

Ref: Williams Gynae 1st/ed, p214; Merck manual online medical library on Internet; Jeffcoate 7th/ed, p531

19. Ans. is b, c and d i.e. Contain hair Teeth, bone & cartilage, Mostly benign, and Torsion is common complication

See the text in for explanation

The only point to note is:

Treatment of dermoid

- Ovarian cystectomy even if only a small amount of ovarian cortex is left
- Laparoscopic Cystectomy is often possible but it is associated with a higher risk of recurrence

20. Ans. is a, i.e. Unilateral *Ref: Shaw 15th/ed, p378; CGDT 9th/ed, p937*

21. Ans. is a and b, i.e. Radiosensitive; and Most common malignant germ cell tumor *Ref: Shaw 15th/ed, p378*

22. Ans. is a, d and e, i.e. Blood spread seen; Bleomycin, etoposide and cisplatin given; and Radiosensitive

Ref: Novak 14th/ed, p1508-9, 1511,15th/ed, p1395-1397

Dysgerminoma:

- It is the second most common *malignant germ cell tumor*Q of ovary.
  They are the most common ovarian malignancy detected during pregnancy.
- Primarily affect ***young women*** (average age of incidence is 20 yearsQ) and not postmenopausal females.
- Usually ***unilateral***Q but they are the only germ cell malignancy with a significant rate of bilateral ovarian involvement – 15 to 20%.
- Pathologically it is a solid neoplasm with *areas of softening*Q due to degeneration. *Ref: CGDT 10th/ed, p875*
- *"Consistency is fleshy"* *Ref: Novak 15th/ed, p1395*
- Unlike other germ cell tumors it ***does not secrete AFP*** and HCG is only rarely secreted, however it ***secretes LDH and placental alkaline phosphate,*** which are used as tumor marker of dysgerminoma.
  M/C, route of spread is via lymphatics (Novaks 15/e,p1396) but hematogenous and direct spread are also seen.
- Dysgerminoma is the *most radio sensitive tumor,*.:Q But treatment of choice is ***surgery*** (unilateral salpingo oophorectomy) ***along with proper surgical staging followed by Bleomycin, Etoposide and Cisplatin (BEP) based chemotherapy*** as fertility can be preserved.

Chemotherapy is helpful in metastatic spread

- They have the best prognosis of all malignant ovarian germ cell variants.

Recurrence rate is high.

23. Ans. is a, i.e. Cisplatin, etoposide, bleomycin *Ref: Novak 14th/ed, p1511, Williams Gynae 3/ed, p766*

Cisplatin is used for dysgerminoma.

Though Dysgerminoma is most radiosensitive tumor known, *treatment of choice is oophorectomy of involved side followed by cisplatin based chemotherapy to preserve fertility, as dysgerminoma is seen in young women with average age incidence being 20 years.*

24. Ans. is b, i.e. Oophorectomy of the involved side *Ref: Devita 7th/ed, p1391; Williams Gynae 1st/ed, p741*

25. Ans. is a, b, c and e, i.e. It is teratoma; Frequently undergo torsion; X-ray is diagnostic; and Contains sebaceous material and hairs

Ref: Shaw 15th/ed, p376-7; Williams Gynae 1st/ed, p214-5

Dermoid cyst: Dermoid cyst is a benign teratoma.

- It is most common *benign tumor of ovary* in reproductive age group.[Q]
- Most common benign neoplasm diagnosed during pregnancy.[Q]

Most common Germ cell tumor.[Q]

It is the commonest tumor to undergo torsion.

- **Characteristically they are unilocular cyst containing hair and cheesy sebaceous material, teeth, bones, thyroid tissue and cartilage.**
- **If teeth or bone are seen in X-ray in adnexal mass, this finding is pathognomonic for teratoma and thus X-ray is diagnostic.**
- *Malignant change in a dermoid cyst occurs in 0.5 – 2% cases in patients > 40 years. Most common malignancy which develops is, squamous cell carcinoma.* *Ref: Textbook of Gynaecology Sheila Balakrishnan 1st/ed, p183*

26. Ans. is a, b, c and d, i.e. Also called endodermal sinus tumor; Always have elevated AFP level; Schiller Duval bodies seen; and Highly malignant

27. Ans. is a, d and e, i.e. Schiller Duval bodies seen; It is seen in young individuals; and It is a malignant tumor

Ref: Williams Gynae 1st/ed, p742; Jeffcoates 7th/ed, p541; Novak 15th/ed, p1403

Endodermal sinus tumor/Yolk sac tumor:

- Endodermal sinus (yolk sac) tumor is third most common malignant germ cell tumor of ovary affecting mostly children or young women. (Age group 14–20 years). *Ref: Novak 15th/ed, p1403*
  (M/C , being Immature teratoma, 2nd M/C dysgerminoma)
- Tumor is *highly malignant* and is *most rapidly growing tumor of whole body.*
- Histologically the pathognomonic finding is *Schiller - Duval bodies*[Q] which is a single papilla lined by tumor cells with a central blood vessel.
- Due to high rate of growth, tumor usually presents with acute abdomen.
- **Unilateral in 100% cases therefore biopsy of opposite ovary is contraindicated.**
- Almost all cases are associated with raised AFP and Alpha 1 antitrypsin.
- **It is the most deadly malignant ovarian germ cell tumor.**
- *Treatment surgery for staging including TAH+BsO followed by:* Chemotherapy (BEP).
- It has a high propensity for rapid growth, peritoneal spread and distant hematogenous dissemination to the lungs.

28. Ans. is a, i.e. Has a rough surface *Ref: Shaw 15th/ed, p425-6*

29. Ans. is b, i.e. Krukenberg tumor *Ref: Shaw 15th/ed, p425-6; CGDT 10th/ed, p877*

Krukenberg tumor:

- Krukenberg tumor by definition ***represent carcinoma of stomach metastasised to ovary***. But the eponym is commonly used to denote any gastric cancer metastatic to ovary
- Tumor arise by *retrograde lymphatic spread*[Q] i.e. carcinoma cells pass from the stomach to the superior gastric lymphnode which also receive lymphatics from ovary.

Characteristics of Krukenberg Tumor:

i. Always bilateral[Q]
ii. Have smooth surface[Q]
iii. No tendency to form adhesions
iv. Freely mobile
v. No infiltration through the capsule.
vi. Histologically tumor has signet ring cells in the background of myxomatous stroma.
vii. They retain the shape of normal ovary.[Q]
viii. Have waxy consistency.[Q]

30. Ans. is c, i.e. Oesophagus *Ref: Novak 14th/ed, p1525-7*

About 5 – 6% of Ovarian tumors are metastatic from other organs. The metastatic tumors can arise from metastasis from the following sites.

Gynaecologic	Gastrointestinal tract	Breast	Lymphoma and Leukemia	Melanoma	Carcinoid Tm
• Tubes (13%)	• Stomach		*(Most common*		
• Endometrium	(Characteristic Krukenberg tumor)		*Burkitt's lymphoma)*		
• Cervix (Rare < 1%)					
• Colon					
• Small intestine					
• Appendix					

Note: M/C tumor to metastasize to ovary-GIT tumor–colon cancer

Second M/C site is Breast tumor.

31. Ans. is a, i.e. Ca ovary *Ref: Jeffcoates 7th/ed, p543; Novaks 15th/ed, p1366*

- M/c age incidence for primary ovarian neoplasms is 40-60 years, peak age incidence being 55–60 years. Ovarian malignancies generally present with vague symptoms like abdominal pain, dyspepsia, and patient may also experience irregular menses and if pelvic mass compresses the bladder or rectum she may have urinary frequency or constipation.

In advanced stages patients have symptoms related to presence of ascites, omental metastasis or bowel metastasis like abdominal distension, dyspnea, bloating, nausea, anorexia or early satiety.

In the patient given in the question all these symptoms are present (which could be seen in other cancers as well) plus her Ca 125 levels are raised, which favors the diagnosis of ovarian cancer in her.

Remember

The most important sign of epithelial ovarian cancer is the presence of a pelvic mass on physical examination.

32. Ans. is d, i.e. Medial surface of thigh *Ref: Lasts Anatomy 10th/ed, p302*

- Ovarian pain is referred along the medial side of thigh
- The obturator nerve during its course, when runs in front of the internal iliac vessels is separated from the normally situated ovary by only the parietal peritoneum lining the pelvic wall, thus pain from the ovary may be referred along the nerve to the skin on the medial side of thigh.

Also Know

- Simpson Pain- colicky pain in patients of Ca Endometrium. It is referred to the hypogastrium or to both iliac fossas. It is not severe and tends to appear at the same time each day lasting only 1–2 hours.

33. Ans. is c and d, i.e. Associated with ascites and pleural effusion; and No treatment required

34. Ans. is d, i.e. Pericardial effusion

35. Ans. is d, i.e. Fibroma *Ref: Comprehensive Gynaecology by Arthus L Herbst 2nd/ed, p533; Jeffcoate 7th/ed, p543*

Meig's syndrome:

- **Ascites and right sided hydrothorax in** association with fibroma of ovary is called as *Meig's syndrome.*
- It can also be seen in Brenner's tumor and Granulosa cell tumor where it is called as *Pseudomeig's syndrome.*
- True meig's syndrome is rare, occurring in < 5 per cent of fibromas.
- Hydrothorax can be bilateral also.
- Ascites is caused by transudation of fluid from the ovarian fibroma. Hydrothorax develops secondary to flow of ascitic fluid into the pleural space via lymphatics of the diaphragm.
- Ascites occurs *(in 50% cases)* when tumor size is > 6 cms.
- Tumors producing Meig's syndrome manifest in *the late childbearing period* i.e., 30–40 years.
- Both ascites and hydrothorax resolve spontaneously after removal of the tumor.

Criteria for diagnosis of Meig's syndrome:

- Tumor must be ovarian, solid and benign.
- Both hydrothorax and ascites must be present.
- Removal of the tumor must result in their spontaneous and permanent cure.

Pseduomeig syndrome:

- Can be seen in association with either benign or malignant tumor.
- Hydrothorax could be a manifestation of pulmonary metastasis.
- Syndrome can result from overstimulation of the ovaries with gonadotropins but, in such cases, the peritoneal exudate is more likely to be caused by an electrolyte imbalance rather than by ovarian tumor.

36. Ans. is a, i.e. Torsion *Ref: Shaw 15th/ed, p382*

Complications of Ovarian tumor (TRIP):

T ***Torsion***

- Most common complication
- Seen in 12% cases
- Most common in benign tumors
- Most common tumor to undergo torsion is dermoid cyst.

R ***Rupture***

- Which can be traumatic or spontaneous.

I ***Infection***

- Rare complication
- Seen following acute salpingitis or during puerperium as a part of an ascending genital tract infection.

P Pseudomyxoma peritonei

- Peritoneal cavity is filled with coagulated mucinous material.

In ovarian Tumors

- Most common in mucinous cystadenoma and mucinous carcinoma.

Also seen in: Mucocoele of appendix.

- Carcinoma of large intestine.
- Appendix cancer overall is the M/C cause of pseudomyxoma peritonei.

37. Ans. is a, i.e. Benign cystic teratoma *Ref: Novak 14th/ed, p510*

"A benign cystic teratoma is the most common neoplasm to undergo torsion, and it to the M/C benign tumor diagnosed during pregnancy." *Ref: Novak 14th/ed, p510*

A benign cystic teratoma is synonymous to dermoid cyst.

38. Ans. is c, i.e. Mucinous cystadenoma

39. Ans. is b, i.e. Mucinous cystadenoma *Ref: Novak 14th/ed, p1462-3*

Pseudomyxoma peritonei is a condition in which the neoplastic epithelium secretes large amounts of gelatinous mucinous material. It is most commonly seen secondary to:

- Appendicular carcinoma (well differentiate carcinoma).
- Ovarian mucinous carcinoma; mucinous cystadenoma.
- Mucocoele of appendix (less commonly seen).

Even after removal of the ovarian tumors, these cells continue to secrete mucin.

Tendency of *recurrence* is present.

Prognosis is Poor.

Management: Hysterectomy with BSO with removal of mucin peritoneal implants along with appendix.

40. Ans. is d, i.e. Carcinoid Tumors of ovary *Ref: Shaw 15th/ed, p378*

Carcinoid tumor of Ovary:

- It is sometimes primary and sometimes metastatic.
- Also called Argentaffinoma.
- Occurs as a malignant change in benign dermoid cyst.
- Presence of solid yellow tumor with histological property of reducing silver salts derived from specialized Kulchitsky cells of intestine.
- It produced 5 - HT which causes attacks of flushing and cyanosis.[Q]

41. Ans. is c, i.e. Staging *Ref: Novak 14th/ed, p1477; Jeffcoate 7th/ed, p550*

"FIGO staging is based on finding at surgical exploration." *Ref: Novak 14th/ed, p1477*

"Whenever malignancy is suspected, a staging laparotomy should be carried out." *Ref: Jeffcoates 7th/ed, p550*

Role of Imaging in Ovarian tumor:

- Used for - delineating the site and size of lesion.
- Characterization of lesion into benign or malignant.
  Detects early metastasis.
- To asses resectability.
- To exclude extraperitoneal metastasis (like liver parenchyma, enlarged pelvic and paraaortic nodes, hydroureter and hydronephrosis)

Role of imaging in ovarian cancer:

"TVS is typically the most useful investigation to differentiate benign tumors and early stage ovarian cancers." In patients with advanced disease, sonography is less helpful. The pelvic sonogram may be particularly difficult to interpret if a large mass encompasses the uterus, adnexa & surrounding structures. Ascites, if present is easily detected but in general abdominal sonography has limited use".

"CT scanning has a primary role in treatment planning for women with advanced ovarian cancer. Preoperatively CB 20). Implants, in the liver, retro peritoneum, omentum other intra-abdominal sites are detected to thereby guide surgical crypto reduction or demonstrate absolutely resectable disease. However, CT is not particularly reliable in detecting intrapertioneal disease small than 1 to 2 cms in diameter. Moreover CT is not useful in differentiating between benign ovarian mass and malignant tumour".

Ref: Williams Gynae 3rd/ed, p742

42. Ans. is b, i.e. Malignant epithelial ovarian tumor *Ref: COGDT 10th/ed, p879*

"Malignant ovarian tumor are often bilateral solid and present with ascites."

Omental caking on CT is also a sign of malignancy.

Physical examination	Benign tumor	Malignant tumor
Mobility	Mobile	Fixed, large and multiloculated
Consistency	Cystic	Solid or firm
Laterality	Unilateral	Bilateral
Cul-de-sac	Smooth on P/V examination	Nodular on P/V examination
Radiography		
Size	Usually < 10 cm size	Any size
Septations	< 2 mm thickness	Multiple septations > 3 mm in size
Calcification	Seen in teratoma	Usually absent
Omental caking	Absent	Seen
Ascites	Absent	Present
Intra operative	Unilateral cyst with no adhesion	Solid areas with adhesion
	Capsule intact	Capsule is breached

Remember

Benign tumors of ovary causing ascites are:
- Ovarian fibroma (Meig's syndrome).
- Theca cell tumor
- Brenner's tumor (Pseudomeig syndrome)
- Granulosa cell tumor (Rarely). *Ref: Shaw 13rd/ed, p403*

43. Ans. is b and c, i.e. Septations; and Bilaterality

44. Ans. is c, i.e. Papillary vegetation *Ref: Sutton 2nd/ed, p1083*

USG features of malignant ovarian tumor:
- Hypoechoic solid area within the mass (highly echogenic solid areas due to fat or calcification are typical of dermoids).
- Thick (more than 3 mm) nodular septations / papillary vegetations
- Size of mass greater than 7 cm, although very large but simple cysts are usually benign cystadenomas.
- Central rather than peripheral vascularity.
- RI less than 0.6. RI greater than 0.8 is suggestive of benign disease but there is an indeterminate range of 0.6 – 0.8.

In Q 42-Presence of papillary vegetation is suggestive of malignancy and hence is an indication for laparotomy.

45. Ans. is c, i.e. Testosterone *Ref: Shaw 15th/ed, p380; Williams Gynae 1st/ed, p391*

"Specifically women with an abrupt onset, typically within several months or sudden worsening of virilising signs should prompt concern for a hormone producing ovarian or adrenal tumor. Serum testosterone levels may be used to exclude these tumors." *Ref: Williams Gynae 1st/ed, p391*

Rapidly developing hirsutism with amenorrhoea and change in voice is suggestive of masculinizing tumor *like Arrhenoblastoma or androblastoma which are invariably associated with raised testosterone (T > 200 ng/dl).*

All ***masculinizing tumor*** have similar presentation *characterized by defeminization such as breast atrophy and amenorrhoea, hirsutism, ache hoarseness of voice, muscular development,* clitoromegaly and receding hair line.

Removal of tumor restores the secondary sexual character but ***hoarseness*** of voice is permanent.

Note:
- Most common cause of hirsutism in young girls - PCOD (80% cases).
- PCOD is not associated with hoarseness and hirsutism is not rapidly developing.
- In PCOD - testosterone levels though raised are less than 200 ng/dl.

Friends here it is important to know that we are measuring the levels of testosterone and not DHEA because main source of DHEA is adrenal gland and not ovary.

46. Ans. is d, i.e. Dermoid cyst *Ref: Sutton 2nd/ed, p1085*

An ovarian mass with radio opaque shadow on X-ray points towards dermoid cyst as the diagnosis.

Causes of Pelvic Calcification are:

i. *Fibroids:* popcorn type
ii. *Dermoid cyst:* it is the commonest ovarian mass to calcify
iii. *Other ovarian masses:* cystadenoma / carcinoma, fibromas
iv. Pseudomyxoma peritonei
v. *Fallopian tube calcification (rare):* suggest TB
vi. *Uterine* i.e. endometrial calcification from chronic endometritis.

47. Ans. is a, i.e. Dysgerminoma *Ref: Novak 15th/ed, p1394, 14th/ed, p1505; Shaw 14th/ed, p338*

M/C tumor in young females is- Germ cell tumor *Ref: Shaw 14th/ed, p555*

Hence in this female it could either be a dysgerminoma, endodermal sinus tumor or malignant terotoma, all of which are germ cell tumors (mucinous cystadenocarcinoma is ruled out)

The mass in this female has solid component as revealed on USG so it is most probably malignant

M/C malignant GCT is teratoma > dysgerminoma, furthermore in the patient- levels of

Alpha-fetoprotein is normal, hence endodermal sinus tumor ruled out

Alkaline phosphatase is elevated hence diagnosis of dysgerminoma is confirmed

"Unlike other germ cell tumors dysgerminoma is not associated with raised AFP and rarely increases HCG, however placental alkaline phosphatase and lactate dehydrogenases are commonly produced by dysgerminoma and may be useful in monitoring the disease."

Ref: Novak 14th/ed, p1505

48. Ans. is b, i.e. Krukenberg tumor *Ref: Shaw 15th/ed, p379*

Already explained.

49. Ans. is d, i.e. Hilus cell tumor *Ref: Shaw 15th/ed, p381*

50. Ans. is a, i.e. Schiller-Duval bodies *Ref: CGDT 9th/ed, p938; Shaw 13rd/ed, p362*

Call exner bodies are small cyst like spaces found in cases of granulosa cell tumor.

Feature	Associated tumor
Call exner bodies & coffee bean nuclei	Granulosa cell tumor
Schiller duval bodies	Endodermal sinus tumor
Reinke's crystal	Hilus cell tumor
Psammoma bodies	Serous epithelial tumors
Walthard cell nest	Brenner tumor
Signet ring cell	Krukenberg tumor
Hobnail cell	Clear cell tumor
Large polygonal cell with lymphocytic	Dysgerminoma
Infiltration and fibrous septa	
Skin, teeth, cartilage	Teratoma

51. Ans. is c, i.e. Serum lactic dehydrogenase *Ref: Novak 14th/ed, p1505; Shaw 15th/ed, p378*

52. Ans. is b, i.e. LDH *Ref: Shaw 15th/ed, p378*

"Unlike other germ cell tumor dysgerminoma is not associated with raised AFP and rarely increase HCG; however placental alkaline phosphate and lactate dehydrogenase are commonly produced by dysgerminomas and may be useful in monitoring the disease." *Ref: Novak 14th/ed, p1505*

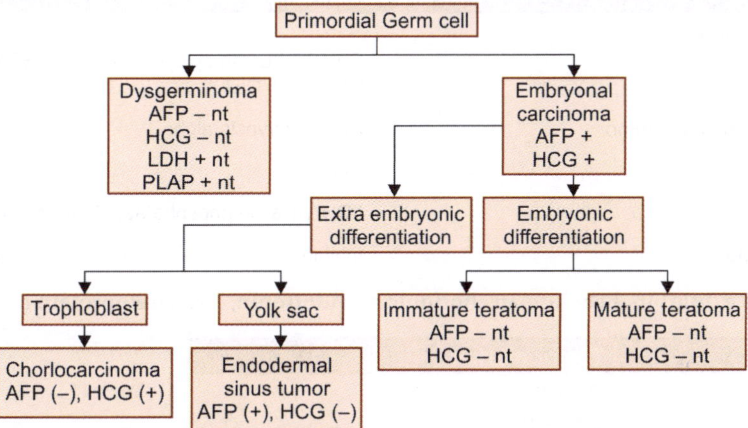

AFP - Alpha Feto Protein

LDH - Lactic Dehydrogenase

HCG - Human Chorionic Gonadotropin

PLAP - Placental Alkaline Phosphatase

53. Ans. is a, i.e. CA - 125 *Ref: Novak 14th/ed, p1505; Shaw 15th/ed, p378, 387*

CA 125 is tumor marker of epithelial cell neoplasm (not for germ cell tumor).

54. Ans. is a, i.e. Carcinoma ovary *Ref: Shaw 15th/ed, p387*

55. Ans. is c, i.e. Ovarian Ca *Ref: Shaw 15th/ed, p387*

56. Ans. is c, i.e. Epithelial cell carcinoma of ovary *Ref: Shaw 15th/ed, p387; Williams Gynae 1st/ed, p722*

- CA - 125 is a glycoprotein secreted by malignant epithelial tumors of ovary. Therefore it is a marker of epithelial cell carcinoma of ovary.
- CA - 125 level correlates with volume of tumor and is elevated in 50% of Stage I tumor and 90% of tumors with Stage II or higher.
- CA - 125 level is also useful for follow up after treatment. Level > 35 units/ml suggests residual tumor.

Remember:

- Two best screening test for ovarian ca are measurement of CA - 125 levels and transvaginal USG.
- CA - 125 is raised in: *Ref: Harrison 16th/ed, p554*

Benign condition	Malignant condition
• Pregnancy	• Endometrial Ca
• PID	• Pancreas Ca
• Endometrioses	• Colon Ca
• Uterine fibroid	• Cervix Ca
• About 1% of normal females	• Fallopian tubes Ca
	• Breast Ca
	• Ovarian epithelial Ca (MC cause)
	• Lung Ca

Mnemonic: **E**ndogenous **P**neumocystis **C**arinii **C**auses **TB** **Of** **L**ungs

- In a postmenopausal women with an asymptomatic pelvic mass and CA - 125 > 65 U/ml is very sensitive for diagnosis of ovarian epithelial tumor.
- Although CA 125 is raised in many cancers it is specific for epithelial ovarian cancer.

57. Ans. is b, i.e. PET *Ref: Novaks Gynae 14th/ed, p1496*

For Recurrence, IOC is PET scan

58. Ans. is d, i.e. Dysgerminoma *Ref: Novak 14th/ed, p1505*

Placental alkaline phosphatase and LDH are tumor markers of dysgerminoma.

59. Ans. is c, i.e. Inhibin *Ref: William Gynae 1st/ed, p747*

Ovarian Tumor	Tumor Marker
• Epithelial ovarian tumors Serous variety Mucinous variety	 CA 125, human epidymal protein (HEP)4 OVA-1 Ca 19 – 9, CEA
• Endodermal sinus/Yolk sac tumor	AFP, antitrypsin alpha 1
• Chorio carcinoma	HCG
• Dysgerminoma	LDH, Alkaline phosphatase (DAL mnemonic)
• Granulosa cell tumor	Inhibin

60. Ans. is a, b, c and e, i.e. Inhibin, Beta human chorionic gonadotropin, Alphafetoprotein (AFP) and NB/70K

Ovarian cancer	Tumor marker
Serous cancer Plucinous cancer	CA 125 CA 19-9
Germ cell tumors	AFP HCG LDH Placental alkaline phosphatase
Granulosa cell tumor	Inhibin

- **Gene NB/70K** are raised in all patients of the pathologic types of early stage, low grade epithelial ovarian cancers (nvbi library)
  - Pax genes play critical roles during fetal development and cancer growth. Pax 7 is associated with alveolar rhabdomyosarcoma.

Note: PAX2 is expressed is ovarian cancer and breast cancer and is expressed in epithelial lining of fallopian tube in females PAX1 is expressed in cervical cancers

61. Ans. is d, i.e. Dermoid cyst *Ref: Williams Gynae 1st/ed, p741*

62. Ans. is a, i.e. Dysgerminoma *Ref: Jeffcoate 6th/ed, p522; Novak 14th/ed, p1519, 1517, 1514*

"Dysgerminomas are the only germ cell malignancy with a significant rate of bilateral involvement 15 to 20%."

Remember:

A ***"Funda"*** – Germ cell tumors are unilateral and maximum bilaterality is seen in dysgerminoma amongst germ cell tumor and that too only in 15 - 20% cases.

So, the other germ cell tumor will obviously be less bilateral therefore our answer to Question 58 is *dermoid cyst.*

Other important fundas:

- Endodermal sinus tumors are unilateral in 100% cases.
- Granulosa cell tumors are U/L in 98% of cases and bilateral in only 2% of cases

In Q 62:

Endodermal sinus tumor as I have said is U/L in 100% cases so it is ruled out, Dysgerminoma is bilateral in 15–20% cases. Lets have a look at embryonal cell carcinoma-

Embryonal cell carcinoma

- The primary lesions tend to be large, and about two thirds are confined to one ovary at the time of diagnosis.

Ref: Novak 14th/ed, p1519

63. Ans. is a, i.e. Granulosa cell tumor *Ref: Shaw 15th/ed, p379-80*

"The metastasis of granulosa cell tumor is interesting because the opposite ovary first become involved, then metastasis develop in the lumber region, secondary deposits become scattered in the mesentery, the liver and mediastinum."

Granulosa cell tumor and theca cell tumor are feminizing tumors that originate from sex cord stroma.

Feminizing Tumors of Ovary:

	Granulosa cell tumor	Theca cell tumor
Incidence	Common	Rare
Age	Occurs at any age but most common after 40 years.	Occur after menopause
Presentation	In prepubertal girls it leads to precocious puberty, hypertrophy[Q] of breast.	Usually presents as postmenopausal bleeding.[Q]
	In adults – leads to amenorrhoea followed by prolonged bleeding (metropathia hemorrhagica)[Q]	
	In postmenopausal women – Causes Postmenopausal bleeding[Q]	
	Metastases to opposite ovary first is characteristic feature.[Q]	
Microscopy	**Exhibits:** Coffee bean nuclei. Call exner bodies.	It has spindle shaped cells together with fat laden cells.

Remember:

- Both these tumors cause endometrial hyperplasia and so, risk of carcinoma endometrium is increased.Q
- Both these tumors can become luteinized to form a luteoma, they may then produce progesterone as well as oestrogen and convert the endometrium to a secretory one.
  Besides granulosa tumor complain other tumor which can show metastasis to opposite ovary is dysgerminoma but it is not very significant. *Ref: Novak 13rd/ed, p1286; 14th/ed, p1509*
- Both these tumors can cause pseudomeig syndrome. *Ref: Dutta Gynae 4th/ed, p277*

64. Ans. is c, i.e. Omental biopsy *Ref: Williams Gynae 1st/ed, p729; Novak 14th/ed, p1478*

Surgical staging is done in all cases of ovarian cancer.

- Typically, the abdominal incision must be adequate to identify and resect any disease that may have been missed on physical examination or imaging tests.
- The operation begin by aspirating free ascitic fluid or collecting peritoneal washing followed by visualization and palpation of all peritoneal surfaces and viscera proceeding in a clockwise manner from cecum.
- Next an extrafascial (simple) hysterectomy and BSO are performed and infracolic omentectomy done.
- In the absence of gross extraovarian disease, peritoneal biopsies are obtained, along with a biopsy or scraping of the right diaphragm.
- Finally, a pelvic and infrarenal para-aortic lymphadenectomy is complete.

Note: Infracolic omentectomy is done: Not omental biopsy

65. Ans. is a, i.e. Stage II b *Ref: Novak Internet-FGO site p427*

From the new staging , given in preceding text it is seen that if there is retroperitoneal or inguinal lymphnode involved, it is in stage IV B, and, pelvic lymphnode involvement is included in stage IIB.

66. Ans. is a, i.e. Stage I *Ref: Novak 14th/ed, p1477; Shaw 15th/ed, p427*

67. Ans. is d, i.e. Stage Ic *Ref: Novak 14th/ed, p1477; Shaw 15th/ed, p427*

Bilateral involvement and malignant ascites is seen in category IC.

- In IC also- according to new classification it is IC 3.

68. Ans. is c, i.e. Stage III *Ref: Shaw 15th/ed, p427*

- Superficial liver metastasis is included in Stage III.
- Metastasis to liver parenchyma is included in Stage IV.

69. Ans. is d, i.e. Multiloculated, sticky, gelatinous fluid *Ref: Shaw 15th/ed, p374; Dutta Gynae 5th/ed, p282*

Serous cystadenoma:

- Most common of cystic neoplasms.
- It accounts for 50% of all ovarian tumors, of these 60% are benign, 15% are borderline, 25% of malignant.
- Occur in 3rd, 4th and 5th decade of life.
- Half cases are bilateral (option "a" and "b" are true)

It is a unilocular cyst.

- Delicate papillary excrescences may be seen on the surface and within the loculi of a benign cyst.
- Histologically – the benign variety shows cystic spaces and the lining of the tumor consists of tall columnar ciliated epithelium resembling the endosalpinx.
- The loculi contain a thin serous straw coloured fluid, which may be blood stained when malignant transformation occurs.

  Rate of malignant transformation-40%
- Option "d" (Dutta Gynae, 5/e, p 282): Mucinous cystadenoma have glistening surface and cut surface shows loculi filled with mucinous material. The content is thick, viscid, and mucin. The cyst is frequently multiloculated.

70. Ans. is c, i.e. Wait and watch *Ref: Novak 14th/ed, p472*

The patient is premenopausal and has a 3 x 4 cm clear ovarian cyst, so she is best managed by giving OC pills for 1–2 cycles and then repeating the USG.

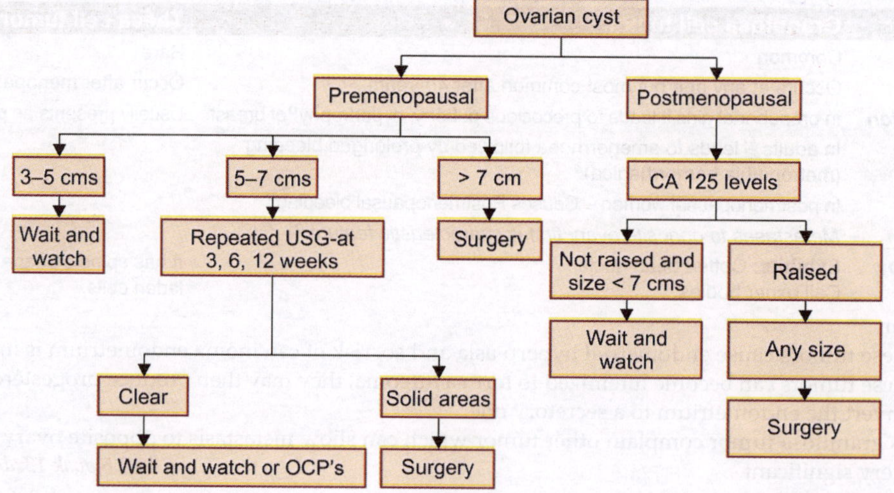

Note: OCP's are not given routinely for ovarian masses as trey decrease the risk of developing new cysts but donot hasten the resolution of existing cyst

71. Ans. is c, i.e. Surgery *Ref: Novak 14th/ed, p472*

As explained in text.

Any ovarian mass with signs of malignancy (B/L and increased vascularity) require surgery irrespective of the size. The exact nature and extent of surgery is only decided intraoperatively, depending upon the frozen section (pathology) report.

72. Ans. is b, i.e. Dermoid cyst

73. Ans. is c, i.e. Dermoid cyst *Ref: Dutta Obs. 6th/ed, p310; Williams Gynae 1st/ed, p214*

74. Ans. is b, i.e. Laparotomy at 14–16 weeks *Ref: Williams obs 23rd/ed, p905-6*

"Dysgerminomas are the most common malignant tumor diagnosed during pregnancy but overall most common is dermoid cyst." *Ref: Williams Gynae 1st/ed, p214*

Ovarian cysts in pregnancy

M/C ovarian cyst diagnosed in pregnancy- Dermoid cyst

M/C ovarian tumor to undergo torsion in pregnancy- Dermoid cyst

M/C time for ovarian cyst to undergo torsion in pregnancy- end of first trimester and/or puerperium.

Management:

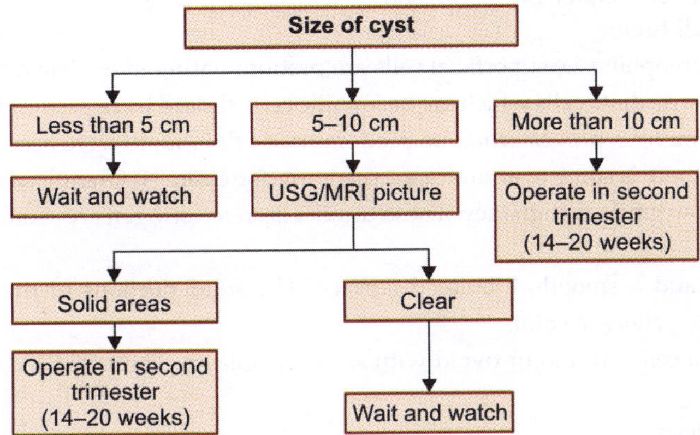

In cases of emergency (e.g., torsion, rupture) do Surgery, irrespective of size and weeks of gestation.

75. Ans. is a, d and e, i.e. Debulking; Chemotherapy; and Cytoreduction.

Ref: Shaw 15th/ed, p428; Dutta Gynae 6th/ed, p378-9

Management of Advanced stage disease (stages III and IV) in ovarian cancer:

- **Advanced stage disease:** Exploratory Laparotomy → Cytoreductive or debulking surgery. This includes: Total abdominal hysterectomy bilateral salpingo-oophorectomy, complete omentectomy, retroperitoneal lymph node sampling and resection of any metastatic tumor. Optimum cytoreductive surgery is aimed to reduce the residual tumor load < 1–2 cm in diameter. Lesser the residual tumor volume (< 1 cm), better is the survival.
- **Chemotherapy:** Chemotherapy is used widely following surgery to improve the result in terms of survival. Drugs are given for five or six cycles at 3–4 weekly interval.
- **Combination chemotherapy:** Paclitaxel (175 mg/m^2) and carboplatin (400 mg/m^2) are commonly used.
- **Neoadjuvant chemotherapy and interval cytoreductive surgery:** Few cycles of chemotherapy followed by interval primary cytoreductive surgery may be done. Indications are: (i) Advanced epithelial ovarian cancer, (ii) High risk for surgery, (iii) Associated comorbid conditions (pleural effusion), (iv) Predicted to be suboptimally resected. Patient should have histological diagnosis of the tumor (biopsy). Benefits of neoadjuvant chemotherapy are: (i) Rapid clinical improvement. (ii) Subsequent surgery is easier and morbidity is reduced, (iii) Optimum cytoreduction with minimal residual disease may be possible.
- **Radiotherapy:** There is very little scope of radiotherapy as an adjunct to surgery because of the advent of chemotherapy.

76. Ans. is d, i.e. Ovarian cyst *Ref: Shaw's Textbook of Gynecology 15th/ed, p79,385*

As described in the examination, the swelling is typically arising from the pelvis as the hand cannot be insinuated. Only an ovarian cyst is a pelvis swelling among the given options.

Abdominal Palpation of pelvic swellings

The sensitive ulnar border of the left hand is used from above downwards to palpate swellings arising from the pelvis. The upper and lateral margins of such swellings can be felt but the lower border cannot be reached, i.e. the hand cannot be insinuated between the mass and the pelvis.

77. Ans. is d and e, i.e. Unilateral salpingo-oophorectomy is generally done and Constitutes 30% of all malignant germ cell tumors.

See the text for explanation. *Ref: Dutta Gyne 5/ed, p367, Nov 14th/ed, p1506-1508*

78. Ans. is b, i.e. Krukenberg tumor *Ref: Shaw's Textbook of Gynecology 15th/ed, p425*

B/L ovarian mass with smooth surface, and mucin secreting cells with signet-ring shaped nuclei indicated Krukenberg tumor.

79. Ans. is b, i.e. Dysgerminoma

The tumor shown in the picture is soft, fleshy with yellow white to pink appearance. On microscopic examination, there are large vesicular cells with clear cytoplasm, well defined cell boundaries and large nuclei with prominent nucleoli. All these leave no doubt towards Dysgerminoma being the answer of choice.

80. Ans. is a, i.e. Mature teratoma

The gross specimen, hair cells, teeth and ovarian mass can be seen. This is typically seen in dermoid cyst of ovary. For details of dermoid cyst, see chapter 14C of the book.

81. Ans. is b, i.e. Granulosa cell tumor

In the pap smear, large eosinophilic, i.e superficial cells are predominating in the late menstrual phase. Although ideally in late menstrual phase-intermediate cells which are basophilic cells should have predominated. This is because in the late menstrual phase, main hormone is progesterone, so predominant cells should have been intermediate cells.

This means in this female, there is some ovarian tumor secreting estrogen. i.e Granulosa cell tumor

Granulosa cell tumor is a low grade malignancy. These tumors secrete estrogen are seen in women of all ages.

They secrete estrogen.

These are rarely bilateral and a smooth, lobulated surface. The solid portions of the tumor are granula, frequently trabeculated, yellow or gray yellow in color.

The classic adult Granulosa cell is round or ovoid with scant cytoplasm. The nucleus contains compact, freely granular chromatin.

They have coffee bean nucleus.

They have call exner bodies.

82. Ans. is a, i.e. Observation and follow up for cyst after 2–3 months

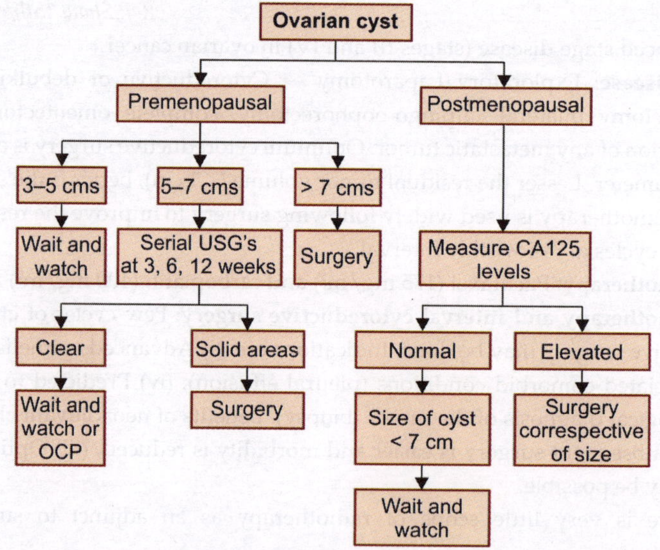

The age of patient is 25 years. The size of ovarian cyst is 5 cm.

Since the size of cyst is 5 cm, we will observe and follow-up the cyst.

Measurement of CA 125 does not hold any significance in young females.

83. Ans. is a, and d, i.e. Schiller Duval body and Spindle shaped cells or myxoid. *Ref: Novaus Gynae 15th/ed, p403*

"Micro scopically the characteristic feature is the Endodermal sinus on the Scheller Duval body. The cystic space is lined with a layer of flattend or irregular endothelium into which projects a glomerulus like tuft with a central vascular core. These structures vary throughout the tumor and the reticular, myxoid elements simulate undifferentiated masoblast. The lining of the papillary infolding and the cavity is irregular, with an occasional cell containing clear, glassy cytoplasm, simulating the libral appearance of the epithelium in clear cell tumors."

REVIEW/PRACTICE QUESTIONS

1. **Most Radiosensitive ovarian tumor:**
   a. Dysgerminoma
   b. Yolk sac Tumor
   c. Teratoma
   d. Epithelial ovarian cancer
2. **Hobnail cells is a feature of:**
   a. Brenner tumor
   b. Clean cell tumor
   c. Embryonal carcinoma
   d. Krukenberg tumor
3. **M/c gene mutation in sex cord tumors**
   a. FOX L-2 b. BRCA – 1
   c. P 53 d. CRAS
4. **All of the following are benign tumors of ovary *except*:**
   a. Brenner tumor
   b. Theca lutein cyst
   c. Dermoid cyst
   d. Serous cyst adenoma
5. **Lutein cysts are seen in all *except*:**
   a. Gestational trophoblastic tumors
   b. Use of OCP's
   c. Clomiphene therapy
   d. Gonadotropin therapy
6. **True about granulosa cell Tumor:**
   a. Bilateral in 20% cases
   b. Most malignant ovarian tumor
   c. Characteristic feature Scheller Duval body
   d. Associated with cancer endometrium
7. **HPE of an ovarian tumor in a 14-years-old girl shows solid disorganised sheets of large anaplastic cells, & papillary structures. The most early diagnosis is:**
   a. Yolk sac tumor
   b. Embryonal carcinoma
   c. Chevs carcinoma
   d. Dysgerminoma
8. **IOC to differentiate between benign and malignant ovarian mass:**
   a. TVS b. TAS
   c. CT scan d. MRI
9. **Malignant tumors are characterized by usually all of the following *except*:**
   a. Large size (>5 cm)
   b. Thick septa
   c. Solid
   d. Uniloculated
10. **All of the following can be used as an ovarian marker in nonmucinous epithelial tumors *except*:**
    a. CA125
    b. OVA 1
    c. Human epididymal protein 4
    d. AFP
11. **Tumor marker for mucinous epithelium ovarian tumors:**
    a. CA 19-9
    b. CEA (carcino embryonic antigen)
    c. Both
    d. None
12. **Maximum nodal metatosis seen in GCT:**
    a. Dysgerminoma
    b. Teratoma
    c. Yolk sac Tumor
    d. Embryonal tumor
13. **M/C cause of pseudomyxoma pertonelli:**
    a. Mucocele of appendix
    b. Appendix cancer
    c. Mucinous cystadenoma
    d. Mucinous cystadenocarcinoma
14. **GCT with worst prognosis:**
    a. Yolk sac Tumor
    b. Embryonal carcinoma
    c. Dysgerminemia
    d. Mature teratoma
15. **M/C symptom of germ cell tumors:**
    a. Bleeding
    b. Irritable Bowel syndrome
    c. Nausea & vomiting
    d. Subacute pain in abdomen
16. **Schiller-Duval bodies are seen in:** *(JIPMER May 2019)*
    a. Endodermal sinus tumour
    b. Embryonal carcinoma
    c. Dermoid cyst
    d. Brenner tumour
17. **Which is/are NOT elevated in dysgerminoma?** *(PGI May 2019)*
    a. Beta-hCG
    b. AFP
    c. CA125
    d. Placental alkaline phosphatase (PLAP)
    e. LDH
18. **True statement(s) about Germ cell tumors:** *(PGI May 2019)*
    a. More common in young adults
    b. Sacrococcygeal chordoma and parachordoma are included in germ cell tumors
    c. Teratocarcinoma is a mixture of teratoma and squamous cell carcinoma
    d. Clear cell tumor is a germ cell
    e. hCG is used as marker

REVIEW/PRACTICE ANSWERS

1. **Ans. is a, i.e. Dysgerminoma**
2. **Ans. is b, i.e. Clean cell tumor**
3. **Ans. is a, i.e. FOX L-2**
   (Its a functional cyst)
4. **Ans. is b, i.e. Theca lutein cyst** *Ref: Williams Gynae 3rd/ed, p219*
5. **Ans. is b, i.e. Use of OCP's**
6. **Ans. is d, i.e. Associated with cancer endometrium** *Ref: Williams Gynae 3rd/ed, p764*
7. **Ans. is b, i. e. Embryonal carcinoma**
8. **Ans. is a, i.e. TVS**
9. **Ans. is d, i.e. Uniloculated** *Ref: Williams gynae 3rd/ed, p742*
10. **Ans. is d, i.e. AFP** *Ref: Williams Gynae 3rd/ed, p742*
11. **Ans. is c, i.e. Both** *Ref: William Gynae 3rd/ed, p742*
12. **Ans. is a, i.e. Dysgerminoma** *Ref: William Gynae 3rd/ed, p763*
13. **Ans. is b, i.e. Appendix cancer**
   " Yolk sac tumors are deadlist malignant GCT"
14. **Ans. is a, i.e. Yolk sac Tumor** *Ref: William Gynae 3rd/ed, p764*
15. **Ans. is d, i.e. Subacute pain in abdomen**
   "Subacute abdominal pain is presenting symptom in 85% patients." *Ref: William Gynae 3rd/ed, p760.*
16. **Ans. is a, i.e. Endodermal sinus tumour** *Ref: Dutta, Textbook of Gynecology, 5th/ed, p368*
   - **Schiller–Duval bodies** are characteristic histological feature of **endodermal sinus tumour.**
   - They are tuft of vascular tissue inside cystic spaces lined by flattened epithelium. For more details see chapter on ovarian tumors.
17. **Ans. is b, i.e. AFP**

   Dysgerminomas: The tumor is neutral and does not secrete either male or female sex hormones but ***placental alkaline phosphatase (PLAP), lactate dehydrogenase (LDH) and*** β-hCG *– Shaw's Gynae 16th/441; 17th/463)*

   "In **dysgerminomas**, diagnosis is usually confirmed by positive immunohistochemical staining for ***LDH, CA-125, β-hCG, PALP, NSE, cytokeratin 18 and S-100 protein"*** *– www.cancerjournal.net*

   Germ cell tumors: Some of these tumors produce elevated levels of human chorionic gonadotropin (hCG), which can lead to isosexual precocious puberty. As with testicular tumors, some of these tumors tend to produce ***AFP (yolk sac tumors)*** or **hCG** (embryonal carcinoma, choriocarcinomas and some ***dysgerminomas***) that are reliable tumor markers" *– Harrison 19th/ed, p594*
18. **Ans. is a and e, i.e. More common in young adults and hCG is used as marker**

   Clear cell (Mesonephroid) tumor is *epithelial cell tumor* of ovary *– Robbins 9th/ed, p1023; Shaw's 17th/ed, p444*

   "**Teratocarcinoma** *refers to germ cell tumor that is a mixture of* ***teratoma with embryonal carcinoma or with choriocarcinoma or with both"*** *– link.springer.com*

   "**Chordomas** are rare malignant tumors of ***notochordal origin*** and are rare locally aggressive ones with a metastatic potential." *– www.hindawi.com*

Ref: Shaw's Gynae 17th/ed, p316; Dutta Gynae 7th/ed, p378-79; radiopaedia.org
Ref: Harrison 20th/ed, p640; Robbins 9th/ed, p1314, 1029, 976, 977; Harshmohan 8th/ed, p782, 777

CHAPTER 14D

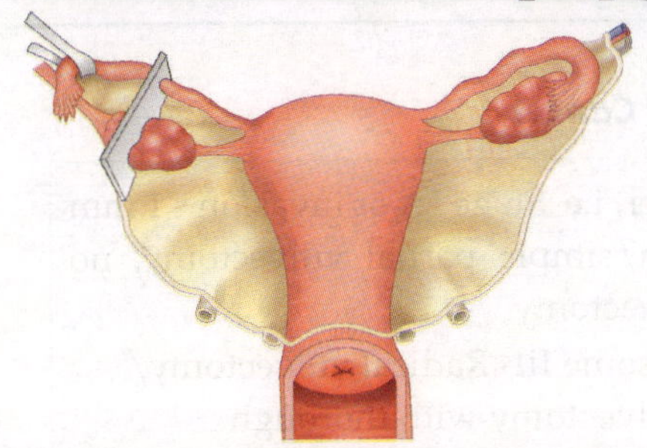

Gynecological Oncology: Miscellaneous Tumors

Vulva

Premalignant Lesions of Vulva

- VIN
- Lichen sclerosis
- Paget's disease
- Squamous hyperplasia/ hyperplastic dystrophy
- Bowen disease erythroplasia of queyrat

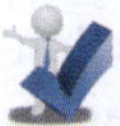

KEY POINTS

Any suspicious lesion of the vulva should be biopsied.

Classification of Epithelial Vulvar Diseases

Non-neoplastic epithelial disorders of skin and mucosa

- Lichen sclerosis
- Squamous hyperplasia (earlier called as hyperplastic dystrophy)

Mixed neoplastic and non-neoplastic epithelial disorders

Intraepithelial neoplasia

Squamous intraepithelial neoplasia	Nonsquamous intraepithelial neoplasia
• VIN 1 • VIN 2 • VIN 3 • VIN 1	• Paget's disease • Tumor of melanocyte and Noninvasive

Invasive tumors

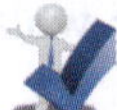

KEY POINTS

Non-neoplastic disorders of vulvar epithelium

Hyperplastic dystrophy (squamous cell hyperplasia)

- Surface thickened and hyperkeratotic
- Most common symptom pruritis seen in post menopausal females
- Treatment-1% fluorinated corticosteroid ointment bid for 6 weeks

Lichen sclerosis

- Subepithelial fat becomes diminished, labia becomes thin and atrophic, labial fusion .
- Symptoms- pruritis, dyspareunia, burning
- Most common in postmenopausal women
- Treatment-ultrapotent topical steroid .05%, clobetasol x 2-4 weeks then taper down.

Paget's Disease of Vulva

Mostly confined to epithelium. It occurs in two forms Intraepithelial Paget's disease and invasive Paget's disease

- M/C in postmenopausal women
- Patients complain of itching, irritation and bleeding
- The lesion has slightly raised margins, it is erythematous, with islands of white epithelium.
- **Histologically, it is characterized by Paget cells,** Velvety red lesion
- 10–15% patients with vulvar Paget's disease have an underlying adenocarcinoma of sweat glands.
- 10% patients of vulvar Paget's disease also have associated breast, colon or genitourinary cancer.
- So workup of Paget's disease should include colonoscopy, cystoscopy, mammography and colposcopy.

Treatment

- Intraepithelial paget – Wide local excision
- Invasive paget – Radical vulvectomy with lymph node dissection
- Recurrence rate is very high.
- Management of recurrence - laser ablation

Treatment of Vulval Intraepithelial Neoplasia

- Treatment of choice – Surgery
  - Wide local excision done in young patient with localized lesion
  - Skinning vulvectomy – (Remove epidermis, not the underlying fibro fatty tissue) done in –Young patient with multicentric lesion
  - Simple vulvectomy done in elderly patient with extensive lesion

- CO_2 laser can be used in multicentric lesions
- Topical 5 Fluorouracil

Vulval Cancer

- M/C variety- Squamous cell carcinoma
- Most common symptom of vulval cancer - pruritis
- Most common site: Labia majora and minora
- Most common type of spread: Lymphatics (First lymph node involved-Superficial Inguinal lymph node, and then Deep inguinal LN and femoral group of lymph nodes).
- For lateral tumors only ipsilateral lymph nodes involved whereas for midline lesions, B/L lymph nodes are involved
- Sentinel lymph node biopsy is helpful in vulval cancer
- Most important prognostic factor- Lymph node status.

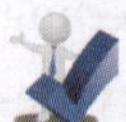

KEY POINTS

HPV 16 and 18 are the most common risk factors for developing vulvar carcinoma:

- Sentinel lymph node for vulvar carcinoma is superficial inguinal lymph node
- Sentinel lymph node biopsy is useful for knowing the spread of vulvar carcinoma
- In vulvar carcinoma both TNM and FIGO staging can be done

Investigations Done in Vulvar Carcinoma

- Physical examination
- Always biopsy
- +/–Colposcopy

FIGO Staging of Vulval Cancer

Stage I – Tumor confined to vulva or perineum (No nodes)
IA – Size ≤ to 2 cms stromal invasion <1 mm
IB – Size > 2 cms stromal invasion > 1 mm

Stage II – Tumor of any size with spreads to lower urethra, lower vagina or anus, with negative nodes.

Stage III – Tumor of any size spread to lower urethra, lower vagina or anus and regional lymph node metastasis (i.e. inguinal, femoral lymphnodes involved)

Stage IVA – Tumor invades upper urethra, upper vagina, bladder mucosa, rectal mucosa or fixed or ulcerated inguinofemoral nodes

Stage IVB – Any distant metastasis including pelvic LN.

Treatment of Vulval Cancer

Microinvasive cancer, i.e. Stage IA or invasion <1 mm Wide local excision/simple partial vulvectomy, no need for lymphadenectomy.
Stage IB and II and some III- Radical vulvectomy/ Modified radical vulvectomy with thorough inguinofemoral lymphadenectomy.
If lesion is central do B/L lymph node dissection otherwise if it is >2 cms from midline do ipsilateral inguinofemoral lymphadenectomy

Postoperative radiotherapy to be given if 2 or more groin nodes involved or disease free margin is <8 cms

Note: In simple partial vulvectomy dissection is carried uptil the superficial layer of urogenital fascia.
In modified radical/radical vulvectomy - dissection done uptil the deep fascia of urogenital diaphragm, i.e. the perineal membrane.

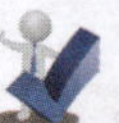

KEY POINTS

Prognosis of Vulvar Carcinoma

- Depends on nodal involvement (single most important predictor followed by tumor size)
- Lesion > 3 cm are associated with poor prognosis
- Overall 5-year survival rate =79%

Vaginal Carcinoma

- Primary cancer of vagina are very rare.
- Most common age group is elderly females > 70 years.
- Most common histologic type is squamous cell carcinoma.
- Most common site is upper third of posterior wall of vagina.

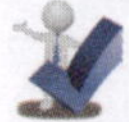

KEY POINTS

Clear cell adenocarcinoma occurs due to DES exposure to mother in first trimester.

Most common lesion due to DES exposure is vaginal adenosis (benign lesion).

Symptoms

- Mostly asymptomatic
- Patient may present with painless abnormal vaginal bleeding (including post coital bleeding).
- Foul smelling discharge per vaginum.

Signs

- On per speculum examination-ulcerative/exophytic growth on vagina.
- Cervix appears normal.

Lymphatic Drainage

- Tumor arising in upper vagina: drains to pelvic lymph node.
- Tumor arising in lower part: drains to inguinal lymph node.

Vaginal cancer staging

Stage 0	Vaginal intraepithelial neoplasia (VAIN)
Stage I	Carcinoma limited to the vaginal wall.
Stage II	Carcinoma extending beyond the vagina, but
Stage	not extending to the pelvic side walls.
III	Carcinoma extends upto the pelvic walls.
	Carcinoma extending beyond the true pelvis/ or involving the bladder and/or rectum, or evidence of distal metastasis.

Management

KEY POINTS

VAIN-Vaginal Intraepithelial Neoplasia

TREATMENT

VAIN 1-No treatment

VAIN 2-Laser

VAIN 3-Surgical excision.

- Stage I – Tumor involving upper 1/3rd vagina – Radical hysterectomy + Radical vaginectomy + bilateral pelvic lymphadenectomy
- Tumor involving lower 1/3rd vagina – Radical vulvectomy + Bilateral inguinofemoral lymphadenectomy + Radical vaginectomy.

Note: Carcinoma involving the distal third of the vagina necessitates dissection of groin nodes.)

- Tumor involving middle 1/3rd of vagina – External Radiotherapy + Brachytherapy
- Stages II and III – Radiotherapy
- Stage IV – Pelvic exenteration + Radiotherapy

NEW PATTERN QUESTIONS

N1. Most common recurrence sites or metastatic sites of malignancy following pelvic surgery are all except:

a. Carcinoma cervix – Lateral pelvic wall and central pelvis
b. Carcinoma ovary – Lung
c. Chorionepithelioma – Suburethral region in anterior vaginal wall
d. Carcinoma body – Vault of vagina

N2. The most common site of vulval cancer:

a. Labia majora
b. Labia minora
c. Prepuce of the clitoris
d. Bartholin's gland

N3. The following statements are related to clear cell carcinoma of the vagina except:

a. Common to those whose mothers were given diethylstilbestrol during early pregnancy
b. Vaginal adenosis may progress to this conditions
c. The middle one-third is the commonest site
d. May be multicentric and may involve even the cervix as well

N4. The following primary tumours are common in the vulva except:

a. Adenocarcinoma
b. Basal cell carcinoma
c. Choriocarcinoma
d. Squamous cell carcinoma

N5. All of the following statements hold true for melanoma of vulva *except*:

a. It is the 2nd M/C vulval cancer
b. M/C site is labia majora
c. May arise from junctional nevus
d. Has a poor prognosis

PREVIOUS YEAR QUESTIONS

1. **Most common vaginal carcinoma is:** *(PGI 99)*
   a. Squamous cell carcinoma
   b. Adenocarcinoma
   c. Botryoid's tumor
   d. Columnar hyperplasia
2. **Involvement of pelvis in a case of vaginal carcinoma of stage:** *(AI 97)*
   a. I b. II
   c. III d. IV
3. **Common differential diagnosis of verrucous carcinoma is:** *(AIIMS 96)*
   a. Condylomata lata b. Condylomata acuminata
   c. Adenocarcinoma d. Tuberculosis
4. **Which is most commonly implicated in genital (vulval) warts?** *(AIIMS May 08)*
   a. HPV 16 b. HPV 18
   c. HPV 31 d. HPV 6
5. **True about Ca vulva associated/predisposed by:** *(PGI 02)*
   a. Paget's disease
   b. Vulval intraepithelial neoplasia
   c. Bowen's disease
6. **Vulval Ca, True statements:** *(PGI Dec 09)*
   a. Squamous hyperplasia predisposes
   b. Paget's disease of vulva predisposes
   c. Lichen sclerosis
   d. Condylomata acuminata
   e. Dystrophy
7. **True about carcinoma vulva:** *(PGI 04)*
   a. Spreads to superficial inguinal nodes
   b. Spreads to iliac nodes
   c. Seen after menopause
   d. Viral predisposition
   e. Radiotherapy given
8. **Brachytherapy is used in:** *(PGI 00)*
   a. Stage Ib Ca cervix
   b. Ovarian Ca
   c. Stage IV Ca vagina
   d. Stage II fallopian tube Ca
9. **All of these secrete hormone, except:** *(AIIMS May 93)*
   a. Granulosa cell tumor
   b. Dysgerminoma
   c. Hilus cell tumor
   d. Theca cell tumor
10. **Pyometra commonly occurs following:** *(AIIMS Dec 94)*
    a. Carcinoma endometrium
    b. Carcinoma cervix
    c. Carcinoma urethra
    d. Senile endometritis
11. **Pyometra is a complication associated with all of the following conditions except:** *(AI 03)*
    a. Carcinoma vulva
    b. Carcinoma cervix
    c. Carcinoma endometrium
    d. Pelvic radiotherapy
12. **Characteristic feature of carcinoma fallopian tube:** *(MAHE 01)*
    a. Watery discharge P/V
    b. Hemorrhage
    c. Pain
    d. Sepsis
13. **Patient diagnosed as squamous cell intraepithelial lesion which of the following has the highest risk for progression to carcinoma:** *(AIIMS Nov 07)*
    a. Low grade squamous intraepithelial neoplasia
    b. High grade squamous intraepithelial neoplasia
    c. Squamous intraepithelial associated with HPV 16
    d. Squamous intraepithelial neoplasia associated with HIV
14. **Sentinel biopsy most effective in:** *(AI 2010)*
    a. Cervix cancer b. Endometrium ca
    c. Vulval ca e. Vaginal ca
15. **The treatment of leukoplakia of vulva is:** *(UPSC 85; PGI 86)*
    a. Irradiation
    b. Simple vulvectomy
    c. Radical vulvectomy
    d. Estrogen cream
16. **All of the following are used for screening cancers in females except:** *(AIIMS Nov 2014)*
    a. CA-125: Ovarian cancer
    b. Office endometrial aspirate: Endometrial carcinoma
    c. Pap smear: Cervical cancer
    d. Mammography: Breast cancer
17. **Which of the following most commonly causes intraorbital metastasis in female?** *(AIIMS Nov 13)*
    a. Breast cancer
    b. Cervical cancer
    c. Ovarian cancer
    d. Endometrial cancer
18. **A 76-year-old female presented with non-healing ulcer on labia majora for 6 months measuring 2 × 3 cm with no palpable lymphadenopathy. Biopsy shows squamous cell carcinoma. Management includes?** *(AIIMS may 2018)*
    a. Radical vulvectomy with unilateral LN dissection
    b. Radical vulvectomy with bilateral LN dissection
    c. Simple vulvectomy
    d. Chemoradiation with resection

ANSWERS TO NEW PATTERN QUESTIONS

N1. Ans. is b, i.e. Carcinoma ovary – Lung *Ref: Dutta Gynae 6th/ed, p360, 354,376*

Endometrial cancer/cancer body uterus *Ref: Dutta Gynae 6th/ed, p360*

Recurrent disease: Common sites for recurrence are the vagina and the pelvis. The extrapelvic metastases are seen in the lung, lymph nodes (aortic), liver, brain and bones. Majority (60%) of recurrences are seen within 2 years of initial therapy.

- Radiation therapy is the choice for isolated recurrence following surgical treatment:
- Exenterative surgery for recurrent endometrial cancer is of limited value.
- Hormonal therapy and chemotherapy have been used depending on the individual case.

Cancer cervix: Recurrent disease *Ref: Dutta Gynae 6th/ed, p354*

Risk factors for recurrent disease are: Large tumor size, lymphovascular space invasion, positive lymph nodes, advanced stage disease.

Most common site of recurrence is pelvic side wall. Features of disease recurrence are: Pain in the pelvis, back, unilateral leg edema, ureteral obstruction, vaginal bleeding, palpable tumor in the pelvis and lymphadenopathy. Single agent or multiagent chemotherapy with cisplatin, paclitaxel or ifosfamide is used. Palliative radiation therapy may be used to those who have been treated initially with surgery.

Follow-up: The majority of the recurrences occur in the first 2 years. As such, the follow-up protocols should be at 3–4 months interval for the first 2 years then at 6 months interval for next 2 years and thereafter annually. Thorough physical examination is done including examination of supraclavicular and inguinal lymph nodes. Cervical or vaginal cytology is performed. Chest X-ray is done annually.

Cancer Ovary *Ref: Dutta Gynae 6th/ed, p376*

Metastasis

The most common sites of metastases are—peritoneum (85%), omentum (70%), contralateral ovary (70%), liver (35%), lung (25%) and uterus (20%). Thus option b is incorrect.

N2. Ans. is a, i.e. Labia majora *Ref: Dutta Gynae 6th/ed, p334*

Sites for vulval cancer

The commonest site is labium majus followed by clitoris and labium minus.

N3. Ans. is c, i.e. The middle one-third is the commonest site *Ref: Dutta Gynae 6th/ed, p339*

Clear cell adenocarcinoma of vagina–

Primary vaginal adenocarcinoma is rare. This is found in adolescent girls who have had history of intrauterine exposure to diethylstilbestrol in the first trimester of pregnancy.

The approximate risk of an offspring to develop the clear cell adenocarcinoma of the vagina following DES exposure is 1 in 1000 or less. These patients are more likely to develop vaginal adenosis but, rarely clear cell adenocarcinoma.

The lesion usually involves the upper-third of the anterior vaginal wall. The cervix may also be involved.

Treatment: Radical hysterectomy, vaginectomy with pelvic lymphadenectomy is the treatment of choice.

Radiotherapy is reserved for advanced cases.

N4. Ans. is c, i.e. Choriocarcinoma *Ref: Dutta Gynae 6th/ed, p334*

Histological types of vulval cancers

- Squamous cell carcinoma–90%
- Melanoma 5%
- Adenocarcinoma (Bartholin's gland)
- Basal cell carcinoma
- Sarcoma

N5. Ans. is b, i.e. M/C site is labia majora *Ref: Dutta Gynae 6th/ed, p337*

Melanoma is the second most common vulval cancer. **The common sites are the clitoris and labia minora.** It may arise from a junctional nevus. Radical vulvectomy and bilateral regional lymphadenectomy (en-block) is the preferred treatment. Pelvic lymphadenectomy does not alter the prognosis. Radiation therapy, adjuvant chemotherapy, or immunotherapy are ineffective. Overall prognosis is poor.

ANSWERS TO PREVIOUS YEAR QUESTIONS

1. **Ans. is a, i.e. Squamous cell carcinoma** *Ref: Dutta Gynae. 4th/ed, p314; Shaw 15th/ed, p398*
2. **Ans. is c, i.e. III** *Ref: Shaw 15th/ed, p399; Table 29.5*

Vaginal carcinoma:

Most common histologic type is squamous cell carcinoma.

Most common site is upper third of posterior wall of vagina.

Lymphatic Drainage:

- Tumor arising in upper vagina: drain to pelvic lymph node.
- Tumor arising in lower part: drain to inguinal lymph node.

Vaginal cancer staging	
Stage 0	Vaginal intraepithelial neoplasia (VAIN)
Stage I	Carcinoma limited to the vaginal wall.
Stage II	Carcinoma extending beyond the vagina, but not extending to the pelvic side walls.
Stage III	Carcinoma extends upto the pelvic walls.
Stage IV	Carcinoma extending beyond the true pelvis/or involving the bladder and/or rectum, or evidence of distal metastasis.

3. **Ans. is b, i.e. Condylomata acuminata** *Ref: Novak 14th/ed, p1412*

Verrucous carcinoma is variant of squamous cell carcinoma of cervix.

"Verrucous carcinomas may resemble giant condyloma accuminatum, are locally invasive and rarely metastasise."

... Novak 14th/ed, p1412

Condylomata accuminata is an STD (due to HPV 6 and HPV 11 infection) and has a verrucous appearance.

4. **Ans. is d, i.e. HPV 6** *Ref: Williams Gynae 1st/ed, p619*

"Low Risk HPV types 6 and 11 cause nearly all genital warts." *... Williams Gynae 1st/ed, p67*

Genital Warts:

- Genital warts are lesion created from productive infection with HPV (most common type 6 and 11).
- They display various morphologies and appearances ranging from flat papules to the classic verrucous, polyphytic lesions, termed "*condyloma acuminata*".
- **Sites**: External genital warts may develop at sites in the lower reproductive tract, urethra, anus, or mouth.
- **Diagnosis**: They are typically diagnosed by clinical infection, and biopsy is nor required unless co-existing neoplasia is suspected. HPV serotyping is not required for routine diagnosis.

Treatment:

- Condyloma acuminata may remain unchanged or resolve spontaneously.
- Effect of treatment on future viral transmission is unclear. However, many women prefer removal, and lesions can be destroyed with sharp or electrosurgical excision, cryotherapy, or laser ablation. In addition, very large, bulky lesions may be managed with cavitational ultrasonic surgical aspiration.

Medical Management of Genital Warts:

- Topical 5-percent imiquimod cream (immunomodulator)
- Podophyllin (antimitotic agent)
- Trichloroacetic acid (proteolytic agent)
- Bichloroacetic acid (proteolytic agent)
- Intralesion injection of interferon

Note: Intralesion injection of interferon has high cost, is painful and is inconvenient to administer, So this therapy is not recommended as a primary modality and is best reserved for recalcitrant cases.

Therapy of choice: No data suggest the superiority of one treatment. Thus in general treatment should be selected based on clinical circumstances and patient and provider preferences.

5. **Ans. is a, b and c, i.e. Paget's disease; Vulvar intraepithelial neoplasia; and Bowen's disease** *Ref: Dutta Gynae. 5th/ed, p307*

Premalignant lesion of vulva:

- Vulvar intraepithelial neoplasia VIN (most common)
- Paget's disease
- Chronic vulvar dystrophies
- Condyloma accuminata
- Lichen sclerosis

- Squamous cell hyperplasia
- Erythoplasia of Queyrat

Bowen's disease is a type of VIN where among the ordinary atypical cells, large bloated cells called Bowen cells are also present.

6. **Ans. is a, b, c, d and e, i.e. All are correct** *Ref: Novak 14th/ed, p591-5; Dutta Gynae 5th/ed, p321-5*

In the past the term *"Chronic vulvar dystrophy"* used to denote disorders of epithelial growth and differentiation which predisposed to vulval cancer.

But the International Society for Study of Vulvar Diseases (ISSVD) recommended that the old dystrophy terminology be replaced by newer classification.

Classification of Epithelial Vulvar Diseases:

Non-neoplastic epithelial disorders of skin and mucosa	
• Lichen sclerosis	
• Squamous hyperplasia (earlier called as hyperplastic dystrophy)	
Mixed neoplastic and non-neoplastic epithelial disorders	
Intraepithelial neoplasia	
Squamous intraepithelial neoplasia	Non-squamous intraepithelial neoplasia
• VIN 1	• **Paget's disease**
• VIN 2	• Tumor of melanocyte, Noninvasive
• VIN 3	
• VIN 1	
Invasive Tumors	

"The malignant potential of the non-neoplastic epithelial disorders is low but patients with lichen sclerosis and concomitant hyperplasia may be at high risk." *... Novak 14th/ed, p591*

So I am taking option "a" and "c" as correct.

Condyloma accuminata (vulvar warts) are caused by HPV type 6 and 11.

Most common site posterior fourchette and lateral areas.

The virus can be transmitted to this site from other parts of body or can be transmitted sexually.

Long standing condyloma can undergo malignant change.

"Malignant change is also associated with chronic inflammatory diseases such as the veneral granulomas and vulvar warts with 20-30 years standing." *... Jeffcoates 7th/ed, p446*

Paget's disease:

- Most cases of vulvar Paget's disease are nonsquamous intraepithelial neoplasia associated with proliferation of atypical glandular cells of the apocrine type.

"Some patients with vulvar paget's disease have an underlying adenocarcinoma, although the precise frequency is difficult to ascertain." *... Novak Gynae 14th/ed, p593*

- The characteristic histological feature is the presence of "Paget cell" in the epidermis - The cells are large round – oval in shape, with abundant pale cytoplasm. Mucopolysaccharide may be present in its cytoplasm.
- It predominantly affects postmenopausal white women and presenting symptom is usually pruritis and vulvar sclerosis. The leison has an eczematoid appearance and usually begins on hair bearing portions of vulva.
- A second synchronous or metachronous primary neoplasm is associated with Paget's disease in 4% cases. Associated carcinomas have been reported in the apocrine sweat gland, Bartholin gland, cervix, colon, bladder, gallbladder and breast.

7. **Ans. is a, b, c, d and e, i.e. Spreads to superficial inguinal nodes; Spreads to iliac nodes; Seen after menopause; Viral predisposition; and Radiotherapy given** *Ref: Shaw 15th/ed, p395; Dutta Gynae. 5th/ed, p321-2; Williams Gynae. 1st/ed, p668-72*

Vulval cancer:

- 2–4% of all malignancies of female genital tract.
- Age: occurs in 6th or 7th decade.
- Most common histologic type is epidermoid cancer (squamous cell CA) seen in 90% cases.
- Nulliparous, women of low parity are predisposed to vulval CA.
- The etiology is same as of carcinoma in situ cervix (that is viral predisposition by viruses - HIV, HPV, HSV-II).
- Most common site – Labia majora (Anterior 2/3rd) followed by clitoris and labia minora.
- Associated with cervical cancer in 20% cases.
- Presents with pruritus and visible lesion. All though pain, bleeding and ulceration also may be the initial complains.
- Spread of tumor – mainly by direct spread and lymphatics.
- First superficial inguinal nodes are involved and then it spreads to deep nodes and via glands of Cloquet to external iliac nodes, obturator and common iliac nodes in late stages.

Staging: Mainly clinical:
- Both FIGO staging and TNM staging are done in case of vulval cancer.
- Recommended is FIGO staging

Note: Vulval cancer is the only genital malignancy which can be staged using TNM staging.[Q]

Treatment:
- Early stages: Radical/Partial Vulvectomy with inguinal nodes dissection.
- Late stages: chemotherapy and radiotherapy.

Prognosis:
- Overall survival rates of women with vulval cancer are excellent.
- Lymphnode involvement is the single most important prognostic factor.
- Presence of inguinal lymphnode metastasis reduces the overall survival rate by 50%.

Note:
- *"Skinning vulvectomy"* refers to removal of only the skin and superficial subcutaneous tissue. This surgery plays no role in the treatment of invasive vulvar cancer but may be used in noninvasive disease such as cases with widespread multifocal VIN 3.
- Sentinel node biopsy – At present, the Gynecologic Oncology Group (GOG) is conducting a multicenter trial to evaluate the benefit of sentinel node biopsy for vulvar cancer.

8. **Ans. is a, i.e. Stage Ib Ca cervix** *Ref: Dutta Gynae. 4th/ed, p352-3, 342; Shaw 15th/ed, p414*
   - Radiotherapy is recommended in advanced stages of Ca cervix i.e. stage IIB onwards.Q
   - Brachytherapy is commonly used.
   - For larger tumors initially external radiation then brachytherapy is given.
   - In small tumors brachytherapy is given first followed by external radiation.
   - For stage IB and IIA – both surgery and radiotherapy yield similar results.
   - There is very little scope of radiotherapy in ovary tumors. Only Granulosa cell tumor and dysgerminoma are radiosensitive and in them also external radiotherapy is instituted for elderly woman. *... Dutta 5th/ed, p365-8*
   - Vaginal squamous cell Ca is only moderately sensitive to irradiation.
   - In all advanced cases exenteration operation is done. *... Shaw 14th/ed, p358*
   - **Fallopian tube carcinoma:** Total hysterectomy with Bilateral Salpingo-oophorectomy along with omentectomy followed by external pelvic radiation is the Treatment of Choice in cancer of Fallopian Tube. *... Dutta Gynae 5th/ed, p356*

9. **Ans. is b, i.e. Dysgerminoma** *Ref: Shaw 15th/ed, p378*

   Dysgerminoma:

   "The tumor is neutral and does not secrete either male or female sex hormones but secretes placental alkaline phosphatase, lactate dehydrogenase and beta hCG.

   Granulosa cell tumor : Secretes estrogen
   Theca cell tumor : Secretes estrogen
   Hilus cell tumor : Secretes androgens

10. **Ans. is a, i.e. Carcinoma endometrium**

11. **Ans. is a, i.e. Carcinoma vulva** *Ref: Jeffcoate 7th/ed, p350*

   Pyometra is collection of pus or mixture of pus and blood within the uterus.

   Causes:
   - Most common cause : Carcinoma endometrium.[Q]
   - 2nd most common cause : Senile endometritis.[Q]

   Other causes:
   - Congenital atresia of the vagina/cervix.
   - Stenosis of cervix/vagina following
     – Operations
     – Burns
     – Radiotherapy
   - Endometritis:
     – Senile
     – Tuberculous
     – Puerperal
   - Carcinoma:
     – Ca endometrium (most common)[Q]
     – Ca cervix
     – Ca corporis

12. Ans. is a, i.e. Watery discharge P/V *Ref: Shaw 15th/ed, p421*

- Fallopian Tube Carcinoma accounts for 0.3% of all cancers of female genital tract.
- Most common site is the ampulla of the tube.
- Most common type is adenocarcinoma.
- The fallopian tube is frequently involved in secondary to carcinoma of ovary, endometrium, gastrointestinal tract, breast and peritoneum.
- Women with mutation in BRCA I and BRCA II have higher risk of developing fallopian tube carcinoma (therefore, a prophylactic surgery in these women should include a complete removal of both tubes along with the ovaries).
- Most common symptom is Vaginal discharge (prominent watery vaginal discharge called as Hydrops tubal profluens). Later due to ulceration – watery discharge becomes blood stained and may take the form of perimenopausal/ postmenopausal bleeding.

Always remember:

- In perimenopausal and postmenopausal women with unusual, unexplained or persistent vaginal discharge, even in absence of bleeding, the clinician should always keep the possibility of occult tubal cancer in mind.
- Triad of:
  - Vaginal discharge
  - Pelvic pain
  - Pelvic mass

  } is seen in 15% of patients

On examination: Pelvic mass may be felt.

Spread: Since the fallopian tube is richly supplied by lymphatics, spread to the pelvic and para-aortic nodes occurs early.

Treatment: *Surgery + chemotherapy + radiotherapy.*

13. Ans. is b, i.e. High grade squamous intraepithelial neoplasia *Ref: Shaw 15th/ed, p402; Williams Gynae 1st/ed, p629*

There are various nomenclatures/classification systems for reporting of Pap smear.

The one which is classically used is by WHO, which uses the terms CIN-I, CIN-II and CIN-III (as discussed in chapter on CIN).

Another system as discussed earlier is Bethesda which classified the disease as LSIL=low grade squamous intraepithelial lesion and HSIL high grade squamous intraepithelial lesion and as discussed in chapter on cancer cervix chances of progressing to cancer are maximum with HSIL which includes CIN11, CIN111 and ca in situ.

14. Ans. is c, i.e. Vulval ca *Ref: Novak 14th/ed, p1425-6, 1562-3*

- The sentinel node is a specific lymph node (or nodes) that is the first to receive drainage from a malignancy and is the primary site of nodal metastasis.
- In theory, the presence or absence of metastatic disease in the sentinel node should reflect the status of the nodal basin as a whole.

Thus a negative sentinel lymph node would allow omission of lymphadenectomy of the whole nodal basin.

- It is detected through perilesional injection of radiolabelled technetium-99 or blue dye followed by intraoperative identification of the sentinel lymph nodes.
- Sentinel lymph node detection has become an integral part of the management strategy for breast cancer and melanoma.

Amongst Gynaecological Cancers:

Preliminary studies suggest that a sentinel node can be identified in most patients of vulval cancer. *...Novak 14th/ed, p1562*

Investigation are being carried out to detect sentinel node in cervical cancer. But at this time – the role of sentinel node detection is purely investigational and complete lymphadenopathy when indicated, remains the standard of care. *...Novak 14th/ed, p1426*

Although in both Ca cervix and Ca vulva, role of sentinel lymph node biopsy is not yet confirmed but vulval cancer is a better bet.

15. Ans. is b and d, i.e. Simple vulvectomy; and Estrogen cream *Ref: Jeffcoate 7th/ed, p403-5*

Treatment of leukoplakia:

Treatment of the cause	General treatment	Emperical measures *(when cause can not be treated)*
• Anemia correction • Folic acid and vit B12 (given in case of deficiency) • Treatment of candidiasis	• Sedatives-to prevent scratching and to ensure sleep • Cold cream application • Washing with 1% sodium bicarbonate • Use of loose and light cotton underclothing	• Corticosteroids (mainstay of therapy)[Q] • Estrogens and testosterone[Q] • Local analgesia • Division of cutaneous nerves; nerve block • Cod liver oil or cream of zinc oxide & olive oil • Local applications • For refractory lesion intralesional injection of triamcinolone acetonide may be tried.

Role of Vulvectomy

- When a non-neoplastic epithelial disorder is localized, local excision or partial vulvectomy may be the best method of biopsy. Otherwise vulvectomy should be reserved for those cases in which atypical epithelial activity is found histologically. In these cases, it need not be accompanied by lymphadenectomy.
- If there is no threat of cancer, empirical vulvectomy should be avoided. It is mutilating and gives poor results. The disorder sooner or later recurs in 50% cases treated by vulvectomy. There is no role of vulvectomy in children and lichen sclerosis.

16. **Ans. b. Office endometrial aspirate: Endometrial carcinoma** *Ref: Novak's 14/e p1348 Harrison 18/e p661-662; Park 21st/129*

Office endometrial aspirate is not used for screening of Endometrial carcinoma.

Transvaginal ultrasound and endometrial sampling have been advocated as screening tests for endometrial cancer but benefit from routine screening has not been shown.

> *"**Screening for endometrial cancer should currently not be undertaken because of lack of an appropriate, cost-effective and acceptable test that reduces mortality.** Routine PAP testing is inadequate test that reduces mortality. Routine PAP testing is inadequate and **endometrial cytology assessment is too insensitive and non-specific to be useful in screening for endometrial cancer even in high-risk population.**" Novak's 14/e p1348*

Screening test	Disease screened
Papanicolaou (Pap's) smear	Cervical cancer
Mammography	Breast cancer
CA-125	Ovarian cancer

Screening test	Disease screened

Screening test is used to search for **an unrecognized disease** or **defect, in apparently healthy individuals,** by means of **rapidly applied tests, examination** or **other procedures.**

Screening test	Disease screened
Papanicolaou (Pap's) smear	**Cervical cancer**[Q]
Mammography	**Breast cancer**[Q]
Bimanual oral examination	Oral cancer[Q]
ELISA	**HIV**[Q]
Urine for sugar, Random blood sugar	Diabetes mellitus[Q]
AFP	Developmental anomalies in fetus[Q]
DRE + PSA	**Prostate cancer**[Q]
Fecal occult blood test	**Colorectal cancer**[Q]
CA-125	**Ovarian cancer**[Q]

17. **Ans. is a, i.e. Breast cancer** *Ref: Journal of head and neck oncology 2011*

Orbital metastasis occurs in 2 to 3% of cancers. Metastasis of breast cancer accounts for majority of ocular and orbital metastasis.

18. **Ans. is a i.e. Radical vulvectomy with unilateral LN dissection**

All details of vulvar cancer are discussed in the appendix at beginning of chapter.

- Tumor size 2 × 3 cm with no palpable nodes means it is stage IB that means management is radical vulvectomy with ***inguinofemoral lymph node dissection. Now the question arises unilateral or bilateral.*** So read following lines of Williams:
- ***"Traditionally both superficial inguinal nodes and deep femoral nodes have been removed for evaluating metastatic disease". These nodes may be excused unilaterally or bilaterally. Traditionally, a unilateral inguinal femoral lymphadenectomy is performed for a lateralized vulvar lesion, namely one that lies > 2 cm beyond midline. Bilateral node excision is recommended for all lesions within 2 cm of midline.***

  This lesion is on Labia majora i.e. > 2 cm away from midline, hence unilateral lymph node removal will be done.
- The answer is further supported by following lines of Novar 15/e, Pg 1440
- **Unilateral versus bilateral groin dissection**
- It is not necessary to perform a bilateral groin dissection if primary lesion is unilateral and ipsilateral lymph nodes are not involved. It is recommended that patients with any bulky or multiple microscopically positive ipsilateral groin lymph nodes undergo contralateral inguinal femoral lymphadenectomy. Bilateral inguinal female lymphadernectomy should be performed for midline lesions (**clitoris, anterior labia minora, posterior fourchette**) or those within 2 cm of the midline because of the more frequent contralateral lymph flow from these region.

CHAPTER 15

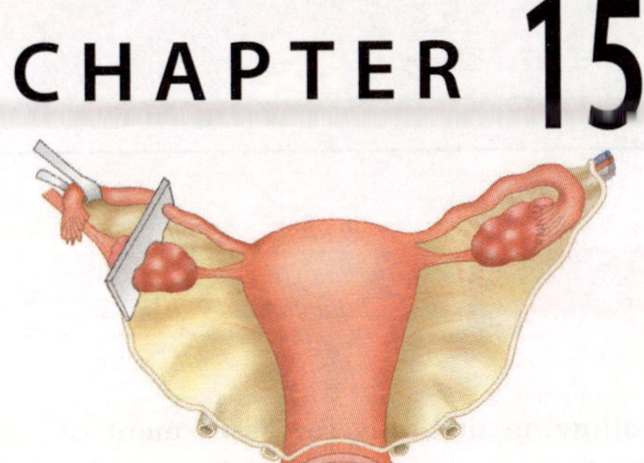

Gynecological Diagnosis and Operative Surgery

NEW PATTERN QUESTIONS

N1. Cryosurgery is effective in all *except*:
a. Chronic cervicitis
b. Squamous intraepithelial lesion (SIL)
c. Condyloma accuminata
d. Cases with severe dysplasia or CIS lesion

N2. Regarding outpatient hysteroscopy all are correct *except*:
a. Abnormal uterine bleeding is an indication
b. Normal saline as distension medium can be used
c. It is less accurate than saline infusion sonography (SIS)
d. It is not reliable to exclude endometrial carcinoma

N3. To minimize ureteric damage, the following preoperative and operative precautions may be taken *except*:
a. Cystoscopy
b. Direct visualization during surgery
c. Ureter should not be dissected off the peritoneum for a long distance
d. Bladder should be pushed downwards and outwards while the clamps are placed near the angles of vagina

N4. Indications of rectal examination in gynecology are all *except*:
a. In cases with Müllerian agenesis
b. In virgin females
c. To differentiate rectocele from enterocele
d. For staging of ovarian malignancy

N5. The advantages of cryosurgery over electrocauterization are all *except*:
a. Less discomfort to the patient
b. Postoperative bleeding is much less
c. Postoperative vaginal discharge is also much less
d. Cervical stenosis is extremely rare

N6. Position of the patient should be as described *except*:
a. Diagnostic laparoscopy—Trendelenburg with about 30° tilt
b. Colposcopy—Lithotomy
c. Transvaginal sonography in gynecology—Lithotomy with full bladder
d. Hysteroscopy—Lithotomy

N7. Posterior colpotomy is done for:
a. Pelvic hematocele
b. Pelvic abscess
c. Ovarian abscess
d. All

PREVIOUS YEAR QUESTIONS

1. **Hysteroscopy means visualization of:** *(PGI June 05)*
   a. Genital tract
   b. Fallopian tube
   c. Uterine cavity
   d. Cervix
   e. Abdominal cavity
2. **For hysteroscopy, following are/is used:** *(PGI Dec 08)*
   a. Distilled Water b. Air
   c. Glycine d. CO_2
3. **Hysteroscopy can diagnose all, *except*:** *(PGI June 98)*
   a. Asherman's syndrome
   b. Septate uterus
   c. Adenomyosis
   d. TB endometritis
4. **Which of the following media is used only in operative hysteroscopy:**
   a. CO_2 b. 0.9% Saline
   c. Ringer lactate d. Mannitol 5%
5. **Asherman's syndrome can be diagnosed by all *except*:**
   a. Hysterosalpingography *(AIIMS Nov 07)*
   b. Saline sonography
   c. Endometrial culture
   d. Hysteroscopy
6. **Best gas used for creating pneumoperitoneum at laparoscopy is:** *(AI 98)*
   a. N_2 b. O_2
   c. CO_2 d. N_2O
7. **Laparoscopy is best avoided in patients with:** *(UPSC 97)*
   a. Hypertension b. Diabetes
   c. Obesity d. COPD
8. **Laparoscopy is contraindicated in:** *(MCI March 11)*
   a. Ectopic pregnancy b. PID
   c. Endometriosis d. Peritonitis
9. **A 26-year-old female with 3 living issues having cervical erosion which bleeds to touch, diagnosis can be done by:** *(PGI Dec 03)*
   a. Pap smear b. Excision biopsy
   c. Hysteroscopy d. Colposcopy
10. **Occurrence of ovulation is indicated by:** *(PGI Dec 03)*
    a. LH
    b. FSH
    c. Estradiol
    d. Progesterone
    e. Cortisol
11. **Time of ovulation is detected by:** *(PGI June 03)*
    a. Urine LH b. Urine FSH
    c. Urine HCG d. Serum Estradiol
    e. BBT
12. **Which of the following methods for assessment of female infertility during a menstrual cycle can best predict timing of ovulation:** *(AI 2010)*
    a. BBT
    b. Fern Test
    c. Spinnbarkeit Phenomenon
    d. Hormonal Study
13. **Best indicator of ovarian reserve is:** *(AIIMS Nov 07)*
    a. FSH
    b. Estradiol
    c. LH
    d. FSH/LH Ratio
14. **Goniometer is used for:** *(AIIMS Nov 07)*
    a. Amount o vaginal secretions
    b. To measure width of genital hiatus
    c. Gonococcal colony count
    d. Urethrovesical angle
15. **Feature of post ovulatory endometrium on ultrasound is:**
    a. Single hyperechoic thin line *(Delhi 03)*
    b. Three line sign
    c. Prominent halo
    d. Prominent posterior enhancement
16. **Luteal phase defect is best diagnosed by:** *(Delhi 97)*
    a. Serum progesterone levels
    b. Endometrial biopsy
    c. Basal body temperature
    d. Ultrasonography
17. **Chassar Moir surgery is done is case of:**
    a. Uterine inversion
    b. VVF repair
    c. Ureterovesical fistula repair
    d. Retroverted uterus
18. **All of the following are advantages of vaginal hysterectomy over abdominal hysterectomy *except*:**
    a. Better tolerated by elderly and obese patients
    b. Lesser risk of postoperative thromboembolism
    c. Other visceral structures can be easily visualized
    d. Corrects prolapse of other organs
19. **Maximum chances of ureteric injury are with:** *(AI 06)*
    a. TAH
    b. Wertheim's hysterectomy
    c. Anterior colporrhaphy
    d. Vaginal hysterectomy
20. **Transcervical endometrial resection (TCRE) is used in:** *(PGI June 99)*
    a. Endometriosis
    b. DUB
    c. Carcinoma endometrium
    d. Submucous fibroid

ANSWERS TO NEW PATTERN QUESTIONS

N1. Ans. is d, i.e. Case with severe dysplasia or CIS lesion *Ref: Dutta Gynae 6th/ed, p591*

Cryosurgery

This is a procedure whereby destruction of the tissue is effective by freezing.

Indications

- Cervical ectopy
- Benign cervical lesions—such as CIN (ideal for minor degree and localized CIN), condyloma acuminata, leukoplakia, etc.
- Condyloma acuminata of vulva and VIN diagnosed colposcopically and not more than 2 cm in size.
- VAIN, condyloma acuminata or vault granulation tissue following hysterectomy.
- As a palliative measure to arrest bleeding in carcinoma cervix or large fungating recurrent vulvar carcinoma.

Principle: It consists of a 'probe', the tip of which is cooled to a temperature below freezing point (–60°C). **Freezing produces cellular dehydration by crystallization of intracellular water and ultimately death of cells.** This is effective by rapid expansion of gas which is passed through it. Carbon dioxide is widely used while nitrous oxide and liquid nitrogen are also used.

The application to the cervix freezes the tissue to a depth of about 3 mm. Healing is complete in 6 to 10 weeks.

N2. Ans. is c, i.e. It is less accurate than saline infusion sonography (SIS)

As discused in Q.5 and 6, abnormal uterine bleeding is an indication for performing hysteroscopy and normal saline can be used as a distention media (i.e. both options a and b are correct).

As far as results of hysteroscopy are concerned, they are comparable with saline infusion sonography (SIS) (i.e. option c is in correct)

A positive hysteroscopy is more reliable and has moral significance than a negative one, hence option d is also correct.

N3. Ans. is a, i.e. Cystoscopy (Read below)

Now this question can be done with common sense as to minimize ureteric damage, all the options given in the questions hold good except cystoscopy. What is the role of visualizing bladder to prevent ureteric surgery.

N4. Ans. is d, i.e. For staging of ovarian malignancy *Ref: Dutta Gynae 6th/ed, p107*

Indication of Rectal examination

- Children or in adult virgins
- Painful vaginal examination
- Carcinoma cervix—to note the parametrial involvement (base of the broad ligament and the uterosacral ligament can only be felt rectally) or involvement of the rectum
- To corroborate the findings felt in the pouch of Douglas by bimanual vaginal examination
- Atresia (agenesis) of vagina
- Patients having rectal symptoms
- To diagnose rectocele and differentiate it from enterocele.

N5. Ans. is c, i.e. Postoperative vaginal discharge is also much less *Ref: Read below*

After cryosurgery there will be profuse vaginal discharge for about 2–3 weeks

N6. Ans. is c, i.e. Transvaginal sonography (TVS) (in gynecology lithotomy with full bladder.

As the position described in the question are correct with respect to the surgery except for TVS.

In TVS, the position is dorsal with legs drawn up and not lithotomy Full bladder may or may not be required.

N7. Ans. is d, i.e. All

ANSWERS TO PREVIOUS YEAR QUESTIONS

1. **Ans. is c, i.e. Uterine cavity**
2. **Ans. is c and d, i.e. Glycine and CO_2**
3. **Ans. is c, i.e. Adenomyosis** *Ref: Novak 14th/ed, p787, 15th/ed, p786-2, Shaw 15th/ed, p494; Wiliams Gynae 1st/ed, p950-1*

- ***Hysteroscopy is the endoscopic technique of visualizing the interior of uterus directly.***[Q]
- It is both diagnostic and therapeutic.

Patient Preparation:

- In premenopausal women, hysteroscopy is ideally performed in the early proliferative phase of menstrual cycle, when endometrium is relatively thin. This allows small masses to be easily identified and removed.
- Alternatively agents like progestins, combined pills, Danazol and GnRH agonist can be administered prior to anticipated surgery.
- Hysteroscope consists of a rigid 4 mm diameter telescope so, cervix has to dilated to 4 mm[Q] for insertion of hysteroscope.

Distension media:

- Because the anterior and posterior uterine walls are in apposition, a distention medium is required to expand the endometrial cavity for viewing.
- Distension media includes CO_2 and low viscous fluids such as sorbitol, mannitol and glycine solutions.
- To expand the cavity, intrauterine pressure of these media must reach 45 to 80 mm of Hg. it should not exceed 100 mg of Hg because high pressure can result in increased intravasation of medium into the patient's circulation and fluid volume overload.

Most common media used for diagnostic purpose – CO_2
Most common media used for therapeutic purpose – Glycine

Contraindications:
- Infection (except in case of misplaced IUCD)
- Pregnancy
- Genital malignancy

Diagnostic Indications of hysteroscopy:

Friends, lets not mug up the diagnostic indications of hysteroscope by any mnemonic but lets understand them.

A hysteroscope can visualize the interior of uterus so, it can diagnose

- *Any congenital malformation of uterus and can also help in differentiating between a bicornuate uterus from a septate uterus.*[Q]
- *Any uterine synechiae (as in Ashermann syndrome).*[Q]
- Misplaced IUCD.[Q]
- Submucous fibroid[Q]

A hysteroscope can visualize the cornua so, it can diagnose

- Any cornual pathology

Hysteroscope can directly visualize the endometrium so, it can diagnose

- Endometrial lesions like – endometrial polyp, endometrial hyperplasia, endometrial cancer, endometrial T.B.[Q]
- Pregnancy-related conditions like: Molar tissue or products of conception.[Q]

Besides these hysteroscopy is also indicated in[Q]**:**

- Unexplained abnormal uterine bleeding[Q]
  - Premenopausal[Q]
  - Postmenopausal[Q]
- Selected infertility cases: In case of
  - Abnormal HSG[Q]
  - Unexplained infertility[Q]
- Recurrent spontaneous abortion

- The therapeutic indications of hysteroscope are (here also don't mug up, just try to understand them).[Q]
- To excise uterine septum[Q]
- To lyse adhesions in Ashermann's syndrome[Q]
- To retrieve lost IUCD[Q]
- Hysteroscopic myomectomy[Q]
- Polypectomy[Q]
- Endometrial ablation for menorrhagia[Q]
- Tubal occlusion for control of fertility[Q]
- Intratubal ballooning in tubal blockage[Q]

As far as adenomyosis is concerned – it can be suspected on hysteroscopy by appearance of diverticuli but definitive diagnosis requires transvaginal ultrasonography.

For management of adenomyosis hysterectomy is the definitive treatment

"Endometrial ablation and resection using hysteroscopy has been used to successfully treat dysmenorrhea and menorrhagia caused by adenomyosis. However, complete eradication is problematic." *... Williams Gynae 1st/ed, p209*

Also know:

Technique for visualization of	
Cervix	Colposcopy
Fallopian tube	
• To see its mucosa	Salpingoscopy
• To see its lumen	Falloscopy
Abdominal cavity	Laparoscopy

4. **Ans. is d, i.e. Mannitol 5%**

This is because electrolyte-poor fluids are commonly used for hysteroscopy, e.g. glycine 1.5%, sorbitol 3% and manitol 5%.

All the electrolyte-poor fluids used in operative hysteroscopy can lead to hyponatremia if a large volume is absorbed. Mannitol differs from others because it is iso-osmolar.

5. **Ans. is c, i.e. Endometrial culture** *Ref: Williams Gynae 1st/ed, p420; Leon Speroff 7th/ed, p419*

Asherman's syndrome:

- It is an acquired uterine defect characterized by the presence of uterine synechiaes and subsequent destruction of the lining endometrium.
- M/C cause for asherman syndrome -Post partum curettage
- 2nd M/C cause - curettage done for MTP
- Other causes - uterine surgery like cesarean section, myomectomy, Sheehan's syndrome
- Infectious causes - TB, Schistosomiasis
- Most characteristic symptom = Hypomenorrhea (scanty bleeding <20 ml or <2 days) or 2° amenorrhea
- Others - Infertility
- Abortion
- **Diagnosis:** *... Williams Gynae 1st/ed, p420-1*
- When Asherman syndrome is *suspected, HSG is indicated. Intrauterine adhesions, characteristically appear as irregular, angulated filling defects* within the uterine cavity.
- At times, *uterine polyps, leiomyomas, air bubbles* and *blood clots* may masquerade as adhesions.
- Transvaginal USG or saline infusion sonography may help clarify these difficult cases.
- A definitive diagnosis requires hysteroscopy. (Investigation of choice)

Treatment:

- Adhesiolysis *via hysteroscopy.*
- Placement of an *intrauterine device* or Pediatric foley's catheter with the bulb filled with 3ml of fluid, to avoid contact between the ends of the adhesions.
- Treatment with *estrogen* to stimulate endometrial growth. (Since estrogen alone can lead to endometrial, cancer. Estrogen and progesterone should be given together).

Prognosis:

- Approximately 70-80% of patients with this condition have achieved successful pregnancy. But pregnancy can be complicated by premature labor, placenta accreta, placenta previa and/or PPH.
- Recurrence rate is high.

6. **Ans. is c, i.e. CO_2**
7. **Ans. is d, i.e. COPD**
8. **Ans. is d, i.e. Peritonitis** *Ref: Williams Gynae 1st/ed, p932,COGDT 10th/ed, p801-2*

Important points to remember on laparoscopy:

- *CO_2 is currently the insufflation gas of choice for laparoscopy. It fulfills most of the requirements for an ideal insufflation gas, being colorless, noninflammable and rapidly excreted from the circulation.*
  Other alternative is N_2O: But it is expensive, less soluble in blood and supports combustion.
- Instrument used for creating pneumoperitoneum is vercess needle.
- It should be inserted at an angle of 45 degrees to the spine.
- Flow rate of CO_2 for creating pneumoperitoneum is 200–2000 ml/min & pressure between 10 – 15 mm of Hg. In many patients, this correlates with an infusion of 2.5 to 3 litres of gas .... *Williams Gynae 1st/ed, p934*

Contraindications of laparoscopy

Absolute	Relative
• Intestinal obstruction[Q]	• Previous periumbilical surgey[Q]
• Generalized peritonitis[Q]	• Cardiac or pulmonary disease[Q]
• Massive hemorrhage[Q]	• Shock[Q]
• Cancer involving anterior abdominal wall[Q]	

9. **Ans. is a, b and d, i.e. Pap smear; Excision biopsy; and Colposcopy**

Ref: Dutta Gynae 5th/ed, p257-9; Jeffcoate 7th/ed, p410-2

Cervical erosion (ectopy) is condition where the squamous epithelium of ectocervix is replaced by columnar epithelium of endocervix.

Etiology:

Congenital	Acquired
Hormonal	Infection
• During pregnancy	• Chronic cervicitis
• In pill users	

Symptoms:

- Mostly asymptomatic
- Patient may present with vaginal discharge - Excessive and mucoid in consistency. It may be mucopurulent, offensive and irritant in presence of infection or may be even blood stained due to premenstrual congestion.
- Contact bleeding specially during pregnancy and "pill use" either following coitus or defecation.
- Associated cervicitis may produce *backache, pelvic pain and infertility.*

Signs:

- On per speculum examination a bright red area is seen surrounding and extending beyond the external os in the ectocervix, **which is neither tender nor bleeds on touch.**

Differential diagnosis:

- Carcinoma cervix[Q]
- Ectropion[Q]
- Tuberculous ulcer[Q]
- Syphilitic and other ulcers of cervix.[Q]

Diagnosis:

"All cases should be subjected to cytological examination from the cervical smear to exclude dysplasia or malignancy. In doubtful cases, colposcopy and/or cervical biopsy should be done." .... *Dutta Gynae 5th/ed, p259*

"Although a cervical smear may be helpful, the diagnosis and distinction (between ectopy and its differential diagnosis) may not be possible except by colposcopy or biopsy." ... *Jeffcoate 7th/ed, p412*

In the given question the female is multiparous and is having cervical erosion which bleeds on touch, which may signify early cervical cancer and therefore pap smear/colposcopy/biopsy all should be done.

10. **Ans. is a, i.e. LH & d, i.e. Progesterone**
11. **Ans. is a, and e, i.e. Urine LH; and BBT**
12. **Ans. is d, i.e. Hormonal study** *Ref: Leon Speroff 8th/ed, p1161–4; Dutta Gynae 5th/ed, p228*

LH Surge

"Evaluation of ovulation is an important part of any female fertility investigation. All of the different methods are useful and no one method is necessarily best. When circumstances require accurate prediction of ovulation as in couples having infrequent intercourse or those who require timely insemination, monitoring urinary LH excretion generally is the most cost-effective and appropriate choice"

Ref: Leon speroff 7th/ed, p1036

"Ovulation predictor kits (LH kits) are noninvasive and widely available, require relatively little time and effort. Their greatest advantage over other methods is the ability to accurately predict when ovulation will occur"

"LH ovulation predictor kits are probably the most convenient home monitoring methods of predicting ovulation"

Ref: Cambridge Guide to Infertility management and Assisted reproduction/68

Note: Ovulation occurs because of LH surge

Onset of LH surge to ovulation = 36 hours

Onset of LH peak to ovulation = 12 hours

Serum Progesterone levels

- It is the simplest method to assess ovulation in a female with regular menstruation

  Test - Should be performed 1 week after LH surge, i.e. on Day 21 if menstrual cycle is of 28 days.

  If serum progesterone levels on day 21 are >3 ng/ml, it indicates ovulation has occured.

13. **Ans. is a, i.e. FSH** *Ref: Novak 14th/ed, p1203-5, Wiliams Gynae 1st/ed, p434; Harrson 17th/ed, p223*

"Best indicator of ovarian reserve is anti-Mullerian hormone. Since it is not given in options, hence we go for day 3 FSH levels."

14. **Ans. is d, i.e. Urethrovesical angle**

Goniometer is used to measure urethrovescical angle.

15. **Ans. is d, i.e. Prominent posterior enhancement** *Ref: Transvaginal Ultrasound by Melvin G. Dodson 1st/ed, p86*

Friends, this is a very important Question

IMPORTANT: I have summarized here the appearances of endometrium on transvaginal ultrasound during different stages of normal menstrual cycle.

A. Just after menstruation (days 3–7)

Single hyperechoic thin lines (central endometrial echo)

B. At the time of ovulation

Halo present

Relatively thin anterior posterior endometrial thickness (< 6 mm)

No posterior enhancement[Q]

Three line sign.Q/Trilaminar appearance

C. Luteal phase

Maximum endometrial thickness

Hyperechoic endometrium

Loss of halo[Q]

Loss of three line sign[Q]

Prominent posterior enhancement[Q]

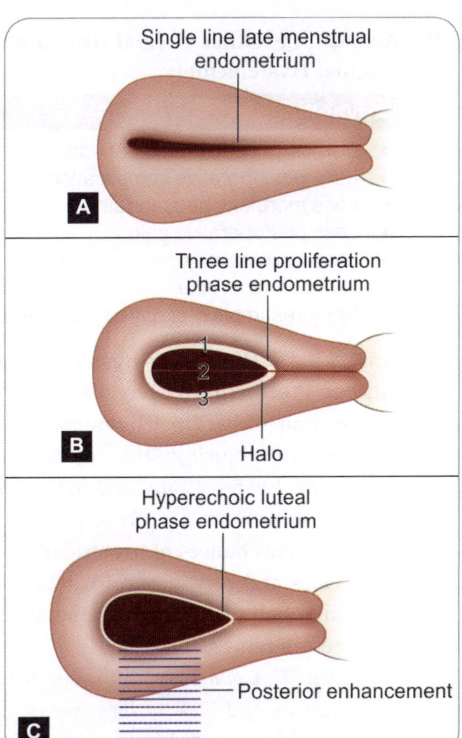

16. Ans. is b, i.e. Endometrial biopsy *Ref: Shaw 14th/ed, p30-1; Dutta Gynae 5th/ed, p230; Novak 15th/ed, p1161*

In luteal phase defect (LPD) as the name suggests there is decreased progesterone secretion which leads to premenstrual spotting and recurrent 1st trimester abortions

Best method of diagnosing – LPD is endometrial biopsy done on day 21 day 23 of cycle (a lag of 48 hrs or more between the chronological dating and histological dating is diagnostic of LPD).

It can also be diagnosed by serum progesterone levels– If serum progesterone done on day 21 of the cycle is < 5 ng/ml-it indicates LPD.

17. Ans. is b, i.e. VVF repair *Ref: Shaw 14th/ed, p168*

Surgery	Done in
1. Kelly stitch/Boney's Test/Marshall Marchetti Krantz Surgery	Stress Urinary Incontinence
2. Chassar Moir Technique/Latzko technique/layer technique	VVF Repair
3. Boari Flap Technique	Uretrovaginal Fistula repair
4. Purandare Sling/Fothergill's Repair/Manchester Repair/Ward Mayo Hysterectomy/Lefort's Colpocleisis	Prolapse Uterus
5. Strassman Unification Surgery	Bicornuate/Didelphic uterus (Indication for operation, if bicornuate or didelphic uterus lead to >3 Abortion)
6. Hysteroscopic Septal Resection (M/c done), Jones/Thompkins/ Williams metroplasty	Septate Uterus
7. McIndoe Vaginoplasty	MRKH Syndrome/Vaginal agenesis (Best time to perform this surgery is just before/just after marriage)
8. Mc Donald/Shirodkar Cerclage	Incompetent Internal os
9. Baldy Webster operation, Modified Gilliams operation, Laparoscopic ventrosuspension	Retroversion of the uterus
10. Haultains Operation(via abdominal route Spinellis operation (via vaginal route)	Inversion of uterus

18. Ans. is c, i.e. Other visceral structures can be easily visualized

Vaginal Hysterectomy

Advantages	Disadvantages
• Can be done in obese patients • Less postoperative complications • Less morbidity and mortality • Less postoperative pain • Less hospital stay • No abdominal scar • Early resumption of day to day activities	• Exploration of abdominal organs and pelvic organs cannot be done • Tubo-ovarian pathologies cannot be simultaneously dealt • Difficult to perform if uterus is >12 weeks size and if pelvic adhesions are present • Concurrent surgical procedures cannot be done

19. Ans. is b, i.e. Wertheims hysterectomy *Ref: COGDT 10th/ed, p779; Dutta Gynae 5th/ed, p408*

Since in Wertheims hysterectomy, we are removing the medial half of cardinal ligament, there are maximum chances of injuring the ureter and furthermore wertheims hysterectomy is done is case of cancers and a lot of adhesions are present during surgery which increases the chances of ureteric injury

- Ureters are very prone to injury during cutting of medial half of cardinal ligaments. But I am sure you need references also

  "About 75% of ureteral injuries result from Gynecological operations and 75% of them occur following abdominal Gynecological procedures" ....*Dutta 5th/ed, p408*

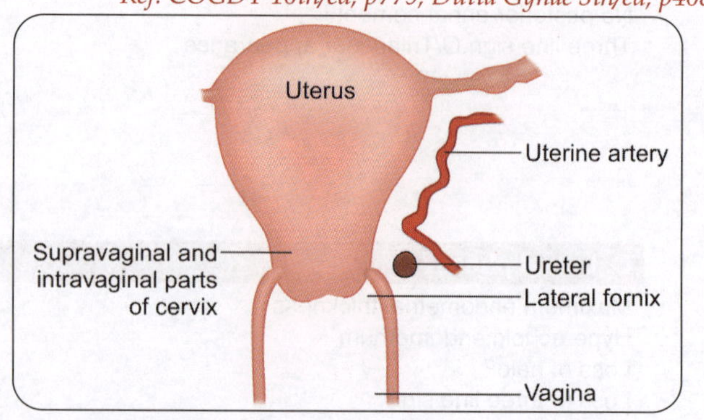

Figure showing the relative position of ureter in relation to uterus and uterine artery

- From the above lines it is clear that, in abdominal operations, ureters are more prone to injury than in vaginal operations (ruling out Options "c" and "d")

"The reported incidence of ureteral injury during Gynecologic procedures ranges from about 0.5% in simple hysterectomies for benign disease upto 1.6% for laparoscopic cases and to as high as 30% for some older series of Wertheim's Radical Hysterectomies."

..... CGDT 10th/ed, p779

Also Know

Piver Rutledge classification of types of hysterectomy

Type I	Total Abdominal Hysterectomy.
Type II	Wertheims hysterectomy
Type III	Radical hysterectomy/Meigs hysterectomy
Type IV	Extended radical hysterectomy
Type V	Complete pelvic extenteration

20. Ans. is b i.e. DUB *Ref: Shaw 15th/ed, p305; Bijoy Sree Sen Gupta 2nd/ed, p151-152; Williams Gynae 1st/ed, p188*

Transcervical endometrial resection (Hysteroscopic endometrial ablation) is a technique for management of DUB.

Aim of the procedure is to produce a therapeutic Asherman's syndrome and produce amenorrhea.

It destroys the endometrium → formation of synchea → Asherman syndrome → amenorrhea.

It is essential to destroy endometrial functionalis and basalis as well as 3 mm of myometrial depth.

Procedure: After appropriate inspection of the landmarks and endometrial cavity, a wire loop electrode is used to resect several strips of endomyometrium, to a depth of 4 mm. Resected tissue is used for pathologic examination and documentation of the absence of cellular atypia. After a few strips are resected initially from the posterior uterine wall, resection of almost all the remaining surface with loop electrode by vaporization is performed. The procedure should be performed soon after menstruation or the woman should be given progesterone, danazol or GnRH to suppress the endometrium.

Result: Short term and long term studies show amenorrhea rates of 20–50%, overall improved bleeding patterns (including amenorrhea) in 85–95%, with failure rates of 5–10% which requires additional surgery i.e. hysterectomy.

Extra Edge

- A COG recommends endometrial sampling prior to ablation surgery. Women with endometrial hyperplasia or cancer should not undergo ablation.
- **Absolute contraindications for endometrial ablation:** *... Williamss Gynae 1st/ed, p188*
  - Genital tract malignancy
  - Women wishing to preserve their fertility
  - Pregnancy
  - Expectation of amenorrhea
  - Acute pelvic infection
  - Prior uterine surgery - Classical cesarean delivery, transmural myomectomy
  - Uterine size > 12 wks

Most Recent Papers

1. NEET 2024
2. NEET 2023
3. NEET 2021
4. INI-CET 2024
5. INI-CET November 2023
6. INI-CET May 2023
7. INI-CET November 2022
8. INI-CET May 2022
9. INI-CET November 2021
10. INI-CET May 2021

NEET 2024

1. **A pregnant woman presents with an IUD in place and the thread is clearly visible. She wishes to continue with the pregnancy. What is the appropriate next step?**
   a. Perform a cesarean section
   b. Remove the IUD gently
   c. Leave the IUD in place
   d. Proceed with medical termination of pregnancy

2. **During sacro-colposuspension surgery, to which bony landmark is the mesh typically attached for suspension?**
   a. Ischial tuberosity
   b. Pubic symphysis
   c. Ischial spine
   d. Sacral promontory

3. **A 30-year-old female, P2L2, with a history of cervical lengthening. What is the recommended surgical option?**
   a. Hysterectomy
   b. Fothergill procedure
   c. Lefort procedure
   d. McCall procedure

4. **What is the most likely diagnosis?**

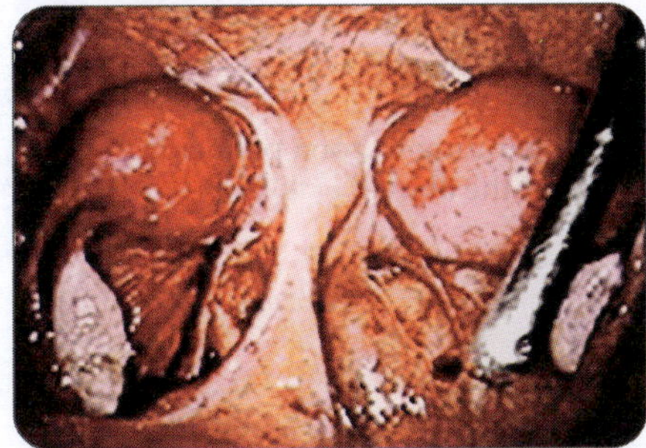

   a. Unicornuate uterus
   b. Septate uterus
   c. Bicornuate uterus
   d. Uterine didelphys

5. **Identify the image.**

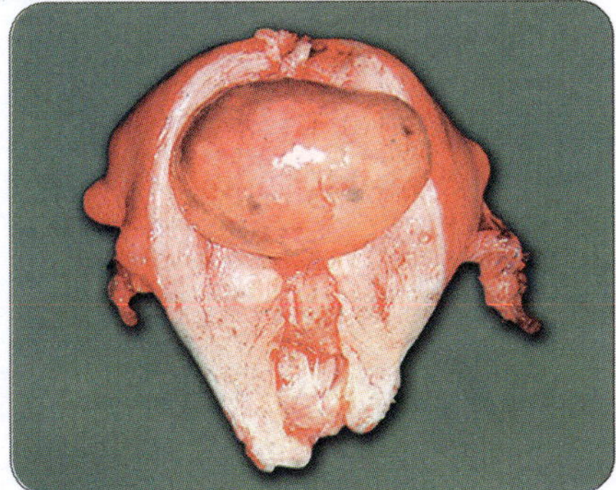

Source: Hiralal Konar. DC Dutta's Textbook of Gynecology, 6th edition; 2013.

   a. Sub-mucosal fibroid
   b. Endometrial polyp
   c. Uterine Malignancy
   d. Pregnancy

6. **At which part of the fallopian tube is a tubectomy typically performed, and why?**
   a. Ampulla because it is the widest
   b. Ampulla as it is the site of fertilization
   c. Isthmus because it has a uniform thickness of muscle
   d. Isthmus because it is the narrowest

7. **What might be the cause of a new 2 cm black nodular mass near an episiotomy scar that is painful and grows larger during menstruation?**
   a. Inclusion cyst
   b. Endometriosis
   c. Foreign body granuloma
   d. Melanoma

8. **What is released during ovulation?**
   a. Primary oocyte arrested in meiosis I
   b. Primary oocyte arrested in meiosis II
   c. Secondary oocyte arrested in meiosis I
   d. Secondary oocyte arrested in meiosis II

9. **After a healthy vaginal delivery, when is the earliest that an intrauterine contraceptive device (IUCD) can be inserted?**
   a. After 6 months
   b. After 3 months
   c. Within 48 hours
   d. After 6 weeks

10. **A teenage girl presents with amenorrhea and an image shows an imperforate hymen. What karyotype would be most appropriate for further evaluation?**
    a. 47,XXY
    b. 46,XY
    c. 45,XO
    d. 46,XX

11. **A 46-year-old woman presents with cervical erosion. What is the most appropriate investigation to perform?**
    a. Cervical biopsy, HBV DNA
    b. Liquid-based cytology, cervical biopsy, HPV testing
    c. Pap smear, HIV DNA
    d. Pap smear, HCV DNA, electrophoresis

12. **A mass is felt on the perineum, the uterus is palpable, and a finger can pass from the os. The patient delivered 20 years ago. What is the likely diagnosis?**
    a. Hypertrophied cervix
    b. Myxomatous polyp
    c. Placental polyp
    d. Uterine inversion

13. **Based on the given image, what could be the possible diagnosis?**

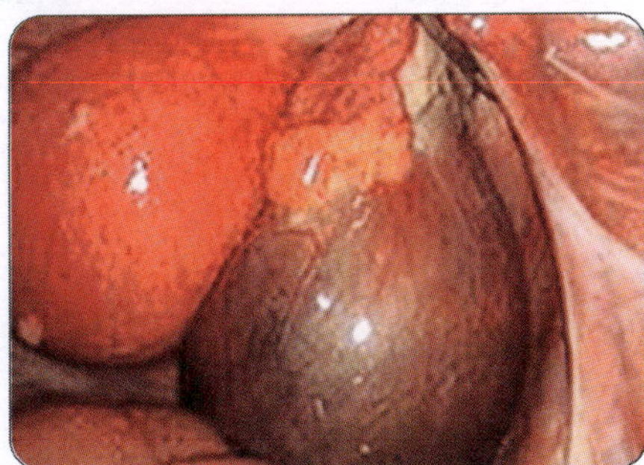

    a. Endometrioma
    b. Germ cell tumor
    c. Endometrial Polyp
    d. Endometrial Ca

14. What is this given image used to assess?

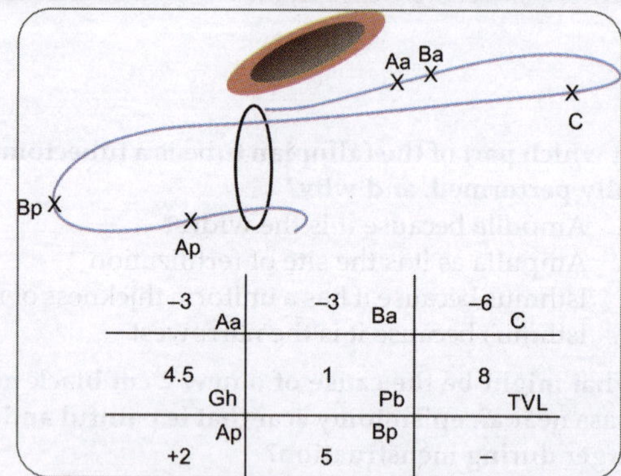

a. Endometrial cancer b. Prolapse
c. Vulvar cancer d. Vesico-vaginal fistula

15. What degree of prolapse is characterized by an organ lying partially outside the pelvis?

a. Second b. Fourth
c. Third d. First

16. Given the karyotype, identify the correct syndrome.

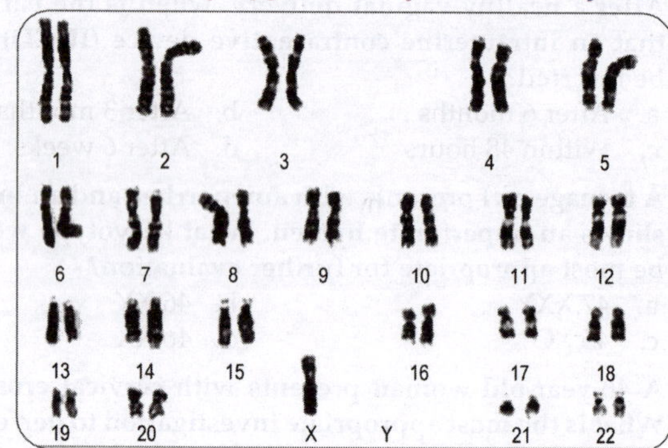

a. Klinefelter syndrome
b. Kallmann syndrome
c. Turner syndrome
d. Androgen insensitivity syndrome

17. At what stage of cervical cancer is hydronephrosis typically observed?

a. Stage 1
b. Stage 2
c. Stage 3
d. Stage 4

18. A patient comes to your clinic with complaints of difficulty conceiving for the past 3 years. Upon further examination, bilateral tubal block was found out on HSG. What will be the next step?

a. Laparoscopic chromopertubation
b. Hysteroscopy
c. IUI
d. Hysterectomy

19. What is the Nugent score used for?

a. Candidiasis
b. Bacterial vaginosis
c. Herpes
d. Trichomonas

20. What mechanism prevents polyspermy by causing structural changes in the zona pellucida during fertilization?

a. Acrosomal reaction
b. Cortical reaction
c. Sperm binding to zona pellucida
d. None of the above

Answer with Explanations

1. **Ans. is b, i.e. Remove the IUD gently** *Ref: DC Dutta's Textbook of Gynae 9th/ed, Ch-30*
   - The pregnancy rate with the device in situ is rare. Lowest pregnancy rates are observed with Cu-T 380A (0.8–HWY) and LNG-IUS (0.2–HWY). When pregnancy occurs with a device in situ, there is risk of ectopic pregnancy (0.02%).
   - *Management of a pregnant woman with device in situ:* If the thread is visible through the cervix it is best to remove the device. This will minimize complications like miscarriage, preterm labor, sepsis, placenta previa, abruption, cesarean delivery, low birth weight baby, including malformations.
   - However, if the thread is not visible, it is better to counsel the patient about the risks involved in continuing pregnancy. Pelvic ultrasound must be carried out to locate the pregnancy.
2. **Ans. is d, i.e. Sacral promontory** *Ref: DC Dutta's Textbook of Gynae 9th/ed, Ch-16*

   As the name says, sacro (means sacrum) colpo (vaginal vault) suspension (to suspend). For vaginal vault prolapse, particularly that which occurs following hysterectomy, the surgical approaches have included a spectrum of techniques applied either vaginally or abdominally. The laparoscopic technique most commonly performed is sacrocolpopexy, where the vaginal apex is loosely attached to the anterior aspect of the sacrum, usually with mesh secured with suture at either end. There is evidence that the abdominal approaches are superior to those performed vaginally and that the laparoscopic technique is associated with equivalent anatomic and functional outcomes at 12 months, equivalent "cures" at about 3 years, with reduced complications and hospital stay.

Type of prolapse and the common surgical repair procedures.

Organ descent	*Clinical condition*	*Type of operation*
Vaginal wall		
Anterior (upper 2/3) or whole	Cystocele/cystourethrocele Paravaginal defect	• Anterior colporrhaphy • Paravaginal defect repair
Posterior (lower 2/3)	Rectocele	• Colpoperineorrhaphy
Posterior (upper 1/3)	Enterocele	• Vaginal repair of enterocele with PFR • McCall culdoplasty • Moskowitz procedure
Combined anterior and posterior	Cystocele and rectocele	• PFR (combined procedure)
Uterovaginal Uterus along with vaginal walls	Uterovaginal prolapse	• Vaginal hysterectomy with PFR (elderly woman, family completed) • Fothergill's operation (preservation of uterus)
Vaginal wall **Following hysterectomy** (Vaginal or abdominal)	Vault prolapse (secondary)	**Vaginal:** • Repair of vaginal vault along with PFR • Sacrospinous colpopexy • Colpocleisis (Le Fort) **Abdominal**: Sacral colpopexy
Uterus (without vaginal walls)	Congenital or nulliparous prolapse (young women)	Cervicopexy or Sling (Purandare's) operation
Pelvic organ prolapse (POP)	POP with stress in continence	• **Vaginal**: TOT operation • **Abdominal**: Burch operation

3. **Ans. is b, i.e. Fothergill procedure** *Ref: DC Dutta's Textbook of Gynae 9th/ed, Ch-16*

   In given case, young 30 years lady with prolapse due to cervical lengthening Fothergill's procedure would be treatment of choice. Others like:
   - Hysterectomy would be done in elderly lady/Postmenopausal patient.
   - Lefort procedure is done in elderly lady who cannot undergo hysterectomy due to other comorbidity and prolonged anaesthesia risk.

- McCall culdoplasty is done for enterocoele repair.

Composite steps of Fothergill's operation.
• Preliminary D&C • Amputation of cervix • Plication of Mackenrodt's ligaments in front of cervix • Anterior colporrhaphy • Colpoperineorrhaphy

4. **Ans. is d, i.e. Uterine didelphys** *Ref: DC Dutta's Textbook of Gynae 9th/ed, Ch-4*

The different types of uterine anomaly are shown in the figure below, classified by AFS (American Fertility Society)

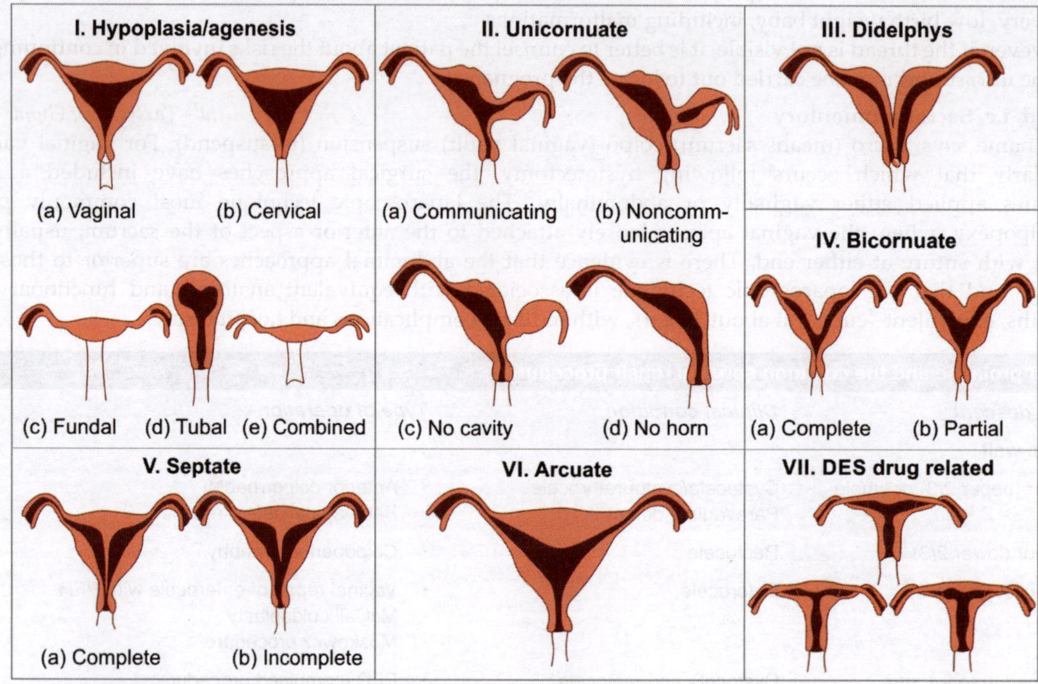

Classification of Mullerian anomalies (Based on classification of American Fertility Society – 1988).

5. **Ans. is b, i.e. Endometrial polyp** *Ref: DC Dutta's Textbook of Gynae 9th/ed, Ch-20*

FIGO classification of fibroid is given below:

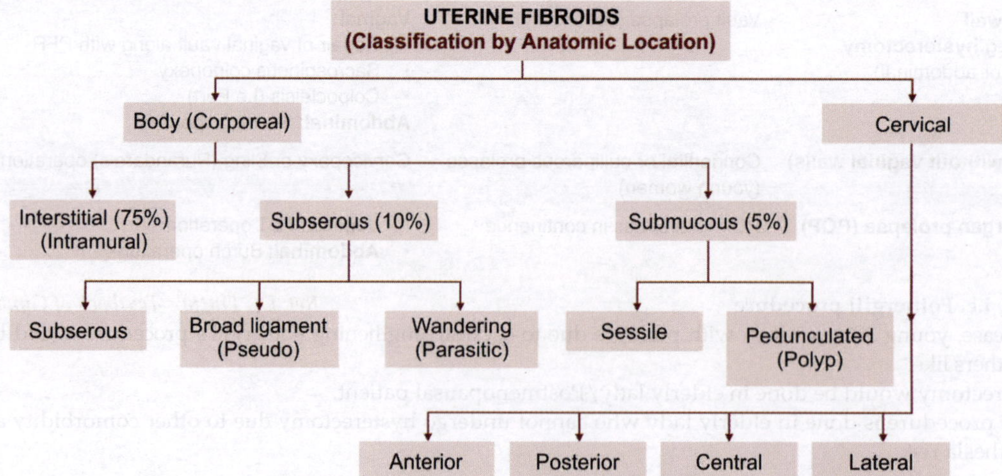

Source: Hiralal Konar. DC Dutta's Textbook of Gynecology, 6th edition; 2013.

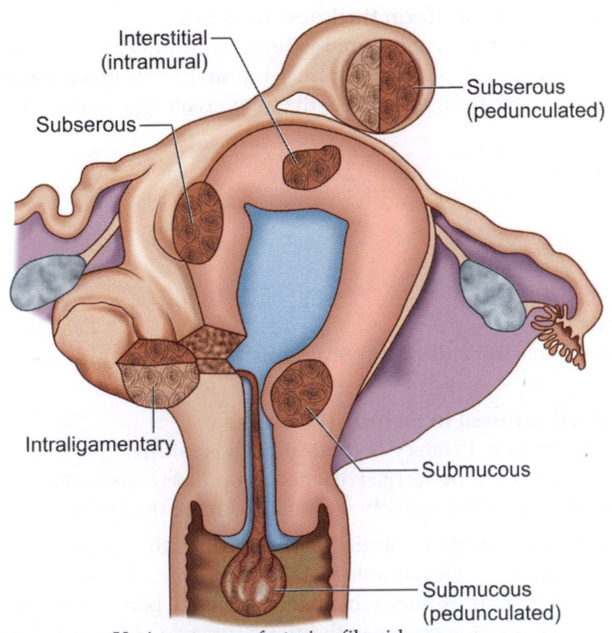

Various types of uterine fibroids.

Source: Hiralal Konar. DC Dutta's Textbook of Gynecology, 6th edition; 2013.

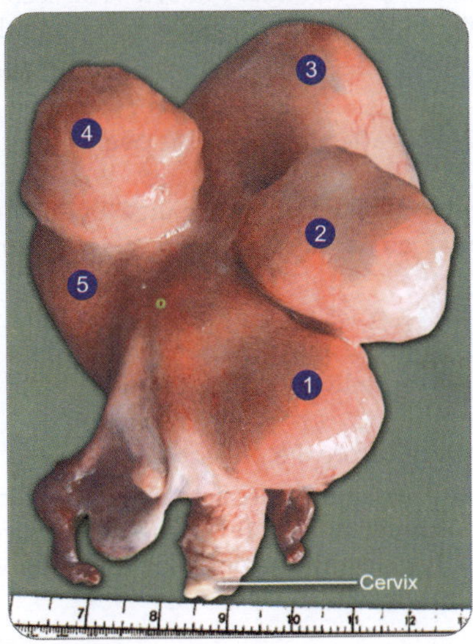

Multiple fibroids causing marked distortion of the uterus. The uterine corpus is almost completely replaced by multiple myomas in subserous, intramural, and submucous positions (Multiple myomas, marked as 1 to 5).

Source: Hiralal Konar. DC Dutta's Textbook of Gynecology, 6th edition; 2013.

SM: Submucosal	0	Pedunculated intracavitary
	1	<50% intramural
	2	≥50% intramural
O: Other	3	Contacts endometrium; 100% intramural
	4	Intramural
	5	Subserosal ≥50% intramural
	6	Subserosal <50% intramural
	7	Subserosal pedunculated
	8	Other (specify, e.g., cervical, parasitic, intraligamentary)

6. **Ans. is c, i.e. Isthmus because it has a uniform thickness of muscle** *Ref: DC Dutta's Textbook of Gynae 9th/ed, Ch-30*
Tubectomy is a sterilisation procedure. Here the mid-isthmic portion of the tube is elevated, allowing the proximal and distal sides of the tube to come together. A single strand of a rapidly absorbable suture (e.g., 1-0 or 0 plain gut suture) is placed around both the proximal and distal portions of the tube, creating a loop or "knuckle" of the fallopian tube above the suture.

Different methods of Tubectomy:
- Pomeroy's:
- Uchida technique:
- Irving method:
- Madlener technique

7. **Ans. is b, i.e. Endometriosis** *Ref: DC Dutta's Textbook of Gynae 9th/ed, Ch-22*
In the given case, 2 cm nodular mass in episiotomy scar which increases in size and painful during menstruation are clear signs of Endometriosis.

8. **Ans. is d, i.e. Secondary oocyte arrested in meiosis II** *Ref: DC Dutta's Textbook of Gynae 9th/ed, Ch-8*
20th week, numbering about 7 million. Primary oocytes at birth is estimated to be about 2 million. The primary oocytes do not finish the first meiotic division until puberty is reached. At puberty, some 400,000 primary oocytes are left behind, the rest being atretic. Out of these, some 400 are likely to ovulate during the entire reproductive period.

Maturation of the oocytes: The essence of maturation is reduction of the number of chromosomes to half. Before the onset of first meiotic division, the primary oocytes double its DNA by replication, so they contain double the amount of normal protein content. There are 22 pairs of autosomes which determine the body characteristics and 1 pair of sex chromosomes, named "XX". The first stage of maturation occurs with full maturation of the ovarian follicle just prior to ovulation but the final maturation occurs only after fertilization.

Ovulation occurs soon after the formation of the secondary oocyte. The secondary oocyte completes the second meiotic division (homotypical) only after fertilization by the sperm in the fallopian tube.

9. **Ans. is c, i.e. Within 48 hours** *Ref: DC Dutta's Textbook of Gynae 9th/ed, Ch-30*
Cu-T insertion:
- **Interval:** It is preferable to insert 2–3 days after the period is over. But it can be inserted any time during the cycle, provided she is not pregnant.
- **Postabortal:** Immediately following termination of pregnancy by suction evacuation or D and E, or following spontaneous abortion. The additional advantage of preventing uterine synechia can help in motivation for insertion.
- **Immediate postpartum:**
  - Post-placental within 10 minutes after expulsion of placenta following vaginal delivery.
  - Intracesarean insertion during cesarean delivery, after removal of the placenta and before closure of the uterine incision.
  - Within 48 hours (MEC-1) after delivery before the patient is discharged from the hospital.

Advantages are: (a) Safe and highly effective; (b) immediate action; (c) long-term protection; (d) special benefit to women having limited access or no access to postpartum care; (e) immediate return to fertility after removal; (f) no need of frequent visits and no further cost; (g) high continuation rates and user satisfaction. However, the expulsion rate is high.

10. **Ans. is d, i.e. 46,XX** *Ref: DC Dutta's Textbook of Gynae 9th/ed, Ch-29*
Gross hymenal abnormality of significance is imperforate hymen. It is due to failure of disintegration of the central cells of the Müllerian eminence that projects into the urogenital sinus which has endodermal epithelium.

As the uterus is functioning normally:
- Cryptomenorrhea: Menstrual blood is pent up inside the vagina behind the hymen
- Hematocolpos: Blood accumulated, it first distends the vagina
- Hematometra: The uterus is next involved and the cavity is dilated

They can present with feature of retention of urine, cause of retention is due to elongation and closure of the urethra.
- Vulvar inspection reveals a tense bulging membrane of bluish coloration.
- Ultrasonography can make the diagnosis of hematometra and hematocolpos.

Treatment: Cruciate incision is made in the hymen.

Note: They do not have any chromosomal abnormality.

11. Ans. is b, i.e. Liquid-based cytology, cervical biopsy, HPV testing *Ref: DC Dutta's Textbook of Gynae 9th/ed, Ch-19*

Cervical ectopy is a condition where the squamous epithelium of the ectocervix is replaced by columnar epithelium, which is continuous with the endocervix. It is not an ulcer.

In the given case, as the lady is 46 years old, with erosion requires thorough investigation to rule out malignancy/ precancerous lesion.

Best would be with:

- PAP/Liquid based cytology
- HPV testing
- Cervical biopsy with colposcopy

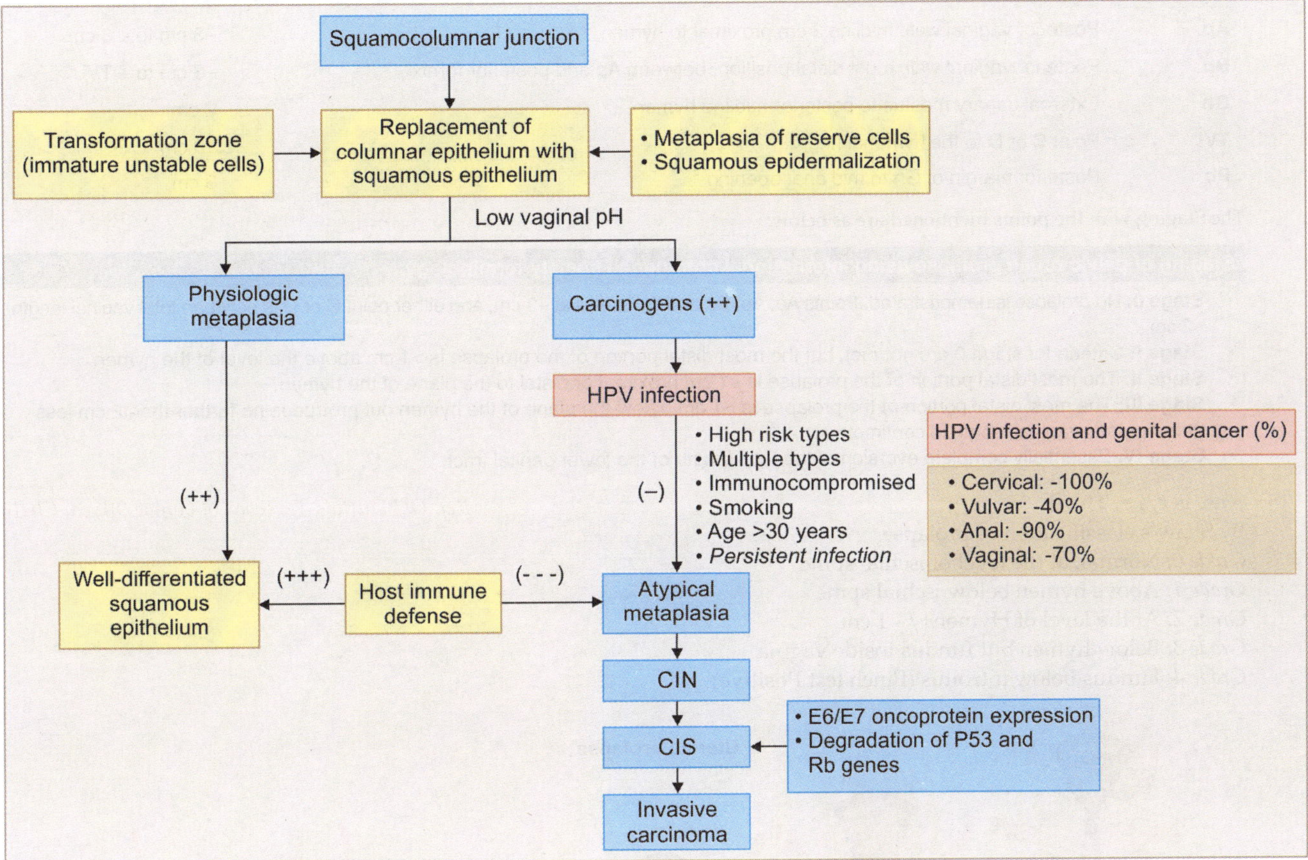

12. Ans. is b, i.e. Myxomatous polyp *Ref: DC Dutta's Textbook of Gynae 9th/ed, Ch-20*

In the given case, symptoms and signs suggest of prolapse:

1. Hypertrophied cervix would not present as prolapse, cervical elongation presents as prolapse.
2. Myxomatous polyp has these features that a polyp arising from uterus hangs down from cervix and vagina presenting as prolapse, and uterus will be palpable with finger (or uterine sound) can pass between polyp stalk and cervical os (which will be not possible in uterine inversion).
3. Placental polyp will be unlikely as history says she delivered 20 years ago.
4. Uterine inversion, unlikely as fingers can pass from the internal os.

13. Ans. is a, i.e. Endometrioma *Ref: DC Dutta's Textbook of Gynae 9th/ed, Ch-22*

The given image shown a chocolate cyst noted in ovary which is typically seen in endometriosis.

The classic lesion of pelvic endometriosis may be as "powder burns" or "match stick" spots on the peritoneum of the pouch of Douglas.

Germ cell tumour like dermoid will have other tissue in ovary like hair follicle, sebaceous gland, teeth, etc.

Endometrial polyp and Ca are ruled out, as image shows ovarian lesion.

14. Ans. is b, i.e. Prolapse *Ref: DC Dutta's Textbook of Gynae 9th/ed, Ch-16*

POP-Q (Pelvic Organ Prolapse Quantification) as name suggest it is used in to grade prolapse.

The pelvic organ prolapse quantification (POP-Q) staging system.

Site	Description	Range
Aa	Anterior vaginal wall, midline 3 cm proximal to hymen	–3 cm to +3 cm
Ba	Anterior vaginal wall, most distal position between Aa and anterior fornix	–3 cm to + TVL
C	Cervix or vaginal vault after total hysterectomy	–
D	Posterior fornix or vaginal apex	–
Ap	Posterior vaginal wall, midline 3 cm proximal to hymen	–3 cm to + 3 cm
Bp	Posterior vaginal wall, most distal position, between Ap and posterior fornix	–3 cm to + TVL
Gh	External urinary meatus to posterior midline hymen	2 cm
TVL	Point C or D to the hymenal ring	10 cm
Pb	Posterior margin of Gh to mid anal opening	3 cm

The Staging with the points mentioned are as below:

Staging of pelvic organ prolapse using international continence society terminology.

- **Stage 0:** No prolapse is demonstrated. Points Aa, Ap, Ba and Bp are all at –3 cm, and either point C or D is between total vaginal length –2 cm.
- **Stage I:** Criteria for stage 0 are not met, but the most distal portion of the prolapse is >1 cm above the level of the hymen.
- **Stage II:** The most distal portion of the prolapse is ≤1 cm proximal or distal to the plane of the hymen.
- **Stage III:** The most distal portion of the prolapse is >1 cm below the plane of the hymen but protrudes no farther than 2 cm less than the total vaginal length in centimeters.
- **Stage IV:** Essentially complete eversion of the total length of the lower genital tract.

15. Ans. is c, i.e. Third *Ref: DC Dutta's Textbook of Gynae 9th/ed, Ch-16*

By Shaw's classification of prolapse:

Grade 0: Normal, at the level of ischial spine
Grade 1: Above hymen below ischial spine
Grade 2: At the level of Hymen+/– 1 cm
Grade 3: Below hymen but fundus inside vagina
Grade 4: Fundus below introitus (Pinch test Positive)

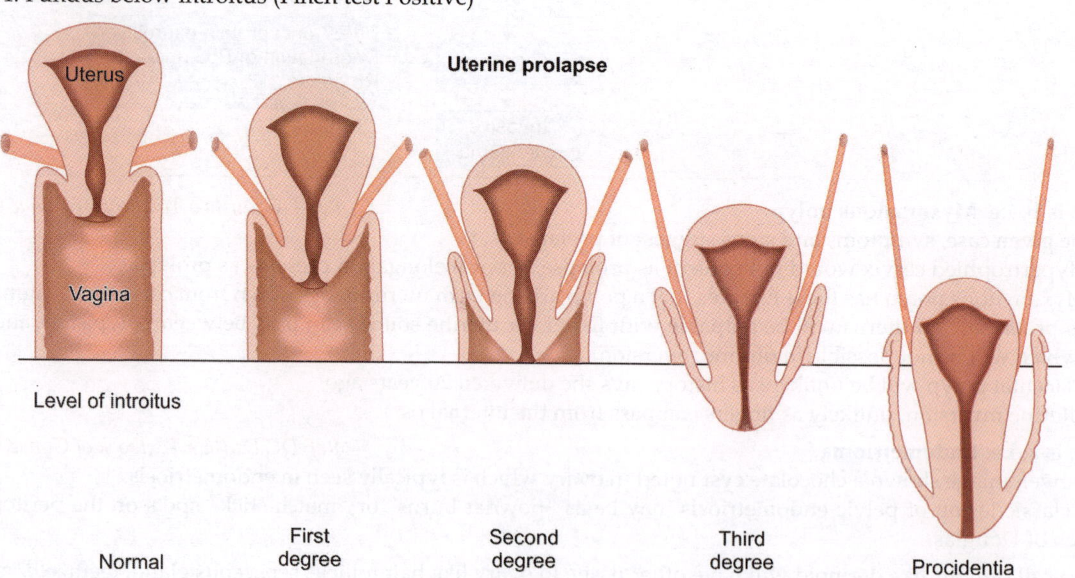

16. Ans. is c, i.e. Turner syndrome *Ref: DC Dutta's Textbook of Gynae 9th/ed, Ch-28*

In the given karyotype, has only one X chromosome (making X0) seen in Turner syndrome

46,XY Disorder of Sexual Development Androgen Insensitivity Syndrome (Testicular Feminization)

Klinefelter's syndrome (47,XXY DSD)

17. Ans. is c, i.e. Stage 3 *Ref: DC Dutta's Textbook of Gynae 9th/ed, Ch-24*

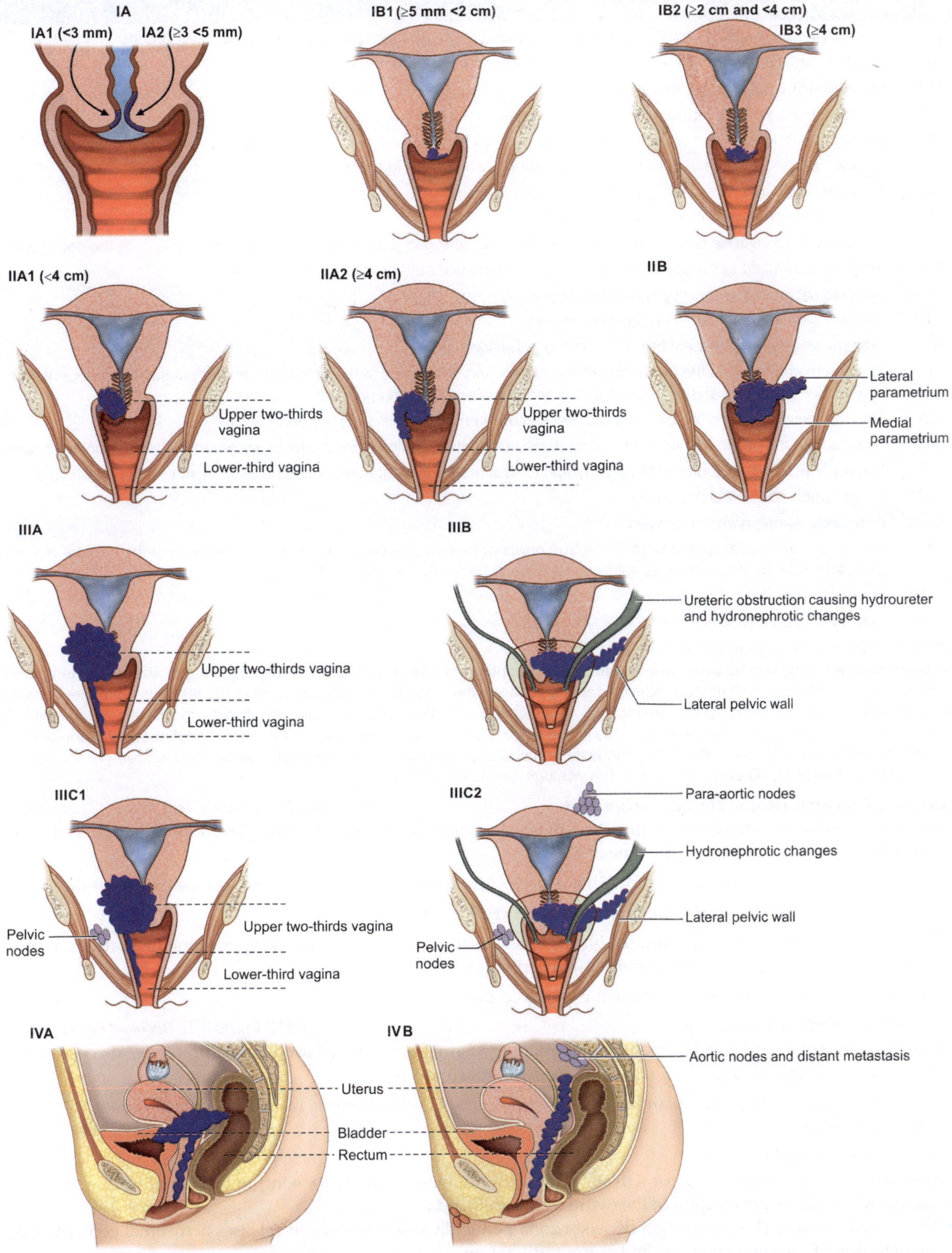

Diagrammatic representation of staging of carcinoma cervix according to FIGO.

Patients with migration failure of GnRH neurons present with hypogonadotropic hypogonadism (Kallmann syndrome) with anosmia.

The given table helps you to remember stages of Ca cervix

FIGO staging of carcinoma of the cervix uteri (2018).	
I	The carcinoma is strictly confined to the cervix (extension to the uterine corpus should be disregarded).
IA	Invasive carcinoma that can be diagnosed only by microscopy with deepest invasion <5 mm[a].
IA1	Measured stromal invasion <3 mm in depth.
IA2	Measured stromal invasion ≥3 mm and <5 mm in depth.
IB	Invasive carcinoma with measured deepest invasion ≥5 mm (greater than stage IA), lesion limited to the cervix uteri[b].
IB1	Invasive carcinoma ≥5 mm depth of stromal invasion, and ≤2 cm in greatest dimension.
IB2	Invasive carcinoma >2 cm and ≤4 cm in greatest dimension.
IB3	Invasive carcinoma >4 cm in greatest dimension.
II	The carcinoma invades beyond the uterus, but has not extended onto the lower third of the vagina or to the pelvic wall.
IIA	Involvement limited to the upper two-thirds of the vagina without parametrial involvement.
IIA1	Invasive carcinoma <4 cm in greatest dimension.
IIA2	Invasive carcinoma ≥4 cm in greatest dimension.
IIB	With parametrial involvement but not up to the pelvic wall.
III	The carcinoma involves the lower third of the vagina and/or extends to the pelvic wall and/or causes hydronephrosis or nonfunctioning kidney and/or involves pelvic and/or para-aortic lymph nodes[c].
IIIA	The carcinoma involves the lower third of the vagina, with no extension to the pelvic wall.
IIIB	Extension to the pelvic wall and/or hydronephrosis or nonfunctioning kidney (unless known to be due to another cause).
IIIC	Involvement of pelvic and/or para-aortic lymph nodes, irrespective of tumor size and extent (with r and p notations)[c].
IIIC1	Pelvic lymph node metastasis only.
IIIC2	Para-aortic lymph node metastasis.
IV	The carcinoma has extended beyond the true pelvis or has involved (biopsy proven) the mucosa of the bladder or rectum. (A bullous edema, as such, does not permit a case to be allotted to stage IV).
IVA	Spread to adjacent pelvic organs.
IVB	Spread to distant organs.

When in doubt, the lower staging should be assigned.

[a]Imaging and pathology can be used, where available, to supplement clinical findings with respect to tumor size and extent, in all stages.

[b]The involvement of vascular/lymphatic spaces does not change the staging. The lateral extent of the lesion is no longer considered.

[c]Adding notation of r (imaging) and p (pathology) to indicate the findings that are used to allocate the case to stage IIIC. Example: If imaging indicates pelvic lymph node metastasis, the stage allocation would be stage IIIC1r, and if confirmed by pathologic findings, it would be stage IIIC1p. The type of imaging modality or pathology technique used should always be documented.

Source: Hiralal Konar. DC Dutta's Textbook of Gynecology, 9th edition; 2024.

18. Ans. is a, i.e. Laparoscopic chromopertubation *Ref: DC Dutta's Textbook of Gynae 9th/ed, Ch-17*

HSG is a screening investigation, confirmation of tubal patency has to be done with chromopertubation as their is chance of false blockage due to spasm at the time of HSG.

Also laparoscopy would help to look for other causes of Infertility and minor ailments can be treated at the same sitting.

Hysteroscopy would not confirm the patency of the peripheral end of the tubes.

IUI is not the treatment of choice in tubal blockage as the egg would not reach the sperm due to anatomical blockage. If confirmed with blockage then may require tubal clipping with IVF.

Hysterectomy is never the choice as patient is yet to conceive.

19. Ans. is b, i.e. Bacterial vaginosis *Ref: DC Dutta's Textbook of Gynae 9th/ed, Ch-12*

Nugent score: It is a 0–10 standardized scale evaluating vaginal microbiota based on the presence/absence of *Lactobacilli* spp., *Gardnerella vaginalis* and *Mobiluncus* spp. bacterial morphotypes.

A lower abundance of Lactobacilli and an increased presence of other bacteria result in a higher Nugent score, suggesting bacterial vaginosis.

20. Ans. is b, i.e. Cortical reaction *Ref: DC Dutta's Textbook of Gynae 9th/ed, Ch-17*

Capacitation results in sperm hyperactivation (an extreme increase in movement) and the ability to release acrosomal contents, which allow penetration of the ovum's zona pellucida.

- *Acrosomal reaction:* This interaction between zona pellucida and acrosome to releases acrosomal contents that permit penetration of the zona pellucida and ovum fertilization.
- Cortical reaction blocks further sperm-oocyte fusion either by sticking at the oolemma or by the induction of a biochemical reaction of the zona pellucida (zona pellucida hardening).

NEET 2023

1. A young female has lower abdomen pain for one month. She reports mild intermenstrual bleeding and dysuria with scanty vaginal discharge which had subsided on its own within a week. She has a history of multiple sexual partners. What is the most likely causative organism?
   a. *Mycobacterium tuberculosis*
   b. *Neisseria gonorrhoeae*
   c. *Candida*
   d. Herpes simplex

2. A 22-year-old female brought by her mother-in-law to the gynecology OPD complaining of inability to conceive for the last six months. She has been cohabiting with her husband without using any contraception. Her BMI is 23 kg/m^2. What will be the management of this patient?
   a. Reassurance for 6 months
   b. Husband's semen analysis
   c. Ovulation analysis
   d. Intrauterine insemination

3. A 15-year-old patient came to the OPD with her mother with a complaint of primary amenorrhea. On physical examination her height is 155 cm, the breasts are developed and there is no pubic or axillary hair. On TVS, the uterus, FT and ovaries are not seen. Inguinal region swellings are noted. What is the most probable diagnosis of the patient?
   a. Turner's syndrome
   b. Complete androgen insensitivity
   c. Mullerian agenesis
   d. Hypergonadotropic hypogonadism

4. A 16-year-old female with primary amenorrhea has cyclical abdominal pain every month. On physical examination she has a suprapubic bulge. P/R examination reveals swelling along the whole length of vagina. What is the diagnosis?
   a. Cervical agenesis
   b. Vaginal agenesis
   c. Transverse vaginal septum in the upper 1/3rd of the vagina
   d. Imperforate hymen

5. A 16-year-old girl's mother had a history of cervical cancer and she was operated for the same. What advice will be given to the girl?
   a. BRCA Gene Testing
   b. PTEN Gene Testing
   c. HPV Vaccine
   d. HPV DNA Testing

6. A female presented to the gynecology OPD with a foul smelling bloody discharge per vagina mixed with mucus. She gives a history of multiple sexual partners. The patient is diagnosed with cervical cancer extending to the left parametrium with lateral wall involvement. What is the treatment of choice for this patient?
   a. Radiotherapy
   b. Chemotherapy
   c. Surgery
   d. Chemoradiation

7. Which of the following cases in the OT will you manage hysteroscopically?
   a. Subserosal fibroid
   b. Tubal ligation
   c. Asherman syndrome
   d. Endocervical polyp

8. A female undergoing treatment for infertility with IVF was given Inj. HMG, presents with a history of vomiting, nausea, and headache. The USG is shown below, what is the diagnosis?

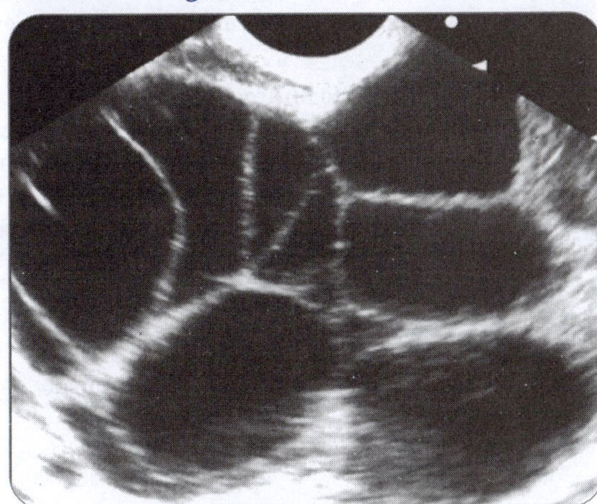

Source: Hiralal Konar. DC Dutta's Textbook of Gynecology, 9th edition; 2024.

   a. Polycystic ovarian syndrome
   b. Theca lutein cysts
   c. Ovarian hyperstimulation syndrome
   d. Granulosa cell tumor

9. A patient underwent hysteroscopic removal of a fibroid. A fluid deficit of 2000 mL is reported. What is the most common immediate complication?
   a. Acute tubular necrosis
   b. DIC
   c. Pulmonary edema
   d. Thromboembolism

Answer with Explanations

1. **Ans. is b, i.e. *Neisseria gonorrhoeae*** *Ref: DC Dutta's Textbook of Gynae 9th/ed, Ch-12 & 13*

All cases of PID are polymicrobial, involving gram-negative and gram-positive aerobic and anaerobic bacteria. PID initiated by Neisseria gonococcus or chlamydia is manifested by the acute onset of pelvic pain that increases with movement, fever, purulent vaginal discharge, and sometimes nausea and emesis.

The most important signs of acute salpingo-oophoritis are cervical motion tenderness and bilateral adnexal tenderness.

Mycobacterium tuberculosis is usually manifested as initial menorrhagia followed by amenorrhea, also they may have symptoms of infertility, Chronic pelvic pain.

Candida infected patients gives history of curdy white discharge associated with pruritis. Also to remember candidial infection is common in immunocompromised patients like diabetic patients, Retroviral positive patients.

Herpes infection would present with painful tender ulcers over the genitalia. To note: With active herpes infection mode of termination will always be LSCS.

2. **Ans. is a, i.e. Reassurance for 6 months** *Ref: DC Dutta's Textbook of Gynae 9th/ed, Ch-17*

Infertility by definition is inability to conceive within 1 or more years of regular unprotected coitus. The interval is however, shortened to 6 months after the age of 35 years of the woman and 40 years of the man.

About 80% of the couples achieve conception if they so desire, within one year of having regular intercourse with adequate frequency (4–5 times a week). Primary denotes those patients who have never conceived. Secondary indicates previous pregnancy but failure to conceive subsequently.

The basic investigations to be carried out are: (a) Semen analysis; (b) Confirmation of ovulation; (c) Confirmation of tubal patency.

3. **Ans. is b, i.e. Complete androgen insensitivity** *Ref: DC Dutta's Textbook of Gynae 9th/ed, Ch-29*

In the given history, 1. Amenorrhea, 2. Normal stature (155 cm), 3. Normal breast development, 4. No pubic/axillary hair, 5. Absent uterus, fallopian tube, ovaries, 6. Inguinal swelling (Testis) all signs are suggestive towards Androgen insensitive/Testicular feminisation syndrome. The table below gives a detailed history of different amenorrhea.

Diagnosis of primary amenorrhea based on clinical examination.

Physical appearance	*External genitalia*	*Internal genitalia*	*Probable diagnosis*
• Secondary sex characters • Stature			
• Normal breast development • Normal sexual hair • Average stature	Normal	• Absence of vagina • Absent uterus	Müllerian agenesis (Mayer-Rokitansky-Küster-Hauser syndrome)
—do—	—do—	Normal	• Unresponsive endometrium—receptor defect (rare) • Uterine synechiae (rare)
• Poor breast development • Scanty pubic hair • Average stature	Underdeveloped	Underdeveloped (vaginal rugosity absent)	Hypogonadotropic hypogonadism
• Tall and lanky	—do—	—do—	Primary ovarian failure
• Poor secondary sex characters • Stature—short • Webbing of the neck and cubitus valgus present • Congenital malformations of cardiac, renal or great vessels (coarctation of aorta) • Phenotypically female	—do—	—do— 'Streak' gonads	Turner's syndrome
• Average height • Delayed secondary sex characters	Normal	Bilateral 'streak' gonads	Pure gonadal dysgenesis
• Normal breast development without areolar pigmentation • Scanty pubic and axillary hair • Average stature	Labial or inguinal gonads (Figs. 27.6 and 27.7)	• Short blind vagina • Absence of uterus	Androgen insensitivity syndrome
• Normal phenotypically female • Average stature	• Labial fusion • Enlargement of clitoris	Normal	Adrenogenital syndrome (late onset)

Contd...

Contd...

Diagnosis of primary amenorrhea based on clinical examination.			
Physical appearance	***External genitalia***	***Internal genitalia***	***Probable diagnosis***
• Features of (hypogonadotropic hypogonadism) – Short stature – Mental retardation – Obesity, retinitis pigmentosa	Underdeveloped	Underdeveloped	• Cretinism due to hypothyroidism • Hypothalamopituitary dysfunction (rare) – Kallmann's syndrome – Prader-Labhart-Willi syndrome – Laurence-Moon-Bardet–Biedl syndrome (rare)

Source: Hiralal Konar. DC Dutta's Textbook of Gynecology, 9th edition; 2024.

4. **Ans. is d, i.e. Imperforate hymen** *Ref: DC Dutta's Textbook of Gynae 9th/ed, Ch-4*

In Mullerian anomaly with imperforate hymen will have these typical symptoms of amenorrhea with cyclical pain every month leading to accumulation of menstrual blood leading to urinary symptoms of frequency/dysuria/retention of urine followed by suprapubic bulge. Vulvar inspection: Bulging membrane with bluish discolouration. Rectal examination bulged vagina. USG: Hematometra/hematocolpos.

Other causes and its differentiating features are mentioned below:

Imperforate hymen	Transverse vaginal septum	Longitudinal vaginal septum
Incidence: 1:1000	1:30,000-50,000	Septum may be partial or complete
Painless initially	Increasing cyclical abdominal	Difficulty with inserting tampons
Painful hematocolpos may affect micturition and defaecation	Pain and absence of menstruation	Dyspareunia, dysmenorrhoea in complete septum
O/E: Blue membrane	O/E: Septum is pink	–
Management: Cruciate incision and drainage	Excision of the septal defect along with end- to-end anastomosis of upper and lower vagina. Patients with a lower 1 /3rd anastomosis → delivery by CS	Excision can be carried out by sharp dissection, diathermy or laser

5. **Ans. is c, i.e. HPV Vaccine** *Ref: DC Dutta's Textbook of Gynae 9th/ed, Ch-24*

The vaccines are prophylactic and not therapeutic. As the girl is 16 and we are preventing her from getting cervical cancer, so best advice for the girl would be HPV vaccine. WHO (2014) recommends HPV vaccine for both the boys and girls between 9 and 14 years: Two doses (0M & 6–12M) are now required. Individual aged >15 years: Three doses (0M 1–2M & 6M) are needed.

HPV DNA testing is required after the onset of sexual activity or after 21 years, even then vaccine should be opted.

BRCA & PTEN is mostly for Ovarian/Breast cancer testing.

6. **Ans. is d, i.e. Chemoradiation** *Ref: DC Dutta's Textbook of Gynae 9th/ed, Ch-24*

The below table gives different management options at different stages of cervical cancer.

Management options of carcinoma cervix.	
Stage	***Management options***
Bulky disease IB3 and IIA2 **IB3:≥4 cm** **IIA1: <4 cm + upper vagina** **IIA2:≥4 cm + upper vagina**	• **Surgery is discouraged due to high morbidity** • Concurrent platinum based chemoradiation therapy (CCRT) • Neoadjuvant chemotherapy (NACT) can be used where radiotherapy facilities are scarce
IIB–IVA	• CCRT is the standard treatment for patients with locally advanced cervical cancer (LACC) • Radiation therapy to cover pelvic and the extended field for stages IIIB and above. Systemic chemotherapy is given for cases stage IIIC2 and above
Stage IVA	• Only central disease without pelvic or side wall recurrence or distant spread: Pelvic exenteration • It has poor prognosis • *Advanced diseases:* Radiotherapy with image based 3D computer dosimetry (p. 331) with reduced toxicity
Stage IVB + **Distant organs**	CCRT may have better response with overall disease free survival (69%). Carboplatin-paclitaxel combination or cisplatin—topotecan, gemcitabine or vinorelbine found to be effective • Palliative chemotherapy • And/or radiotherapy/supportive care (hospice)

7. **Ans. is c, i.e. Asherman syndrome** *Ref: DC Dutta's Textbook of Gynae 9th/ed, Ch-36*

In hysteroscopy the camera is inserted via cervical canal to look inside the Uterine Cavity, Among the given options Only Asherman's syndrome has Cavitary abnormality with intrauterine adhesions requiring Operative hysteroscope to look inside and treat. Whereas Subserosal fibroid is in serial layer requiring Laparoscope to see and treat. Tubal ligation also we use Laparoscope with Falope ring applicators for Sterilisation Sx. Endocervical polyp will be see on Speculum examination, entering the uterine cavity with hysteroscope is not required.

8. **Ans. is c, i.e. Ovarian hyperstimulation syndrome** *Ref: DC Dutta's Textbook of Gynae 9th/ed, Ch-17*
In the given history key points are: (1) Infertility, (2) On IVF treatment; (3) Ovulation stimulation with Injection HMG; (4) Has nausea vomiting and finally the photo which shows multiple follicles has been stimulated, all of them clearly suggest hyperstimulation of ovary leading to ovarian hyperstimulation syndrome (OHSS). Theca lutein cyst are seen in conditions with high levels of β-hCG like molar pregnancy, twin pregnancy. Polycystic ovarian syndrome, the follicles are arranged peripherally and have pearl of chain appearance.

9. **Ans. c, i.e Pulmonary edema** *Ref: DC Dutta's Textbook of Gynae 9th/ed, Ch-36*
   - A fluid deficit of more than 1000 mL should be used as threshold to define fluid overload when using hypotonic solutions glycine 1.5%, sorbitol 3% in healthy women of reproductive age. A fluid deficit of 2500 mL should be used as threshold to define fluid overload when using isotonic solutions (Normal saline) in healthy women of reproductive age. Surgery is immediately stopped on reaching these limits. (ACOG 2013 Guidelines)

Distension Media

Because the anterior and posterior uterine walls lie in apposition, a distension medium is required to expand the endometrial cavity for viewing. Fluid media include saline, and low-viscous fluids, such as sorbitol, mannitol, and glycine solutions **(Table 1)**. Historically, carbon dioxide was used for diagnostic hysteroscopy but is infrequently employed today. Each group has distinct advantages and properties. To expand the cavity, intrauterine pressures of these media must reach 45 to 80 mm Hg. Rarely is more than 100 mm Hg required. Moreover, because for most women, mean arterial pressure approximates 100 mm Hg, higher pressures can result in increased intravasation of media into the patient's circulation to create fluid volume overload.

Table 1: Hysteroscopic Media

Medium	Properties	Indications	Risks	Safety Measures
Gas				
Carbon dioxide	Colorless gas	Diagnostic	Gas embolism	Avoid Trendelenburg Keep flflow <100 mL/min Intrauterine pressure <100 mm Hg
Electrolyte fluid				
0.9% saline	Isotonic 380 mOsm/kg H_2O	Diagnostic Operative w/ bipolar tools	Volume overload	Plan to complete procedure at 750 mL deficit Stop procedure at 2.5 L deficit End earlier in patients with comorbidities or elderly
Lactated Ringer	Isotonic 273 mOsm/kg H_2O	Same as above	Volume overload	Same as above
Electrolyte-poor fluid				
Sorbitol 3%	Hypoosmolar 178 mOsm/kg H_2O	Operative w/ monopolar tools	Volume overload Hyponatremia Hypoosmolality Hyperglycemia	Plan to complete procedure at 750 mL deficit Stop procedure at 1-1.5L deficit End earlier in patients with comorbidities or elderly
Mannitol 5%	Isoosmolar 280 mOsm/kg H_2O	Operative w/ monopolar tools	Volume overload Hyponatremia	Same as above
Glycine 1.5%	Hypoosmolar 200 mOsm/kg H_2O	Operative w/ monopolar tools	Volume overload Hyponatremia Hypoosmolality Hyperammonemia	Same as above

Data from Cooper, 2000; American Association of Gynecologic Laparoscopists, 2013; American College of Obstetricians and Gynecologists, 2011.

Carbon Dioxide

This gaseous distension medium, when used under pressure, tends to flatten the endometrium and provides excellent visibility. A continuous flow is necessary to replace any gas lost through the tubes, and typically flow rates of 40 to 50 mL/min are adequate. Rates higher than 100 mL/min are associated with increased risks for gas embolism and therefore discouraged. Importantly, because *laparoscopic* insufflating machines can permit flow rates >1000 mL/min, these should not be used for hysteroscopy.

Disadvantages to CO_2 include its tendency, when mixed with blood or mucus, to form visually obstructive gas bubbles. Accordingly, prior to hysteroscope insertion, blood and mucus are carefully removed from the cervical os with a dry swab (Sutton, 2006). Similarly, use of CO_2 with thermal energy sources is avoided as smoke production prohibits adequate viewing. Because of these limitations, CO_2 is best used in cases in which minimal bleeding is anticipated, such as diagnostic hysteroscopy. The most serious complication associated with CO_2 use is venous gas embolism.

Fluid Media

Bleeding is common with operative hysteroscopy procedures. Thus rather than CO2, fluid media are typically selected because of their optical clarity and ability to mix with blood. The main risk of fluid distension media, however, involves increased fluid absorption and circulatory fluid volume overload.

Fluid distension media can be divided according to their viscosity and electrolyte status. In general, low-viscosity fluids are used in modern hysteroscopy. An appropriate medium is selected based on its compatibility with electrosurgical instrumentation.

Low-viscosity Electrolyte Fluids

Normal saline and lactated Ringer solutions are isotonic, electrolyte fluids. They are readily available in the operating room and are frequently used for diagnostic hysteroscopy. However, these fluids cannot be used with monopolar electrosurgery. Specifically, these solutions conduct current; thus, dissipate the energy; and thereby render the instrument useless.

These electrolyte-containing, isotonic fluids have lower associated risks of hyponatremia compared with hypoosmolar fluids, described in the next section. Still, rapid absorption can lead to pulmonary edema. In general, when using isotonic medium in a healthy patient, a surgeon should consider terminating the procedure when the fluid deficit nears 2500 mL (American Association of Gynecologic Laparoscopists, 2013; American College of Obstetricians and Gynecologists, 2011).

Low-viscosity, Electrolyte-poor Fluids

Of other available media, 1.5-percent glycine, 3-percent sorbitol, and 5-percent mannitol are all low-viscosity, electrolyte-poor fluids. Because they are nonconducting, these media are used for electrosurgery involving monopolar instruments. Unfortunately, these fluids can create volume overload with con-current development of hyponatremia and hypoosmolality and the potential for cerebral edema and death (American College of Obstetricians and Gynecologists, 2011). Mechanistically, sorbitol is a six-carbon sugar and is metabolized following absorption. This effectively leaves free water in the intravascular space. Normal serum sodium levels are 135 to 145 mEq/L, and levels significantly below this may lead to seizure followed by respiratory arrest. In addition, hypokalemia and hypocalcemia can often develop concurrently. Five-percent mannitol, also a six-carbon sugar, is isoosmolar and so has diuretic properties but does not lead to serum osmolality changes (American Association of Gynecologic Laparoscopists, 2013).

In cases in which large fluid volume deficits are calculated, measurement of serum electrolyte levels is warranted. If a serum sodium level lower than 125 mEq/L is reached, postoperative care should be continued in a critical care setting. Treatment includes stimulation of diuresis with furosemide (Lasix), 20 to 40 mg given intravenously. Correction of hyponatremia is achieved with 3-percent sodium chloride, administered at a rate of 0.5 to 2 mL/kg/hr. In those with acute neurologic symptoms, 3-percent saline can instead be given in a 100 mL infusion over 30 minutes and repeated an additional two times. The goal of therapy is to reach a serum sodium level of 135 mEq/L within 24 hours. Overcorrection is avoided to prevent additional cerebral effects.

To assist with intraoperative fluid volume calculation, most operative hysteroscopes contain continuous flow systems that allow fluid deficits to be calculated. Calculation of deficits is performed every 15 minutes during procedures. If deficits of a hypotonic solution reach 1000 mL, a surgeon should consider procedure termination, measure electrolytes, and give diuretics as indicated (American Association of Gynecologic Laparoscopists, 2013). At the end of every hysteroscopic procedure, a final deficit is determined, and this value is recorded in the operative note.

NEET 2021

1. **Which of the following is least common in Didelphys uterus?**
   a. Preterm labour
   b. Transverse lie
   c. Endometriosis
   d. Abortions

2. **A lady with primary infertility was diagnosed to have 2 uterine fibroids in the cornual region. Right side is 7 × 5 cms and left side is 5 × 4 cms. On HSG both the tubes are found to be blocked. What is your management if you are told that the woman is ovulating and the semen analysis of her partner is normal?**
   a. Myomectomy
   b. ART
   c. Hysterectomy
   d. Hysteroscopic cannulation of tubes

3. **A 32-years-old female presents to the hospital with cannon ball appearance on the chest X-ray. Patient had a history of molar evacuation. Which of the following is the best management?**
   a. Hysterectomy
   b. EMACO regimen
   c. Single agent chemotherapy like methotrexate
   d. Radiotherapy

4. **A 25-years-old female with primary infertility came to the hospital with USG finding of uterine anomaly. Which of the following is used to confirm the diagnosis?**
   a. TVS
   b. Hysteroscopy and laparoscopy
   c. Laparoscopy
   d. HSG

5. **A 25-years-old female present to the hospital with midline septum in uterus. Which of the following is the management of this condition?**
   a. Laparoscopic metroplasty
   b. Hysteroscopic septoplasty
   c. Uterine metroplasty
   d. Septoplasty

6. **A 28-year-old married female, anxious about conception with complaints of profuse white discharge with no h/o itching presented on 12th day of LMP. Which of the following is the most probable diagnosis?**
   a. Candida
   b. Trichomonas
   c. Bacterial vaginosis
   d. Physiological

7. **A 55-years-old multigravida with history of frequently micturating due to coughing laughing & sneezing what type of urinary incontinence does she likely have?**
   a. Urge incontinence
   b. Stress incontinence
   c. Neurogenic bladder
   d. Urinary Tract Infection

8. **A 18 years old girl with Partial transverse vaginal septum presents with hospital with dysmenorrhea and chronic pelvic pain. Which of the following is the most common complication?**
   a. Endometriosis
   b. Tubo-ovarian abscess
   c. Dermoid cyst
   d. Theca luteal cyst

Answer with Explanations

1. **Ans. is b, i.e. Transverse lie** *Ref: DC Dutta's Textbook of Gynae 9th/ed, Ch-4*

Uterine didelphys is a mullerian anomaly where both the mullerian ducts have not fused at all giving a 2 separate uterus, cervix and vagina as shown in the image. Where chances of reproductive complications are high due to anomalous uterus. Complications like infertility, subfertility, recurrent mid trimester abortions, preterm labour, IUGR, breech presentation. But to note transverse lie is unlikely as there is no enough anatomical space to accommodate foetus in the position.

Reproductive outcome is best in Septate uterus and poor in unicornuate uterus among different uterine anomalies.

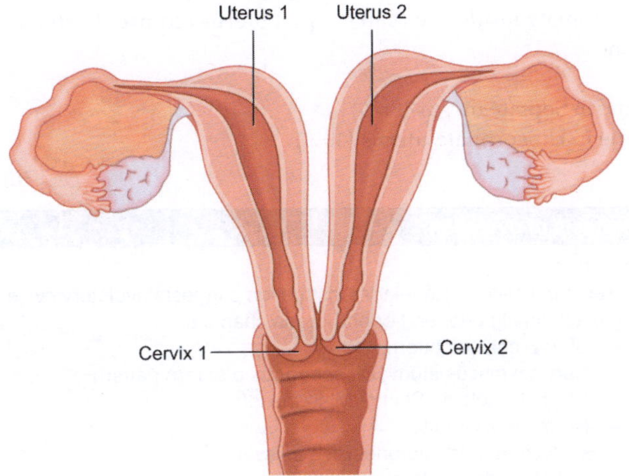

2. **Ans. is a, i.e. Myomectomy** *Ref: DC Dutta's Textbook of Gynae 9th/ed, Ch-17*

As the lady is having 2 uterine corneal fibroids blocking the Ostia of fallopian tube preventing sperm to meet ovum for fertilisation. Which is shown in HSG saying blocked tubes. As mentioned ovulating rules out ovarian causes of infertility and Normal semen analysis rules out Male partner related causes of infertility. Hence we are left with two options: (1) Myomectomy and (2) ART. Myomectomy is first treatment of choice as the size of fibroids mentioned are pretty big which will distort the anatomy of uterus leading to failure of implantation. Hence even if you do ART like IVF as anatomy is distorted their will be high chance of failure.

3. **Ans. is c, i.e. Single agent chemotherapy like methotrexate** *Ref: DC Dutta's Textbook of Gynae 9th/ed, Ch-24*

Here the Lady had Molar pregnancy (GTD) which has now become gestational trophoblastic neoplasia due to recurrence of Disease. Here the mode of treatment depends upon the Risk factors associated, as mentioned in this case: Age 32 years score 0 + molar pregnancy again score 0 + Lung metastasis score 0. As mentioned in the table below score of less than 6 suggest low risk and requires only single agent chemotherapy like methotrexate. If ever score was more may require multi dose regime like MAC or EMACO (etoposide, methotrexate, actinomycin D, cyclophosphamide and vincristine) regime.

FIGO scoring system.

FIGO scoring	*0*	*1*	*2*	*4*
Age (years)	<40	≥40	–	–
Antecedent pregnancy	Mole	Abortion (including miscarriage)	Birth	–
Interval months from end of index pregnancy to treatment	<4	4 to <7	7 to <13	≥13
Pretreatment serum hCG (IU/l)	$<10^3$	10^3 to $<10^4$	10^4 to $<10^5$	$\geq10^5$
Largest tumour size, including uterus (cm)	<3	3 to <5	≥5	–
Size of metastases	Lung	Spleen, kidney	Gastrointestinal	Liver, brain
Number of metastases	–	1–4	5–8	>8
Previous failed chemotherapy	–	–	Single drug	Two or more drugs

4. **Ans. is b, i.e. Hysteroscopy and laparoscopy** *Ref: DC Dutta's Textbook of Gynae 9th/ed, Ch-17*

As the question is about Confirmation of diagnosis, it is by Surgical method - Hysteroscopy with laparoscopy.

Hysteroscope is to look for cavity related anomalies like Septum/Bicornuate, etc. also to look for Uterine cavity, endometrium and Ostia of the tubes. Laparoscope to look for structural anomalies like fibroid/Arcuate uterus, also to look for fallopian tube anomalies and Ovaries. With chromopertubation can also look for tubal patency. Whereas other given options like TVS/HSG are only used for diagnosis but not confirmatory investigations.

5. **Ans. is b, i.e. Hysteroscopic septoplasty** *Ref: DC Dutta's Textbook of Gynae 9th/ed, Ch-4*

Uterine anomalies have effect on reproductive outcome, requiring surgical treatment:

- **Septate Uterus:** Hysteroscopic metroplasty/Septoplasty
- Unicornuate uterus having rudimentary horn - Excision
- **Bicornuate uterus:** Strassman, Jones and Jones/Abdominal metroplasty

Remember in case of uterine anomaly inside cavity like septet uterus requires hysteroscopy, whereas in bicornuate uterus laparoscopic approach in done.

To note:

- Best reproductive Outcome in Septate uterus (86%)
- Poor reproductive outcome in Unicornuate uterus (40%)

6. **Ans. is d, i.e. Physiological** *Ref: DC Dutta's Textbook of Gynae 9th/ed, Ch-17*

Diagnosis of ovulation.

Indirect:

- Menstrual history: Regular menstruation suggests ovulatory cycle
- Evaluation of peripheral or end-organ changes
  - BBT: Biphasic pattern
  - Cervical mucus study: Disappearance of fern pattern
  - Vaginal cytology: Shift of MI to the left
  - Hormone estimation
    - Serum progesterone: Rise in level
    - Serum IH: Midcycle surge
    - Serum estradiol: Midcycle rise
    - Urine IH
  - Endometrial biopsy (secretory phase)
  - Sonography (TVS)

Direct: Laparoscopy	Conclusive: Pregnancy

Given symptoms like profuse white discharge during ovulation (12th day), with no itching all suggest towards Physiological discharge during ovulation.

Characteristics of common vaginal infections.

Category	*Complaint*	*Discharge*	*KOH "Whiff Test"*	*Vaginal pH*	*Microscopic findings*
Normal	None	White, clear	–	3.8–4.2	NA
BV	Odor, increased after intercourse and/or menses	Thin, gray or white, adherent, often increased	+	>4.5	Clue cells, bacteria clumps (saline wet prep)
Candidiasis	Itching, burning, discharge	White, curdy	–	<4.5	Hyphae and buds (10-percent KOH solution wet prep)
Trichomoniasis	Frothy discharge, odor, dysuria, pruritus, spotting	Green-yellow, frothy, adherent, increased	±	>4.5	Motile trichomonads (saline wet prep)
Bacterial[a]	Thin, watery discharge, pruritus	Purulent	–	>4.5	Many WBCs

[a] Streptococcal, staphylococcal, or *Escherichia coli.*

BV = bacterial vaginosis; KOH = potassium hydroxide; NA = not applicable; WBC = white blood cell

7. Ans. is b, i.e. Stress incontinence *Ref: DC Dutta's Textbook of Gynae 9th/ed, Ch-25*

The table given below, differentiates different clinical symptoms for different incontinence. Here as mentioned coughing, laughing, sneezing are different types of stress during which patient complaints of leakage of urine making it stress incontinence.

Differences in clinical presentation.		
Stress *incontinence*	***Urge incontinence (sensory)***	***Overactive bladder (OAB)***
• Leakage of urine coincides with stress • No prior urge to void • Amount—small • Patient—fully aware of it • Micturition—normal	• Unable to control the escape of urine, once there is urge to void • Amount—large • Patient—aware of the urge • Urgency and frequency	• The incontinence may occur abruptly even without a full bladder or a clinical cause • Amount—large • Patient—not aware of it • Frequency and nocturia

8. Ans. is a, i.e. Endometriosis *Ref: DC Dutta's Textbook of Gynae 9th/ed, Ch-22*

As given partial vaginal septum is a type of mullerian anomaly, leading to improper/incomplete drainage of menstrual blood causing menstrual blood accumulation in uterus and retrograde implantation. Which is proven theory for endometriosis and common in patients with Mullerian anomaly having noncommunicating horn where outflow of menstrual blood is not happening. Other complications in mullerian anomalies like:

Gynecological	Obstetric
Infertility, dysmenorrhea, dyspareunia, hematometra, primary amenorrhea, chronic pelvic pain	Second trimester miscarriage, RPL, cervical incompetence, rudimentary horn pregnancy, malpresentation, preterm labor, IUGR, IUD, prolonged labor

INI-CET 2024

1. Select the correct dose of Antara:

a. 300 mg
b. 200 mg
c. 250 mg
d. 150 mg

2. A 19-year-old female presented to you with primary amenorrhea and secondary sexual characteristics are normal. Karyotype is 46XX. FSH levels are 5.5 IU and LH level is 10 IU. Choose the correct diagnosis:

a. Gonadal dysgenesis
b. Mullerian agenesis
c. Androgen insensitivity syndrome
d. Kallmann syndrome

3. A 13-year-old girl has come to you with acute retention of urine, and she complains about cyclical pain in abdomen. A tense blue swelling is seen on local examination and suprapubic bulge is seen on PR examination. What is her condition as per the examination?

a. Cervical agenesis
b. Transverse vaginal septum
c. Imperforate hymen
d. Longitudinal vaginal septum

4. The mineral required for fertility is —

a. Copper
b. Zinc
c. Iron
d. Selenium

5. Most potent form of estrogen seen in a reproductive female is:

a. Estriol
b. Estradiol
c. Esterone
d. Conjugated estrogen

Answer with Explanations

1. **Ans. is d, i.e. 150 mg** *Ref: DC Dutta's Textbook of Gynae 9th/ed, Ch-30*

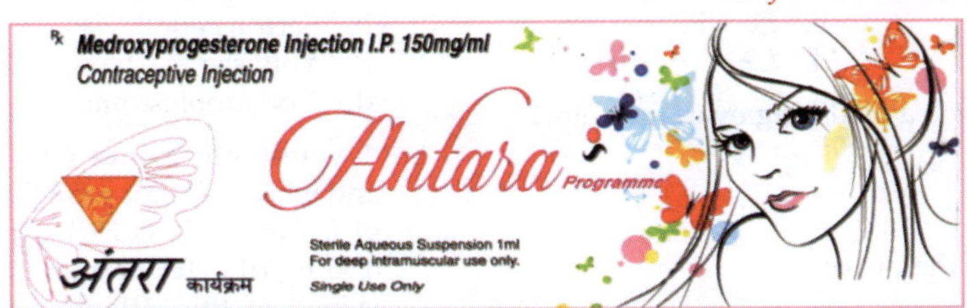

The preparations commonly used are Depo Medroxy Progesterone Acetate (DMPA) and Norethisterone Enanthate (NET-EN). Both are administered intramuscularly (deltoid or gluteus muscle) within 5 days of the cycle. The injection should be deep, Z-tract technique and the site not to be massaged. DMPA in a dose of 150 mg every 3 months (WHO, 4 months) or 300 mg every 6 months; NET-EN in a dose of 200 mg given at 2 monthly intervals.

2. **Ans. is b, i.e. Mullerian agenesis** *Ref: DC Dutta's Textbook of Gynae 9th/ed, Chs-28 &29*

In the given case 46XX rules out Androgen insensitivity, other differentiating factors are mentioned in below table:

Differentiation between androgen insensitivity syndrome (AIS) and Müllerian agenesis (MRKH).

Characters	*Androgen insensitivity syndrome*	*Müllerian agenesis (MRKH syndrome)*
Sexual hair (pubic and axillary)	Absent or sparce	Normal female
Primary amenorrhea	Present	Present
Vagina	Short and blind	Absent
Clitoris	Enlarged	Normal as in female
Gonads: • Structure • Location	• Testes • Inguinal, labial or abdominal	• Ovary • Abdominal
Breasts	Developed	Developed
Serum testosterone level	Slightly elevated	Normal as in female
Müllerian system (uterus)	Absent	Absent or rudimentary
Wolffian system	Absent	Absent
Karyotype	46,XY	46,XX
Associated anomalies	Rare	Skeletal 12% and urological (renal) 47%
Pregnancy	Incomplete	Possible

Normal FSH and LH rules out Gonadal dysgenesis.

3. **Ans. is c, i.e. Imperforate hymen** *Ref: DC Dutta's Textbook of Gynae 9th/ed, Ch-5*

In the given case: (1) Cyclical abdominal pain rules out longitudinal vaginal septum and cervical agenesis causes; (2) Blue swelling rules out Transverse vaginal septum which would look like a Thick Pink Septum on examination.

The given signs are classics for Imperforate hymen: (1) Cyclical abdominal pain; (2) Amenorrhea; (3) Blue swelling on local examination; (4) Suprapubic bulge on PR examination. Treatment is Cruciate incision and drainage.

4. **Ans. is b, i.e. Zinc** *Ref: DC Dutta's Textbook of Gynae 9th/ed, Ch-17*

Studies have shown the Zinc and folic acid have shown to increase the Sperm concentration and morphology. Hence exogenous administration of Zinc and folic acid is recommended.

5. **Ans. is b, i.e. Estradiol** *Ref: DC Dutta's Textbook of Gynae 9th/ed, Ch-32*

Most potent estrogen:

- Before puberty and after menopause: Estrone
- Reproductive age: Estradiol
- Pregnancy: Estriol

INI-CET November 2023

1. **Recombinant HPV vaccine has which protein?**
    a. E1 + E2
    b. E6 + E7
    c. L1
    d. L2

2. **Which of the following is a virilizing ovarian tumor?**
    a. Theca cell tumor
    b. Brenner's tumor
    c. Arrhenoblastoma
    d. Carcinoid tumor of the ovary

3. **A woman was taking DMPA regularly as contraception. But now, she has come 14 days late with respect to the due date for DMPA.**

    What should be the advice to her?
    a. Give DMPA and advise her to use back up method for 7 days
    b. Give DMPA and no back up is needed
    c. After doing UPT give DMPA
    d. DMPA from next menstrual cycle

4. **Which of the following risk factors is associated with borderline ovarian tumor?**
    a. OCP intake
    b. Functional ovarian cyst
    c. PCOS
    d. Low parity

5. **Image of Reinke's crystal. Which tumor?**

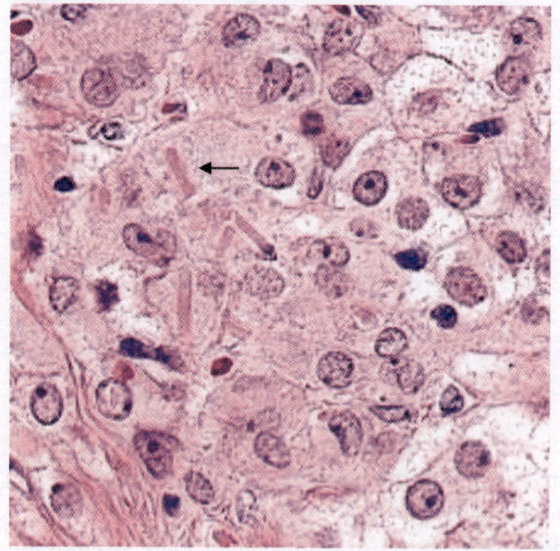

    a. Leydig cell tumor
    b. Sertoli cell
    c. Yolk sac
    d. Gonadoblastoma

6. **A young girl comes with menstrual irregularity, acne, and increased hair growth with Ferriman-Gallwey score of 6. Her BMI is 29 kg/m^2 and testosterone level was 0.36 ng/dL. Her mother is diabetic and on medication. Which of the following will not be recommended to her?**
    a. OCP
    b. OCP plus antiandrogen
    c. Lifestyle modification
    d. Counsel her about the risk of Metabolic syndrome

7. **A 58-year-old female presented with ovarian mass with ascites. Further investigations (CT scan) showed omental caking and peritoneal carcinomatosis. What is the management for this patient?**
    a. Chemotherapy followed by debulking surgery
    b. Debulking surgery followed by chemotherapy
    c. Debulking surgery followed by Radiotherapy
    d. Staging laparotomy

Answer with Explanations

1. **Ans. is c, i.e. L1** *Ref: DC Dutta's Textbook of Gynae 9th/ed, Chs-23 & 24*
   - Prophylactic HPV vaccine is approved to all school girls (12–18 years) and women (16–25 years). (Bivalent, Quadrivalent, nonavalent).
   - Prepared from purified virus like particles(VLP) of the major capsid L1 Vaccine induced neutralizing antibodies (IgG, IgA) works locally (cervix) by preventing the attachment of the virus to the cervical epithelium
   - By CDC: 9-14 years – 2 doses, >15 years – 3 doses WHO SAGE: 1 or 2 doses 9-20 years, >21 years 2 doses
   - Bivalent vaccines (cervarix) against HPV types 16, 18 Quadrivalent (Gardasil) against HPV types 16, 18, 6, 11
   - Nonavalent against HPV 6,11,16,18, 31, 33, 45, 52 and 58
   - Helps in Genital warts, Condyloma accuminata, Precancerous lessions, Ca cervix, Vulval ca, vaginal ca, anal ca, oropharynx ca.
2. **Ans. is c, i.e. Arrhenoblastoma** *Ref: DC Dutta's Textbook of Gynae 9th/ed, Ch-24*
   - 75% are associated with sexual pseudoprecocity because of the estrogen secretion.
   - For women of reproductive age, most patients have menstrual irregularities or secondary amenorrhea, and cystic hyperplasia of the endometrium
   - For postmenopausal women, abnormal uterine bleeding is frequently the initial symptom.
   - Sex Cord-Stromal Tumors
   - Granulosa –stromal cell tumors
   - Sertoli – stromal cell tumors
   - Gynandroblastoma
   - Sex – cord tumor with annular tubules
   - Unclassified sex-cord tumors Steroid cell tumors - arrhenoblastoma
   - Granulosa cell tumor
   - Typically post-menopausal patients
   - May produce estrogen leading to PMB, endometrial hyperplasia/endometrial ca Typically have a yellow color due to lipid accumulation
   - Tumor marker: Inhibin
   - Tend to have recurrences, Role of adjuvant uncommon tumors of the ovary, usually low-grade cancers, usually produce hormones that lead to symptoms, Surgical treatment with tumor resection and surgical staging, therapy.
3. **Ans. is b, i.e. Give DMPA and no back up is needed.** *Ref: DC Dutta's Textbook of Gynae 9th/ed, Ch-30*
   - A medical history to assess the contraindications.
   - Women aged <18 years – DMPA can be used as first-line contraception after consideration of other methods.
   - Women using DMPA who wish to continue – review every 2 years to assess individual situations and discuss the benefits and potential risks.
   - Use may continue to age 50 years.
   - POIC can be safely used by women who are breastfeeding.
   - Women can start a POIC up to day 21 postpartum to provide immediate contraceptive protection. If started after that time, advise another method of contraception or abstinence for 7 days.
   - POIC may be given following miscarriage or termination. If started within 5 days after the miscarriage/termination, then additional contraceptive or abstinence is not required
   - Repeat injection of DMPA every 12 weeks (or every 8 weeks for NET-EN). If necessary, a repeat POIC can be given up to 2 weeks early.
   - A repeat injection of POIC can be given up to 2 weeks late (i.e., 14 weeks since the last DMPA and 10 weeks for NET-EN) without additional contraception.
4. **Ans. is d, i.e. Low parity** *Ref: DC Dutta's Textbook of Gynae 9th/ed, Chs-21 & 24*
   - Risk factors have to do with more number of ovulations, which traumatize the epithelial lining of the ovary
   - Low parity
   - Infertility
   - Early menarche
   - Late menopause
   - Family History

5. Ans. is a, i.e. Leydig cell tumor *Ref: DC Dutta's Textbook of Gynae 9th/ed, Ch-24*

Ovarian tumor	Specific cell
Serous carcinoma	Psammoma bodies
Clear cell carcinoma	Both clear and "hobnail"
Krukenberg tumor	Signet ring cell
Yolk sac tumor	Schiller-duval body
Granulosa cell tumor	Call-exner bodies coffee bean" appearance
Leydig cell tumor	Reinke crystalloid

6. Ans. is b, i.e. OCP plus antiandrogen *Ref: DC Dutta's Textbook of Gynae 9th/ed, Ch-32*

Ferriman Gallwey Scoring System:

To quantify the degree of hirsutism for research purposes. The Ferriman-Gallwey scoring:

- 0 - no hair growth
- 1–4 - extensive hair growth 8-15 - Mild Hirsutism
- >15 - Moderate and severe Hirsutism

Androgen levels:

- Male 300–1000 ng/dL
- Female 15–70 ng/dL
- In the given history the FG score is normal and Testosterone levels too are normal hence not indicating to give Antiandrogens.

7. Ans. is b, i.e. Debulking surgery followed by chemotherapy *Ref: DC Dutta's Textbook of Gynae 9th/ed, Ch-24*

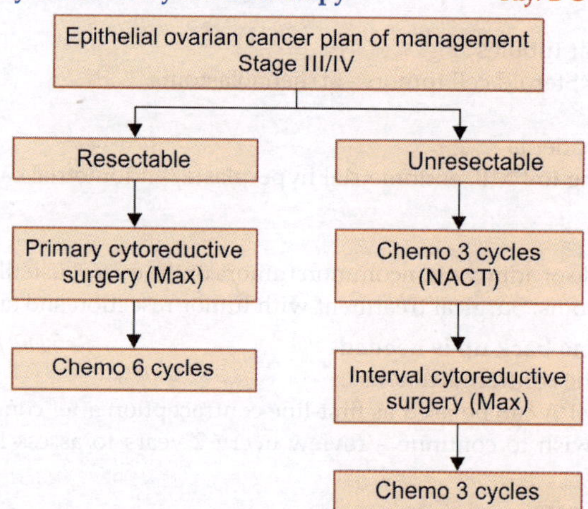

Ovarian cancer with peritoneal carcinomatosis (spread of cancer to the peritoneum) is often staged as advanced (stage III or IV). In these cases, the primary goal is to achieve maximal tumor reduction to allow chemotherapy to be most effective. Options a and c are incorrect because chemotherapy is typically given after surgery, not before (option a) or in combination with radiation (option c, as radiation is not standard for ovarian cancer management). Option d (staging laparotomy) is outdated in this context, as current management usually involves a combination of imaging (CT scan) and biopsy for staging, rather than the invasive laparotomy approach.

INI-CET May 2023

1. Where is the SRY gene located?

a. Long arm of Y Chromosome
b. Short arm of Y Chromosome
c. Long arm of X Chromosome
d. Short arm of X Chromosome

2. In cases of complete gonadal dysgenesis, what type of mutation will be seen in the SRY Gene?

a. Point mutation
b. Deletion
c. Inversion
d. Translocation

3. Which of the following statements is incorrect?

a. At 8-week gestation, zygote is bipotential
b. DHT is necessary for development of external genitalia
c. MIS inhibits the formation of Mullerian Ducts
d. Wolffian Duct forms the male internal genitalia

4. A patient presents to the clinic with clitoromegaly, prepubertal breasts and Tanner 2 Pubic Hair and a blind ending vagina. The karyotype is 46 XY and testosterone levels are in the range of a male. Which of the following is the probable diagnosis?

a. Complete AIS
b. Swyer syndrome
c. 5 alpha reductase deficiency
d. 17 alpha Hydroxylase deficiency

5. A 26-year-old woman with a BMI of 40 presents to the clinic. She also has a history of infertility for the past 6 years. On physical examination hirsutism is noted. What is the best next step?

a. Weight reduction + Metformin + Ovulation induction with urinary gonadotrophins
b. Weight reduction + Metformin + Ovulation induction with clomiphene
c. Finasteride + Metformin and wait for spontaneous conception
d. Finasteride + Metformin and ovulation induction

6. Which is the most common cause of Abnormal Uterine Bleeding in pubertal girls?

a. Endometriosis
b. Anovulation
c. Malignancy
d. Bleeding disorder

7. A patient who is a known case of Fibroid Uterus presents with acute abdomen, fever and leukocytosis in the 24th week of gestation. What is the most likely diagnosis?

a. Torsion
b. Red degeneration in pregnancy
c. Infection
d. Preterm labor

8. A 27-year-old female presents with painful bleeding during menses and pain while having intercourse. On physical examination there is adnexal tenderness, and the uterus is retroverted. Which investigation would be done to confirm the diagnosis?

a. TVS
b. Diagnostic laparoscopy
c. Laparotomy
d. HSG

9. Which of the following is the feature of primary dysmenorrhea?

a. Pain is present for the first 48 hours and then it subsides
b. Dyspareunia
c. Post coital bleeding
d. Non-cyclical pain

10. A female presented to the Gynecology OPD with complaints of vaginal discharge. Upon further investigation, clue cells were found in microscopy. What are these clue cells?

a. Gardnerella vaginalis rods accumulated
b. Epithelial cells studded with bacteria
c. Macrophage which have phagocytosed doderlein bacilli
d. None of the above

11. A woman presents to the clinic with complaints of non-foul smelling white vaginal discharge. On further investigations, pH is found to be acidic and normal lactobacillus count is found. There is no pruritus and inflammation. Which is the probable cause?

a. Physiological discharge
b. Candida
c. Chlamydia
d. Bacterial vaginosis

12. Which of the following is incorrectly matched?

a. Colpo suspension - Cystocele
b. Sacrospinous fixation - Vault prolapse
c. Vaginal hysterectomy - Uterine prolapse
d. Posterior perineal colporrhaphy – Rectocele

13. A semen analysis shows absent fructose. Which of the following is the probable cause?

a. Absent seminal vesicle
b. Obstruction of ejaculatory duct
c. Both of the above
d. Testicular carcinoma

14. Which of the following is a true statement for HRT?

a. Decreases breast cancer
b. Decreases endometrial cancer
c. Decreases colon cancer
d. Increases osteoporosis

15. Which of the following drugs is not used in the management of Endometriosis?

a. Leuprolide
b. Estradiol
c. Medroxyprogesterone acetate
d. Clomiphene

Answer with Explanations

1. **Ans. is b, i.e. Short arm of Y Chromosome** *Ref: DC Dutta's Textbook of Gynae 9th/ed, Ch-3*
2. **Ans. is a, i.e. Point mutation** *Ref: DC Dutta's Textbook of Gynae 9th/ed, Ch-3*
3. **Ans. is a, i.e. At 8-week gestation, zygote is bipotential** *Ref: DC Dutta's Textbook of Gynae 9th/ed, Ch-3*
   - SRY gene located on the short arm of Y chromosome directly controls the differentiation of testis from the bipotential gonad
   - Apart from SRY, autosomal genes are also essential for differentiation of the gonads. Absence of SRY gene leads to female sex differentiation
   - Second gene involved in development of testis is SOX9 and anti-Müllerian hormone (produced by Sertoli cells). DAXI gene expression is involved in ovarian differentiation. DAXI antagonizes the action of SRY gene
   - It is thought to be due to point mutation in SRY gene at the Y chromosome
   - Testicular Regression Syndrome (Swyer syndrome)
   - The individual presents with primary amenorrhea. External genitalia are female.
   - Internal genital organs are female. Secondary sexual characters are absent. Karyotype 46, XY.
   - Gonads are fibrous due to failure of development or regression.
4. **Ans. is c, i.e. 5 alpha reductase deficiency** *Ref: DC Dutta's Textbook of Gynae 9th/ed, Ch-5*

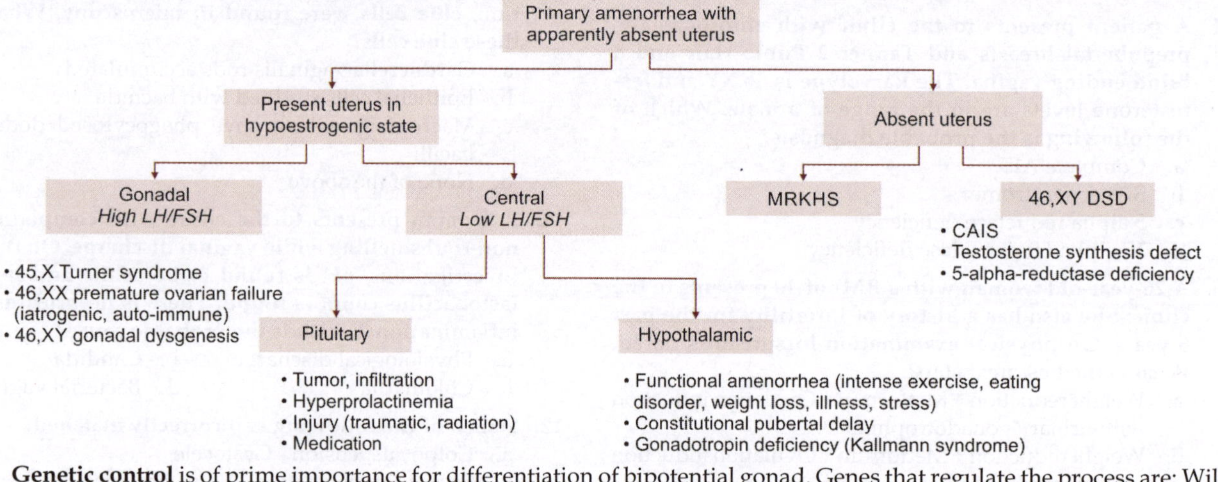

Genetic control is of prime importance for differentiation of bipotential gonad. Genes that regulate the process are: Wilms' tumor gene (WTI), FTZI and SRY

5. **Ans. is b, i.e. Weight reduction+ Metformin+ Ovulation Induction with clomiphene** *Ref: DC Dutta's Textbook of Gynae 9th/ed, Ch-16*

Treatment with metformin (insulin sensitizer) is found to reduce hyperinsulinemia and hyperandrogenemia.
Finasteride— It inhibits 5 alpha-reductase activity. It improves hirsutism significantly without any side effects. Daily dose is 5 mg. CI in pregnancy as it can cause male antiandrogen effect and cause ambiguous genitalia.

6. **Ans. is b, i.e. Anovulation** *Ref: DC Dutta's Textbook of Gynae 9th/ed, Ch-14*

The newer classification system is known by the acronym PALM–COEIN
Dysfunctional uterine bleeding (95%). Anovulatory cycles → unopposed estrogen → endometrial hyperplasia →prolonged and heavy periods. In the absence of growth limiting progesterone due to anovulation, the endometrial growth is under the influence of estrogen throughout the cycle.

Classification of AUB (FIGO-2011).

Structural causes (PALM)		*Nonstructural systemic causes (COEIN)*	
Polyp	AUB-**P**	**C**oagulopathy	AUB-**C**
Adenomyosis	AUB-**A**	**O**vulatory dysfunction	AUB-**O**
• **L**eiomyoma • **S**ubmucosal myoma	AUB-**L** AUB-**L SM**	**E**ndometrial	AUB-**E**
Other myoma	AUB-**LO**	**I**atrogenic	AUB-**I**
Malignancy and hyperplasia	AUB-**M**	**N**ot yet identified	AUB-**N**

7. **Ans. is b, i.e. Red degeneration in pregnancy** *Ref: DC Dutta's Textbook of Gynae 9th/ed, Ch-19*

Secondary changes in uterus

- Degenerations, Atrophy, Necrosis, Infection, Vascular changes, Sarcomatous change
- Degenerations
- Hyaline
- ***Cystic:*** Formed by liquefaction of the areas with hyaline changes
- ***Fatty degeneration:*** Fat globules are deposited mainly in the muscle cells
- ***Calcific degeneration:*** Precipitation of calcium carbonate or phosphate within the tumor. When whole of the tumor is converted into a calcified mass, it is called "womb stone"
- Red degeneration (corneous degeneration) occurs in a large fibroid mainly during second half of pregnancy and puerperium

8. **Ans. is b, i.e. Diagnostic laparoscopy** *Ref: DC Dutta's Textbook of Gynae 9th/ed, Ch-14*

Endometriosis: Presence of functioning endometrium (glands and stroma) in sites other than uterine mucosa is called endometriosis

Diagnosis

- Clinical diagnosis is by the classic symptoms of progressively increasing secondary dysmenorrhea, dyspareunia and infertility.
- *Imaging:* USG, MRI, CT, Colonoscopy
- Laparoscopy is the gold standard. Confirmation is done by double puncture laparoscopy
- Complications of endometriosis
- Endocrinopathy – This may be mostly responsible for infertility
- Rupture of chocolate cyst
- Infection of chocolate cyst
- Obstructive features:
  - Intestinal obstruction
  - Ureteral obstruction → hydroureter→ hydronephrosis → renal infection
  - Malignancy(adenoacanthoma)

9. **Ans. is a, i.e. Pain is present for the first 48 hours and then it subsides** *Ref: DC Dutta's Textbook of Gynae 9th/ed, Ch-14*

Characteristics	Primary dysmenorrhea	Secondary dysmenorrhea
AKA	Spasmodic	Congestive
Cause	No obvious cause	Presence of pelvic pathology
Time of onset and duration	With onset or just before menstruation	Pain starts 7–10 days before the onset of menstruation
Examination	Normal	Cause may be found on investigation

10. **Ans. is b, i.e. Epithelial cells studded with bacteria** *Ref: DC Dutta's Textbook of Gynae 9th/ed, Chs-10 & 12*

Bacterial Vaginosis

Amsel's four diagnostic criteria are: (1) Homogeneous vaginal discharge. (2) Vaginal pH >4.5 (litmus paper test); (3) Positive whiff tests; (4) Presence of clue cells (>20% of cells).

Clue cells: A smear of vaginal discharge is prepared with drops of normal saline on a glass slide and is seen under a microscope. Vaginal epithelial cells are seen covered with these coccobacilli and the cells appear as stippled or granular. At times, the cells are so heavily stippled that the cell borders are obscured.

These stippled epithelial cells are called "clue cells". Presence of clue cells (>20% of cells) are diagnostic of BV.

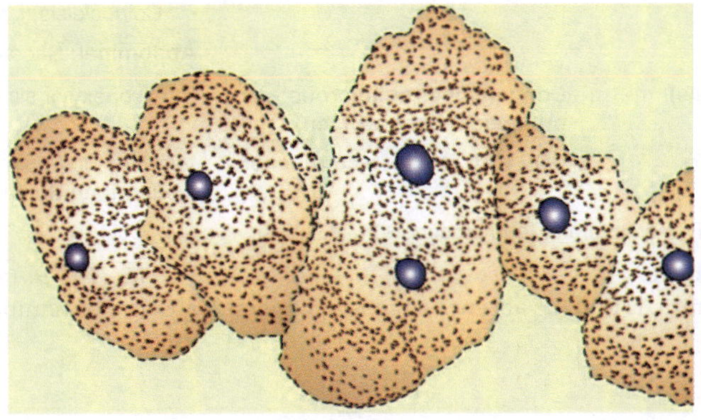

11. **Ans. is a, i.e. Physiological discharge** *Ref: DC Dutta's Textbook of Gynae 9th/ed, Ch-10*
In the given case clear discharge, non-foul smelling with acidic Ph in Mid cycle suggestive of Ovulatory or Normal Vaginal discharge.

Differential diagnosis of vaginal discharge.

Characteristics	*Trichomoniasis*	*Candidiasis*	*Bacterial vaginosis*	*Chlamydia*	*Normal vaginal discharge*
Color	Gray, yellow or green	Curdy white	Gray white to green yellow white	Mucopurulent	White, clear
Consistency	Thin, frothy, adherent, mal odor	Thick, no odor	Thin, adherent homogeneous	Thick	Thin
Whiff test (p. 143)	Negative has unpleasant odor	Negative	Positive (Fishy amine)	Negative	Negative
pH	≥4.5	<4.5	≥4.5	<4.5	<4–4.5
Pruritus	+++, dysuria	++	Nonirritating	–	–
Diagnosis (Wet mount microscopy)	• Motile trichomonas (p. 102) • Increased white cells	Hyphae and buds, spores	Clue cells (>20%) (p. 143), amine odor after adding KOH to wet mount; ↓ lactobacilli	*Chlamydia* NAAT (p. 140)	–
Treatment	Metronidazole 500 mg PO BID × 7 days Or 200 mg TID × 7 days	• Clotrimazole intravaginal 1–3 days • Fluconazole 150 mg PO weekly for 6 weeks	Metronidazole 500 mg PO BID × 7day	Azithromycin 1g orally single dose	–

12. **Ans. is a, i.e. Colpo suspension - Cystocele** *Ref: DC Dutta's Textbook of Gynae 9th/ed, Ch-15*
Colposuspension done at bladder neck for Stress urinary incontinence.

Type of prolapse and the common surgical repair procedures (ACOG-2019).

Organ descent	*Clinical condition*	*Type of operation*
Vaginal wall		
Anterior (upper 2/3) or whole	**Cystocele/cystourethrocele Paravaginal defect**	• Anterior colporrhaphy • Paravaginal defect repair
Posterior (lower 2/3)	**Rectocele**	Colpoperineorrhaphy
Posterior (upper 1/3)	**Enterocele**	• Vaginal repair of enterocele with PFR • McCall culdoplasty • Moskowitz procedure
Combined anterior and posterior	**Cystocele and rectocele**	PFR (combined procedure)
Uterovaginal Uterus along with vaginal walls	**Uterovaginal prolapse**	• Vaginal hysterectomy with PFR (elderly woman, family completed) • Fothergill's operation (preservation of uterus)
Vaginal wall		
Following hysterectomy (vaginal or abdominal)	**Vault prolapse (secondary)**	**Vaginal:** • Repair of vaginal vault along with PFR • Sacrospinous colpopexy • Colpocleisis (Le Fort) **Abdominal:** Sacral colpopexy
Uterus (without vaginal walls)	**Congenital or nulliparous prolapse (young women)**	Cervicopexy or sling (Purandare's) operation
Pelvic organ prolapse (POP)	**POP with stress in continence**	**Vaginal:** TOT operation (midurethral sling) **Abdominal:** Burch operation

(PFR: pelvic floor repair; TOT: transobturator tape procedure)

13. **Ans. is c, i.e. Both of the above** *Ref: DC Dutta's Textbook of Gynae 9th/ed, Ch-16*
Fructose content in the seminal fluid: Its absence suggests congenital absence of seminal vesicle or portion of the ductal system or both.

Sperm production
Testis → Maturation in epididymis → Vas deference → Seminal vesicle → Prostate → during ejaculation bulbourethral gland secretes mucus for lubrication.

14. Ans. is c, i.e. Decreases colon cancer *Ref: DC Dutta's Textbook of Gynae 9th/ed, Ch-6*

The HRT is indicated in menopausal women to overcome the short-term and long-term consequences of estrogen deficiency

Indications
- Relief of menopausal symptoms.
- Prevention of osteoporosis.
- To maintain the quality of life in menopausal years.

Benefits of hormone replacement therapy (HRT)
- Improvement of vasomotor symptoms (70– 80%)
- Improvement urogenital atrophy
- Increase in bone mineral density (2–5%)
- Decreased risk in vertebral and hip fractures (25–50%) Reduction in colorectal cancer (20%) possibly cardioprotection

Risks of hormone replacement therapy
- Endometrial cancer
- Breast cancer.
- Venous thromboembolic (VTE) disease
- Coronary heart disease (CHD)
- Lipid metabolism
- Dementia, Alzheimer

15. Ans. is b, i.e. Estradiol *Ref: DC Dutta's Textbook of Gynae 9th/ed, Ch-21*

Presence of functioning endometrium (glands and stroma) in sites other than uterine mucosa is called endometriosis
Cyclic hormones stimulate growth but continuous hormones suppress it.
Treatment options for Pelvic Endometriosis :
Expectant Management (observation only)
Medical therapy:
- Hormones
- Others

Surgery:
- Conservative
- Definitive

Combined therapy:
- Medical and surgical
- The mechanism of endometrial atrophy by 'pseudopregnancy' - combined oral pills 'pseudo menopause' - Danazol
- 'medical oophorectomy' - GnRH agonists.

INI-CET November 2022

1. **All are long term reversible methods of contraception except:**
   a. Progestin injection
   b. Female sterilisation
   c. Levonorgestrel and copper containing intrauterine devices
   d. Subcutaneous progestin implants

2. **What is the age group distribution of vulval cancer?**
   a. 35-55 years
   b. 45-85 years
   c. No specific age groups
   d. Both A and B

3. **Steps of D & C**

   i. Serial dilatation

   ii. Curettage

   iii. Uterine sound

   iv. Assessment of uterine size and direction

   a. iv, iii, i, ii
   b. iv, iii, ii, i
   c. iv, ii, iii, i
   d. iv, i, ii, iii

4. **All the following are risk factors of vulval cancers except:**
   a. Vulval dystrophy
   b. Vulval hamartoma
   c. Smoking
   d. Vulval warts

5. **The non contraceptive uses of oral contraceptives include all except:**
   a. Protects against STDs including HIV
   b. Reduces the risk of Ovarian cancer
   c. Reduces the risk of ectopic pregnancy
   d. Reduces the risk of endometrial cancer

6. **Which statement is not true about the image shown below?**

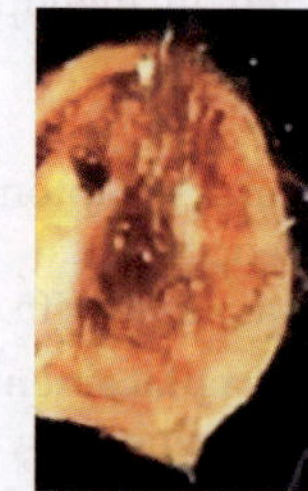

   a. Bilateral in 80%
   b. Low risk of malignancy
   c. Highest risk of torsion
   d. None of the above

7. **True about ovarian cancer recurrence:**
   a. Platinum susceptible if recurrence is <6 months
   b. Partially platinum resistant if recurrence is 6–12 months
   c. Platinum resistant if recurrence is >12 months
   d. Platinum resistant if recurrence occurs at <6 months

8. **Cancer caused by DESA.**
   a. Sarcoma botryoides
   b. Squamous cell cancer of vagina
   c. Paget's disease of vagina
   d. Clear cell cancer of vagina

9. **Which part of virus is used to make HPV vaccine:**
   a. E6 b. E7
   c. L1 d. E1

10. **Your next patient is a 55-year-old G2P2 who has been referred from a primary care provider for yeast vaginitis. While reviewing her outside medical records, it shows 5 episodes of vulval pruritus that are treated with oral and vaginal antifungal medication. The patient says these helped but her pruritus has persisted for more than a year. Her Wet prep shows a pH of 5.5, rare pseud-hyphae, no lactobacillus, no WBC or RBC and rare clue cells. What is the diagnosis?**
    a. Angioma of vulva b. Lichen Planus
    c. Lichen Sclerosus d. None of the above

Answer with Explanations

1. **Ans. is b, i.e. Female sterilisation** *Ref: DC Dutta's Textbook of Gynae 9th/ed, Ch-30*

   Long acting reversible contraceptives (larcs): are designed to be used for at least 1 year. LARC methods are cost effective compared to shorter acting methods. Commonly 2 types of IUD are available: (a) Nonhormonal and (b) Hormonal. LNG-IUS, CU IUD, progesterone only injectables and implant. Pregnancy rates are extremely low with LARCs. These are user independent methods. The women need to do nothing until the method has expired.

   Sterilisation: is a permanent method of contraception.

2. **Ans. is b, i.e. 45-85 years** *Ref: DC Dutta's Textbook of Gynae 9th/ed, Ch-24*

   Following are the common risk factors for vulval cancer, advance age being the common age group of presentation.

Risk factors for vulvar cancer
• Infection with high risk oncogenic HPV • Non-neoplastic chronic epithelial disorders (lichen sclerosis 4–7%) • Immunocompromised state • Smoking • Advanced age • Immune deficiency • Presence of cervical neoplasia • Melanoma • Paget's disease • Presence of VIN (5–96%)

3. **Ans. is a, i.e. iv, iii, i, ii** *Ref: DC Dutta's Textbook of Gynae 9th/ed, Ch-35*

   Dilatation and curettage:

   Indication:

   Procedure:

   - Empty the bladder and patient is made to placed in lithotomy position
   - Bimanual examination is done to access uterine size and position
   - Vaginal wall is retracted using Sim's speculum
   - Uterine sounding done to measure
   - UCL (UteroCervical Length)
   - Serial dilatation done at internal os using Hawkin-Ambler dilator or Hegar dilator
   - In benign lesion, sharp curette and in suspected malignancy, blunt curette is used.

Indications of D&C
• **Diagnostic** – Infertility (for dating of endometrium) – Abnormal uterine bleeding (AUB) – Pathologic amenorrhea – Endometrial tuberculosis – Endometrial carcinoma – Postmenopausal bleeding – Chorionepithelioma • **Therapeutic** – Dysfunctional uterine bleeding (DUB) – Endometrial polyp – Removal of IUD – Incomplete abortion • **Combined** – DUB – Endometrial polyp

4. Ans. is b, i.e. Vulval hamartoma *Ref: DC Dutta's Textbook of Gynae 9th/ed, Ch-24*

Following are the common risk factors for vulval cancer, advance age being the common age group of presentation.

Risk factors for vulvar cancer
Infection with high risk oncogenic HPV
Non-neoplastic chronic epithelial disorders (lichen sclerosis 4–7%)
Immunocompromised state
Smoking
Advanced age
Immune deficiency
Presence of cervical neoplasia
Melanoma
Paget's disease
Presence of VIN (5–96%)

5. Ans. is a, i.e. Protects against STDs including HIV *Ref: DC Dutta's Textbook of Gynae 9th/ed, Ch-30*

Noncontraceptive health benefits: Improvement of menstrual abnormalities – (1) Regulation of menstrual cycle; (2) Reduction of dysmenorrhea (40%); (3) Reduction of menorrhagia (50%); (4) Reduction of PMS; (5) Reduction of Mittelschmerz syndrome; (6) Protection against iron-deficiency anemia. Protection against health disorders; (7) PID (thick cervical mucus); (8) Ectopic pregnancy; (9) Endometriosis; (10) Fibroid uterus; (11) Hirsutism, acne and PCOD; (12) Functional ovarian cysts; (13) Benign breast disease; (14) Osteopenia and postmenopausal osteoporotic fractures; (15) Autoimmune disorders of thyroid; (16) Rheumatoid arthritis; (17) Increases bone mineral density. Prevention of malignancies; (18) Endometrial cancer (50%); (19) Epithelial ovarian cancer (50%); (20) Colorectal cancer (40%).

6. Ans. is a, i.e. Bilateral in 80% *Ref: DC Dutta's Textbook of Gynae 9th/ed, Ch-21 & 24*

In the image shown, hair follicle is seen very evident making it a mature Ovarian Teratoma.

Important Features of a Dermoid Cyst

- Germ cell ovarian tumor
- >90% of all germ cell tumors
- 30% of all ovarian tumors
- Bilateral: 15–20%
- Contains elements of three germ cell layers
- Many contain thyroid tissues (struma ovarii)
- Symptomatic (50%)
- Torsion is common (15–20%)
- Risk of malignancy is low (1–2%).
- *Serum tumor markers:* CA19-9 (common) and CA125 are elevated.

7. Ans. is d, i.e. Platinum resistant if recurrence occurs at <6 months *Ref: DC Dutta's Textbook of Gynae 9th/ed, Ch-24*

Platinum based treatment are the drug of choice for ovarian cancers. Hence in resistant cases Der is high chance of recurrence.

New platinum based treatment regimens in advanced stage ovarian cancer (FIGO: III -IV All residuum, EOC or PPC international), all regimens: 8 cycle (2009).
Drugs and Therapy Schedule
Paclitaxel: 175 mg/m², 3 hrs + Carboplatin AUC 5 mg/mL. min (IV)
Topotecan 1.5 mg/m², day 1–3 + Carboplatin AUC 5 mg/mL. min day 3 → then Paclitaxel 175 mg/m², 3 hr + Carboplatin AUC 6 mg/mL. min (IV)
Gemcitabine 1000 mg/m² day 1 by 8 + Carboplatin AUC 6 mg/mL. min, day 8 → then Paclitaxel 175 mg/m², 3 hr + Carboplatin AUC 6 mg/mL. min (IV)

8. Ans. is d, i.e. Clear cell cancer of vagina *Ref: DC Dutta's Textbook of Gynae 9th/ed, Ch-24*

Diethylstilbestrol (DES) is related with clear cell adenocarcinoma of the vagina. This is found in those who had history of intrauterine exposure to diethylstilbestrol.

9. Ans. is c, i.e. L1 *Ref: DC Dutta's Textbook of Gynae 9th/ed, Ch-23*

- The vaccines are prophylactic and not therapeutic. As the girl is 16 and we are preventing her from getting cervical cancer, so best advice for the girl would be HPV vaccine. WHO (2014) recommends HPV vaccine for both the boys and girls between 9 and 14 years: Two doses (0M & 6–12M) are now required. Individual aged >15 years: Three doses (0M 1–2M & 6M) are needed.
- HPV DNA testing is required after the onset of sexual activity or after 21 years, even then vaccine should be opted.

Characteristic	Bivalent (2V HPV)	Quadrivalent (4V HPV)	9 Valent (9V HPV)
Brand name	Cervarix	Gardasil	Gardasil-9
HPV subtypes	16, 18	6, 11, 16, 18	6, 11, 16, 18, 31, 33, 45, 52, 58
Protects against	CIN, Ca cervix	Anogenital warts, CIN, Ca cervix	Anogenital warts CIN, Ca cervix, vulva intraepithelial neoplasia, vaginal intraepithelial neoplasia
Manufacturing	Trichoplusia insect line infected with L1 encoding baculovirus	Saccharomyces cerevisiae expressing L1	Saccharomyces cerevisiae expressing L1
Adjuvant	500 mcg aluminium hydroxide with monophosphoryl lipid A	225 mcg Al(OH) PO_4SO_4	500 mcg Al(OH) PO_4SO_4
Dose	0.5 mL	0.5 mL	0.5 mL
Administration	1/m	1/m	1/m
Administered to males or females	Both males and females	Both males and females	Both males and females
Age in females ideal age range	11-12 years 9-26 years	11-12 years 9-26 years	11-12 years 9-26 years
Age in males ideal age range	11-12 years 9-26 years	11-12 years 9-26 years	11-12 years 9-15 years—FDA approved 9-26 years—ACIP recommendation

10. Ans. is b, i.e. Lichen Sclerosus *Ref: DC Dutta's Textbook of Gynae 9th/ed, Ch-18*

In the given case persistent pruritic with rare pseudohyphae and no lactobacilli suggests non infective causes like lichen plants or sclerosis. Important differentiating factor is Lichen sclerosis affects only vulva as mentioned in this case. Whereas lichen plants can affect both vulva and vagina including oral mucosa.

INI-CET May 2022

1. A couple already has 3 children and have been trying for another child since the past 1 year. On investing for infertility, the male partner was found to have hypo-gonadotropic hypogonadism. Which of the following are associated with this condition?

a. Azoospermia/oligospermia
b. Low LH, low FSH
c. High FSH, low LH
d. Low testosterone
e. Low prolactin

2. All the following statements about anti-Mullerian hormones are true, *except:*

a. It is best tested in the fasting state on day 2 of menstrual cycle
b. Lipopeptide secreted from granulosa cell of early antral follicle
c. Correlates with pregnancy rate of IVF cycle
d. It decreases sensitivity of the pre-antral follicles to FSH

3. Seminal vesicles and vas deferens would be bilaterally absent, congenitally in which of the following conditions?

a. Cystic fibrosis
b. Klinefelter's syndrome
c. Kallman syndrome
d. Kartagener's syndrome

4. Recommended HPV vaccine schedule for 9 to 14 years old according to WHO SAGE guidelines is:

a. 1 or 2 doses
b. 2 doses
c. 1 dose
d. 3 doses

Answer with Explanations

1. Ans. is a, b, d i.e. Azoospermia/oligospermia; Low LH, low FSH; Low testosterone

Ref: DC Dutta's Textbook of Gynae 9th/ed, Ch-16

In the given history the cause for infertility is mentioned as male partner having Hypogonadotropic hypogonadism. The normal pathway of spermatogenesis (Hypothalamus GnRh → Pituitary → FSH and LH → Testes → Testosterone (has negative feedback on LH and FSH) → Spermatogenesis → Sperms enter epididymis) is altered. That is hypogonadism causes reduced FSH, LH leading to reduced Testosterone and finally reduced/nil sperm count.

Pretesticular	Testicular	Post-testicular drugs	
Genetic • 47, XXY • Microdeletion (Y chromosome, Yq) • Single gene mutations • Sperm DNA fragmentation **Endocrine** • Gonadotropin deficiency (Kallmann's syndrome) • Obesity • Thyroid dysfunction • Hyperprolactinemia **Psychosexual** • Erectile dysfunction • Impotence	• Immotile cilia (Kartagener) syndrome • Cryptorchidism • Infection (mumps orchitis) • Toxins: Drugs, smoking, radiation • Varicocele • Immunologic • Sertoli-cell-only syndrome • Primary testicular failure • Oligoasthenoteratozoospermia • Undescended testis (depressed spermatogenesis) • Immunologic • Idiopathic	**Obstruction of efferent duct** **Congenital:** • Congenital absence of bilateral vas deferens (CABVD) (cystic fibrosis) • Young's syndrome **Acquired infection:** • Tuberculosis • Gonorrhoea • **Others** • Ejaculatory failure • Retrograde ejaculation • Hypospadias • Bladder neck surgery • Surgical • Herniorrhaphy • Vasectomy	• Antihypertensives • Antipsychotics • Impair spermatogenesis: radiation, cytotoxic drugs, nitrofurantoin • Antiandrogenic effects: Cimetidine, spironolactone • Erectile dysfunction: Beta-blockers (metoclopramide) • Ejaculatory failure: Antidepressants, alpha-blockers • Pituitary suppression: GnRH analogs

2. Ans. is b, i.e. Lipopeptide secreted from granulosa cell of early antral follicle

Ref: DC Dutta's Textbook of Gynae 9th/ed, Ch-16

- It is a peptide produced by the granulosa cells of primordial follicles (<6 mm). It causes Müllerian duct regression during male sexual differentiation.
- AMH levels reflect the number of growing follicles in the ovary and it helps oocyte maturation and follicular development.
- Low levels of AMH is observed with rise of FSH and E2 levels and also with increasing age of the women (as the follicle number declines).
- Estimation of serum AMH is used as a screening test of ovarian reserve
- Low levels of AMH is observed with rise of FSH and E2 levels and also with increasing age of the women (as the follicle number declines).
- Estimation of serum AMH is used as a screening test of ovarian reserve
- Other markers for ovarian reserve
- S. FSH (>10IU/L)
- Estradiol >80 pg/mL
- Antral follicle count (2–10, normal) Ovarian volume

3. Ans. is a, i.e. Cystic fibrosis *Ref: DC Dutta's Textbook of Gynae 9th/ed, Ch-16*

Cystic fibrosis

Absence of Vas deference

Klinefelter's Syndrome

The patients are eunuchoid in build, infertile with small penis, testis and varying degrees of gynecomastias. The features at times become confusing when first seen in adolescence. Sex chromatin is positive. Karyotype is XXY or XXXY. Genitalia—small and infantile. Genital ducts are Wolffian. Serum gonadotrophins are elevated.

Kallmann syndrome

Embryologically GnRH neurones develop in the ectodermal olfactory placode before they migrate finally to the hypothalamus. GnRH neurones are absent due to partial or complete agenesis of olfactory bulb (olfactogenital dysplasia). This disorder is characterized by hypogonadotropic hypogonadism, anosmia and color blindness. There may be associated cleft lip and palate. Patients present with primary amenorrhea. Mode of inheritance is due to a variety of genetic mutations in the KAL gene (X linked) or as an autosomal dominant or recessive fashion. Menstruation can be induced with combined estrogen and progestin therapy. Induction of ovulation is successful with exogenous gonadotropins. Kartagener syndrome (autosomal disease)— there is loss of ciliary function and sperm motility.

4. **Ans. is a, i.e. 1 or 2 doses** *Ref: DC Dutta's Textbook of Gynae 9th/ed, Ch-18*
   - Prophylactic HPV vaccine is approved to all school girls (12–18 years) and women (16–25 years). Three doses are to be given (Bivalent 0–2–6 months, Quadrivalent 0–1–6 months nonvalent). Bivalent vaccines (cervarix) against HPV types 16, 18
   - Quadrivalent (Gardasil) against HPV types 16, 18, 6, 11 Nonvalent against HPV 6, 11, 16, 18
   - WHO SAGE:1or 2 doses 9-20 years
   - >21 years 2 doses
   - Vaccine induced neutralizing antibodies (IgG, IgA) works locally (cervix) by preventing the attachment of the virus to the cervical epithelium

   Helps in:
   - Genital warts
   - Precancerous lesions
   - Ca cervix
   - Condyloma accuminata

INI-CET November 2021

1. What is the probable diagnosis from the clinical image?

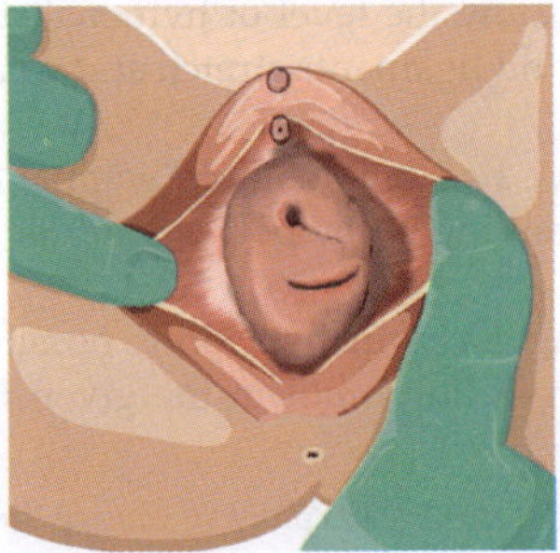

a. Cervical carcinoma
b. Uterine inversion
c. Uterocervical prolapse
d. Fibroid polyp

2. A 26-year-old woman who has had 2 children through normal delivery presents with a dull aching pain over the abdomen, with irregular menses. Per vaginal examination revealed a mass felt through the posterior fornix. A USG showed a clear ovarian cyst of size 5 x 5 cm. What is the next best step?

a. Measure CA 125 levels
b. Follow up after 6 weeks
c. Laparoscopy
d. CT pelvis

3. What is the fixative used for a pap smear?

a. Formalin
b. Air dried
c. Normal saline
d. 95% ethanol

4. What should be the ideal percentage for normal sperm morphology in a seminal fluid analysis?

a. 10%
b. 4%
c. 6%
d. 8%

5. Match the following:

Section A	Section B
1. Yolk sac tumor	A. Epithelial cell tumor LDH
2. Dysgerminoma	B. Beta-hCG
3. Choriocarcinoma	C. AFP
	D. CA-125

a. 1-A, 2-C, 3-B, 4-D
b. 1-C, 2-A, 3-B, 4-D
c. 1-C, 2-A, 3-D, 4-B
d. 1-A, 2-C, 3-D, 4-B

6. A 17-year-old girl was brought by her mother to the outpatient department with primary amenorrhea. She had normal breast development and pubic hair. On examination, the vagina was blind-ending, and the uterus was not palpable. What is the most probable diagnosis?

a. Mullerian agenesis
b. Gonadal dysgenesis
c. Turner syndrome
d. Testicular feminization syndrome

7. An 18-year-old girl presented with amenorrhoea. On examination, she had normal genitalia and normal breast development. Her test reveals a 5 alpha-reductase deficiency. What could be the probable diagnosis?

a. Concealed sex
b. True hermaphrodite
c. Female pseudo hermaphroditism
d. Male pseudo hermaphroditism

8. Which of the following emergency contraceptive is used in India?

a. Misoprostol 400 mcg
b. Ethinyl oestradiol 600 mcg
c. Ulipristal 30 mg
d. Levonorgestrel 1.5 mg

9. Match the following disorders causing secondary amenorrhoea with their respective lab findings.

Condition	Lab markers
1. Sheehan's syndrome	A. Normal FSH, Normal LH, Normal estradiol.
2. Premature ovarian	B. High LH, Low FSH, High estradiol
3. PCOS	C. Low LH, Low FSH, Low estradiol
4. Asherman's syndrome	D. High LH, High FSH, Low estradiol

a. 1-C, 2-B, 3-D, 4-A
b. 1-D, 2-B, 3-C, 4-A
c. 1-C, 2-D, 3-B, 4-A
d. 1-A, 2-B, 3-D, 4-C

10. Which of the following investigations is used to diagnose unicornuate uterus?

1. Falloposcopy
2. Laparoscopy
3. HSG
4. X-ray

a. 2, 4
b. 1, 2
c. 1, 3
d. 2, 3

11. A 62-year-old patient with a history of diabetes and hypertension came with post-menopausal bleeding. Which of the following you will do to evaluate the cause?

a. Pap smear
b. Visual inspection with iodine
c. Colposcopy
d. Endometrial sampling

12. A couple presents to the infertility clinic with a normal hysterosalpingogram and a semen analysis report with azoospermia. Which of the following test is useful to differentiate between an obstructive and a testicular cause?

a. Serum FSH levels
b. Serum testosterone levels
c. Testicular biopsy
d. Serum LH level

Answer with Explanations

1. **Ans. is c, i.e. Uterocervical prolapse** *Ref: DC Dutta's Textbook of Gynae 9th/ed, Ch-16*
   - In the given photo it is clearly seen as that uterus and cervix is lying below the level of hymenal ring suggestive of uterine prolapse. Uterine prolapse occurs when the pelvic floor muscles and ligaments stretch and weaken, causing the uterus to slip down into or protrude out of the vagina.
   - Uterine prolapse is most common in people after menopause who have had one or more vaginal deliveries. It can cause symptoms such as tissue bulging out of the vagina, heaviness or pulling in the pelvis, bladder problems, bowel movement difficulties, and discomfort during sexual activity.
   - To differentiate from uterine inversion we can do **uterine sounding** i.e, which is only possible with Uterine Prolapse and not in Inversion. Note Uterine sounding is possible even in Polyp but in the given image their is no polyp seen.

2. **Ans. is b, i.e. Follow up after 6 weeks** *Ref: DC Dutta's Textbook of Gynae 9th/ed, Chs-9 and 24*

   In the given case, it is mentioned: Young lady, immediate postpartum, irregular cycles, and USG showing clear cyst: all suggest a Benign Ovarian Lesion. Hence next best step is to do a followup after 6 weeks to check for the size, number or change to complex cyst.

   Cysts that are simple, unilocular, <8 cm in diameter with normal serum CA-125—can be managed conservatively. Women should be under follow up with ultrasound scan and serum CA-125 at an interval of 4 months

   However if the same case mentioned an elderly <post menopausal, complex cyst or size >5 cm then it would require further investigation with measuring CA 125 levels.

   To access the risk of malignancy, we can do a

   Risk of malignancy index (RMI):

   RMI = U × M × CA125;

   U = USG score (one point each for: Multilocular cyst; solid areas; metastasis; ascites; bilateral lesions), U = 3 (for score 2–5)

   M = 3 (postmenopausal women) CA-125 level in U/mL.

   The risk of cancer is 20%

   with the score of 25 and 250 and it is 75% when the RMI value is >250.

3. **Ans. is d, i.e. 95% ethanol** *Ref: DC Dutta's Textbook of Gynae 9th/ed, Ch-9*

   The fixative used for a Pap smear (Papanicolaou smear or Pap test) is typically 95% ethanol.

   Ethanol is used to fix and preserve the cellular material collected during the Pap smear so that it can be adequately prepared, stained, and examined under a microscope for the detection of abnormal cervical cells, which may indicate cervical cancer or precancerous changes.

   Fixation and Staining

   The material so collected should be immediately spread over a microscopic slide and at once fixed with ethyl alcohol (95%) before drying. After fixing of the slide sent to the laboratory. The slide so sent is stained either with Papanicolaou's or Sorr's method and examined by a trained cytologist.

   Benefits: The objective of screening is to reduce the incidence and mortality from cervical cancer. The lifetime risk of developing cervical cancer by the age of 74 is 0.9% in developed countries compared to 1.6% in low and middle income countries (LMICs). Lifetime risk of death from cervical cancer is 0.3% in developed countries compared to 0.9% in LMICs.

4. **Ans. is b, i.e. 4%** *Ref: DC Dutta's Textbook of Gynae 9th/ed, Ch-17*

   The ideal percentage for normal sperm morphology in a seminal fluid analysis, as per the World Health Organization (WHO) guidelines, is typically 4% or higher.

   However, it's important to note that other factors, such as sperm count, motility, and volume, also play a significant role in male fertility.

Semen analysis (WHO reference values, 2010 and 2021).		
Semen analysis	***Normal reference values***	
	2010	***2021***
Volume	1.5 mL	≥1.4 mL
pH	7.2–7.8	≥7.2
Sperm concentration	15-16 million/mL	≥15 million/mL
Total sperm number	39 million per ejaculate	≥39 million per ejaculate
Motility (%)	Total motility: 40% (Progressive motility = 32%)	Total motility: ≥42% (Non-progressive motility: ≥1%, Progressive motility: ≥30%, Immobile sperms: ≥20%)
Normal morphology (%)	4%	≥4%
Viability	58%	≥54% live spermatozoa
WBCs	Less than 1 million/mL	
Round cells	<5 million/mL	
Sperm agglutination	<10% spermatozoa with adherent particles	

5. Ans. is b, i.e. 1-C, 2-A, 3-B, 4-D *Ref: DC Dutta's Textbook of Gynae 9th/ed, Ch-31*

The correct match is:

1. Yolk sac – C. AFP
2. Dysgerminoma – A. LDH
3. Choriocarcinoma – B. Beta-Hcg
4. Epithelial cell tumor – D. CA-125

Other tumor markers and associated conditions are mentioned in the below table.

Commonly used gynecological tumor markers.	
Marker	***Tissue of origin of cancer***
Human chorionic gonadotropin **(hCG)**	Trophoblastic and some germ cell tumor (dysgerminoma, embryonal carcinoma)
Alpha fetoprotein **(AFP)**	Germ cell tumor (yolk sac, immature teratoma tumor), dysgerminoma and others: Gastric, lung cancers
CA-125	Ovarian epithelial tumors (benign and malignant), endometrial carcinoma, endometriosis, PID, fibroid, salpingitis Pancreatitis, normal women, non-ovarian cancers: Breast, pancreas, stomach, liver
HE 4 (glycoprotein)	Serous epithelial ovarian cancer, urologic cancer, lung cancer, endometrial cancer
Carcinoembryonic antigen **(CEA)**	Ovarian (serous, endometrioid), cervical carcinoma (squamous cell), endometrial cancer, colon and pancreatic cancers
Tumor associated glycoprotein-72 **(TAG-72)**	Epithelial ovarian tumor (EOT)
Macrophage colony stimulating factor **(M-CSF)**	Epithelial ovarian tumor (EOT)
Squamous cell carcinoma antigen **(SCC)**	Carcinoma cervix, vulvar and vaginal squamous cell carcinoma
Lactate dehydrogenase **(LDH)**	Ovarian germ cell tumors (dysgerminoma)
CA 15–3, **OVX 1, OVX 2, CA19-9** **HER-2/neu (oncogene product) HE 4**	Ovarian epithelial carcinoma
Galactosyltransferase associated with tumor **(GAT)**	To differentiate ovarian cancer from endometriosis
Estrogen **Progesterone** **Testosterone**	Gonadal stromal tumors
Inhibin, anti-Müllerian hormone **(AMH)**	Granulosa cell tumor, mucinous and endometrioid cancers
Cell free DNA	Epithelial ovarian carcinoma (EOC)
Glycodelin	Serous ovarian cancer
CYFRA 21-1	Endometrial cancer, ovarian and cervical cancer

Serum Biomarkers and Organ Malignancy

- Circulating methylated DNA in ovarian cancer.
- Cell–Free DNA–Epithelial ovarian carcinoma (EOC).
- Risk of ovarian malignancy algorithm **(ROMA):** Combines HE4 and CA125
- Risk of malignancy index **(RMI)** combines USG score, serum CA125 and menopausal status.

6. Ans. is a, i.e. Mulleran agenesis *Ref: DC Dutta's Textbook of Gynae 9th/ed, Ch-28 &29*

In the given case it is to differentiate between MRKH and Testicular feminizing syndrome. The following features can be used for the same.

Differentiation between androgen insensitivity syndrome (AIS) and Müllerian agenesis (MRKH).		
Characters	***Androgen insensitivity syndrome***	***Müllerian agenesis (MRKH syndrome)***
Sexual hair (pubic and axillary)	Absent or sparce	Normal female
Primary amenorrhea	Present	Present
Vagina	Short and blind	Absent
Clitoris	Enlarged	Normal as in female
Gonads: • Structure • Location	• Testes • Inguinal, labial or abdominal	• Ovary • Abdominal
Breasts	Developed	Developed
Serum testosterone level	Slightly elevated	Normal as in female
Müllerian system (uterus)	Absent	Absent or rudimentary
Wolffian system	Absent	Absent
Karyotype	46, XY	46, XX
Associated anomalies	Rare	Skeletal 12% and urological (renal) 47%
Pregnancy	Incomplete variety-possible	Possible

7. Ans. is d, i.e. Male pseudo hermaphroditism *Ref: DC Dutta's Textbook of Gynae 9th/ed, Ch-28*

The probable diagnosis in this case is Male pseudohermaphroditism.

As in given case their is 5 alpha reductase deficiency, which is required for conversion of testosterone to active form i.e, Dihydrotestosterone. Dihydrotestosterone is further required for development of male internal and external genitalia. Lack of which is leading to by default development of female internal and external genitalia.

Entity, clinical presentation, diagnosis and possible reproductive outcome of an individual with DSD.			
Characters (DSD)	***Clinical presentation***	***Diagnostic criteria***	***Reproductive outcome***
Adrenogenital syndrome 46 XX DSD (androgen excess)	Ambiguity of sex at birth	• Sonographic evaluation of internal genital organs • Karyotype 46, XX • Serum 17 hydroxyprogesterone ↑ • Urinary pregnanetriol ↑ >5 µg/100 mL	Pregnancy possible
Gonadal dysgenesis Turner's syndrome sex chromosome DSD	• Primary amenorrhea • Poor secondary sexual characters • Short stature • Webbing of neck • Cubitus valgus • Genitalia underdeveloped	• Karyotype 45, XO • Bilateral 'streak' gonads • Serum: E2 ↓ and FSH ↑	Pregnancy with donor oocyte
Mosaic turner syndrome sex chromosome DSD	• Primary/secondary amenorrhea • Average height • Poor secondary sexual characters • Genitalia underdeveloped	• Karyotype 45, XO/46, XX • Bilateral 'streak' gonads	Pregnancy possible
Pure gonadal dysgenesis 46 XX or 46 XY DSD	• Primary amenorrhea • Delayed secondary sexual characters • Average height • Genitalia underdeveloped	• Karyotype—46, XX or 46, XY • Bilateral 'streak' gonads	Rare
Mixed gonadal dysgenesis 45 X/46 XY DSD	• At birth: Ambiguous sex • At puberty: – Virilism with amenorrhea – External genitalia—partial masculinization – Internal genitalia may have unilateral Müllerian development	• Karyotype —45 XO/46 XY • Gonads—testis on one side and on the other side a 'streak'	Depends on anatomic sex

Contd...

Contd...

Entity, clinical presentation, diagnosis and possible reproductive outcome of an individual with DSD.			
Characters (DSD)	***Clinical presentation***	***Diagnostic criteria***	***Reproductive outcome***
Androgen insensitivity syndrome (46 XY DSD)	• Primary amenorrhea • Infertility • Phenotypically female • Breast development—good • External genitalia—female	• Axillary and pubic hair scanty or absent • Short, blind vagina • Gonads—labial, inguinal or abdominal • Karyotype—46, XY • Gonads are testes	Incomplete variety: Possible
Sex chromosome DSD (Klinefelter's syndrome)	• Eunuchoid • Infertility (azoospermia) • Gynecomastia	• External genitalia—male • Genital ducts—Wolffian • Gonads—testes (small) • Sex chromatin—positive • Karyotype—47, XXY	May be possible with ICSI
Complete gonadal dysgenesis (Swyer syndrome) 46 XY DSD	• Amenorrhea • Secondary sex characters absent • External genitalia female	• Karyotype 46 XY • Gonadal–fibrous tissues • Internal genitalia female	Rare with IVF and donor oocytes

8. Ans. is d, i.e. Levonorgestrel 1.5 mg *Ref: DC Dutta's Textbook of Gynae 9th/ed, Ch-30*

- In India, one of the emergency contraceptives commonly used is Levonorgestrel 1.5 mg.
- Levonorgestrel is available over the counter in many countries, including India, for emergency contraception and is considered a safe and effective option when taken within a specified time frame after unprotected intercourse to prevent pregnancy. It is often marketed under brand names like "i-pill" and "Unwanted 72" in India.
- Levonorgestrel works in three different ways:
  - It prevents ovulation, prevents fertilization of the egg by sperm (if the egg is already released), and stops the egg from binding to the lining of the womb (if the egg is already fertilized). Other Emergency contraceptives are mentioned below:

Emergency contraceptives.						
Method/ drug	***Dose***	***Timing of use***	***Failure rate***	***Individual: Obese/enzyme inducing drugs (+)***	***Breast feeding***	***Contraindication***
Cu IUCD	—	**Up to 120 hours of UPSI or within 5 days of ovulation; whichever is later**	**<0.1%**	Ideal	Uterine perforation	—
UPA	30 mg	**Up to 120 hours of UPSI**	**1–2%**	Less effective	No breast-feeding up to 1 week	Asthma, glucocorticoid use
LNG	1.5 mg	**Up to 72 hours of UPSI (ineffective after 96 hours of UPSI)**	**0.6–2.6%**	Double the dose (3 mg) [Less effective]	Nil effect	Concurrent use of UPA and LNG to be avoided.

*UPSI: Unprotected Sexual Intercourse.

9. Ans. is c, i.e. 1-C, 2-D, 3-B, 4-A

Sheehan's syndrome: C. Low LH, Low FSH, Low estradiol

- Sheehan's syndrome is characterized by pituitary infarction often due to postpartum hemorrhage. It leads to a deficiency of pituitary hormones, including luteinizing hormone (LH), follicle- stimulating hormone (FSH), and estradiol.

Premature ovarian failure (POF): D. High LH, high FSH, Low estradiol.

- The triad for diagnosis of premature ovarian failure include amenorrhea, raised gonadotropins and low serum estradiol. Karyotype should be done for younger (<30 years) age group. Serum antibodies are positive in autoimmune variety.
- Ovarian biopsy is not essential to the diagnosis.

Polycystic ovary syndrome (PCOS): B. High LH, Low FSH, High estradiol.

- Polycystic ovarian syndrome is a syndrome manifested by amenorrhea, hirsutism, and obesity associated with enlarged polycystic ovaries.
- The serum values in it are - LH level is elevated and/or the ratio LH: FSH is >3:1. Raised level of estradiol and estrone—the estrone level is markedly elevated. SHBG level is reduced.
- Asherman's syndrome: A.Normal FSH, Normal LH, Normal estradiol.

- Asherman's syndrome, also known as intrauterine adhesions (IUA) or intrauterine synechiae, is an acquired uterine condition that occurs when scar tissue forms inside the uterus and/or the cervix.
- This scar tissue can build up, decreasing the amount of open space inside the uterus. Since the primary problem in Asherman's Syndrome is of a structural nature, rather than an endocrine

10. Ans. is d, i.e. 2, 3 *Ref: DC Dutta's Textbook of Gynae 9th/ed, Ch-4*

- A unicornuate uterus is a rare congenital irregularity where a person has only one fallopian tube and an abnormally shaped uterine cavity. It is formed from one of the paired Müllerian ducts while the other Müllerian duct does not develop or only develops in a rudimentary fashion. The uterus may have a single horn linked to the ipsilateral fallopian tube that faces its ovary.
- For exact diagnosis of the malformation, internal as well as external architecture of the uterus must be visualized. For this reason, several investigations in different combinations are done. Three-dimensional (3D) ultrasonography are helpful in most cases. Other investigations are: Hysterography, hysteroscopy, laparoscopy, ultrasonography (vaginal probe). Magnetic resonance imaging (MRI) is the gold standard for the diagnosis of such anomalies. 3D ultrasonography and MRI are noninvasive procedures. Urological tract is also evaluated at the same time. The renal tract abnormality in association with Müllerian abnormality is about 40%.Skeletal system anomaly (12%) is also associated.

11. Ans. is d, i.e. Endometrial sampling

- Post-menopausal bleeding can be a symptom of vaginal dryness, polyps, or other changes in the reproductive system. In about 10% of women, bleeding after menopause is a sign of uterine cancer.

Common causes of postmenopausal bleeding.	
Senile endometritis (60–80%)	***Decubitus ulcer***
Genital malignancy	Retained pessary or IUCD
Endometrial hyperplasia	Urethral caruncle

(DUB: dysfunctional uterine bleeding; IUCD: intrauterine contraceptive device)

- In a post-menopausal woman presenting with abnormal vaginal bleeding, including post-menopausal bleeding, one of the primary investigations to evaluate the cause is endometrial sampling.
- Endometrial sampling, also known as an endometrial biopsy, is a procedure in which a sample of the tissue lining the uterus (endometrium) is collected and examined. It is an important diagnostic tool for assessing the cause of abnormal uterine bleeding in post- menopausal women. The goal is to rule out or diagnose potential underlying conditions such as endometrial hyperplasia or endometrial cancer, which can present with post- menopausal bleeding.

Note: Corpus cancer syndrome - Obesity, Hypertension and diabetes are common risk factors in Postmenopausal bleeding patient to develop Endometrial cancer.

12. Ans. is c, i.e. Testicular biopsy *Ref: DC Dutta's Textbook of Gynae 12th/ed*

Testicular biopsy: Either open or percutaneous testicular biopsy is done to differentiate primary testicular failure from obstructive cause of azoospermia or severe oligospermia.

Common Causes of Azoospermia:

- *Hypogonadotropic hypogonadism:* Could be treated with pulsatile GnRH, hCG or therapy with gonadotropins.
- *Iatrogenic:* Due to the use of testosterone. This could be treated with stopping the testosterone and treatment with clomiphene citrate, hCG and/or FSH.
- *Testicular azoospermia:* Gonadal failure due to radiation, chemotherapy, orchitis (mumps), testicular maldescent.

INI-CET May 2021

1. **What is the normal uterocervical length?**
   a. 3 cm
   b. 5 cm
   c. 7 cm
   d. 10 cm
2. **Which of the following is not a cause of secondary amenorrhea?**
   a. Sheehan syndrome
   b. Asherman's syndrome
   c. Turner syndrome
   d. Kallmann syndrome
3. **Symptoms seen in endometriosis are:**
   1. Unexplained infertility
   2. Dysmenorrhea
   3. Abnormal vaginal discharge
   4. Vaginal bleeding
   a. All 4
   b. 1,2 and 4
   c. 1,2
   d. 2 and 4
4. **What should be the lower reference value for normal semen morphology in a semen analysis?**
   a. 4%
   b. 6%
   c. 10%
   d. 8%
5. **Match the following disorders causing secondary amenorrhea with their appropriate lab findings.**
   a. 1-C, 2-D, 3-B, 4-A
   b. 1-C, 2-B, 3-D, 4-A
   c. 1-D, 2-B, 3-C, 4-A
   d. 1-A, 2-B, 3-D, 4-C
6. **Which of the following best measures ovarian reserve?**
   a. Luteal phase LH.
   b. Postle luteal phase LH
   c. FSH in follicular phase
   d. Anti Mullerian hormone (AMH)
7. **An 18-year-old girl represented with amenorrhea. On examination she had normal genitalia and normal breast development. Her test revealed a 5-Alpha reductase deficiency. What could be the probable diagnosis?**
   a. Concealed sex
   b. True Hermaphroditism.
   c. Female pseudo hermaphroditism.
   d. Male Pseudo-hermaphroditism.
8. **What is the probable diagnosis from the given clinical image?**

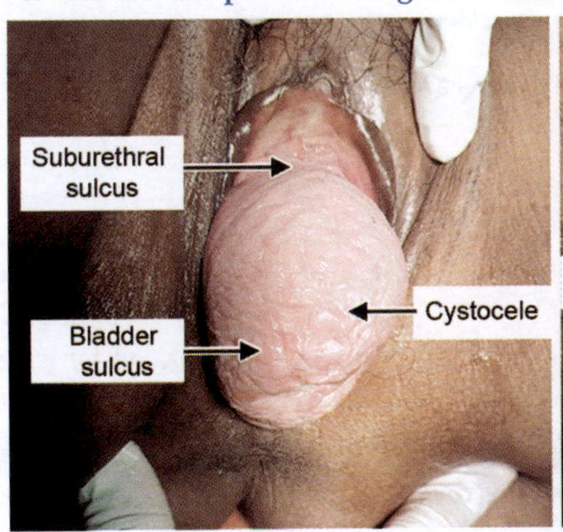

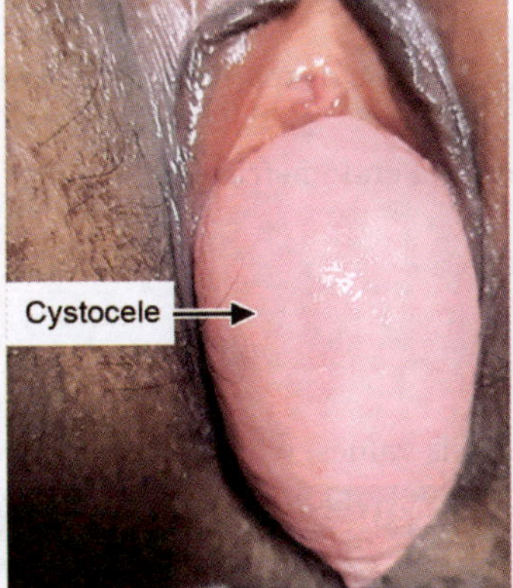

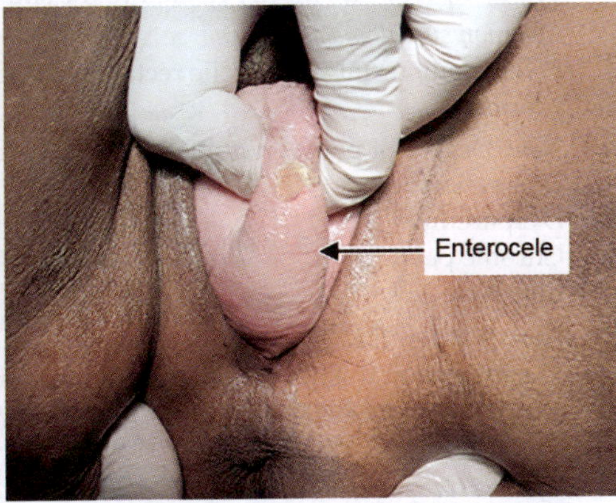

Source: Hiralal Konar. DC Dutta's Textbook of Gynecology, 9th edition

   a. Fibroid polyp.
   b. Uterine inversion.
   c. Utero cervical prolapse.
   d. Cancel cervix
9. **A 26 years old female who has two kids through normal delivery presents with a dull aching pain over the abdomen with irregular menses. Per vaginal examination revealed a mass was felt through the posterior fornix. A USD showed a clear ovarian cyst of 5 x 5 centimeters. What is the next best step?**
   a. Measure CA 125 levels
   b. Follow-up after 6 weeks
   c. Laparoscopy
   d. CT pelvis
10. **Arrange the following in sequential order with regards to steps of collection of samples for pap smear testing:**
    1. Use a posterior vaginal wall retractor.
    2. Take the sample
    3. Make smear on a slide
    4. Fix the smear
    a. 1, 2, 4, 3
    b. 2, 1, 3, 4
    c. 3, 1, 2, 4
    d. 1, 2, 3, 4
11. **Fixative in Pap Smear:**
    a. 10% Formalin
    b. 95% Ethyl alcohol
    c. Air dried
    d. Normal saline
12. **All of the following investigations are done to diagnose Unicornuate uterus?**
    a. Laparoscopy and HSG.
    b. HSG and X-Ray
    c. Falloposcopy and USG
    d. X-Ray and laparoscopy

Answer with Explanations

1. **Ans. is c, i.e. 7 cm** *Ref: DC Dutta's Textbook of Gynae 9th/ed, Ch-1 & 5*
   - The cavity of the uterine body is triangular on coronal section with the base above and the apex below. It measures about 3.5 cm. There is no cavity in the fundus. The cervical canal is fusiform and measures about 2.5 cm.
   - Thus, the normal length of the uterine cavity including the cervical canal is usually 6–7 cm
   - UCL is measured using Uterine Sound.
   - The uterine body and the cervix ratio at birth 1:2, at menarche 1:1
   - Thereafter, the enlargement of the body occurs rapidly, so that the ratio soon becomes 2:1
2. **Ans. is d, i.e. Kallmann syndrome** *Ref: DC Dutta's Textbook of Gynae 9th/ed, Ch-29*
   Kallmann syndrome - Embryologically GnRH neurons develop in the ectodermal olfactory placode. Such individual presents with hypogonadotropic, hypogonadism, leading to primary Amenorrhea.

Common causes of secondary amenorrhea.

Hypothalamus	*Pituitary*	*Ovary*	*Uterine*	*Systemic*
• Stress • *Pott pill* • *Weight:* Either too much loss or too much gain • *Drugs:* Psychotropic and antihypertensive drugs	• Adenoma • Sheehan's syndrome	• Polycystic ovary syndrome (PCOS) • Premature ovarian failure	Synechiae (Spontaneous or induced)	• Malnutrition • Hypothyroid state • Diabetes

3. **Ans. is c, i.e. 1,2** *Ref: DC Dutta's Textbook of Gynae 9th/ed, Ch-22*
   Presence of functioning endometrium (glands and stroma) in sites other than uterine mucosa is called endometriosis
   Symptoms
   About 25% of patients with endometriosis have no symptom
   The symptoms are mostly related to the site of lesion.
   Common symptoms are:
   Pelvic pain, rectal pain, cyclic rectal bleeding, diarrhea, dyspareunia. Midline lesions are more symptom producing.
   Note: Degree of pain is not related to the severity of endometriosis.
   Dysmenorrhea
   Dyspareunia
   Chronic pelvic pain.
   Infertility
4. **Ans. is a, i.e. 4%** *Ref: DC Dutta's Textbook of Gynae 9th/ed, Ch-17*
   It is important to know the normal semen analysis values, which are as follows:

Semen analysis (WHO reference values, 2010 and 2021).

	Normal reference values	
Semen analysis	***2010***	***2021***
Volume	1.5 mL	≥1.4 mL
pH	7.2-7.8	≥7.2
Sperm concentration	15-16 million/mL	≥15 million/mL
Total sperm number	39 million per ejaculate	≥39 million per ejaculate
Motility (%)	Total motility: 40% (Progressive motility = 32%)	Total motility: ≥42% (Non-progressive motility: ≥1%, Progressive motility: ≥30%, Immobile sperms: ≥20%)
Normal morphology (%)	4%	≥4%
Viability	58%	≥54% live spermatozoa
WBCs	Less than 1 million/mL	
Round cells	<5 million/mL	
Sperm agglutination	<10% spermatozoa with adherent particles	

5. **Ans. is a, i.e. 1-C, 2-D, 3-B, 4-A** *Ref: DC Dutta's Textbook of Gynae 9th/ed, Ch-29*
   1. *Sheehan's syndrome:* C. Low LH, Low FSH, Low estradiol Sheehan's syndrome is characterized by pituitary infarction often due to postpartum hemorrhage. It leads to a deficiency of pituitary hormones, including luteinizing hormone (LH), follicle-stimulating hormone (FSH), and estradiol.

2. *Premature Ovarian Failure (POF):* D. High LH, high FSH, Low estradiol The triad for diagnosis of premature ovarian failure include amenorrhea, raised gonadotropins and low serum estradiol. Karyotype should be done for younger (<30 years) age group. Serum antibodies are positive in autoimmune variety.
Ovarian biopsy is not essential to the diagnosis.
3. *Polycystic Ovary Syndrome (PCOS):* B. High LH, Low FSH, High estradiol. Polycystic ovarian syndrome is a syndrome manifested by amenorrhea, hirsutism, and obesity associated with enlarged polycystic ovaries.

Condition Lab markers.
1. Sheehan Syndrome A. Low -LH, FSH, Estradiol
2. Premature ovarian Failure B. LH-High, FSH-Low, Estradiol-low
3. PCOS C. LH-low. FSH-Low, Estradiol-Low
4. Asherman syndrome D. LH-high, FSH-high, Estradiol-low

The serum values in it are - LH level is elevated and/or the ratio LH: FSH is >3:1. Raised level of estradiol and estrone—the estrone level is markedly elevated.

SHBG level is reduced.

4. *Asherman's syndrome:* A. Normal FSH, Normal LH, Normal estradiol.
Asherman's syndrome, also known as intrauterine adhesions (IUA) or intrauterine synechiae, is an acquired uterine condition that occurs when scar tissue forms inside the uterus and/or the cervix. This scar tissue can build up, decreasing the amount of open space inside the uterus. Since the primary problem in Asherman's Syndrome is of a structural nature, rather than an endocrine dysfunction, hormone levels in these patients, including LH, FSH, and estradiol, are normal.

6. Ans. is d, i.e. Anti Mullerian hormone (AMH). *Ref: DC Dutta's Textbook of Gynae 9th/ed, Ch-32*

Detection of diminished ovarian reserve (DOR):

Tests for detection of DOR can identify the women who are likely to have poor response with gonadotropin and lower pregnancy rate:

- Levels of cycle D3 serum FSH >10–15 IU/L.
- Levels of D3 serum estradiol >60–80 pg/mL.
- Clomiphene citrate challenge test
- Levels of serum anti-Müllerian hormone (AMH)—low (0.2–0.7 ng/mL).
- Levels of basal serum inhibin B—low (<40 pg/mL).
- Antral follicle count (AFC)

Ovarian volume measurement (OVM)

Best among these would be AMH measurement.

7. Ans. is d, i.e. Male Pseudo-hermaphroditism. *Ref: DC Dutta's Textbook of Gynae 9th/ed, Ch-28*

- The probable diagnosis in this case is Male pseudohermaphroditism.
- As in given case their is 5 alpha reductase deficiency, which is required for conversion of testosterone to active form i.e, Dihydrotestosterone.
- Dihydrotestosterone is further required for development of male internal and external genitalia. Lack of which is leading to by default development of female internal and external genitalia.

Entity, clinical presentation, diagnosis and possible reproductive outcome of an individual with DSD.

Characters (DSD)	*Clinical presentation*	*Diagnostic criteria*	*Reproductive outcome*
Adrenogenital syndrome 46 XX DSD (androgen excess)	Ambiguity of sex at birth	• Sonographic evaluation of internal genital organs • Karyotype 46, XX • Serum 17 hydroxyprogesterone ↑ • Urinary pregnanetriol ↑ >5 µg/100 mL	Pregnancy possible
Gonadal dysgenesis Turner's syndrome sex chromosome DSD	• Primary amenorrhea • Poor secondary sexual characters • Short stature • Webbing of neck • Cubitus valgus • Genitalia underdeveloped	• Karyotype 45, XO • Bilateral 'streak' gonads • Serum: E_2 ⁻ and FSH ↑	Pregnancy with donor oocyte
Mosaic turner syndrome sex chromosome DSD	• Primary/secondary amenorrhea • Average height • Poor secondary sexual characters • Genitalia underdeveloped	• Karyotype 45, XO/46 XX • Bilateral 'streak. gonads	Pregnancy possible

Contd...

Contd...

Entity, clinical presentation, diagnosis and possible reproductive outcome of an individual with DSD.			
Characters (DSD)	***Clinical presentation***	***Diagnostic criteria***	***Reproductive outcome***
Pure gonadal dysgenesis 46 XX or 46 XY DSD	• Primary amenorrhea • Delayed secondary sexual characters • Average height • Genitalia underdeveloped	• Karyotype—46, XX or 46, XY • Bilateral 'streak' gonads	Rare
Mixed gonadal dysgenesis 45 X/46 XY DSD	• At birth: Ambiguous sex • At puberty: – Virilism with amenorrhea – External genitalia—partial masculinization – Internal genitalia may have unilateral Mullerian development	• Karyotype—45 XO/46 XY • Gonads—testis on one side and on the other side a 'streak'	Depends on anatomic sex
Androgen insensitivity syndrome (46 XY DSD)	• Primary amenorrhea • Infertility • Phenotypically female • Breast development—good • External genitalia—female	• Axillary and pubic hair scanty or absent • Short, blind vagina • Gonads—labial, inguinal or abdominal • Karyotype—46, XY • Gonads are testes	Incomplete variety: Possible
Sex chromosome DSD (Klinefelter's syndrome)	• Eunuchoid • Infertility (azoospermia) • Gynecomastia	• External genitalia—male • Genital ducts—Wolffian • Gonads—testes (small) • Sex chromatin—positive • Karyotype—47, XXY	Maybe possible with ICSI
Complete gonadal dysgenesis (Swyer syndrome) 46 XY DSD	• Amenorrhea • Secondary sex characters absent • External genitalia female	• Karyotype 46 XY • Gonadal-fibrous tissues • Internal genitalia female	Rare with IVF and donor oocytes

8. Ans. is c, i.e. Utero cervical prolapse. *Ref: DC Dutta's Textbook of Gynae 9th/ed*

- In the given photo it is clearly seen as that uterus and cervix is lying below the level of hymenal ring suggestive of uterine prolapse. Uterine prolapse occurs when the pelvic floor muscles and ligaments stretch and weaken, causing the uterus to slip down into or protrude out of the vagina. Uterine prolapse is most common in people after menopause who have had one or more vaginal deliveries. It can cause symptoms such as tissue bulging out of the vagina, heaviness or pulling in the pelvis, bladder problems, bowel movement difficulties, and discomfort during sexual activity.
- To differentiate from uterine inversion we can do uterine sounding i.e, which is only possible with Uterine Prolapse and not in Inversion. Note Uterine sounding is possible even in Polyp but in the given image their is no polyp seen.

9. Ans. is b, i.e. Follow-up after 6 weeks *Ref: DC Dutta's Textbook of Gynae 9th/ed, Ch-21 & 24*

- In the given case, it is mentioned: Young lady, immediate post partum, irregular cycles, and USG showing clear cyst: all suggest a Benign Ovarian Lesion. Hence next best step is to do a followup after 6 weeks to check for the size, number or change to complex cyst.
- Cysts that are simple, unilocular, <8 cm in diameter with normal serum CA-125—can be managed conservatively.
- Women should be under follow up with ultrasound scan and serum CA-125 at an interval of 4 months
- However if the same case mentioned an elderly <post menopausal, complex cyst or size >5 cm then it would require further investigation with measuring CA 125 levels.

To access the risk of malignancy, we can do a Risk of malignancy index (RMI):

RMI = U × M × CA125;

U = USG score (one point each for: Multilocular cyst; solid areas; metastasis; ascites; bilateral lesions),

U = 3 (for score 2–5)

M = 3 (postmenopausal women)

CA-125 level in U/mL.

The risk of cancer is 20% with the score of 25 and 250 and it is 75% when the RMI value is >250.

10. Ans. is d, i.e. 1, 2, 3, 4 *Ref: DC Dutta's Textbook of Gynae 9th/ed, Ch-9*

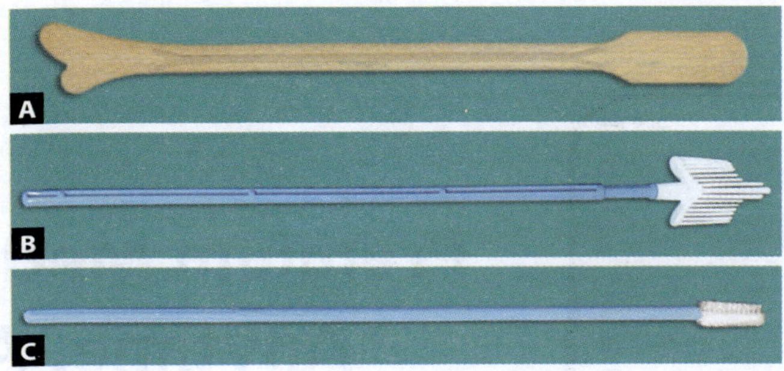

(A) Ayre spatula; (B) Rocket endocervical broom-it is for both ecto- and endocervical smear. It has conical shape with plastic bristles; (C) Endocervical brush.

Pap Testing Procedure

- Transformation zone is the squamocolumnar junction, which is the area of meeting point for the squamous epithelium of the ectocervix with the columnar epithelium of the endocervix. Smear is collected by a plastic spatula from the ectocervix. The endocervical cells are collected using an endocervical brush or using the broom. The sample is placed on a glass slide and fixed with ethyl alcohol.
- This liquid medium is also used for HPV DNA testing.
- Cervical cytology reporting by The Bethesda system.

11. Ans. is b, i.e. 95% Ethyl alcohol *Ref: DC Dutta's Textbook of Gynae 9th/ed, Ch-9*

- The fixative used for a Pap smear (Papanicolaou smear or Pap test) is typically 95% ethanol. Ethanol is used to fix and preserve the cellular material collected during the Pap smear so that it can be adequately prepared, stained, and examined under a microscope for the detection of abnormal cervical cells, which may indicate cervical cancer or precancerous changes.
- Fixation and Staining
- The material so collected should be immediately spread over a microscopic slide and at once fixed with ethyl alcohol (95%) before drying. After fixing of the slide sent to the laboratory. The slide so sent is stained either with Papanicolaou's or Sorr's method and examined by a trained cytologist.
- *Benefits:* The objective of screening is to reduce the incidence and mortality from cervical cancer. The lifetime risk of developing cervical cancer by the age of 74 is 0.9% in developed countries compared to 1.6% in low and middle income countries (LMICs).
- Lifetime risk of death from cervical cancer is 0.3% in developed countries compared to 0.9% in LMICs.

12. Ans. is a, i.e. Laparoscopy and HSG. *Ref: DC Dutta's Textbook of Gynae 9th/ed, Ch-4*

- A unicornuate uterus is a rare congenital irregularity where a person has only one fallopian tube and an abnormally shaped uterine cavity. It is formed from one of the paired Müllerian ducts while the other Müllerian duct does not develop or only develops in a rudimentary fashion. The uterus may have a single horn linked to the ipsilateral fallopian tube that faces its ovary.
- For exact diagnosis of the malformation, internal as well as external architecture of the uterus must be visualized. For this reason, several investigations in different combinations are done. Three-dimensional (3D) ultrasonography are helpful in most cases. Other investigations are: Hysterography, hysteroscopy, laparoscopy, ultrasonography (vaginal probe). Magnetic resonance imaging (MRI) is the gold standard for the diagnosis of such anomalies. 3D ultrasonography and MRI are noninvasive procedures. Urological tract is also evaluated at the same time. The renal tract abnormality in association with Müllerian abnormality is about 40%. Skeletal system anomaly (12%) is also associated.

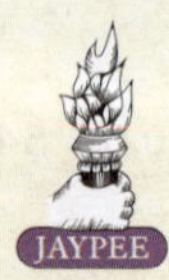

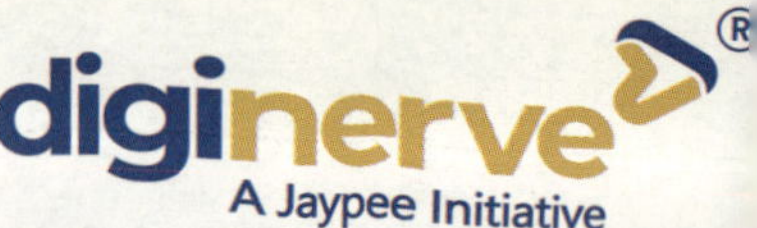

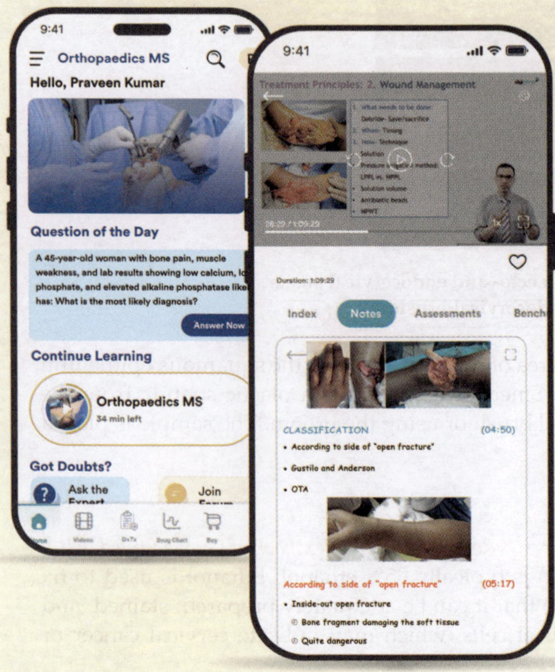

Premium Medical Content, Anytime, Anywhere

Trusted by 150K+ Users

20+ Courses

3600+ Hrs of Video Content

790+ Mentors

A host of features for **UnderGrads, PostGrads** and **Professionals**

Video Lectures

Notes

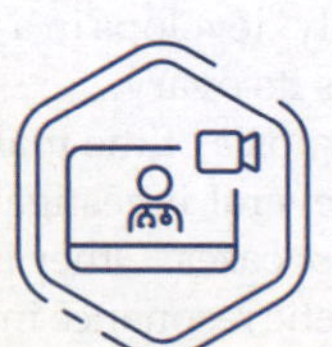

OSCEs

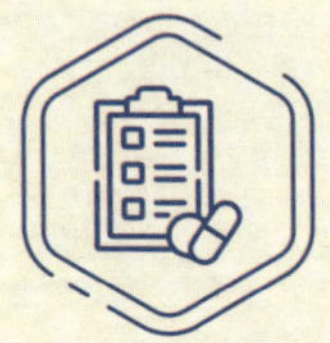

Drug Chart

Question Bank

Dr. Wise AI Chatbot

+91-8800-418-418 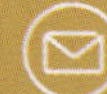 marketing@diginerve.com